Peripheral Neuropathy

By 78 Authorities

VOLUME I

edited by

PETER JAMES DYCK, M.D.
Mayo Clinic, Rochester, Minnesota

P. K. THOMAS, M.D., D.Sc., F.R.C.P.
The Royal Free Hospital, London, England

EDWARD H. LAMBERT, M.D., Ph.D.
Mayo Clinic, Rochester, Minnesota

1975

W. B. SAUNDERS COMPANY Philadelphia, London, Toronto

W. B. Saunders Company: West Washington Square
Philadelphia, P.A. 19105

12 Dyott Street
London, WC1A 1DB

833 Oxford Street
Toronto, Ontario M8Z 5T9, Canada

Library of Congress Cataloging in Publication Data

Main entry under title:

Peripheral neuropathy.

Includes index.

1. Nerves, Peripheral — Diseases.   I. Dyck, Peter James.
   II. Thomas, Peter Kynaston.   III. Lambert, Edward
   Howard, 1915–   [DNLM: 1. Peripheral nerve diseases.
   2. Peripheral nerves — Pathology. WL500 P445]

RC409.P47   616.8'3   73–81830

ISBN 0–7216–3270–X (v. 1)
     0–7216–3271–8 (v. 2)

Peripheral Neuropathy

Vol I: 0-7216-3270-X
Vol II: 0-7216-3271-8

Last digit is the print number: 9   8   7   6   5   4   3   2   1

CONTRIBUTORS

ALBERT J. AGUAYO, M.D., F.R.C.P.(C.)

Experimental Pathology of Unmyelinated Fibers, Compression and Entrapment
Associate Professor of Neurology and Neurosurgery, McGill University Faculty of
Medicine, Montreal, Quebec, Canada. Associate Physician, Department of Medicine, Montreal General Hospital, Montreal, Quebec, Canada.

BARRY G. W. ARNASON, M.D.

Serum Sickness, Inflammatory Polyradiculoneuropathies
Associate Professor of Neurology, Harvard Medical School, Boston, Massachusetts.
Associate Neurologist, Massachusetts General Hospital, Boston, Massachusetts.

ARTHUR K. ASBURY, M.D.

Schwann Cells, Uremic and Hepatic Neuropathy
Professor and Chairman of the Department of Neurology, University of Pennsylvania School of Medicine, Philadelphia, Pennsylvania.

J. RICHARD BARINGER, M.D.

Herpes
Associate Professor of Neurology and Pathology and Vice Chairman of the Department of Neurology, University of California School of Medicine, San Francisco,
California. Chief of the Neurology Service, San Francisco Veterans Hospital, San
Francisco, California.

JAMES A. BASTRON, M.D., M.S.

Thyroid Neuropathy
Associate Professor of Neurology, Mayo Medical School, Rochester, Minnesota.

FRIEDRICH BEHSE, M.D.

Sensory Potentials
Associate Professor of Neurophysiology, University of Copenhagen Institute of
Neurophysiology, Copenhagen, Denmark.

MERRILL D. BENSON, M.S., M.D.

Amyloid Neuropathy
Assistant Professor of Medicine, Boston University School of Medicine, Boston,
Massachusetts. Assisting Physician and Head, Allergy-Immunology Clinic, Boston
City Hospital, Boston, Massachusetts.

ALBERT BISCHOFF, M.D.

Microscopic Anatomy of Myelinated Fibers, Leukodystrophies
Professor of Neurology, University of Berne School of Medicine, Berne, Switzerland. Co-director of the Neurology Department, Inselspital, Berne, Switzerland.

WALTER GEORGE BRADLEY, M.A., B.Sc., D.M., M.R.C.P.

Anterior Horn Cells, Spinal Roots
Professor of Experimental Neurology, The University of Newcastle-upon-Tyne,
Newcastle-upon-Tyne, England. Honorary Consultant Neurologist, Newcastle Area
Health Authority (Teaching) Hospitals, Newcastle-upon-Tyne, England.

ROSCOE O. BRADY, M.D.

Fabry's Disease
Chief, Developmental and Metabolic Neurology Branch, National Institute of
Neurological Diseases and Stroke, National Institutes of Health, Bethesda, Maryland.

GARTH M. BRAY, M.D., F.R.C.P.(C.)

Experimental Pathology of Unmyelinated Fibers
Assistant Professor of Neurology and Neurosurgery, McGill University Faculty of
Medicine, Montreal, Quebec, Canada. Associate Physician, Department of Medi-
cine, Montreal General Hospital, Montreal, Quebec, Canada.

DONAL BROOKS, M.A., M.B., R.Ch., F.R.C.S., F.R.C.S.I.

Peripheral Nerve Tumors
Consultant Orthopaedic Surgeon, University College Hospital, Royal National
Orthopaedic Hospital; Civilian Consultant in Hand Surgery to the Royal Navy and
Royal Air Force, London, England.

FRITZ BUCHTHAL, M.D.

Sensory Potentials
Professor of Neurophysiology, University of Copenhagen Institute of Neurophysiology, Copenhagen, Denmark. Head of the Department of Clinical Neurophysiology, University Hospital, Copenhagen, Denmark.

MARY BARTLETT BUNGE, Ph.D.

Tissue Culture
Associate Professor of Anatomy, Washington University School of Medicine, St.
Louis, Missouri.

RICHARD PAUL BUNGE, M.D.

Tissue Culture
Professor of Anatomy, Washington University School of Medicine, St. Louis,
Missouri.

JOHN R. CALVERLEY, M.D.

Lumbosacral Plexus
Professor and Chairman, Department of Neurology, The University of Texas
Medical Branch, Galveston, Texas.

JOHN B. CAVANAGH, M.D., F.R.C.P.

Physical Agents
Professor of Applied Neurobiology, Institute of Neurology, University of London,
London, England. Consultant Pathologist, National Hospitals, Queen Square,
London, England.

ALAN S. COHEN, M.D.

Amyloid Neuropathy
Conrad Wesselhoeft Professor of Medicine, Boston University School of Medicine,
Boston, Massachusetts. Chief of Medicine and Director, Thorndike Memorial
Laboratory, Boston City Hospital, Boston, Massachusetts.

DOYT L. CONN, M.D.

Angiopathic Neuropathy in Connective Tissue Disease
Assistant Professor of Medicine, Mayo Medical School, Rochester, Minnesota. Consultant in Rheumatology and Internal Medicine, Mayo Clinic, Rochester, Minnesota.

JASPER R. DAUBE, M.D.

Peripheral Vascular Diseases
Assistant Professor of Neurology, Mayo Medical School, Rochester, Minnesota. Consultant in Neurology and Electromyography, Mayo Clinic, Rochester, Minnesota.

J. NEWSOM DAVIS, M.A., M.D., F.R.C.P.

Ninth, Tenth, Eleventh, and Twelfth Cranial Nerves
Honorary Lecturer, Institute of Neurology, University of London, London, England. Consultant Neurologist to the National Hospitals for Nervous Diseases and The Royal Free Hospital, London, England.

JOHN E. DESMEDT, M.D.

Cerebral Evoked Potentials
Professor and Director, Brain Research Unit, Brussels University Faculty of Medicine, Brussels, Belgium.

ELLIS DOUEK, F.R.C.S.

Eighth Cranial Nerve
Chairman, Guy's Hearing Research Group, and Consultant Otologist, Guy's Hospital, London, England.

PETER JAMES DYCK, M.D.

Pathologic Alterations in Man, Biopsy, Compound Action Potentials, Quantitation of Sensation, Peripheral Vascular Diseases, Definition and Classification of Hereditary Neuropathy, Hereditary Motor and Sensory Neuropathy, Angiopathic Neuropathy in Connective Tissue Disease, Metal Neuropathy
Professor of Neurology, Mayo Medical School, Rochester, Minnesota. Consultant in Neurology, Mayo Clinic and Mayo Foundation, Rochester, Minnesota.

LORENTZ ELDJARN, M.D., Dr. med.

Refsum's Disease
Professor and Chairman, Institute of Clinical Biochemistry, Rikshospitalet, University of Oslo, Oslo, Norway.

SVEN GUSTAV ELIASSON, M.D., Ph.D.

Diabetic Neuropathy
Professor of Neurology, Washington University School of Medicine, St. Louis, Missouri. Associate Neurologist, Barnes Hospital; Visiting Neurologist, City Hospital; and Consultant Neurologist, Long Term Care Division, Jewish Hospital, St. Louis, Missouri.

ANDREW GEORGE ENGEL, M.D.

Motor Endplate
Professor of Neurology, Mayo Medical School, Rochester, Minnesota. Consultant in Neurology, Mayo Clinic, Rochester, Minnesota.

MICHEL P. FARDEAU, M.D.

Refsum's Disease
Maître de Recherche, Centre National de la Recherche Scientifique, Hôpital de la Salpétrière, Paris, France.

ERNEST DEAN GARDNER, M.D.

Gross Anatomy
Professor of Neurology, Orthopaedic Surgery, and Anatomy, University of California School of Medicine, Davis, California. Member, Department of Neurology, Sacramento Medical Center, Sacramento, California.

NORMAN P. GOLDSTEIN, M.D.

Metal Neuropathy
Professor of Neurology, Mayo Medical School, Rochester, Minnesota. Consultant in Neurology, Mayo Clinic and Mayo Foundation, Rochester, Minnesota.

M. SPENCER HARRISON, M.D., F.R.C.S., F.R.C.P.(Edinburgh)

Ninth, Tenth, Eleventh, and Twelfth Cranial Nerves
Honorary Lecturer, Institute of Neurology, University of London, London, England. Consultant Surgeon to the Department of Neuro-otology at the National Hospitals for Nervous Diseases, London, England.

ANTHONY P. HOPKINS, M.D.

Pathophysiology of Unmyelinated Fibers, Toxic Industrial Agents
Consultant Neurologist, The Royal Hospital of Saint Bartholomew, London, England.

FELIX JERUSALEM, M.D.

Motor Endplate
Associate Professor of Neurology, University of Zürich, Zürich, Switzerland.

WILLIAM E. KARNES, M.D.

Seventh Cranial Nerve
Assistant Professor of Neurology, Mayo Medical School, Rochester, Minnesota. Consultant and Section Head in Neurology, Mayo Clinic and Mayo Foundation, Rochester, Minnesota.

FRANK M. KING, M.D.

Fabry's Disease
Chief, Division B, Air Force Institute of Pathology, Washington, District of Columbia.

THOMAS TYRRELL KING, M.B., B.S., F.R.C.S.

Tumors of Cranial Nerves and Spinal Roots
Consultant Neurosurgeon, The London Hospital, Whitechapel, London, England.

ROMAN S. KOCEN, T.D., M.B., F.R.C.P.

Diphtheritic Neuropathy
Sub-Dean, Institute of Neurology, London, England. Physician, National Hospitals for Nervous Diseases, Queen Square and Maida Vale, London, England. Consultant Neurologist, Edgware General Hospital, Edgware, Middlesex, England.

WILHELM KRÜCKE, M.D.

Introduction
Professor of Neuropathology, Institute of Neurology (Edinger Institute) of the Johann Wolfgang Goethe University, Frankfurt-Am-Main, West Germany. Department of Neuropathology, Max Planck Institute for Brain Research, Frankfurt-Am-Main, West Germany.

EDWARD H. LAMBERT, M.D., Ph.D.

Compound Action Potentials
Professor of Physiology, Mayo Graduate School of Medicine, University of Minnesota, Rochester, Minnesota. Head of Section of Clinical Electromyography, Mayo Clinic, Rochester, Minnesota.

PAMELA M. Le QUESNE, D.M., B.Sc., F.R.C.P.

Drug Neuropathy
Member M.R.C. Toxicology Unit, Carshalton, Surrey, England. Honorary Consultant Neurologist, The Middlesex Hospital, London, England.

ERIC P. LOFGREN, M.D.

Biopsy
Assistant Professor of Surgery, Mayo Medical School, Rochester, Minnesota.

JOHN T. McCALL, Ph.D.

Metal Neuropathy
Associate Professor of Biochemistry and Laboratory Medicine, Mayo Medical School, Rochester, Minnesota. Consultant, Department of Laboratory Medicine, Mayo Clinic and Mayo Foundation, Rochester, Minnesota.

WILLIAM IAN McDONALD, Ph.D.(N.Z.), F.R.C.P., F.R.A.C.P.

Diphtheritic Neuropathy
Professor of Clinical Neurology, Institute of Neurology, Queen Square, London, England. Honorary Physician, National Hospitals, Queen Square and Maida Vale, London, England. Honorary Physician (Neurologist), Moorfield's Eye Hospital, City Road, London, England.

JAMES G. McLEOD, M.B., B.S., D.Phil.(Oxon.), B.Sc.(Med.), M.R.C.P., F.R.A.C.P.

Paraproteinemias and Dysproteinemias, Carcinomatous Neuropathy, Lymphomas and Reticuloses
Professor of Medicine, University of Sydney, Sydney, Australia. Honorary Physician, Royal Prince Alfred Hospital and Sydney Hospital, Sydney, Australia.

CHARLES DAVID MARSDEN, M.Sc., M.R.C.P.

Hereditary Motor Neuropathy
Professor of Neurology, Institute of Psychiatry and Kings College Hospital Medical School, London, England. Consultant Neurologist at The Bethlem Royal Hospital, The Maudsley Hospital, and King's College Hospital, London, England.

W. B. MATTHEWS, D.M., F.R.C.P.

Sarcoid Neuropathy
Professor of Clinical Neurology, Oxford University, Oxford, England. Consultant Neurologist, The Churchill Hospital and Radcliffe Infirmary, Oxford, England.

DONALD WILLIAM MULDER, M.D.

Motor Neuron Disease
Professor of Neurology, Mayo Medical School, Rochester, Minnesota. Consultant in Neurology at Mayo Clinic, St. Mary's, and Methodist Hospitals, Rochester, Minnesota.

PIERRE NOËL, M.D.

Cerebral Evoked Potentials
Assistant, Brain Research Unit, Brussels University Medical Faculty, Brussels, Belgium.

JOSÉ L. OCHOA, M.D., Ph.D.

Microscopic Anatomy of Unmyelinated Fibers
Assistant Professor of Neurology, Dartmouth Medical School, Hanover, New Hampshire.

SIDNEY OCHS, Ph.D.

Axoplasmic Transport
Professor of Physiology, Indiana University School of Medicine, Indianapolis, Indiana.

MICHIYA OHTA, M.D.

Hereditary Sensory Neuropathy
Associate Professor of Neuropathology, Faculty of Medicine, Kyushu University, Fukuoka, Japan.

YNGVE OLSSON, M.D.

Microscopic Anatomy of Connective Tissue, Vascular Permeability
Associate Professor in Neuropathology, University of Uppsala, Uppsala, Sweden.

DAVID ELLIOTT PLEASURE, M.D.

Structural Proteins, Abetalipoproteinemia, Tangier Disease
Associate Professor of Neurology and Pediatrics, University of Pennsylvania School of Medicine, Philadelphia, Pennsylvania. Director of Research in Pediatric Neurology, Children's Hospital of Philadelphia, Philadelphia, Pennsylvania.

JOHN W. PRINEAS, M.D.

Pathology of the Nerve Cell Body
Professor of Neuroscience, College of Medicine and Dentistry of New Jersey, New Jersey Medical School, Newark, New Jersey. Attending Neurologist at Veterans Administration Hospital, East Orange, New Jersey, and at Martland Hospital, Newark, New Jersey.

HENRY J. RALSTON, III, M.D.

Microscopic Anatomy of the Spinal Cord
Professor and Chairman, Department of Anatomy, University of California School of Medicine, San Francisco, California.

SIGVALD REFSUM, M.D., Ph.D.

Refsum's Disease
Professor of Neurology, University of Oslo Medical School, Oslo, Norway. Chief Physician, Department of Neurology, Rikshospitalet, University of Oslo Hospitals, Oslo, Norway.

ALAN RIDLEY, M.D., Ph.D., M.R.C.P.

Porphyric Neuropathy
Consultant Physician, Neurological Department, The London Hospital, Whitechapel, London, England.

ANNELISE ROSENFALCK, M.Sc.

Sensory Potentials
Associate Professor of Neurophysiology, University of Copenhagen Institute of Neurophysiology, Copenhagen, Denmark.

THOMAS D. SABIN, M.D.

Leprosy
Assistant Professor of Neurology, Tufts University School of Medicine, and Lecturer, Harvard Medical School, Boston, Massachusetts. Associate Director, Neurological Unit, Boston City Hospital, Boston, Massachusetts. Formerly Deputy Chief, Rehabilitation Branch, U.S. Public Health Service Hospital, Carville, Louisiana.

J. MICHAEL SCHRÖDER, Prof. Dr. med.

Degeneration and Regeneration of Myelinated Fibers
Professor at the Johannes Gutenberg University, Mainz, West Germany. Head of the Department of Neuropathology, Institute of Pathology, Hospital of the Johannes Gutenberg University, Mainz, West Germany.

GEORGE SELBY, M.D., F.R.C.P., F.R.C.P.(Ed.), F.R.A.C.P.

Fifth Cranial Nerve
Lecturer in Medicine (Neurology), University of Sydney, Sydney, Australia. Honorary Neurologist, The Royal North Shore Hospital and Hornsby and District Hospitals, Sydney, Australia.

RICHARD S. SMITH, M.D.

Muscle Spindle
Associate, Medical Research Council of Canada. Associate Professor of Surgery, University of Alberta Faculty of Medicine, Edmonton, Alberta, Canada.

J. M. K. SPALDING, D.M., F.R.C.P.

Ninth, Tenth, Eleventh, and Twelfth Cranial Nerves
Senior Research Fellow, St. Peter's College, Oxford University, Oxford, England. Consultant Neurologist, United Oxford Hospitals, Oxford, England.

PETER S. SPENCER, Ph.D.

Pathology of the Nerve Cell Body
Assistant Professor of Pathology and Joseph P. Kennedy Fellow in the Neurosciences, Albert Einstein College of Medicine of Yeshiva University, The Bronx, New York.

J. CLARKE STEVENS, M.D., F.R.C.P.(C.)

Biopsy
Instructor of Neurology, Mayo Medical School, Rochester, Minnesota. Consultant in Neurology, Mayo Clinic, Rochester, Minnesota.

G. KEITH STILLWELL, M.D., Ph.D.

Rehabilitation
Professor of Physical Medicine and Rehabilitation, Mayo Medical School, Rochester, Minnesota. Chairman, Department of Physical Medicine and Rehabilitation, Mayo Clinic and Mayo Foundation, Rochester, Minnesota.

ODDVAR STOKKE, M.D., Dr. med.

Refsum's Disease
Department of Clinical Chemistry, Rikshospitalet, University of Oslo, Oslo, Norway.

THOMAS R. SWIFT, M.D.

Leprosy
Assistant Professor of Neurology, Medical College of Georgia, Augusta, Georgia. Director, Electromyography Laboratory, Eugene Talmadge Memorial Hospital, Augusta, Georgia. Formerly Deputy Chief, Rehabilitation Branch, U.S. Public Health Service Hospital, Carville, Louisiana.

VIRGINIA M. TENNYSON, M.S., Ph.D.

Microscopic Anatomy of Dorsal Root and Sympathetic Ganglia
Associate Professor, Department of Pathology, Division of Neuropathology, Columbia University College of Physicians and Surgeons, New York, New York.

PETER KYNASTON THOMAS, M.D., D.Sc., F.R.C.P.

Microscopic Anatomy of Myelinated Fibers and Connective Tissue; Clinical Features; Differential Diagnosis; Ninth, Tenth, Eleventh, and Twelfth Cranial Nerves; Physical Agents; Diabetic Neuropathy
Professor of Neurology in the University of London at The Royal Free Hospital School of Medicine and the Institute of Neurology, Queen Square, London, England. Consultant Neurologist, The Royal Free Hospital, National Hospital for Nervous Diseases, and Royal Orthopaedic Hospital, London, England.

JEANNETTE J. TOWNSEND, M.D.

Herpes
Fellow in Neuropathology, University of California, San Francisco, California. Fellow in Neuropathology, San Francisco Veterans Hospital, San Francisco, California.

JAMES C. TRAUTMANN, M.D.

Third, Fourth, and Sixth Cranial Nerves
Assistant Professor of Ophthalmology, Mayo Medical School, Rochester, Minnesota. Consultant in Ophthalmology, Mayo Clinic and Mayo Foundation, Rochester, Minnesota.

PETER TSAIRIS, M.D.

Brachial Plexus
Assistant Professor of Neurology, Cornell University Medical College, New York, New York. Director of Neurology, The Hospital for Special Surgery, and Assistant Attending Neurologist, The New York Hospital, New York, New York.

MITSUHIRO TSUJIHATA, M.D.

Motor Endplate
Assistant Professor of Medicine, Faculty of Medicine, Nagasaki University, Nagasaki, Japan.

HENRY URICH, M.D., F.R.C.P., F.R.C.Path.

Pathology of Tumors
Professor of Neuropathology, University of London, London, England. Consultant Neuropathologist, The London Hospital, Whitechapel, London, England.

MAURICE VICTOR, M.D.

Nutritional Deficiency and Alcoholism
Professor of Neurology, Case Western Reserve University School of Medicine, Cleveland, Ohio. Director, Neurology Service, Cleveland Metropolitan General Hospital, Cleveland, Ohio.

JOHN C. WALSH, M.D., B.Sc.(Med.), F.R.A.C.P.

Paraproteinemias and Dysproteinemias, Lymphomas and Reticuloses
Staff Neurologist, Royal Prince Alfred Hospital, Sydney, Australia.

HENRY deF. WEBSTER, M.D.

Development of Myelinated and Unmyelinated Fibers
Head, Section on Cellular Neuropathology, Laboratory of Neuropathology and Neuroanatomical Sciences, National Institute of Neurological Diseases and Stroke, National Institutes of Health, Bethesda, Maryland.

PREFACE

This collaborative work on peripheral neuropathy was written to meet the need for a comprehensive up-to-date textbook on the scientific basis and clinical features of peripheral nerve diseases. Although some earlier writings, particularly those of Ramón y Cajal, of Woltman, and of Krücke, on more limited aspects of peripheral nerve disorders were masterpieces, there remained a need not only for a broader coverage but for inclusion of much recently acquired information. The opening section of the book on the biology of the peripheral nervous system reflects in part the great increase in scientific information bearing on the subject of peripheral neuropathy.

Until about 20 years ago, peripheral nerve disorders did not receive the attention from clinical neurologists and neuropathologists that they deserve, although during the Second World War the necessities of the time yielded an impressive body of work on peripheral nerve injury, notably by J. Z. Young and his collaborators at Oxford and Paul Weiss and his co-workers in Chicago. A significant aspect of these studies was the use of quantitative methods, to which peripheral nerves are singularly amenable, and also the application of animal models in the study of the mechanisms of nerve injury and repair.

The interest in peripheral nerve disorders that began in the mid 1950's had its origins in several related developments. Peripheral nerves have the advantage of accessibility to biopsy, and the application of the quantitative histometric methods developed during the Second World War to the study of human neuropathies was an obvious extension, as was the use of electron microscopy, then being employed to examine the ultrastructure of normal peripheral nerve by Fernández-Morán, Sjöstrand, Geren, Robertson, and others. At approximately the same time, the feasibility of using nerve conduction studies for the investigation of peripheral nerve disorders, which had been raised by the observations of Hodes, Larrabee, and German in 1949 on nerve injuries, was exploited initially by Simpson and Gilliatt in Britain and by Lambert in the United States. This immediately raised questions of a morphologic nature, for example, concerning the localized and generalized reductions in nerve conduction velocity that were detected in a variety of peripheral nerve disorders and for which no good explanation in pathologic terms was available at that time. The answers have slowly been emerging since then from correlated electrophysiologic and morphologic observations in both human neuropathies and animal models.

The extensive amount of work that has accumulated from these several approaches has so far not been assembled into a single presentation. The aim of this collective work on peripheral neuropathy has been to achieve a comprehensive account of the pathology, clinical neurophysiology, clinical features, and treatment of peripheral nerve disorders, preceded by a survey of the general biology of peripheral nerves. As editors, we have been fortunate in securing the collaboration of many of the workers who have remolded the concepts in this field during the past two decades, although the responsibility for the selection of the topics included and excluded is solely that of the editors. For a variety of reasons, projected chapters on the conduction of the nerve impulse, on motor nerve conduction in neuropathies, and on peripheral nerve lipids have had to be excluded.

The editors are deeply conscious of the influence and stimulation of their families, teachers, and collaborators. Peter Dyck acknowledges with gratitude the help of his father, Jacob, his wife, Isabelle, and his children, James and Katherine; of Professor D. S. Rawson, on whose limnobiology survey party at Lac la Ronge he first learned the methodology of sampling and measurement useful in the study of nerve; of Professor Jerzy Olszewski, who aroused his interest in cell biology; and of his past and present collaborators at the Mayo Clinic. P. K. Thomas wishes to express his appreciation to J. Z. Young, who first kindled his interest in peripheral nerves in the period immediately following the Second World War; to J. David Robertson, from whom he learned electron microscopy at the time the ultrastructure of peripheral nerve was first being defined; to R. W. Gilliatt for an introduction to clinical neurophysiology during the period when he and T. A. Sears were applying the nerve conduction techniques developed by G. D. Dawson to the study of peripheral neuropathies; and finally to B. G. Cragg, with whom he collaborated in his earlier experimental studies on peripheral nerve. E. H. Lambert acknowledges his introduction to neuromuscular disorders to Lee M. Eaton and stimulating association with many residents and graduate students at the Mayo Clinic.

The editors gratefully acknowledge their indebtedness to the staff of the W. B. Saunders Company, in particular to Miss Ruth Barker for her forbearance and scrupulous attention to setting this material in order for printing, and to Mr. Kendall S. McNally, Mr. Raymond Kersey, and Mr. Herbert J. Powell for administrative and production excellence. Peter Dyck and P. K. Thomas are particularly indebted to Mrs. Karen Oviatt and Miss Vivienne Tippet, respectively, for meticulous secretarial work.

CONTENTS

SECTION III
Pathology of the Peripheral Nervous System

SECTION IV
Nerve Conduction and Measurement of Cutaneous Sensation in Diseases of the Peripheral Nervous System

SECTION V
Diseases of the Peripheral Nervous System

PART A
Symptomatology and Differential Diagnosis of Peripheral Neuropathy

PART B
Diseases of the Cranial Nerves

PART C
Diseases of Spinal Cord, Spinal Roots, and Limb Girdle Plexuses

PART D
Neuropathy Due to Ischemia and Physical Agents

PART E
Inherited Peripheral Neuropathy

PART G
Infectious, Postinfectious, and Inflammatory Neuropathy

PART H
Neuropathy Due to Toxic Agents and Drugs

PART I
Neuropathy Associated With Neoplasms

SECTION VI
Rehabilitative Procedures

SECTION I

Introduction

Chapter 1

INTRODUCTION

Wilhelm Krücke

In 1970, for the first time, the pathology of the peripheral nerves and end organs was one of the main themes of discussion at an International Congress of Neuropathology; now, also for the first time, an independent, comprehensive volume on biology, pathology and clinical disorders of the peripheral nervous system is going to appear in which a larger than ever number of contributors have covered their various special disciplines.

At the beginning of this century Edinger was already convinced that no longer could one person alone do justice to the whole field of brain research; this view was restated by Penfield in 1932 in *Cytology and Cellular Pathology of the Nervous System*. Today the same applies to the relatively small field of the peripheral nervous system, which up till now has been regarded as easily surveyable. I have on two occasions reviewed the pathology of the peripheral nervous system single-handedly and know that such a task is no longer possible without the help of other specialists in the field.

In a short survey of the historical development of knowledge regarding the pathology of peripheral nerves, one is reminded of the new epoch that began for microscopic histology and histopathology when it was discovered that every organ of all organisms, plant and animal, was made up of cells (Schwann, 1839). By means of numerous microscopic investigations new facts soon came to light. The new methods, however, too enthusiastically applied by many inexperienced in general pathology, were almost discredited. Only through the work of experienced pathologists did histopathology develop into cellular

pathology (Virchow, 1858) and thus become an indispensable tool in medical science.

Fundamental discoveries were made at an early time on peripheral nerve tissue since it was readily accessible for microscopic examination: the recognition of the cellular structure of the nerve fiber, and of the Schwann cell (Schwann, 1839); the fact that the neuron was a trophic center and that transection of its process led to degeneration (Waller, 1850, 1852); the histology and physiology of the segmentation of nerve fibers into internodes and their degeneration and regeneration (Ranvier, 1871–1872, 1875, 1878); and their demyelination (névrite segmentaire périaxile) (Gombault, 1880–1881).

The significance of many of the newly discovered morphologic findings for the interpretation of function and of disorders of the nerves remained obscure in many instances, as is true even today. Some of the cellular constituents or proliferations discovered at that time, such as the π and μ granules of Schwann cells (Reich, 1903, 1907), the Elzholz bodies, the Renaut bodies and the "cellules godronnées" of Renaut (1881) and Langhans (1892), or the melanin-containing cells in the spinal root ganglia, remain even now subjects for investigation with newer methods and for discussion concerning their role in physiology or pathology.

Initially, the histopathologic changes had to be analyzed and grouped according to morphologic characteristics (Nissl, 1892; Alzheimer, 1904; Spielmeyer, 1922). The term "Äquivalentbild" that Nissl coined at the time, however, retains its validity also for the newer methods:

Wenn wir unter den gleichen Bedingungen der Technik an normalem Material immer die gleichen Bilder bekommen, so dürfen wir sie als gleichwertig dem lebenden Gewebe ansehen (Spielmeyer, 1922).

When the same histologic features are consistently obtained in normal material by the use of the same techniques, these features may be viewed as equivalent to [what exists] in the living tissue.

Whatever deviates from this norm may be regarded as pathologic, provided that only such methods are used as will give consistent results; for this reason Spielmeyer did not include the "inconsistent" silver impregnation methods among the most useful techniques in the study of histopathology. Spielmeyer further stipulated the necessity of a thorough knowledge of every fixation schedule and staining artifact that may occur.

It should be mentioned at this juncture that silver impregnation methods have proved most valuable both for the understanding of normal structure and for demonstration of segmental demyelination of the nerve fiber. It should also not be forgotten that, on the basis of a critical survey of the results obtained by silver methods, Waldeyer (1891) coined the well-chosen term "neurone" as an equivalent to the term "cell" in other organs. The "neurone theory" permitted the first well-founded statements about the connection between structure and function of the nervous system (see Cajal, 1935). Only today, however, do we realize the complexity of the connections between the central and the peripheral nervous systems and their functional "plasticity"; how much more we know now than was indicated in the old models and how little we understand, even today, about the interrelation between sensory and motor innervation.

Utilizing the methods and concepts of the early era of neuropathology, it was possible to delimit a number of the more complex reactions of the nerve cell; such as retrograde cell change (Nissl, 1892), chromatolysis after interruption of the axon, and the primary change of the nerve fiber after crushing of a nerve, resulting in swelling of the interrupted axon proximal and distal to the site of the lesion (Stroebe, 1893). It is interesting to observe the fate of these two discoveries. While Nissl's findings met with general recognition, Stroebe's were ignored to the point of rejec-

tion, although he had shown the sprouting of new axons from the central stump of axis cylinders in a regenerating nerve (as shown earlier by Ranvier, 1875, and Vanlair, 1882) and the process of regrowth, "neurotization," of a regenerating nerve via old degenerated nervous pathways. The doctrine, popular at the time among many authors, of autogenic regeneration and discontinuity of the nerve fiber, which was thought to be composed of segmental neuroblasts, completely displaced both the ingenious concept of Waller and its histopathologic proof by Vanlair, Ranvier, and Stroebe, Cajal (1905) noted this phenomenon as follows:

Paradoxical as it may appear, it is certain that in the problem with which we are dealing, contrary to the usual course of science, error is modern while truth is ancient.

And thus the struggle between autogenists and monogenists had commenced, finally to be resolved only in our own day.

Stroebe's further discovery of the swelling of the axon proximal and distal to a crushed region of the nerve provided the basis for experimental studies at a much later stage that suggested a proximodistal axoplasmic flow (Weiss and Hiscoe, 1948; Weiss and Mayr, 1971a, 1971b). According to the latest findings, however, this concept has to be amended since there is, apparently, an additional retrograde axoplasmic transport toward the perikaryon (Kristensson and Olsson, 1973). This would explain Stroebe's original finding regarding the axonal swelling of the distal stump. Interruption of this retrograde axoplasmic flow may provide the signal for the retrograde and chromatolytic reaction of the perikaryon to set in.

Doinikow (1911), in his classic studies on the morbid anatomy of neuritis and polyneuritis, failed to give a satisfactory classification of different types of nerve fiber degeneration. Nevertheless, his studies with their many new results provided the first comprehensive description of the cellular pathology of the peripheral nerves, and he also refuted the doctrine of peripheral neuroblasts. Doinikow's summary was disappointing, since he postulated that the segmental demyelination of the nerve fibers was to be interpreted only as a precursor of wallerian degeneration, which represented the end result of neuritis. The parallel processes of parenchymal degeneration and inflammatory reaction of the sheaths were supposed to influence each other, with sometimes the former and sometimes the latter reaction governing the histopathologic changes and thus creating the polymorphic pathologic picture of neuritis. This was confusing when a clear-cut subdivision of the clinical manifestations was aimed at. As recently as 1935, the term "neuritis" was even used for traumatic and parenchymatous lesions of the nerve, just as in former times the term "encephalitis" was used for almost any disease of the brain. Out of this confusion, the aim of morphologic analysis was directed toward a comprehensive study of the character and spread of the pathologic changes in the various diseases of the human peripheral nervous system and toward a comparison of the results with those produced experimentally. In this way it was hoped to delimit the fundamental differences of the various degenerative processes within the nerve fiber. There were, to begin with, only few examples in which the dominance of a specific feature, be it demyelination, wallerian degeneration, or a third type of disease that includes the peripheral neuron or a neuronal degeneration or atrophy starting nucleo-distally, was sufficiently clear to be determined by its morphologic characteristics (Krücke, 1955, 1959, 1961).

Nowadays whenever a discussion centers around the classification of the various nerve fiber diseases into morphologic types, and the relationship of these types to different human neurologic diseases, everyone familiar with the early struggles and misunderstandings is surprised and pleased about the ease with which neuropathologists talk about demyelination and neuronal degeneration or neuronal atrophy. It is also a gratifying thought that within the last 15 years a large number of experimental models representing different types of nerve fiber changes have been worked out (see that of Peter Dyck, Chapter 16 in this volume, among others). The results of this experimental work are encouraging and should stimulate further studies not only toward an analysis and subdivision of the etiologically and pathogenetically different processes of demyelination, but also toward a better understanding of the apparently diverse causative mechanism underlying neuronal degeneration and atrophy.

The lack of direct studies in man and in some disease entities can be partly compensated for by the results in animal experiments since, in principle, the degenerative and regenerative processes are the same in small laboratory animals as they are in man. Nevertheless,

certain differences between species do exist; these were first shown by Doinikow when he produced lead neuropathy whose morphologic picture differed in rabbits and guinea pigs.

The new quantitative methods, which, thanks to the improved embedding and cutting techniques, clearly demonstrate every nerve fiber, permit a more exact correlation with physiologic findings and will not only help in our understanding of the diseases, but possibly also lead toward a better appreciation of function within the nervous system as a whole. C. J. Herrick (1943) published a survey entitled: "The cranial nerves. A review of 50 years." His words may conclude this introduction:

It is obvious that there can be no understanding of the operations of the brain without accurate knowledge of the nerves which connect this central adjustor with the peripheral apparatus through which we have our only contacts with environment. It may be that we shall find, after all, that the peripheral nerves contain the thread of Ariadne which will guide our steps through the labyrinths of the brain.

REFERENCES

Alzheimer, A.: Histologische Studien zur Differentialdiagnose der progressiven Paralyse. *In* Histologische und histopathologische Arbeiten (Nissl-Alzheimer). Vol. 1. Jena, Fischer, 1904, pp. 1–299.

Cajal, S. R.: Mecanismo de la regeneración de los nervios. Trab. Lab. Invest. Biol., *4*:119–210, 1905–1906.

Cajal, S. R.: Die Neuronenlehre. *In* Bumke, O., and Foerster, O., (eds.): Handbuch der Neurologie. Vol. 1. Berlin, Julius Springer, 1935, pp. 887–994.

Doinikow, B.: Beiträge zur Histologie und Histopathologie des peripheren Nerven. *In* Histologische und histopathologische Arbeiten (Nissl-Alzheimer). Vol. 4. Jena, Fischer, 1911, pp. 445–630.

Edinger, L.: Wege und Ziele der Hirnforschung. Die interakademischen Hirnforschungsinstitute. Naturwissenschaften, *1*:441–444, 1913.

Elzholz, A.: Zur Histologie alter Nervenstümpfe in amputierten Gliedern. Jb. Psychiatr. Neurol., *19*:78–105, 1900.

Gombault, A.: Contribution à l'étude anatomique de la névrite parenchymateuse subaiguë et chronique. Névrite segmentaire péri-axile. Arch. Neurol. (Paris), *1*:11–38, 177–190, 1880–1881.

Herrick, C. J.: The cranial nerves. A review of fifty years. J. Sci. Lab., *38*:41–51, 1943.

Kristensson, K., and Olsson, Y.: Uptake and retrograde axonal transport of protein tracers in hypoglossal neurons. Acta Neuropathol. (Berl.), *23*:43–47, 1973.

Krücke, W.: Erkrankungen der peripheren Nerven. *In* Lubarsch, O., Henke, F., and Rössle, R., (eds.): Handbuch der speziellen pathologischen Anatomie und Histologie. Part 13/5. Berlin, Göttingen, Heidelberg, Springer, 1955, pp. 1–248.

Krücke, W.: Histopathologie der Polyneuritis und Polyneuropathie. Dtsch. Z. Nervenheilkd., *180*:1–39, 1959.

Krücke, W.: Die Erkrankungen der peripheren Nerven. *In* Staemmler, M. (ed.): Lehrbuch der speziellen pathologischen Anatomie. Part 3/2. Berlin, Walter de Gruyter & Co., 1961, pp. 750–793.

Langhans, T.: Über Veränderungen in den peripheren Nerven bei Cachexia thyreopriva des Menschen und Affen, sowie bei Cretinismus. Virchows Arch. Pathol. Anat., *128*:318–408, 1892.

Nissl, F.: Über die Veränderung der Ganglienzellen am Facialiskern des Kaninchens nach Ausreissung des Nerven. Allg. Z. Psychiatr., *48*:197–198, 1892.

Penfield, W.: Preface. *In* Penfield, W. (ed.): Cytology and Cellular Pathology of the Nervous System. Vol. 1. New York, P. and B. Hoeber, 1932.

Ranvier, L.: L'histologie et la physiologie des nerfs. Arch. Physiol. Norm. Pathol., *4*:427–446, 1871–1872a.

Ranvier, L.: Recherches sur l'histologie et la physiologie des nerfs. Arch. Physiol. Norm. Pathol., *4*:129–149, 1871–1872b.

Ranvier, L.: De la régénération des nerfs sectionnés. C. R. Acad. Sci. (Paris), *76*:491–495, 1875.

Ranvier, L.: Leçons sur l'histologie du système nerveux. Vol. II. Paris, Savy, 1878.

Reich, F.: Zur feineren Anatomie der Nervenzellen. Neurol. Zbl., *22*:138–139, 1903.

Reich, F.: Über den zelligen Aufbau der Nervenfasern auf Grund mikrohistochemischer Untersuchungen. I. Teil: Die chemischen Bestandteile des Nervenmarks, ihr mikrochemisches und färberisches Verhalten. J. Psychol. Neurol. (Leipzig), *8*:244–273, 1907.

Renaut, M. J.: Recherches sur quelques points particuliers de l'histologie des nerfs. Arch. Physiol. Norm. Pathol. II. ser. (Paris), *8*:161–190, 1881a.

Renaut, M. J.: Système hyalin de soutènement des centres nerveux et de quelques organes des sens. Arch. Physiol. Norm. Pathol. II. ser. (Paris), *8*:845–860, 1881b.

Schwann, T.: Mikroskopische Untersuchungen über die Übereinstimmung in der Struktur und dem Wachstum der Tiere und Pflanzen. Berlin, 1839. Reprinted by F. Hünseler, Ostwalds Klassiker 176, Leipzig, 1910.

Spielmeyer, W.: Histopathologie des Nervensystems. Part 1. Berlin, Springer, 1922.

Stroebe, H.: Experimentelle Untersuchungen über Degeneration peripherer Nerven nach Verletzungen. Beitr. Pathol. Anat., *13*:160–278, 1893.

Vanlair: 1882 (Cited by Stroebe, Beitr. Pathol. Anat., *13*:160–278, 1893.

Virchow, R.: Die Cellularpathologie in ihrer Begründung auf physiologische und pathologische Gewebslehre. Berlin, August Hirschwald, 1858.

Waldeyer, W.: Über einige neuere Forschungen im Gebiete der Anatomie des Centralnervensystems. Dtsch. Med. Wochenschr., Nr. 44–50, 1891.

Waller, A.: Experiments on the section of the glossopharyngeal and hypoglossal nerves of the frog, and observations of the alterations produced thereby in the structure of their primitive fibres. Philos. Trans. R. Soc. Lond. B., *140*:423–429, 1850.

Waller, A.: Sur la réproduction des nerfs et sur la structure et les functions des ganglions spinaux. Arch. Anat. Physiol. Wiss. Med., 392–401, 1852.

Weiss, P. A., and Hiscoe, H. B.: Experiments on the mechanism of nerve growth. J. Exp. Zool., *107*:315–395, 1948.

Weiss, P. A., and Mayr, R.: Neuronal organelles in neuroplasmic ("axonal") flow, I. Mitochondria. *In* Friede, R. L., and Seitelberger, F. (eds.): Symposium on pathology of axons and axonal flow. Acta Neuropathol. (Berl.), Suppl. V, 187–197, 1971a.

Weiss, P. A., and Mayr, R.: Neuronal organelles in neuroplasmic ("axonal") flow, II. Neurotubules. *In* Friede, R. L., and Seitelberger, F. (eds.): Symposium on pathology of axons and axonal flow. Acta Neuropathol. (Berl.), Suppl. V, 198–206, 1971b.

SECTION II

Biology of the
Peripheral Nervous System

Chapter 2

GROSS ANATOMY OF THE PERIPHERAL NERVOUS SYSTEM

Ernest Gardner

By common definition, the peripheral nervous system includes the cranial nerves, the spinal nerves with their roots and rami, the peripheral nerves, and the peripheral components of the autonomic nervous system. This chapter presents the principles of organization and distribution of the peripheral nervous system, and outlines its major gross anatomical features; the cranial nerves and their autonomic components are considered in other chapters. Books and atlases that provide more detailed information, most of which have valuable bibliographies (Gardner, Gray, and O'Rahilly, 1969; Hollinshead, 1968, 1969, 1971; Hovelacque, 1927; von Lanz and Wachsmuth, 1953–1972; Pernkopf, 1963; Pitres and Testut, 1925; Schadé, 1966; and Warwick and Williams's Gray's Anatomy, 1973), are included in the references. Illustrations are limited to those that present concepts of the arrangement and distribution of spinal and peripheral nerves. The terminology used follows the *Nomina Anatomica* (1966) translated into English where appropriate.

GENERAL FEATURES

Spinal and Peripheral Nerves

The dorsal and ventral roots are attached to the spinal cord by a series of filaments. Each root enters a dural pouch, or sac, and then a dural sheath, the sac being subdivided by a septum. Immediately peripheral to the spinal ganglion of the dorsal root, corresponding dorsal and ventral roots form a spinal nerve. The dural sheaths become confluent at the ganglion, and then merge with the epineurium of the spinal nerve. Each spinal nerve quickly divides into a dorsal and a ventral (primary) ramus. The dorsal rami supply the back; the ventral rami supply the limbs and ventrolateral part of the body wall. In the cervical and lumbosacral regions, the ventral rami intermingle and form plexuses from which the major peripheral nerves emerge (the term peripheral nerve also refers to cranial nerves, to the direct continuations of the thoracic ventral rami, and to various branches of dorsal rami).

Although the funicular organization and connective tissue elements of nerves are described in other chapters, some general aspects are worth noting here. The sheaths convey the intrinsic blood and lymphatic vessels, and the nervi nervorum, which supply the connective tissue and vessels with sensory and autonomic fibers. The sheaths also impart strength, especially against tensile stresses. Spinal nerves have thinner and less well-defined sheaths and are, therefore, more fragile. The funicular arrangement of nerves is a matter of considerable importance, especially in connection with injury, surgical repair, and regeneration. Sunderland (1968) has described these arrangements in detail, especially with respect to the variation in number and size of funiculi, their intraneural course, and their redistribution through the formation of funicular plexuses.

A number of classifications of nerve fibers have been proposed, based on their various properties. One that is in common use is based chiefly on comparative studies and has proved useful in clarifying our concepts, especially of cranial nerves. It describes seven different kinds of fibers or functional components, of which four are present in spinal nerves: somatic efferent (motor to skeletal muscle), general visceral efferent (autonomic), general somatic afferent (sensory from skin, muscles, joints, and deep tissues), and general visceral afferent (sensory from viscera). This classification, however, is more detailed than necessary for this chapter and the terms "motor," "sensory," and "autonomic" are used, with clarification or elaboration where necessary.

Cranial nerves differ significantly from spinal nerves, especially in their mode of embryologic development and their relation to the special senses, and because some cranial nerves supply branchial arch structures. They are attached to the brain at irregular rather than regular intervals; they are not formed of dorsal and ventral roots; some have more than one ganglion, whereas others have none; and the optic nerve is a fiber tract and not a true peripheral nerve. Cranial nerves vary in the number of functional components present, and some cranial nerves contain functional components not present in spinal nerves. These are: (1) special visceral efferent (motor to branchiomeric muscles), (2) special visceral afferent (taste, a special sense associated with visceral functions), and (3) special somatic afferent (the other special senses).

DISTRIBUTION OF SPINAL AND PERIPHERAL NERVES

When the ventral ramus of a spinal nerve enters a plexus and joins other such rami, its component funiculi ultimately enter several of the peripheral nerves emerging from the plexus. Thus, as a general principle, each ramus entering a plexus contributes to several peripheral nerves, and each such peripheral nerve contains fibers derived from several ventral rami. Thus, each spinal nerve has a pattern of ultimate distribution referred to as segmental or dermatomal, in contrast to that characteristic of peripheral

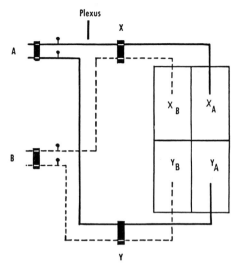

Figure 2–1 Schematic diagram of spinal and peripheral nerve distribution. Only sensory fibers to the skin are represented. Two nerve fibers of spinal nerve A are shown entering a plexus. One of the fibers joins peripheral nerve X, and the other joins peripheral nerve Y. Two fibers of spinal nerve B also join the two peripheral nerves. Thus, the areas supplied by the two spinal nerves are different from the areas supplied by the two peripheral nerves, as shown in the subdivided rectangle. (From Gardner, E., Gray, D. J., and O'Rahilly, R.: Anatomy. 3rd Ed. Philadelphia, W. B. Saunders Co., 1969.)

nerves (Fig. 2–1) (Hansen and Schliack, 1962; Haymaker and Woodhall, 1953; Sunderland, 1968). The term "segmental" refers to the fact that the longitudinal extent of spinal cord to which a right and left pair of spinal roots is attached constitutes a segment of the spinal cord. The term "dermatome" refers to skin, and a dermatome is the area of skin supplied by the sensory fibers of a single dorsal root through the dorsal and ventral rami of its spinal nerve. It is evident, then, that since most dorsal rami have cutaneous branches, the area of skin supplied by just a ventral ramus is usually not a complete dermatome.

The mixture of nerve fibers in plexuses is such that it is difficult, if not impossible, to trace their course by dissection, and dermatomal distribution has been determined by physiologic experimentation and by studying disorders and surgical sections of spinal roots and nerves. The results of such studies have yielded complex maps, chiefly because of variation, overlap, and differences in method. Variation results from intrasegmental rootlet anastomoses adjacent to the cervical and lumbosacral spinal cord (Pallie, 1959) and from individual differences in plexus formation and peripheral nerve distribution. Overlap is such that section of a single root does not produce complete anesthesia in the area supplied by that root; at the most, some degree of hypalgesia may result. Overlap is greater for touch than for pain, hence the more common occurrence of hypalgesia rather than hypesthesia after section of a single root. Problems of interpretation result from differences in method:

As pointed out by Pearson et al. (1966), the fundamental problem is one of segmentation and involves the question: Do certain dermatomes extend as a series of bands from the median plane of the back into the limbs, and are these bands of dermatomes arranged in an uninterrupted sequence? A full discussion of this problem and its embryologic basis is beyond the scope of this chapter. Nevertheless, it is important to note that the maps published by Keegan and Garrett (1948) indicate that all dermatomes, from C2 to S1, form an uninterrupted, simply arranged series extending from the median plane of the back. Their data were based largely on the detection of hypalgesia following compression of a single nerve root by a herniated nucleus pulposus. The degree of compression was usually not verified. Valuable as their maps might be as diagnostic aids in such disorders, it must be emphasized that their methods yield zones of hypalgesia that are not complete dermatomes. Moreover, as Pearson et al. (1966) point out, the discussion presented by Keegan and Garrett (1948) contains significant conceptual defects, and some of their data are at serious odds with anatomical arrangements. In contrast, Foerster (1933, 1936) published data on dermatomes that, while admittedly incomplete, derived from studies based on sound physiologic methods, as follows: (1) Method of residual sensitivity—a single root was left intact, as contiguous roots above and below were divided. This gave the total distribution of the intact dorsal root. (2) Constructive method— a series of contiguous roots was divided; consequently, the superior border of the resulting anesthesia represented the inferior border of the dermatome corresponding to the next higher intact root, and the inferior border of the anesthetic area represented the superior border of the next lower intact root. (3) Stimulation of dorsal roots—electrical stimulation yielded vasodilatation in areas of skin that were smaller than the dermatomes determined by the residual method, but that

were similar in shape and general location. These areas resembled the zones reported by Head and Campbell (1900) in their classic study of the distribution of herpes zoster.

The maps shown in Figures 2–2 and 2–3 are based on Foerster's study of a large number of human patients in which he used combinations of the methods just outlined; they have been shown to be useful clinically (Fender, 1939; Foerster, 1933, 1936). It must, however, be emphasized that the maps depict presumably normal dermatomes, not areas of sensory deficit. This statement is qualified because spinal cord sensitivity may be altered by root sections in such a way as to affect the size of the dermatome being tested by peripheral stimulation.

It is of interest that there is little correspondence between dermatomes and underlying muscles. Many tables have been published that list the segmental supply of muscles or of the segments controlling movements at joints. Schemes have been proposed that attempt to bring some logical proximodistal order into the segmental supply of limb muscles (Last, 1949). These tables and schemes, however, tend to be limited in value because of variation, overlap, and incomplete information about segmental motor origin and distribution. The general arrangement is that the more rostral segments of the cervical and lumbosacral enlargements supply the more proximal limb muscles (note, however, that segments C5 to C8 are involved in shoulder movements), and that the more caudal segments supply the more distal muscles (T1 is the chief motor supply of the intrinsic muscles of the hand). A muscle usually receives fibers from each of the spinal nerves that enter the peripheral nerve supplying it (although one spinal nerve may be its chief supply), and section of a single spinal nerve weakens but does not usually paralyze a muscle. Finally, published diagrams that illustrate the segmental sensory supply of bones and joints are based chiefly on dissections and clinical observations. Their clinical value is doubtful, especially in view of the diffuse and often referred nature of pain from these deep structures.

The distribution of peripheral nerves in the limbs is fundamentally different from that of spinal nerves, as shown in Figures 2–4 and 2–5. These enable one to contrast cutaneous supply with the dermatomes of Figures 2–2 and 2–3 (in the trunk, however, peripheral and spinal nerves are usually identical in their

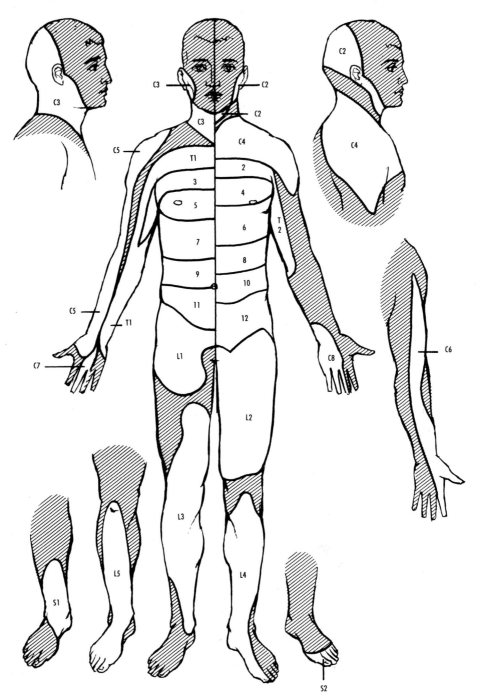

Figure 2–2 Front view of dermatomal distribution, based on Foerster's data (1933, 1936). The right and left halves show the total distribution of alternating dermatomes, thereby illustrating the degree of overlap. In some regions, however, overlap is very great and more than two dermatomes may be involved. Hence, additional figures (insets) are necessary to show the total distribution of certain dermatomes. (From Gardner, E., Gray, D. J., and O'Rahilly, R.: Anatomy. 3rd Ed. Philadelphia, W. B. Saunders Co., 1969.)

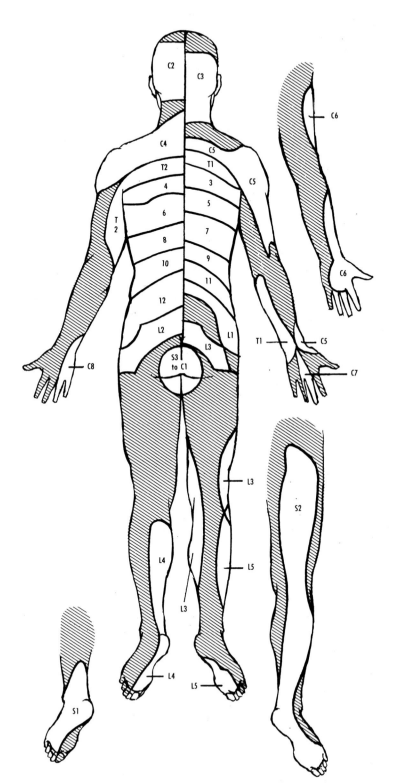

Figure 2–3 Back view of dermatomes, based on Foerster's data (1933, 1936) as explained in legend for Figure 2–2.

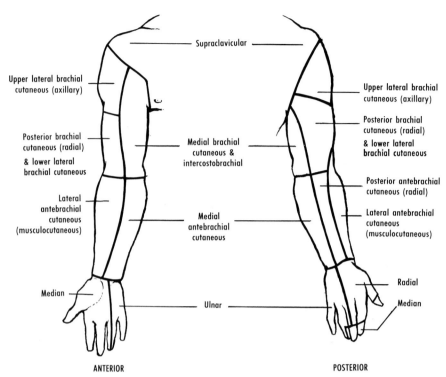

Figure 2–4   Approximate areas of cutaneous nerve distribution to the upper limb. Neither variation nor overlap is shown. (From Gardner, E., Gray, D. J., and O'Rahilly, R.: Anatomy. 3rd Ed. Philadelphia, W. B. Saunders Co., 1969.)

cutaneous distribution). Peripheral nerves to the limbs also overlap, but to a lesser extent than do spinal nerves. Thus, if a peripheral nerve is cut, the muscles supplied by the nerve are greatly weakened or completely paralyzed, autonomic dysfunction occurs, and sensation is lost in the central part of the area of distribution of the nerve and diminished at the edges of its area of supply. The last is due to overlap from adjacent peripheral nerves; the overlap is less than in the case of spinal nerves and is often less for touch than for pain. Peripheral nerves vary in their course and distribution, and adjacent nerves may communicate with each other (variations of individual nerves are discussed in Gardner, Gray, and O'Rahilly, 1969, and in Hollinshead, 1968, 1969, 1971). Such communications sometimes account for unexpected residual sensation or movement after section of a nerve.

Whatever the pattern of distribution, major peripheral nerves usually have five general kinds of branches: (1) muscular (motor, sensory, and autonomic fibers; the sensory fibers are from muscle fibers and associated connective tissue and tendons, and sometimes joints), (2) cutaneous or mucosal

(each has sensory and autonomic fibers; the cutaneous branches often include fibers from subjacent joints, ligaments, and tendons, especially in the case of digital nerves), (3) articular (arising when the nerve crosses a joint, and containing sensory and autonomic fibers), (4) vascular (sensory and autonomic to adjacent blood vessels), and (5) terminal (one, several, or all of the foregoing).

Also of importance, in addition to peripheral distribution, are the order and site of origin of individual branches, including distances to the muscles they supply, as well as the order in which structures are innervated, and the nature and extent of variations (Sunderland, 1946; Sunderland and Hughes, 1946; Sunderland and Ray, 1946). Moreover, in many instances peripheral nerves pass through osteofibrous canals where they may be subject to compression. The chief sites of compression and related literature are summarized by Smorto and Basmajian (1972).

Autonomic Nervous System

Certain general principles of organization are presented here to clarify the relationships

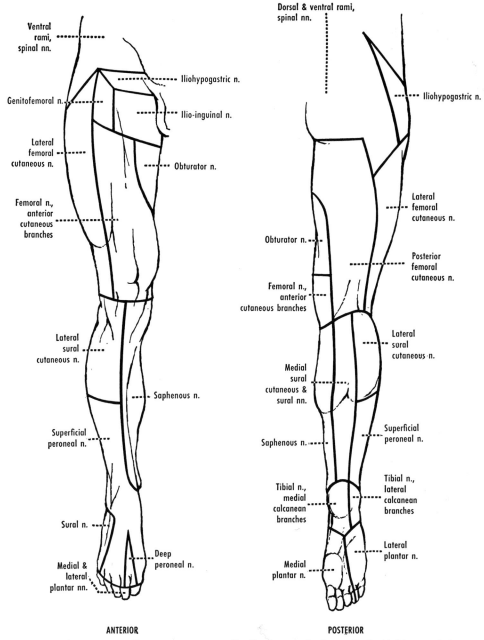

Figure 2–5   Approximate areas of cutaneous nerve distribution to the lower limb. Neither variation nor overlap is shown. (From Gardner, E., Gray, D. !., and O'Rahilly, R.: Anatomy. 3rd Ed. Philadelphia, W. B. Saunders Co., 1969.)

of spinal and peripheral nerves with the autonomic nervous system.

By classic anatomical definition, the autonomic nervous system, sometimes called the visceral or vegetative nervous system, is that system of motor nerve fibers that supplies cardiac muscle, smooth muscle, and glands, and that consists, in its simplest form, of a pathway of two succeeding nerve cells. The

first cell is located in the brain or spinal cord, the second in a ganglion outside the brain and spinal cord. Anatomically and functionally, however, the autonomic nervous system is much more complex than the simplistic definition just given would indicate, to a degree far beyond the scope of this chapter.

The autonomic pathway or outflow begins with certain nerve cells in the brain stem and

spinal cord. The axons of these cells, termed
preganglionic fibers, leave the brain stem and
spinal cord over certain cranial nerves and
ventral roots, and synapse in peripheral
autonomic ganglia (including the suprarenal
medullae and certain chromaffin cells). The
axons of the ganglion cells are termed postganglionic fibers and are distributed to
cardiac muscle, smooth muscle, and certain
gland cells. The locations, arrangements,
connections, and patterns of distribution of
the preganglionic and postganglionic autonomic fibers are grouped, on the basis of an
anatomical classification or subdivision of the
pathways, into *sympathetic* and *parasympathetic
systems* or *divisions.* Most viscera are supplied
by both systems, which furnish what might be
termed opposing functions.

Works cited in the references, several of
which contain valuable bibliographies, provide additional information about the autonomic nervous system (Delmas and Laux,
1952; Hovelacque, 1927; Kuntz, 1953; Mitchell, 1953; Pick, 1970).

SYMPATHETIC (THORACOLUMBAR) SYSTEM

This part of the autonomic nervous system
comprises the preganglionic fibers that issue
from the thoracic and upper lumbar levels
of the spinal cord. These fibers travel in
ventral roots and spinal nerves to reach
peripheral sympathetic ganglia where they
synapse with ganglion cells. The locations of
these ganglia are related to the embryonic
migration of cells from the neural tube and
neural crest, which form the ganglia of the
sympathetic trunk and prevertebral plexuses.

SYMPATHETIC TRUNK AND GANGLIA

Most preganglionic fibers leave the spinal
nerves or ventral rami and reach the adjacent
sympathetic trunk and ganglia by way of rami
communicantes (Fig. 2–6). The sympathetic
trunks are long nerve strands, one on each
side of the vertebral column, extending from
the base of the skull to the coccyx. Each
usually contains 21 to 25 ganglia of varying
sizes, but broader ranges have been recorded.

Many of the preganglionic fibers that enter
the sympathetic trunks synapse in the ganglia
of the trunks and in accessory ganglia; those

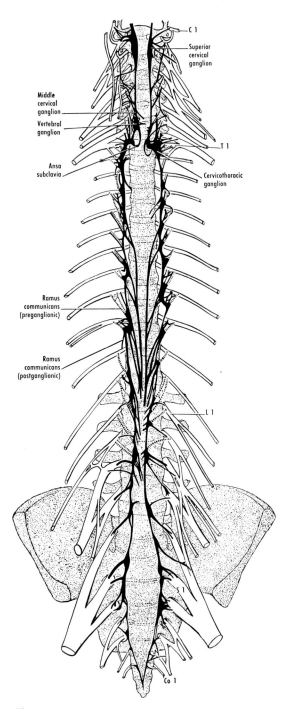

Figure 2–6 The sympathetic trunks. Preganglionic
rami communicantes are shown as interrupted lines,
postganglionic rami as solid black. Based on studies by
Pick and Sheehan (1946). From Gardner, E., Gray, D. J.,
and O'Rahilly, R.: Anatomy. 3rd Ed. Philadelphia, W. B.
Saunders Co., 1969.)

that do not synapse continue through and reach ganglia of the prevertebral plexuses. Of the postganglionic fibers arising in the trunk ganglia, some go directly to adjacent viscera and blood vessels; the others return to spinal nerves and dorsal and ventral rami by way of rami communicantes. The fibers in these rami eventually supply secretory fibers to sweat glands, motor fibers to the smooth muscle of the hair follicles (arrectores pilorum), and motor fibers to the smooth muscle of the blood vessels of the limbs and walls of the trunk. However, some of the postganglionic fibers to the back and to the proximal parts of the limbs reach these parts by accompanying blood vessels.

Each trunk ganglion has one to four rami communicantes, which connect it with the corresponding nerve and often with the nerve above or below. The ramus or rami containing the most postganglionic fibers tend to connect with the corresponding nerve (each spinal nerve or one of its rami receives such fibers). In the thorax, the rami containing the most preganglionic fibers are more oblique in direction (coming from the spinal nerve above or below), and they are more lateral in position, that is, farther from the spinal cord (Pick and Sheehan, 1946).

PREVERTEBRAL PLEXUSES AND GANGLIA AND CHROMAFFIN SYSTEM

Many embryonic ganglion cells migrate to a position in front of the vertebral column where they form ganglionic masses that are named according to adjacent viscera or blood vessels. The preganglionic fibers that enter these ganglia are those that traverse the sympathetic trunks without synapsing. They reach the prevertebral ganglia by way of branches termed splanchnic nerves (the term splanchnic is also applied to certain visceral branches in the pelvis). These nerves may contain ganglia along their course. The postganglionic fibers from these various ganglia go directly to adjacent viscera and blood vessels. These ganglia, their preganglionic and postganglionic fibers, and the thoracic and abdominal branches of the vagus nerves, form what are termed the prevertebral plexuses. Many sensory fibers from viscera (for pain as well as reflexes) traverse these plexuses and reach the spinal cord by way of splanchnic nerves, rami communicantes, and dorsal roots, or the brain stem by way of the vagus nerves.

Some of the migrating embryonic cells form the chromaffin system, in particular the medullae of the adrenal glands. Correspondingly, some of the preganglionic fibers in the splanchnic nerves end in relation to these cells.

ACCESSORY GANGLIA

Some of the migrating embryonic cells stop along spinal nerves, ventral rami, and rami communicantes, especially in the cervical, lower thoracic, and upper lumbar levels. Here they form scattered sympathetic cells, which often are collected into definite accessory (intermediate) ganglia (Skoog, 1947; Wrete, 1943). The postganglionic fibers from these cells continue in their associated nerves; hence sympathectomies in these regions may not be completely effective (Monro, 1959).

PARASYMPATHETIC (CRANIOSACRAL) SYSTEM

This part of the autonomic system comprises the preganglionic fibers that issue from the brain stem by way of the third, seventh, ninth, tenth, and eleventh cranial nerves, and from the sacral cord by way of its second and third or third and fourth ventral roots. The ganglion cells are usually in or near the organ to be innervated, hence the postganglionic fibers are short. Moreover, none seem to go to the blood vessels, smooth muscle, or glands of the limbs or body walls.

The cranial nerves are described elsewhere, but it is worth noting that the parasympathetic ganglia of the third, seventh, and ninth cranial nerves form what are termed the cephalic or cranial parasympathetic ganglia (ciliary, pterygopalatine, otic, and submandibular). Their postganglionic fibers supply the eye, lacrimal and salivary glands, and mucous and serous glands of the oral and nasal cavities. The preganglionic fibers of the eleventh nerve are distributed with the vagus nerves; the ganglion cells are near or in the walls of the viscera of the neck, thorax, and abdomen. As mentioned earlier, vagal branches contribute to the prevertebral plexuses.

The sacral preganglionic parasympathetic fibers leave the sacral plexus as pelvic splanchnic nerves, enter the inferior hypogastric plexus, and reach ganglion cells in the walls of pelvic organs.

GROSS ANATOMY

The gross anatomy of the peripheral nervous system of each region of the body and the distribution and branching of nerves are outlined here, with emphasis on certain regional or topographical features. Additional special details are to be found in references dealing with peripheral nerve injuries (Haymaker and Woodhall, 1953; Seddon, 1972; Smorto and Basmajian, 1972; Sunderland, 1968).

Head and Neck and Upper Limb

CERVICAL PLEXUS

The ventral rami of the upper four cervical nerves unite to form the cervical plexus; those of the lower four, together with the greater part of that of the first thoracic, join to form the brachial plexus. (The distribution of the dorsal rami of the cervical nerves is described later.) Each cervical ramus receives one or more rami communicantes (containing postganglionic fibers) from a cervical sympathetic ganglion, and often from the vertebral nerve and plexus as well.

The cervical plexus is arranged as an irregular series of loops located in front of the levator scapulae and scalenus medius, under cover of the sternocleidomastoid muscle and internal jugular vein. The branches of the loops are superficial (to the skin of the back of the head, the neck, and the shoulder) and deep (to certain neck muscles and the diaphragm).

SUPERFICIAL BRANCHES

These cutaneous branches emerge near the middle of the posterior border of the sternocleidomastoid. They include: the *lesser occipital nerve*, which ascends behind the ear and supplies some of the skin on the side of the head and on the cranial surface of the ear; the *great auricular nerve*, which ascends obliquely across the sternocleidomastoid to supply the skin over the parotid gland, over the mastoid process, and on both surfaces of the ear; the *transverse cervical nerves*, which supply the skin on the side and front of the neck; and the *supraclavicular nerves*, derived from a common trunk that divides into anterior, middle, and posterior supraclavicular nerves, which supply the skin over the shoulder and the front of the thorax.

DEEP BRANCHES

These are the ansa cervicalis, the phrenic nerve, and muscular branches to the sternocleidomastoid, trapezius, levator scapulae, scalene, and prevertebral muscles. There are also small communicating branches to the tenth, eleventh, and twelfth cranial nerves.

The *ansa cervicalis* (ansa hypoglossi) is a loop formed by fibers of the first three (or the second and third) cervical nerves. It presents a superior root (the so-called descending branch of the hypoglossal nerve), which connects it with the hypoglossal nerve, but which consists of fibers from the second or first cervical nerve, and an inferior root (nervus descendens cervicalis), which connects it with branches from the second and third cervical nerves. The ansa cervicalis supplies the infrahyoid muscles. The thyrohyoid, however, receives its cervical fibers by way of the hypoglossal nerve.

The *phrenic nerve*, which supplies the diaphragm, arises chiefly from the fourth cervical nerve, but commonly has a root from the fifth as well, and sometimes from the third. Rarely, it may arise entirely from the accessory phrenic nerve. It descends in front of the scalenus anterior, enters the thorax, and descends between the pericardium and mediastinal pleura. The right phrenic nerve passes in front of the root of the right lung, pierces the diaphragm near the opening for the inferior vena cava (or traverses the opening for that vessel), and distributes most of its motor fibers from below. The left phrenic nerve passes in front of the root of the left lung and pierces the diaphragm immediately to the left of the pericardium.

Each nerve carries motor fibers to the diaphragm and sensory and autonomic fibers for the diaphragm, pleura, and peritoneum. Referred pain from the area of supply of a phrenic nerve is commonly felt in the skin over the trapezius (C4 and C5). Pain is sometimes referred to the region of the ear; this is probably related to a contribution from the third cervical nerve.

The *accessory phrenic nerve* is present in about one third of instances. It usually arises from the fifth cervical nerve through the nerve to the subclavius, but may arise from the cervical plexus or from a cardiac branch of a cervical sympathetic ganglion. The accessory nerve runs a variable course before joining the phrenic nerve in the thorax. If such a nerve is present, section of the phrenic nerve in the neck will not paralyze the corresponding half of the diaphragm completely.

BRACHIAL PLEXUS

The brachial plexus, which is situated partly in the neck and partly in the axilla, is formed by the ventral rami of the lower four cervical nerves and the greater part of the ventral ramus of the first thoracic nerve. These rami lie first between the scalenus anterior and the scalenus medius, and then in the posterior triangle of the neck. Here the plexus is situated above the clavicle, posterior and lateral to the sternocleidomastoid. It lies above and behind the third part of the subclavian artery and is crossed by the inferior belly of the omohyoid. In this situation, the plexus may be injected with a local anesthetic. The general features of the plexus are discussed in greater detail by Fenart (1958), Harris (1904, 1939), and Kerr (1918).

The plexus descends behind the concavity of the medial two thirds of the clavicle, and accompanies the axillary artery under cover of the pectoralis major. It is enclosed with the axillary vessels in the axillary sheath, and its cords are arranged around the second part of the axillary artery behind the pectoralis minor. The terminal branches of the plexus arise at the inferolateral border of the pectoralis minor. The brachial plexus can be marked on the surface by a line from the posterior margin of the sternocleidomastoid at the level of the cricoid cartilage to the midpoint of the clavicle. The plexus can be palpated both above and below the omohyoid, in the angle between the clavicle and the sternocleidomastoid.

The common, though not invariable, arrangement of branches is as follows. The ventral rami of the fifth and sixth cervical nerves unite to form the upper trunk, that of the seventh remains single as the middle trunk, and the eighth cervical and first thoracic rami form the lower trunk. Each trunk then divides into an anterior and a posterior division (for the front and back of

the limb respectively). The anterior divisions of the upper and middle trunks unite to form the lateral cord, the anterior division of the lower trunk forms the medial cord, and the three posterior divisions form the posterior cord. The terminal branches arise from the three cords. The brachial plexus is thus composed successively of (1) ventral rami and trunks that lie in the neck in relation to the subclavian artery (the lowest trunk lies on the first rib behind the subclavian artery), (2) divisions that lie behind the clavicle, and (3) cords and branches that lie in the axilla in relation to the axillary artery.

VARIATIONS

The brachial plexus frequently receives contributions from the fourth cervical or the second thoracic nerve also, or from both. When the contribution from the fourth cervical is large and that from the first thoracic small, the plexus is described as being prefixed in relation to the vertebral column. When the contributions from the first and second thoracic nerves are large, the plexus is termed postfixed; this latter situation is prominent when the first rib is rudimentary (Cave, 1929; Dow, 1925). It is, however, uncommon to find prefixation or postfixation in the sense of a complete shift in which a full nerve is gained at one end while one is completely lost at the other end. Other variations (in gross form, component arrangements, and branching) are common.

BRANCHES OF THE VENTRAL RAMI

These are the dorsal scapular and long thoracic nerves, and twigs to the scalene and longus colli muscles.

The *dorsal scapular nerve* (chiefly C5) sometimes supplies the levator scapulae but is distributed chiefly to the rhomboids. The *long thoracic nerve* arises by three roots from C5 to C7, descends behind the brachial plexus, and enters the external surface of the serratus anterior.

BRANCHES OF THE TRUNKS

These are the nerve to the subclavius and the suprascapular nerve, and occasionally medial and lateral pectoral nerves also.

The *nerve to the subclavius* (C5) descends behind the clavicle, in front of the brachial plexus to supply the subclavius muscle and the sternoclavicular joints. It often sends fibers to the phrenic nerve by a communicating branch, the accessory phrenic nerve described earlier. The *suprascapular nerve* (C5, C6) passes through the scapular notch, supplies the acromioclavicular and shoulder joints and the supraspinatus muscle, and then passes through the spinoglenoid notch to end in the infraspinatus.

BRANCHES OF THE CORDS

These include a number of cutaneous and muscular branches, and the important terminal branches, namely, the median, ulnar, radial, musculocutaneous, and axillary nerves.

Several *lateral pectoral nerves* (C5 to C7) arise from the lateral cord (or upper and middle trunks) and supply both pectoral muscles as well as the acromioclavicular and shoulder joints. *Medial pectoral nerves* (C8, T1) from the medial cord (or lower trunk) supply both pectoral muscles. Also arising from the medial cord is the *medial antebrachial cutaneous nerve* (C8, T1), which descends with the brachial artery to the lower part of the arm where it becomes cutaneous. It divides into anterior and ulnar branches, which supply the skin of the medial half of the forearm. The *medial brachial cutaneous nerve* (chiefly T1), also a branch of the medial cord, is a small nerve that supplies the medial and posterior aspects of the arm and communicates with the intercostobrachial nerve.

From the posterior cord, there arise the *upper subscapular nerve* (or nerves) (C5), for the subscapularis; the *thoracodorsal nerve* (C7, C8), for the latissimus dorsi; and the *lower subscapular nerve* (or nerves) (C5, C6), for the subscapularis and teres major.

The *median nerve* (C5, C6 to C8, T1) arises from the medial and lateral cords by medial and lateral roots, which unite in a variable fashion (Fig. 2–7). Descending as a part of the neurovascular bundle, it enters the cubital fossa where it lies under cover of the bicipital aponeurosis and supplies the elbow joint. It then passes between the two heads of the pronator teres and descends on the deep surface of the flexor digitorum superficialis. It is indicated on the surface by a line down the middle of the forearm to the midpoint between the styloid processes. Just above the

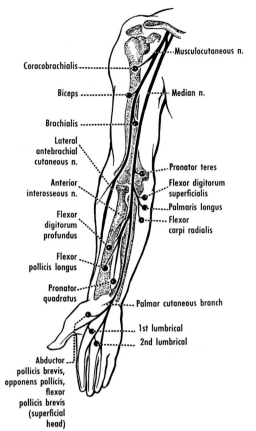

Figure 2–7 Schematic representation of the sequences of muscular and cutaneous branches of the musculocutaneous and median nerves. The black dot in each instance represents a muscle or a muscle group. The sequences of muscular branches are the more common ones. Based on studies by Sunderland and Ray (1946). (From Gardner, E., Gray, D. J., and O'Rahilly, R.: Anatomy. 3rd Ed. Philadelphia, W. B. Saunders Co., 1969.)

flexor retinaculum, it is quite superficial in the interval between the flexor carpi radialis and palmaris longus tendons, and completely so if the latter muscle is absent. The median nerve enters the hand by passing through the carpal canal, behind the flexor retinaculum. It then spreads out in an enlargement and divides into its terminal branches under cover of the palmar aponeurosis and the superficial palmar arch. Usually it divides first into lateral and medial portions or divisions.

The median nerve has no muscular branches in the arm. In the forearm, it supplies all the muscles of the front of the forearm except the flexor carpi ulnaris and the medial half of the flexor digitorum profundus. In the cubital fossa, a bundle of muscular branches is given to the pronator teres, flexor carpi radialis, palmaris longus, and flexor digitorum superficialis. The anterior interosseous nerve also arises in the cubital fossa. It descends on the front of the interosseous membrane, supplies the flexor pollicis longus and flexor digitorum profundus (lateral part), passes behind and supplies the pronator quadratus, and ends in twigs to the wrist and intercarpal joints. In the lower part of the forearm, the median nerve gives off an inconstant palmar branch for the supply of a small area of the skin of the palm. The median and ulnar nerves may communicate in the forearm, and the anterior interosseous nerve may communicate with the ulnar nerve.

In the hand, the lateral division gives off an important muscular branch (recurrent branch) for the abductor pollicis, flexor pollicis brevis, and opponens pollicis, which anastomoses with the deep branch of the ulnar nerve (Harness and Sekeles, 1971). The lateral division then divides in such a way as to furnish three palmar digital nerves for both sides of the thumb and the lateral aspect of the index finger and the first lumbrical. The medial division divides in such a way as to furnish four palmar digital nerves for the adjacent sides of the index and middle fingers, middle and ring fingers, and the second lumbrical. All digital nerves, near their terminations, send branches dorsally to the backs of the distal parts of the fingers, and all digital nerves, in both hand and foot, supply ligaments, joints, and tendons of the digits, as well as skin. Rarely the median nerve supplies the first dorsal interosseous or the adductor pollicis. As a general rule, the median nerve tends to supply the thenar muscles, and the ulnar nerve the remainder. However, the dividing line between the two distributions is variable, and either nerve may invade the territory of the other.

The *ulnar nerve* (C7, C8, T1) arises from the medial cord, but usually has a lateral root also from the lateral cord, which carries the C7 fibers (Fig. 2–8). It descends with the neurovascular bundle, pierces the medial intermuscular septum and descends behind the medial epicondyle, between the two heads of the flexor carpi ulnaris. Here it supplies the elbow joint. It then descends on the flexor digitorum profundus to the middle of the forearm and then along the lateral side of the ulnar artery. Both enter the hand by passing

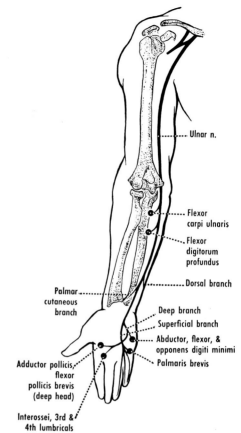

Figure 2–8 Schematic representation of the sequence of muscular and cutaneous branches of the ulnar nerve. The sequences of muscular branches are the more common ones. Based on studies by Sunderland and Hughes (1946). (From Gardner, E., Gray, D. J., and O'Rahilly, R.: Anatomy. 3rd Ed. Philadelphia, W. B. Saunders Co., 1969.)

in front of the flexor retinaculum, a slip of which covers them, between the pisiform and the hook of the hamate. The nerve then divides into its superficial and deep terminal branches. The course of the nerve in the forearm may be indicated on the surface by a line from the front of the medial epicondyle to the lateral margin of the pisiform.

There are no muscular branches in the arm. In the upper forearm, muscular branches are given to the flexor carpi ulnaris and the medial part of the flexor digitorum profundus. In the middle of the forearm, the large cutaneous dorsal branch arises and then descends to the back of the hand. In the lower part of the forearm, a variable palmar branch is given to the skin on the medial side of the palm.

In the hand, the dorsal branch gives twigs to the skin of the back of the hand and then

ganglion gives rami communicantes to the upper cervical ventral rami and the last four cranial nerves, twigs to the carotid body and sinus and to the pharyngeal plexus, and cervical cardiac nerves to the heart. Several branches form a plexus along the external carotid artery (Gardner, 1943), with some of the fibers reaching the salivary glands. One or more large branches form an internal carotid nerve (Kuntz et al., 1957), which ascends with the internal carotid artery to supply the eye, orbit, and intracranial structures by forming first an internal carotid plexus and then subsidiary plexuses along the branches of the artery, and by giving twigs to various nerves (tympanic, greater petrosal, and third, fourth, fifth, and sixth cranial) and to the ciliary ganglion.

The *middle cervical ganglion* is quite variable and is often fused with either the superior or the vertebral ganglion. It usually lies just above the arch formed by the inferior thyroid artery (along which twigs form a plexus), at the level of the sixth cervical vertebra. Rami are given to cervical nerves, usually C4 to C6, as well as a branch to the heart.

The *vertebral ganglion* usually lies in front of the vertebral artery, just below the arch of the inferior thyroid artery, and about at the level of the seventh cervical vertebra. As the sympathetic trunk extends downward from the vertebral to the stellate (or inferior cervical) ganglion it forms two or more cords, which pass on each side of the vertebral artery. Rami from the ganglion reach some of the lower cervical nerves and thereby enter the brachial plexus. Twigs are given to the vertebral plexus (discussed later), and a cord termed the ansa subclavia loops in front of and below the first part of the subclavian artery to the stellate (or inferior cervical) ganglion. Branches of the ansa contribute to a plexus along the subclavian artery.

The *cervicothoracic (stellate) ganglion* has two parts: the inferior cervical and the first thoracic (occasionally a second and third also). These ganglia may be completely fused (Jamieson et al., 1952). The ganglionic mass lies usually at the level of the seventh cervical and first thoracic vertebrae, in front of the eighth cervical and first thoracic nerves, the seventh cervical transverse process and neck of the first rib, and behind the vertebral artery. The stellate ganglion receives preganglionic fibers from the first, or first and second, thoracic nerves. Its postganglionic

fibers supply chiefly the upper limb by way of rami to the lower cervical and upper thoracic nerves, and branches to the subclavian and vertebral arteries.

Branches of the vertebral and stellate ganglia form a vertebral plexus, which accompanies the vertebral artery into the posterior cranial fossa. During its course, postganglionic fibers are given to the lower cervical nerves (Sunderland and Bedbrook, 1949). Some fibers ascend separately, behind the artery, as a distinct vertebral nerve, which extends to the level of the axis or atlas. Postganglionic fibers in it are given to the cervical nerves and spinal meninges.

Thorax

THORACIC NERVES

Each of the twelve thoracic nerves gives off a meningeal branch and then, after emerging from an intervertebral foramen, divides into a dorsal and a ventral ramus. The meningeal branches and dorsal rami are described with the back. Each ventral ramus is connected to the sympathetic trunk by a variable number of rami communicantes, and each runs a separate course forward, supplying the skin, muscles, and serous membranes of the thoracic and abdominal walls. The ventral rami of the first 11 nerves are called intercostal nerves; that of the twelfth is the subcostal nerve.

TYPICAL INTERCOSTAL NERVES

The fourth, fifth, and sixth *intercostal nerves* are typical intercostal nerves and supply only the thoracic wall (Fig. 2–10). Each passes below the neck of the numerically corresponding rib and enters the costal groove below the posterior intercostal vessels. At the anterior end of the intercostal spaces, the nerves turn forward through the overlying muscles and, as anterior cutaneous branches, are distributed to the skin of the front of the thorax. Here they give off medial mammary branches. At the angle of the rib, each nerve supplies the external intercostal muscle and gives off a collateral and a lateral cutaneous branch. The collateral branch passes forward in the intercostal space and ends anteriorly as a lower anterior cutaneous nerve. The lateral cutaneous branch pierces the overlying

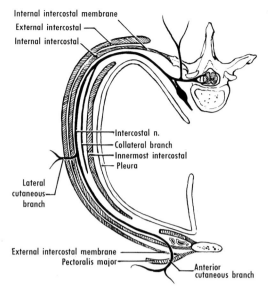

Figure 2–10 Diagrammatic representation of the nerves of the thoracic wall. The thickness of the intercostal muscles is exaggerated. (From Gardner, F., Gray, D. J., and O'Rahilly, R.: Anatomy. 3rd Ed. Philadelphia, W. B. Saunders Co., 1969.)

muscles and divides into anterior and posterior branches that supply the skin of the thorax. Some of the anterior branches form lateral mammary branches. The intercostal nerves supply the intercostal, subcostal, serratus posterior superior, and transversus thoracis muscles.

SPECIAL INTERCOSTAL NERVES

The first, second, and third intercostal nerves are special in that they supply the arm as well as the thorax. The first thoracic nerve is the largest of the thoracic spinal nerves. It divides into a larger upper and a smaller lower part. The upper joins the brachial plexus, and the lower becomes the *first intercostal nerve*. Its distribution is like that of a typical intercostal nerve (Cave, 1929), except that its lateral cutaneous branch supplies the skin of the axilla, and may communicate with the intercostobrachial nerve. The *second intercostal nerve*, which often contributes to the brachial plexus, also has a distribution like that of a typical intercostal nerve, except that its lateral cutaneous branch passes into the arm as the intercostobrachial nerve. This nerve pierces the overlying muscles and supplies the skin on the back and medial side of the arm as far as the elbow. It usually anastomoses with

the posterior and medial brachial cutaneous nerves and supplies the axillary arch when that muscle is present. The *third intercostal nerve* likewise has a distribution like that of a typical intercostal nerve, but its lateral cutaneous branch often gives a twig to the medial side of the arm.

The *seventh to eleventh intercostal nerves* are also special in that they supply the abdominal wall as well as the thorax (Fig. 2–11). Known as *thoracoabdominal nerves*, they course forward and downward to the anterior ends of the intercostal spaces. They continue between the transversus and internal oblique muscles, and then between the rectus abdominis and the posterior wall of its sheath. Here, each nerve divides into two branches. The larger one forms a plexiform arrangement that gives twigs to the rectus and from which an anterior cutaneous branch pierces the rectus to supply the overlying skin. The smaller branch also supplies the rectus, and may pierce the rectus and become cutaneous. During its course,

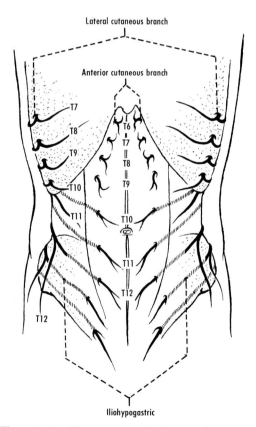

Figure 2–11 The cutaneous distribution of the thoracoabdominal nerves. (From Gardner, E., Gray, D. J., and O'Rahilly, R.: Anatomy. 3rd Ed. Philadelphia, W. B. Saunders Co., 1969.)

each thoracoabdominal nerve gives off a lateral cutaneous branch that pierces the external oblique and divides into anterior and posterior branches. These supply the back, side, and front of the abdominal wall. The thoraco-abdominal nerves also supply intercostal, subcostal, serratus posterior inferior, transversus abdominis, external and internal oblique, and rectus abdominis muscles, and give sensory twigs to adjacent diaphragm, pleura, and peritoneum.

The ventral ramus of the twelfth thoracic nerve is special in that it is subcostal rather than intercostal in position and is known as the *subcostal nerve*. It enters the abdomen, courses downward and laterally behind the kidney, pierces the transversus abdominis, and passes between this muscle and the internal oblique. It then enters the sheath of the rectus, turns forward, and becomes cutaneous between the umbilicus and the pubic symphysis. Its lateral cutaneous branch supplies the skin of the gluteal region and upper thigh as far down as the greater trochanter. Muscular branches are given to the transversus, oblique, and rectus muscles. Sensory twigs are given to the adjacent peritoneum.

AUTONOMIC NERVE SUPPLY

The parasympathetic supply of the thoracic viscera is furnished by the vagus nerves.

SYMPATHETIC TRUNK AND GANGLIA

The sympathetic trunks enter the thorax from the neck, descend in front of the heads of the ribs and the posterior intercostal vessels and accompanying nerves, and enter the abdomen by piercing the crura of the diaphragm or by passing behind the medial arcuate ligaments (see Fig. 2–6). In the thorax, each trunk usually has 11 or 12 separate ganglia of varying size (occasionally 10 or 13). As described earlier, the first thoracic ganglion is often fused with the inferior cervical to form the cervicothoracic or stellate ganglion. The trunk itself may be very slender between two adjacent ganglia; sometimes it is double.

Each ganglion has one to four rami communicantes whose distinguishing characteristics were described under general features. Preganglionic fibers for the thoracic and ab-dominal walls and back arise from all levels of the thoracic spinal cord and reach the sympathetic trunk by way of rami communicantes. The postganglionic fibers return to the spinal nerves by way of rami communicantes and are distributed by way of dorsal and ventral rami and in the meningeal branches of the spinal nerves.

The postganglionic fibers for thoracic and abdominal viscera are distributed by visceral branches. These include cardiac branches of the ansa subclavia, stellate ganglion, and the upper four or five thoracic ganglia; and pulmonary branches of the upper four or five thoracic ganglia. Scattered filaments of the trunk are also given to the aortic and esophageal plexuses. The major visceral branches, however, are the three splanchnic nerves.

The *greater splanchnic nerve* is formed by three or four large roots and an inconstant number of smaller ones, all of which arise in a variable fashion from the trunk and ganglia; the upper and lower limits are usually the fifth and tenth. The nerve pierces the diaphragm or passes through its aortic opening and ends in the celiac ganglion and plexuses. It and the other splanchnic nerves contain sensory as well as preganglionic fibers, and a relatively large splanchnic ganglion is usually present along the nerve near the diaphragm.

The *lesser splanchnic nerve*, which may be absent, usually arises from the lower thoracic ganglia by one to three rootlets. Descending slightly lateral to the greater splanchnic nerve, it pierces the diaphragm and joins the aorticorenal ganglion and celiac plexus.

The *lowest splanchnic nerve*, which also may be absent, usually arises from the lowest thoracic ganglion. Descending medial to the sympathetic trunk, it enters the abdomen and joins the aorticorenal ganglion and adjacent plexus.

More detailed information about the sympathetic trunks, ganglia, and branches is available in the reports of Mitchell (1956), Jit and Mukerjee (1960), and Pick and Sheehan (1946), as well as the references cited under General Features.

PREVERTEBRAL PLEXUSES

These are formed by the branches of the vagus nerves and sympathetic trunks that supply the thoracic viscera and blood vessels.

The *cardiac plexus* may be considered as

comprising interconnected aortic arch, right and left coronary, and right and left atrial plexuses, all lying in adventitia or under epicardium (Mizeres, 1963). The sympathetic components reach the plexuses by way of cervical, cervicothoracic, and thoracic cardiac nerves (the preganglionic fibers arise from the upper four to five or six segments of the thoracic spinal cord). A variable number of cardiac ganglia occur along the cervicothoracic nerves.

The *pulmonary plexuses*, which are usually described as anterior and posterior (with respect to the root of the lung), are essentially continuous with the cardiac plexus. Lying mostly posterior to the root of the lung and formed chiefly by the vagus nerves, the plexuses receive branches directly from the upper four to five or six segments of the thoracic spinal cord.

The *esophageal plexus* is formed in a variable fashion by the vagus nerves after they leave the pulmonary plexuses. Lying in the fibrous wall of the esophagus, the plexus receives filaments from the sympathetic trunks and greater splanchnic nerves; the preganglionic fibers arise mainly from the lower segments of the thoracic spinal cord.

The *thoracic aortic plexus* receives filaments from the vagus nerves and sympathetic trunks (the preganglionic fibers arise from the upper thoracic segments) that ramify in its adventitia and form a delicate plexus that continues for a short distance along the branches of the aorta. The plexus is also continuous through the aortic opening of the diaphragm with the abdominal aortic and celiac plexuses.

Abdomen, Pelvis, and Lower Limb

LUMBAR PLEXUS

The dorsal rami of the lumbar nerves, which provide part of the nerve supply of the back, are described later. The ventral rami enter the psoas major muscle when they combine in a variable fashion to form the lumbar plexus (a division into anterior and posterior divisions that then combine, as occurs in the trunks of the brachial plexus, has been described but is difficult to demonstrate). Within the muscle they are connected to the lumbar sympathetic trunk by rami communicantes. Strictly speaking, the second to fourth nerves are usually (in about three fourths of instances) described as forming the lumbar plexus proper. However, the lower part of the fourth lumbar nerve and all of the fifth enter the sacral plexus (the combined trunk is known as the lumbosacral trunk or furcal nerve), and the two plexuses are commonly known as the *lumbosacral plexus;* the fourth lumbar is then the one ventral ramus common to both plexuses. Moreover, the branches of the first lumbar nerve also are usually described with the lumbar plexus. The general features of the lumbar plexus are discussed further by Bardeen and Elting (1901), Horwitz (1939), and Webber (1961).

VARIATIONS

As in the case of the brachial plexus, prefixation and postfixation of the lumbosacral plexus in the sense of complete shifts upward or downward are uncommon. Nevertheless, the plexus is often spoken of as prefixed when the upper level is the eleventh or twelfth thoracic nerve, and postfixed when the lower border is the fifth sacral or first coccygeal nerve. The total range may therefore be from the eleventh thoracic to the first coccygeal. The rami supplying the limbs, exclusive of the cutaneous branches of T12 and L1, can range from the first lumbar to the third sacral. Moreover, minor variations in pattern are common, and the plexuses are often asymmetrical with respect to right and left.

BRANCHES

Direct branches (L1 to L4) are given to the quadratus lumborum, psoas major, and psoas minor muscles. The first lumbar nerve has variable connections with the subcostal nerve and with the second lumbar, and gives twigs to adjacent muscles. It resembles an intercostal nerve in giving off a collateral branch, the ilioinguinal nerve, and then continuing as the iliohypogastric nerve, which has lateral and anterior cutaneous branches (Davies, 1935). The terminal branches of the lumbar plexus are the lateral femoral cutaneous and the femoral nerves, which emerge laterally from the psoas major, the genitofemoral nerve, which emerges from its front, and the obturator and sometimes the accessory obturator nerve, which emerge medially.

The *iliohypogastric nerve* emerges from the lateral side of the psoas major, runs behind the kidney, pierces the transversus above the iliac crest, and divides into lateral and anterior cutaneous branches. The lateral supplies the skin over the side of the buttock, the anterior the skin above the pubis (see Fig. 2–11). Muscular branches, if any, are probably sensory. A motor branch is occasionally given to the pyramidalis.

The *ilioinguinal nerve* runs a similar course to the iliac crest. Here it pierces the transversus and internal oblique, accompanies the spermatic cord through the inguinal canal, emerges from the superficial ring, and gives cutaneous branches to the thigh and anterior scrotal or anterior labial branches.

The *lateral femoral cutaneous nerve* (L2, or L2 and L3, or L1 and L2) runs obliquely across the iliacus toward the anterior superior iliac spine and enters the thigh by passing behind the inguinal ligament. It divides into anterior and posterior branches that supply the skin of the anterior and lateral aspects of the thigh.

The *femoral nerve* (chiefly L4, plus L2 and L3) is the largest branch of the lumbar plexus (Fig. 2–12). It descends between the psoas and iliacus and enters the thigh behind the middle of the inguinal ligament in the muscular compartment lateral to the femoral vessels. Entering the femoral triangle, it breaks up into a number of terminal branches.

In the iliac fossa it supplies the iliacus and the femoral artery. The nerve to the pectineus arises here (or in the femoral triangle), and passes behind the femoral sheath to supply the pectineus and the hip joint.

The terminal branches of the femoral nerve are sometimes classified into an anterior division (anterior cutaneous and a branch to the sartorius) and a posterior division (muscular and saphenous). The muscular branch of the anterior division goes directly to the sartorius. The anterior cutaneous branches of the same division are subdivided into the intermediate and medial cutaneous nerves. The intermediate nerve, which is usually double, gives branches to the sartorius and supplies the skin on the front of the thigh; distally it contributes to the patellar plexus. The medial nerves supply the skin on the medial side of the thigh and contribute to the subsartorial and patellar plexuses. The muscular branches of the posterior division supply the rectus femoris (a twig from this is given to the hip joint); the vastus medialis (a branch continues to the knee joint); the

vastus intermedius (branches continue to the articularis genus and the knee joint); and the vastus lateralis (a branch continues to the knee joint). The saphenous nerve can be regarded as the termination of the femoral nerve. It descends with the femoral vessels through the femoral triangle and subsartorial canal, crosses the femoral artery from lateral to medial, and then becomes cutaneous. It descends in the leg with the large saphenous vein and supplies the skin on the medial side of the leg and foot. It gives a branch to the knee joint and takes part in the subsartorial and patellar plexuses. The saphenous nerve may be joined by filaments constituting an accessory femoral nerve. This is a common variant that arises from the lumbar plexus, runs a separate course into the thigh, and usually ends by joining one of the cutaneous branches of the femoral nerve.

The subsartorial plexus, which lies in the adductor canal deep to the sartorius, is formed by branches from the medial femoral cutaneous, saphenous, and obturator nerves. The patellar plexus, which lies in front of the knee, is formed by branches of the lateral, intermediate, and medial femoral cutaneous and saphenous nerves.

The *genitofemoral nerve* (L2, or L1 and L2, occasionally L3) descends on the front of the psoas major and divides into genital and femoral branches. The genital branch enters the inguinal canal through the deep ring, supplies the cremaster, and continues to supply the scrotum (or labium majus) and the adjacent part of the thigh. The femoral branch enters the femoral sheath, lateral to the artery, and turns forward to supply the skin of the femoral triangle.

The *obturator nerve* (L3, L4, sometimes L2 or L5 also) emerges from the medial side of the psoas major at the inlet of the pelvis (see Fig. 2–12). It runs downward and forward on the lateral wall of the pelvis to the obturator groove, where it divides into anterior and posterior branches. These pass through the obturator foramen into the thigh, where they are separated by the adductor brevis. Branches to the hip joint arise from the trunk and from one or both branches. The anterior branch lies in front of the adductor brevis, behind the pectineus and adductor longus. It descends along the latter muscle, supplies it and the gracilis, adductor brevis, and sometimes the pectineus also, and ends as a filament to the femoral artery and subsartorial plexus; twigs from it supply the overlying skin

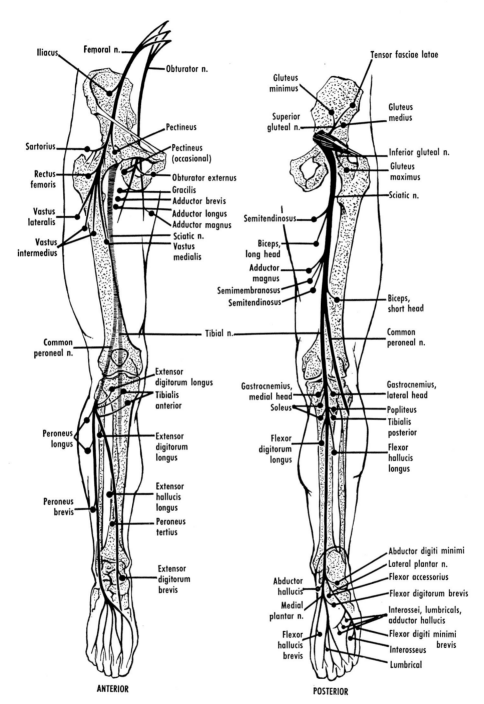

Figure 2–12 The sequences of branches of the sciatic, tibial, and common peroneal nerves, based on studies by Sunderland and Hughes (1946). The sequences of branches of the femoral and obturator nerves are based on studies by Pitres and Testut (1925). (From Gardner, E., Gray, D. J., and O'Rahilly, R.: Anatomy. 3rd Ed. Philadelphia, W. B. Saunders Co., 1969.)

and occasionally the knee joint. The posterior branch pierces the obturator externus and descends behind the adductor brevis, in front of the magnus. It then pierces the magnus and accompanies the popliteal artery to the back of the knee joint. It supplies the obturator externus, adductor magnus, and sometimes the adductor brevis.

The *accessory obturator nerve* (L3, L4), which is present in nearly 10 per cent of cases, descends medial to the psoas and enters the thigh deep to the pectineus (Woodburne, 1960). It supplies the hip joint and pectineus.

SACRAL PLEXUS

The dorsal rami of the sacral nerves are described with the back. The ventral rami of the first four sacral nerves emerge from the sacral canal through the pelvic sacral foramina. The fourth then divides into an upper and lower division; the upper division and the first three ventral rami combine with the lumbosacral trunk to form the sacral plexus. Anterior and posterior divisions of the first three rami have been described, but, as in the case of the lumbar plexus, they are difficult to demonstrate. Each ramus contributing to the sacral plexus is connected to a single ganglion of the sacral sympathetic trunk by one or more rami communicantes.

The sacral plexus lies in front of the piriformis, separated from the internal iliac vessels and ureter anteriorly by the parietal pelvic fascia. From the complex and variable union of the ventral rami, 12 named branches arise. Five supply pelvic structures; the remainder are distributed to the buttock and lower limb.

BRANCHES TO PELVIC STRUCTURES

The chief branch is the *pudendal nerve* (S2, S3, S4), which supplies most of the perineum. It passes through the greater sciatic notch below the piriformis and, after crossing the back of the ischial spine, enters the perineum through the lesser sciatic notch, accompanied by the internal pudendal artery. Running forward in the pudendal canal in the ischiorectal fossa, it gives off the inferior rectal nerve and then divides into the perineal nerve and the dorsal nerve of the penis (or clitoris). The inferior rectal nerve (which may arise separately from S3 and S4 of the sacral

plexus) pierces the medial wall of the pudendal canal and divides into branches that traverse the ischiorectal fossa. They supply the skin around the anus, the sphincter ani externus, and the anal mucosa as far upward as the pectinate line. The perineal nerve divides into superficial and deep branches. The superficial branch gives off two posterior scrotal (labial) nerves (medial and lateral), which pierce the superficial and deep perineal fasciae and run forward to supply the scrotum (or labium majus). The deep branch of the perineal nerve gives twigs to the sphincter ani externus and levator ani and then enters the superficial perineal space to supply the bulbospongiosus, ischiocavernosus, superficial transversus perinei, and bulb of the penis. The dorsal nerve of the penis (or clitoris), the other terminal branch of the pudendal nerve, pierces the posterior edge of the urogenital diaphragm. As it runs forward, it supplies the deep transversus perinei and sphincter urethrae. It then pierces the inferior fascia of the diaphragm, gives a branch to the corpus cavernosum penis (or clitoris), and then runs forward on the dorsum of the penis (or clitoris) to supply the skin, prepuce, and glans.

In addition to the pudendal nerve, the sacral plexus gives the following additional branches to pelvic structures: the *nerve to the piriformis* (S1, S2), the *nerve to the levator ani and coccygeus* (S3, S4), the *nerve to the sphincter ani externus* (perineal branch of S4), and the *pelvic splanchnic nerves* (S2, S3 and S4, S5), which contain parasympathetic preganglionic as well as sensory fibers and which enter the inferior hypogastric plexus.

BRANCHES TO THE BUTTOCK AND LOWER LIMB

These are seven in number. The *superior gluteal nerve* (L4, L5, S1) passes backward through the greater sciatic notch, above the piriformis. An upper branch supplies the gluteus medius, and a lower branch supplies the gluteus medius, minimus, tensor fasciae latae, and hip joint. The *inferior gluteal nerve* (L5, S1, S2) passes through the greater sciatic foramen below the piriformis and supplies the gluteus maximus. The *nerve to the obturator internus* (L5, S1, S2) leaves the pelvis below the piriformis, supplies the superior gemellus, and then passes through the lesser sciatic foramen to the obturator internus. The *nerve to the quadratus femoris* (L4, L5, S1) leaves the pelvis below the piriformis in front of the sciatic nerve. It supplies the inferior gemellus, the quadratus femoris, and the hip joint. The *posterior femoral cutaneous nerve* (S1 to S3) leaves the pelvis below the piriformis. It descends in company with the sciatic nerve, becomes superficial near the popliteal fossa, and accompanies the small saphenous vein to the middle of the calf. Its branches are inferior clunial nerves (gluteal branches) to the skin of the buttock, perineal branches to the skin of the genitalia, and femoral and sural branches to the skin on the back of the thigh and calf. The *perforating cutaneous (inferior medial clunial) nerve* (S2, S3) pierces the sacrotuberous ligament and supplies the skin over the lower part of the buttock.

The *sciatic nerve* (L4, L5, S1 to S3), the largest nerve in the body, consists of peroneal and tibial parts, which are usually bound together, leaving the pelvis through the greater sciatic foramen, below the piriformis (see Fig. 2–12) (Beaton and Anson, 1937). Sometimes they leave separately, the peroneal portion piercing the piriformis, and the tibial portion passing below it. The exit of the sciatic nerve from the pelvis is indicated by the superior point of trisection of a line from the posterior superior iliac spine to the ischial tuberosity. Its downward course is indicated by a line down the middle of the back of the thigh (from the midpoint of a line between the greater trochanter and ischial tuberosity). The sciatic nerve descends under cover of the gluteus maximus, between the greater trochanter and ischial tuberosity. In the thigh it lies anteriorly on the adductor magnus and is accompanied by the posterior femoral cutaneous nerve and the companion artery. In the lower third of the thigh the nerve separates into its two components, the tibial and common peroneal nerves (the separation may occur at any level in the gluteal region or thigh). Its branches arise mostly on the medial side and supply the semitendinosus, semimembranosus, long head of the biceps, adductor magnus (all by the tibial nerve), and short head of the biceps (by the common peroneal nerve).

The *tibial* (medial popliteal) *nerve* (L4 to S3) descends separately through the popliteal fossa (see Fig. 2–12). It then lies on the popliteus muscle, under cover of the gastrocnemius, and at the lower border of the popliteus passes deep to the fibrous arch of the soleus to reach the back of the leg. Here it descends first on the tibialis posterior and flexor digitorum longus and then on the tibia. Then, becoming more superficial and crossing the posterior tibial artery posteriorly to gain its lateral side, it ends by dividing into medial and lateral plantar nerves under cover of the flexor retinaculum.

In the thigh, muscular branches arise as listed with the sciatic nerve. In the popliteal fossa, branches are given to the knee joint, and muscular branches to the gastrocnemius, soleus, plantaris, popliteus, and tibialis posterior. A branch of the nerve to the popliteus, the interosseous nerve of the leg, descends on the interosseous membrane. The medial sural cutaneous nerve joins the peroneal communicating branch of the common peroneal nerve to form the sural nerve. The sural nerve descends in company with the small saphenous vein, gives lateral calcanean branches to the skin of the back of the leg and lateral aspect of the foot and heel, twigs to the ankle joint and adjacent intertarsal joints, and continues forward along the lateral side of the little toe as the lateral dorsal cutaneous nerve. In the leg the tibial nerve gives muscular branches to the soleus, tibialis posterior, flexor hallucis longus, and flexor digitorum longus. Medial calcanean branches supply the skin of the heel and sole, and a twig is given to the ankle joint. The course of the tibial nerve in the leg is indicated on the surface by a line from about the level of the tibial tuberosity downward to the midpoint between the medial malleolus and the heel.

The medial plantar nerve, the larger of the two terminal branches of the tibial nerve, at first lies deep to the abductor hallucis. It then runs forward in the sole between the abductor and the flexor digitorum brevis. It supplies these muscles and the skin on the medial side of the sole. Its terminal branches are four plantar digital nerves for muscles (flexor hallucis and first lumbrical) and for the medial side of the big toe and the adjacent sides of the first and second, second and third, and third and fourth toes. The nerves extend on to the dorsum and supply the nail beds and tips of the toes.

The lateral plantar nerve runs forward and laterally between the quadratus plantae and the flexor digitorum brevis and divides into superficial and deep branches. During its course it supplies the quadratus plantae and abductor digiti minimi and the skin of the lateral side of the sole. The superficial branch supplies the flexor digiti minimi brevis and the lateral side of the sole and little toe and, by plantar digital nerves, the adjacent sides of the fourth and fifth toes. The deep branch turns medially, supplies the interossei, the second, third, and fourth lumbricals, and the adductor hallucis, and gives off articular twigs.

The *common peroneal* (lateral popliteal) *nerve* (L4 to S2) descends through the popliteal fossa, following the medial edge of the biceps closely (see Fig. 2–12). It crosses the lateral head of the biceps, gains the back of the head of the fibula, and winds around the neck of that bone (where it is often palpable, and where it is susceptible to injury) under cover of the peroneus longus. Here it divides into its terminal branches, the superficial and deep peroneal nerves.

While a part of the sciatic nerve, it supplies the short head of the biceps and sometimes the knee joint also. In the popliteal fossa, it supplies the knee joint and gives rise to a branch that divides into the lateral sural cutaneous nerve (for the skin on the lateral side of the leg), and the peroneal communicating branch (which joins the medial sural cutaneous nerve to form the sural nerve). At the neck of the fibula it gives off a small recurrent branch that supplies the knee and tibiofibular joints and the tibialis anterior. The common peroneal nerve sometimes supplies the peroneus longus or extensor digitorum longus or both.

The *superficial peroneal* (musculocutaneous) *nerve,* one of the two terminal branches of the common peroneal, descends in front of the fibula, between the peronei and the extensor digitorum longus. Muscular branches supply the peroneus longus and brevis; the branch to the latter is often prolonged to the extensor digitorum brevis and adjacent joints and is termed the accessory deep peroneal nerve (Lambert, 1969; Winckler, 1934). In the lower part of the leg, the superficial peroneal nerve divides into medial and intermediate dorsal cutaneous nerves. These pass in front of the extensor retinacula, the medial supplying the skin and joints of the medial side of the big toe and (by dorsal digital nerves) the adjacent sides of the second and third toes; the intermediate nerve (by dorsal digital nerves) supplies the adjacent sides of the third and fourth, and the fourth and fifth toes.

As in the hand, the territories of distribution of the cutaneous nerves of the foot show considerable variation in size and overlap, and reciprocal changes in size (Jones, 1949).

The *deep peroneal nerve* continues the winding course of the common peroneal around the neck of the fibula, then pierces the anterior intermuscular septum and extensor digitorum longus and descends on the interosseous membrane. It meets the anterior tibial artery, and both pass deep to the extensor retinacula. Branches are given to the tibialis anterior, extensor hallucis longus, extensor digitorum longus, peroneus tertius, and ankle joint. In the foot, where it lies about midway between the malleoli, the nerve divides into its terminal branches, medial and lateral. The medial gives dorsal digital nerves for the adjacent sides of the first and second toes, and the lateral supplies the extensor digitorum brevis and adjacent joints. It may also send twigs (probably afferent) to the first three dorsal interossei.

COCCYGEAL PLEXUS

The ventral ramus of the fifth sacral nerve enters the pelvis between the sacrum and coccyx; that of the coccygeal nerve passes forward below the rudimentary transverse process of the first piece of the coccyx. The coccygeal (or sacrococcygeal) plexus is formed by these two ventral rami, together with the lower division of the ventral ramus of the fourth sacral (Sicard and Bruézière, 1950). The plexus supplies the coccyx, the sacrococcygeal joint, and the skin over the coccyx.

AUTONOMIC NERVE SUPPLY

The parasympathetic supply of the abdominal viscera is furnished chiefly by the vagus nerves. The descending and sigmoid colons and the pelvic viscera are supplied by the sacral parasympathetics.

SYMPATHETIC TRUNK AND GANGLIA

The two trunks enter the abdomen by piercing the diaphragm or by passing behind the medial arcuate ligaments (see Fig. 2–6). In descending on the vertebral column, adjacent to the psoas major muscles, the right trunk lies behind the inferior vena cava, the left one beside the aorta. The trunks continue into the pelvis, where they lie on the pelvic surface of the sacrum, medial to the upper three pelvic sacral foramina and usually in front of the fourth. They end by uniting in front of the coccyx to form an enlargement, the ganglion impar.

In the lumbar region, the two trunks are seldom symmetrical and the ganglia are irregular in size, number, and position. There are usually four or five ganglia (three or four, according to Webber, 1958), but there may be from two to six, and occasionally a trunk is an elongated ganglionic mass. The variations are such as to make identification of the proper level of a specific ganglion very difficult. Nor can counting from the highest lumbar ganglion be depended upon. When the first lumbar ganglion is present, it lies between the crus of the diaphragm and the vertebral column, is difficult to reach, and is often overlooked. Rami communicantes are a better means of identification.

In the pelvis, the number of ganglia is variable, but there are usually three or four.

Each lumbar ganglion has two or more rami communicantes to two or more spinal nerves. The lowest ramus at upper levels contains the most preganglionic fibers and is the clue to the identification of a ganglion. For example, the second lumbar ganglion is connected to the first and second lumbar nerves; hence the lowest ramus (from the second nerve) leads to the second ganglion. Nevertheless, the identification of ganglia during surgical procedures remains an uncertain and difficult task. The second lumbar nerve is usually the lowest one to contain preganglionic sympathetic fibers.

Each sacral ganglion tends to be connected by rami communicantes with only one spinal nerve.

The postganglionic fibers in the lumbar and sacral rami communicantes are for the supply of the lower part of the abdominal wall and back, the anal canal and perineum and external genitalia, and the lower limb by way of the lumbosacral and coccygeal plexuses. The preganglionic fibers for the lower limbs arise from the lower thoracic and upper lumbar levels of the spinal cord and descend in the trunks to the lumbar and sacral ganglia where they synapse.

The preganglionic fibers for abdominal viscera descend mostly in the thoracic splanchnic nerves. Some, however, descend in the sympathetic trunks and leave by way of visceral branches. These consist of four or more *lumbar splanchnic nerves* of variable size, which, depending upon level, join the celiac or intermesenteric and adjacent plexuses or the superior hypogastric plexus (Kuntz, 1956). These nerves also contain preganglionic

and sensory fibers, and some of their postganglionic fibers reach pelvic viscera by way of the hypogastric plexuses, and the iliac fossa and upper thigh by way of the aortic plexus.

The preganglionic fibers for pelvic viscera arise in the upper lumbar levels of the spinal cord. They descend and synapse in lumbar and sacral ganglia. The postganglionic fibers reach pelvic viscera by way of rami communicantes or lumbar splanchnic nerves (just described), and by way of *sacral splanchnic nerves*. These last are a variable number of fine visceral branches of the sacral sympathetic trunks that join the inferior hypogastric plexus.

More detailed information about the sympathetic trunks and ganglia is available in the references cited under General Features and in the reports of Pick and Sheehan (1946) and Labbok (1937).

PREVERTEBRAL PLEXUSES

In the abdomen, these are best considered as a single great plexus formed by the splanchnic nerves, branches of both vagus nerves, and masses of ganglion cells, with various parts named according to the arteries with which they are associated. The plexus lies in front of the upper part of the abdominal aorta. Its chief ganglia are the irregularly shaped celiac ganglia at the origin of the celiac trunk, each lying on the corresponding crus of the diaphragm. The inferolateral extensions of the ganglia are termed the aorticorenal ganglia. The superior mesenteric ganglion (or ganglia) is usually fused with the celiac ganglia. Smaller ganglia, for example, phrenic and renal, are often found along the smaller subsidiary plexuses.

The *celiac* and *superior mesenteric plexuses* lie on the front and sides of the aorta at the origins of the celiac trunk and the superior mesenteric and renal arteries. They contain the celiac, aorticorenal, and superior mesenteric ganglia, and many smaller unnamed masses. Branches of the plexuses extend along arteries and are named accordingly, for example, hepatic, gastric, phrenic, suprarenal, renal, ureteric, and testicular or ovarian. Downward continuations of the prevertebral plexus form the aortic and inferior mesenteric plexus.

The *aortic plexus* consists of a variable number of interconnected strands that, as they descend along the aorta, receive branches from the lumbar splanchnic nerves. The part of the plexus between the origins of the superior and inferior mesenteric arteries is also known as the *intermesenteric plexus*, and below the bifurcation of the aorta the aortic plexus becomes the superior hypogastric plexus. Some filaments from the aortic plexus accompany the lumbar arteries and provide a pathway for postganglionic fibers to the abdominal wall and back. Other filaments, together with branches of the lumbar splanchnic nerves, form a plexus along the common and external iliac arteries. This plexus is reinforced by a branch of the femoral nerve and continues into the thigh along the femoral artery.

The *inferior mesenteric plexus* is a continuation of the aortic plexus along the inferior mesenteric plexus. It contains one or more inferior mesenteric ganglia and it forms the superior rectal plexus, which supplies the rectum with sympathetic and sensory fibers.

In the pelvis, in front of the fifth lumbar vertebra, the aortic plexus becomes the *superior hypogastric plexus* (or *presacral nerve*). This then divides in front of the sacrum into two elongated narrow networks termed the *right* and *left hypogastric nerves*. Each of these nerves descends on the side of the rectum (or rectum and vagina) and is joined by the pelvic splanchnic nerves to form the right and left *inferior hypogastric* (or *pelvic*) *plexuses*. Each plexus contains small, scattered pelvic ganglia and each is joined by the sacral splanchnic nerves from the sympathetic trunk. Many branches of the inferior hypogastric plexus supply the rectum, with some of them forming a middle rectal plexus. Large portions of the inferior hypogastric plexuses form either the prostatic plexus (which continues forward as the cavernous nerves of the penis and from which is derived the vesical plexus) or the uterovaginal plexus (fibers from the lowermost part of this plexus continue as the cavernous nerves of the clitoris).

The inferior hypogastric plexuses carry sensory, postganglionic sympathetic, and preganglionic parasympathetic fibers. Some of the preganglionic parasympathetic fibers supply the descending and sigmoid colons, usually by a single ascending branch of the hypogastric nerve (Woodburne, 1956). Some of the sensory fibers are pain fibers that reach the spinal cord by way of the superior hypogastric plexuses and lumbar splanchnic nerves as well as by way of pelvic splanchnic nerves. The other sensory fibers, concerned with reflexes and visceral sensations, reach the spinal cord by way of the pelvic splanchnic nerves.

Back

The nerve supply of the back is provided by the meningeal branches and dorsal rami of spinal nerves.

Each spinal nerve gives off a meningeal branch (or sinuvertebral nerve), which is often connected with adjacent sympathetic ganglia and which reenters the vertebral canal and supplies dura mater, posterior longitudinal ligament, periosteum, and epidural and intraosseous blood vessels (Pedersen et al., 1956). The meningeal branches of the upper three cervical nerves give off branches that ascend through the foramen magnum and supply the dura mater of the floor of the posterior cranial fossa (Kimmel, 1961).

The dorsal rami arise after the spinal nerves emerge from the intervertebral foramina (sacral nerves divide within the sacrum, and the dorsal rami pass backward through the dorsal sacral foramina). They contain motor, sensory, and autonomic fibers (Dass, 1952) and run backward to supply the muscles, bones, joints, and skin of the back. Most divide into medial and lateral branches, which descend as they run dorsally, each supplying muscles and each anastomosing with nerves above and below to form a plexus in the muscles. In the upper half of the trunk the medial branches supply skin, whereas in the lower half the lateral branches become cutaneous. However, the level of shift is variable (see Thoracic Dorsal Rami).

CERVICAL DORSAL RAMI

The connecting loops between the dorsal rami of the first three or four cervical nerves form what is termed the posterior cervical plexus (Cave, 1937), which gives branches to adjacent muscles. The dorsal ramus of the first cervical nerve, which usually lacks cutaneous fibers, is known as the *suboccipital nerve*. It emerges above the posterior arch of the atlas, below the vertebral artery, and supplies the semispinalis capitis and the muscles of the suboccipital triangle. The dorsal ramus of the second cervical nerve supplies the obliquus capitis inferior and then divides into medial and lateral branches. The medial branch, termed the *greater occipital nerve,* pierces the semispinalis capitis and trapezius, and then accompanies the occipital artery and supplies the skin of the scalp as far forward as the vertex. The medial branch of the dorsal ramus of the third cervical nerve continues as the *third occipital nerve,* piercing the trapezius and supplying the skin on the back of the head. The dorsal rami of C6, C7, and C8 usually have no cutaneous branches (Cave, 1937; Johnston, 1908; Pearson et al., 1966), hence the C5 dermatome is adjacent to T1 and, with overlap, C4 meets T2. This junction marks what might be called the dorsal axial line (from about the spine of CV7 to near the deltoid insertion).

THORACIC DORSAL RAMI

Each ramus passes backward, supplying the deeply placed muscles, and divides into a medial and a lateral cutaneous branch, which are separated by slips of the longissimus thoracis. The medial branches pass backward and downward, supplying the erector spinae and its divisions. The medial branches of the upper thoracic nerves (T1 to T3) also become cutaneous. The lateral branches supply the levatores costarum, the longissimus thoracis, and the iliocostalis thoracis. They have a long downward course (Johnston, 1908), the lower ones (T9 to T12) piercing the latissimus dorsi and supplying the skin of the back as far down as the gluteal region. In what might be termed a transitional zone, both medial and lateral branches of T4 to T8 give cutaneous twigs.

LUMBAR, SACRAL, AND COCCYGEAL DORSAL RAMI

The lateral branches of the upper lumbar rami give rise to the superior clunial nerves, which supply the skin of the buttock. The lateral branches of the lower lumbar rami, together with those of the sacral dorsal rami, form the dorsal sacral plexus. The dorsal rami of the first four sacral nerves pass backward through the dorsal sacral foramina, whereas those of the fifth sacral and the coccygeal emerge through the sacral hiatus. The medial branches of the first dorsal rami supply the erector spinae. The lateral branches, together with those of the lower lumbar and a contribution from the fifth sacral, form the dorsal sacral plexus immediately behind the sacrum

and coccyx (Horwitz, 1939). Loops of this plexus give off two or three middle clunial nerves (though not invariably), which pierce the overlying gluteus maximus and supply the skin of the buttock. The dorsal rami of the fifth sacral and coccygeal nerves lack medial and lateral branches; they communicate (often forming a single nerve) and supply adjacent ligaments and overlying skin.

REFERENCES

Bardeen, C. R., and Elting, A. W.: A statistical study of the variations in the formation and position of the lumbo-sacral plexus in man. Anat. Anz., *19*:124, 209, 1901.

Beaton, L. E., and Anson, B. J.: The relation of the sciatic nerve and of its subdivisions to the piriformis muscle. Anat. Rec., *70*:1, 1937.

Cave, A. J. E.: The distribution of the first intercostal nerve and its relation to the first rib. J. Anat., *63*:367, 1929.

Cave, A. J. E.: The innervation and morphology of the cervical intertransverse muscles. J. Anat., *71*:497, 1937.

Dankmeijer, J., and Waltman, J. M.: Sur l'innervation de la face dorsale des doigts humains. Acta Anat., *10*:377, 1950.

Dass, R.: Sympathetic components of the dorsal primary divisions of human spinal nerves. Anat. Rec., *113*: 493, 1952.

Davies, F.: A note on the first lumbar nerve (anterior ramus). J. Anat., *70*:177, 1935.

Davies, F., and Laird, M.: The supinator muscle and the deep radial (posterior interosseous) nerve. Anat. Rec., *101*:243, 1948.

Delmas, J., and Laux, G.: Système Nerveux Sympathique. Paris, Masson et Cie, 1952.

Dow, D. R.: The anatomy of rudimentary first thoracic ribs with special reference to the arrangement of the brachial plexus. J. Anat., *59*:166, 1925.

Fenart, R.: La morphogénèse du plexus brachial, ses rapports avec la formation du cou et du membre supérieur. Acta Anat., *32*:322, 1958.

Fender, F. A.: Foerster's scheme of the dermatomes. Arch. Neurol. Psychiatry, *41*:688, 1939.

Foerster, O.: The dermatomes in man. Brain, *56*:1, 1933.

Foerster, O.: Symptomatologie der Erkankungen des Rückenmarks und seiner Wurzeln. *In* Bumke, O., and Foerster, O.: Handbuch der Neurologie. Vol. 5. Berlin, J. Springer, 1936.

Gardner, E.: Surgical anatomy of the external carotid plexus. Arch. Surg., *46*:238, 1943.

Gardner, E., Gray, D. J., and O'Rahilly, R.: Anatomy. 3rd Ed. Philadelphia, W. B. Saunders Co., 1969.

Hansen, K., and Schliack, H.: Segmentale Innervation. Stuttgart, Georg Thieme Verlag, 1962.

Harness, D., and Sekeles, E.: The double anastomotic innervation of thenar muscles. J. Anat., *109*:461, 1971.

Harris, W.: The true form of the brachial plexus, and its motor distribution. J. Anat., *38*:399, 1904.

Harris, W.: The Morphology of the Brachial Plexus. London, Humphrey Milford, 1939.

Haymaker, W., and Woodhall, B.: Peripheral Nerve

Injuries. 2nd Ed. Philadelphia, W. B. Saunders Co., 1953.

Head, H., and Campbell, A. W.: The pathology of herpes zoster and its bearing on sensory localisation. Brain, 23:353, 1900.

Hollinshead, H.: Anatomy for Surgeons. 2nd Ed. New York, Hoeber Medical Division, Harper & Row, 1968, 1969, 1971.

Horwitz, M. T.: The anatomy of (A), the lumbosacral nerve plexus—its relation to variations of vertebral segmentation, and (B), the posterior sacral nerve plexus. Anat. Rec., 74:91, 1939.

Hovelacque, A.: Anatomie des nerfs cranien et rachidiens et du système grande sympathique chez l'homme. Paris, Gaston Doin et Cie, 1927.

Jamieson, R. W., Smith, D. B., and Anson, B. J.: The cervical sympathetic ganglia. Bull. Northwest. Univ. Med. Sch., 26:219, 1952.

Jit, I., and Mukerjee, R. N.: Observations on the anatomy of the human thoracic sympathetic chain and its ganglia; with an anatomical assessment of operations for hypertension. J. Anat. Soc. India, 9:55, 1960.

Johnston, H. M.: The cutaneous branches of the posterior primary divisions of the spinal nerves, and their distribution in the skin. J. Anat., 43:80, 1908.

Jones, F. W.: The Principles of Anatomy as Seen in the Hand. 2nd Ed. London, Baillière, Tindall, & Cox, 1942.

Jones, F. W.: Structure and Function as Seen in the Foot. 2nd Ed. London, Baillière, Tindall, & Cox, 1949.

Kaplan, E. B.: Functional and Surgical Anatomy of the Hand. 2nd Ed. Philadelphia, J. B. Lippincott Co., 1965.

Keegan, J. J., and Garrett, F. D.: The segmental distribution of the cutaneous nerves in the limbs of man. Anat. Rec., 102:409, 1948.

Kerr, A. T.: The brachial plexus of nerves in man, the variations in its formation and branches. Am. J. Anat., 23:285, 1918.

Kimmel, D. L.: Innervation of spinal dura mater and dura mater of the posterior cranial fossa. Neurology, (Minneap.) 11:800, 1961.

Kuntz, A.: The Autonomic Nervous System. 4th Ed. Philadelphia, Lea & Febiger, 1953.

Kuntz, A.: Components of splanchnic and intermesenteric nerves. J. Comp. Neurol., 105:251, 1956.

Kuntz, A., Hoffman, H. H., and Napolitano, L. M.: Cephalic sympathetic nerves. Arch. Surg., 75:108, 1957.

Labbok, A.: Anatomische Untersuchungen und Typen des Kreuzabschnittes der Trunci sympathici. Anat. Anz., 85:14, 1937.

Lambert, E. H.: The accessory deep peroneal nerve. Neurology (Minneap.), 19:1169, 1969.

von Lanz, T., and Wachsmuth, W.: Praktische Anatomie. Some parts in 2nd edition. Berlin, J. Springer, 1953–1972.

Last, R. J.: Innervation of the limbs. J. Bone Joint Surg., 31-B:452, 1949.

Learmonth, J. R.: A variation in the distribution of the radial branch of the musculo-spiral nerve. J. Anat., 53:371, 1919.

Mitchell, G. A. G.: Anatomy of the Autonomic Nervous System. Edinburgh, E. & S. Livingstone, 1953.

Mizeres, N. J.: The cardiac plexus in man. Amer. J. Anat., 112:141, 1963.

Monro, P. A. G.: Sympathectomy. London, Oxford University Press, 1959.

Nomina Anatomica. 3rd Ed. Amsterdam, Excerpta Medica Foundation, 1966.

Pallie, W.: The intersegmental anastomoses of posterior spinal rootlets and their significance. J. Neurosurg., 16:188, 1959.

Pearson, A. A., Sauter, R. W., and Buckley, T. F.: Further observations on the cutaneous branches of the dorsal primary rami of the spinal nerves. Am. J. Anat., 118:891, 1966.

Pedersen, H. E., Blunck, C. F. J., and Gardner, E.: The anatomy of lumbosacral posterior rami and meningeal branches of spinal nerves (sinu-vertebral nerves). J. Bone Joint Surg., 38-A:377, 1956.

Pernkopf, E.: Atlas of Topographical and Applied Human Anatomy. Ed., H. Ferner, transl., H. Monsen. Philadelphia, W. B. Saunders Co., 1963.

Pick, J.: The Autonomic Nervous System. Philadelphia, J. B. Lippincott Co., 1970.

Pick, J., and Sheehan, D.: Sympathetic rami in man. J. Anat., 80:12, 1946..

Pitres, A., and Testut, L.: Les nerfs en schémas. Paris, Gaston Doin et Cie, 1925.

Schadé, J. P.: The Peripheral Nervous System. Amsterdam, Elsevier Publishing Co., 1966.

Seddon, H.: Surgical Disorders of the Peripheral Nerves. Edinburgh, Churchill Livingstone, 1972.

Sicard, A., and Bruézière, J.: Le plexus sacro-coccygien. Arch. Anat. Histol. Embryol., 33:43, 1950.

Skoog, T.: Ganglia in the communicating rami of the cervical sympathetic trunk. Lancet, 253:457, 1947.

Smorto, M. P., and Basmajian, J. V.: Clinical Electroneurography. Baltimore, Williams & Wilkins Co., 1972.

Stopford, J. S. B.: The variation in distribution of the cutaneous nerves of the hand and digits. J. Anat., 53:14, 1918.

Sunderland, S.: Metrical and non-metrical features of the muscular branches of the radial nerve. J. Comp. Neurol., 85:93, 1946.

Sunderland, S.: Nerves and Nerve Injuries. Baltimore, Williams & Wilkins Co., 1968.

Sunderland, S., and Bedbrook, G. M.: The relative sympathetic contribution to individual roots of the brachial plexus in man. Brain, 72:297, 1949.

Sunderland, S., and Hughes, E. S. R.: Metrical and non-metrical features of the muscular branches of the ulnar nerve. J. Comp. Neurol., 85:113, 1946.

Sunderland, S., and Hughes, E. S. R.: Metrical and non-metrical features of the muscular branches of the sciatic nerve and its medial and lateral popliteal divisions. J. Comp. Neurol., 85:205, 1946.

Sunderland, S., and Ray, L. J.: Metrical and non-metrical features of the muscular branches of the median nerve. J. Comp. Neurol., 85:191, 1946.

Warwick, R., and Williams, P. L., (eds.): Gray's Anatomy. 35th Ed. London, Longmans, Green & Co., Ltd., 1973.

Webber, R. H.: A contribution on the sympathetic nerves in the lumbar region. Anat. Rec., 130:581, 1958.

Webber, R. H.: Some variations in the lumbar plexus of nerves in man. Acta Anat., 44:336, 1961.

Winckler, G.: Le nerf péronier accessoire profond. Arch. Anat. Histol. Embryol., 18:181, 1934.

Woodburne, R. T.: The accessory obturator nerve and the innervation of the pectineus muscle. Anat. Rec., 136:367, 1960.

Woodburne, R. T.: The sacral parasympathetic innervation of the colon. Anat. Rec., 124:67, 1956.

Wrete, M.: Die intermediären vegetativen Ganglien der Lumbalregion beim Menschen. Z. Mikrosk. Anat. Forsch., 53:122, 1943.

Chapter 3

DEVELOPMENT OF PERIPHERAL MYELINATED AND UNMYELINATED NERVE FIBERS

Henry deF. Webster

The mechanisms involved in nerve fiber development, growth, ensheathment, myelination, and ending formation are among the most fascinating and important topics in contemporary cytologic research. Observations germane to these topics have been reported for more than a century and currently are widely scattered in an ever expanding number of periodicals. An excellent introduction to this complex subject is Billings's review (1971) of the concepts of nerve fiber development from 1839 until 1930, when the outgrowth theory was generally accepted. Here, our survey of nerve fiber development emphasizes recent morphologic research in vertebrates; it proceeds from the cellular to the tissue level, and reflects the interests of the author. Several books and the other literature cited should provide adequate bibliographies for additional reading and chronologic documentation (see Hughes, 1968; Wolstenholme and O'Connor, 1968; Himwich, 1969; Jacobson, 1970; Davison and Peters, 1970). The final section deals with human nerve fiber development. Since substantially less is known, the survey is shorter and much more complete. It is hoped that use of the same topic sequence will help readers identify major areas of ignorance, especially those that deserve future exploration.

Since developmental patterns vary, some may find it helpful to review the cellular morphology and relationships of mature nerve fibers, as well as the neurons from which they originate (see Chapters 4 through 7) as well as

Peters et al., 1970; Asbury, 1974; Webster 1974). Briefly, fibers in roots and nerves include axons of somatic and visceral multipolar neurons in the central nervous system, axons of neurons in autonomic ganglia, and both central and peripheral processes of sensory neurons in cranial and spinal ganglia. The plasma membranes covering these fibers are trilaminar and measure about 9 nm. Surface specializations are apparent at the initial segment of multipolar neurons in the central nervous system, at all nodes of Ranvier, and at synaptic endings (Palay et al., 1968; Kelly and Zacks, 1969; Pappas and Waxman, 1972). Within the axoplasm, microtubules, neurofilaments, mitochondria, and profiles of agranular endoplasmic reticulum predominate; also, there are occasional multivesicular bodies, ribosomes, and vesicles that vary in size and density.

Rows of Schwann cells are arranged longitudinally along nerve fibers, forming sheaths around them. A carbohydrate-rich basal lamina covers the Schwann cell's surface membrane, which may include pinocytotic invaginations along its external and axonal surfaces (Waxman, 1968). A long ellipsoidal nucleus is usually located midway between the ends of a Schwann cell. Cisternae of granular endoplasmic reticulum, the Golgi complex, mitochondria, and lysosomes surround the nucleus and are less numerous elsewhere; filaments, microtubules, and profiles of agranular endoplasmic reticulum are more evenly distributed. Myelinated and unmyelinated fibers have different relationships with the Schwann cells that surround them. These relationships are established during development and include the process of myelination. How this is accomplished is considered in the section following the discussion of the formation and growth of neuronal processes.

DEVELOPMENT OF NEURONAL PROCESSES

The formation and elongation of neurites and the transport required to sustain growth are dynamic activities. Therefore, it seems appropriate to describe the action in living neurons, to consider their morphology after fixation, and finally to review what has been learned about the mechanisms involved by attempting to change these events experimentally.

Observations on Living Neurons

Neuronal process formation and elongation are intimately associated with growth cones, the structures first so named by Cajal in 1890.

Each fiber of this commissural fascicle terminates at a variable distance, proportional to its degree of development. The terminal structure is a conical swelling studded with very irregular spiny processes. This terminal swelling, which we call the growth cone, clearly demarcates the extremity of every developing nerve fiber.

(Translated by L. Guth, 1960)

Since then, many investigators have observed living neurons directly in order to characterize the dynamic activity of growth cones and to study how neuronal processes originate and grow (see reviews by Harrison, 1935; Speidel, 1964; Murray, 1965; Pomerat et al., 1967).

When dissociated neurons are explanted, new fiber formation can be identified, traced, and measured with far greater certainty since the neurons appear rounded, with few neurite remnants, when they are first observed. In an early study, Nakai (1956) described dissociated dorsal root ganglion neurons cultured in Maximov slide assemblies. The initial events included rocking movements of the neuron, loss of its smooth contour, and emergence and retraction of multiple fine processes before the eventual establishment

and dominance of one or two major neurites within a few hours. During subsequent development, only one neuronal process had a typical large growth cone with multiple filopodia or microspikes on its surface. They protruded or retracted at rates of from 6 to 10 μm per minute, measured about 0.3 μm in diameter, were usually between 10 and 20 μm long, and contained no vacuoles, mitochondria, or granules. Contact with a cell or a variety of foreign particles was associated with focal extension of many other filopodia that made surface contact, then adhered or retracted as though they functioned as antennae in guiding neurite growth (Nakai and Kawasaki, 1959). Growth cones also contained pinocytotic vacuoles that moved about and then traveled proximally in processes at from about 1 to 5 μm per minute (Nakai, 1956). Neurites elongated at variable rates (50 to 350 μm per day) and some lengthening was observed between the perikaryon and branch points. Fascicles of parallel fibers were formed by active association that involved adhesion of a growth cone's filopodia to a neighboring process followed by forceful pulling together of the fibers (Nakai, 1960). Collaterals were formed frequently and often grew back toward the cell body.

The sympathetic neurons studied by Bray (1973) were isolated and grown in the presence of nerve growth factor (NGF). Fine spicules projected occasionally from the rounded neurons as they moved and then settled on coverslips placed in dishes. Shortly thereafter, growth cones appeared as fiber formation began. Two types of motion were observed in growth cones, which were present on the tips of all neuronal processes. Rapid, flamelike extensions and retractions of microspikes were superimposed upon a much slower linear advance of the cone as a whole. In almost all cases, branches were formed by bifurcation of a growth cone that had broadened initially. Retraction took place between two or three areas of ruffling membrane that then became the growth cones of the newly formed branches. All the growth cones of a neuron advanced at a relatively constant rate (about 40 μm per hour), while the distances between the cell body and the fibers' branch points remained fixed; this indicated that growth was carefully regulated and occurred at least partially by the addition of new material at the fibers' tips. Branching angles were smaller for thinner processes, and the final growth pattern achieved under these conditions resembled the dendrites of sympathetic neurons in the animal; axon formation was not observed. Nevertheless, these direct observations define some developmental growth characteristics of these neurons that are independent of their cellular environment; they also emphasize the importance of growth cones in fiber formation, branching, and elongation. Fascicles of neurites, similar to those described by Nakai (1960) in dorsal root ganglion neurons, were not present.

In another study of isolated dorsal root ganglion neurons, Okun (1972) found that the neurite growth patterns and rates were similar in most respects to those just described. He also studied the function of processes that were, by visual criteria, fully isolated from any other cells. Responses could be evoked from processes soon after outgrowth, and most spike propagation rates were from 0.1 to 0.2 m per second. Responses recorded from regions within 50 to 100 μm of the growing tips of processes indicated that these membrane areas were active also, but more susceptible to damage.

Explants of dorsal root ganglia have been used to study other features of process growth. If segments of the central and peripheral processes of the neurons are preserved in the explants, they exhibit different growth characteristics (Filogamo, 1969). The distal processes were thicker, grew more slowly, had a greater tendency to form fascicles and associate with fibroblasts, and had larger growth cones with undulating membranes. The central processes were thinner, formed fewer bundles, and had simpler, tuftlike expansions with longer filopodia at their tips. Finally, when dorsal root ganglia were cultured under conditions that inhibited fasciculation, growth cones retracted when they contacted other processes and then elongated in another direction. This produced a radial pattern of growth by a reaction termed "contact inhibition of extension" (Dunn, 1971).

Processes of living neurons contain moving mitochondria, vacuoles, and particles that reflect the transport of cellular constituents between the cell body and its endings. As Pomerat and his collaborators emphasize in their review (1967), the movements are bidirectional and their velocities are highly variable. Mitochondria, for example, moved in either direction at about 10 μm per minute. Recently, Berlinrood, McGee-Russell, and Allen (1972) studied patterns of particle movement in amphibian neurites and analyzed them by photokymography. They found that particles 1.0 to 1.5 μm in diameter moved bidirectionally in a series of jumps (saltatory motion). Some particles reversed direction, and any region of a given fiber contained those moving at a variety of velocities. Also, a particle's instantaneous velocity often differed during successive jumps and ranged from about 0.1 to 2.0 μm per second in the species studied. Most particles moved between 10 and 20 μm per jump, but the distance traveled by a particle in one jump was not related to its velocity. These patterns of movement need to be considered in hypotheses used to characterize transport in neural processes (see Chapter 12).

Fine Structure of Developing Neuronal Processes

The fine structure of growth cones and process elongation have been studied in the developing embryo by Tennyson (1970) and in isolated sympathetic neurons grown in vitro by Bunge (1973) under the same conditions as those observed by Bray (1973).

In rabbit embryos at about 11 days of gestation, the centrally directed neurites (axons) of both the small dark and large light neuroblasts in the dorsal root ganglion were identified and traced (Tennyson, 1970). The initial segments of the latter contained many more neurofilaments; both had numerous microtubules. As in mature dorsal root ganglion neurons (Palay et al., 1968), the initial segments lacked a plasmalemmal undercoating and fascicles of microtubules. Axons were 0.4 to 1.5 μm in diameter and could be followed for up to 60 μm. In addition to randomly dispersed tubules, they contained profiles of agranular reticulum that were often found near the axolemma, clusters of ribosomes, mitochondria, and a variable number of neurofilaments. Close to the endings of neurites, there were occasional fine projections that resembled microspikes and contained dense filamentous material. The enlarged tips of axons (growth cones) included a thickened central cytoplasmic core (varicosity) and a thin, irregular expansion of cytoplasm (filopodium) that contained a fine filamentous matrix similar to that found in the projections. Varicosities had numerous profiles of smooth endoplasmic reticulum;

this extensive membrane network was thought to be important in the formation of the pinocytotic vacuoles observed in living growth cones. Numerous vesicles, mitochondria, and subsurface collections of fine filaments were present also.

After the growth histories and motion of cultured sympathetic neuronal processes were documented photographically, Bunge (1973) showed that movement ceased abruptly within five minutes of initiating aldehyde fixation. A comparison of light and electron micrographs of the same regions before and after fixation and sectioning showed no changes in size, shape, or organelle content. The tips of spikes and leading edges of ruffling membranes in cones during active growth contained a network of microfilaments, some as thin as 3 nm. A similar network was present in filopodia along with pinocytotic vacuoles. Thicker regions of cones were filled with numerous agranular membranous elements embedded in a filamentous matrix. Many dense-cored vesicles and variable numbers of mitochondria, membranous tubules, pinocytotic vacuoles, dense bodies, other lysosomal profiles, ribosomes, and microtubules were present also. An area fixed during retraction contained a large myelin figure and other profiles suggesting autophagic vacuole formation. Evidence to be presented in a subsequent section has shown that the motion in growth cones depends on the integrity of their microfilamentous network, and it is of interest that a protein resembling actin has been isolated from growing nerve cells (Fine and Bray, 1971). Bunge's other observations strongly suggest that the agranular reticulum in growth cones plays an active role in the formation of new surface membrane that accompanies process growth. Lysosomal profiles that participate in the breakdown of membrane during retraction and remodeling of fiber tips probably are also formed locally by the agranular reticulum in growth cones. Another function suggested for this organelle in sympathetic neurons is the formation of dense-cored vesicles (see also Teichberg and Holtzman, 1973).

Transport of cellular components along neuronal processes is required for their survival and growth. Since this topic is covered in detail in Chapter 12, only those observations that concern development are included here. Present evidence strongly suggests that microtubules and their lateral projections participate in axonal transport. They are present in initial outgrowths of neuronal processes and as axons increase in diameter during development, the number of microtubules per unit area of transversely sectioned axon decreases (Friede and Samorajski, 1970). During development, Lasek (1970) found that transport's slow component was two to three times faster than in adult fibers (about 1 mm per day). Finally, uptake and distoproximal transport of protein from muscle into nerves and spinal cord was observed in suckling mice; no uptake into nerves occurred in mature mice (Kristensson, 1970). Thus, much remains to be learned about developmental factors that influence axonal transport mechanisms, rates, and barriers.

Experimental Alterations of Neuronal Process Growth

Since its discovery in 1954, nerve growth factor (NGF) has commanded the attention of many investigators. Here, we can include only a brief summary prepared from reviews by Levi-Montalcini (1966), Levi-Montalcini and Angeletti (1968), Angeletti and co-workers (1968), and Frazier and co-workers (1972) and also mention a few recent observations.

Nerve growth factor is a protein with a molecular weight of about 44,000. Some of its structural and functional properties resemble those of insulin, suggesting a common evolutionary precursor. Mouse submaxillary glands and snake venoms contain relatively large amounts, and the nerve growth factors isolated from these sources are related immunologically (Angeletti, 1971). Nerve growth factor is a normal constituent of sympathetic neurons throughout life, is present in embryonic dorsal root ganglia, and is found in much smaller amounts in serum and other organs. Both in vivo and in vitro, it has dramatic, specific effects on the growth of neurons in sympathetic and embryonic dorsal root ganglia. The growth increase is dose related and is characterized, in sympathetic neurons, by early nuclear changes, then by neuronal enlargement, hypertrophy of the granular endoplasmic reticulum, abundance of ribosomes, and the presence of interlacing bundles of neurofilaments (Angeletti et al., 1971). The metabolic effects on receptor neurons include an increase in both ribonucleic acid and net protein synthesis, enhanced lipid biosynthesis, and an increase in glucose metabolism via direct oxidative pathways. A major increase in outgrowth of neuronal processes also occurs. This has recently been studied quantitatively in cultured dorsal root ganglion neurons (Blood, 1972).

Variations in culture conditions may partially explain differences observed when drugs were used to explore the mechanisms for nerve growth factor stimulation of neurite outgrowth. Yamada and Wessells (1971) suggested that it might stimulate the production or activity of growth cones; they did not observe an increase in total protein or in the accumulation of microtubule protein during early outgrowth. Later experiments suggested that the embryo extract included in their culture media may have masked the increase in microtubule protein produced (Hier et al., 1972). Treatment of nerve growth factor–stimulated sympathetic ganglia with actinomycin D showed that initiation of outgrowth did not require ribonucleic acid synthesis; its inhibition of subsequent fiber elongation resembled that produced by cyclohexamide and paralleled the reduction in protein synthesis observed with both drugs (Partlow and Larrabee, 1971). Finally, administration of nerve growth factor antiserum to newborn animals destroys sympathetic neurons (Levi-Montalcini, 1966) and produces degeneration of their axons and some of the Schwann cells that surround them (Aguayo et al., 1972).

Adenosine 3',5'monophosphate (cyclic AMP) is another normal tissue constituent that affects a variety of cellular activities including aggregation, differentiation, and locomotion. Since changes in chick dorsal root ganglion explant size, neurite number, length, diameter, and degree of branching were variable and independent of each other, Roisen and his collaborators (1972a) compared the effects of 5' AMP, dibutyryl cyclic AMP, cyclic AMP and nerve growth factor on these parameters by using more than 100 explants to test each substance. Cultures treated with 5' AMP were similar to controls; cyclic AMP produced a significant increase in area of outgrowth, numbers of neurites, their lengths, and degree of branching. A still larger and similar increase was produced by dibutyryl cyclic AMP and nerve growth factor. Simultaneous treatment with both demecolcine (Colcemid) and dibutyryl cyclic AMP produced neurite growth

similar to that observed with the latter alone. These observations suggest that nerve growth factor may stimulate microtubule formation by assembly from preexisting subunits via a cyclic AMP intermediary (Roisen et al., 1972b).

During the past five years, the systematic study of growth patterns and fine structure of cultured neurons treated with cytochalasin B, colchicine, and cyclohexamide has defined some of the major parameters of growth cone movement and process elongation (Yamada et al., 1970, 1971; review by Wessells et al., 1971). Cytochalasin B alters microfilaments. Within from 30 seconds to three minutes after its addition to cultured dorsal root ganglion neurons, microspikes protruding from growth cones wilted and retracted. Peristaltic waves progressed proximally in many axons, which became thinner and disappeared. The length of axons that remained was unchanged. Electron microscopic study showed that relatively few microspikes were present. They were curved and short; their elongated polygonal network of microfilaments was collapsed and partially disrupted. Replacement of the drug by control medium was associated with the formation of new microspikes and growth cones. Axon elongation began again within four hours, and a similar pattern of early recovery was observed in the presence of cyclohexamide, an inhibitor of protein synthesis. Further studies have correlated differences in the arrangement of microfilaments in cultured dorsal root ganglia neurons and glia (presumably Schwann cells) with their patterns of locomotion (Spooner et al., 1971; Luduena and Wessells, 1973). In neurons, microfilaments were found only in areas that moved—namely, in growth cones, their areas of ruffled membrane, and in microspikes. The microfilaments were arranged in lattices with focal variation in their orientation. They are responsible for the advance of growth cones across a substrate surface while the positions of a neuron and its proximal branches remain relatively fixed. Similar lattices were found in ruffled membranes on leading edges of migratory glial (Schwann) cells. They also contained, however, a subplasmalemmal sheath of microfilaments oriented parallel to the long axis of the cell and its direction of migratory locomotion.

Colchicine and vinca alkaloids disrupt microtubules. When added to cultured neurons, colchicine produced concentration-dependent, reversible inhibition of the total length of a neuron's processes (Daniels, 1972), and during the initial stages of shortening, growth cone and microspike activity were unaltered (Yamada et al., 1970, 1971). When examined electron microscopically, the processes of colchicine-treated neurons contained fewer microtubules and many more 7 to 10 nm filaments (Daniels, 1973); also, the changes were not associated with an inhibition of protein synthesis.

Thus, present evidence shows that growth cones and their lattices of microfilaments are involved in the formation of processes, the locomotion of their tips, and branching. The agranular endoplasmic reticulum in growth cones has a major role in adding surface membrane constituents for process growth and recycling those in retracting tips. Assembly of microtubules is also required for fiber elongation. In addition, these elements probably also are important in the transport required for maintenance of neuronal processes.

Neuronal Process Growth in Developing Neural and Limb Tissue

Cellular and tissue interactions that influence fiber growth in the intact nervous system are complex. Autonomic neurons and those in anterior horns and dorsal root ganglia each have different patterns of differentiation, migration, process growth, and ending formation. In mammals, many of these interactions occur during gestation and have been difficult to study experimentally. As expected, amphibian and chick embryos have been used in most investigations. Several books and reviews include useful summaries of most of the available evidence (Speidel, 1964; Kollros, 1968; Hughes, 1968; Jacobson, 1970; Schmitt, 1970).

Observations on transplants that have been rotated or on neurons with aberrant process growth suggest that a neuron's polarity, the direction of its axonal outgrowth, and the pattern of its dendritic branching are genetically determined. How, then, do neuronal processes grow over long distances and arrive in relatively small, specific terminal regions? Mechanical and chemical (neurotrophic) influences have been suggested, but their nature remains poorly defined. Recently, Nornes and Das (1972) have shown that as axons appear on differentiating neuroblasts in the spinal cord's ventral horn, there are oriented interfaces to help facilitate their subsequent ventral and longitudinal growth. Interactions of cell surfaces similar to those implicated in cell recognition may also play a role (Goldschneider and Moscona, 1972). In addition neurite growth probably is influenced by the contents of the extracellular matrix. Collagens found in extracellular fibrils and in cell coats provide contact guidance for growing processes in the periphery. A similar effect seems likely in the central nervous system also, since Cohen and Hay (1971) have shown that epithelial cells in the embryonic spinal cord also secrete collagens. Since neurite outgrowth within both the central and peripheral nervous systems occurs before the appearance of either glia or Schwann cells, neither appears to have a major role in this process. Also, it seems unlikely that functional activity of a neurite or neighboring cells influences its growth, since no changes have been observed during long periods of anesthesia.

Once in the periphery, some aspects of neuronal process growth can be observed directly in favorable locations such as the tailfins and limb buds of living tadpoles. Many years ago, Speidel showed that single pioneer sprouts grew out among mesenchymal cells toward the skin (see 1964 review). Before the arrival of Schwann cells, small fascicles were formed as other axons followed in the same paths. Nerve sprouts are also found in limb buds as they form, and when a frog's hind limb bud is less than 1 mm long, the major limb nerves can be recognized (Taylor, 1943). At this early stage, muscle and bone are represented only by condensing mesenchyme. When neuronal processes arrive in regions where they terminate, both branching and ending formation may be profuse and highly variable before the mature pattern is established.

Numerous studies have shown that as development proceeds, both neurons and their processes in roots or nerves degenerate (see, for example, Hughes, 1968; Reier and Hughes, 1972a; Aguayo et al., 1973). Initial overproduction with subsequent fallout of cells and fibers that fail to establish terminal connections has seemed like a reasonable explanation, but this has been difficult to demonstrate quantitatively. One study that includes counts of ventral root fibers to the lower limb showed that after an initial rapid tenfold increase in the number of unmyelinated fibers, about three fourths of those that still were unmyelinated at a later stage suddenly degenerated. Subsequently, the numbers of ventral root fibers and ventral horn neurons were in the same range and there was little further change (Prestige and Wilson, 1972).

Recently, New and Mizell (1972) have shown that opossum fetuses can be grown in culture. This model system offers a number of possible advantages for the investigation of cellular interactions in intact mammalian tissue during the development of the peripheral nervous system. For example, are there trophic effects of nerves, similar to those present in amphibia, that influence limb differentiation and permit regeneration following limb amputation (Guth, 1969; Drachman, 1974)?

Formation of Endings

Few endings are of greater clinical importance than the neuromuscular junction. Recent studies pertaining to its development have attempted to correlate the morphologic and functional events that accompany endplate formation and differentiation. In intercostal muscles of rats at 16 days gestational age, junction-like complexes were found between adjacent membranes of axons and myotubes (Kelly and Zacks, 1969). Then, groups of axons were located within depressions of myotube walls; focal thickening in myotube membranes with some overlying basal lamina was thought to represent primitive motor endplate differentiation. By 18 days, axon terminals contained vesicles and the plasmalemmas of large myotubes resembled postsynaptic membranes. At birth, intercostal muscles were formed by separate myofibrils with motor endplates that contained rudimentary primary and secondary synaptic clefts. Junctions resembling those in mature muscle were observed at age 10 days. Physiologic studies have shown that in rat fetuses, nerve stimulation produced muscle contraction at 16 days (Straus and Weddell, 1940), and that at 17 days discrete transmitter release at sites where junctions subsequently appeared could be identified by intracellular recording (Diamond and Miledi, 1962).

The correlation of these morphologic, functional, and pharmacologic events has been pursued at the cellular level by studying them in vitro. In cord-myotome explants, axons arborized among muscle fibers and developed characteristic bulbous endings that stained with acetylcholinesterase (Bornstein et al., 1968). Stimulation of the cord in these explants produced widespread synchronized muscle twitches that could be blocked by curare (Crain, 1970). Robbins and Yonezawa (1971) have shown that excitatory junctional potentials were present within hours or one or two days of nerve-muscle contact. Contractility and transmission developed independently and the latter could be identified in young noncontractile myotubes with only three nuclei. It is also of interest that initially dissociated spinal cord neurons and muscle cells can also form functional neuromuscular junction in vitro (Fischbach, 1970). The minimal structural requirements for early chemical transmission have not been described.

Relatively little is known about cellular structure and functional relationships during the development of other endings in the peripheral nervous system. Recently, Landon (1972) found that sensory terminals resembling mature annulospiral endings were present in spindles of gastrocnemius muscles from 18 day rat fetuses. The axoplasm contained 40 to 60 nm vesicles (a few with dense cores), many small mitochondria, and some amorphous material. The axon terminals were not covered by Schwann cells, and the gap between adjacent axoterminal and sarcolemmal membranes did not contain junctional complexes or a basal lamina.

SCHWANN CELLS AND NERVE FIBER DEVELOPMENT
Origin of Schwann Cells

The cells described by Schwann have had a long and interesting history (see, for example, Chapter 11 as well as Schwann, 1847; Causey, 1960; Jacobson, 1970). Like certain areas of the world, they have been involved in controversy since their discovery, and only a few of the important disputes have been settled. In 1924 Harrison showed that the neural crest provides most of the Schwann cells for developing nerve fibers. Although this conclusion was disputed, it was reexamined when radioautographic techniques made it possible to label neural crest cells, transplant them, and follow their subsequent differentiation.

Both Johnston (1966) and Noden (1974) showed that virtually all satellite cells that surrounded neurons, their processes, and terminals in the cranial portion of the peripheral nervous system were derived from the neural crest. It was clear that neural crest cells also participated in the formation of bone, cartilage, connective tissue, and skeletal muscle. Finally, these experiments also documented the great migratory capacity of neural crest cells, a characteristic exemplified by the occasional presence of spinal ganglion neurons in the sciatic nerve (Metz et al., 1958). Since Schwann cells begin migrating early and proliferate extensively before differentiating, their origin has again been reexamined with a new biologic marker that is not diluted during cell division (Douarin, 1973). Cells in the chick and Japanese quail are compatible and can be distinguished by differences in chromatin pattern that continue to replicate. This technique has provided additional, convincing evidence for the neural crest origin of Schwann cells and has also been useful in identifying new crest derivatives (Johnston et al., 1974).

Migration and Early Association With Axons

As noted in the previous section, experiments using explants of dissociated neurons have added to the evidence showing that neither glia nor Schwann cells are required by neurons during the elongation of their processes or the formation of functional endings. Nevertheless, in the developing peripheral nervous system, outgrowth of neurites is soon followed by the appearance of Schwann cells. Their behavior in vivo was described in detail by Speidel (1932), who later correlated his own observations with in vitro and electron microscopic studies of others (Speidel, 1964). In the transparent tailfins of lightly anesthetized tadpoles, Schwann cells migrated out along the naked pioneer nerve sprouts that were growing toward the skin. Actively migrating cells moved about 60 μm a day; however, the rate was highly variable and some Schwann cells remained stationary for days. Mitotic division occurred as Schwann cells moved distally along pioneer sprouts, which provided paths for the "myelin emergent" axons that usually grew out later. As migration and proliferation continued, trans-fer of Schwann cells to "myelin-emergent" fibers began. Usually, this occurred within the same small fascicle of axons. Some Schwann cells, however, developed small pseudopods before migrating laterally to establish contact with a fiber in a different bundle. The preferential attraction of "myelin-emergent" axons for Schwann cells seemed to be quite specific, since transfer from these fibers to those that remained unmyelinated was rarely observed.

More recently, these observations have been extended by correlating in vivo observations with the electron microscopic appearance of developing nerve fibers in tadpoles (Webster and Billings, 1972; Billings-Gagliardi et al., 1974). When examined with the differential interference (Nomarski) microscope, Schwann cells seen moving freely between fibers were ovoid in shape and had several long processes ending in blunt expansions. In the electron microscope, these Schwann cells showed no basal lamina. Ruffled areas were found along the plasmalemma, but there was no conspicuous microfilamentous sheath beneath it. The organelles were similar to those found in Schwann cells that had settled down and had begun to spread along one or several axons. Later, they became more spindle-shaped and acquired a basal lamina, a morphologic sign, perhaps, of a more permanent axon–Schwann cell relationship. In our material, individual axons that could be followed for long distances were almost always accompanied by one or several others. Schwann cell nuclei were easily located in vivo, but their cytoplasmic margins and the branches of each axon could not be traced with certainty. Thus, it was not possible for us to characterize the dynamic geometry of the relationships between Schwann cells and axons in these small fascicles before myelination. They are, however, probably more complex than Speidel's descriptions and diagrams indicate.

Although tissue culture methods have been used for more than 60 years to study the pattern of neurite outgrowth and Schwann cell migration, there are few observations that characterize their relationships before myelination. Peterson and Murray (1955) showed that Schwann cells that surrounded axons were long, thin, and veil-like. Prior to myelin formation, their attachment seemed firm and their position along axons relatively fixed. Occasionally, small refractile granules were seen in the perinuclear region. Myelination was observed in these cultures and a later light and electron microscopic study showed that after long-term maintenance in vitro, the Schwann cell–axon relationships were similar to those found in mature nerves (Bunge et al., 1967).

Recently, the structural basis of migratory motion has been studied in dissociated glial cells from embryonic chick dorsal root ganglia (Spooner et al., 1971; Luduena and Wessells, 1973). These cells, some of which resemble Schwann cells, contained a sheath of actin-like microfilaments oriented parallel to the direction of movement. When cultures of these cells were treated with cytochalasin B, migration ceased; the microfilaments were disrupted while other organelles, including microtubules, remained intact. Though not yet described, similar sheaths or aggregates of microfilaments may be present in actively migrating Schwann cells within developing nerves or dorsal root ganglia cultures.

Early Schwann Cell–Axon Relationships in Nerves

In developing nerves, the relationships between Schwann cells and axons change rapidly. During this complex sequence of events, axons are sorted into a population of fibers that becomes myelinated and into another that remains unmyelinated. At present, little is known about the surface interactions of the cells, and most of our concepts are based on electron microscopic observations.

Peters (1961) showed that newly formed nerves in amphibian limb buds contained small naked axons, all of which were surrounded by a single layer of Schwann cells. Then larger axons appeared, and Schwann cell processes began invading the central core of axons. A similar appearance had also been described in the digital nerves of rat embryos (Peters and Muir, 1959). Schwann cell processes separated all the nerve's axons into large bundles that were subsequently subdivided as the Schwann cells multiplied rapidly. Some of the larger axons were segregated in separate furrows of Schwann cell cytoplasm. Single Schwann cells surrounded other larger axons and this 1:1 relationship preceded myelin formation. Nuclear counts in this study showed that mitoses were numerous and that

the increase in the nerve's Schwann cell population before birth could have occurred by division of those already present in the nerve at 16½ days of gestation. This initially high rate of Schwann cell division and its decrease during myelination have also been demonstrated radioautographically (Asbury, 1967); in neonatal mouse sciatic nerves, Schwann cells were dividing every 24 hours and about 25 per cent stopped dividing during the cycle he studied.

Recently some geometric and quantitative aspects of these changing relationships were examined in skip serial sections of a fiber population found at the margin of the sciatic nerve's posterior tibial fascicle (Fig. 3–1) (Webster et al., 1973; Martin and Webster, 1973). At birth, none of this region's axons was myelinated and almost all of its transverse area was occupied by "Schwann cell families," a term we used to describe all the axons and processes of different Schwann cells located within a common basal lamina (Fig. 3–2). Big axon bundles were located in the center of each family, and larger axons were found more commonly at the edge of a bundle, segregated in a separate furrow, or in a 1:1 relationship with a Schwann cell located on the family's outer surface. This concentric arrangement, which persisted during axon bundle subdivision and the onset of myelination, suggested that radial sorting of axons destined to be myelinated occurred in sheaths formed by longitudinal columns of Schwann cell families (Fig. 3–3). The sorting sequence included initial surface contact with a Schwann cell process, segregation in a separate furrow of a family sheath, Schwann cell division, and establishment of a 1:1 relationship with one of the daughter Schwann cells, which then became isolated from the family sheath before myelination began.

Counts during the week after birth also showed that Schwann cell families did the sorting in this population of fibers and permitted us to estimate rates for axon bundle subdivision, segregation of larger axons in separate furrows, and establishment of 1:1 relationships. With time, families decreased greatly in size and increased in number. These changes were associated with a dramatic decrease in the size of the axon bundles. Each family, however, continued to contain about the same number of bundles and larger axons in segregated furrows or in a 1:1 relationship. Since approximately half the

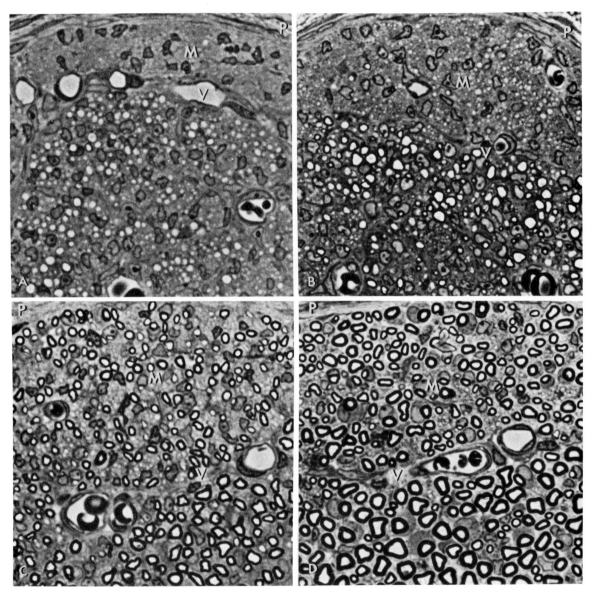

Figure 3–1 In these transverse sections of rat sciatic nerves, fibers in the marginal bundle (M) are shown at the same magnification. The perineurium (P) of the posterior tibial fascicle is at the top of each figure and a row of endoneurial fibroblasts and vessels (V) is above the larger, more centrally located fibers. At birth (A) there are no compact sheaths and at three days (B), there is only one in the marginal bundle. At age seven days (C), there are many myelinated fibers; they are more numerous and larger at age 16 days (D). × 900.

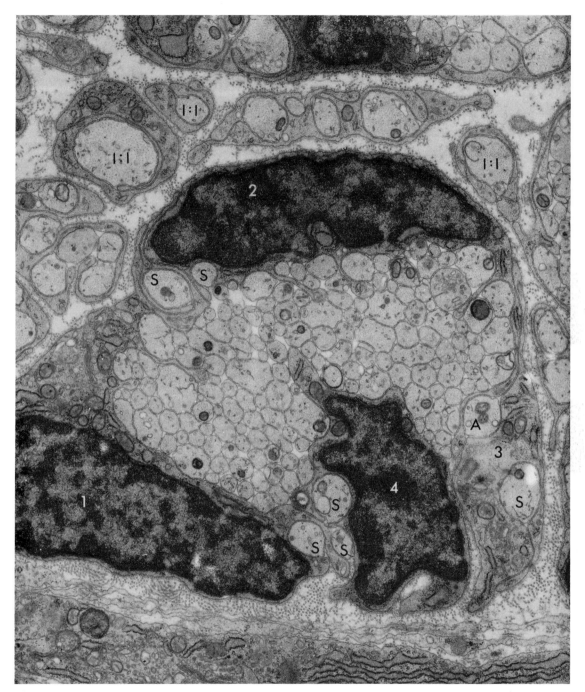

Figure 3–2 Transverse section of marginal bundle of rat sciatic nerve at birth. A common basal lamina surrounds a family of four Schwann cells (1 to 4) and three of them surround more than 100 axons in a single bundle. Six other axons (S) are segregated in separate furrows. One axon (A) indents adjacent surfaces of two Schwann cells. At other levels, the segregated axon (S) at the lower right is in a 1:1 relationship. Above the family sheath, there are several axons (1:1), each surrounded by a Schwann cell that is isolated from its neighbors by endoneurial collagen. × 15,000.

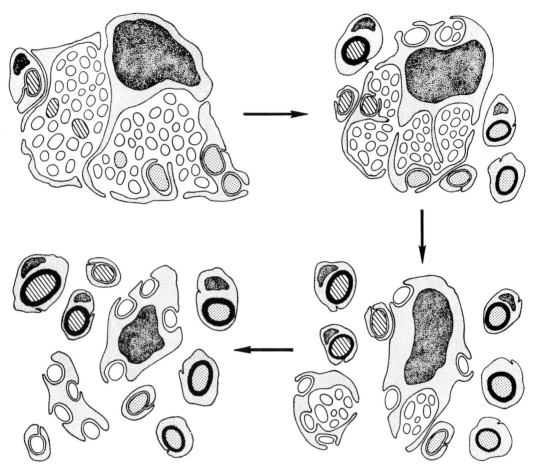

Figure 3–3   Radial sorting by Schwann cell sheaths during axon bundle subdivision. Axons to be myelinated progress radially from a bundle to a segregated furrow and then to a 1:1 relationship at the sheath's outer margin. Family sheaths containing multiple Schwann cells become smaller and more numerous as axon bundles are subdivided (compare Figs. 3–2 and 3–7A). When sorting is completed, chains of individual Schwann cells form the sheaths that surround the myelinated and unmyelinated axons. (From Webster, H. de F., Martin, J. R., and O'Connell, M. F.: The relationships between interphase Schwann cells and axons before myelination: a quantitative electron microscopic study. Dev. Biol., 32:401, 1973. Reprinted by permission.)

Schwann cells that surrounded axon bundles also enveloped larger axons in separate furrows, this process of segregation was thought to be an essential intermediate step in the establishment of the 1:1 relationship that preceded myelination.

In order to understand better the geometry and dynamics of this sorting process, the relationships of dividing Schwann cells were examined also (Martin and Webster, 1973). In newborn rat sciatic nerves, virtually all the mitotic Schwann cells were located in the family sheaths just described (Fig. 3–4). As mitosis began, the radial extent of the processes that surrounded axons decreased. By the end of prophase, the Schwann cell was spindle-shaped and remained so through metaphase

and much of anaphase (Figs. 3–5 and 3–6). The axis of mitosis was parallel to the long axis of the cell, and cytoplasmic division occurred between daughter nuclei that had formed proximally and distally to each other in the nerve. In anaphase, cytoplasmic outgrowth was thought to begin with the appearance of two new slender axial processes that contained longitudinally oriented microtubules. These processes originated at the level of each spindle pole, arched over, and grew longitudinally beside and beyond the dividing nucleus in opposite directions as shown in Figure 3–6. These axial processes were thought to play a role in reestablishing the longitudinal symmetry of the daughter cells. Radial processes that surrounded axons

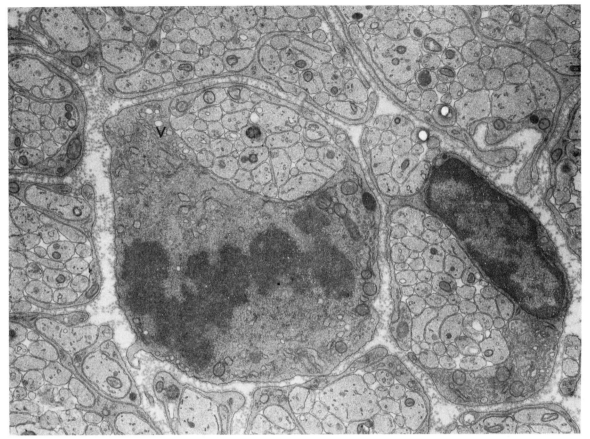

Figure 3–4   Transverse section of marginal bundle of rat sciatic nerve at birth. A family sheath surrounds a bundle of axons enclosed by two Schwann cells. The lower one, in metaphase, has no radial processes that surround axons (see Figs. 3–5 and 3–6); it also contains a few vesicles (V) at the upper left. × 13,500.

reappeared in telophase and extended along processes of neighboring interphase Schwann cells or the basal lamina that enclosed the family. The rapid reduction in surface membrane area associated with radial process retraction was accompanied by the appearance of numerous 100 nm vesicles in the cytoplasm from late prophase to telophase. They probably were derived from the surface membrane since they disappeared as the radial processes were reextended. The nature of the Schwann cell–axon interactions that are associated with this sorting process are still undefined, but the shape changes that occur during mitosis may help increase the contact rate. Also, glycoprotein membrane components, similar perhaps to those recently identified in central nervous system myelin (Quarles et al., 1972), may prove to be important in the cellular recognition and segregation of axons to be myelinated.

Formation and Growth of Myelin Sheaths

Although the resolution of the light microscope is insufficient to demonstrate and trace membranes, the basic relationships between Schwann cells, myelin sheaths, and axons have been known for almost a century (Ranvier, 1878). When living nerve fibers were observed while developing in vivo or in vitro, thin segments of myelin were found first in the perinuclear regions of Schwann cells (Speidel, 1932; 1964; Peterson and Murray, 1955). How these segments were formed remained obscure until the electron microscopic observations and hypothesis of Geren (1954) clearly established the basic morphologic parameters of peripheral myelination. The mesaxon, which is continuous with the Schwann cell surface membrane, grows and forms a spiral sheet around the axon. Further

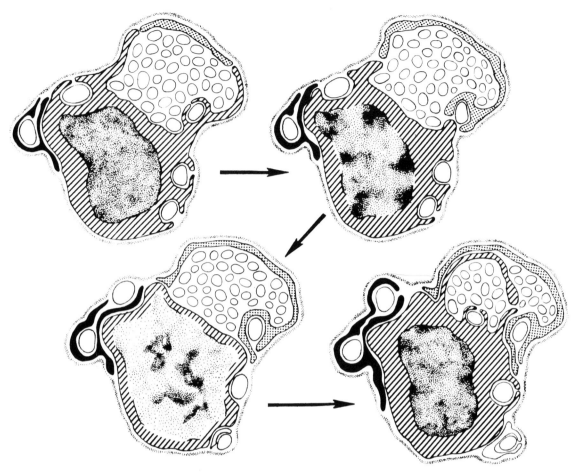

Figure 3–5   Family axon relationships during Schwann cell division. In prophase and early metaphase; radial processes that surround axons retract. Some axons are temporarily enclosed by processes of other Schwann cells in the family sheath that later guide the mitotic cell's processes as they re-extend during telophase. (From Martin, J. R., and Webster, H. de F.: Mitotic Schwann cells in developing nerve: their changes in shape, fine structure and axon relationships. Dev. Biol., 32:417, 1973. Reprinted by permission.)

growth and apposition of the spiral layers occur as the myelin sheath matures. Since then, Geren's observations have been confirmed and extended by many investigators (reviewed by Robertson, 1962; Sjostrand, 1963; Peters and Vaughn, 1970; Mokrasch et al., 1971; see also, Matthews, 1968; Friede and Samorajski, 1968; Uzman and Hedley-Whyte, 1968). In general, they agreed that the Schwann cell, or part of its surface, moves around the axon during growth of the myelin spiral. Two other observations that could not be explained by any simple rotation mechanism have also been discussed. The contour of the myelin spiral is not uniform along the internode; complex variations occur (Webster and Spiro, 1960; Webster, 1964; Rosenbluth, 1966). Second, after the

compact sheath is formed, its internal circumference increases to accommodate the growing axon (Geren, 1956; Robertson, 1962; Rosenbluth, 1966; Friede and Samorajski, 1968).

Since little was known about the geometry and dimensions of the myelin spiral as it formed and grew in a Schwann cell, these parameters were studied in skip serial sections of the fiber population shown in Figure 3–1 (Webster, 1971). Since all these fibers were unmyelinated at birth, the onset and duration of myelination were easily established. At appropriate intervals, approximate dimensions for the bundle and its largest fibers were measured and calculated at the same relative level in litter mates' nerves. These data showed that the myelin membrane's area and trans-

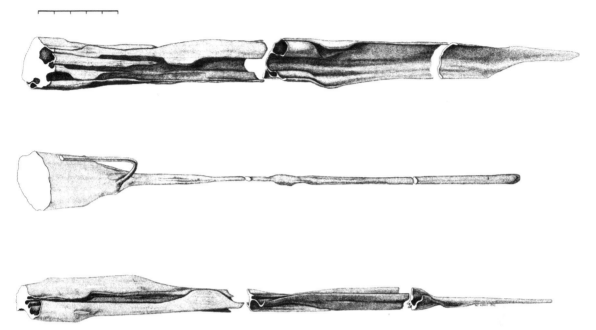

Figure 3–6   Three dimensional reconstruction of half lengths of three mitotic Schwann cells identified in 28 consecutive levels, approximately 2 μm apart (one subdivision of the 10 μm scale at the upper left). Axons and nuclei are not shown. *Top.* At the left end of the early prophase cell, radially extended processes at the midnuclear level form five furrows; farther to the right, three become confluent and their axons form a common bundle. Along the top of the cell, another radial process begins to surround a different bundle, completes the enclosure (top of first cut) and disappears distally. All axons then lie in a common compartment and are surrounded mostly by processes of adjacent cells. *Center.* Late anaphase cell with a slender new axial process that originates at the level of the spindle pole, arches over, and runs beyond the midnuclear level shown at the left. There, the cell's diameter is greatest; it decreases in excessive paranuclear levels and varies slightly along the main axial process. *Bottom.* Beginning at the midinternuclear level, a telophase cell's radial processes surround a bundle of axons through nuclear and paranuclear levels. Farther to the right, the radial processes diminish in extent and ultimately disappear. A slender axial process, similar to the one in the anaphase cell, is behind the rear surface and is not shown in this view. It originates at the spindle pole and runs toward the left edge of the figure. (From Martin, J. R., and Webster, H. de F.: Mitotic Schwann cells in developing nerve: their changes in shape, fine structure and axon relationships. Dev. Biol., *32*:417, 1973. Reprinted by permission.)

verse length increased exponentially with time; the growth rate increased rapidly during the formation of the first four to six spiral layers and remained relatively constant during the subsequent enlargement of the compact sheath.

As others had noted, the minimum diameter of axons that Schwann cells began myelinating was about 1 μm (Fig. 3–7*A*) (cf. Duncan, 1934; Matthews, 1968). During the formation of the first spiral turn, the mesaxon's length and configuration varied when it was studied at different levels in the same Schwann cell (Fig. 3–7*B*). The position of the mesaxon's termination shifted while its origin, at the Schwann cell surface, remained relatively constant. Along myelin internodes composed of two to six spiral turns, there were many variations in the number of lamellae and their

contour; near the mesaxon's origin, longitudinal strips of cytoplasm separated the myelin layers (Fig. 3–7*A* and *C* and Fig. 3–8). Thicker sheaths were larger in circumference, more circular in transverse sections, and more uniform at different levels. Separation of lamellae by cytoplasm was discontinuous and occurred at Schmidt-Lanterman clefts (Friede and Samorajski, 1969). Variations in sheath contour similar to those described earlier by Webster and Spiro (1960) were confined to the paranodal region. Junction-like complexes similar to those present at nodes of Ranvier were also occasionally found along mesaxons or the outer or inner myelin lamellae (Fig. 3–9).

The observations in our study suggested that the spiral form and initial enlargement of the myelin sheath can be explained, in part,

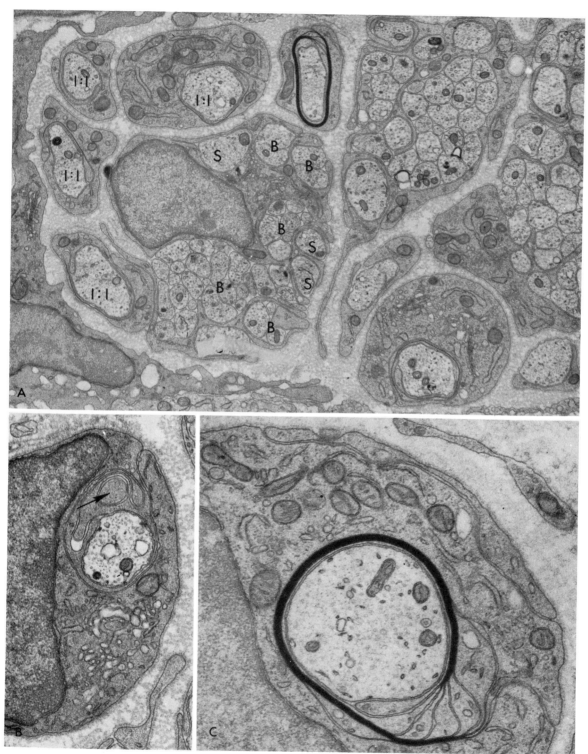

Figure 3–7 Transverse section, marginal bundle of rat sciatic nerve at age seven days. *A.* The family sheath shown at the left includes two Schwann cells that surround the family's five axon bundles (B) and four segregated axons (S). The family's third Schwann cell surrounds a single axon (1:1) at the lower left. Other axons (1:1) and their Schwann cells probably were part of this family at earlier stages in the radial sorting process (see Fig. 3–3). × 13,000. *B.* There is a large redundant loop in the mesaxon's first spiral turn that partially surrounds a projection (arrow) of the Schwann cell's surface. × 21,000. *C.* In the myelin sheath shown, cytoplasm containing organelles separates the layers of compact myelin near the mesaxon's origin. When traced in three dimensions, these cytoplasmic zones form continuous longitudinal strips (see Fig. 3–10). Part of the cell's surface is also covered by a thin band of projecting cytoplasm. × 29,000.

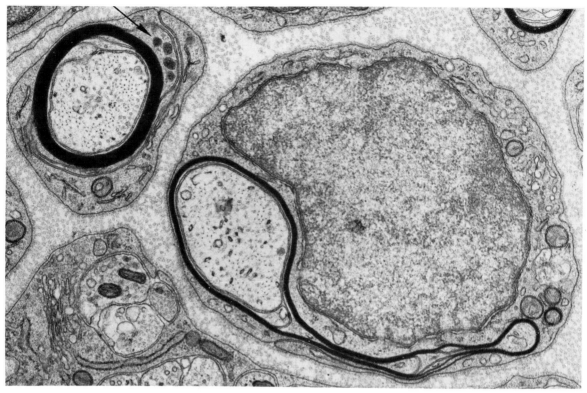

Figure 3–8   Transverse section of marginal bundle of rat sciatic nerve at age seven days. A large loop is present in the lower myelin sheath. The thicker sheath is circular; four dense bodies (arrow) that resemble lysosomes are present in a patch of cytoplasm inside the sheath's outer layer. × 25,000.

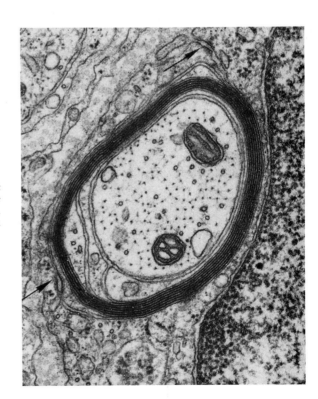

Figure 3–9   Transverse section of neonatal rat sciatic nerve. Junctional complexes (arrows), similar to those found at nodes of Ranvier and Schmidt-Lanterman clefts, are present at the mesaxon's origin and in the myelin spiral's outer layer. × 42,000.

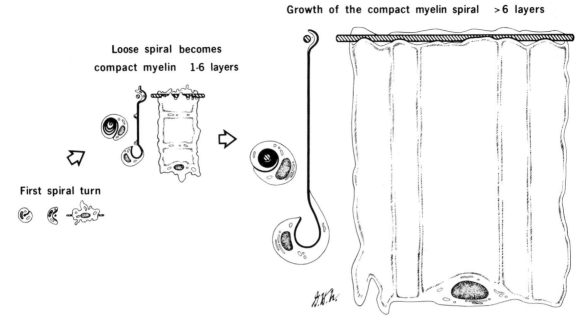

Growth of the compact myelin spiral   > 6 layers

Loose spiral becomes compact myelin   1-6 layers

First spiral turn

Figure 3–10 A diagram of myelin formation in a Schwann cell that shows how the location and relative size of the myelin membrane's cytoplasmic interfaces change during the sheath's growth. The Schwann cell's appearance in cross sections is supplemented by transverse and face views of the "unrolled" cell. To facilitate comparison, the three stages are drawn at the same magnification. After the sheath becomes compact, the initial increase in its circumference is facilitated by the presence of the longitudinal cytoplasmic strips shown in the center. (From Webster, H. de F.: The geometry of peripheral myelin sheaths during their formation and growth in rat sciatic nerves. J. Cell Biol., *48*:348, 1971. Reprinted by permission.)

by developmental events that impose limits on the geometry of the rapid membrane growth that occurs in these Schwann cells (Webster, 1971). In the cellular columns that surround and subdivide axon bundles, the arrangement of processes is consistent with a relatively free pattern of surface growth. After mitosis, a daughter cell in a 1:1 relationship acquires a complete basal lamina and becomes surrounded by endoneurial collagen, both of which probably limit radial spread and favor growth along and around the axon. Cellular elongation predominates until proximal and distal Schwann cells meet at nodes of Ranvier. Then the major site for membrane expansion shifts from the Schwann cell's external and axonal surfaces to the membrane pair that connects them, the mesaxon. Initially, the position of its outer edge is relatively fixed while its inner edge remains free to rotate around the axon. These conditions seem consistent geometrically with a situation that would favor spiral growth of the mesaxon regardless of where new membrane material were added. Periaxonal movement of the Schwann cell nucleus may occur as Murray

(1965) observed, but it does not seem to be an essential prerequisite for spiral formation. The mesaxon's growth rate increases rapidly. The spiral sheet enlarges, becomes more compact, and the relative area of myelin membrane that is covered by cytoplasm begins to decrease. As these surface relationships change, the rate of membrane growth levels off and the geometry of the sheath becomes more regular.

The greatest increase in myelin membrane area probably occurs at a relatively constant rate while the sheath is a compact lamellar spiral (Fig. 3–10). Its length and internal circumference become larger; the number of turns also increases. How this happens remains poorly understood. Our data indicated that the mesaxons, the incisures, and the sheath's outer and inner layers provide large enough interfaces for the addition of new membrane material from the cytoplasm at the rate required for the sheath's growth. As others have suggested, the positions of the layers and their components probably change continuously to achieve the best packing arrangement for the changing molecular constituents of the growing sheath (cf. Robertson, 1962;

Rosenbluth, 1966; Uzman and Hedley-Whyte, 1968; Friede and Samorajski, 1968; Friede, 1972). As the number of spiral turns increases, the origin of the external mesaxon and the nucleus probably move around the axon. Rotation, in the opposite direction, of the sheath itself and the internal mesaxon may also occur.

From a functional standpoint, the three most important dimensions of a nerve fiber are the axon diameter and both the thickness and the length of its myelin sheath. Are developmental changes in these dimensions related to each other and are similar patterns of change found throughout the peripheral nervous system? Generally, elongation of myelin internodes parallels growth of the part that contains the nerve fibers (Vizoso and Young, 1948; Thomas, 1955; Schlaepfer and Myers, 1973). Although longer myelin sheaths are usually thicker and surround larger axons in mature nerves, developmental increases in axon caliber and myelin sheath thickness do not parallel body growth throughout the peripheral nervous system.

In a recent series of studies, Friede and his collaborators have suggested that axon caliber controls the onset and rate of myelin formation (Friede and Samorajski, 1967, 1968; Friede and Martinez, 1970; Friede and Miyagishi, 1972; Friede, 1972). In transverse sections of sciatic nerves removed from rats at intervals from ages one day to four months, they found a linear relationship between the circumference of an axon and the number of layers in its myelin sheath. Adjustments of compact sheaths to changes in axon caliber were demonstrated by applying ligatures to sciatic nerves at age two weeks and examining the proximal and distal regions during long-term constriction and subsequent recovery. Proximally, there were swollen axons surrounded by relatively few myelin lamellae; during recovery, the size of the axons decreased to control values and their sheaths increased proportionately in thickness. If the measurements at one transverse level were representative of those along entire myelin internodes, substantial slipping of layers must have occurred to maintain the sheaths' compact structure during swelling and recovery. Distally, the nerve fibers' growth rate was decreased during compression since axons and their myelin sheaths became progressively smaller than controls. Again, recovery to normal values occurred rapidly; this sug-

gested that the abnormally high rate of enlargement associated with the release of dammed axoplasm could also greatly accelerate myelin membrane biosynthesis in the Schwann cells that surrounded them.

These observations are of interest, but the evidence presented by Friede and Samorajski (1968) seems insufficient to support the contention that axon caliber controls the initiation of myelination, that mesaxons grow because they are stretched by enlarging axons, and that new turns are added to the sheath by a threefold increase in transverse length of mesaxon membranes as they fuse to form the major dense line. Values for the time required for one complete turn of myelin lamella (hours), the increase in axon circumference during the given time (arbitrary units), and the average speed of advancement of the free edge of myelin lamella (per cent of initial speed) are presented (Friede and Samorajski's Table 1), but their validity remains questionable because of the assumptions included in the calculations and the presence of different fiber populations in the sciatic nerve. The growth rate is also shown in a confusing graph (Friede and Samorajski's Fig. 7). The length of the myelin lamella (arbitrary units) is plotted against age in days; this should be a rising sigmoid curve that levels off at maturity. Instead, the curve shown is labeled "increase in length of the myelin lamella per day"; it is bell-shaped and probably represents the slope of the curve expected by the reader. Finally, neither the model nor the rates just noted are consistent with data obtained from more uniform fiber populations. When axon diameters and myelin sheath thicknesses in developing sensory and motor fibers were compared, different growth patterns were found (Williams and Wendell-Smith, 1971). From birth to age eight weeks, the period of marked limb growth, the diameters and growth rates of axons in rabbit sural (sensory) and medial gastrocnemius (motor) nerves were similar, but the myelin sheaths surrounding the motor axons were thicker at each interval. After eight weeks, the sensory axons and their sheaths stopped growing while the motor axons and their sheaths continued to enlarge. Also, a more recent statistical analysis of developing anterior root fibers has shown that myelination began around fibers that varied greatly in circumference (Fraher, 1972). A linear relation between axon caliber and myelin sheath thickness was not found during the initial stages of myelination and was not clearly established until age 17 days, when more than half the sheaths examined had 30 turns or more. The available evidence, then, indicates that axon caliber may influence myelin sheath thickness after its growth pattern is established, but it certainly is not the major determinant of either the growth rate or the final area of the myelin sheath's compact, spirally wrapped membrane sheet.

Biochemistry of Peripheral Myelination

In mammalian experimental animals, the chemical composition and metabolism of peripheral myelin sheaths have been difficult to study during their formation and growth. The available data suggest that myelin is not made de novo (see recent reviews by Davison, 1970; Mokrasch et al., 1971). Instead, the initial turns of the mesaxon spiral probably are similar biochemically to the Schwann cell's plasmalemma. Compared to mature myelin, this early or "myelin-like" membrane probably has a higher protein to lipid ratio and contains more phosphatidyl choline, less cerebroside, and almost no sulfatide or basic protein. As the myelin spiral becomes compact and grows, the basic protein, cerebroside, and sulfatide content increases and the amount of phosphatidyl choline decreases.

Electron microscopic radioautography has been used to study the sites of incorporation and subsequent distribution of myelin precursors and components. When myelinating dorsal root ganglia cultures were exposed to tritiated choline, radioactivity appeared all along the internode (Hendelman and Bunge, 1969). The distribution within the developing spiral could not be determined, and there was no preferential site of initial incorporation in the Schwann cell. When tritiated cholesterol was injected intraperitoneally into five day old mice and their sciatic nerves were examined, the labeled cholesterol was found predominantly in myelin (Hedley-Whyte et al., 1969). The growing sheaths were uniformly labeled in a radial direction after 3 hours, 24 hours, and seven weeks. This diffuse distribution of radioactivity suggested that incorporation also occurred at multiple sites and that there was continuous exchange of cholesterol along and between the spiral layers during myelination.

Recently, peripheral myelin biosynthesis has been studied in vitro by Pleasure and Prockop (1972). When incubated in a simple medium, sciatic nerves of chick embryos incorporated labeled sulfate into myelin sulfatide. They also found that a transport lipoprotein was required to transfer the labeled sulfate from the nerve's microsomal subfraction to myelin.

Experimental Alterations Affecting Schwann Cells and Myelination

Added insight into the mechanisms underlying Schwann cell differentiation and myelin biosynthesis has been provided by studying abnormal developmental patterns.

Genetically induced metabolism disturbances in three neurologic mutations of the mouse are also associated with abnormal peripheral myelination (Meier and MacPike, 1972). In quaking mice a quantitative electron microscopic study has shown that many myelin sheaths had about half as many layers as did sheaths that surrounded axons of the same caliber in control animals (Samorajski et al., 1970). The lamellar structure of these thin sheaths appeared normal, as did the axons they surrounded. Abnormalities in sphingolipid fatty acids of central myelin have also been found in sciatic nerves (Kishimoto, 1971), suggesting that the hypomyelination may be due to a defect in chain elongation of fatty acids.

Undernutrition and inhibitors of cholesterol biosynthesis also selectively affect Schwann cells and myelination. In the former condition, the Schwann cell mitotic rate, the relationships associated with the initiation of myelination, and axonal growth were normal; the growth of myelin sheath thickness, however, was slower than that found in controls (Clos and Legrand, 1970; Hedley-Whyte and Meuser, 1971). Inhibitors of cholesterol biosynthesis delayed the initiation of myelination in addition to slowing the growth of those cells formed prior to drug administration (Rawlins and Uzman, 1970a, 1970b).

In contrast to the foregoing conditions, neonatal hypothyroidism produces little change in the early development of myelinated fibers (Clos and Legrand, 1970; Reier and Hughes, 1972b). Quantitative data in the latter study, however, showed that the maturation of nonmyelinated fiber bundles was retarded; growth of these unmyelinated axons and the Schwann cells that surrounded them was decreased, slowing the rate of axon bundle subdivision (Reier and Hughes, 1972b). These changes, which could be reversed by thyroid hormone treatment, suggested that Schwann cells might be especially sensitive to hormone deficiency at specific stages in their relationships with axons during the sorting process that precedes myelination.

DEVELOPMENT OF HUMAN NERVE FIBERS

In Vitro Observations

When human embryonic neurons were explanted and maintained in vitro, the formation and motion of growth cones were similar to those already described (Nakai, 1960; Pomerat, 1967). Comparable patterns of process outgrowth, fasciculation, and branching have also been observed. Movements of particles, mitochondria, and pinocytotic vacuoles usually were saltatory and variable in both rate and direction. Recently, with Nomarski optics, axoplasmic flow has also been observed directly in sural nerve biopsy specimens (Kirkpatrick and Stern, 1973). Mitochondria and spherical particles that were identified in electron micrographs as vesicles of agranular reticulum generally moved distally in a series of variable jumps at a velocity of slightly less than 1 μm per second. This rate falls within the range recorded for the fast component of axoplasmic transport.

Human spinal cord, with and without attached dorsal root ganglia, can be explanted from six week embryos; during long-term maintenance, complex bioelectric activity was observed. Although peripheral myelin did not form in these cultures (Peterson et al., 1965), it has been observed and described in cultures of human dorsal root ganglia (Yonezawa, 1965, cited by Peterson et al., 1965).

The formation of neuromuscular junctions in vitro has not been described. During a survey of fetuses nine to sixteen weeks old, however, motor endplates were identified in the tenth week, when muscle fibers were still in the myotube stage (Fidziańska, 1971). It is also of interest that explants of fetal rodent spinal cord will establish functional connections in vitro with adjacent explants of human muscle (Crain et al., 1970).

Nerve Fibers in Nerves — Early Development

The electron microscopic appearance of developing fibers has been studied in brachial plexuses and sciatic, ulnar, radial, sural, and cutaneous nerves removed from fetuses aged 9 to 22 weeks (Cravioto, 1965; Davison et al., 1973; Gamble and Breathnach, 1965; Gamble, 1966; Dunn, 1970; Ochoa, 1971). Transverse sections have been used for almost all observations. Even though the three-dimensional relationships of Schwann cells and axons have not been studied yet, the available data from the nerves just listed indicate that the major developmental events are similar and resemble the patterns found in other mammals. The description here is based on findings in the sural nerve (Ochoa, 1971), since diameters and counts of axons are included and because biopsies of it are often performed after birth.

In nine week fetuses, each of the sural nerve's small fascicles contained large axon bundles surrounded by Schwann cell processes that also segregated a few bigger axons in separate furrows. A basal lamina covered the surfaces of Schwann cell processes. The narrow clefts between processes surrounding the bundles contained collagen but no blood vessels, fibroblasts, or mast cells. The perineurial cells contained glycogen and were observed in mitosis. At 16 weeks, the major changes were a decrease in axon bundle size and an increase in their number. More Schwann cells were present also, and many of their processes participated in subdividing bundles and segregating larger axons. In the histogram, the maximum axon diameter increased to 2.4 μm, a minor peak appeared at 0.7 μm, and the minimum diameter and major peak were unchanged.

Myelination

The onset of myelination was found at age 18 weeks in sural nerves (Ochoa, 1971). Many axons, 1.0 to 3.2 μm in diameter, were in a 1:1 relationship with Schwann cells that had formed mesaxons and small spirals. Compact sheaths with from 3 to 15 layers were observed. The lamellar arrangement was consistent with the presence of longitudinal cytoplasmic strips between layers (Webster, 1971); irregularities in contour were observed also. In the histogram, the major peak shifted to 0.4 μm, the minor peak at 0.7 μm was larger. In agreement with the data of Fraher (1972), there was a rather large overlapping range for diameters of myelinated and unmyelinated axons. The smallest in the former group were 0.9 μm, and the largest of the latter were more than three times as large (3.2 μm). Coincident with the onset of myelination, the amount of perineurial glycogen decreased and both blood vessels and fibroblasts had appeared in the endoneurial compartment. Similar changes in glycogen have been described by others also (Gamble and Eames, 1964; Duckett and Scott, 1972), and it is of interest that insulin secretion increases substantially between 15 and 24 weeks of age, a growth period characterized by rapid cell division (Ashworth et al., 1973).

During postnatal growth, the number of myelinated fibers in the sural nerve increases from 4000 to about 12,000 by age five years (Gutrecht and Dyck, 1970). These investigators found a linear relationship between the total fiber diameter (axon and myelin sheath) and the internodal length. The frequency distribution was unimodel at birth, became bimodel by the seventh month, and reached adult values by five years of age.

Before myelin began forming, the only lipids present in fetal sciatic nerves were phospholipids and cholesterol (Davison et al., 1973). Cerebrosides and sulfatides were first identified during the onset of myelination at 17 to 18 weeks, and a week later, nerve extracts contained lecithin, ethanolamine phospholipid, phosphatidylserine, phosphatidylinositol, and sphingomyelin. The adult type of basic protein was not identified electrophoretically until age 20 weeks, when substantially more axons were surrounded by compact myelin sheaths.

Finally, Rexed's comprehensive histologic survey of postnatal developmental changes in nerve fiber size in the human peripheral nervous system will be of interest to those concerned with the appraisal of pathologic material (Rexed, 1944).

References

Aguayo, A. A., Martin, J. B., and Bray, G. M.: Effects of nerve growth factor antiserum on peripheral unmyelinated nerve fibers. Acta Neuropathol. (Berl.), 20:288, 1972.

Aguayo, A. A., Terry, L. C., and Bray, G. M.: Spontaneous loss of axons in sympathetic unmyelinated nerve fibers of the rat during development. Brain Res., 54:360, 1973.

Angeletti, P. U., Levi-Montalcini, R., and Calissano, P.: The nerve growth factor (NGF): chemical properties and metabolic effects. Adv. Enzymol., 31:51, 1968.

Angeletti, P. U., Levi-Montalcini, R., and Caramia, F.: Ultrastructural changes in sympathetic neurons of newborn and adult mice treated with nerve growth factor. J. Ultrastruct. Res., 36:24, 1971.

Angeletti, R. H.: Immunological relatedness of nerve growth factors. Brain Res., 25:424, 1971.

Asbury, A. K.: Schwann cell proliferation in developing mouse sciatic nerve. J. Cell Biol., 34:735, 1967.

Asbury, A. K.: Peripheral nerves. In Haymaker, W., and Adams, R. D. (eds.): Histology and Histopathology of the Nervous System. Springfield, Ill., Charles C Thomas, 1974.

Ashworth, M. A., Leach, F. N., and Milner, R. D. G.: Development of insulin secretion in the human fetus. Arch. Dis. Child., 48:151, 1973.

Berlinrood, M., McGee-Russell, S. M., and Allen, R. D.: Patterns of particle movement in nerve fibers in vitro—an analysis by photokymography and microscopy. J. Cell Sci., 11:875, 1972.

Billings, S. M.: Concepts of nerve fiber development, 1839–1930. J. Hist. Biol., 4:275, 1971.

Billings-Gagliardi, S. M., Webster, H. deF., and O'Connell, M. F.: In vivo and electron microscopic observations in developing tadpole nerve fibers. Dev. Biol., 1974, in press.

Blood, L. A.: Some quantitative effects of nerve growth factor on dorsal root ganglia of chick embryos in culture. J. Anat., 112:315, 1972.

Bornstein, M. B., Iwanami, H., Lehrer, G. M., and Breitbart, L.: Observations on the appearance of neuromuscular relationships in cultured mouse tissues. Z. Zellforsch. Mikrosk. Anat., 92:197, 1968.

Bray, D.: Branching patterns of individual sympathetic neurons in culture. J. Cell Biol., 56:702, 1973.

Bunge, M. B.: Fine structure of nerve fibers and growth cones of isolated sympathetic neurons in culture. J. Cell Biol., 56:713, 1973.

Bunge, M. B., Bunge, R. P., Peterson, E. R., and Murray, M. R.: A light and electron microscope study of long-term organized cultures of rat dorsal root ganglia. J. Cell Biol., 32:439, 1967.

Cajal, S. R.: Studies on Vertebrate Neurogenesis. (Translated by L. Guth.) Springfield, Ill., Charles C Thomas, 1960.

Causey, G.: The Cell of Schwann. Edinburgh, E. & S. Livingstone, Ltd., 1960.

Clos, J., and Legrand, J.: Influence de la déficience thyroïdienne et de la sousalimentation sur la croissance et la myélinisation des fibres nerveuses du nerf sciatique chez le jeune rat blanc. Étude au microscope électronique. Brain Res., 22:285, 1970.

Cohen, A. M., and Hay, E. D.: Secretion of collagen by embryonic neuroepithelium at the time of spinal cord–somite interaction. Dev. Biol., 26:578, 1971.

Crain, S. M.: Bioelectric interactions between cultured fetal rodent spinal cord and skeletal muscle after innervation in vitro. J. Exp. Zool., 173:353, 1970.

Crain, S. M., Alfei, L., and Peterson, E. R.: Neuromuscular transmission in cultures of adult human and rodent skeletal muscle after innervation in vitro by fetal rodent spinal cord. J. Neurobiol., 1:471, 1970.

Cravioto, H.: The role of Schwann cells in the development of human peripheral nerves. An electron microscopic study. J. Ultrastruct. Res., 12:634, 1965.

Daniels, M. P.: Colchicine inhibition of nerve fiber formation in vitro. J. Cell Biol., *53*:164, 1972.

Daniels, M. P.: Fine structural changes correlated with colchicine inhibition of nerve fiber formation in vitro. J. Cell Biol., *58*:463, 1973.

Davison, A. N.: The biochemistry of the myelin sheath. *In* Davison, A. N., and Peters, A. (eds.): Myelination. Springfield, Ill., Charles C Thomas, 1970.

Davison, A. N., and Peters, A. (eds.): Myelination. Springfield, Ill., Charles C Thomas, 1970.

Davison, A. N., Duckett, S., and Oxberry, J. M.: Correlative morphological and biochemical studies of the human fetal sciatic nerve. Brain Res., *57*:327, 1973.

Diamond, J., and Miledi, R.: A study of foetal and new-born rat muscle fibres. J. Physiol., *162*:393, 1962.

Douarin, N.: A biological labelling technique and its use in experimental embryology. Dev. Biol., *30*:217, 1973.

Drachman, D. B.,: Trophic functions of the neuron. Ann. N.Y. Acad. Sci., *228*:160–176, 1974.

Duckett, S., and Scott, T.: Glycogen in human fetal sciatic nerve. Rev. Can. Biol., *31*:147, 1972.

Duncan, D.: A relation between axone diameter and myelination determined by measurement of myelinated spinal root fibers. J. Comp. Neurol., *60*:437, 1934.

Dunn, G. A.: Mutual contact inhibition of extension of chick sensory nerve fibres in vitro. J. Comp. Neurol., *143*:491, 1971.

Dunn, J. S.: Developing myelin in human peripheral nerve. Scot. Med. J., *15*:108, 1970.

Fidziańska, A.: Electron microscopic study of the development of human foetal muscle, motor end-plate and nerve. Acta Neuropathol. (Berl.), *17*:234, 1971.

Filogamo, G.: Some factors that regulate neuronal growth and differentiation, in Cellular Dynamics of the Neuron (S. H. Barondes, ed.), New York and London, Academic Press, 1969.

Fine, R. E., and Bray, D.: Actin in growing nerve cells. Nature, *234*:115, 1971.

Fischbach, G.: Synaptic potentials recorded in cell cultures of nerves and muscle. Science, *169*:1331, 1970.

Fraher, J. P.: A quantitative study of anterior root fibres during early myelination. J. Anat., *112*:99, 1972.

Frazier, W. A., Angeletti, R. H., and Bradshaw, R. A.: Nerve growth factor and insulin structural similarities indicate an evolutionary relationship reflected by physiological action. Science, *176*:482, 1972.

Friede, R. L.: Control of myelin formation by axon caliber (with a model of the control mechanism). J. Comp. Neurol., *144*:233, 1972.

Friede, R. L., and Martinez, A. J.: Analysis of the process of sheath expansion in swollen nerve fibers. Brain Res., *19*:165, 1970.

Friede, R. L., and Miyagishi, T.: Adjustment of the myelin sheath to changes in axon caliber. Anat. Rec., *172*:1, 1972.

Friede, R. L., and Samorajski, T.: Relation between the number of myelin lamellae and axon circumference in fibers of vagus and sciatic nerves of mice. J. Comp. Neurol., *130*:223, 1967.

Friede, R. L., and Samorajski, T.: Myelin formation in the sciatic nerve of the rat. J. Neuropathol. Exp. Neurol., *27*:546, 1968.

Friede, R. L., and Samorajski, T.: The clefts of Schmidt-Lantermann: a quantitative electron microscopic study of their structure in developing and adult sciatic nerves of the rat. Anat. Rec., *165*:89, 1969.

Friede, R. L., and Samorajski, T.: Axon caliber related to neurofilaments and microtubules in sciatic nerve fibers of rats and mice. Anat. Rec., *167*:379, 1970.

Gamble, H. J.: Further electron microscope studies of human fetal peripheral nerves. J. Anat., *100*:487, 1966.

Gamble, H. J., and Breathnach, A. S.: An electron-microscope study of human foetal peripheral nerves. J. Anat., *99*:573, 1965.

Gamble, H. J., and Eames, R. A.: An electron microscope study of the connective tissues of human peripheral nerves. J. Anat., *98*:655, 1964.

Geren, B. B.: The formation from the Schwann cell surface of myelin in the peripheral nerves of chick embryos. Exp. Cell Res., 7:558, 1954.

Geren, B. B.: Structural studies of the formation of myelin sheath in peripheral nerve fibers. *In* Rudnick, D. (ed.): Cellular Mechanisms in Differentiation and Growth. Princeton, N.J., Princeton University Press, 1956.

Goldschneider, I., and Moscona, A. A.: Tissue-specific cell surface antigens in embryonic cells. J. Cell Biol., *53*:435, 1972.

Guth, L.: "Trophic" effects of vertebrate neurons. Neurosci. Res. Prog. Bull., *7*:1, 1969.

Gutrecht, J. A., and Dyck, P. J.: Quantitative teased fiber and histologic studies of human sural nerve during postnatal development. J. Comp. Neurol., *138*:117, 1970.

Harrison, R. G.: Neuroblast versus sheath cell in the development of peripheral nerves. J. Comp. Neurol., *37*:123, 1924.

Harrison, R. G.: On the origin and development of the nervous system studied by the methods of experimental embryology. Proc. R. Soc. Lond. [Biol.], *118*:155, 1935.

Hedley-Whyte, E. T., and Meuser, C. S.: The effect of undernutrition on myelination of rat sciatic nerve. Lab. Invest., *24*:156, 1971.

Hedley-Whyte, E. T., Rawlins, F. A., Salpeter, M. M., and Uzman, B. G.: Distribution of cholesterol-1, 2-H^3 during maturation of mouse peripheral nerve. Lab. Invest., *21*:536, 1969.

Hendelman, W. J., and Bunge, R. P.: Radioautographic studies of choline incorporation into peripheral nerve myelin. J. Cell Biol., *40*:190, 1969.

Herschkowitz, N., Vassella, F., and Bischoff, A.: Myelin differences in the central and peripheral nervous system in the Jimpy mouse. J. Neurochem., *18*:1361, 1971.

Hier, D. B., Arnason, B. G. W., and Young, M.: Studies on the mechanism of action of nerve growth factor. Proc. Natl. Acad. Sci., U.S.A., *69*:2268, 1972.

Himwich, W. (ed.): Developmental Neurobiology. Springfield, Ill., Charles C Thomas, 1969.

Hughes, A. F. W.: Aspects of Neural Ontogeny. London, Logos Press, Ltd., 1968.

Jacobson, M.: Developmental Neurobiology. New York, Holt, Rinehart & Winston, 1970.

Johnston, M. C.: A radioautographic study of the migration and fate of cranial neural crest cells in the chick embryo. Anat. Rec., *156*:143, 1966.

Johnston, M. C., Bhakdinaronk, A., and Reid, Y. C.: An expanded role of the neural crest in oral and pharyngeal development. *In* Bosma, J. F. (ed.): Oral Sensation and Perception—Development in the Fetus and Infant. Washington, D.C., U.S. Government Printing Office, 1974.

Kelly, A. M., and Zacks, S. I.: The fine structure of motor endplate morphogenesis. J. Cell Biol., *42*:154, 1969.

Kirkpatrick, J. B., and Stern, L. Z.: Axoplasmic flow in human sural nerve. Arch. Neurol., 28:308, 1973.

Kishimoto, Y.: Abnormality in sphingolipid fatty acids from sciatic nerve and brain of quaking mice. J. Neurochem., 18:1365, 1971.

Kollros, J. J.: Order and control of neurogenesis (as exemplified by the lateral motor column). Dev. Biol., Suppl. 2:274, 1968.

Kristensson, K.: Transport of fluorescent protein tracer in peripheral nerves. Acta Neuropathol. (Berl.), 16:293, 1970.

Landon, D. N.: The fine structure of the equatorial regions of developing muscle spindles in the rat. J. Neurocytol., 1:189, 1972.

Lasek, R. J.: Axonal transport of proteins in dorsal root ganglion cells of the growing cat: a comparison of growing and mature neurons. Brain Res., 20:121, 1970.

Levi-Montalcini, R.: The nerve growth factor: its mode of action on sensory and sympathetic nerve cells. Harvey Lect., 60:217, 1966.

Levi-Montalcini, R., and Angeletti, P. U.: Nerve growth factor. Physiol. Rev., 48:534, 1968.

Luduena, M. A., and Wessells, N. K.: Cell locomotion, nerve elongation and microfilaments. Dev. Biol., 30:427, 1973.

Martin, J. R., and Webster, H. deF.: Mitotic Schwann cells in developing nerve: their changes in shape, fine structure and axon relationships. Dev. Biol., 32:417, 1973.

Matthews, M. A.: An electron microscopic study of the relationship between axon diameter and the initiation of myelin production in the peripheral nervous system. Anat. Rec., 161:337, 1968.

Meier, H., and MacPike, A. D.: Myelin hypoplasia including peripheral neuropathy caused by three mutations of the mouse. Exp. Neurol., 37:643, 1972.

Metz, G. E., Judice, R. C., and Finerty, J. C.: Occurrence of neurons in the sciatic nerves of albino rats. Anat. Rec., 130:197, 1958.

Mokrasch, L. C., Bear, R. S., and Schmitt, F. O.: Myelin: a report based on an NRP work session. Neurosci. Res. Prog. Bull., 9:443, 1971.

Murray, M. R.: Nervous tissue in vitro. In Cells and Tissues in Culture. Vol. 2. London, Academic Press, 1965.

Nakai, J.: Dissociated dorsal root ganglia in tissue culture. Am. J. Anat., 99:81, 1956.

Nakai, J.: Studies on the mechanism determining the course of nerve fibers in tissue culture. II. The mechanism of fasciculation. Z. Zellforsch. Mikrosk. Anat., 52:427, 1960.

Nakai, J., and Kawasaki, Y.: Studies on the mechanism determining the course of nerve fibers in tissue culture. I. The reaction of the growth cone to various obstructions. Z. Zellforsch. Mikrosk. Anat., 51:108, 1959.

New, D. A. T., and Mizell, M.: Opossum fetuses grown in culture. Science, 175:533, 1972.

Noden, D. M.: An analysis of the migratory behavior of avian cephalic neural crest cells. Dev. Biol., 42:106, 1975.

Nornes, H. O., and Das, G. D.: Temporal pattern of neurogenesis in spinal cord: cytoarchitecture and directed growth of axons. Proc. Natl. Acad. Sci. U.S.A., 69:1962, 1972.

Ochoa, J.: The sural nerve of the human foetus: electron microscope observations and counts of axons. J. Anat., 108:231, 1971.

Okun, L. M.: Isolated dorsal root ganglion neurons in culture: cytological maturation and extension of electrically active processes. J. Neurobiol., 3:111, 1972.

Palay, S. L., Sotelo, C., Peters, A., and Orkand, P. M.: The axon hillock and the initial segment. J. Cell Biol., 38:193, 1968.

Pappas, G. D., and Waxman, S. G.: Synaptic fine structure: morphological correlates of chemical and electrotonic transmission. In Pappas, G. D., and Purpura, D. P. (eds.):Structure and Function of Synapses. New York, Raven Press, 1972.

Partlow, L. M., and Larabee, M. G.: Effects of a nerve growth factor, embryo age and metabolic inhibitors on growth of fibres and on synthesis of ribonucleic acid and protein in sympathetic ganglia. J. Neurochem., 18:2101, 1971.

Peters, A.: The development of peripheral nerves in Xenopus Laevis. In Electron Microscopy in Anatomy. London, Edward Arnold, 1961.

Peters, A., and Muir, A. R.: The relationship between axons and Schwann cells during development of peripheral nerves in the rat. Q. J. Exp. Physiol., 64:117, 1959.

Peters, A., and Vaughn, J. E.: Morphology and development of the myelin sheath. In Davison, A. N., and Peters, A. (eds.): Myelination. Springfield, Ill., Charles C Thomas, 1970.

Peters, A., Palay, S. L., and Webster, H. deF.: The Fine Structure of the Nervous System. The Cells and Their Processes. New York, Harper & Row, 1970.

Peterson, E. R., and Murray, M. R.: Myelin sheath formation in cultures of avian spinal ganglia. Am. J. Anat., 96:319, 1955.

Peterson, E. R., Crain, S. M., and Murray, M. R.: Differentiation and prolonged maintenance of bioelectrically active spinal cord cultures (rat, chick, human). Z. Zellforsch. Mikrosk. Anat., 66:130, 1965.

Pleasure, D. E., and Prockop, D. J.: Myelin synthesis in peripheral nerve in vitro: sulfatide synthesis requires a transport lipoprotein. J. Neurochem., 19:283, 1972.

Pomerat, C. M., Hendelman, W. J., Raiborn, C. W., and Massay, J. F.: Dynamic activities of nervous tissue in vitro. In Hyden, H. (ed.): The Neuron. Amsterdam, Elsevier, 1967.

Prestige, M. C., and Wilson, M. A.: Loss of axons from ventral roots during development. Brain Res., 41:467, 1972.

Quarles, R. H., Everly, J. L., and Brady, R. O.: Demonstration of a glycoprotein which is associated with a purified myelin fraction from rat brain. Biochem. Biophys. Res. Commun., 47:491, 1972.

Ranvier, M. L.: Leçons sur Histologie du Système Nerveux. Paris, F. Savy, 1878.

Rawlins, F. A., and Uzman, B. G.: Effect of AY-9944, a cholesterol biosynthesis inhibitor on peripheral nerve myelination. Lab. Invest., 23:184, 1970a.

Rawlins, F. A., and Uzman, B. G.: Retardation of peripheral nerve myelination in mice treated with inhibitors of cholesterol biosynthesis. A quantitative electron microscopic study. J. Cell Biol., 46:505, 1970b.

Reier, P. J., and Hughes, A.: Evidence for spontaneous axon degeneration during peripheral nerve maturation. Am. J. Anat., 135:147, 1972a.

Reier, P. J., and Hughes, A. F.: An effect of neonatal radiothyroidectomy upon nonmyelinated axons and associated Schwann cells during maturation of the mouse sciatic nerve. Brain Res., 41:263, 1972b.

Rexed, B.: Contributions to the knowledge of the postnatal development of the peripheral nervous system in man. Acta Psychiatr. Neurol., Suppl. *33*:1, 1944.

Robbins, N., and Yonezawa, T.: Developing neuromuscular junctions: first signs of chemical transmission during formation in tissue culture. Science, *172*:395, 1971.

Robertson, J. D.: The unit membrane of cells and mechanisms of myelin formation. *In* Korey, S. R., Pope, A., and Robins, E. (eds.): Ultrastructure and Metabolism of the Nervous System. Proc. Ass. Res. Nerv. Ment. Dis., Vol. 40. Baltimore, The Williams & Wilkins Co., 1962.

Roisen, F. J., Murphy, R. A., and Braden, W. G.: Neurite development in vitro. I. The effects of adenosine 3'5'-cyclic monophosphate (cyclic AMP). J. Neurobiol., *4*:347, 1972a.

Roisen, F. J., Murphy, R. A., and Braden, W. G.: Dibutyryl cyclic adenosine monophosphate stimulation of colcemid-inhibited axonal elongation. Science, *177*:809, 1972b.

Rosenbluth, J.: Redundant myelin sheaths and other ultrastructural features of the toad cerebellum. J. Cell Biol., *28*:73, 1966.

Samorajski, T., Friede, R. L., and Reimer, P. R.: Hypomyelination in the quaking mouse. J. Neuropathol. Exp. Neurol., *29*:507, 1970.

Schlaepfer, W. W., and Myers, F. K.: Relationship of myelin internode elongation and growth in the rat sural nerve. J. Comp. Neurol., *147*:255, 1973.

Schmitt, F. O. (ed.): The Neurosciences, Second Study Program. New York, Rockefeller University Press, 1970.

Schwann, T.: Microscopical Researches into the Accordance in the Structure and Growth of Animals and Plants. Translated by Henry Smith. London, Sydenham Society, 1847.

Sjostrand, F. S.: The structure and formation of the myelin sheath. *In* Rose, A. S., and Pearson, C. M. (eds.): Mechanisms of Demyelination. New York, McGraw-Hill Book Co., 1963.

Speidel, C. C.: Studies of living nerves. I. The movements of individual sheath cells and nerve sprouts correlated with the process of myelin-sheath formation in amphibian larvae. J. Exp. Zool., *61*:279, 1932.

Speidel, C. C.: In vivo studies of myelinated nerve fibers. Int. Rev. Cytol., *16*:173, 1964.

Spooner, B. S., Yamada, K. M., and Wessells, N. K.: Microfilaments and cell locomotion. J. Cell Biol., *49*:595, 1971.

Straus, W. L., and Weddell, G.: Nature of the first visible contractions of the forelimb musculature in rat fetuses. J. Neurophysiol., *3*:358, 1940.

Taylor, A. C.: Development of the innervation pattern in the limb bud of the frog. Anat. Rec., *87*:379, 1943.

Teichberg, S., and Holtzman, E.: Axonal agranular reticulum and synaptic vesicles in cultured embryonic chick sympathetic neurons. J. Cell Biol., *57*:88, 1973.

Tennyson, V. M.: The fine structure of the axon and growth cone of the dorsal root neuroblast of the rabbit embryo. J. Cell Biol., *44*:62, 1970.

Thomas, P. K.: Growth changes in the myelin sheath of peripheral nerve fibers in fishes. Proc. R. Soc. [Biol.], *143*:380, 1955.

Uzman, B. G., and Hedley-Whyte, E. T.: Myelin: dynamic or stable? J. Gen. Physiol., *51*:85, 1968.

Vizoso, A. D., and Young, J. Z.: Internode length and fibre diameter in developing and regenerating nerves. J. Anat., *82*:110, 1948.

Waxman, S. G.: Micropinocytotic invaginations in the axolemma of peripheral nerves. Z. Zellforsch. Mikrosk. Anat., *86*:571, 1968.

Webster, H. deF.: Some ultrastructural features of segmental demyelination and myelin regeneration in peripheral nerve. Progr. Brain Res., *13*:151, 1964.

Webster, H. deF.: The geometry of peripheral myelin sheaths during their formation and growth in rat sciatic nerves. J. Cell Biol., *48*:348, 1971.

Webster, H. deF.: Peripheral nerve structure. *In* Hubbard, J. I. (ed.): The Vertebrate Peripheral Nervous System. New York, Plenum Press, 1974.

Webster, H. deF., and Billings, S. M.: Myelinated nerve fibers in *Xenopus* tadpoles; in vivo observations and fine structure. J. Neuropathol. Exp. Neurol., *31*:102, 1972.

Webster, H. deF., and Spiro, D.: Phase and electron microscopic studies of experimental demyelination. I. Variations in myelin sheath contour in normal guinea pig sciatic nerve. J. Neuropathol. Exp. Neurol., *19*:42, 1960.

Webster, H. deF., Martin, J. R., and O'Connell, M. F.: The relationships between interphase Schwann cells and axons before myelination: a quantitative electron microscopic study. Dev. Biol., *32*:401, 1973.

Wessells, N. K., Spooner, B. S., Ash, J. F., Bradley, M. R., Luduena, M. A., Taylor, E. L., Wrenn, J. T., and Yamada, K. M.: Microfilaments in cellular and developmental processes. Science, *171*:135, 1971.

Williams, P. L., and Wendell-Smith, C. P.: Some additional parametric variations between peripheral nerve fibre populations. J. Anat., *109*:505, 1971.

Wolstenholme, G. E. W., and O'Connor, M.: Growth of the Nervous System. Boston, Little, Brown & Co., 1968.

Yamada, K. M., and Wessells, N. K.: Axon elongation. Effect of nerve growth factor on microtubule protein. Exp. Cell Res., *66*:346, 1971.

Yamada, K. M., Spooner, B. S., and Wessells, N. K.: Axon growth: roles of microfilaments and microtubules. Proc. Natl. Acad. Sci. U.S.A., *66*:1206, 1970.

Yamada, K. M., Spooner, B. S., and Wessells, N. K.: Ultrastructure and function of growth cones and axons of cultured nerve cells. J. Cell Biol., *49*:614, 1971.

Chapter 4

MICROSCOPIC ANATOMY OF THE SPINAL CORD

Henry J. Ralston, III

The motor neurons of the spinal cord and the neurons of the adjacent spinal ganglia are the sources of nerve fibers innervating the somatic periphery. This chapter deals with the organization of the mammalian spinal cord, the termination of afferent fibers within the cord, and, briefly, with some of the methods used for analyzing the neuronal organization within the cord.

The adult spinal cord retains the basic organization that appeared in the nervous system during development. The cells lining the small central canal were once the site of neuronal proliferation during the histogenesis of spinal neurons. The surrounding gray matter, roughly in an H-shaped configuration, is the locus of the nerve cell bodies of the adult cord. External to the gray matter is the white substance of the spinal cord, which carries both long fiber systems and propriospinal fiber systems interconnecting adjacent segments of the cord. The spinal gray matter can be readily subdivided into dorsal and ventral horns. The dorsal horns are primarily associated with sensory systems in that they receive the majority of incoming afferent fibers from the periphery and give rise to many of the ascending sensory systems.

The ventral horns are the locus of motor neurons innervating extrafusal muscle fibers, the alpha motor neurons, and the fibers of muscle spindles, the gamma motor neurons. At thoracic levels there is an accumulation of motor neurons that are clustered into a lateral horn and give rise to preganglionic fibers of the sympathetic component of the autonomic nervous system.

We tend to view different sectors of the cord as being largely the recipients of various long fiber systems, whether they are from the periphery or from higher centers of the brain. It is, however, becoming increasingly evident that the vast majority of information processing in the spinal cord occurs locally within each spinal segment. The vast majority of synaptic interconnections between spinal neurons arise from neurons in the immediate vicinity, and the major fiber systems contribute but a small percentage of the total synaptic population of the cord.

THE DORSAL HORN

The neurons of the dorsal horn are arranged into horizontal laminae that are

Figure 4–1 *A.* Nissl-stained section of cells of the upper dorsal horn of the cat. The cellular laminae of Rexed (1952) are indicated by Roman numerals I to V. Lamina II is the substantia gelatinosa. Some of the cells of lamina I have been shown to send axons into the spinothalamic tract, as have lamina IV cells. × 120. *B.* Laminae I, II, and III of the upper dorsal horn of the squirrel monkey spinal cord five days following dorsal root section. Degenerating dorsal root axons (arrows), stained by the Nauta method, are shown coursing across lamina I, descending in cascades through II (substantia gelatinosa), and distributed in large numbers in III. × 300.

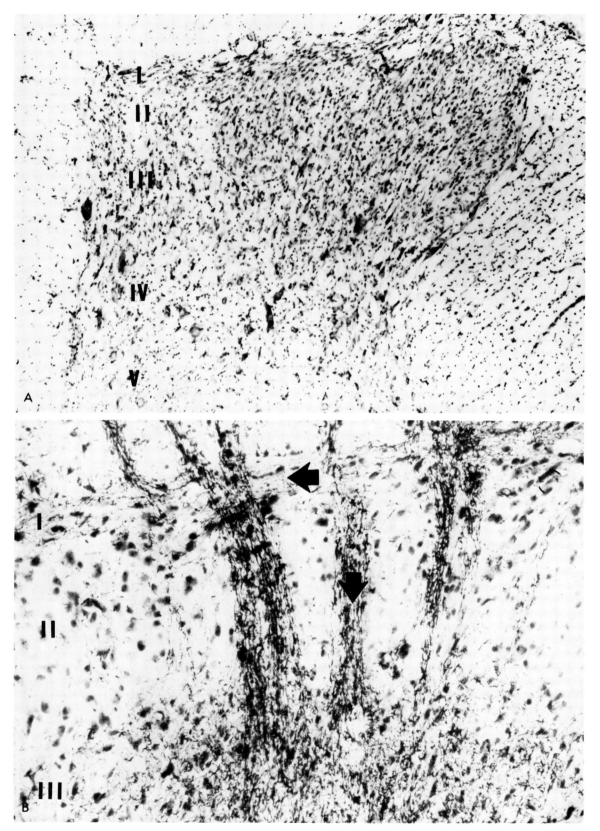

Figure 4–1 *See opposite page for legend.*

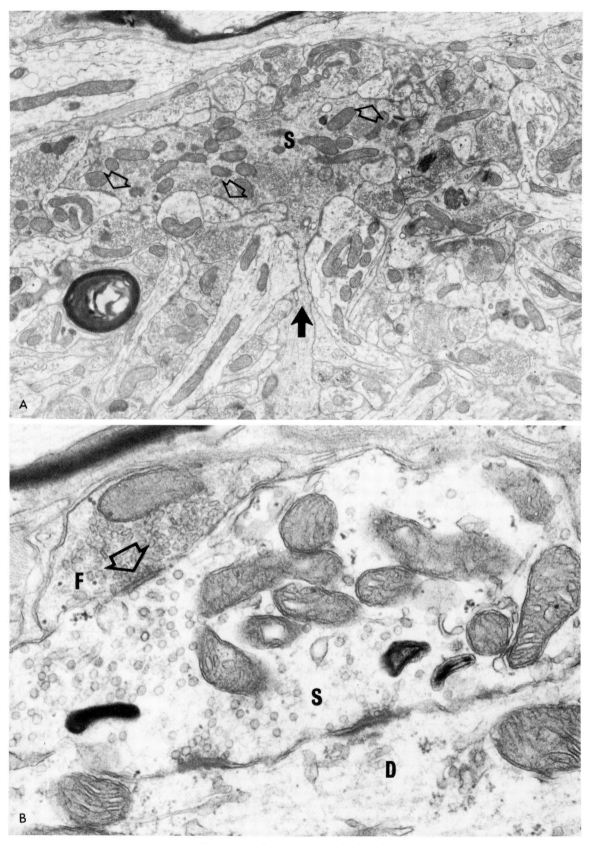

Figure 4–2 *See opposite page for legend.*

parallel to the dorsal surface of the spinal cord. This laminar arrangement was first noted in the cat by Rexed (1952) and has been noted by many investigators in the cord of primates, including man, since that time (Fig. 4–1*A*). There are six cellular laminae of the dorsal horn, which are numbered sequentially from the dorsalmost part of the horn to approximately the level of the central canal. Lamina I, the uppermost cellular lamina of the cord, is also called the marginal cell layer. Lamina II is best known as the substantia gelatinosa because of its rather clear appearance on freshly cut spinal cord, owing to the numerous small neurons that it contains and the small number of large nerve fibers. Lamina III, immediately below the substantia gelatinosa, also contains many small nerve cells but also exhibits many more nerve fibers. These upper three laminae of the cord, especially laminae I and III, receive a major input from the dorsal roots. Some of the cells of lamina I contribute to the ascending spinothalamic tract (Christensen and Perl, 1970). There is no direct evidence at the present time that the spinothalamic tract arises from neurons of lamina II (the substantia gelatinosa) or lamina III. Laminae IV, V, and VI constitute the bulk of the dorsal horn and contain many large neurons, up to 45 μm in diameter, interspersed with medium-sized to small neurons. These laminae also receive many incoming dorsal root fiber projections. It is likely that several of the neurons of the deeper layers of the dorsal horn contribute their axons to the contralateral spinothalamic tract (Dilly et al., 1968; Trevino et al., 1972).

Another major locus of dorsal root termination within the cord is the large neurons of Clarke's column, which are located at the medial base of the dorsal horn in the thoracic and upper lumbar segments of the spinal cord. Clarke's column neurons are among the largest of the spinal cord and receive input both from muscle spindles and from other cutaneous and deep afferent sources. The Clarke's column neurons in turn give rise to the ipsilateral dorsal spinal cerebellar tract, which is an important system involved with the coordination of movement by the cerebellum.

The electron microscope has yielded a great amount of information about the spinal cord, as it has about so many other areas of the brain. Different regions of the cord can be distinguished under the electron microscope because of certain characteristics of synaptic structures found within the laminae of the dorsal horn. For instance, laminae I, II, and III are characterized by innumerable bundles of nonmyelinated axons, many less than 0.1 μm in diameter, which arborize extensively throughout these laminae and give rise to synaptic contacts upon dorsal horn neurons (Fig. 4–2*A*) (Ralston, 1968a). Following section of dorsal roots proximal to the dorsal root ganglia, one can demonstrate those axons within the cord that are derived from dorsal roots as they undergo degeneration (cf. Fig. 4–6) (Ralston, 1968b). It can be shown by degeneration methods that many of the small nonmyelinated axons of the upper dorsal horn are derived from peripheral nerve fibers that enter the cord via the dorsal roots. These fine fibers bring information about painful stimuli, other types of mechanical stimuli such as movement of hairs, touch or pressure upon the skin, and thermal stimuli as well (Iggo, 1960; Hensel et al., 1960). Information conveyed by fine fiber systems is ultimately transferred to higher brain centers by the spinothalamic tract (Bishop, 1959).

The large fibers of the dorsal roots arborize extensively throughout the spinal gray, especially in the deeper levels of the dorsal horn and upon interneurons and motor neurons of the ventral horn (Figs. 4–2*B* and 4–3*A*). Many of the larger dorsal root fibers ascend the dorsal columns upon entering the spinal cord and project to the dorsal column nuclei, carrying information about well-localized mechanical stimuli to the skin and deep tissues as well as information concerning positions of the joints. Large dorsal root fibers also project to Clarke's column cells to relay muscle and cutaneous information to the cerebellum.

It was previously thought that afferent information concerning painful stimuli was relayed in the substantia gelatinosa and that the substantia gelatinosa neurons in turn sent their axons to the opposite side of the spinal cord to give rise to the spinothalamic tract.

Figure 4–2 *A.* Electron micrograph of lamina II of the cat dorsal horn. A stem axon (dark arrow) widens to form a large synaptic terminal (S), which makes many synaptic contacts with other profiles (open arrows). × 15,000. *B.* Cat dorsal horn, lamina V. A large synaptic terminal (S) makes contact with a dendrite (D). An adjacent synaptic terminal (F) in turn contacts S (arrow) and may thus modify the latter's activity. × 60,000.

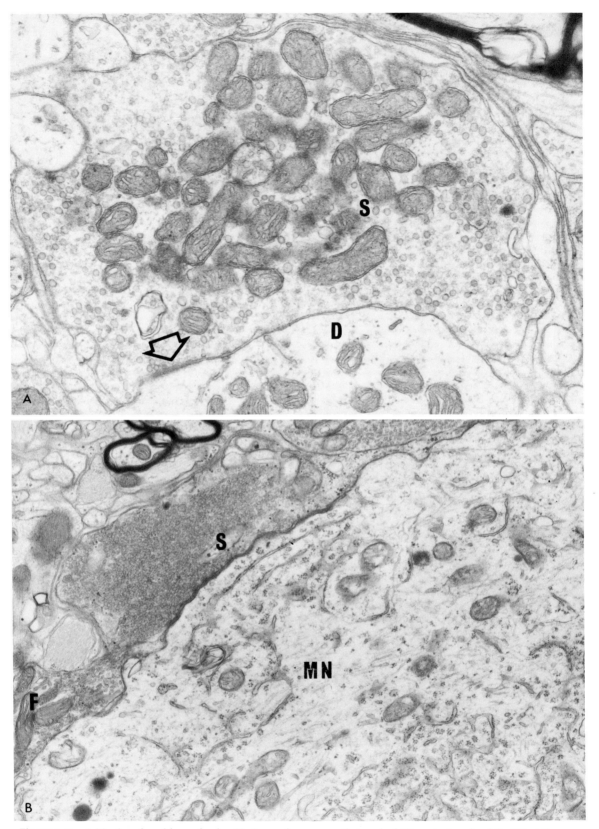

Figure 4–3 *A.* Monkey dorsal horn, lamina V. A very large synaptic terminal (S) contacts a dendrite (D) at the arrow. It can be shown that this type of synapse undergoes degeneration following dorsal root section. × 50,000. *B.* Cat ventral horn. Two different synaptic profiles (S and F) are in contact with a motor neuron (MN). There is a total of seven morphologically distinct types of synapse that contact motor neurons. × 20,000.

66

This view of the central pain pathway is now no longer tenable. It has been found, by means of antidromic invasions of cells of the spinal cord following stimulation of axons of the spinothalamic tract, that many neurons giving rise to the spinothalamic tract are located deep in the dorsal horn or even in the ventral horn (Trevino et al., 1972). There is now much evidence to suggest that several synapses may be intercalated between the incoming dorsal root fibers and the neurons that form the spinothalamic tract. A multi-synaptic system lends itself to modification of afferent information by local neuronal circuits. For instance, it is apparent that the central nervous system has mechanisms for monitoring afferent information and either focusing attention upon or dampening the information by a variety of synaptic inhibitory mechanisms (Andersen et al., 1964). The inhibition of sensory information within the spinal cord may play a role in the ability of individuals to undergo very painful procedures without being debilitated by the pain, such as in the use of acupuncture in place of surgical anesthesia. Attempts are now being made to analyze experimentally the local circuits within the spinal cord with both physiologic and anatomical means in order to better understand how the transfer of sensory information may be modified once it reaches the central nervous system.

THE VENTRAL HORN

The characteristic cell type of the ventral horn is the spinal motor neuron, the axon of which exits via the ventral roots and ultimately supplies skeletal muscle of the periphery. The motor neurons are subdivided into two major classes: the larger supplying extrafusal muscle fibers (alpha motor neurons) and the smaller supplying intrafusal muscle fibers (gamma motor neurons). The location of alpha motor neurons within the spinal gray has been mapped out by several investigators using retrograde chromatolysis to identify neurons supplying particular muscles after crushing the motor nerves to those muscles. Gamma motor neurons have been much more difficult to identify, as these smaller cells do not exhibit chromotolysis in the adult animal following injury to a muscle nerve. Recently, Bryan, Trevino, and Willis (1972) have been able to inject gamma motor neurons with a fluorescent dye (procion yellow) following electrophysiologic identification of these cells and found that the gamma motor neurons are scattered among the larger alpha motor neurons.

Alpha motor neurons are very large cells with dendrites that frequently extend 1 to 3 mm away from the cell body, both in a rostral-caudal direction within the ventral horn and in a transverse plane extending up into the base of the dorsal horn. The vast majority of input to motor neurons is upon their dendritic tree, and estimates of the total number of synapses impinging upon one cell range up to 10,000. When the ventral horn is viewed with the electron microscope the extraordinary feature is the wide morphologic diversity of synapses ending upon motor neurons (Fig. 4–3B) (McLaughlin, 1972a). These synapses range in size from less than 1 μm up to 7 or 8 μm and appear to be derived from many different sources. A surprising finding in two recent studies is that direct dorsal root projections to spinal motor neurons, which mediate monosynaptic reflexes such as the knee jerk, constitute less than 1 per cent of the total number of synapses upon motor neurons (Conradi, 1969; McLaughlin, 1972b). When the spinal cord is transected, thus interrupting all descending projections to motor neurons, one finds that the vast majority of synapses upon these cells survive the transection (McLaughlin, 1972c). Thus it appears that synaptic inputs to motor neurons are derived primarily from neurons in the immediate vicinity: that is, within the segment in which the particular neuron is located. There is, therefore, much information processing at the local level of the spinal cord, which then can be influenced by major afferent sensory pathways or descending pathways from higher centers that impinge upon motor neurons.

When viewed under the electron microscope, normal spinal neurons are seen to have an extensive perinuclear cytoplasm containing stacks of granular endoplasmic reticulum (the Nissl bodies of light microscopy), numerous mitochondria, microtubules, and neurofilaments (Fig. 4–4). When the axons of motor neurons are damaged following section of the ventral roots, chromatolysis of the motor neurons develops between 6 and 10 days following the injury in the cat. The lysis of Nissl bodies viewed by light microscopy is

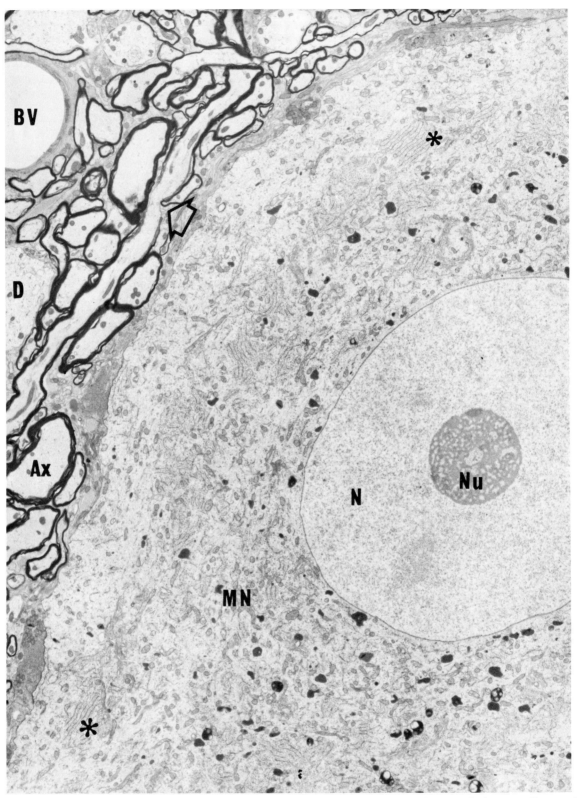

Figure 4–4 A cat spinal motor neuron (MN), which contains a nucleus (N) and a prominent nucleolus (Nu). Clusters of granular endoplasmic reticulum (*) correspond to the "Nissl bodies" of light microscopy. Nearby there are myelinated axons (Ax), one of which reveals a node of Ranvier (arrow). A blood vessel (BV) and several dendrites (D) are also present. × 4,000.

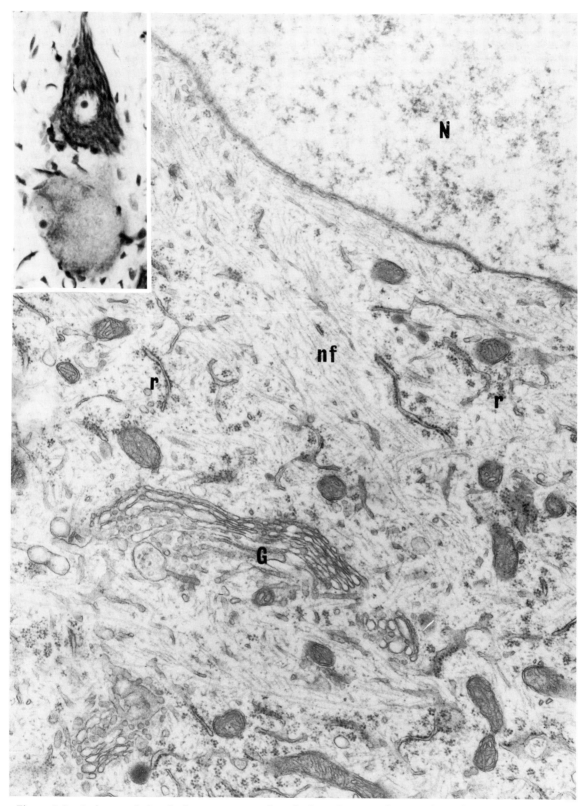

Figure 4–5 A chromatolytic spinal motor neuron of cat six days after ventral root section. There is a marked increase in neurofilaments (nf), and a loss of the membraneous elements of the granular endoplasmic reticulum. Most ribosomes (r) are not membrane bound. The nucleus (N) is eccentric. There are many prominent elements of the Golgi apparatus (G). The inset shows, by light microscopy, a chromatolytic cell and a normal cell from the same specimen. × 25,000.

manifested under the electron microscope by loss of the membranous elements of the endoplasmic reticulum and scattering of ribosomes into randomly distributed polysomes or single ribosomes throughout the cytoplasm. There is also a marked increase in the number of neurofilaments within the cytoplasm of the chromatolytic motor neuron (Fig. 4–5). These neuronal changes following axonal injury are somewhat similar to those that Bodian (1964) has described in motor neurons subsequent to poliovirus infection in the monkey, except that infected neurons undergoing chromatolysis exhibit vacuolation and an increase in free ribosomes.

ANALYSIS OF NEURONAL ORGANIZATION IN THE SPINAL CORD

The analysis of neuronal organization is based first on the demonstration of the normal form and structure of the spinal cord. This can be done by a variety of traditional methods such as cellular staining by Nissl dye techniques that demonstrate the sizes and distribution of the constituent neurons of the cord. Golgi techniques may be used to examine neurons in order to demonstrate the dendritic organization and the axonal distributions about neurons. Neurofibrillar methods are of value in revealing sizes and distributions of the axons of the cord and the character of boutons ending upon spinal neurons. The electron microscope may be used to reveal the fine details of neuronal organelles and the character of synaptic populations found in various regions of the cord.

Because of the great complexity of neuronal circuitry within the spinal cord, experimental analysis of the origins and terminations of particular fiber systems originating or terminating within the cord must be used. Wallerian degeneration subsequent to a lesion in a particular fiber pathway such as the dorsal root may be studied in order to analyze the distribution of a given fiber system. Under the light microscope, modern techniques such

as the Nauta or Fink-Heimer methods allow one to stain degenerating axoplasm selectively, and the resultant axonal degeneration products stand out clearly in a relatively unstained background. This permits the investigator to analyze the precise fields of termination of particular pathways. Wallerian degeneration methods may also be used with the electron microscope, as degenerating synapses appear significantly different from their normal neighbors (Fig. 4–6B). This allows a very detailed analysis of synaptic input to a neuronal system and a subsequent comparison with electrophysiologic studies so that we may better understand the neuronal substrates of functional mechanisms within the spinal cord.

Recently developed techniques may also be used to trace connections between neuronal systems. These techniques make use of the fact that materials are transported within the axon. In one case one may present labeled amino acids—for instance, tritiated leucine or proline—to neurons by injecting the radioactive amino acid into the area of clusters of nerve cell bodies. This labeled amino acid is taken up by nerve cell bodies, incorporated into protein, and transported out the axon to the terminal branches of the axon ending upon other nerve cells (Cowan et al., 1972). The labeled protein is then identified by autoradiographic methods. This technique has the advantage over wallerian degeneration methods in that amino acids apparently are not transported by axons passing through a given region into which the labeled amino acids are injected. Thus one may inject amino acids into a particular region of the nervous system, and they will be incorporated and transported only by neurons in that vicinity and not transported by axons arising from neurons elsewhere that happen to be passing through that region of the brain. Another use of axonal transport mechanisms involves the retrograde transport of horseradish peroxidase from axonal terminations back to the cell bodies of origin of the axons. For instance, it has been shown that horseradish peroxidase injected into striated muscle will be incorporated into the nerve ending

Figure 4–6 *A*. A degenerating axon (dAx) and a normal axon (Ax) in the ventral horn of a cat four days after dorsal root section. In the degenerating axon, several mitochondria are visible in the dense axoplasm. × 25,000. *B*. A degenerating synapse (dS) in lamina I of cat dorsal horn five days after dorsal root section. The synapse contacts other profiles (arrows), one of which contains synaptic vesicles (sv). × 40,000.

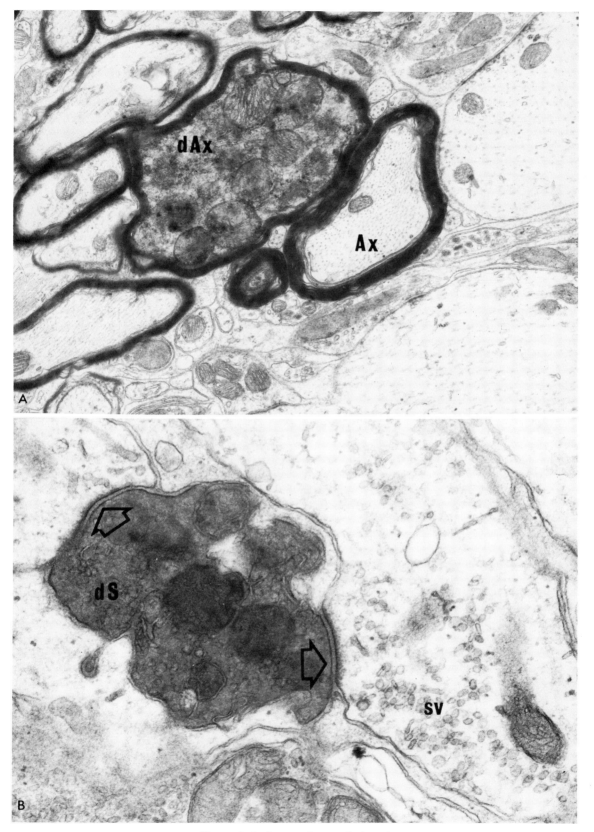

Figure 4–6 *See opposite page for legend.*

upon striated muscle fibers and transported in a retrograde fashion all the way back to motor neurons in the spinal cord (Kristensson and Olsson, 1971). These two different methods of studying transport mechanisms, one using orthograde transport of radioactive amino acids incorporated into protein and the other using retrograde transport of horseradish perioxidase, add significantly to the neuroanatomist's ability to analyze precisely the circuitry of the spinal cord as well as other regions of the central nervous system.

Another recently developed technique, that of dye injection into physiologically identified neurons (Stretton and Kravitz, 1968), is proving to be a powerful method for the analysis of neuronal organization. In these techniques neurons are impaled with microelectrodes in the form of micropipettes filled with a conducting solution that also contains a fluorescent dye such as procion yellow that can be injected into the neuron in very small amounts. This dye has the ability to diffuse widely throughout the neuron, and often it may be transported out the axon as well. Later, when viewed under the fluorescent microscope, the dye is readily seen among the uninjected neurons. Recent investigators have used this technique to label precisely the location of gamma motor neurons, which had heretofore escaped definite morphologic localization (Bryan et al., 1972), and also the Renshaw cell, an important interneuron mediating inhibitory feedback upon motor neurons (Jankowska and Lindstrom, 1971). Other dye injection techniques currently being developed for use under the electron microscope would permit analysis of synaptic input to the dendritic tree of injected physiologically identified neurons.

SUMMARY

The spinal cord is an elaborate array of neuronal systems receiving sensory information from the somatic periphery from the spinal dorsal roots and giving rise to motor fibers to skeletal muscles that will ultimately determine the behavior of the individual as manifested by motor activity. The spinal cord is by no means a simple input-output circuit of neurons, but is proving to be a site where much information processing of sensory stimuli takes place as well as providing a mechanism for modifying motor behavior under the control of higher neural centers. Disorders of peripheral nerves will of necessity influence the spinal cord, either by modifying or destroying sensory input to the cord or by damaging the motor neurons that send their axons out of the cord via the ventral roots. Modern neuroanatomical and neurophysiologic methods will very likely yield substantial new information about the details of neural circuitry within the cord. An improved understanding of the mechanisms underlying the function of the spinal cord will permit those engaged in the care of patients with disorders involving the cord or peripheral nerves to analyze better and eventually treat more successfully those patients suffering from these disorders.

Acknowledgments: Some of the work reported here was supported by grants NS–06279 and NS–09167 from the United States Public Health Service. I am indebted to Diane Ralston for her experimental neurosurgical assistance and her printing of photographic materials, and to Peter V. Sharp for his neurohistologic skills.

REFERENCES

Andersen, P., Eccles, J. C., and Sears, T. A.: Cortically evoked depolarization of the primary afferent fibers in the spinal cord. J. Neurophysiol., *27*:63–77, 1964.

Bishop, G. H.: The relation between nerve fiber size and sensory modality: phylogenetic implications of the afferent innervation of cortex. J. Nerv. Ment. Dis., *128*:89–114, 1959.

Bodian, D.: An electron-microscopic study of the monkey spinal cord. III. Cytologic effects of mild and virulent poliovirus infection. Bull. Johns Hopkins Hosp., *114*:13–119, 1964.

Bryan, R. N., Trevino, D. L., and Willis, W. D.: Evidence for a common location of alpha and gamma motoneurones. Brain Res., *38*:193–196, 1972.

Christensen, B. N., and Perl, E. R.: Activation of spinal cells in the dorsal horn by cutaneous nociceptors and thermoreceptors. J. Neurophysiol., *33*:293–307, 1970.

Conradi, S.: Ultrastructure of dorsal root boutons on lumbosacral motoneurons of the adult cat, as revealed by dorsal root section. Acta Physiol. Scand., Suppl. 332, 85–115, 1969.

Cowan, W. M., Gottlieb, D. I., Hendrickson, A. E., Price, J. L., and Woosley, T. A.: An autoradiographic demonstration of axonal connections in the central nervous system. Brain Res., *37*:21–51, 1972.

Dilly, P. N., Wall, P. D., and Webster, K. E.: Cells of origin of the spinothalamic tract in the cat and rat. Exp. Neurol., *21*:550–562, 1968.

Hensel, H., Iggo, A., and Witt, I.: A quantitative study of sensitive cutaneous thermoreceptors with C afferent fibers. J. Physiol., *153*:113–126, 1960.

Iggo, A.: Cutaneous Mechanoreceptors with Afferent C Fibers. J. Physiol., *152*:337–353, 1960.

Jankowska, E., and Lindstrom, S.: Morphological identification of Renshaw cells. Acta Physiol. Scand., *91*:428–430, 1971.

Kristensson, K., and Olsson, Y.: Retrograde axonal transport of protein. Brain Res., *29*:363–365, 1971.

McLaughlin, B. J.: The fine structure of neurons and synapses in the motor nuclei of the cat spinal cord. J. Comp. Neurol., *144*:429–460, 1972a.

McLaughlin, B. J.: Dorsal root projections to the motor nuclei in the cat spinal cord. J. Comp. Neurol., *144*:461–474, 1972b.

McLaughlin, B. J.: Propriospinal and supraspinal projections to the motor nuclei in the cat spinal cord. J. Comp. Neurol., *144*:475–500, 1972c.

Ralston, H. J. III.: The fine structure of neurons in the dorsal horn of the cat spinal cord. J. Comp. Neurol., *132*:275–302, 1968a.

Ralston, H. J. III.: Dorsal root projections to dorsal horn neurons in the cat spinal cord. J. Comp. Neurol., *132*:303–330, 1968b.

Rexed, B.: The cytoarchitectonic organization of the spinal cord in the cat. J. Comp. Neurol., *96*:415–496, 1952.

Stretton, A. O. W., and Kravitz, E. A.: Neuronal geometry: determination with a technique of intracellular dye injection. Science, *162*:132–134, 1968.

Trevino, D. L., Maunz, R. A., Bryan, R. N., and Willis, W. D.: Location of cells of origin in the spinothalamic tract in the lumbar enlargement of cat. Exp. Neurol., *34*:64–77, 1972.

Chapter 5

LIGHT AND ELECTRON MICROSCOPY OF DORSAL ROOT AND SYMPATHETIC GANGLIA

Virginia M. Tennyson

DORSAL ROOT GANGLIA

The dorsal root ganglia, also called spinal ganglia, are part of the peripheral sensory nervous system. The ganglia are associated with all the spinal nerves except the first cervical nerve, which often lacks a dorsal root, and with certain coccygeal nerves (Crosby et al., 1962). The ganglion is a collection of somatic and visceral sensory nerve cells and their processes, which form an ovoid enlargement on the dorsal root. The axons of the dorsal root originate from the cell bodies in the ganglion and carry sensory impulses to the spinal cord through lateral and medial divisions of the dorsal root. These nerve fibers are anatomically and functionally axons. The nerve bundle, which exits from the peripheral pole of the ganglion, joins the ventral roots of the spinal cord to form the spinal nerve trunk. The peripheral sensory nerve brings afferent impulses from visceral receptors and somatic receptors located in the skin, muscles, tendons, and joints. The peripheral sensory nerve fibers, therefore, are functionally dendritic, but they are called axons because they have the morphologic characteristics of axons.

Histology

The ganglion has a thick connective tissue capsule, which is continuous with the epineurium and perineurium of the spinal nerves. The perineurium acts as a diffusion barrier to the passage of many substances into the

nerve and ganglion (see Chapter 9). Delicate vascular connective tissue penetrates into the ganglion, forming a framework for the nerve cells and nerve fibers. The dorsal root neurons are arranged in rows or in groups and are concentrated at the periphery of the ganglion (Fig. 5–1A). The central portion of the ganglion contains primarily large bundles of nerve fibers. The perikarya of the dorsal root neurons are globular (Fig. 5–1A and B), pear-shaped, or mushroom-shaped. They vary in diameter from less than 20 to over 100 μm (Truex and Carpenter, 1969). Crosby et al. (1962) propose that the smallest cells in the ganglion, which have spherical cell bodies, may be the neurons that transmit impulses set up by painful stimuli. The small nerve cells have small nerve fibers. Some small to medium-sized neurons are presumed to receive impulses from the viscera. The larger, more differentiated neurons have thicker axons and transmit temperature, tactile, and proprioceptive impulses (Crosby et al., 1962).

Dorsal root neurons have a central or paracentral pale nucleus with a prominent nucleolus. The size of the nucleus relative to the cell volume varies in different species (Häggqvist and Lindberg, 1961). The neurons lack true dendritic expansions; thus they are unipolar (Figs. 5–1C and D). A capsule of satellite cells, which are ectodermal cells and sometimes called amphicytes, surrounds the individual neurons (Fig. 5–1B). The large space between the satellite cells and the neuron is an artifact of the preparation, as can be seen by comparison with specimens prepared

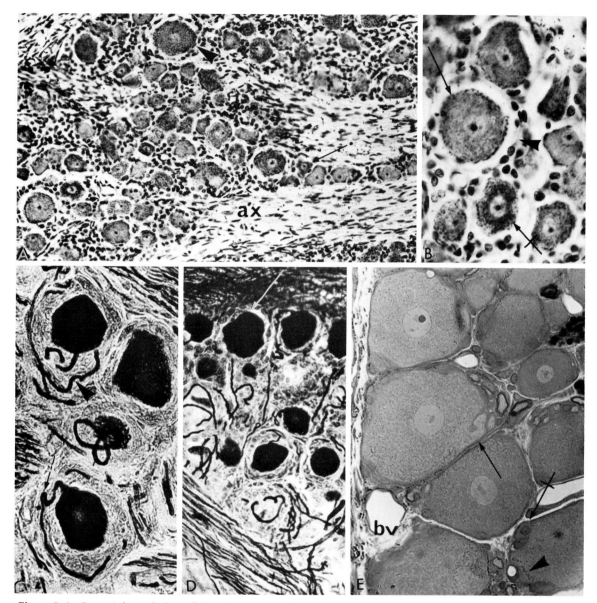

Figure 5–1   Parts *A* through *D* are light micrographs of dorsal root ganglia of the human infant prepared by conventional light microscopy techniques (slides courtesy of Dr. Charles Noback). *E* is a light micrograph of a semithick section of a dorsal root ganglion of an adult rabbit prepared by methods used for electron microscopy. *A.* The sensory neurons may be very small (arrow) or large (arrowhead) and have centrally located nuclei with prominent nucleoli. Their axons (ax) form large bundles, which course through the central portion of the ganglion. The small dense nuclei encircling neuronal perikarya are satellite cell nuclei. Elsewhere in the ganglion, the dense nuclei belong to Schwann cells or connective tissue cells. Nissl stain. × 180. *B.* The large pale neuron (arrow) has smaller Nissl bodies than the moderate-size neuron (crossed arrow). The large space between the nuclei of the satellite sheath (arrowhead) and the large neuron is an artifact due to shrinkage. Nissl stain. × 430. *C.* The proximal portion of an axon forms a loop (arrow) then partially encircles the perikaryon. Another axon (arrowhead) appears to be more convoluted, but is not continuous in this section. The grayish tissues surrounding the neurons and their axons are the satellite and Schwann cell sheaths, which are not well stained by this method. Cajal silver. × 430. *D.* The unipolar axon of a neuron (arrow) bifurcates a short distance from the cell body. Cajal silver. × 270. *E.* Large and moderate-sized granular neurons, as well as a small neuron with homogeneous moderately dense cytoplasm, are seen. A pale axon (arrow), which is surrounded by darker sheath cytoplasm is evident. There is no obvious space between satellite sheath cells (crossed arrow) and their perikarya. Collections of dense granules (arrowhead) are probably lipofuscin. The very dense structures are myelin sheaths. The dense smudge in the neuron with a prominent nucleolus is an artifact. Blood vessel (bv). Glutaraldehyde-osmium fixation, cresyl violet stain. × 430.

for electron microscopy (Fig. 5–1*E*; also see section on electron microscopy). The satellite cells are continuous with the Schwann cells of the axon. Satellite cells and Schwann cells in the dorsal root ganglia have been considered to be variants of a single cell type (Pineda et al., 1967). Silver impregnations reveal that the axon of the larger neurons may wind circuitously around its perikaryon (Fig. 5–1*C*), or it may coil forming a glomerulus close to the cell body (see Cajal, 1909; Scharf, 1958, for illustrations of the complexity of these convolutions). It has been stated that the axon may give off recurrent collaterals that terminate in end disks situated close to the ganglion cells or their capsule (Crosby et al., 1962), but confirmatory electron microscopic evidence of vesicle-filled axonal boutons in this location has not yet been reported. After leaving the dorsal root neuron, the single axon usually extends for some distance from the cell, where it bifurcates into a T or Y-shaped division (Fig. 5–1*D*). The bifurcation occurs at a node of Ranvier and may take place in the vicinity of the cell body or in the central portion of the ganglion. The centrally directed process is thinner than the peripherally directed process. Thin axons in the ganglion may be either unmyelinated or myelinated, but thicker axons have myelin. There is a spatial progression in the degree of myelination as the axon leaves the unmyelinated glomerular region, i.e., initially there are unusually thin layers of myelin (Spencer et al., 1973), which are followed by thicker myelin in segments close to the axonal bifurcation (Ha, 1970).

Nissl granules, a Golgi network, mitochondria, neurofibrillae, and pigment granules have been observed in sensory neurons by light microscopy. The pattern and intensity of the basophilic Nissl staining differs from one neuron to another. The darker homogeneously staining neurons, which are usually the smaller cells, have very fine powdery Nissl particles densely distributed throughout their cytoplasm. The lighter cells, which may be either small or large (Fig. 5–1*B*), have small or large clumps of Nissl substance separated by pale areas of cytoplasm. Electron microscopy has shown that neurofilaments are present in the pale cytoplasmic areas, as is discussed later in the section on electron microscopy. The Golgi apparatus appears as black or gray irregular bodies and connecting threadlike strands after silver or osmium preparations (see Scharf, 1958, and Malhotra,

1959, for discussion of early references, techniques, and controversies concerning the results). Although Malhotra (1959) pointed out the similarity of the distribution of his preparations of the Golgi apparatus to the distribution of the endoplasmic reticulum in electron micrographs, the Golgi complex and the endoplasmic reticulum are currently considered to be different and distinct organelles. It is possible, however, that there are interconnections between the two systems. Mitochondria appear as fine curved threads that are as long as 4 μm is fixed preparations. These organelles are readily seen by phase contrast microscopy in living neurons in tissue culture (Pomerat et al., 1967). Mitochondria are capable of independent movement in the living cell and reproduce themselves by division. Since mitochondria contain enzyme systems involved in oxidation-reduction reactions of the citric acid cycle, they are probably the organelles responsible for the intracellular formazan deposits in neurons and satellite cells of cerebrospinal and sympathetic ganglia after treatment with tetrazolium salts (Wolf et al., 1956). Neurofibrillae are seen in many neurons after silver impregnations. They form large or small loops within the cell body and extend out into the processes. Dark brown melanin pigment has been found in some dorsal root neurons, and larger lipofuscin granules that stain with carbolfuchsin and are acid fast are found in others, but the two pigments have not been seen in the same dorsal root neuron (Wolf and Pappenheimer, 1945). The lipofuscin granule is insoluble in the usual lipid solvents used for histology. After hematoxylin and eosin staining or Nissl staining, lipofuscin granules are unaltered and have a yellowish color. They are blackened by osmic acid and stain red with scharlach R.

For more details and illustrations and for reference to the early literature the reader is referred to Scharf (1958).

AUTONOMIC GANGLIA

The autonomic ganglia are part of the visceral motor system. They include the sympathetic chain ganglia (paravertebral ganglia) and their trunks, the celiac ganglion, and the superior and inferior mesenteric ganglia (collateral or prevertebral ganglia), which are found in the mesenteric nerve plexuses surrounding the abdominal aorta, and the parasympathetic ganglia (terminal ganglia), which are located within or close to the structures they innervate (Truex and Carpenter, 1969). The autonomic ganglia receive preganglionic fibers from cranial nerves III, VII, IX, and X, from the intermediolateral nucleus of the thoracolumbar spinal cord, and from the sacral autonomic nuclei of the spinal cord. The thoracolumbar division is sympathetic and its effects are mediated by norepinephrine. The craniosacral division is parasympathetic. Its terminals are generally thought to be cholinergic, but there is evidence that nerve fibers of both sympathetic and parasympathetic origin reach the myenteric plexus (see Gabella, 1972, for references).

Histology

The sympathetic chain ganglia have a thin connective tissue capsule, but there is no sharp delimiting capsule between the collateral ganglia and the connective tissue of the surrounding area (Crosby et al., 1962). The sympathetic chain neurons are intermingled with myelinated and nonmyelinated fibers throughout the ganglion (Fig. 5–2A and B). Some of these nerve fibers originate from the sympathetic neurons and some of them are axons of preganglionic neurons that will terminate in the ganglion. Others are visceral efferent fibers in passage and originate from cell bodies in the dorsal root or cranial ganglia (Crosby et al., 1962). The parasympathetic ganglia are usually embedded within the connective tissue between the fibers of smooth muscle of an organ (Fig. 5–2C). The ganglia do not have a distinct connective tissue capsule.

The sympathetic and parasympathetic neurons are multipolar and their diameters vary from 20 to 60 μm (Figs. 5–2D and E). In general the cells are smaller and of more equal size than those of the dorsal root ganglion (compare Fig. 5–1A and E with Fig. 5–2A and F). The nucleus of the sympathetic neuron is pale and it is frequently eccentrically located. Binucleate cells (discussed in the section on fluorescence microscopy) are seen. The neurons of the sympathetic chain are surrounded by a capsule of satellite cells (Fig. 5–2B). As in the dorsal root ganglion, the wide space between the capsule and the neuron is not present after fixation procedures used for electron microscopy (Fig. 5–2F). The dendrites of the sympathetic neurons may be short and ramify between the perikaryon and the satellite cell capsule (Fig. 5–2D). Longer dendrites pierce the capsule and end within the intercellular plexuses (Fig. 5–2E). Preganglionic cholinergic axonal boutons may make synaptic contact with the perikaryon or with intracapsular and extracapsular dendrites. The entire complex is surrounded by a sheath. The axon of the sympathetic chain neuron is usually thin and unmyelinated, particularly within the ganglion. The axon is surrounded by a Schwann cell sheath.

Autonomic nerve cells have organelles similar to those described in the section on the dorsal root neurons. The Nissl substance is generally diffusely scattered, i.e., a dustlike pattern, but sometimes small Nissl bodies are present (Fig. 5–2B). The Golgi complex may be quite uniformly distributed as a network in the cell body, or it may be aggregated in the perinuclear zone (Sulkin and Kuntz, 1952). Lipofuscin pigment is common in sympathetic neurons (Sulkin, 1953; Kuntz, 1953), and it has a pronounced autofluorescence (Mytilineou et al., 1963; also see the following section on fluorescence microscopy). Melanin granules, similar to those in the substantia nigra, were not demonstrable in sympathetic ganglia by histochemical methods (Sulkin, 1953; Mytilineou et al., 1963), but dense conglomerates in large vesiculated pigment bodies seen by electron microscopy might be melanin clumps below the level of resolution of the light microscope (Pick, 1967).

For more details and illustrations of the sympathetic and parasympathetic ganglia, and for references to the early literature, the reader is directed to Kuntz (1953) and Stohr (1957).

Fluorescence Microscopy

Cells having catecholamines (norepinephrine, epinephrine, dopamine) or serotonin can be studied with fluorescence microscopy by the Falck-Hillarp technique (Falck et al., 1962). The tissue is quick-frozen, dried, and treated with formaldehyde gas at 80° C. Catecholamines and serotonin are converted to isoquinolines and β-carbolines respectively, which fluoresce when excited by ultraviolet

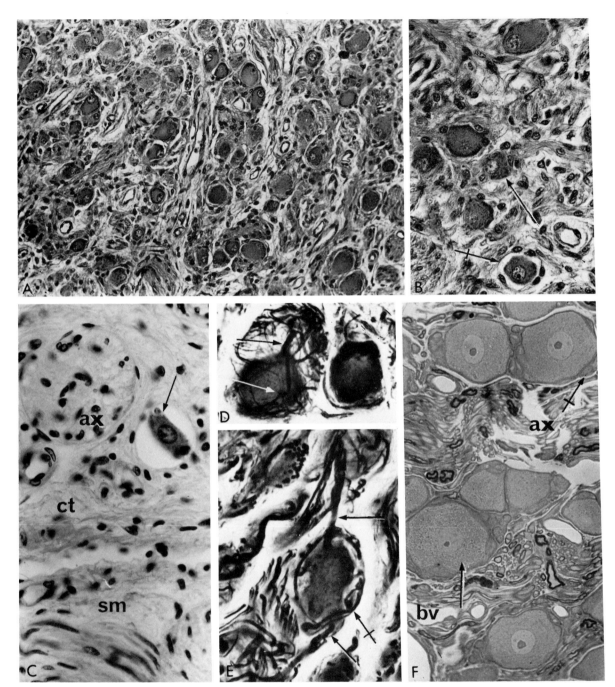

Figure 5–2   Parts *A* through *E* are light micrographs of autonomic ganglia of the human prepared by conventional light microscopy techniques (slides courtesy of Drs. Edward Dempsey and Charles Noback). *F* is a light micrograph of a semithick section of a sympathetic ganglion of an adult rabbit prepared by methods used for electron microscopy. *A*. The sympathetic neurons are small to moderate in size and have eccentrically located nuclei with prominent nucleoli. Their axons course in small groups among the neurons. The small dense nuclei surrounding the neurons are sheath cell nuclei. Others belong to Schwann cells and connective tissue cells. Nissl stain, thoracic ganglion. × 180. *B*. The cytoplasm of the sympathetic neurons usually has a homogeneous moderately dense appearance, although some fine Nissl granules are evident (arrow). A continuous satellite sheath (crossed arrow) surrounds the neurons. Nissl stain, thoracic ganglion. × 380. *C*. Terminal parasympathetic neurons of Auerbach's plexus are usually small and ovoid (arrow), and they are found in the connective tissue area (ct) between the longitudinal and circular smooth muscle (sm). This section passes through only one neuron, but they usually occur in small groups. They do not have a complete neuroectodermal en-

Figure 5–2 legend continued on opposite page.

light. Sympathetic ganglia and their terminals contain norepinephrine as well as dopamine (Euler, 1956, 1971; Laverty and Sharman, 1965). Sympathetic nerve cells and an intraganglionic system of varicose axons exhibit a catecholamine-induced fluorescence (Eränkö and Härkönen, 1963; Norberg and Hamberger, 1964; Jacobowitz and Woodward, 1968). These findings are illustrated in Figure 5–3*A*, *B*, and *C*. A large number of the sympathetic neurons have a slight to moderate greenish yellow fluorescence (Fig. 5–3*A* and *B*) that is attributable to norepinephrine. The fluorescence is diffusely distributed throughout the perikaryon and sometimes appears as dustlike particles. Both large and small neurons may be fluorescent, but not all neurons in the ganglion exhibit catecholamine fluorescence (Fig. 5–3*B*). It is not known whether this is a reflection of physiologic depletion in some cells or whether some neurons lack norepinephrine entirely. A few adrenergic varicose axons and terminals are seen randomly distributed in the ganglion (Fig. 5–3*C*). Satellite cells and connective tissue cells in the ganglion do not exhibit fluorescence. Some neurons have large or small orange autofluorescent granules, which are lipofuscin granules (Fig. 5–3*B*). The lipid in the lipofuscin granule fluoresces on exposure to ultraviolet light without formaldehyde treatment, and thus should not be confused with catecholamine-induced fluorescence. Lipofuscin granules are particularly numerous in specimens from older individuals, as is illustrated in the ganglion from a 48 year old human.

Sympathetic neurons grown in tissue culture also exhibit a catecholamine-induced fluorescence (Sano et al., 1967; Burdman, 1968; England and Goldstein, 1969). When these cultures are labeled with tritiated catecholamines and later examined by radioautography, the label has been taken up only by sympathetic neurons and their processes and not by satellite cells or fibroblasts in the culture

(Burdman, 1968; England and Goldstein, 1969).

In addition to the principal postganglionic sympathetic neurons, there is another population of small intensely fluorescent (SIF) cells that are sparsely distributed in the sympathetic ganglion (Fig. 5–3*C*) (Norberg and Hamberger, 1964; Norberg et al., 1966; Jacobowitz and Woodward, 1968). These cells have a fluorescence intensity that is much higher than that of the principal cells. Although early reports suggested that the fluorescence was due to serotonin or norepinephrine, microspectrofluorimetric studies indicate that these cells contain dopamine (Björklund et al., 1970). The SIF cells are very small, 6 to 12 μm in diameter, and they have both long and short processes. Although they may be seen alone, they usually occur in small groups, often near blood vessels or nerve bundles. Recent studies have shown that administration of hydrocortisone causes a tenfold increase in the number of SIF cells in newborn rats, presumably from poorly differentiated weakly fluorescent stem cells in the ganglion (Eränkö and Eränkö, 1972.) Hydrocortisone injections in adult rats, however, did not induce dramatic changes in the sympathetic ganglia.

Grillo (1966) pointed out that the small intensely fluorescent cell might correspond to a cell type seen by electron microscopy that has the characteristics of both a neuron and a chromaffin cell. They have long processes, which synapse with cells of their own type as well as with the principal sympathetic neuron. They receive preganglionic terminals. Unlike most neurons, they contain numerous large dense-core granules that resemble those in the adrenal medulla, but are smaller. The fine structure of the SIF cells has been described in detail in a number of species as well as in tissue culture (Siegrist et al., 1968; Williams and Palay, 1969; Matthews and Raisman, 1969; Masurovsky et al., 1972). These cells may be intraganglionic interneurons, which

---

Figure 5–2 *Continued.*
sheathment. The space surrounding the neuron is an artifact. A bundle of axons (ax) is nearby. Hematoxylin and eosin, esophagus. × 410. D. Multiple processes (arrows) emerge from this sympathetic neuron and enter the pericellular plexus. Pyridine silver, sympathetic ganglion. × 750. E. Processes (arrows) extend from both poles of this sympathetic neuron through the satellite sheath (crossed arrow) to enter the intercellular plexus of nerve fibers. Pyridine silver, sympathetic ganglion. × 750. F. Moderate-sized and small neurons with centrally located nuclei, are present in the sympathetic ganglion of the rabbit. Although some of the neurons have granular cytoplasm (arrow), most of them have a rather homogeneous moderately dense cytoplasm. The satellite sheath cells (crossed arrow) are closely apposed to the perikarya. Both myelinated and unmyelinated axons (ax) are present among the neurons. Blood vessel (bv). Glutaraldehyde-osmium fixation, cresyl violet stain. × 450.

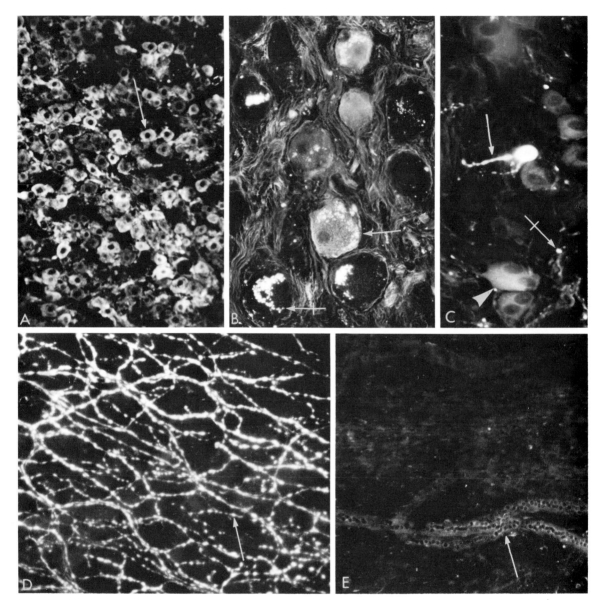

Figure 5–3 Fluorescence micrographs prepared according to the Falck-Hillarp technique to locate catecholamines in tissue (slides courtesy of Drs. Catherine Mytilineou and Robert E. Barrett). *A.* Sympathetic nerve cells (arrow) of the superior cervical ganglion of a rat show weak to moderate fluorescence intensity attributable to norepinephrine. The nuclei, which lack fluorescence, appear as central black spheres. × 150. *B.* Lipofuscin appears as autofluorescent granules (arrow) superimposed on the diffuse cytoplasmic fluorescence of norepinephrine-containing neurons, but are more readily seen in neurons that do not exhibit catecholamines (crossed arrow). Lumbar sympathetic chain ganglia, 48 year old human. × 350. *C.* Small intensely fluorescent cells with processes (arrow) are found among the principal cells. Some fluorescent (arrowhead) and nonfluorescent cells with two nuclei are present. Fluorescent terminals (crossed arrow) are seen. Superior cervical ganglion, 21 day postnatal rabbit. × 350. *D.* Plexus of intensely fluorescent varicose adrenergic terminal axons (arrow). Iris, rat. × 350. *E.* No fluorescence is apparent in the axons of this iris from a rat treated with reserpine (10 mg. per kilogram) 20 hours prior to sacrifice. Autofluorescence permits visualization of red blood cells (arrow) in blood vessels. × 350.

are interposed between some of the preganglionic axons and the principal sympathetic neurons. The SIF cells may play a role in the control of inhibitory mechanisms of transmission through the ganglion via synaptic junctions or by functioning as an endocrine structure. They lack a complete satellite sheath; thus they may act by liberating active substances into the extracellular space or into blood vessels in the ganglion (Siegrist et al., 1968).

Although there are a small number of fluorescent axons in the sympathetic nerve trunks, the great majority of the axons lack fluorescence throughout most of their preterminal extent. Presumably the catecholamine content is too small to be visible by this method. The terminal portions of the sympathetic axons, however, have intensely fluorescent varicosities such as are seen in the iris (Fig. 5–3D) (Falck, 1962; Malmfors, 1965). Treatment with reserpine, which markedly reduces the norepinephrine content of the iris, results in the elimination of its fluorescence (Fig. 5–3E) (Malmfors, 1965). At least a portion of the norepinephrine in fluorescent varicosities is contained in a population of small dense-core vesicles in the nerve ending; these vesicles lose their density after reserpine treatment, as discussed in the section on electron microscopy. Administration of an analogue of dopamine, i.e., 6-hydroxydopamine, causes destruction of norepinephrine-containing nerve terminals (Tranzer and Thoenen, 1968). When examined by fluorescent microscopy, the axons initially appear as large fluorescent ovoids, which are fragmenting terminal axons; ultimately the fluorescence disappears as the axons degenerate (Malmfors and Sachs, 1968).

FINE STRUCTURE OF GANGLION CELLS

The fine structure of the organelles within the dorsal root and autonomic neurons is similar; therefore, the cytologic features of these cells are considered together and significant differences noted. References to original observations are given in the text, but also recommended are articles on the ultrastructure of the various ganglia by Bunge and co-workers (1967), Matthews and Raisman (1969), Peters, Palay, and Webster (1970), Pick (1970), and Gabella (1972).

Portions of a typical small neuron and a large neuron from a dorsal root ganglion, and of a medium sized neuron from a sympathetic ganglion are illustrated (Figs. 5–4, 5–5, and 5–6). The same types of cytoplasmic organelles are present in these cells, but the number and distribution differ. These differences are probably responsible for variations in staining seen by light microscopy. It is well known that the Nissl substance stained by cresyl violet corresponds to the granular endoplasmic reticulum of neurons (Figs. 5–4, 5–5, and 5–6 er) (Palay and Palade, 1955; Cervós-Navarro, 1959; Andres, 1961a), and that the ribosomes are responsible for the basophilia. The quantity and distribution of the granular endoplasmic reticulum and associated ribosomes, as well as the presence or absence of neurofilaments that are not stained by cresyl violet, determine whether a neuron exhibits discrete Nissl clumps or a diffuse basophilia. For instance, the cell in Figure 5–5, which has clumps of endoplasmic reticulum (er) separated by large areas containing numerous neurofilaments (f), would appear as a light cell having discrete Nissl granules. It is likely that the sparsity of filaments and the abundance of endoplasmic reticulum that appears in clumps as well as throughout the cell in Figure 5–4 would result in a rather diffuse Nissl stain. Other variations should be noted, but their significance is not known at this time. The cisternae of endoplasmic reticulum in Figures 5–4 and 5–6 are arranged roughly parallel to one another, whereas they are in random arrays in Figure 5–5. The Golgi complex is rather small and the number of its sites are few in Figure 5–4 whereas long curvilinear arrays occur in numerous areas in Figure 5–6. The mitochondrial matrix is denser in Figures 5–5 and 5–6 than in Figure 5–4. Since these specimens came from the same rabbit, it is unlikely that fixation alone could cause this result.

The neuronal nucleus is usually spherical, but sometimes shallow indentations are present (Fig. 5–4). The chromatin material is finely dispersed throughout the nucleus. The nucleolus is large and has a dense coiled nucleolonema, which is formed of very fine filaments called the pars fibrosa, and granules called the pars granulosa (Fig. 5–7A). The granules are smaller than cytoplasmic ribo-

Text continued on page 85.

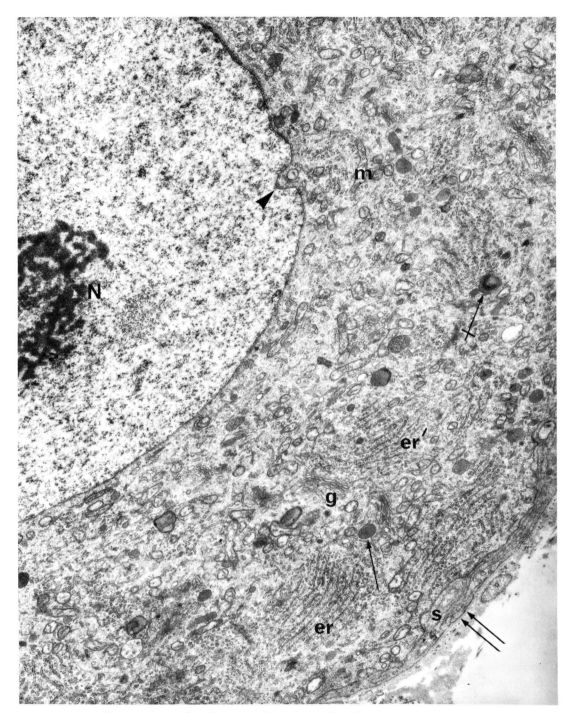

Figure 5–4   A small neuron from a dorsal root ganglion. The ovoid nucleus has shallow indentations (arrowhead) and a prominent nucleolus (N) with a coiled nucleolonema. The cytoplasm appears dense owing to the sparsity of neurofilaments and microtubules. Parallel stacks of endoplasmic reticulum (er) form a small Nissl body separated from another Nissl body (er') by elements of the Golgi complex (g) and other organelles. Mitochondria (m), lysosomes (arrow), and heterogeneous bodies (crossed arrow) are present. Thin layers of the satellite sheath (s) are closely apposed to the neuronal cell membrane. A basement membrane (double arrows) coats the surface of the sheath facing the extracellular space. × 11,250. Electron micrograph is from dorsal root ganglion of an adult rabbit perfused with a buffered glutaraldehyde-formaldehyde solution and further fixed in osmium tetroxide. The tissue was block stained in uranyl acetate and thin sections were stained additionally with uranyl acetate and with lead citrate.

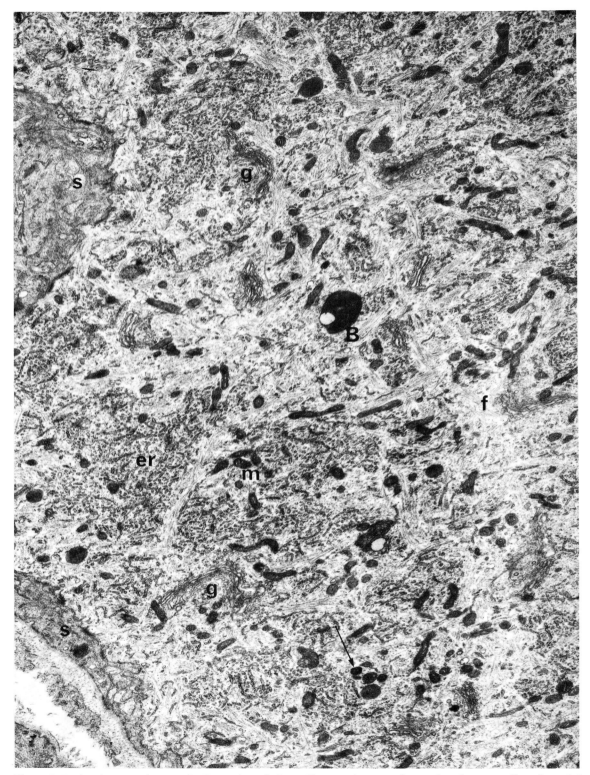

Figure 5–5 An electron micrograph of a portion of a large filamented neuron from a dorsal root ganglion of an adult rabbit. Numerous bundles of neurofilaments (f) wind throughout the cytoplasm separating collections of endoplasmic reticulum (er), mitochondria (m), and Golgi areas (g) from one another. A large body (B), which is probably a lipofuscin granule, and smaller heterogeneous bodies (arrow) are present. Satellite cell sheath (s). × 10,000. Animal was perfused with a buffered glutaraldehyde-formaldehyde solution and further fixed in osmium tetroxide. The tissue was block stained in uranyl acetate, and thin sections were stained additionally with uranyl acetate and with lead citrate.

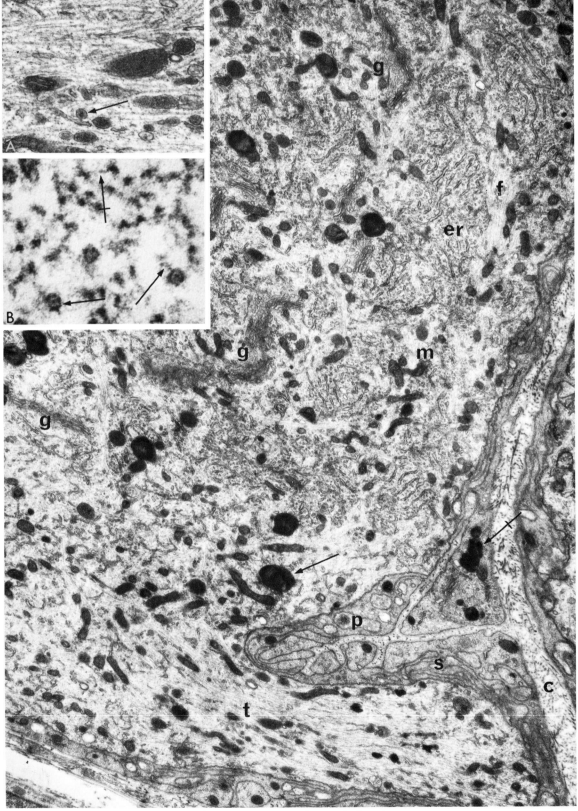

Figure 5–6 *See opposite page for legend.*

somes. Both parts contain ribonucleoprotein. The less dense zone in the interstices of the coiled threads is karyoplasm and may contain some chromatin material. A peculiar structure called an intranuclear rodlet has been described in the nuclei of avian sympathetic neurons (Masurovsky et al., 1970). The rodlets are formed of proteinaceous filaments associated with a spheroidal body and seem to be related to the nucleolus. The nucleus of neurons is surrounded by a double-layered nuclear envelope, which fuses to form pores (Fig. 5–7B). The pores have a diaphragm with fibrous material on both sides, and seem to be a likely spot for the passage of substances between the nucleus and cytoplasm, but further studies are needed before this can be stated with certainty about all cells. The inner nuclear membrane is fairly smooth, but the outer one shows slight undulations. Sometimes ribosomes are attached to the outer nuclear membrane.

The Nissl substance or endoplasmic reticulum of neurons consists of flattened ribosome-studded cisternae of endoplasmic reticulum and clusters of ribosomes called polyribosomes (Fig. 5–7C). The cisternae frequently show connections, and study of serial sections shows that they form an interconnected reticulum through the cell (Palay and Palade, 1955). As mentioned, the cisternae may be oriented parallel to one another or may be disposed at random (cf. Figs. 5–4 and 5–5). Studies of other cells have shown that the endoplasmic reticulum and polyribosomes are the sites of protein synthesis in the cell. Subsurface cisternae, a type of endoplasmic reticulum in neurons, are flattened saccules closely apposed to the inner aspect of the plasma membrane (Fig. 5–7C) (Rosenbluth, 1962). Ribosomes may be present on their cytoplasmic surface. Although the functional relationship of the subsurface cisternae to the plasma membrane is unknown, Rosenbluth has suggested two possibilities: they may be

areas that exhibit selective permeability, which could alter mobility and effective concentration of ions at the cell surface, thereby affecting electrophysiologic behavior at the neuronal surface; or it may be that material entering a neuron in these regions is channeled directly into the granular endoplasmic reticulum by connections between them and the subsurface cisternae.

In addition to the well known sites of cytoplasmic ribonucleoprotein just discussed, peculiar inclusion bodies called nematosomes have been found in the cytoplasm of sympathetic neurons of the rat (Grillo, 1970). The nematosome has the appearance of the coiled fibrous component of the nucleolus. It contains protein and some ribonucleic acid, but no cytoplasmic ribosomes.

Certain enzymes have been localized in the endoplasmic reticulum of dorsal root and sympathetic neurons by electron microscopic cytochemistry, such as glucose-6-phosphatase and inosine diphosphatase and acetylcholinesterase (Teichberg and Holtzman, 1973; Koelle and Foroglou-Kerameos, 1965; Novikoff et al., 1966; Brzin et al., 1966). The end product of acetylcholinesterase activity is found on the inner surface of the endoplasmic reticulum (Fig. 5–7D), in subsurface cisternae, and in the nuclear envelope as well as in the agranular reticulum of the axon. The role that acetylcholinesterase plays in the reticulum is unknown. Fukuda and Koelle (1959) suggested that acetylcholinesterase synthesized in the endoplasmic reticulum could be transported via its canaliculi to the surface of the cell and its processes. The assumption was supported by Kása and Csillik (1968), but confirmatory evidence that enzyme-containing agranular reticulum was deposited at the external axonal surface was not apparent in a study of acetylcholinesterase development in the rabbit embryo (Tennyson and Brzin, 1970). It has been suggested that the presence of acetylcholinesterase in some neurons of the

Figure 5–6 A medium-sized sympathetic neuron from the superior cervical ganglion. Narrow bundles of neurofilaments (f) and microtubules separate clumps of endoplasmic reticulum (er), mitochondria (m), and extensive Golgi areas (g) from one another. Heterogeneous dense bodies (arrow) are found in the neuron and in the satellite cell (crossed arrow). Microtubules (t) are particularly numerous in the axon hillock and initial segment of the process. Small neural processes (p) are partially or completely enveloped by the sheath cell (s), which forms interdigitating layers as it surrounds the perikaryon. Collagen (c). × 10,200. *Inset A.* A higher magnification of the process showing microtubules and large and small dense bodies (arrow). × 30,400. *Inset B.* Microtubules sectioned transversely frequently exhibit a central density and projections from their surface (arrows). Neurofilaments are irregular in cross section and often have projections (crossed arrow). × 164,000. Electron micrograph is of sympathetic ganglion of an adult rabbit perfused with a buffered glutaraldehyde-formaldehyde solution and further fixed in osmium tetroxide. The tissue was block stained in uranyl acetate and thin sections were stained additionally with uranyl acetate and with lead citrate.

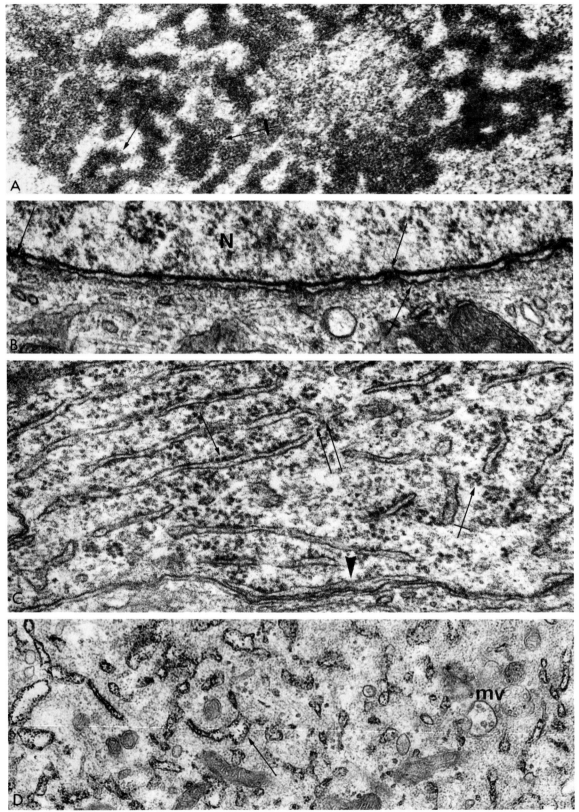

Figure 5–7 *See opposite page for legend.*

sympathetic ganglia indicates that these cells are cholinergic neurons (Koelle and Koelle, 1959). The great majority of neurons in frog dorsal root and sympathetic ganglia exhibit acetylcholinesterase activity in their endoplasmic reticulum (Brzin et al., 1966); therefore it is unlikely that such a large population in both ganglia are cholinergic. It has been hypothesized that acetylcholinesterase in the axonal membrane plays a role in membrane permeability (Nachmansohn, 1970); a similar permeability mechanism may be utilized by the membranes of the endoplasmic reticulum during their normal synthetic functions in the cell body.

The Golgi complex may be small and occupy relatively few areas in some neurons, but it is usually a conspicuous organelle (Figs. 5–4 and 5–6). It is common to find the Golgi complex curved into a C-shaped configuration (Figs. 5–5 and 5–8A). The Golgi apparatus consists of closely packed flattened saccules and vesicles. There is less cytoplasm between these elements than between the cisternae of the endoplasmic reticulum. Although the saccules may ramify and their branches join up with one another, there is very little anastomosis between saccules at different levels in the stack (Peters et al., 1970). Grazing sections of the saccules reveals fenestrations in their walls (Fig. 5–8A). Ribosomes are not attached to the Golgi membranes, but connections are sometimes seen between them and the cisternae of endoplasmic reticulum via a system of agranular reticulum. Glycogen granules have been found in association with a system of smooth membranes in spinal ganglia of the guinea pig and rabbit (Pannese, 1969), but large areas of glycogen occur alone in the cytoplasmic ground substance in sympathetic neurons of the frog (Yamamoto, 1963).

Coated vesicles having a spiked or furry outer surface are commonly found in the Golgi region (Fig. 5–8A). They sometimes appear to be coalescing with or budding off the saccules. A similar but larger coated vesicle seen at the cell surface appears to be a pinocytosis vesicle and can incorporate marker substances into the cell and transport them to multivesicular bodies for digestion (Rosenbluth and Wissig, 1964; Holtzman et al., 1973). Examples of multivesicular bodies are seen in Figure 5–7D.

Various types of single membrane-bound dense bodies, multivesicular bodies, multilaminar bodies, and lipofuscin granules are found throughout the cell (Figs. 5–7D and 5–8A to D). Many of these organelles, as well as some of the coated vesicles, exhibit acid phosphatase activity and are assumed to be part of an intracellular degradation process, i.e., the lysosome or autophagic vacuole system (Holtzman et al., 1967). Lysosomes and autophagic vacuoles increase in neurons that are reacting to injury, and they appear to be formed in association with the Golgi-related region of smooth reticulum (Holtzman et al., 1967). The lipofuscin granule may arise from the coalescence of a number of lysosomes, presumably those that are no longer as active in intracellular digestion as in earlier stages. As is well known, lipofuscin granules increase with age; thus, they may be residual bodies of the intracellular digestion system. The matrix of the lipofuscin granule exhibits a complex structure (Fig. 5–8D). The vacuoles probably represent the sites of former lipid droplets that have been removed by the preparative procedures (Fig. 5–8C and D). The fine structure of these granules in sympathetic neurons of an older human being has been examined (Pick, 1967); they closely resemble those illustrated here.

Large (80 to 100 nm) dense-core granules may be found in the Golgi region where they are presumed to be formed (Fig. 5–8A) (Holtz-

---

Figure 5–7. A. The nucleolonema of the nucleolus consists of filamentous material (arrow) and granules (crossed arrow) about 15 nm in diameter. × 33,000. B. The nucleus (N) is surrounded by a double membrane in which pores (arrows) are present. A diaphragm and filamentous material cover the pores. The membrane facing the cytoplasm is undulated (crossed arrow). × 56,000. C. Ribosomes (arrow) are attached to the surface of the cisternae of the endoplasmic reticulum and rosettes of ribosomes (crossed arrow) are present in the intervening cytoplasm. Connections (double arrows) are frequently seen between the cisternae. A subsurface cistern (arrowhead) is closely apposed to the cell surface, which is adjacent to another cell in the lower part of the micrograph. × 64,000. (Parts A through C are electron micrographs from dorsal root ganglia of an adult rabbit perfused with a buffered glutaraldehyde-formaldehyde solution and further fixed in osmium tetroxide. The tissue was block stained in uranyl acetate, and thin sections were stained additionally with uranyl acetate and with lead citrate.) D. The dense particles within the endoplasmic reticulum (arrow) are the cytochemical end product of acetylcholinesterase activity. Two single membrane-bound bodies containing a varied population of vesicles are multivesicular bodies (mv). Ribosomes are poorly defined in this preparation. Incubated in copper glycinate using acetylthiocholine as substrate, followed by conversion of end product to copper sulfide. Frog, sympathetic ganglion. × 28,000.

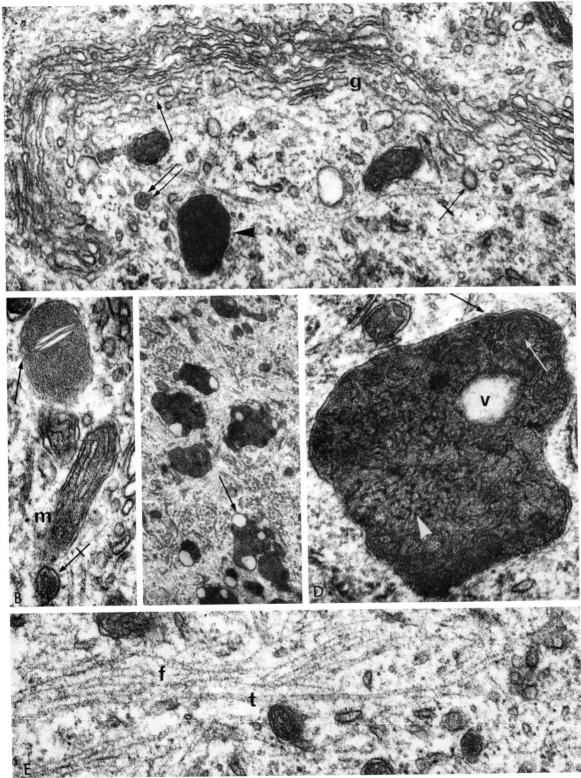

Figure 5–8 *See opposite page for legend.*

man et al., 1967), as well as elsewhere in the perikarya and in the processes of both dorsal root and sympathetic neurons (Figs. 5–8B and 5–6, inset A). The smaller (50 to 60 nm) dense-core vesicles, which are typical of sympathetic nerve terminals (discussed in the section on axonal terminals), have been reported in the perikarya of sympathetic neurons, usually after fixation in potassium permanganate (Grillo, 1966; Bunge et al., 1967; Hokfelt, 1969). In general only clear vesicles are seen after the usual glutaraldehyde-osmium fixation.

The long threadlike mitochondria seen by light microscopy are usually sectioned obliquely when examined by electron microscopy; thus they appear ellipsoidal or rodlike (Fig. 5–8B). They have an outer limiting membrane and an inner membrane that is folded into platelike cristae. The cristae may be parallel, perpendicular, or oblique to the long axis of the mitochondrion. The matrix of the mitochondrion may vary in density.

Neurofilaments are common in the large light neurons, where they course between collections of endoplasmic reticulum and other organelles (Figs. 5–8E and 5–5). They increase greatly in number in the axon hillock (Fig. 5–9A). The abundance of neurofilaments and the sparsity of polyribosomes and granular endoplasmic reticulum account for the absence of basophilia of this region in Nissl stains. Neurofilaments are the predominant organelle in the initial segment of the axon of the dorsal root neuron, but some microtubules, mitochondria, and agranular reticulum are also present (Fig. 5–9A and B). The neurofilaments are about 10 nm in diameter and exhibit a hollow core in optimal cross sections at high magnification (Fig. 5–9C). Neurofilaments have irregular contours due to short spinelike projections from their surface (Figs. 5–6B, and 5–9B). Microtubules are

scattered sparsely among the neurofilaments in neural perikarya, but they are abundant in the processes of sympathetic neurons (Figs. 5–8E and 5–6 and inset A). The term "process" is used here because it is difficult to distinguish between the axon and dendrites of a sympathetic neuron by electron microscopy (Elfvin, 1963a). Microtubules are about 23 nm in diameter and are circular in cross section. They usually have a core of low density, but sometimes they contain a central dot (Fig. 5–6, inset B). Projections or side arms can be seen extending from the microtubules under optimal conditions (Figs. 5–6, inset B and 5–9B). Neurofilaments and microtubules may be involved in the fast transport of substances along axons via their side arms (see Chapter 12 for discussion).

Sheath Cells

Dorsal root and sympathetic neurons are completely ensheathed by a capsule of satellite cells, which have long thin sheetlike processes that often interdigitate with one another (Figs. 5–4, 5–5, 5–6, and 5–9A) (Wyburn, 1958; Cervós-Navarro, 1960). The sheath is usually directly apposed to the neuronal cell bodies and follows any irregularities in the neuronal surface (Pannese, 1960; Rosenbluth, 1963). There is usually only a space of about 20 nm intervening between the surface of the neuron and its sheath. Sometimes an axon or dendrite runs along the surface of its perikaryon before exiting from the capsule; in some species, such as the frog, preganglionic axons and their terminals enter the capsule to end on the cell body or its dendrites. In these cases, the entire complex is surrounded by the capsule. As the axons and dendrites of the ganglionic neurons leave the capsule, they

Figure 5–8 *A.* The Golgi complex (g) is usually a curved array of closely packed small vesicles and agranular saccules, which are roughly parallel to one another. Grazing sections of the saccules reveals fenestrations in their walls (arrow). Vesicles with a furry coat (crossed arrow), a large 100 nm granular vesicle (double arrows), and a single membrane-bound dense body (arrowhead), which is probably a lysosome, are present. × 38,400. *B.* A single membrane-bound dense body showing lamination (arrow) is probably derived from a lysosome. A large 100 nm granular vesicle (crossed arrow) exhibits a less dense zone beneath its limiting membrane. The cristae of the mitochondrion (m) are aligned parallel to its long axis. × 60,000. *C.* Lipofuscin granules are large irregularly shaped bodies with a dense matrix and vacuolated areas (arrow) that probably contained lipid in vivo. × 10,500. *D.* The lipofuscin granule is bounded by a single membrane (black arrow) and there are curvilinear patterns (white arrow) and superimposed dense material (arrowhead) in its matrix. Lipid vacuole (v). × 60,000. *E.* Numerous neurofilaments (f) about 10 nm in diameter and microtubules (t) about 23 nm in diameter are present in this area of perikaryal cytoplasm. The fuzzy contours of the neurofilaments suggest the possibility of surface projections. × 60,000. Electron micrographs are from dorsal root ganglia of an adult rabbit perfused with a buffered glutaraldehyde-formaldehyde solution and further fixed in osmium tetroxide. The tissue was block stained in uranyl acetate, and thin sections were stained additionally with uranyl acetate and with lead citrate.

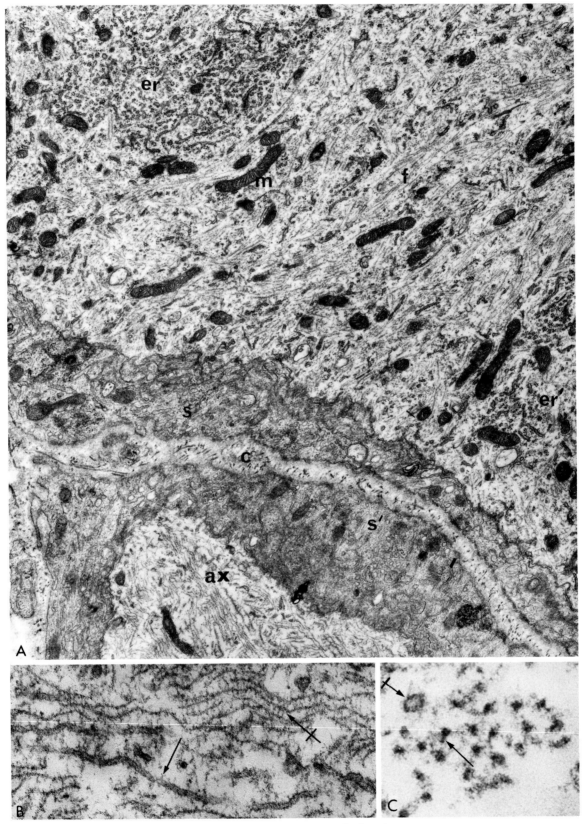

Figure 5–9 *See opposite page for legend.*

are surrounded by a sheath of Schwann cells, which are morphologically similar to the satellite cells and are continuous with them (Fig. 5–9A). The ensheathment of the ganglion cell processes extends throughout their course in the ganglion and into the nerve trunks. The satellite cells and Schwann cells are coated by a basement membrane on their outer surface facing the extracellular space. The narrow spaces between the wrappings of satellite cell cytoplasm appear to represent patent aqueous channels, since ferritin (particle size 10 nm) introduced into the extracellular space of a toad spinal ganglion can traverse these clefts (Rosenbluth and Wissig, 1964). Adenosinetriphosphatase activity and acetylcholinesterase activity have been demonstrated in the clefts between the interdigitating processes of satellite cell and Schwann cell cytoplasm, as well as between these sheaths and their respective perikarya and axons (Brzin et al., 1966; Novikoff et al., 1966; Schlaepfer and Torack, 1966; Schlaepfer, 1968). The cytoplasm of the sheath cell often appears denser than the adjacent neuronal cytoplasm (Figs. 5–6 and 5–9A). The usual organelles are concentrated near the nucleus and in thicker layers of cytoplasm, but they are sparse in the thin interdigitating processes. Peroxisomes, which are membrane-limited ovoid bodies with a moderately dense matrix, have been identified in satellite and Schwann cells of rat dorsal root ganglia (Citkowitz and Holtzman, 1973). Peroxisomes contain the enzyme catalase, but not acid phosphatase, the enzyme that is characteristic of lysosomes.

Preganglionic Axonal Terminals

The preganglionic axon may enter the satellite cell capsule of the sympathetic neuron to form axosomatic junctions (Fig. 5–10A). This mode of termination is common in sympathetic ganglia of the frog and in the ciliary ganglion of the chick (Taxi, 1961; de Lorenzo, 1960). In mammals, the preganglionic axons usually synapse with dendrites of the neuron in the intercellular plexuses outside of the ganglion cell capsule (Elfvin, 1963b). In an electron microscopic study of serial sections of the sympathetic ganglion of the cat, Elfvin (1963b) showed that the preganglionic axons run parallel to the dendrites and wind around them establishing synapses "en passant" at several points. There is usually an increase in thickness and density of the junctional membranes at both axosomatic and axodendritic synapses. The terminals contain mitochondria, a few large, moderately dense granular vesicles about 70 to 100 nm in diameter, and a large population of clear vesicles about 40 to 60 nm in diameter (Fig. 5–10A). These are cholinergic boutons and exhibit a precipitate due to acetylcholinesterase activity at their surface after cytochemical incubation (Fig. 5–10B) (Brzin et al., 1966).

Postganglionic Terminals

The centrally directed axons of the dorsal root neurons project to the dorsal horn of the spinal cord. Synapses in this region have been studied by electron microscopy (Ralston, 1968a), but it is not possible to identify a particular bouton as originating from a dorsal root neuron in normal preparations. Following extensive section of the dorsal roots, Ralston (1968b) found two types of degenerating boutons in the dorsal horn, i.e., a small electron-dense knob and a large knob filled with neurofilaments. The relationship of the degenerating knobs to the postsynaptic element varied depending on the lamina in which they terminated, but degenerating knobs were seen at axodendritic, axosomatic, and axoaxonic junctions.

The preterminal postganglionic axons of

Figure 5–9 *A.* A near-serial thin section of the axon hillock and initial axonal segment of the large neuron seen in the phase micrograph (Fig. 5–1E, arrow). The plane of section no longer passes through the junction of the axon and perikaryon here. Neurofilaments (f) fill most of the cytoplasm of the axon hillock and the axon (ax), although mitochondria (m) are present as well. Clumps of endoplasmic reticulum (er, er') border the axon hillock. The sheath cell cytoplasm surrounding the cell body (s) and axon (s') appear morphologically similar to each other. Collagen (c) in the extracellular space. × 13,950. *B.* Projections are seen at the surface of neurofilaments (crossed arrow) and microtubules (arrow). Initial segment of the axon in Figure 5–9A. × 60,000. *C.* A cross section of an axon showing the hollow core and projection of a neurofilament (arrow). Microtubule with projections (crossed arrow). × 208,000. Electron micrographs from dorsal root ganglia of an adult rabbit perfused with a buffered glutaraldehyde-formaldehyde solution and further fixed in osmium tetroxide. The tissue was block stained in uranyl acetate, and thin sections were stained additionally with uranyl acetate and with lead citrate.

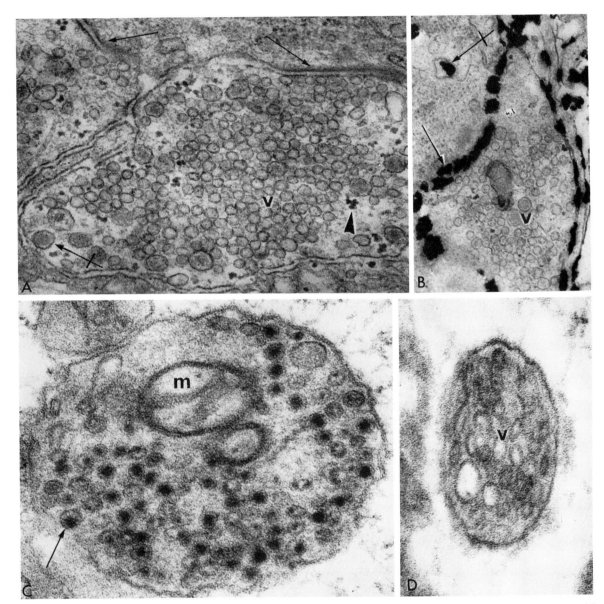

Figure 5–10   *A.* An electron micrograph of preganglionic axonal terminals that form synaptic junctions (arrows) with the perikaryon of a sympathetic neuron. The presynaptic and postsynaptic membrane are slightly increased in density and thickness. The boutons have clear vesicles (v), large moderately dense granules (crossed arrow) and some particles of glycogen (arrowhead). Frog. × 56,000. *B.* An electron micrograph showing that a very dense precipitate (arrow) due to acetylcholinesterase activity surrounds this preganglionic axonal bouton and its thin sheath cell layer. End product (crossed arrow) is also present in the endoplasmic reticulum of the sympathetic neuron. Axonal vesicles (v). Incubated in copper glycinate using acetylthiocholine as substrate, followed by conversion of end product to copper sulfide. Frog, sympathetic ganglion. × 44,000. *C.* An electron micrograph of a sympathetic axonal varicosity from the pineal gland of a rat. Small vesicles having very dense cores (arrow) that partially or completely fill them are characteristic. A few clear vesicles, large moderately dense granular vesicles, and mitochondria (m) are present. Sodium permanganate fixation. × 90,000. *D.* Twenty hours after the administration of reserpine to a rat, the small vesicles (v) of sympathetic varicosities are depleted of their dense cores. Rat, pineal gland. Sodium permanganate fixation. × 90,000.

both the parasympathetic and sympathetic nervous systems have numerous varicosities along their length that probably represent synapses "en passant" (Richardson, 1964). Although the terminals may be closely apposed to the indentations of smooth muscle of the effector organ, as noted in the vas deferens by Richardson (1962), there is frequently a rather wide extracellular space separating the nerve and the muscle. This suggests that the transmitters of the autonomic nervous system may have to traverse a much wider area than do those at the motor endplate and those at cerebral synapses. Moreover, there does not seem to be any specialization of the smooth muscle surface in the contact zone of sympathetic junctions (Richardson, 1962, 1964). Although axons of the sympathetic nerve trunks are ensheathed by Schwann cells, at least a portion of the surface of the varicose terminal lacks a sheath. The transmitter, therefore, can be discharged directly into the extracellular space.

The varicosities of postganglionic sympathetic axons contain a mixed population of small clear vesicles about 40 to 60 nm in diameter, as well as small dense-core vesicles of about the same size (Fig. 5–10*C*) (Grillo and Palay, 1962; Richardson, 1962, 1964). Autoradiographic evidence suggests that norepinephrine is stored in the small dense-core vesicles and sympathetic varicosities exhibit a catecholamine-induced fluorescence (Wolfe et al., 1962) (discussed earlier in the section on fluorescence microscopy). The possibility that the clear vesicles of sympathetic terminals contain acetylcholine has been discussed, but recent studies using potassium permanganate fixation have shown that most of the vesicles retain a dense core after this treatment (Fig. 5–10*C*) (Richardson, 1964, 1966; Hökfelt, 1969). This suggests that large numbers of clear vesicles in sympathetic boutons may represent artifacts. It is possible that the few vesicles that remain clear after potassium permanganate fixation are norepinephrine-type vesicles that are only partially filled or have been depleted physiologically (Tranzer and Thoenen, 1967a). It should be pointed out, however, that acetylcholinesterase activity has been demonstrated along the surface of sympathetic axons and varicosities containing dense-core vesicles in the pineal gland of the rat (Eränkö et al., 1970).

It is generally assumed that the cell body is a

source of the newly formed norepinephrine, but the axonal terminals have an important function in conserving this neurotransmitter. Biochemical and pharmacologic evidence shows that norepinephrine released by sympathetic nerve terminals is then picked up by the same axons to help to replenish their supply (Axelrod, 1971). The importance of the axon in the uptake of substances is illustrated by autoradiographic studies of sympathetic neurons in tissue culture labeled with tritiated norepinephrine (England and Goldstein, 1969). A denser concentration of label was found over the axons than over the cell bodies. 5-Hydroxydopamine, a compound that increases the density of vesicles in catecholamine nerve terminals in the cat when administered intraperitoneally, is also picked up by sympathetic nerve terminals in tissue culture (Tranzer and Thoenen, 1967b; Holtzman et al., 1973). These data suggest that some dense-core vesicles are formed in the terminals, as well as in the perikaryon. Recent electron microscopic studies of sympathetic axonal growth cones grown in tissue culture support this assumption and indicate that the agranular reticulum of the axon takes part in dense-core vesicle formation (Bunge, 1973; Teichberg and Holtzman, 1973).

The sympathetic innervation to the iris and pineal gland provides a model system for studying the anatomical, physiologic, and pharmacologic characteristics of norepinephrine nerve terminals by fluorescence and electron microscopy. Administration of appropriate doses of reserpine to an animal depletes norepinephrine in these axons and results in degeneration of the dense-core vesicles (Fig. 5–10*D*) (Pellegrino de Iraldi et al., 1965; Duffy and Markesbery, 1970). Irises depleted of catecholamines by reserpine have been used to study the uptake of substances that may act as "false transmitters," such as α-methyl norepinephrine, 5-hydroxydopamine, and tetrahydroisoquinolines (Hökfelt, 1968; Tranzer et al., 1969; Cohen et al., 1972; Tennyson et al., 1973). These compounds refill the depleted vesicles with a dense core, thereby demonstrating the incorporation of the false transmitter. The tetrahydroisoquinolines, which are formed in vitro by the condensation of acetaldehyde and catecholamines, may be involved in some of the manifestations of alcoholism (Cohen et al., 1972; Tennyson et al., 1973).

It is beyond the scope of this chapter to

describe the fine structure of the peripheral sensory nerve endings of the dorsal root neurons; for this the reader is referred to the following studies: pacinian corpuscle (Pease and Quilliam, 1957), Merkel's corpuscle (Munger, 1965), neuromuscular spindle (Chapter 8 of this volume; Scalzi and Price, 1972; Banker and Girvin, 1972; Karlsson, 1972).

Parasympathetic Ganglia

The terminal ganglia of the parasympathetic nervous system exhibit certain differences in their fine structure from those of other ganglia. In the myenteric plexus of the ileum, the ganglia consist of a compact group of nerve cell bodies and their nerve plexuses, which are isolated from the surrounding connective tissue and blood vessels by a basement membrane (Gabella, 1972). The ganglion lacks large areas of extracellular space, such as is found in sympathetic and dorsal root ganglia. Moreover, parasympathetic ganglia do not have a complete capsular ensheathment. A portion of the surface of many of the large neurons lies at the edge of the ganglion immediately adjacent to the basement membrane facing the extracellular space. Many of the axons in the ganglion exhibit synapses "en passant" (Gabella, 1972). A large population of the synapses in terminal ganglia have clear spherical vesicles and form junctions on the cell bodies (Taxi, 1959, 1965; Gabella, 1972). The parasympathetic nerve terminals to the sphincter pupillae muscle of the rabbit iris are uniformly populated with clear vesicles (Richardson, 1964). Similar cholinergic axons and boutons in the guinea pig heart show end product of acetylcholinesterase activity at their surfaces after cytochemical incubation (Hirano and Ogawa, 1967). There are a number of other types of boutons in terminal ganglia. Some of the axonal varicosities contain flattened clear vesicles. Spherical clear vesicles have been associated with excitatory synapses, whereas flattened vesicles are linked to inhibitory synapses (Bodian, 1966). Boutons with a mixture of clear vesicles and the large, moderately dense-core granule are common in terminal ganglia. In addition, typical sympathetic varicosities containing small dense-core vesicles are found that innervate approximately half the neurons in the myenteric ganglion (Gabella, 1972).

Alterations in Ganglion Cells

Profuse chromatolytic changes appear in spinal ganglia following section or crush of the peripheral spinal nerve (see Scharf, 1958; Carmel and Stein, 1969, for references to early literature) and in sympathetic ganglia after section of the postganglionic nerves (see Stöhr, 1957, for review). Chromatolytic cells are swollen and have eccentric nuclei and pale cytoplasm with the Nissl substance displaced to the periphery. Chromatolytic changes can be produced by irradiation of an animal or of ganglion cells grown in tissue culture (Andres, 1963a; Pick, 1965; Masurovsky et al., 1967). When chromatolytic neurons are examined by electron microscopy (Smith, 1961; Andres, 1961b, 1963a; Pannese, 1963; Härkönen, 1964; Mackey et al., 1964; Holtzman et al., 1967; Lentz, 1967; Masurovsky et al., 1967; Zelená, 1971; Matthews and Raisman, 1972), the following changes have been found depending on the cell and the stage of chromatolysis. The nucleus may be indented, and there may be nucleolar changes and margination of the nuclear chromatin. The clear central zone seen by light microscopy often has large collections of dense bodies and a prominent Golgi apparatus. The peripherally displaced Nissl substance usually consists of swollen cisternae of endoplasmic reticulum, which are randomly oriented and have few attached ribosomes. Instead of the normal polyribosomal clusters consisting of multiple ribosomal units in close aggregation, single ribosomes (probably the result of disintegration of the polyribosomes) are common in the intervening cytoplasm. It is generally accepted that polyribosomes are the functioning protein synthesizing unit rather than the single free ribosome. There is often a marked increase in vacuoles, lipofuscin granules, autophagic vacuoles, and membranous bodies. The autophagic bodies contain the lysosomal enzyme, acid phosphatase (Holtzman et al., 1967). Unusually large mitochondria and abnormal accumulations of filaments and glycogen occur in some cells.

The axon also exhibits changes after section or crush. With the exception of the granular endoplasmic reticulum, many components of the perikaryon leave it and traverse the axon by the process of axonal flow (see Chapter 12 for details). The organelles collect in the swollen portion of the axon proximal to the nerve section or crush. Histo-

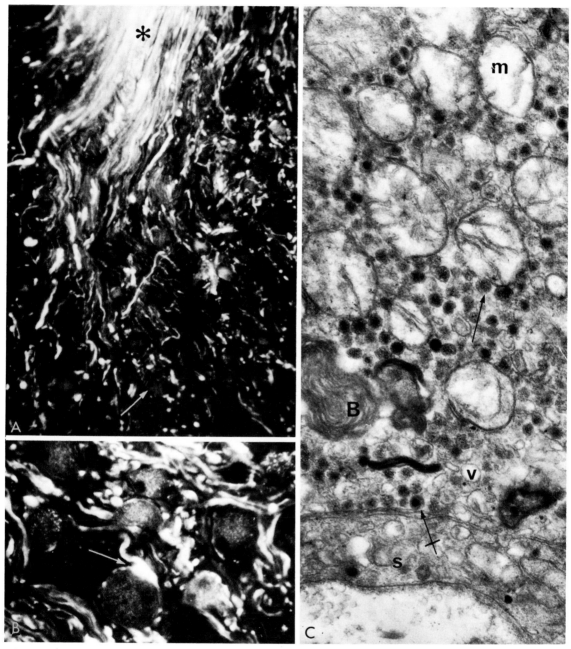

Figure 5–11 Parts *A* and *B* are fluorescence micrographs; *C* is an electron micrograph showing the effects of ligation of the sympathetic nerve trunks of the cat just proximal to the entrance into the carotid canal. (Courtesy of Drs. Robert E. Barrett and Adam Bender). *A.* The large bundle of intensely fluorescent axons (*) is about 1.0 mm proximal to the site of the ligature of the sympathetic trunk. Scattered fluorescent axons and some weakly fluorescent cell bodies (arrow) are nearer to the ganglion. × 150. *B.* There is only weak to moderate fluorescence in the sympathetic perikarya, but there is intense fluorescence in the axon hillock (arrow), in the initial axonal segment, and in other nerve fibers in the ganglion. × 370. *C.* About 0.5 mm from the ligature, the axons are grossly swollen. They contain swollen mitochondria (m) having few disarranged cristae, multilaminar bodies (B), clear vesicles (v), agranular reticulum, and large granular vesicles having a moderately dense (arrow) or very dense (crossed arrow) core. Schwann cell (s). × 38,000.

chemical studies have demonstrated acetyl-cholinesterase and norepinephrine (Lubińska, 1964; Härkönen, 1964; Dahlström, 1965; Kapeller and Mayor, 1967; Jacobowitz and Woodward, 1968). Electron microscopic studies of the proximal nerve stump reveal accumulations of vesicles, agranular reticulum, enlarged mitochondria, heterogeneous bodies, tangled filaments, and in sympathetic axons, large and small dense-core vesicles (Andres, 1963b; Holtzman and Novikoff, 1965; Kapeller and Mayor, 1967; Zelená, 1968; Zelená et al., 1968; Matthews and Raisman, 1972; Matthews, 1973). The changes that take place in the sympathetic ganglion and its trunk after ligation of the trunk close to the carotid canal are illustrated by fluorescence microscopy and electron microscopy (Fig. 5–11). On the second postoperative day, most of the neural peri-karya showed a decreased fluorescence intensity, although intensely fluorescent material was present in the axon hillock and in axons throughout the ganglia (Fig. 5–11B). There were scattered fluorescent axons along the postganglionic nerve trunk up to about 1.5 mm from the constriction, where there was an enormous accumulation of fluorescent material in all axons visible (Fig. 5–11A). This massive amount of fluorescence was present up to the ligature. Axons 0.5 mm proximal to the constriction contained swollen mitochondria, heterogeneous multilaminated bodies, vesicles, agranular reticulum, and large dense core granules about 100 to 120 nm in diameter (Fig. 5–11C). The material in the core varied from moderately dense to very dense.

DEVELOPING GANGLION CELLS

Embryonic Dorsal Root Ganglia

Dorsal root and sympathetic nerve cells and their sheaths originate from the neural crest, i.e., a wedge-shaped group of cells found in the dorsal midline of the neural tube just after closure of the neural folds in the trunk region of the embryo (see reviews by Hörstadius, 1950, and Weston, 1970). The dorsal root neuroblast starts to migrate ventrally to its position lateral to the neural tube during day 9 of gestation in the rabbit (Fig. 5–12A) (Tennyson, 1965, 1970a). These cells appear to be undifferentiated. Early somites appear to play a role in the differentiation of the migrating neural crest derivatives into neuroblasts. Spinal ganglia from early chick embryos will differentiate and form myelinated nerves in vitro only when somites are included in the explant (Peterson and Murray, 1955). By day 10 of gestation in the rabbit, the primordia of the dorsal root ganglia contain a few spindle-shaped neuroblasts that have neurites extending from opposite poles of the cells. Poly-ribosomes are abundant in the cytoplasm of these bipolar neuroblasts, but initially there is little granular endoplasmic reticulum. Presumptive sheath cells are present, but they too are undifferentiated and do not encircle the neuroblast. The growth cone of the centrally directed axon enters the dorsal portion of the neural tube at this stage. The axonal growth cone has a central core and thin veil-like filopodial processes in vitro (Pomerat et al., 1967). The bulbous core contains mitochondria, agranular reticulum, microtubules, neurofilaments, and heterogeneous dense bodies, whereas the filopodial process is filled with a finely filamentous matrix material (Tennyson, 1970a, b).

Similar filamentous material has been seen in the filopodia of dorsal root neurons and sympathetic neurons grown in tissue culture (Yamada et al., 1971; Bunge, 1973). The filamentous material is made up of microfilaments, which are probably responsible for the locomotory behavior of the undulating filopodium of the growth cone (Yamada et al., 1971). Treatment of tissue cultures with cytochalasin B, which alters the fine structure of the microfilaments, also changes the shape of the filopodium and prevents axonal elongation (Yamada et al., 1971). As the neuroblast matures, cytoplasm accumulates in the cell center and the cell assumes a bell shape. The nucleus is eccentric, and the neurites exit from the opposite side of the perikaryon, but close to each other. There is a considerable increase in granular endoplasmic reticulum, and a conspicuous Golgi complex occupies the cell center. The presumptive satellite cells are star-shaped and fill the interstices between the neuroblasts. The ganglion is almost a continuous epithelium at this stage. The processes of a single satellite cell are apposed to several neuroblasts. The unipolar process of the young neuron arises by constriction and elongation of the base of the perikaryon adjacent to the exiting neurites (Cajal, 1909).

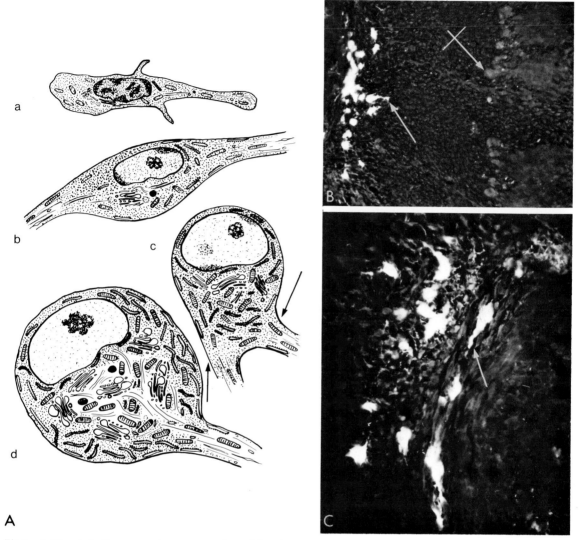

Figure 5–12 *A.* A diagrammatic representation of the changes occurring during the differentiation of the neuroblast of the dorsal root ganglion of the embryonic rabbit. (a) Presumptive neuroblast migrating from the neural crest. (b) Spindle-shaped bipolar neuroblast, which is found in the primordium of the ganglion. (c) Bell-shaped bipolar neuroblast. A constriction occurs (arrows) resulting in the formation of the unipolar process. (d) Early unipolar neuron. (From Tennyson, V. M.: Electron microscopic study of the developing neuroblast of the dorsal root ganglion of the rabbit embryo. J. Comp. Neurol. *124*:267, 1965. Reprinted by permission.) *B.* A sagittal section showing a collection of fluorescent cells (arrow) dorsolateral to the aorta in an 11 day gestation rabbit. Dorsal root ganglia and their emerging peripheral axons (crossed arrow) lie dorsal to fluorescent cells. (Courtesy of Dr. Catherine Mytilineou.) × 215. *C.* The elongated perikaryon of the sympathoblast extends out into processes (arrow). The nucleus is obscured by the intense cytoplasmic fluorescence. Rabbit, 11 days' gestation. (Courtesy of Dr. Catherine Mytilineou.) × 550.

The original neurites, therefore, become the bifurcations of the unipolar process. By the time the unipolar process has emerged, one or more satellite cells are related to a single neuron and form a sheath completely surrounding the perikaryon.

Two topographically distinct cell groups can be recognized in the dorsal root ganglion of the chick at the end of day 8 of incubation (Hamburger and Levi-Montalcini, 1949). There are large lightly staining neurons in the cup-shaped ventrolateral region and small darker staining neurons in a mediodorsal position. Amputation of the limb bud in three-day chick embryos results in massive degeneration of the ventrolateral neurons, but only moderate atrophy of the mediodorsal cells (Levi-Montalcini, 1966).

Embryonic Sympathetic Ganglia

Sympathetic neuroblasts (sympathoblasts) migrate from the neural crest of the chick a few hours earlier than the dorsal root neuroblasts (Levi-Montalcini, 1966). They migrate ventrally and form two columns of cells, the primary sympathetic chains, which are located along the dorsolateral aspect of the aorta. After further migration and differentiation, these cells give rise to the anlage of the sympathetic ganglia (the secondary sympathetic chain), the paraganglia (chromaffin tissue), and the adrenal medulla. The anlagen are formed during a very short period in embryonic life. In the human, primitive fluorescing sympathetic tissue is present as early as seven weeks of gestation (Hervonen, 1971). Within the next two weeks, fluorescing cells form primitive ovoid paraganglia. At the end of this period fluorescing cells invade the cords of presumptive adrenal cortical tissue (Hervonen, 1971). The paraganglia are prominent during fetal life, but they undergo fibrotic degeneration in the human shortly after birth (Brundin, 1966).

Sympathoblasts do not exhibit catecholamine fluorescence in the neural crest or during their initial ventral migration, but they are fluorescent in the region of the primary sympathetic chain (Enemar et al., 1965; de Champlain et al., 1970; Cohen, 1972; Mytilineou, 1973). The primary sympathetic chain of an 11 day gestation rabbit is illustrated in the fluorescence micrograph (Fig. 5–12B). The cells have elongated cell bodies and short axons (Fig. 5–10C). Biochemical assays of chick embryos have shown that the catecholamine present is norepinephrine (Enemar et al., 1965). The enzymes involved in norepinephrine synthesis are induced in the chick in the sequence needed for the proper metabolic step in the biosynthetic pathway (Ignarro and Shideman, 1968). The first enzyme needed, i.e., tyrosine hydroxylase, is present well before the neural crest can be recognized as a morphologic entity. Aromatic-L-amino acid decarboxylase appears after the sympathoblasts have started to migrate. Dopamine-β-oxidase appears by the time the primary sympathetic chain is formed and when fluorescence can first be detected (Ignarro and Shideman, 1968). Cohen (1972) has shown by ablation experiments that somites, and to some extent the ventral neural tube, promote the differentiation of neural crest cells into catecholamine-containing cells.

The sympathoblasts of the primary sympathetic chain collect in groups near the segmental aortic branches and develop into segmental enlargements. At first, only thin strands of fluorescent cells and fibers extend dorsally from the chain toward the dorsal root ganglia; then accumulations of cells migrate along the same route and come to rest near the ventral ramus of the spinal nerve where they form the secondary sympathetic chain (the primordia of the adult sympathetic chain ganglia). As the sympathoblasts mature, they develop long fluorescent axons that run in the intercostal nerves. The sympathetic trunk also contains fluorescent axons during the early period of fetal life (Enemar et al., 1965; de Champlain et al., 1970; Mytilineou, 1973). Presumably, large amounts of catecholamines are transported at this time through the axoplasm to the terminals. The fluorescence intensity decreases in the sympathetic neurons and their processes with increasing maturation. In the adult, the cells exhibit only a weak to moderate fluorescence, and the axons in the sympathetic trunk usually lack fluorescence. Small intensely fluorescent cells have been reported in sympathetic ganglia of the human fetus and in the postnatal rabbit as shown by fluorescent microscopy (Fig. 5–3C) (Hervonen, 1971; Hervonen and Kanerva, 1972; Mytilineou, 1973).

Ultrastructural studies of sympathetic ganglia in the human fetus have been reported from the thirteenth week to the seventeenth week of gestation, as well as in the chick and the rabbit (Pick et al., 1964; Hervonen and Kanerva, 1972; Wechsler and Schmekel, 1966; Tennyson, 1973). Most of the cells in the primary sympathetic chain are relatively immature. They contain numerous polyribosomes, but little granular endoplasmic reticulum. At first their processes are simple extensions of perikaryal cytoplasm, but with further differentiation, well-defined axons with microtubules and neurofilaments appear. The perikaryon of the sympathoblast contains centrioles, lysosomes, mitochondria, and a small Golgi complex. Unlike the dorsal root neuroblast, the sympathoblast has large numbers of large and small dense-core vesicles. As the cells mature, they become globular with eccentric nuclei. Immature dendrites appear. At this stage the ganglion consists of closely packed epithelial cells, many of which are linked by desmosomes. The dense-core vesicles persist in the perikarya at this stage, but they become sparser as the sympathoblast develops into a young nerve cell with a complete satellite sheath. Presumably, the dense-core vesicles have been transported to the axonal endings. Dense-core vesicles have been reported in growth cones of cultured sympathetic neurons, but at least some of them appear to be formed locally (Bunge, 1973). Large quantities of agranular reticulum are also present in the growth cone; these structures may play a role in the assembly or degradation of the surface membrane of the filopodia. A few primitive synaptic junctions have been seen in sympathetic ganglia of the human at 15 weeks and 17 weeks of gestation and in the late fetal rabbit (Pick et al., 1964; Hervonen and Kanerva, 1972; Tennyson, 1973). The small intensely fluorescent cell has been identified ultrastructurally in the human fetal sympathetic ganglion (Hervonen and Kanerva, 1972). These cells contain very large 200 to 300 nm dense-core vesicles.

Alterations in Young Neurons

Nerve growth factor, a protein isolated from the mouse salivary gland, causes hypertrophic and hyperplastic responses of sensory and sympathetic ganglia when injected into chick embryos (Levi-Montalcini, 1966). Immunosympathectomy, i.e., treatment of newborn mice with antisera to nerve growth factor, results in destruction of some of the sympathetic neuroblasts by affecting the nuclear and nucleolar compartments (Levi-Montalcini et al., 1969).

Newborn animals are more sensitive to some drugs than adult animals. Although 6-hydroxydopamine causes a dramatic degeneration of sympathetic nerve terminals in the adult, apparently it does not damage the perikarya (Tranzer and Thoenen, 1968). Administration of this drug to newborn animals, on the other hand, results in the permanent destruction of sympathetic nerve cells (Angeletti and Levi-Montalcini, 1970). Cytoplasmic vacuolization appears in the more differentiated cells as an early change, but after one week, all nerve cells are destroyed.

The adrenergic blocking agent, bretylium tosylate, also results in degenerative changes in neonatal sympathetic neurons, but discontinuation of the treatment is followed by partial recovery (Caramía et al., 1972). The altered neurons contain enormously enlarged mitochondria, which appear almost empty.

REFERENCES

Andres, K. H.: Untersuchungen über den Feinbau von Spinalganglien. Z. Zellforsch. Mikrosk. Anat., 55:1, 1961a.

Andres, K. H.: Untersuchungen über morphologische Veränderungen in Spinalganglien während der retrograden Degeneration. Z. Zellforsch. Mikrosk. Anat., 55:49, 1961b.

Andres, K. H.: Elektronenmikroskopische Untersuchungen über Strukturveränderungen im Zytoplasma von Spinalganglienzellen der Ratte nach Bestrahlung mit 185 MEV-Protonen. Z. Zellforsch. Mikrosk. Anat., 60:633, 1963a.

Andres, K. H.: Elektronenmikroskopische Untersuchungen über. Strukturveränderungen an den Nervenfasern in Rattenspinalganglien nach Bestrahlung mit 185 MeV-Protonen. Z. Zellforsch. Mikrosk. Anat., 61:1, 1963b.

Angeletti, P. U., and Levi-Montalcini, R.: Sympathetic nerve cell destruction in newborn mammals by 6-hydroxydopamine. Proc. Natl. Acad. Sci. U.S.A., 65:114, 1970.

Axelrod, J.: Noradrenaline: Fate and control of its biosynthesis. Science, 173:598, 1971.

Banker, B. Q., and Girvin, J. P.: The ultrastructural features of the normal and de-efferented mammalian muscle spindle. In Banker, B. Q., Przybylski, R. J., Van der Meulen, J. P., and Victor, M. eds.: Research in Muscle Development and the Muscle Spindle. Princeton, N. J.: Excerpta Medica Foundation, 1972, pp. 267–296.

Björklund, A., Cegrell, L., Falk, B., Ritzén, M., and Rosengren, E.: Dopamine-containing cells in sympathetic ganglia. Acta Physiol. Scand., 78:334, 1970.

Bodian, D.: Synaptic types on spinal motoneurons: An electron microscopic study. Bull. Johns Hopkins Hosp., 119:16, 1966.

Brundin, T.: Studies on the preaortal paraganglia of newborn rabbits. Acta Physiol. Scand., 70:5, Suppl. 290, 1966.

Brzin, M., Tennyson, V. M., and Duffy, P.: Acetylcholinesterase in frog sympathetic and dorsal root ganglia. A study by electron microscope cytochemistry and microgasometric analysis with the magnetic diver. J. Cell Biol., 31:215, 1966.

Bunge, M. B.: Fine structure of nerve fibers and growth cones of isolated sympathetic neurons in culture. J. Cell Biol., 56:713, 1973.

Bunge, M. B., Bunge, R. P., Peterson, E. R., and Murray, M. R.: A light and electron microscope study of long-term organized cultures of rat dorsal root ganglia. J. Cell Biol., 32:439, 1967.

Burdman, J. A.: Uptake of [³H] catecholamines by chick embryo sympathetic ganglia in tissue culture. J. Neurochem., 15:1321, 1968.

Cajal, S. Ramón y.: Histologie du Systèm Nerveux de l'Homme et des Vertébrés. Vol. I. 1909. Translated by Azoulay, L. Paris, Maloine, 1952, pp. 420–460.

Caramía, F., Angeletti, P. U., Levi-Montalcini, R., and

Carratelli, L.: Mitochondrial lesions of developing sympathetic neurons induced by bretylium tosylate. Brain Res., *40*:237, 1972.

Carmel, P. W., and Stein, B.: Cell changes in sensory ganglia following proximal and distal nerve section in the monkey. J. Comp. Neurol., *135*:145, 1969.

Cervós-Navarro, J.: Elektronenmikroskopische Untersuchungen an Spinalganglien. I. Nervenzellen. Arch. Psychiat. Z. Gesamte Neurol., *199*:643, 1959.

Cervós-Navarro, J.: Elektronenmikroskopische Untersuchungen an Spinalganglien. II. Satellitenzellen. Arch. Psychiat. Z. Gesamte Neurol., *200*:267, 1960.

Citkowitz, E., and Holtzman, E.: Peroxisomes in dorsal root ganglia. J. Histochem. Cytochem. *21*:34, 1973.

Cohen, A. M.: Factors directing the expression of sympathetic nerve traits in cells of neural crest origin. J. Exp. Zool., *179*:167, 1972.

Cohen, G., Mytilineou, C., and Barrett, R.: 6,7-Dihydroxytetrahydroisoquinoline: Uptake and storage by peripheral sympathetic nerve of the rat. Science, *175*:1269, 1972.

Crosby, E. C., Humphrey, T., and Lauer, E.: Correlative Anatomy of the Nervous System. New York, Macmillan, 1962, pp. 14–19.

Dahlström, A.: Observations on the accumulation of noradrenaline in the proximal and distal parts of peripheral adrenergic nerves after compression. J. Anat., *99*:677, 1965.

de Champlain, J., Malmfors, T., Olson, L., and Sachs, C.: Ontogenesis of peripheral adrenergic neurons in the rat: Pre- and postnatal observations. Acta Physiol. Scand., *80*:276, 1970.

de Lorenzo, A. J.: The fine structure of synapses in the ciliary ganglion of the chick. J. Biophys. Biochem. Cytol., *7*:31, 1960.

Duffy, P. E., and Markesbery, W. R.: Granulated vesicles in sympathetic nerve endings in the pineal gland: Observations on the effects of pharmacologic agents by electron microscopy. Am. J. Anat., *128*:97, 1970.

Elfvin, L. G.: The ultrastructure of the superior cervical sympathetic ganglion of the cat. I. The structure of the ganglion cell processes as studied by serial sections. J. Ultrastruct. Res., *8*:403, 1963a.

Elfvin, L. G.: The ultrastructure of the superior cervical sympathetic ganglion of the cat. II. The structure of the preganglionic end fibers and the synapses as studied by serial sections. J. Ultrastruct. Res., *8*:441, 1963b.

Enemar, A., Falck, B., and Håkanson, R.: Observations on the appearance of norepinephrine in the sympathetic nervous system of the chick embryo. Dev. Biol., *11*:268, 1965.

England, J. M., and Goldstein, M. N.: The uptake and localization of catecholamines in chick embryo sympathetic neurons in tissue culture. J. Cell Sci., *4*:677, 1969.

Eränkö, L., and Eränkö, O.: Effects of hydrocortisone on histochemically demonstrable catecholamines in the sympathetic ganglia and extra-adrenal chromaffin tissue of the rat. Acta Physiol. Scand., *84*:125, 1972.

Eränkö, O., and Härkönen, M.: Histochemical demonstration of fluorogenic amines in the cytoplasm of sympathetic ganglion cells of the rat. Acta Physiol. Scand., *58*:285, 1963.

Eränkö, O., Rechardt, L., Eränkö, L., and Cunningham, A.: Light and electron microscopic histochemical observations on cholinesterase-containing sympathetic nerve fibers in the pineal body of the rat. Histochem. J., *2*:479, 1970.

Euler, U. S., von: Noradrenaline. Chemistry, Physiology, Pharmacology and Clinical Aspects. Springfield, Ill., Charles C Thomas, 1956. pp. 133–168.

Euler, U. S., von: Adrenergic neurotransmitter functions. Science, *173*:202, 1971.

Falck, B.: Observations on the possibilities of the cellular localization of monoamines by a fluorescence method. Acta Physiol. Scand., *56*:Suppl. 197, 1, 1962.

Falck, B., Hillarp, N. Å., Thieme, G., and Torp, A.: Fluorescence of catecholamines and related compounds condensed with formaldehyde. J. Histochem. Cytochem., *10*:348, 1962.

Fukuda, T., and Koelle, G.: The cytological localization of intracellular neuronal acetylcholinesterase. J. Biophys. Biochem. Cytol., *5*:433, 1959.

Gabella, G.: Fine structure of the myenteric plexus in the guinea-pig ileum. J. Anat., *111*:69, 1972.

Grillo, M.: Electron microscopy of sympathetic tissues. Pharmacol. Rev., *18*:387, 1966.

Grillo, M.: Cytoplasmic inclusions resembling nucleoli in sympathetic neurons of adult rats. J. Cell Biol., *45*:100, 1970.

Grillo, M., and Palay, S. L.: Granule-containing vesicles in the autonomic nervous system. *In* Breese, S. S. (ed.): Electron Microscopy. New York, Academic Press, 1962, Vol. 2, p. U-1.

Ha, H.: Axonal bifurcation in the dorsal root ganglion of the cat. A light and electron microscopic study. J. Comp. Neurol., *140*:227, 1970.

Häggqvist, G., and Lindberg, J.: Über die Grösse der Kerne resp. Zellen in den Spinalganglien. Z. Mikrosk. Anat. Forsch., *67*:529, 1961.

Hamburger, V., and Levi-Montalcini, R.: Proliferation, differentiation and degeneration in the spinal ganglia of the chick embryo under normal and experimental conditions. J. Exp. Zool., *111*:457, 1949.

Härkönen, M.: Carboxylic esterases, oxidative enzymes and catecholamines in the superior cervical ganglion of the rat and the effect of pre- and post-ganglionic nerve division. Acta Physiol. Scand., *63*:Suppl. 237, 9, 1964.

Hervonen, A.: Development of catecholamine-storing cells in human fetal paraganglia and adrenal medulla. Acta Physiol. Scand., Suppl. *368*, 3, 1971.

Hervonen, A., and Kanerva, L.: Cell types of human fetal superior cervical ganglion. Z. Anat. Entwicklungsgesch., *137*:257, 1972.

Hirano, H., and Ogawa, K.: Ultrastructural localization of cholinesterase activity in nerve endings in the guinea pig heart. J. Electron Microsc., *16*:313, 1967.

Hökfelt, T.: In vitro studies on central and peripheral monoamine neurons at the ultrastructural level. Z. Zellforsch. Mikrosk. Anat., *91*:1, 1968.

Hökfelt, T.: Distribution of noradrenaline storing particles in peripheral adrenergic neurons as revealed by electron microscopy. Acta Physiol. Scand., *76*:427, 1969.

Holtzman, E., and Novikoff, A. B.: Lysosomes in the rat sciatic nerve following crush. J. Cell Biol., *27*:651, 1965.

Holtzman, E., Novikoff, A. B., and Villaverde, H.: Lysosomes and GERL in normal and chromatolytic neurons of the rat ganglion nodosum. J. Cell Biol., *33*:419, 1967.

Holtzman, E., Teichberg, S., Abrahams, S. J., Citkowitz, E., Crain, S. M., Kawai, N., and Peterson, E. R.: Notes on synaptic vesicles and related structures, endoplasmic reticulum, lysosomes and peroxisomes in nervous tissue and the adrenal medulla. J. Histochem. Cytochem., *21*:349, 1973.

Hörstadius, S.: The Neural Crest. New York, Oxford University Press, 1950.

Ignarro, L. J., and Shideman, F. E.: Appearance and concentrations of catecholamines and their biosynthesis in the embryonic and developing chick. J. Pharmacol. Exp. Ther., *159*:38, 1968.

Jacobowitz, D., and Woodward, J. K.: Adrenergic neurons in the cat superior cervical ganglion and cervical sympathetic nerve trunk. A histochemical study. J. Pharmacol. Exp. Ther., *162*:213, 1968.

Kapeller, K., and Mayor, D.: The accumulation of noradrenaline in constricted sympathetic nerves as studied by fluorescence and electron microscopy. Proc. Roy. Soc. [Biol.] *167*:282, 1967.

Karlsson, U. L.: The frog muscle spindle: Ultrastructure and intrafusal stretch characteristics. *In* Banker, B. Q., Przybylski, R. J., Van der Meulen, J. P., and Victor, M. (eds.): Research in Muscle Development and the Muscle Spindle. Princeton, N.J., Excerpta Medica, 1972, pp. 299–332.

Kása, P., and Csillik, B.: AChE synthesis in cholinergic neurons: electron histochemistry of enzyme translocation. Histochemie, *12*:175, 1968.

Koelle, G. B., and Foroglou-Kerameos, C.: Electron microscopic localization of cholinesterases in a sympathetic ganglion by a gold-thiolacetic acid method. Life Sci., *4*:417, 1965.

Koelle, W. A., and Koelle, G. B.: The localization of external or functional acetylcholinesterase at the synapses of autonomic ganglia. J. Pharmacol. Exp. Ther., *126*:1, 1959.

Kuntz, A.: The Autonomic Nervous System. Philadelphia, Lea & Febiger, 1953, pp. 46–68 and 371–392.

Laverty, R., and Sharman, D. F.: The estimation of small quantities of 3,4-dihydroxy-phenylethylamine in tissues. Br. J. Pharmacol., *24*:538, 1965.

Lentz, T. L.: Fine structure of sensory ganglion cells during limb regeneration of the newt *Triturus.* J. Comp. Neurol., *131*:301, 1967.

Levi-Montalcini, R.: The Nerve Growth Factor: its mode of action on sensory and sympathetic nerve cells. Harvey Lect., Series *60*:217, 1966.

Levi-Montalcini, R., Caramía, F., and Angeletti, P. U.: Alterations in the fine structure of nucleoli in sympathetic neurons following NGF-antiserum treatment. Brain Res., *12*:54, 1969.

Lubińska, L.: Axoplasmic streaming in regenerating and in normal nerve fibers. *In* Singer, M., and Schadé, J. P. (eds.): Mechanisms of Neural Regeneration, Progress in Brain Research. Amsterdam, Elsevier, 1964, Vol. 13, pp. 1–71.

Mackey, E. A., Spiro, D., and Wiener, J.: A study of chromatolysis in dorsal root ganglia at the cellular level. J. Neuropathol. Exp. Neurol., *23*:508, 1964.

Malhotra, S. K.: What is the "Golgi apparatus" in its classical site within the neurons of vetebrates? J. Microsc. Sci., *100*:339, 1959.

Malmfors, T.: Studies on adrenergic nerves. Acta Physiol. Scand., *64*:Suppl. 248, 1, 1965.

Malmfors, T., and Sachs, C.: Degeneration of adrenergic nerves produced by 6-hydroxydopamine. Eur. J. Pharmacol., *3*:89, 1968.

Masurovsky, E. B., Benitez, H. H., Kim, S. U., and Murray, M. R.: Origin, development, and nature of intranuclear rodlets and associated bodies in chicken sympathetic neurons. J. Cell Biol., *44*:172, 1970.

Masurovsky, E. B., Benitez, H. H., and Murray, M. R.: Development of interneurons in long-term, organotypic cultures of rat superior cervical and stellate ganglia. J. Cell Biol., *55*:166a, 1972 abs.

Masurovsky, E. B., Bunge, M. B., and Bunge, R. P.: Cytological studies of organotypic cultures of rat dorsal root ganglia following x-radiation in vitro. I. Changes in neurons and satellite cells. J. Cell Biol., *32*:467, 1967.

Matthews, M. R.: An ultrastructural study of axonal changes following constriction of postganglionic branches of the superior cervical ganglion in the rat. Philos. Trans. R. Soc. Lond. [Biol. Sci.], *264*:479, 1973.

Matthews, M. R., and Raisman, G.: The ultrastructure and somatic efferent synapses of small granule-containing cells in the superior cervical ganglion. J. Anat., *105*:255, 1969.

Matthews, M. R., and Raisman, G.: A light and electron microscopic study of the cellular response to axonal injury in the superior cervical ganglion of the rat. Proc. R. Soc. Lond. [Biol.], *181*:43, 1972.

Munger, B. L., and Roth, S. I.: The intraepidermal innervation of the snout skin of the opossum. A light and electron microscope study, with observations on the nature of Merkel's *Tastzellen.* J. Cell Biol., *26*:79, 1965.

Mytilineou, C.: Fluorescence microscopic studies of sympathetic ganglia of the fetal, postnatal, and adult rabbit. Anat. Rec., *175*:395, 1973.

Mytilineou, C., Issidorides, M., and Shanklin, W. M.: Histochemical reactions of human autonomic ganglia. J. Anat., *97*:533, 1963.

Nachmansohn, D.: Proteins in excitable membranes. Science, *168*:1059, 1970.

Norberg, K. A., and Hamberger, B.: The sympathetic adrenergic neuron. Acta Physiol. Scand., *63*:Suppl. 238, 1964.

Norberg, K. A., Ritzén, M., and Ungerstedt, U.: Histochemical studies on a special catecholamine-containing cell type in sympathetic ganglia. Acta Physiol. Scand., *67*:260, 1966.

Novikoff, A. B., Quintana, N., Villaverde, H., and Forschirm, R.: Nucleoside phosphatase and cholinesterase activities in dorsal root ganglia and peripheral nerve. J. Cell Biol., *29*:525, 1966.

Palay, S. L., and Palade, G. E.: The fine structure of neurons. J. Biophys. Biochem. Cytol., *1*:69, 1955.

Pannese, E.: Observations on the morphology, submicroscopic structure and biological properties of satellite cells (S.C.) in sensory ganglia of mammals. Z. Zellforsch. Mikrosk. Anat., *52*:567, 1960.

Pannese, E.: Investigations on the ultrastructural changes of the spinal ganglion neurons in the course of axon regeneration and cell hypertrophy. II. Changes during cell hypertrophy and comparison between the ultrastructure of nerve cells of the same type under different functional conditions. Z. Zellforsch. Mikrosk. Anat., *61*:561, 1963.

Pannese, E.: Unusual membrane-particle complexes within nerve cells of the spinal ganglia. J. Ultrastruct. Res., *29*:334, 1969.

Pease, D. C., and Quilliam, T. A.: Electron microscopy of the Pacinian corpuscle. J. Biophys. Biochem. Cytol., *3*:331, 1957.

Pellegrino de Iraldi, A., Zieher, L. M., and De Robertis, E.: Ultrastructure and pharmacological studies of nerve endings in the pineal organ. *In* Kappers, J. A., and Schadé, J. P. (eds.): Structure and Function of the Epiphysis Cerebri, Progress in Brain Research. New York, Elsevier, 1965, Vol. 10, pp. 389–422.

Peters, A., Palay, S. L., and Webster, H. de F.: The Fine Structure of the Nervous System. New York, Harper & Row, 1970.

Peterson, E. R., and Murray, M. R.: Myelin sheath formation in cultures of avian spinal ganglia. Am. J. Anat., 96:319, 1955.

Pick, J. P.: The fine structure of sympathetic neurons in x-irradiated frogs. J. Cell Biol., 26:335, 1965.

Pick, J.: Pigment, abnormal mitochondria and laminar bodies in human sympathetic neurons. Z. Zellforsch. Mikrosk. Anat., 82:118, 1967.

Pick, J.: The Autonomic Nervous System. Morphological, Comparative, Clinical and Surgical Aspects. Philadelphia, J. B. Lippincott, 1970.

Pick, J., Gerdin, C., and Delemos, C.: An electron microscopical study of developing sympathetic neurons in man. Z. Zellforsch. Mikrosk. Anat., 62:402, 1964.

Pineda, A., Maxwell, D. S., and Kruger, L.: The fine structure of neurons and satellite cells in the trigeminal ganglion of cat and monkey. Am. J. Anat., 121:461, 1967.

Pomerat, C. M., Hendelman, W. J., Raiborn, C. W., Jr., and Massey, J. F.: Dynamic activities of nervous tissue in vitro. In Hydén, H. (ed.): The Neuron. New York, Elsevier, 1967, pp. 119–178.

Ralston, H. J., III.: The fine structure of neurons in the dorsal horn of the cat spinal cord. J. Comp. Neurol., 132:275, 1968a.

Ralston, H. J., III.: Dorsal root projections to dorsal horn neurons in the cat spinal cord. J. Comp. Neurol., 132:303, 1968b.

Richardson, K. C.: The fine structure of autonomic nerve endings in smooth muscle of the rat vas deferens. J. Anat., 96:427, 1962.

Richardson, K. C.: The fine structure of the albino rabbit iris with special reference to the identification of adrenergic and cholinergic nerves and nerve endings in its intrinsic muscles. Am. J. Anat., 114:173, 1964.

Richardson, K. C.: Electron microscopic identification of autonomic nerve endings. Nature (Lond.), 210:756, 1966.

Richardson, K. C.: The fine structure of autonomic nerves after vital staining with methylene blue. Anat. Rec., 164:359, 1969.

Rosenbluth, J.: Subsurface cisterns and their relationship to the neuronal plasma membrane. J. Cell Biol., 13:405, 1962.

Rosenbluth, J.: Contrast between osmium-fixed and permanganate-fixed toad spinal ganglia. J. Cell Biol., 16:143, 1963.

Rosenbluth, J., and Wissig, S. L.: The distribution of exogenous ferritin in toad spinal ganglia and the mechanism of its uptake by neurons. J. Cell Biol., 23:307, 1964.

Sano, Y., Odake, G., and Yonezawa, T.: Fluorescence microscopic observations of catecholamines in cultures of the sympathetic chains. Z. Zellforsch. Mikrosk. Anat., 80:345, 1967.

Scalzi, H. A., and Price, H. M.: Electron-microscopic observations of the sensory region of the mammalian muscle spindle. In Banker, B. Q., Przybylski, R. J., Van der Meulen, J. P., and Victor, M. (eds.): Research in Muscle Development and the Muscle Spindle. Princeton, N.J., Excerpta Medica, 1972, pp. 254–263.

Scharf, J. H.: Sensible Ganglien. In Handbuch der mikroskopischen Anatomie des Menschen. Vol. 4, pt. 3. Berlin, Springer-Verlag, 1958.

Schlaepfer, W. W.: Acetylcholinesterase activity of motor and sensory nerve fibers in the spinal nerve roots of the rat. Z. Zellforsch. Mikrosk. Anat., 88:441, 1968.

Schlaepfer, W. W., and Torack, R. M.: The ultrastructural localization of cholinesterase activity in the sciatic nerve of the rat. J. Histochem. Cytochem., 14:369, 1966.

Siegrist, G., Dolivo, M., Dunant, Y., Foroglou-Kerameos, C., de Ribaupierre, F., and Rouiller, C.: Ultrastructure and function of the chromaffin cells in the superior cervical ganglion of the rat. J. Ultrastruct. Res., 25:381–407, 1968.

Smith, K.: The fine structure of neurons of dorsal root ganglia after stimulating or cutting the sciatic nerve. J. Comp. Neurol., 116:103, 1961.

Spencer, P. S., Raine, C. S., and Wisniewski, H.: Axon diameter and myelin thickness—unusual relationships in dorsal root ganglia. Anat. Rec., 176:225, 1973.

Stöhr, P., Jr.: Mikroskopische Anatomie des vegetativen Nervensystems. In Handbuch der mikroskopischen Anatomie des Menschen. Vol. 4, pt. 5. Berlin, Springer-Verlag, 1957, pp. 30–103.

Sulkin, N. M.: Histochemical studies of the pigments in human autonomic ganglion cells. J. Gerontol., 8:435, 1953.

Sulkin, N. M., and Kuntz, A.: Histochemical alterations in autonomic ganglion cells associated with aging. J. Gerontol., 7:533, 1952.

Taxi, J.: Sur la structure des travées du plexus d'Auerbach: Confrontation des données fournies par le microscope ordinaire et par le microscope électronique. Ann. Sci. Natur. Zool., Series 12, 571, 1959.

Taxi, J.: Cytologie. Étude de l'ultrastructure des zones synaptiques dans les ganglions sympathiques de la Grenouille. C. R. Acad. Sci., 252:174, 1961.

Taxi, J.: Contribution à l'étude des connexions des neurones moteurs du système nerveux autonome. Ann. Sci. Natur. Zool., 7:413, 1965.

Teichberg, S., and Holtzman, E.: Axonal agranular reticulum and synaptic vesicles in cultured embryonic chick sympathetic neurons. J. Cell Biol., 57:88, 1973.

Tennyson, V. M.: Electron microscopic study of the developing neuroblast of the dorsal root ganglion of the rabbit embryo. J. Comp. Neurol., 124:267, 1965.

Tennyson, V. M.: The fine structure of the axon and growth cone of the dorsal root neuroblast of the rabbit embryo. J. Cell Biol., 44:62, 1970a.

Tennyson, V. M.: The fine structure of the developing nervous system. In Himwich, W. A. (ed.): Developmental Neurobiology. Springfield, Ill., Charles C Thomas, 1970b, pp. 47–116.

Tennyson, V. M.: Ultrastructural studies of sympathetic ganglia of the fetal, postnatal, and adult rabbit. Anat. Rec., 175:456, 1973.

Tennyson, V. M., and Brzin, M.: The appearance of acetylcholinesterase in the dorsal root neuroblast of the rabbit embryo. J. Cell Biol., 46:64, 1970.

Tennyson, V. M., Cohen, G., Mytilineou, C., and Heikkila, R.: 6-7-Dihydroxytetrahydroisoquinoline: Electron microscopic evidence for uptake into the amine-binding vesicles in sympathetic nerves of rat iris and pineal gland. Brain Res., 51:161, 1973.

Tranzer, J. P., and Thoenen, H.: Significance of "empty vesicles" in postganglionic sympathetic nerve terminals. Experientia, 23:123, 1967a.

Tranzer, J. P., and Thoenen, H.: Electronmicroscopic localization of 5-hydroxydopamine (3, 4, 5-trihydroxy-phenyl-ethylamine) a new "false" sympathetic transmitter. Experientia, 23:743, 1967b.

Tranzer, J. P., and Thoenen, H.: An electron microscopic study of selective, acute degeneration of sympathetic nerve terminals after administration of 6-hydroxydopamine. Experientia, 24:155, 1968.

Tranzer, J. P., Thoenen, H., Snipes, R. L., and Richards, J. G.: Recent developments on the ultrastructural aspects of adrenergic nerve endings in various experimental conditions. *In* Akert, K., and Waser, P. G. (eds.): Mechanisms of Synaptic Transmission, Progress in Brain Research. Vol. 31. New York, Elsevier, 1969, pp. 33–46.

Truex, R. C., and Carpenter, M. B.: Human Neuro-anatomy. Baltimore, Williams & Wilkins Co., 1969, pp. 164–172 and 216–235.

Wechsler, W., and Schmekel, L.: Elektronenmikroskopischer Nachweis spezifischer Grana in den Sympathicoblasten der Grenzstrangganglien von Hühnerembryonen. Experientia, *22*:296, 1966.

Weston, J. A.: The migration and differentiation of neural crest cells. *In* Abercrombie, H., Brachet, J., and King, T. (eds.): Advances in Morphogenesis. Vol. 8. New York, Academic Press, 1970, pp. 41–114.

Williams, T. H., and Palay, S. L.: Ultrastructure of the small neurons in the superior cervical ganglion. Brain Res., *15*:17, 1969.

Wolf, A., Cowen, D., and Antopol, W.: Reduction of neotetrazolium in the satellite cells of the cerebrospinal and sympathetic ganglia. J. Neuropathol. Exp. Neurol., *15*:384, 1956.

Wolf, A., and Pappenheimer, A. M.: Occurrence and distribution of acid-fast pigment in the central nervous system. J. Neuropathol. Exp. Neurol., *4*: 402, 1945.

Wolfe, D. E., Potter, L. T., Richardson, K. C., and Axelrod, J.: Localizing tritiated norepinephrine in sympathetic axons by electron microscopic autoradiography. Science, *138*:440, 1962.

Wyburn, G. M.: The capsule of spinal ganglion cells. J. Anat., *92*:528, 1958.

Yamada, K. M., Spooner, B. S., and Wessells, N. K.: Ultrastructure and function of growth cones and axons of cultured nerve cells. J. Cell Biol. *49*:614–635, 1971.

Yamamoto, T.: Some observations on the fine structure of the sympathetic ganglion of bullfrog. J. Cell Biol., *16*:159, 1963.

Zelená, J.: Bidirectional movements of mitochondria along axons of an isolated nerve segment. Z. Zellforsch. Mikrosk. Anat., *92*:186, 1968.

Zelená, J.: Neurofilaments and microtubules in sensory neurons after peripheral nerve section. Z. Zellforsch. Mikrosk. Anat., *117*:191, 1971.

Zelená, J., Lubińska, L., and Gutmann, E.: Accumulation of organelles at the ends of interrupted axons. Z. Zellforsch. Mikrosk. Anat., *91*:200, 1968.

Chapter 6

MICROSCOPIC ANATOMY OF MYELINATED NERVE FIBERS

Albert Bischoff *and* P. K. Thomas

The term "nerve fiber" may denote either the axon or the axon together with its associated satellite cells. Here the latter usage has been adopted. The morphologic peculiarities of nerve fibers relate to their function in transmitting precise information between fixed points in the organism. The information may be transmitted extremely rapidly, as it is in the propagated nerve impulse, in which the velocities range between 1 and 100 m per second. The axon also functions as a chemical transport system so that material can be transported both centrifugally and centripetally. A fast centrifugal system has been identified moving material at a rate of about 410 mm per day, with a slower retrograde rate of 230 mm per day (Ranish and Ochs, 1972). Less clearly defined slower transport of substances occurs (see Chapter 12), and particulate material is also known to move in both directions along axons (Lubińska, 1964), but the concept of a bulk flow of axoplasm, originally propounded by Weiss and Hiscoe (1948), is now open to question (Spencer, 1972). While some of the axonal transport is no doubt concerned with the metabolic maintenance of these very long cell processes, translocation of material along axons is involved in their neurosecretory activity, and axonal transport mechanisms are possibly important in the "trophic" signaling to other cells such as muscle fibers as discussed in Chapter 12.

In mammalian unmyelinated axons, the conduction velocity of the propagated nerve impulse is of the order of 1 m per second. Substantially faster velocities can be achieved in unmyelinated axons, but only if diameter is greatly increased, as in the giant axons of invertebrates. The structural specializations of myelinated axons are largely related to achieving fast conduction velocities without such very large increases in axon diameter, and probably also to the transmission of impulses at high frequencies. It is of interest that myelination has evolved independently in invertebrates and vertebrates, and that the mechanisms of myelin formation are not identical. This discussion is limited to the structure of mammalian myelinated nerve fibers.

THE STRUCTURE OF MYELINATED NERVE FIBERS

Transverse sections through peripheral nerve trunks stained for fat or with aniline dyes and viewed by light microscopy reveal the myelin sheath as a tube, surrounding the axon and interrupted at the nodes of Ranvier (Fig. 6–1*A* and *B*). The myelin sheath extends along the nerve fiber from a point near the cell body, excluding the initial segment, and ceases at about 1 to 2 μm from the axon terminals at the periphery. The myelin sheath therefore consists of a succession of cylindrical segments, each being termed an internode. The myelin is derived from a chain of supporting cells, the cells of Schwann, which lie end to end, their junctions being represented by the nodes of Ranvier. The Schwann cell cytoplasm is visible as a narrow layer external

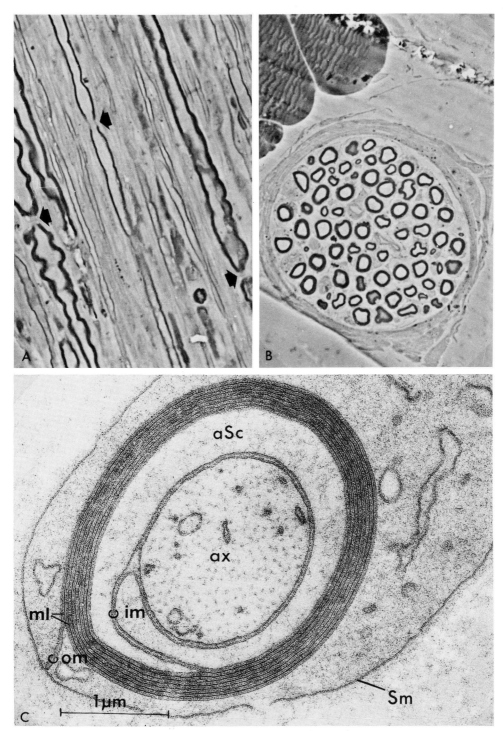

Figure 6–1 *A.* Phase contrast micrograph of longitudinal section through mouse sciatic nerve. Thick and thin myelinated fibers are distinguishable. Three nodes of Ranvier are present (arrows). *B.* Phase contrast micrograph of transverse section through a fascicle from mouse peroneal nerve. A population of large and small myelinated fibers is evident. *C.* Electron micrograph of transverse section through a myelinated nerve fiber from a five day postnatal mouse sciatic nerve. The outer (om) and inner (im) mesaxons are easily visible. The major dense lines (ml) of the myelin arise by the fusion of the inner surfaces of the Schwann cell surface membrane (Sm). The axon (ax) is surrounded by a conspicuous layer of adaxonal Schwann cell cytoplasm (aSc).

to the myelin sheath. It contains an elongated nucleus that is situated approximately at the midpoint of the internode. This often indents the myelin, as shown in Figure 6–2A, and is surrounded by a local accumulation of cytoplasm. A further narrow zone of Schwann cell cytoplasm, Mauthner's layer, is visible internal to the myelin sheath where it surrounds the axon, and there is a local accumulation in the paranodal region. When peripheral myelinated axons extend into the central nervous system, the transition from peripheral to central myelin takes place abruptly at the nodes of Ranvier at the Obersteiner-Redlich zone (see Chapter 9).

The Axon

The axon is bounded by a surface membrane, the axolemma, which on electron microscopy is seen to be a trilaminar membrane 7 to 8 nm in thickness (Robertson, 1957). In the region of the nodes of Ranvier, the axolemma is specialized in that it possesses a granular undercoating (cf. Figs. 6–12 and 6–14) (Elfvin, 1961). This is also present in the initial segment of the axon as it arises from the cell body (Peters and Vaughn, 1970). The specialization of the axolemma related to the termination of the myelin lamellae is discussed later. Waxman (1968) has drawn attention to the occasional presence of coated micropinocytotic axolemmal invaginations.

Fixed silver-stained preparations of peripheral nerve viewed by light microscopy show longitudinally oriented fibrillar material. The existence of a regular longitudinal organization in life was confirmed by the studies of Bear, Schmitt, and Young (1937), which demonstrated a positive birefringence with respect to length. Electron microscopy subsequently established the presence of both neurofilaments and microtubules (neurotubules) (see Fig. 6–13). Axonal microtubules are cylindrical structures 25 nm in diameter with a wall 5 nm in thickness surrounding a hollow core. As in other tissues, they provide a cytoskeleton for the axon and may be involved in axonal transport mechanisms (see Chapter 12). Neurofilaments are unbranched structures 6 to 10 nm in diameter. Their chemical composition and molecular organization are considered in Chapter 13. The number of microtubules is not constant in a given axon and its branches. In the accessory

nerve of the rat, the number of microtubules in the branches of a single axon exceeds that in the parent axon, indicating that they may be formed locally in the branches (Zenker and Hohberg, 1973). Branching of axonal microtubules has never been observed. They possibly arise by polymerization of preexisting tubular protein (Auclair and Siegal, 1966); during cooling of nerve, microtubules have been observed to disaggregate and to become reconstituted on rewarming (Rodriguez Echandía and Piezzi, 1968).

The axoplasm also contains mitochondria, which tend to be elongated in the length of the axon, together with vesicles or elongated profiles of smooth endoplasmic reticulum and, in autonomic nerves, occasional dense-cored vesicles. Free ribosomes and granular endoplasmic reticulum are not present. Even in normal axons, dense lamellar bodies and multivesicular bodies, similar to those that accumulate during wallerian degeneration (Webster, 1962) and that are probably lysosomal in nature (Holtzman and Novikoff, 1965) are sometimes observed. They may indicate a normal turnover of axonal organelles.

The Schwann Cell

The portion of the Schwann cell internal to the myelin sheath forms a narrow layer, the adaxonal Schwann cell cytoplasm, which is traversed by the inner mesaxon and which contains few organelles. It tends to be wider in fibers of small diameter (Fig. 6–1C). It is in communication with the Schwann cell cytoplasm external to the myelin through the Schmidt-Lanterman clefts and at the nodes of Ranvier. The Schwann cell surface membrane is separated from the axolemma by a gap of 10 to 20 nm.

The cytoplasmic layer external to the myelin is also small in amount except in the perinuclear region and adjacent to the nodes of Ranvier, and is traversed by the external mesaxon. In other regions the cytoplasm is generally reduced to a thin rim, or the outer Schwann cell surface membrane may be in intimate contact with the outermost lamella of the myelin sheath (Fig. 6–3B). Cytoplasmic lips, however, always remain on either side of the outer mesaxon. The nucleus possesses clumped peripheral chromatin, as shown in Figures 6–2A and 6–3B, and is elongated in

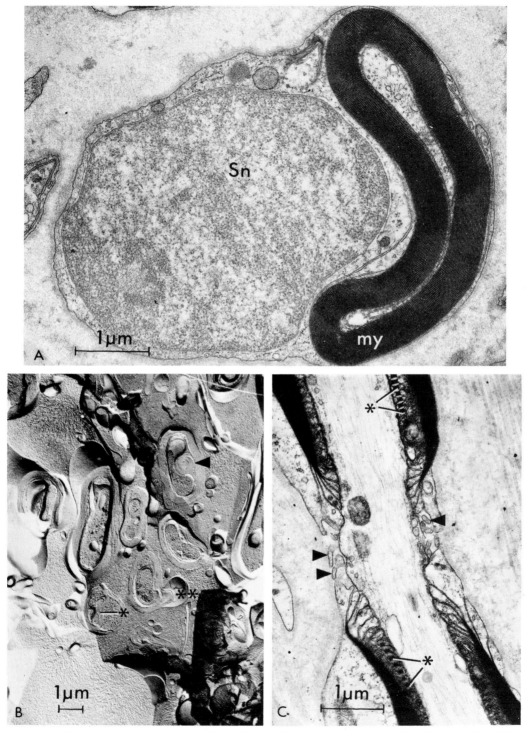

Figure 6–2 *A.* Electron micrograph of normal myelinated fiber transversely sectioned at the level of the Schwann cell nucleus (Sn). The nucleus strongly indents the myelin sheath (my) and the axon. *B.* Cross fractured peripheral nerve fibers prepared by the freeze-etching method. The electron micrograph shows several types of variation in the myelin sheath, including loops of myelin lamellae protruding into the axon (*) and outward into the Schwann cell cytoplasm (**) and one circular island of myelin at the inner aspect of the myelin sheath (arrow). *C.* Electron micrograph of a longitudinal section through a node of Ranvier. The nodal axolemma is surrounded by finger-like Schwann cell nodal processes (arrows). The paranodal terminal myelin loops show serial desmosome-like densities (*).

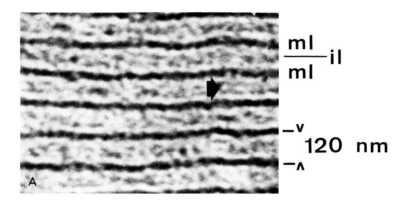

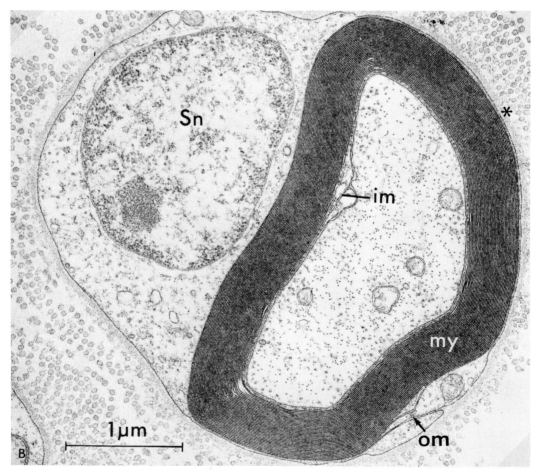

Figure 6–3 *A.* High-resolution electron micrograph of myelin from adult mouse sciatic nerve, stained by osmium tetroxide. The major dense line (ml) is clearly distinguishable from the intraperiod line (il). The latter is irregularly separated into two faint densities (arrow). *B.* Electron micrograph of myelinated nerve fiber sectioned at the level of the Schwann cell nucleus (Sn), which indents the myelin sheath (my). The outer mesaxon (om) shows a desmosome-like structure (arrow). The Schwann cell surface membrane lies in close contact with the myelin sheath (*) except in the region of the outer mesaxon, where two lips of cytoplasm are formed. The same is true at the inner mesaxon (im).

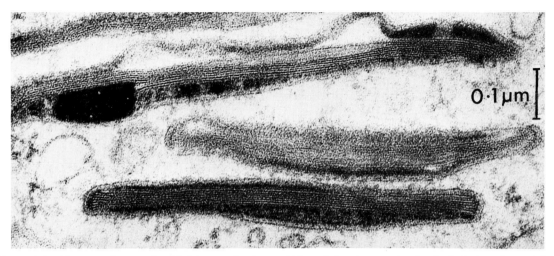

Figure 6–4   Electron micrograph of Reich granules from rabbit peripheral nerve showing both the lamellar and dense amorphous components.

the length of the axon. The perinuclear Schwann cell cytoplasm contains a profusion of organelles, including rough endoplasmic reticulum, Golgi membranes, mitochondria, lipid vacuoles, and Reich granules.

The π granules described by Reich (1903) are small rod-shaped bodies approximately 1 μm in length that are stained metachromatically by toluidine blue, thionin, and methylene blue. The metachromasia is due to the presence of phosphatide or sulphatide (Noback, 1953). They gradually accumulate with age. Ultrastructural studies reveal them to be membrane-bound lamellated bodies, sometimes associated with densely osmiophilic amorphous material (Fig. 6–4) (Thomas and Slatford, 1964; Tomonaga and Sluga, 1970). The lamellar component in human Schwann cells has been shown to be composed of stacks of membranes with a periodicity of 5 to 6 nm (Tomonaga and Sluga, 1970). More complex lamellar arrangements are sometimes observed (Thomas and Slatford, 1964). Reich granules are associated with acid phosphatase activity and can therefore be classified as lysosomes (Weller and Herzog, 1970). These authors suggested that they are analogous to the lipofuscin granules that accumulate in other nondividing cells. It is of interest that lipofuscin accumulates with age in Schwann cells associated with unmyelinated axons, as reported by Sharma and Thomas (1975), but not in those associated with myelinated axons. A further type of inclusion is the Elzholz body, which is a Marchi-positive lipid droplet. Although most numerous in the perinuclear

region, the π granules of Reich and the Elzholz bodies are also encountered in the paranodal region.

The Schwann cell contains numerous filaments 7 to 10 nm in diameter, often grouped in small bundles and oriented predominantly in the long axis of the cell. Less numerous microtubules are also present with a similar orientation.

The Schwann cell is invested by a basal lamina that is continuous across the nodes of Ranvier and thus forms a tubular investment for the fiber (cf. Fig. 6–12). The organization of the endoneurial connective tissue sheaths is considered in Chapter 9. The surface features of isolated fixed myelinated nerve fibers as revealed by scanning electron microscopy have been considered by Spencer and Lieberman (1971) (Fig. 6–5).

The Myelin Sheath

In electron micrographs of transverse sections through myelinated nerve fibers, the myelin sheath is characterized by a highly regular construction composed of concentrically arranged lamellae. Each lamella represents a repeating unit of alternate dark and light layers with a radial periodicity of 12 to 17 nm in fixed material, depending upon the method of fixation and embedding. The periodicity is 16 to 19 nm when measured in fresh nerve by x-ray diffraction (see Finean, 1958). The initial concept of Fernán-

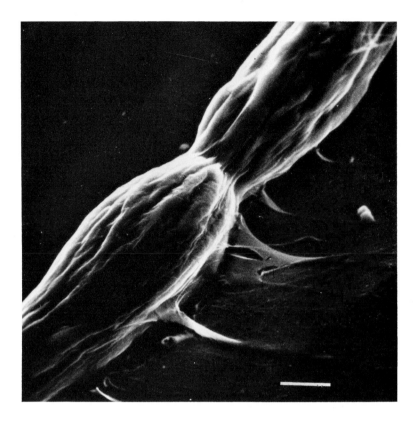

Figure 6–5 Scanning electron micrograph of a normal isolated nerve fiber at the level of a node of Ranvier showing the asymmetry in the size of the paranodal bulbs. Scale marker represents 10 μm. (From Spencer, P. S., and Lieberman, A. R.: Scanning electron microscopy of isolated peripheral nerve fibers: normal surface structure and alterations proximal to neuromas. Z. Zellforsch. Mikrosk. Anat., *119*:534, 1971. Berlin–Heidelberg–New York, Springer. Reprinted by permission.)

dez-Morán (1952) and Sjöstrand (1953) was of alternating dark lines, the major dense lines, approximately 2.5 nm in thickness, separated by a light interspace bisected by a less dense line, the intermediate or intraperiod line. In some instances, the intraperiod line appears as a pair of faint lines that are irregularly separated by a gap of 2 to 3 nm (Fig. 6–3*A*) (Bischoff and Moor, 1967b; Napolitano and Scallen, 1969; Revel and Hamilton, 1969).

About a century ago, it was demonstrated that the main constituents of brain myelin were lipids (Thudichum, 1884) and proteins (Ewald and Kühne, 1877). Later, this chemical composition was found to be consistent with the polarization optical findings on the myelin sheath as provided by Schmidt (1936) and with the results of x-ray diffraction studies by Schmitt and Clark (1935). Both investigations provided a new insight into the macromolecular structure of myelin. They indicated that the myelin sheath consists of alternating cylindrical layers of lipid and protein. In this arrangement, the lipid molecules were considered to form a bimolecular leaflet and to be radially oriented with the hydrophobic ends directed toward the center and with the hydrophilic polar ends extended outward

and sandwiched between monolayers of protein. The observation that on fixation for electron microscopy by osmium tetroxide, the heavy atomic nucleus of osmium becomes attached to the polar groups and thus makes these structures electron-opaque, was interpreted as indicating that the dark electron-dense line is to be identified with the polar region where lipid and protein interact, whereas the light, electron-lucent interspace represents the hydrophobic hydrocarbon chains of the bimolecular lipid leaflet.

This concept of the myelin sheath configuration received further support from the ontogenetic studies of myelin in chick embryos by Geren (1954) and the high-resolution electron microscopic analyses by Robertson (1955) (see Chapter 3). These authors established that the myelin sheath is a membrane system, and demonstrated that each individual lamella arises by the spiral wrapping of Schwann cell plasma membrane around the axon during myelination. The fainter intraperiod line is derived by the approximation of the external surfaces of the paired membranes of a spiral Schwann cell process, while the uniting of the cytoplasmic inner surfaces of the plasma membranes of the process produces the more conspicuous major dense line. The differences in the electron density of the two regions of apposition could be explained by an asymmetry in the molecular structure of the inner and outer surfaces of the Schwann cell plasma membrane (Finean, 1960; Robertson, 1960; Bischoff and Moor, 1967a). Alternatively, it might be related to molecular reorganization consequent upon the fusion or close adherence of the inner surfaces of the plasma membrane. Previous views as to the macromolecular organization of the myelin sheath may, however, require revision in terms of more recent concepts of membrane structure advanced by Vanderkooi (1972) and Singer (1972), in which globular protein molecules are inserted into a lipid bilayer, rather than the proteins being in an extended or fibrous conformation on either side of the bilayer.

In the mature myelin sheath, the connection of the outer end of the spiral with the surface membrane of the Schwann cell persists, as well as the connection between the innermost lamella and the Schwann cell surface membrane that surrounds the axon. These connections are represented by the outer and inner mesaxons, shown in Figure 6–1C, which are composed of paired membranes separated by a narrow channel with a width of 12 nm. The term "mesaxon" was introduced by Gasser (1952), who indicated the similarity with the mesentery suspending the intestine. Although convenient, this term is not entirely satisfactory as it displaces the emphasis from the mode of formation of myelin, which involves the encircling of the axon by a flattened spiral Schwann cell process. As already emphasized, myelination is achieved by the compaction of this process by obliteration of the contained cytoplasm and apposition of the cytoplasmic surfaces of its enclosing plasmalemma. At the junction of the outer mesaxon with the surface of the Schwann cell, the paired membranes are usually closely joined and in some instances are tightened by a desmosome-like structure, while a visible gap may exist in the section between this point and the myelin spiral.

In fixed nerves prepared by conventional techniques, but also in freeze-etched preparations made rigid exclusively by physical means as illustrated in Figure 6–2B, the myelin sheath can deviate from the regular cylindrical appearance and display appearances that have no pathologic significance. Often these variations occur as outfoldings of the myelin sheath that indent the axoplasm or protrude into the outer Schwann cell cytoplasm. Such irregularities are particularly common in the juxtanodal portion of the myelin (Webster and Spiro, 1960). More rarely there exist, in transverse section, isolated balls of myelin, located in the cytoplasm of the Schwann cell external to the myelin sheath. They represent aberrant contorted lamellae thrusting out from the sheath and exhibiting, in an electron micrograph, the typical myelin lamellar structure. Occasionally, redundant loops of myelin sheath may also bulge into the axon (Fig. 6–2B).

Fixed nerve examined by light microscopy after appropriate preparative procedures exhibits a reticular proteinaceous network in the myelin sheath that has been referred to as the "neurokeratin network" (Ewald and Kühne, 1877). This appearance is a fixation artifact resulting from the selective loss of myelin lipids from certain areas during tissue preparation (Fig. 6–6) (Spencer and Lieberman, 1971).

Schmidt-Lanterman Incisures

Despite reports that the incisures of Schmidt (1874) and Lanterman (1877) are present in living nerve fibers (e.g., Ranvier, 1876; Nageotte, 1910), doubts persisted until recent years about whether these biconical clefts in the myelin sheath were genuine structures or artifactually induced shearing defects. The presence of the spiral apparatus of Golgi-Rezzonico demonstrable after silver impregnation (Golgi, 1881; Rezzonico, 1881) in these clefts could have provided a clue to the spiral structure of myelin: it was interpreted by Young (1945) as representing the broken edges of the myelin lamellae in defects of the myelin sheaths arising because of mechanical stresses.

It is now established that the incisures are part of the normal structure of myelinated nerve fibers. Their number is directly related to myelin thickness (Wulfhekel and Düllmann, 1971), approximately 25 being present per internode in the largest fibers of the sciatic nerve of the rat (Hiscoe, 1947). They tend not to be present in the paranodal region (Hiscoe, 1947; Webster, 1965). Hiscoe considered that they were slightly more numerous in developing and regenerating fibers. Although Friede

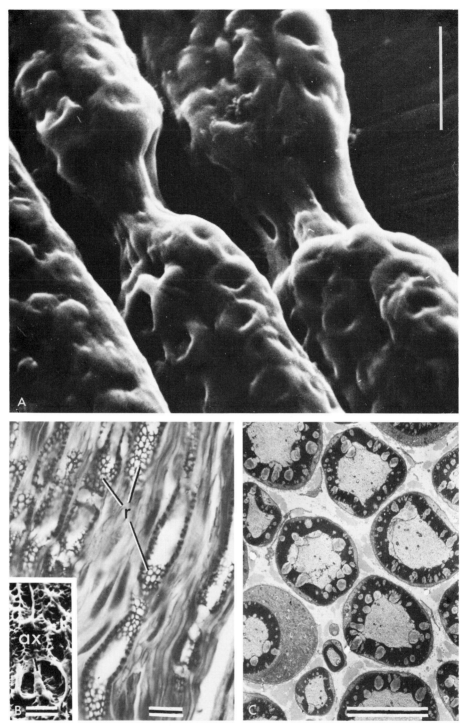

Figure 6–6 *A.* Scanning electron micrograph of three normal myelinated nerve fibers, two of which possess nodes of Ranvier. Their surfaces, which have been stripped of endoneurial collagen, display multiple pits, probably equivalent to the interstices of the "neurokeratin network" of light microscopy. Scale marker represents 5 μm. *B.* Light micrograph of rabbit peripheral nerve fibers stained with methosol fast blue and cresyl violet to demonstrate the reticulated "neurokeratin network" (r). Scale marker represents 5 μm. The inset shows a scanning electron micrograph of part of a deparaffinized 5 μm section originally processed for light microscopy; it displays a shrunken axon (ax) and reticulation of the myelin. Scale marker represents 5 μm. *C.* Transmission electron micrograph of transversely sectioned myelinated fibers showing multiple focal defects in the myelin sheath probably equivalent to the "neurokeratin" artifact. Collapse of the surface of the fibers during preparation for scanning electron microscopy is the likely explanation of the pitted surfaces of the fibers shown in *A.* Scale marker represents 5 μm. (From Spencer, P. S., and Lieberman, A. R.: Scanning electron microscopy of isolated peripheral nerve fibres: normal surface structure and alterations proximal to neuromas. Z. Zellforsch. Mikrosk. Anat., *119*:534, 1971. Berlin–Heidelberg–New York, Springer. Reprinted by permission.)

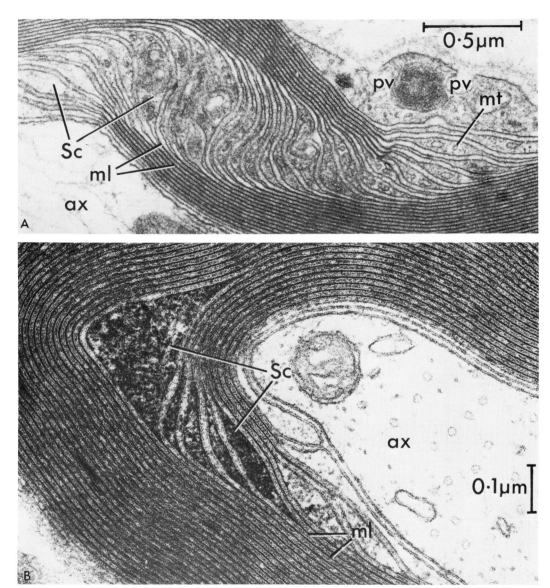

Figure 6–7   *A.* Electron micrograph of Schmidt-Lanterman incisure. The major dense lines of the myelin (ml) open to enclose pockets of Schwann cell cytoplasm (Sc) that contain microtubules (mt). The Schwann cell surface membrane external to the myelin shows pinocytotic vesicles (pv); ax, axon. *B.* Electron micrograph through partial Schmidt-Lanterman incisure. The myelin lamellae (ml) open to enclose pockets of densely stained Schwann cell cytoplasm (Sc). ax, Axon. (Micrographs kindly provided by Dr. R. H. M. King.)

and Samorajski (1969) did not observe them before the twelfth day of postnatal development in rats, Hall and Williams (1970) found them to be present at the first postnatal day in mice.

Their ultrastructural features were first examined by Robertson (1958) and have been the subject of a detailed study by Hall and Williams (1970). In the incisures, the major dense lines open to enclose a variable quantity of granular Schwann cell cytoplasm that frequently is intensely osmiophilic in glutaraldehyde-fixed material (Fig. 6–7). They may extend through the whole width of the myelin layer or involve only a few lamellae. The surfaces of the cleft subtend an angle of approximately 9 degrees to the plane of the myelin lamellae (Friede and Samorajski, 1969). In some instances they are oriented in the shape of an arrow with the apex toward the nearer end of the myelin segment. Friede and Samorajski stated that incisures are not ob-

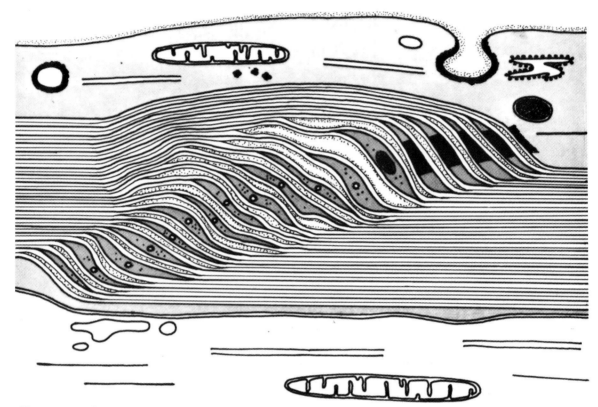

Figure 6–8 Diagrammatic representation of the ultrastructural features of the Schmidt-Lanterman incisure. The major dense lines of the myelin lamellae open to enclose pockets of Schwann cell cytoplasm that contain microtubules and a dense body. The cytoplasm of the outer portion of the incisure (upper right) possesses desmosome-like densities. There is also some separation of the intermediate lines of the myelin. The Schwann cell cytoplasm external to the myelin (upper part of figure) contains a coated vesicle, and there is a coated pinocytotic vesicle related to the Schwann cell surface membrane. (From Hall, S. M., and Williams, P. L.: Studies on the "incisures" of Schmidt and Lanterman. J. Cell Sci., 6:767, 1970. Reprinted by permission.)

served in fibers with less than 20 lamellae, whereas Hall and Williams found them in myelin sheaths composed of only five compact lamellae. They can be seen in remyelinating nerve fibers when only two or three lamellae are present (R. H. M. King, unpublished observations).

The cytoplasm of the incisures frequently contains a single helical microtubule (Fig. 6–7*A*), and occasional dense bodies, multi-vesicular bodies, and electron-dense granules are also observed. The outer portions of the incisures may show stacks of "desmosomoid" densities. Hall and Williams (1970) also commented upon the presence of coated smooth-walled vesicles in the Schwann cell cytoplasm adjacent to the outer termination of the incisures. These various features have been presented diagrammatically in Figure 6–8. The incisures have been shown by Pinner, Davison, and Campbell (1964) to be associated with acid phosphatase activity, and Glees

(1942) has claimed that alongside them there is a thickening of the inner endoneurial sheath.

The function of the incisures remains obscure. Robertson (1958) believed that they were shearing defects and suggested that they were part of a dynamic process in which the myelin lamellae were repeatedly parting and coming together in response to physiologic stresses. Friede and Samorajski (1969) proposed that the incisures allow for some plasticity in the myelin sheath, so that the internodes are able to elongate. They calculated that each cleft could permit a change in length amounting to 9 per cent of the fiber diameter and that it would tolerate changes in axon volume of up to 22 per cent. Singer and Bryant (1969) reported in vitro observations on fibers in which the incisures were thought to open and close rhythmically at a slow rate and to move progressively along the fibers. He postulated that they may be involved in a pulsatile flow of axoplasm across the myelin layer and in peristaltic activity along the fiber. The in vivo observations of Hall and Williams (1970) and their documentation of the effects of hypotonic and hypertonic solutions failed to support this contention. The assumed cytoskeletal role of microtubules supports the view that incisures may have a great deal more structural permanency than supposed by Robertson and Singer, although their dimensions may alter between a widened or "opened" state, and a narrowed or "closed" state. Hall and Williams questioned whether they might be involved in fiber growth and in the passage of substances between the abaxonal and adaxonal Schwann cell cytoplasm. Singer and Salpeter (1966) have provided some radio-autographic evidence for the transfer of labeled amino acids across the myelin sheath, although transport through the incisures was not demonstrated in the radioautographic studies of Friede and Samorajski (1969).

The Nodes of Ranvier

In his original paper Louis Ranvier (1871) described the structure that came to bear his name as "un étranglement annulaire du tube . . . d'une forme élégante." When he examined preparations stained by picric acid carmine, he observed that the myelin sheath was indented at regular intervals. It was later appreciated that the essential feature of the nodes was a complete interruption of the myelin. On the smaller fibers, the terminal part of the myelin approaches the nodal axon at an acute angle. On the larger fibers, the ends of the myelin segments form bulbous expansions and the terminal myelin approaches the axon more steeply, sometimes being recurved so that it forms an angle in excess of 90 degrees. The axon becomes narrowed at the nodes, the relative degree of narrowing being greater for the larger fibers (Hess and Young, 1952).

Quantitative observations on the dimensions of the node of Ranvier indicate that the length of the nodal gap and the diameter of the nodal axon are in inverse proportion (Hess and Young, 1952; Berthold and Skoglund, 1967). The longitudinal extent of the gap in nerve fibers of small caliber is up to six times as great as in those of large caliber. In measurements on electron micrographs of 20 nodes

from the mouse sciatic nerve, the gap distance varied from 0.3 μm to 2 μm and displayed a strict inverse relationship to the diameter of the nodal axon (A. Bischoff, unpublished observations). When the surface area of the axon in the nodal region was calculated, 15 of the 20 nodes gave values that fell between 4 and 6 μm^2. This result supports the conclusion that despite variations in the length of the nodal gap, because of its inverse relationship to nodal axon diameter, the surface area of the excitable membrane and thus its capacitance remain within certain narrow limits. This is of importance in relation to theoretical considerations concerning impulse transmission (Rushton, 1951).

The myelin of the bulbous paranodal expansions has a fluted arrangement because of the presence of a series of ridges, from three to six in number, which extend in a low spiral for a distance of approximately 40 μm from the node on large mammalian fibers (Figs. 6–9 and 6–10) (Hess and Young, 1952). The axon within the paranodal expansion conforms to the shape of the myelin fluting. The troughs between the myelin ridges on the outer aspect of the myelin layer contain Schwann cell cytoplasm within which there are very large numbers of mitochondria (Williams and Landon, 1963; Berthold and Skoglund, 1967).

It is of interest that the bulbous paranodal myelin expansions are asymmetrical (cf. Fig. 6–5) (Lubińska and Lukaszewska, 1956). These authors found that the paranodal bulb is larger on the proximal side, that is, nearer to the cell body. A more detailed study by Williams and Kashef (1968) confirmed that this relationship exists in most peripheral nerve trunks with the notable exception of the recurrent laryngeal nerve. The usual relationship obtains in the descending part of that nerve, whereas in the ascending part the polarity is reversed so that the distal nodal bulb is the larger. Lubińska and Lukaszewska (1956) originally questioned whether the nodal asymmetry could be the result of a damming by the constricted nodal axon of the proximodistal axoplasmic flow postulated by Weiss and Hiscoe (1948). This suggestion was later withdrawn by Lubińska (1958) on the basis of her observations on intercalated segments. Williams and Kashef (1968) have argued that the asymmetry probably depends upon local growth patterns.

The electron microscope revealed a degree

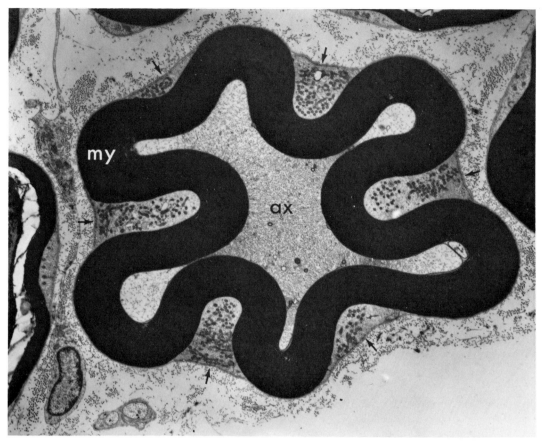

Figure 6–9 Electron micrograph of transverse section through paranodal region of a large myelinated nerve fiber from cat ventral root, about 15 μm from the node. The myelin sheath (my) is highly crenated. Accumulations of Schwann cell cytoplasm (arrows) contain large numbers of mitochondria. The axon (ax) is "fluted." × 3500. (From Berthold, C.-H.: Ultrastructure of the node-paranode region of mature feline ventral lumbar spinal-root fibres. Acta Soc. Med. Upsal. 73:Suppl. 9:37, 1968. Reprinted by permission.)

of structural complexity at the nodes that was unsuspected from studies by light microscopy (cf. Fig. 6–10). Early descriptions were provided by Uzman and Nogueira-Graf (1957), Robertson (1959), Elfvin (1961), and others, and further details were provided by Landon and Williams (1963), Williams and Landon (1963) and Berthold (1968). As the myelin lamellae approach the axolemma, the major dense lines, in longitudinal section, open to form terminal "cytoplasmic pockets" (Figs. 6–2C, 6–11, and 6–12). These are sections through a helical rim of cytoplasm linking the adaxonal Schwann cell cytoplasm with the cytoplasm on the external aspect of the myelin layer. Harkin (1964) and Bunge and associates (1967) have drawn attention to the occasional presence of a series of desmosome-like densities within these cytoplasmic pockets linking the pairs of membranes (see Fig. 6–2C).

In longitudinal section they are seen to have a spiral configuration.

It is evident from the studies on nerve compression by Ochoa, Fowler, and Gilliatt (1972) that the terminal cytoplasmic rim of the myelin lamellae is firmly adherent to the axolemma at either side of the node. The axolemma at the junction with the helical rim is specialized. The outer leaflet of the axolemma possesses a helical series of ridges that come into close contact with the outer leaflet of the Schwann cell membrane of the terminal cytoplasmic rim (Fig. 6–13). This structural specialization was first observed in peripheral nerve fibers by Bargmann and Lindner (1964) and examined in greater detail in central nodes by Peters (1966) and Laatsch and Cowan (1966), and in peripheral nodes by Livingston and co-workers (1973). Studies with lanthanum as a tracer by Hirano and

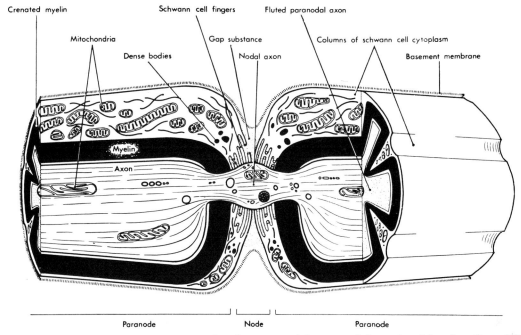

Figure 6–10   Diagrammatic representation of the ultrastructural features of the node of Ranvier. (From Williams, P. L., and Landon, D. N.: The energy source of the nerve fibre. New Scientist, *21*:166, 1963. Reprinted by permission.)

Dembitzer (1969) demonstrated that there is a narrow helical path, 25 to 30 nm in width, between the spiral ridging on the axolemma, which links the extracellular nodal space with the periaxonal space. Functionally, besides providing a mechanical consolidation, this structural arrangement may be involved in other interactions between the axon and the Schwann cell (Livingston et al., 1973).

On the larger fibers, not all the terminal

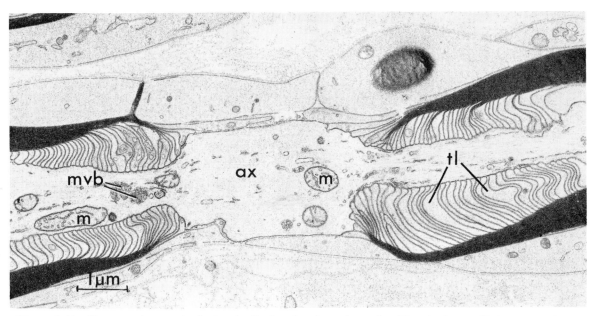

Figure 6–11   Electron micrograph of a longitudinal section through a node of Ranvier from a 10 day postnatal mouse sciatic nerve. The paranodal structural organization is clearly depicted, with the terminal loops of Schwann cell cytoplasm (tl) attached to the axolemma. The axon (ax) contains mitochondria (m) and multivesicular bodies (mvb).

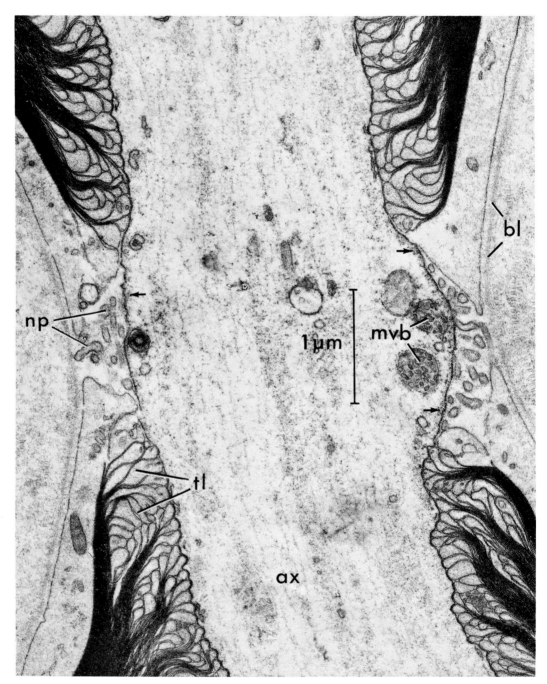

Figure 6–12   Electron micrograph of a longitudinal section through a node of Ranvier in an adult mouse sciatic nerve. The arrangement of the terminal myelin loops (tl) is less regular than in Figure 6–11, as not all the loops make contact with the axolemma. The axon (ax) contains multivesicular bodies (mvb), and the nodal axolemma is surrounded by Schwann cell nodal processes (np). The "undercoating" of the nodal axolemma is indicated by the arrows. The node is ensheathed by a basal lamina (bl).

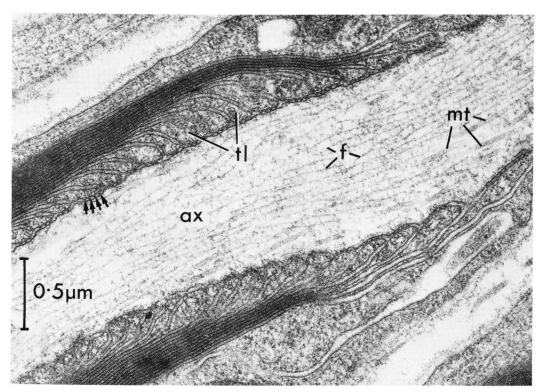

Figure 6–13   Electron micrograph of longitudinal section through portion of a node of Ranvier from guinea pig dorsal root. The terminal loops (tl) of the myelin lamellae are attached to the axolemma by specialized contacts. The axolemma possesses a series of helical ridges seen as dots (arrows) in transverse section. The axon (ax) contains filaments (f) and microtubules (mt). (Micrograph kindly provided by Dr. R. H. M. King.)

loops of the myelin lamellae reach the axolemma. Groups of them may terminate at some distance from the axolemma, forming double rows at right angles to the axon. Several such rows may be present symmetrically on both sides of the axon when observed in transverse section, with intervening lamellae terminating in cytoplasmic loops attached to the axon as shown in Figure 6–12. This occurrence is probably responsible for the histologic appearance known as the "spinous bracelets of Nageotte" (Berthold, 1968). In material stained by the Altmann acid fuchsin technique, Nageotte (1910) had observed a ring of "spines" extending into the terminations of the myelin at the nodes, curved backward in the direction of the nodal myelin.

On the nodal side of the myelin terminations, the Schwann cell cytoplasm external to the myelin gives rise to a collar that overlaps in an irregular manner the collar from the adjacent Schwann cell. As is true of the Schwann cell cytoplasm in the clefts in the paranodal bulbs, these nodal collars also contain numerous mitochondria. The collars

give rise to multiple finger-like nodal processes, 70 to 100 nm in diameter, which extend into the nodal gap and become closely approximated to the axolemma with a separation of approximately 5 nm (Figs. 6–2C, 6–12, and 6–14) (Berthold, 1968). On large fibers, the nodal processes form a regular hexagonal array with a separation of about 50 nm. They contain four to eight longitudinal filaments (Berthold, 1968).

The nodal collars of the Schwann cells are bounded externally by the basal lamina that invests the node (Fig. 6–12). The interval between the myelin bulbs external to the basal lamina may be termed the perinodal space (Hess and Young, 1952). It contains the collagen fibrils of the inner endoneurial sheath that are inflected at the nodes. In large fibers with deep perinodal spaces, the outer portion of the spaces contains a system of interwoven microvilli-like processes from the adjacent Schwann cells, which are surrounded by a basal laminal ensheathment (Berthold, 1968). Similar tufts of processes may project externally from the paranodal Schwann cell

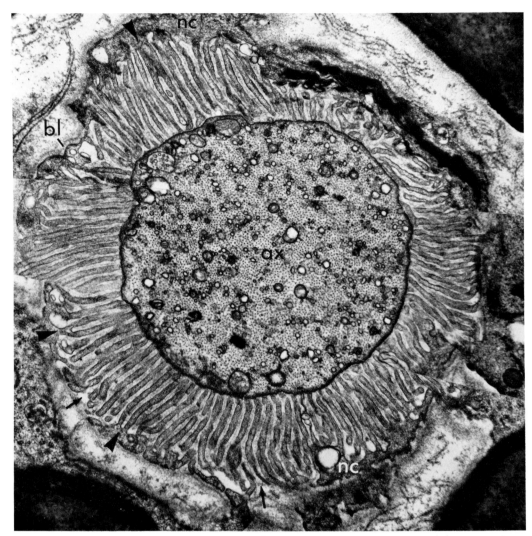

Figure 6–14　Electron micrograph of transverse section through node of Ranvier from a large myelinated nerve fiber from cat ventral root (montage from three sections through the same node). The axon (ax) is surrounded by closely packed and radially arranged nodal processes (arrow heads) derived from the nodal collar of the Schwann cell (nc). Arrows indicate regions where the nodal gap appears to lack a covering nodal collar and is directly invested by the basal lamina (bl). The axon contains a dense population of neurofilaments and microtubules, together with mitochondria and profiles of smooth endoplasmic reticulum. Note the electron-dense undercoating of the axolemma. × 1800. (From Berthold, C.-H.: Ultrastructure of the node-paranode region of mature feline ventral lumbar spinal-root fibres. Acta Soc. Med. Upsal. *73*: Suppl. *9*:37, 1968. Reprinted by permission.)

surface on smaller fibers. Their significance is uncertain.

The nodal processes evidently constitute a specialized form of contact between the Schwann cells and the axon. Landon and Williams suggested that they may provide a pathway for metabolic exchanges between the mitochondrion-rich paranodal Schwann cell cytoplasm and the nodal axon, which is relatively poorly endowed with mitochondria (Landon and Williams, 1963; Williams and Landon, 1964). The Schwann cell might thus provide the energy supplies for the axolemmal ionic pump. In this connection, it is of interest that during development the appearance of adult physiologic characteristics, such as the ability to transmit impulses at high frequencies, coincides with the accumulation of paranodal Schwann cell mitochondria (Berthold and Skoglund, 1967).

The space between the nodal processes that is bounded externally by the basal laminal ensheathment of the node contains material of moderate electron density with a granular or mottled appearance (Berthold, 1968). This has been termed the "gap substance" (Landon and Williams, 1963). It is equivalent to the "cementing disc" as defined by Hess and Young (1952) in their perspicacious light microscope study when they raised the possibility that the particular staining qualities of this zone might be related to a function as a region of active ionic interchanges. Abood and Abul-Haj (1956) showed that it contains non-sulphated mucopolysaccharides. Subsequently, Herbst (1965) and Gerebtzoff and Mladenov (1967) demonstrated that the "cementing disc" has a great affinity for a variety of metallic salts. A series of histochemical studies by Langley and Landon (1967, 1969) and Langley (1969, 1970) established that the node is surrounded by polyanionic material that provides a cation exchange reservoir at the node. This was considered to be composed predominantly of protein-linked carboxylated mucopolysaccharides. Landon and Langley (1969, 1971) confirmed by electron microscope histochemical observations that this activity resides in the gap substance. They postulated that the presence of such ion-binding material around the nodal axolemma could be important in regulating the ionic movements that accompany the propagated nerve action potential.

Berthold (1968) noted the occasional presence of multiple axonal compartments that lie embedded in the adaxonal Schwann cell cytoplasm in the paranodal region of large fibers. The cytoplasm of the intervening Schwann cell partitions is often obliterated so that their membranes are apposed to form a single layer. The axonal processes tend to contain multiple mitochondria and dense lamellar bodies, and the adjacent Schwann cell cytoplasm frequently contains debris. Such appearances may be seen in normal fibers, but are particularly evident in fibers central to an amputation neuroma (Spencer, 1971) and in experimental acrylamide neuropathy (Prineas, 1969; R. S. Kocen and P. K. Thomas, unpublished observations). Spencer (1971) has shown that these appearances arise by the ingrowth of processes from the adaxonal Schwann cell cytoplasm and has suggested that they represent a "scavenger" activity by the Schwann cell, whereby effete organelles or damaged portions of axoplasm are sequestered and removed.

MORPHOMETRIC FEATURES OF MYELINATED NERVE FIBERS

Myelinated Fiber Size Distribution

The analysis of the distribution of fiber size in peripheral nerves dates back to Sherrington (1894). Eccles and Sherrington (1930) and O'Leary, Heinbecker, and Bishop (1934) established that there was a bimodal distribution of motor fibers to the calf muscles in the cat, and Lloyd and Chang (1948) and Rexed and Therman (1948) found that three groups of afferent fibers could be identified. An extensive study on cat nerves with a detailed analysis of the significance of these groups was undertaken by Boyd and Davey (1968). Fernand and Young (1951) surveyed fiber size distribution in a wide variety of motor nerves in the rabbit and showed that in a number of instances, such as in the nerves to the laryngeal muscles, the distribution was unimodal with a single small-fiber peak. Species differences exist: Wulfhekel and Düllmann (1971) found the distribution to be trimodal in the sciatic nerve of the Rhesus monkey, whereas Friede and Samorajski (1967) found it to be unimodal in the mouse.

Myelinated nerve fibers in human peripheral nerve trunks range in diameter between 2 and 22 μm. Early observations on the distribution of fiber size in human nerves were made by Ranson and co-workers (1935), Greenfield and Carmichael (1935) and Aring and associates (1941), and later by Sunderland, Laverack, and Ray (1949), Laverack, Sunderland, and Ray (1951), Tomasch and Schwarzacher (1952), Tomasch and Britton (1956), and Garven, Gairns, and Smith (1962). More detailed observations on larger series of subjects at different ages are available for the anterior tibial nerve (Swallow, 1966), the radial nerve at the wrist (O'Sullivan and Swallow, 1968), the sural nerve at the ankle (Dyck, 1966; O'Sullivan and Swallow, 1968; Dyck et al., 1968, 1972) and the peroneal nerve (Stevens et al., 1973). In both the radial and the sural nerves, the fiber size distribution is bimodal, with peaks at 3 to 6 μm and 9 to 13 μm (Fig. 6–15) (O'Sullivan and Swallow, 1968). Peaks at slightly smaller values were reported by Dyck and associates (1968), the difference probably being related to differences in fixation and embedding procedures. A bimodal distribution was also shown for the great

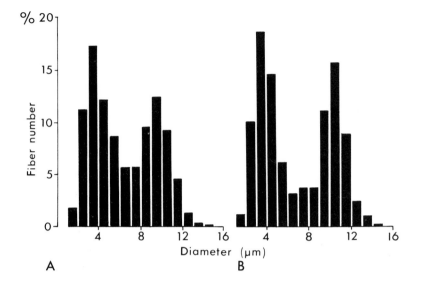

Figure 6–15 Size frequency distributions for myelinated fibers in the radial nerve at the wrist (*A*) and sural nerve at the ankle (*B*) in control subjects aged 28 and 30 respectively. (Data from O'Sullivan, D. J., and Swallow, M.: The fibre size and content of the radial and sural nerves. J. Neurol. Neurosurg. Psychiatry, *31*:464, 1968.)

auricular nerve (Dyck et al., 1965). The extensive observations of Rexed (1944) on the postnatal changes in fiber size in the spinal roots indicate that the roots with a distribution to the limb girdle and the proximal portions of the limbs possess a greater diameter than those to the distal parts of the limbs. Fiber size has a unimodal distribution in the recurrent laryngeal nerve (Scheuer, 1964). Adult fiber size is achieved during the second half of the first decade of life (Rexed, 1944; Gutrecht and Dyck, 1970).

Relationship Between Internodal Length and Fiber Diameter

Ranvier (1875) drew attention to the fact that the nodes that he had observed on myelinated nerve fibers were spaced at longer intervals on larger than on smaller fibers. This relationship was confirmed by all subsequent observers, including those who have examined human nerves, except for certain special instances (Vizoso, 1950; Lascelles and Thomas, 1966; Arnold and Harriman, 1970; Gutrecht and Dyck, 1970). The nature of the relationship has been variously described. Most commonly, a simple rectilinear correlation has been assumed, although a curvilinear relationship has at times seemed more appropriate (e.g., Rushton, 1951), and more complex mathematical descriptions have also been adopted (e.g., Schuchardt, 1947; Thomas, 1955).

In adult human nerve trunks, internodal

length ranges from about 0.1 mm on the smallest myelinated fibers to 1.8 mm on the largest. Measurement of the length of consecutive internodes along individual fibers shows that in young adult subjects the scatter is limited. The regular relationship between internodal length and fiber diameter becomes less precise with aging (Vizoso, 1950; Lascelles and Thomas, 1966; Arnold and Harriman, 1970). This is related both to the occurrence of segmental demyelination and remyelination and to axonal degeneration and regeneration, and involves an increased variability both between successive internodes along individual fibers and between fibers (Lascelles and Thomas, 1966). This can be specified by using a "coefficient of variation" (see Chapter 15).

Ranvier (1872) was quick to point out that internodal length is greater in larger than in smaller specimens of an animal. This suggested a relationship to growth. From observations on developing nerve fibers, Speidel (1932) noted that Schwann cells become spaced at approximately regular intervals along the fibers. Hiscoe (1947) appreciated that it was this spacing that determined the initial value for internodal length. Studies on developing mammalian nerves have indicated that at the time of initial myelination, internodal length is approximately 0.2 to 0.3 mm. Internodal length increases progressively during growth, as does the slope of the line relating internodal length and fiber diameter (Vizoso and Young, 1948). Comparison of the change in internodal length with changes in the length of the part in which the nerve lies indicates that both in man (Vizoso, 1950) and in other species (Thomas, 1955; Schlaepfer and Myers, 1973), there is a close correlation between the two. This implies that the number of Schwann cells does not normally alter during growth and that, as elongation of the nerve takes place, the internodes undergo a corresponding increase in length. The direct relationship between internodal length and fiber diameter could be explained if the fibers that ultimately achieve the largest diameter become myelinated first so that their internodes are therefore subjected to the greatest elongation during growth (Thomas and Young, 1949; Thomas, 1955). There is evidence in many nerves that this is so (Thomas, 1956), although Friede and Samorajski (1968) believed that myelination begins approximately simultaneously in all fibers destined to become myelinated in the rat sciatic nerve. The relationship between internodal length and fiber diameter is not always very precise, and the exact form of the relationship may be influenced by a certain amount of remodeling during development in which some internodes are eliminated and others are extended (Berthold and Skoglund, 1967; see also Chapter 11).

The relationship between internodal length and fiber diameter varies between different nerves in man, with a less steep slope in the facial nerve than in the ulnar and peroneal nerves (Vizoso, 1950). This can be related to the disparate growth rates of the parts through which these nerves run (Shepherd et al., 1949). Although observations are not available in man, internodal length may be considerably shorter in profusely branched skin plexuses than the usual minimum value of 0.2 mm found in the nerve trunk (Whitear, 1952). The possible significance in relation to nerve conduction of such variations in the relationship between internodal length and fiber diameter has recently been considered by Waxman (1972).

Relationship Between Myelin Thickness and Axon Diameter

Studies on the consequences of cross anastomosis between myelinated and unmyelinated nerves have indicated that it is the axon that provides the stimulus for the Schwann cell to produce myelin (Simpson and Young,

1945; Hillarp and Olivecrona, 1946). An anastomosis between the proximal stump of a transected myelinated nerve and the distal stump of an unmyelinated nerve results in the appearance of myelinated axons in the reinnervated distal stump. Conversely, if an unmyelinated proximal stump is anastomosed to a formerly myelinated distal stump, myelination of the regenerating axons in the distal stump does not occur. Furthermore, myelin thickness bears a definite relationship to axon diameter, and the information transferred from the axon to the Schwann cell evidently determines the number of myelin lamellae that are produced. The nature of the axonal influences on the Schwann cell is unknown, but possible mechanisms that have been suggested are considered later.

Early observations on the correlation subsisting between myelin thickness and axon diameter date back to Donaldson and Hoke (1905), who reported that in a wide range of species there was an approximately one-to-one relationship between the cross sectional area of the axon and that of the myelin sheath over the whole range of fiber sizes. Boughton (1906) found that this relationship was present throughout the postnatal growth period in the rat, but Dunn (1912) and Donaldson and Nagasaka (1918) later considered that it did not become established until some time during the postnatal growth period.

The numerous observers who have studied myelin thickness in more recent years have reached a wide variety of conclusions. Sanders (1948) found that a direct plot of myelin thickness against axon diameter gave the most easily interpretable presentation. The majority of workers have found either a direct rectilinear correlation between myelin thickness and axon diameter (e.g., Schwarzacher, 1954; Dyck, 1966; Williams and Wendell-Smith, 1971) or a relatively greater myelin thickness for fibers of smaller diameter (e.g., Sanders, 1948; Evans and Vizoso, 1951; Thomas, 1955; Sunderland and Roche, 1958). By contrast, Buchthal and Rosenfalck (1966) found that myelin thickness was proportionately greater in larger fibers.

Williams (1959), Wendell-Smith and Williams (1959), and Williams and Wendell-Smith (1960, 1971) have considered the possible causes for such wide divergences in the published results. These include dimensional changes occurring during tissue preparation when measurements on transverse sections from fixed and stained material are employed,

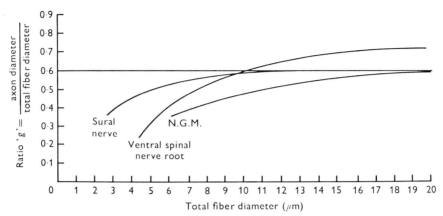

Figure 6–16 Curves showing the relationship between the ratio "g" and total fiber diameter (D) for the nerve to the medial head of the gastrocnemius muscle (N.G.M.), the sural nerve and a ventral spinal nerve root (seventh lumbar) from mature rabbits. (From Williams, P. L., and Wendell-Smith, C. P.: Some additional parametric variations between peripheral nerve fibre populations. J. Anat., *109*:505, 1971. Reprinted by permission.)

the magnifying effect of the refractile myelin layer when observations are made on fresh isolated fibers, and the use of mixed nerves containing both muscle and cutaneous components. They themselves therefore examined fresh frozen sections by polarization microscopy (Williams and Wendell-Smith, 1971). In a variety of rabbit nerves they found a positive rectilinear correlation between myelin thickness and axon diameter. There were consistent differences, both in the rate of increase of myelin thickness with axon diameter and in the absolute thickness of the myelin sheath, between the nerves examined. Fibers in the nerve to the medial head of the gastrocnemius muscle were found to be more heavily myelinated than those in the sural nerve, and the rate of increase of myelin thickness with axon diameter was less in spinal roots than in these two peripheral nerve trunks (Fig. 6–16). More widespread sampling of nerves is likely to reveal a wide range of different patterns of myelination.

The understanding of the ultrastructural organization of the myelin sheath led to the conclusion that the width of the myelin sheath is determined by the number of myelin lamellae, and that counting the number of lamellae therefore provides a precise way of assessing sheath thickness (Bischoff, 1965). This approach was adopted by Friede and Samorajski (1967) and Dyck and co-workers (1970, 1971). The number of myelin lamellae was counted and the axon circumference measured in transverse electron microscope sections. A direct rectilinear relationship between axon circumference and the number

of lamellae was utilized in the vagus and sciatic nerves of mice by Friede and Samorajski (1967), in the human sural nerve by Dyck and his associates (1971), and in the rat tibial nerve (N. Muenthongchin, unpublished observations). This procedure has the disadvantage that fixed and embedded material is used, but has the advantage that direct measurement of axon size can be substituted for adoption of the inner diameter of the myelin sheath as equivalent to axon diameter, as must be done in light microscope preparations. Errors introduced by separation of the myelin lamellae or unrecognized Schmidt-Lanterman incisures are also avoided.

Schmitt and Bear (1937) made observations on the total fiber diameter (D) and axon diameter (d) and designated the ratio d/D as g. This ratio has been found useful in theoretical treatments relating to saltatory conduction. Rushton (1951) predicted that a value of 0.6 to 0.7 for g would be optimal for conduction velocity, and this was subsequently reiterated by Hodgkin (1964) and Deutsch (1969) in further theoretical treatments and derived by Smith and Koles (1970) in a computer simulation.

Schmitt and Bear (1937) found that in adult amphibian nerves, g increased progressively with increasing axon diameter until a value of 9 μm was reached, above which it remained relatively constant. A similar pattern was reported by Sanders (1948), Evans and Vizoso (1951), and Williams and Wendell-Smith (1971). Although it is clear that g departs from the theoretical optimal value for conduction velocity for the smaller fibers in all these studies, g tends to approach the predicted value of 0.6 to 0.7 for fibers of larger size. Other relationships have also been reported. Sunderland and Roche (1958) found that g continued to rise with increasing axon diameter without the plateau for the higher values. The measurements obtained by Friede and Samorajski (1967) show an approximately constant value of g (at about 0.7 to 0.8) over the whole diameter range. This is also true of the rat tibial nerve, although there is a slight positive correlation with diameter (Fig. 6–17) (N. Muenthongchin, unpublished observations). Buchthal and Rosenfalck (1966), on the other hand, found smaller values of g for fibers of larger size. In certain special situations, relationships have been described between myelin thickness and axon diameter that differ substantially from those usually observed. A striking example is provided by the fibers in the glomeruli of the dorsal root ganglia, which possess abnormally thin myelin sheaths, with g values of as high as 0.95 (Spencer et al., 1973).

The mechanisms involved in the initiation and control of myelination remain uncertain. Duncan (1934) suggested that there was a critical axon diameter of about 1 μm above which myelin developed. Friede (1972) has proposed a mechanism for the control of the growth of the myelin sheath by postulating two phases of growth. The first consists of an elongation of the plasma membranes of the internal mesaxon, which lengthen in proportion to the degree of stretch imposed by the underlying axon; the second consists of the compaction of the myelin by obliteration of the cytoplasm from the spiral Schwann cell

process. The extent of myelin compaction in the second phase is determined by the length of the spiral formed in the first phase. This model requires that slippage must occur between adjacent lamellae to allow for axonal expansion.

There are substantial difficulties in accepting the Friede model. The model was partly based upon observations on the effects of experimental constrictions applied to nerves, the interpretation of which is open to question (Spencer, 1972; Spencer and Thomas, 1975). Friede and Samorajski (1967) found no overlap between the diameter of the axons of the thickest unmyelinated and the thinnest myelinated fibers, but this was not confirmed by Ochoa and Mair (1969), who detected a significant degree of overlap. Moreover, the correlation between axon size and the onset of myelination is poor (Fraher, 1972, 1973). Factors other than axon size must be involved in the control of myelin thickness. These are necessary to account for the differences in myelination between muscle and cutaneous nerves reported by Williams and Wendell-Smith (1971), shown in Figure 6–16, and in fibers close to dorsal root ganglion cells, to which reference has already been made, that possess unusually thin myelin sheaths (Spencer et al., 1973). It is also difficult to explain in terms of this model the aberrant myelination observed by Ballin and Thomas (1968) in experimental allergic neuritis and occasionally encountered during regeneration after wallerian degeneration, shown in Figure 6–18, and even in normal nerves. Here Schwann cells in contact with axons override each other at the nodes of Ranvier. The portion of the

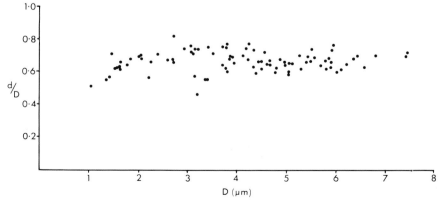

Figure 6–17 Relationship between the ratio of axon diameter (d) to total fiber diameter (D), designated as "g," and total fiber diameter (D), for tibial nerve of rat. Measurements based on counts of number of myelin lamellae and on axon circumference in electron micrographs. (Plotted from data provided by Dr. N. Muenthongchin.)

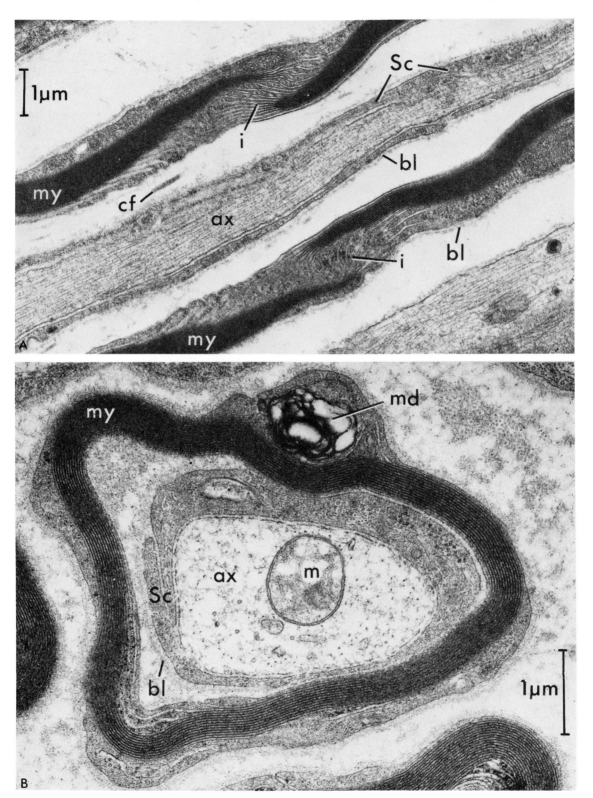

Figure 6–18 Electron micrographs showing aberrant myelination following regeneration in the rabbit recurrent laryngeal nerve after a crush lesion of the cervical vagus nerve in the neck. *A.* In a longitudinal section, a central axon (ax) is covered with a Schwann cell ensheathment (Sc) and is bounded by basal lamina (bl). This is surrounded by a myelin ensheathment (my) possessing a Schmidt-Lanterman incisure (i), with an intervening space containing collagen fibrils (cf). *B.* In transverse section, a central axon (ax) that contains an enlarged mitochondrion (m) is enclosed by a Schwann cell process (Sc) surrounded by basal lamina (bl). As in *A.* this is enclosed by a myelin sheath (my) with an intervening extracellular space. The Schwann cell associated with this myelin contains myelin debris (md).

Schwann cell that overrides the other and that is therefore not in contact with the axon nevertheless may produce myelin.

The alternative suggestion that, rather than being a mechanical influence by the axon, the stimulus to the Schwann cell is chemical in nature has been proposed by Spencer (1971) and Singer and Steinberg (1972), but no critical experiment has so far been devised to test this hypothesis.

Dr. Bischoff's investigation was supported by grant No. 3.747.72 of the Swiss National Fund.

REFERENCES

Abood, L. G., and Abul-Haj, S. F.: Histochemistry and characterization of hyaluronic acid in axons of peripheral nerve. J. Neurochem., *1*:119, 1956.

Aring, C. D., Bean, W. B., Roseman, E., Rosenbaum, M., and Spies, T. D.: The peripheral nerves in cases of nutritional deficiency. Arch. Neurol., *45*:772, 1941.

Arnold, N., and Harriman, D. G. F.: The incidence of abnormality in control human peripheral nerves studied by single axon dissection. J. Neurol. Neurosurg. Psychiatry, *33*:55, 1970.

Auclair, W., and Siegal, B.: Cilia regeneration in the sea urchin embryo; evidence for a pool of ciliary proteins. Science, *154*:913, 1966.

Ballin, R. H. M., and Thomas, P. K.: Demyelination and remyelination in experimental allergic neuritis. II. Remyelination. J. Neurol. Sci., *8*:225, 1968.

Bargmann, W., and Lindner, E.: Ueber den Feinbau des Nebennierenmarkes des Igels (Erinaceus europaeus L.). Z. Zellforsch. Mikrosk. Anat., *64*:868, 1964.

Bear, R. S., Schmitt, F. O., and Young, J. Z.: Investigations of the protein constituents of nerve axoplasm. Proc. R. Soc. Lond. [Biol.], *833*:520, 1937.

Berthold, C.-H.: Ultrastructure of postnatally developing feline peripheral nodes of Ranvier. Acta Soc. Med. Upsal., *73*:145, 1968.

Berthold, C.-H., and Skoglund, S.: Histochemical and ultrastructural demonstration of mitochondria in the paranodal region of developing feline spinal roots and nerves. Acta Soc. Med. Upsal., *72*:37, 1967.

Bischoff, A.: Problèmes et possibilités de l'exploration de l'ultrastructure du système nerveux périphérique. Rev. Neurol. (Paris), *112*:377, 1965.

Bischoff, A., and Moor, H.: The ultrastructure of the difference factor in the myelin. Z. Zellforsch. Mikrosk. Anat., *81*:571, 1967a.

Bischoff, A., and Moor, H.: Ultrastructural differences between the myelin sheaths of peripheral nerve fibers and CNS white matter. Z. Zellforsch. Mikrosk. Anat., *81*:303, 1967b.

Boughton, T. H.: The increase in the number and size of the medullated fibers in the oculomotor nerve of the white rat and of the cat at different ages. J. Comp. Neurol., *16*:153, 1906.

Boyd, I. A., and Davey, M. R.: Composition of Peripheral Nerves. Edinburgh, E. & S. Livingstone, 1968.

Buchthal, F., and Rosenfalck, A.: Evoked action potentials and conduction velocity in human sensory nerves. Brain Res., *3*:1, 1966.

Bunge, M. B., Bunge, R. P., Peterson, E. R., and Murray, M. R.: A light and electron microscope study of long-term organized cultures of rat dorsal root ganglia. J. Cell Biol., *32*:439, 1967.

Deutsch, S.: The maximization of nerve conduction velocity. IEEE Trans. Systems Sci. Cybernetics, *5*:86, 1969.

Donaldson, H. H., and Hoke, G. W.: On the areas of the axis cylinder and medullary sheath as seen in cross sections of the spinal nerves of vertebrates. J. Comp. Neurol., *15*:1, 1905.

Donaldson, H. H., and Nagasaka, G.: On the increase in the diameters of nerve-cell bodies and of the fibers arising from them during the later stages of growth (Albino rat). J. Comp. Neurol., *29*:529, 1918.

Duncan, D.: A relation between axon diameter and myelination determined by measurement of myelinated spinal root fibers. J. Comp. Neurol., *60*:437, 1934.

Dunn, E. H.: The influence of age, sex, weight, and relationship upon the number of medullated fibers and on the size of the largest fibers in the ventral root of the second cervical nerve of the albino rat. J. Comp. Neurol., *22*:131, 1912.

Dyck, P. J.: Histologic measurements and fine structure of biopsied sural nerve: normal and in peroneal muscular atrophy, hypertrophic neuropathy and congenital sensory neuropathy. Mayo Clin. Proc., *41*: 742, 1966.

Dyck, P. J., and Lais, A. C.: Electron microscopy of teased nerve fibers: method permitting examination of repeating structure of same fiber. Brain Res., *23*:418, 1970.

Dyck, P. J., Beahrs, O. H., and Miller, R. H.: Peripheral nerves in hereditary neural atrophies: number and diameters of myelinated fibers. Proceedings. Sixth International Congress of Electroencephalography and Clinical Neurophysiology, Vienna, 673, 1965.

Dyck, P. J., Lambert, E. H., and Nichols, P. C.: Quantitative measurement of sensation related to compound action potential and number and sizes of myelinated and unmyelinated fibers of sural nerve in health, Friedreich's ataxia, hereditary sensory neuropathy, and tabes dorsalis. *In* Cobb, W. A. (ed.): Handbook of Electroencephalography and Clinical Neurophysiology. Vol. 9. Amsterdam, Elsevier Publishing Co., 1972, p. 83.

Dyck, P.J., Lambert, E. H., Sanders, K., and O'Brien, P. C.: Severe hypomyelination and marked abnormality of conduction in Dejerine-Sottas hypertrophic neuropathy: myelin thickness and compound action potential of sural nerve in vitro. Mayo Clin. Proc., *46*:433, 1971.

Dyck, P. J., Gutrecht, J. A., Bastron, J. A., Karnes, W. E., and Dale, A. J. D.: Histologic and teased-fiber measurements of sural nerve in disorders of lower motor and primary sensory neurons. Mayo Clin. Proc., *43*:81, 1968.

Eccles, J. C., and Sherrington, C. S.: Numbers and contraction values of individual motor units examined in some muscles of the limb. Proc. R. Soc. Lond. [Biol.], *106*:326, 1930.

Elfvin, L. G.: The ultrastructure of the nodes of Ranvier in cat sympathetic nerve fibers. J. Ultrastruct. Res., *5*:374, 1961.

Evans, D. H. L., and Vizoso, A. D.: Observations on the mode of growth of motor nerve fibers in rabbits during postnatal development. J. Comp. Neurol., *95*:429, 1951.

Ewald, A., and Kühne, W.: Ueber einen neuen Bestand-teil des Nervensystems. Verh. Naturh. Med. Ver. Heidelb., *1*:457, 1877.

Fernand, V. S. V., and Young, J. Z.: The sizes of the nerve fibres of muscle nerves. Proc. R. Soc. Lond. [Biol.], *139*:38, 1951.

Fernández-Morán, H.: The submicroscopic organization of vertebrate nerve fibers. Exp. Cell Res., *3*:282, 1952.

Finean, J. B.: X-ray diffraction studies of the myelin sheath in peripheral and central nerve fibers. Exp. Cell Res., Suppl, *5*:18, 1958.

Finean, J. B.: X-ray diffraction analysis of nerve myelin. *In* Cumings, J. N. (ed.): Modern Scientific Aspects of Neurology. London, E. Arnold, 1960, p. 232.

Fraher, J. P.: A quantitative study of anterior root fibres during early myelination. J. Anat., *112*:99, 1972.

Fraher, J. P.: A quantitative study of anterior root fibres during early myelination. II. Longitudinal variation in sheath thickness and axon circumference. J. Anat., *115*:421, 1973.

Friede, R. L.: Control of myelin formation by axon caliber (with a model of the control mechanism). J. Comp. Neurol., *144*:233, 1972.

Friede, R. L., and Samorajski, T.: Relation between the number of myelin lamellae and axon circumference in fibers of vagus and sciatic nerves of mice. J. Comp. Neurol., *130*:223, 1967.

Friede, R. L., and Samorajski, T.: Myelin formation in the sciatic nerve of the rat. J. Neuropathol. Exp. Neurol., *27*:546, 1968.

Friede, R. L., and Samorajski, T.: The clefts of Schmidt-Lantermann: a quantitative electron microscopic study of their structure in developing and adult sciatic nerves of the rat. Anat. Rec., *165*:89, 1969.

Garven, H. S. D., Gairns, F. W., and Smith, G.: The nerve fibre populations of the nerves of the leg in chronic occlusive arterial disease in man. Scott. Med. J., *7*:250, 1962.

Gasser, H. S.: The hypothesis of saltatory conduction. Cold Spring Harbor Symp. Quant. Biol., *17*:32, 1952.

Gerebtzoff, M. A., and Mladenov, S.: Affinity for metallic salts and acetylcholinesterase activity at Ranvier nodes. Acta Histochem., *26*:318, 1967.

Geren, B.: The formation from the Schwann cell surface of myelin in the peripheral nerves of chick embryos. Exp. Cell Res., *7*:558, 1954.

Glees, P.: Observations on the structure of the connective tissue sheaths of cutaneous nerves. J. Anat., *77*:153, 1942.

Golgi, C.: Sulla struttura della fibre nervose midollate periferiche e centrali. Arch. Sci. Med. (Torino), *4*:221, 1881.

Greenfield, J. G., and Carmichael, E. A.: The peripheral nerves in cases of subacute combined degeneration of the cord. Brain, *58*:483, 1935.

Gutrecht, J. A., and Dyck, P. J.: Quantitative teased-fiber and histologic studies of human sural nerve during post-natal development. J. Comp. Neurol., *138*:117, 1970.

Hall, S. M., and Williams, P. L.: Studies on the "incisures" of Schmidt and Lanterman. J. Cell Sci., *6*:767, 1970.

Harkin, J. C.: A series of desmosomal attachments in the Schwann sheath of myelinated mammalian nerves. Z. Zellforsch. Mikrosk. Anat., *64*:189, 1964.

Herbst, F.: Untersuchungen über Metallreaktionen an der Ranvierschen Schnürringen. Acta Histochem. (Jena), *22*:223, 1965.

Hess, A., and Young, J. Z.: The nodes of Ranvier. Proc. R. Soc. Lond. [Biol.], *140*:301, 1952.

Hillarp, N. Å., and Olivecrona, H.: The role played by the axon and the Schwann cells in the degree of myelination of the peripheral nerve fibre. Acta Anat. (Basel), *2*:17, 1946.

Hirano, A., and Dembitzer, M.: The transverse bands as a means of access to the periaxonal space of the central myelinated nerve fiber. J. Ultrastruct. Res., *28*:141, 1969.

Hiscoe, H. B.: Distribution of nodes and incisures in normal and regenerated nerve fibers. Anat. Rec., *99*:447, 1947.

Hodgkin, A. L.: The Conduction of the Nervous Impulse. Springfield, Ill., Charles C Thomas, 1964.

Holtzman, E., and Novikoff, A. B.: Lysosomes in the rat sciatic nerve following crush. J. Cell Biol., *27*:651, 1965.

Laatsch, R. H., and Cowan, W. M.: A structural specialization at nodes of Ranvier in the central nervous system. Nature (Lond.), *210*:757, 1966.

Landon, D. N., and Langley, O. K.: Cationic binding at the node of Ranvier. J. Anat., *105*:196, 1969.

Landon, D. N., and Langley, O. K.: The local chemical environment of nodes of Ranvier: a study of cation binding. J. Anat., *108*:419, 1971.

Landon, D. N., and Williams, P. L.: The ultrastructure of the node of Ranvier. Nature (Lond.), *199*:575, 1963.

Langley, O. K.: Ion exchange at the node of Ranvier. Histochem. J., *1*:295, 1969.

Langley, O. K.: The interaction between peripheral nerve polyanions and alcian blue. J. Neurochem., *17*:1535, 1970.

Langley, O. K., and Landon, D. N.: Light and electron histochemical approach to the node of Ranvier and myelin of peripheral nerve. J. Histochem. Cytochem., *15*:722, 1967.

Langley, O. K., and Landon, D. N.: Copper binding at nodes of Ranvier: a new electron histochemical technique for the demonstration of polyanions. J. Histochem. Cytochem., *17*:66, 1969.

Lanterman, A. J.: Ueber den feineren Bau der mark-haltigen Nervenfasern. Arch. Mikrosk. Anat. Entwicklungsmech., *13*:1, 1877.

Lascelles, R. G., and Thomas, P. K.: Changes due to age in internodal length in the sural nerve in man. J. Neurol., Neurosurg., Psychiatry, *29*:40, 1966.

Laverack, J. O., Sunderland, S., and Ray, L. J.: The branching of nerve fibers in human cutaneous nerves. J. Comp. Neurol., *94*:293, 1951.

Livingston, R. B., Pfenninger, K., Moor, H., and Akert, K.: Specialized paranodal and interparanodal glial-axonal junctions in the peripheral and central nervous system: a freeze-etching study. Brain Res., *58*:1, 1973.

Lloyd, D. P. C., and Chang, H. T.: Afferent fibers in muscle nerves. J. Neurophysiol., *11*:199, 1948.

Lubińska, L.: Short internodes "intercalated" in nerve fibres. Acta Biol. Exp. (Wars.), *18*:117, 1958.

Lubińska, L.: Axoplasmic streaming in regenerating and in normal nerve fibres. Progr. Brain Res., *13*:1, 1964.

Lubińska, L., and Lukaszewska, I.: Shape of myelinated nerve fibres and proximo-distal flow of axoplasm. Acta Biol. Exp. (Wars.), *17*:115, 1956.

Nageotte, J.: Incisures de Schmidt-Lanterman et proto-plasma des cellules de Schwann. C. R. Acad. Sci. (Paris), *68*:39, 1910.

Napolitano, L., and Scallen, T. J.: Observations on the

fine structure of peripheral nerve myelin. Anat. Rec., *163*:1, 1969.

Noback, C. R.: The protagon (π) granules of Reich. J. Comp. Neurol., *99*:91, 1953.

Ochoa, J., Fowler, T. J., and Gilliatt, R. W.: Anatomical changes in peripheral nerves compressed by a pneumatic tourniquet. J. Anat., *113*:433, 1972.

Ochoa, J., and Mair, W. G. P.: The normal sural nerve in man. I. Ultrastructure and numbers of fibres and cells. Acta neuropathol., *13*:197, 1969.

O'Leary, J., Heinbecker, P., and Bishop, G. H.: Analysis of function of a nerve to muscle. Am. J. Physiol., *110*:636, 1934.

O'Sullivan, D. J., and Swallow, M.: The fibre size and content of the radial and sural nerves. J. Neurol. Neurosurg. Psychiatry, *31*:464, 1968.

Peters, A.: The node of Ranvier in the central nervous system. J. Exp. Physiol., *51*:229, 1966.

Peters, A., and Vaughn, J. E.: Morphology and development of the myelin sheath. *In* Davison, A. N., and Peters, A. (eds.): Myelination. Springfield, Ill., Charles C Thomas, 1970, p. 3.

Pinner, B., Davison, J. F., and Campbell, J. B.: Alkaline phosphatase in peripheral nerves. Science, *145*:936, 1964.

Prineas, J.: The pathogenesis of dying-back polyneuropathies. II. An ultrastructural study of experimental acrylamide intoxication in the cat. J. Neuropathol. Exp. Neurol., *28*:598, 1969.

Ranish, N., and Ochs, S.: Fast axoplasmic transport of acetylcholinesterase in mammalian nerve fibers. J. Neurochem., *19*:2641, 1972.

Ranson, S. W., Droegemueller, W. H., Davenport, K., and Fisher, C.: Number, size and myelination of the sensory fibers in the cerebrospinal nerves. Proc. Ass. Res. Nerv. Ment. Dis., *15*:3, 1934.

Ranvier, L.: Recherches sur l'histologie et la physiologie des nerfs. Arch. Physiol., I. Sér., *4*:129, 1871.

Ranvier, L.: Des étranglements annulaires et des segments interannulaires chez les Raies et les Torpilles. C. R. Acad. Sci. (Paris), *75*:1129, 1872.

Ranvier, L.: Traité Technique d'Histologie. Paris, Savy, 1875.

Ranvier, L.: Leçons sur l'Histologie du Système Nerveux, Paris, Savy, 1876.

Reich, F.: Ueber eine neue Granulation in der Nervenzellen. Arch. Anat. Physiol., Physiol. Abt., p. 208, 1903.

Revel, J. P., and Hamilton, D. W.: The double nature of the intermediate dense line in peripheral nerve myelin. Anat. Rec., *163*:7, 1969.

Rexed, B.: Contributions to the knowledge of the postnatal development of the peripheral nervous system in man. Acta Psychiatr. Scand. [Suppl.] 33, 1944.

Rexed, B., and Therman, P. O.: Caliber spectra of motor and sensory nerve fibers to flexor and extensor muscles. J. Neurophysiol., *11*:133, 1948.

Rezzonico, G.: Sulla struttura delle fibre nervose del midollo spinale. Arch. Sci. Med. (Torino), *4*:78, 1881.

Robertson, J. D.: The ultrastructure of adult vertebrate peripheral myelinated nerve fibers in relation to myelinogenesis. J. Biophys. Biochem. Cytol., *1*:271, 1955.

Robertson, J. D.: New observations of the ultrastructure of the membrane of frog peripheral nerve fibers. J. Biophys. Biochem. Cytol., *3*:1043, 1957.

Robertson, J. D.: The ultrastructure of Schmidt-Lanter-

man clefts and related shearing defects of the myelin sheath. J. Biophys. Biochem. Cytol., *4*:39, 1958.

Robertson, J. D.: Preliminary observations on the ultrastructure of nodes of Ranvier. Z. Zellforsch. Mikrosk. Anat., *50*:553, 1959.

Robertson, J. D.: The molecular structure and contact relationships of cell membranes. Progr. Biophys., *10*:343, 1960.

Rodriguez Echandía, E., and Piezzi, R.: Microtubules in the nerve of the toad *Bufo arenarum* Hensel. Effects of low temperature on the sciatic nerve. J. Cell Biol., *39*:491, 1968.

Rushton, W. A. H.: A theory of the effects of fibre size in medullated nerve. J. Physiol. (Lond.), *115*:101, 1951.

Sanders, F. K.: The thickness of the myelin sheath of normal and regenerating peripheral nerve fibres. Proc. R. Soc. Lond. [Biol.], *135*:323, 1948.

Scheuer, J. L.: Fibre size frequency distribution in human laryngeal nerves. J. Anat., *98*:99, 1964.

Schlaepfer, W. W., and Myers, F. K.: Relationship of myelin internode elongation and growth in the rat sural nerve. J. Comp. Neurol., *147*:255, 1973.

Schmidt, H. D.: On the construction of the dark or double-bordered nerve fibre. Mon. Microsc. J. (Lond.), *11*:200, 1874.

Schmidt, W. J.: Doppelbrechung und Feinbau der Markscheide der Nervenfasern. Z. Zellforsch. Mikrosk. Anat., *23*:657, 1936.

Schmitt, F. O., and Bear, R. S.: Optical properties of the axon sheaths of crustacean nerves. J. Cell Comp. Physiol., *9*:275, 1937.

Schmitt, F. O., and Clark, G. L.: X-ray diffraction studies on nerve. Radiology, *25*:131, 1935.

Schuchardt, E.: Der Zusammenhang zwischen Faserdurchmesser und Länge der interanulären Segmente bei Fasern des Nervus ischiadicus von Fröschen verschiedener Wachstumsstadien. Anat. Anz., *96*:241, 1948.

Schwarzacher, H. G.: Markscheidendicke und Achsenzylinderdurchmesser in peripheren menschlichen Nerven. Acta Anat., *21*:26, 1954.

Sharma, A. K., and Thomas, P. K.: Quantitative studies on age changes in unmyelinated nerve fibres in the vagus nerve in man. *In* Kunze, K., and Desmedt, J. (eds.): Studies on Neuromuscular Diseases. Proceedings of the International Symposium on Neuromuscular Diseases, April 1973, in Giessen. Basel, S. Karger, 1975.

Shepherd, R. H., Sholl, D. A., and Vizoso, A. D.: The size relationships subsisting between body length, limbs and jaws in man. J. Anat., *83*:296, 1949.

Sherrington, C. S.: On the anatomical constitution of nerves of skeletal muscles: with remarks on recurrent fibres in the ventral roots. J. Physiol. (Lond.), *17*:211, 1894.

Simpson, S. A., and Young, J. Z.: Regeneration of fibre diameter after cross-unions of visceral and somatic nerves. J. Anat., *79*:48, 1945.

Singer, S. J.: A fluid lipid-globular protein mosaic model of membrane structure. Ann. N.Y. Acad. Sci., *195*:16, 1972.

Singer, M., and Bryant, S. V.: Movement in the myelin Schwann sheath of the vertebrate axon. Nature (Lond.), *221*:1148, 1969.

Singer, M., and Salpeter, M. M.: The transport of ^{3}H-L-histidine through the Schwann and myelin sheath into the axon, including a re-evaluation of myelin function. J. Morphol., *120*:281, 1966.

Singer, M., and Steinberg, M. C.: Wallerian degeneration: a reevaluation based on transected and colchicine-poisoned nerves in the amphibian, Triturus. Am. J. Anat., *133*:51, 1972.

Sjöstrand, F. S.: The lamellated structure of the nerve myelin sheath as revealed by high resolution electron microscopy. Experientia, *9*:68, 1953.

Smith, R. S., and Koles, Z. J.: Myelinated nerve fibers: computed effect of myelin thickness on conduction velocity. Am. J. Physiol., *219*:1256, 1970.

Speidel, C. C.: Studies of living nerves. I. J. Exp. Zool., *61*:279, 1932.

Spencer, P. S.: Light and electron microscopic observations on localized peripheral nerve injuries. Ph.D. thesis, University of London, 1971.

Spencer, P. S.: A reappraisal of the model for "bulk axoplasmic flow." Nature [New Biol.], *240*:283, 1972.

Spencer, P. S., and Lieberman, A. R.: Scanning electron microscopy of isolated peripheral nerve fibers: normal surface structure and alterations proximal to neuromas. Z. Zellforsch. Mikrosk. Anat., *119*:534, 1971.

Spencer, P. S., and Thomas, P. K.: Electron microscope observations on the effects of constriction on regenerating axons. To be published, 1975.

Spencer, P. S., Raine, C. S., and Wisniewski, H.: Axon diameter and myelin thickness—unusual relationships in dorsal root ganglia. Anat. Rec., *176*:225, 1973.

Stevens, J. C., Lofgren, E. P., and Dyck, P. J.: Histometric evaluation of branches of peroneal nerve: technique for combined biopsy of muscle nerve and cutaneous nerve. Brain Res., *52*:37, 1973.

Sunderland, S., Laverack, J. O., and Ray, L. J.: The caliber of nerve fibers in human cutaneous nerves. J. Comp. Neurol., *91*:87, 1949.

Sunderland, S., and Roche, A.: Axon-myelin relationships in peripheral nerve fibres. Acta Anat., *33*:1, 1958.

Swallow, M.: Fibre size and content of the anterior tibial nerve of the foot. J. Neurol. Neurosurg. Psychiatry, *29*:205, 1966.

Thomas, P. K.: Growth changes in the myelin sheath of peripheral nerve fibres in fishes. Proc. R. Soc. Lond. [Biol.], *143*:380, 1955.

Thomas, P. K.: Growth changes in the diameter of peripheral nerve fibres in fishes. J. Anat., *90*:5, 1956.

Thomas, P. K., and Slatford, J.: Lamellar bodies in the cytoplasm of Schwann cells. J. Anat., *98*:691, 1964.

Thomas, P. K., and Young, J. Z.: Internode lengths in nerves of fishes. J. Anat., *83*:336, 1949.

Thudichum, J. L.: A Treatise of the Chemical Constitution of the Brain. London, Baillière, Tindall and Cox, 1884.

Tomasch, J., and Britton, W. A.: On the individual variability of fibre composition in human peripheral nerves. J. Anat., *90*:337, 1956.

Tomasch, J., and Schwarzacher, H. G.: Die innere Struktur peripherer menschlicher Nerven im Lichte faseranalytischer Untersuchungen. Acta Anat. (Basel), Suppl., *16*:315, 1952.

Tomonaga, M., and Sluga, E.: Zur Ultrastruktur der π-Granula. Acta Neuropathol., *15*:56, 1970.

Uzman, B. G., and Nogueira-Graf, G.: Electron microscope studies of the formation of nodes of Ranvier in mouse sciatic nerves. J. Biophys. Biochem. Cytol., *3*:589, 1957.

Vanderkooi, G.: Molecular architecture of biological membranes. Ann. N.Y. Acad. Sci., *195*:6, 1972.

Vizoso, A. D.: The relationship between internodal length and growth in human nerves. J. Anat., *84*: 342, 1950.

Vizoso, A. D., and Young, J. Z.: Internode length and fibre diameter in developing and regenerating nerves. J. Anat., *82*:110, 1948.

Waxman, S. G.: Micropinocytotic invaginations in the axolemma of peripheral nerves. Z. Zellforsch. Mikrosk. Anat., *86*:571, 1968.

Waxman, S. G.: Regional differentiation of the axon: a review with special reference to the concept of the multiplex neuron. Brain Res., *47*:269, 1972.

Webster, H. de F.: Transient, focal accumulation of axonal mitochondria during the early stage of Wallerian degeneration. J. Cell Biol., *12*:361, 1962.

Webster, H. de F.: The relationship between Schmidt-Lantermann incisures and myelin segmentation during Wallerian degeneration. Ann. N.Y. Acad. Sci., *122*:29, 1965.

Webster, H. de F., and Spiro, D.: Phase and electron microscopic studies of experimental demyelination. I. Variations in myelin sheath contour in normal guinea pig sciatic nerve. J. Neuropathol. Exp. Neurol., *19*:42, 1960.

Weiss, P., and Hiscoe, H. B.: Experiments on the mechanism of nerve growth. J. Exp. Zool., *107*:315, 1948.

Weller, R. O., and Herzog, I.: Schwann cell lysosomes in hypertrophic neuropathy in normal human nerves. Brain, *93*:347, 1970.

Wendell-Smith, C. P., and Williams, P. L.: The use of teased preparations and frozen sections in quantitative studies of mammalian peripheral nerve. Q. J. Microsc. Sci., *100*:499, 1959.

Whitear, M.: Internode length in the skin plexuses of fish and the frog. Q. J. Microsc. Sci., *93*:307, 1952.

Williams, P. L.: Sections of fresh mammalian nerve trunks for quantitative studies: a rapid freezing technique. Q. J. Microsc. Sci., *100*:425, 1959.

Williams, P. L., and Kashef, R.: Asymmetry of the node of Ranvier. J. Cell Sci., *3*:341, 1968.

Williams, P. L., and Landon, D. N.: Paranodal apparatus of peripheral myelinated nerve fibres of mammals. Nature (Lond.), *198*:670, 1963.

Williams, P. L., and Landon, D. N.: The energy source of the nerve fibre. New Scientist, *21*:166, 1964.

Williams, P. L., and Wendell-Smith, C. P.: The use of fixed and stained sections in quantitative studies of peripheral nerve. Q. J. Microsc. Sci., *101*:43, 1960.

Williams, P. L., and Wendell-Smith, C. P.: Some additional parametric variations between peripheral nerve fibre populations. J. Anat., *109*:505, 1971.

Wulfhekel, U., and Düllmann, J.: Quantitative Untersuchungen an den Markscheiden im N. ischiadicus des Frosches und des Rhesusaffen unter besonderer Berücksichtigung der Schmidt-Lantermanschen Einkerbungen. Z. Anat. Entwicklungsgesch., *134*: 298, 1971.

Young, J. Z.: The history of the shape of a nerve fibre. *In* Le Gros Clark, W. E., and Medawar, P. B. (eds.): Essays on Growth and Form. Oxford, Oxford University Press, 1945.

Zenker, W., and Hohberg, E.: A-α-nerve fibre: number of neurotubules in the stem fibre and in the terminal branches. J. Neurocytol., *2*:143, 1973.

Chapter 7

MICROSCOPIC ANATOMY OF UNMYELINATED NERVE FIBERS

José Ochoa

Knowledge of the biology of unmyelinated fibers has progressed at a slow pace as a consequence of their very small size.* Their slender axons are perhaps the extreme example of disproportion between length and thickness among cell processes. Scrutiny of a number of structural parameters, which in myelinated fibers were satisfactorily accessible to light microscopy, had to await electron microscopy in unmyelinated fibers. Equally, those evasive electrical properties of unmyelinated fibers that are dependent on axon size have retarded electrophysiologic research. Consequently, some structural and functional properties that were defined decades ago for myelinated fibers are currently being resolved in unmyelinated fibers. This may be the reason why reference to them is sometimes omitted in articles on composition of peripheral nerves, despite the fact that they are the most numerous components of both sensory and autonomic nerves.

By definition, axons covered by satellite cells that have not produced myelin around them are "unmyelinated." In a broad sense, this category includes all axons at an early stage of development or regeneration, certain portions of mature myelinated axons adjoining the cell body and nerve endings, demyelinated axons, and finally the large group of mature, small nerve fibers that are

normally not myelinated. Strictly, only the latter are referred to as unmyelinated fibers. Although the classification of fibers as unmyelinated is made on the basis of a negative structural feature that may be to some extent circumstantial, such fibers constitute a fairly well-defined group in terms of their phylogenesis, electrophysiologic properties, and subservience to certain functional modalities, and perhaps also in terms of particular metabolic features as far as can be speculated from the occurrence of disease processes that affect unmyelinated fibers or their neurons specifically or predominantly.

In this chapter emphasis is laid on the structural features of somatic rather than autonomic unmyelinated fibers, with special reference to man.

HISTORICAL BACKGROUND

It seems unlikely that Antonius van Leeuwenhoek who first saw nerve fibers through his newly invented microscope in the seventeenth century may have seen the unmyelinated fibers. Dedicated histologists of the eighteenth century like Felice Fontana, who in 1781 made a remarkable description of what was later called the myelinated fiber, may have seen unmyelinated fibers, but there is no record to indicate that such slender nerve cell processes had been recognized by anyone before Robertus Remak wrote of his "observationes anatomicae et microscopicae" in Germany in the 1830's. Remak's material consisted

---

*The term "unmyelinated fiber" is employed to describe the structure made up by one or more unmyelinated axons and their associated satellite cells (see also Chapter 17).

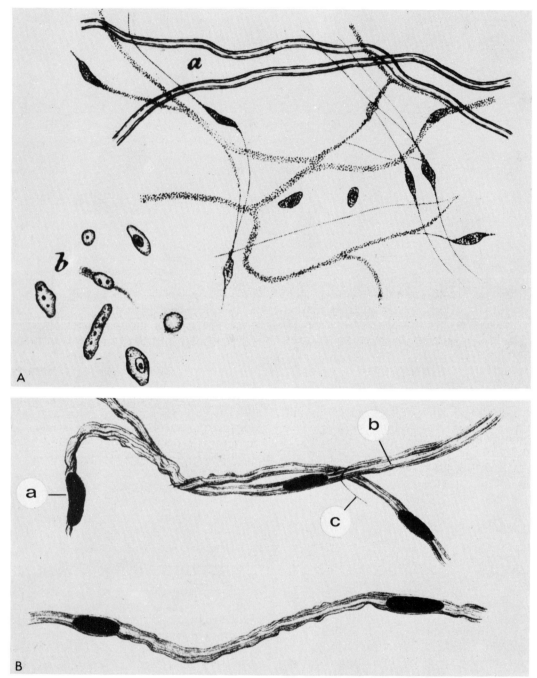

Figure 7–1   *A.* "Fibrae organicae from a sympathetic nerve from the ox, with two thin tubuli primitivi (a) and several nucleated and nonnucleated corpuscles (b) intervening between the fibrae organicae." (From Remak, R.: Observationes anatomicae et microscopicae de systematis nervosi structura. Berlin, Sumptibus et Formis Reimerianis, 1838.) *B.* "Fibres of Remak from the carotid canal of a rabbit: teased in aqueous humour, fixed in 1 per cent osmic acid. Grubler's haematoxylin and eosin in glycerine. These fibres, being somewhat flattened through teasing and crushing, show how the sheath breaks into fibrils: a, nucleus; b, core of the fibre; c, sheath." (From Tuckett, I. L.: On the structure and degeneration of non-medullated nerve fibres. J. Physiol. (Lond.), *19*:267, 1895.)

of autonomic nerves and his technique, the only available at the time, was the examination of fibers from freshly excised nerves teased apart in water. Among the myelinated fibers ("tubuli primitivi"), Remak saw and illustrated delicate fibers both in man and in animals that he called fibrae organicae (Fig. 7–1*A*). Although he specifically pointed at nucleated corpuscles that were present in relation to nerve fibers, according to the review by Münzer (1939), Remak did not quite realize that they were cells. Only a year after Remak's classic monograph, Theodor Schwann (1839) elaborated upon the concept of the cell and reported on his discovery of the cell that we name after him. Although acknowledged by Schwann, it is not generally appreciated today that Remak (1837) was in fact the discoverer of the axis cylinder in myelinated fibers; he failed, however, to notice that unmyelinated fibers also contain axis cylinders.

It was Ivor Tuckett, working in Cambridge, who in 1895 was the first to describe the unmyelinated fibers as composed of sheath cells surrounding cores (Fig. 7–1*B*). In the same report, Tuckett advanced an accurate description of the gross changes in unmyelinated fibers following nerve transection.

Santiago Ramón y Cajal might have written more about unmyelinated fibers if his silver technique for axon impregnation had allowed him to visualize them better. The introduction by Ranson of the pyridine-silver modification of Cajal's technique in the first decade of this century was a significant advance that permitted him and his colleagues to demonstrate the profusion of unmyelinated fibers in somatic nerves of man and animals, and to demonstrate the origin of most of them in the small neurons of the dorsal root ganglia (Fig. 7–2*A*) (Ranson, 1911, 1912). This new information immediately placed Ranson and his co-workers in a favorable position to attempt to relate peripheral nerve fiber types and functions. Their report, "Unmyelinated nerve fibres as conductors of protopathic sensation," published in 1915, stands in many ways unchallenged. Ranson's early view that the vast majority of unmyelinated fibers in peripheral nerves arise from the dorsal root ganglia and are afferent was eventually questioned by Bishop et al. (1933), who attributed to them an efferent function and singled them out as an exception to the Bell-Magendie law of organization of nerve fiber systems. Subsequent work by Ranson and his

associates (1935) vindicated their original view, since accepted universally.

When Jean Nageotte developed a method for dissociating myelinated fibers by treating the nerves with weak acid after alcohol fixation, he noticed that unmyelinated fibers became particularly accessible to examination. By using this technique Nageotte (1922) felt he had achieved authority to "elucidate some controversial or unknown aspects of the structure of unmyelinated fibres." He stressed that unmyelinated fibers are composite, that is, each fiber contains several axons, and made the point that although fibers are arranged in interlacing trabeculae that branch and reunite, it is only their satellite apparatus that anastomoses; their axons are merely exchanged. Having settled this delicate matter, Nageotte nevertheless remained convinced that Schwann cells of unmyelinated fibers form a syncytium, a misconception that was due to the limited microscopic resolution then available and that was not rectified by early electron microscopists in the field.

A decisive step toward defining the finer structural features of unmyelinated fibers was made by Herbert Gasser, who turned his attention to morphology in order to increase his understanding of the electrophysiology of nerve fibers. Initially, using phase microscopy of fresh preparations, Gasser (1950) confirmed that frequently each unmyelinated fiber contains a bundle of axons. Later, by electron microscopy, Gasser (1952, 1955) further penetrated the fine details of the surface relations of unmyelinated axons and satellite cells in nerves of the cat. He pointed out that the axons are limited by well-defined walls, to which the metallic particles become attached after silver impregnation (Fig. 7–2*B* and *C*). In 1952, Gasser still entertained the rather primitive concept that unmyelinated axons are floating within the cytoplasm of the Schwann cell, attached on one side to the sheath by a delicate ligament that he called the "mesaxon." Gasser also endorsed Nageotte's view that the Schwann cell sheath is syncytial. That the unmyelinated axons are outside of the satellite cells, and that the mesaxon is an infolding of the plasma membrane of such cells, was eventually shown by Gasser (1955) a year after Geren (1954) had demonstrated this same basic relationship in nerve fibers during development.

Although the chief morphologic difference between myelinated and unmyelinated axons

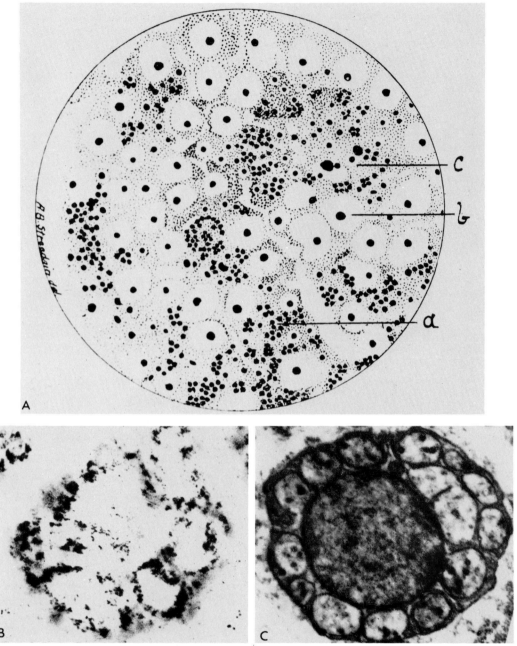

Figure 7–2 *A.*"From a transverse section of a human sciatic nerve. Cajal's method. a, non-medullated fibers; b, large medullated fibers; c, small medullated fiber." *B.* "Electron microscope picture of C fibers in the saphenous nerve of the cat, stained with silver by the Ranson method. Note the silver precipitation about the fibers. To derive the better-known light pictures with this stain, it should be borne in mind that in sections 10 to 20 times as thick (1 to 2 μ) the granules about the fibers would form a continuous ring. Without special precautions in microphotography the rings are caused to appear as solid black dots as the result of light diffraction" (Gasser, 1950). *C.* "Electron micrograph of Schwann cell sheath containing unmyelinated axons in the hypogastric nerve of the cat." (*A* from Ranson, S. W.: Non-medullated nerve fibers in the spinal nerves. Am. J. Anat., *12*:67, 1911. *B* and *C* from Gasser, H. S.: Properties of dorsal root unmedullated fibers on the two sides of the ganglion. J. Gen. Physiol., *38*:709, 1955. Reprinted by permission.)

These figures illustrate the abundance of unmyelinated fibers in peripheral nerves, their distribution within nerve trunks, and the improvement in image resolution afforded by the electron microscope: *B* and *C* would appear as dots in *A*.

is in a sense quantitative and ultimately dependent on the degree of orderly growth of the Schwann cell tongues that define the mesaxon, there is no question of such a growth process ever taking place in unmyelinated fibers; their axons remain completely bare of myelin. Some confusion in this area arose from earlier polarized light microscopic studies from which it was maintained that unmyelinated axons were thinly coated by myelin. Fernández-Morán (1952), involved by Hess and Lansing (1953) in this issue, did, however, make it quite clear that

... unmyelinated fibers* from spinal cords ... and sympathetic trunks ... consist of uniform filaments, approximately 100Å in diameter ... which are tightly packed together ... and show a thin sheath consisting of a *single granular membrane* ... which envelops the dense bundle of filaments.

INTRANEURAL AND TERMINAL DISTRIBUTION OF PERIPHERAL UNMYELINATED FIBERS

Arrangement of Unmyelinated Fibers Within Nerve Trunks

From the early transverse sections of nerves stained with pyridine-silver shown in Figure 7–2A, it was clear that unmyelinated fibers are not confined to exclusive compartments of the nerves, but are instead widely dispersed between myelinated fibers. Improved morphologic techniques have consistently shown that the compound unmyelinated fibers (bundles of axons) are assembled in groups rather than being scattered randomly in the endoneurium. Further, there is a consistent tendency for small-caliber myelinated fibers to be mixed in such groups (Fig. 7–3A). This close relationship of small myelinated fibers and unmyelinated fibers in adult nerves is reminiscent of that which prevails, in developing nerves, between fibers that have already acquired myelin and those without it; here the newly myelinated fibers, just segregated from the groups of primitive axons devoid of myelin, maintain a close space relation to such groups (Peters and Muir, 1959; Cravioto, 1965; Gamble, 1966; Friede and Samorajski, 1968; Allt, 1969; Ochoa, 1971; Webster, 1971).

Since the small-diameter myelinated fibers in a nerve are those that become myelinated last (Boughton, 1906), they would be expected to sustain in their definitive pattern the closest relationship to the unmyelinated fibers, which are the vestiges of the primitive bundles of axons.

Normally in mature peripheral nerves in various species, the relation between small myelinated fibers and genuine unmyelinated fibers is distinctly different from that which prevails in clusters of regenerated fibers containing sprouts before and after myelination (Thomas, 1968; Schröder, 1968; Ochoa, 1970a, 1970b; Spencer, 1971). In these clusters the myelinated and future myelinated axons are closely applied to each other, with little intervening collagen, in such a way that the profile of the group in cross section is neatly rounded or oval (Fig. 7–3B). Further, a common basal lamina, which covered the original fiber before degeneration and regeneration, may still enclose the elements of the cluster. No matter how closely associated myelinated and unmyelinated fibers may be, whether in the normal adult, in the developing nerve, or in regenerating clusters, myelinated axons are not seen sharing a satellite cell with other axons except in very rare instances.

Another interesting association of myelinated and unmyelinated fibers that does not occur normally is seen in the complexes that result from the orientation of unmyelinated fibers along myelinated fibers. Such a curious event was reported by Evans and Murray (1954) and confirmed on electron microscopy by King and Thomas (1971) in the context of regenerating autonomic axons that become misdirected toward a myelinated branch of the nerve. Ochoa and Mair (1969b) and Ochoa (1970c) maintained that the same ill-understood tropism may attract unmyelinated fibers to myelinated fibers in some human neuropathies, and explain a variant of hypertrophic "onion bulb" formation characterized by a core fiber surrounded by a whorl of genuine unmyelinated fibers or their denervated Schwann cell bands. (For further details, see Chapter 17.)

The differences between the various patterns of association of myelinated and unmyelinated fibers gain relevance when one is dealing with abnormal nerves in which regenerating fibers frequently occur and thus confuse the identification of the nerve fiber types.

---

*"Fibers" obviously refers to axons.

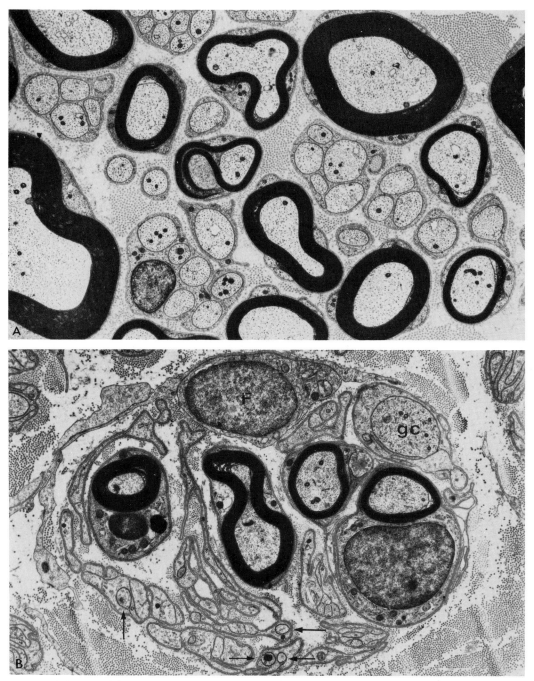

Figure 7–3   *A.* An area rich in unmyelinated fibers and in myelinated fibers of small caliber from a transverse section of the medial popliteal nerve of a normal baboon. These two categories are rarely found independently of each other. Glutaraldehyde perfusion fixation, osmium tetroxide. × 7400. *B.* Cross section of a cluster of regenerated fibers from the sural nerve of a patient with isoniazid neuropathy. Within the unit there are small myelinated fibers and axons devoid of myelin (arrows) suspended in their Schwann cells. A "growth cone" (gc) also occurs. The various subunits and the fibroblast (F) fit to complement an oval pattern. Osmium tetroxide immersion fixation. × 7200.

Course of Axons Within Unmyelinated Nerve Fibers

The course of axons within the anastomosing systems of unmyelinated fibers along the nerve trunks caught the interest of Gasser in the 1950's. He became concerned with the possibility of electrical interaction of neighboring unmyelinated axons, an echo of Katz and Schmitt's (1940) interest in the interaction of myelinated fibers. In this respect it was important to determine the lengths along which neighboring axons ran in parallel, since on theoretical grounds a more or less critical distance could be established beyond which electrical interaction could be predicted from the spike durations of the action currents and the conduction velocities of unmyelinated axons. After trying unsuccessfully to follow the course of axons in teased preparations and in longitudinal sections for electron microscopy, Gasser (1955) decided to "embark upon the laborious but certain method of building up the sheath from cross sections." From reconstructions, he managed to follow 54 axons over a distance of 500 μm in the saphenous nerve of the cat and found that the composition of the bundles kept continuously changing so that it would be unlikely for a pair of neighboring axons to run in close association for more than a short distance. Gasser therefore concluded that interaction sufficient to result in excitation of one axon by another was improbable in the bundles of unmyelinated fibers. As shown later in this chapter, the particular arrangement of unmyelinated axons in cutaneous nerves in man probably makes interaction even less likely: this is in keeping with the conclusions of Torebjörk and Hallin (1970), who recorded single C fiber units intraneurally from nerves in man.

Branching and Terminal Distribution of Unmyelinated Axons

It is uncertain whether unmyelinated axons branch within the nerve trunks. From the quantitative studies of Davenport and Bothe (1934) using silver stains, it was argued by Ranson et al. (1935) that dichotomization of unmyelinated axons was the likeliest explanation for the larger numbers of unmyelinated axons present in nerves than in their corresponding roots. In view of the limitations of light microscopic counts of axons impregnated with silver and the fact that unmyelinated axons are more closely packed in roots than in peripheral nerves, the author considers that the studies just mentioned cannot be regarded as conclusive. An alternative way of attacking the problem would be the direct observation of intraneural branching of unmyelinated axons; however, light microscopic observations might again give rise to legitimate controversy, and confirmation, by electron microscopic studies of serial sections, does not appear to be available.

The ultimate distribution of unmyelinated fibers in cerebrospinal nerves is a function of the system to which they belong (Ranson et al., 1935). A small contingent of sensory unmyelinated fibers enters the deep nerves to supply the periosteum, the joints, and the connective tissue of striated muscle; the blood vessels in the latter also receive a rich supply of vasomotor autonomic unmyelinated fibers. The largest proportion of sensory unmyelinated fibers derived from dorsal root ganglia enter cutaneous nerves to reach the skin. A similar course is followed by the autonomic efferent fibers concerned with the innervation of cutaneous appendages; indeed, the area of cutaneous distribution is the same for autonomic and sensory nerve fibers coursing along any given nerve. Clinical use of this coincidence is possible in cases of acute nerve lesions in which the area of sensory loss can be graphically outlined from the area of sweat loss (Guttmann, 1940; Moberg, 1958).

The pattern of distribution of myelinated and unmyelinated fibers in the skin has been extensively studied by, among others, Weddell and associates, using methylene blue intravitally and silver stains, and Cauna, who has examined the fine structure of nerve terminals and nerve endings with the electron microscope (Weddell, 1941, 1966; Weddell et al., 1954; Cauna, 1968). Although convincing illustrations are hard to find in the literature, it seems established that, like most myelinated axons, unmyelinated axons undergo terminal branching in the skin. To establish this event is difficult because myelinated axons lose their myelin preterminally and also, near the end organs, both types of axons may intermingle. Terminal branching probably occurs in autonomic as well as in somatic unmyelinated axons and is taken to constitute the anatomical basis for some cutaneous "axon reflexes" involving pain fibers and autonomic fibers (Bruce, 1910; Lewis, 1927; Celander and Folkow, 1953; Lewis and Landis, 1929; Rothman and Coon, 1940). There is also indirect electrophysiologic evidence of branching of sensory unmyelinated axons in human skin (Hallin and Torebjörk, 1971).

ULTRASTRUCTURE OF UNMYELINATED FIBERS

Spatial Relationship Between Axons, Schwann Cells, and Collagen

The way in which the Schwann cells in an unmyelinated fiber handle the axons in the bundle varies in different nerves and species. The most primitive pattern is usually exemplified in olfactory nerves. Here many axons in contact with each other are packed in a common compartment limited by enveloping Schwann cell tongues. This crowded situation, which is commonplace in developing nerves, may also be retained in part in adult somatic nerves (Fig. 7–4A).

Some axonal isolation is achieved when Schwann cell tongues partition the bundles and separate individual axons. Although several axons continue to cohabit in a compact and well-defined fiber, delicate septa prevent their axonal surfaces from contacting those of their fellows. This is actually the pattern that was first publicized with the early electron micrographs of unmyelinated fibers and is common in autonomic nerves and in deeply situated somatic nerves (Fig. 7–4B; see also Figs. 7–2C and 7–3A).

Greater independence of unmyelinated axons, whether necessary in terms of function or not, does occur in cutaneous nerves (Fig. 7–4C). Gamble and Eames (1964) noticed this pattern in cutaneous nerves in man where, remote from the perinuclear region of the satellite cell, the bundles branch to form simpler cords, each containing one or sometimes two axons. Such arrangement permits the distinguishing of genuine unmyelinated fibers from regenerated clusters before myelination of the sprouts they contain and has been utilized for differential quantitative estimations of unmyelinated axons in aging and in neuropathies in man (Ochoa and Mair, 1969b; Ochoa, 1970b, 1970c).

In material prepared by chemical fixation for conventional electron microscopy there is a discernible gap of the order of 10 to 15 nm separating the osmiophilic components of the surface membranes of axon and Schwann cell. Such space is, of course, not empty; its regularity would be highly surprising should it not contain a substance of definite width mediating contact. A special technique to reveal "intercellular substance" was first introduced by Doggenweiler and Frenk (1965), who used lanthanum either prior to or during fixation to achieve differential staining of the external coating of the plasma unit membrane. Thus the gap between unmyelinated axons and Schwann cells appeared enhanced, as did the "intercellular substance" in other neural tissues. Similar results have been obtained with ruthenium red and violet (Bondareff, 1967; Luft, 1971). It has become clear that such "intercellular substance" is in fact part of the "greater" cell membrane of apposing cells (Revel and Ito, 1967; see also Schmitt and Samson, 1969). Tight as the adhesion may be, the space can be permeated by extracellular markers such as ferritin (Hall and Williams, 1971).

More frequently than not the whole surface of unmyelinated axons in normal mature somatic nerves is invested by Schwann cell processes (Fig. 7–5A; see also Figs. 7–4B and C and Fig. 7–7A). When a Schwann cell process fails to cover part of the surface of a peripheral axon, there is still the layer of basal lamina separating the axon from the endoneurium. The position of the Schwann cell processes in relation to the axon is not a fixed one. As a result of anoxia (and also following inadequate fixation procedures), the Schwann cell tongues may retract and expose more of the axonal surface than they do under normal circumstances (Ochoa, unpublished data, 1972). The Schwann cell tongues that encircle an unmyelinated axon and whose apposing surface membranes define the "mesaxon" may overlap, but rarely does one surmount the other by more than one turn. More numerous uncompacted turns are a feature of myelinating axons; similar occurrences in "collagen pockets" allow speculation on the question of a possible inhibitory influence of the unmyelinated axon on the winding initiative of the Schwann cells (Fig. 7–5B).

"Collagen pockets" were described by Gamble (1964) and Gamble and Eames (1964) in peripheral nerves of rat and man, and

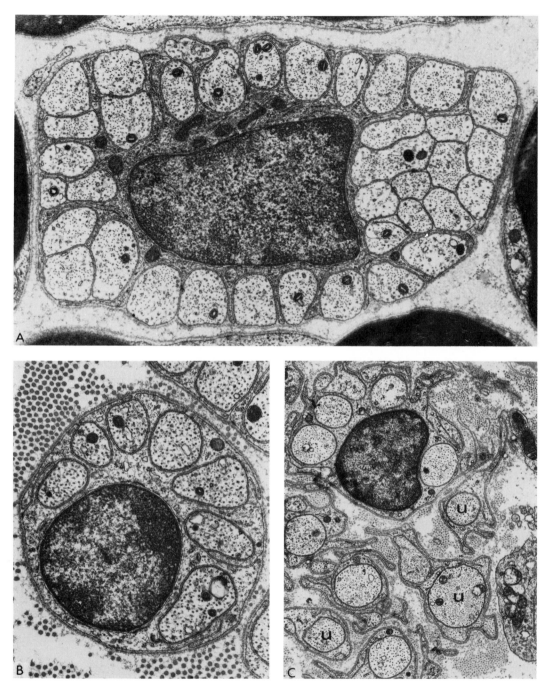

Figure 7–4 *A.* Section from a spinal nerve root of adult cat. Toward the right, a dozen axons are crowded together, their contours being mutually adapted. Most of the axons elsewhere are individually held by Schwann cell tongues; some show part of their surfaces covered by basal lamina only. Glutaraldehyde perfusion fixation followed by osmium tetroxide perfusion fixation. × 16,000. *B.* Section from the medial popliteal nerve of a normal baboon. The axons are completely enveloped by apposing Schwann cell tongues. The complex of axons and satellite cell form a well-defined unit. Glutaraldehyde perfusion fixation; osmium tetroxide. × 15,500. *C.* Section from the sural nerve of a young adult woman. Characteristic arrangement of normal unmyelinated fibers in cutaneous nerves in man. A fiber, dispersed into subunits (u), retains axonal aggregation at the nuclear region. Glutaraldehyde immerson fixation, osmium tetroxide. × 7300.

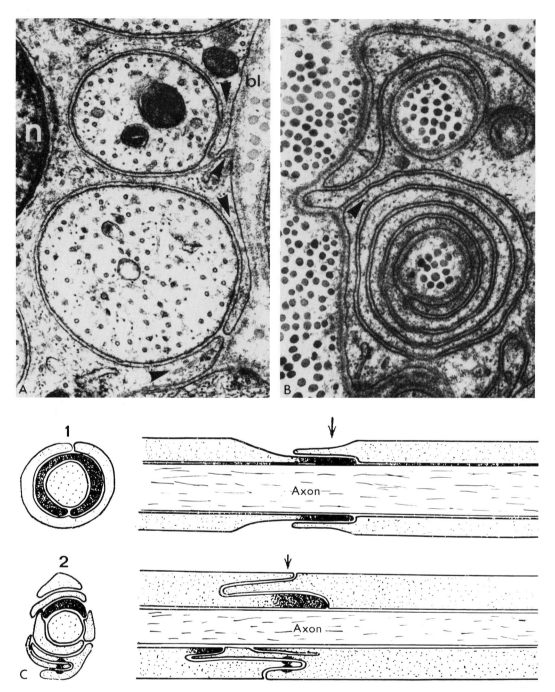

Figure 7–5   *A.* Section from the medial popliteal nerve of a normal baboon. Two unmyelinated axons independently and completely invested by Schwann cell tongues (arrowheads). An extremely narrow gap of uniform width separates the osmiophilic components of the unit surface membranes of axon and Schwann cell. n, Nucleus of the Schwann cell. bl, Basal lamina. Glutaraldehyde perfusion fixation, osmium tetroxide. × 41,600. *B.* Section from the sural nerve of an adult patient suffering from hypertrophic neuropathy. Part of an unmyelinated fiber with two collagen pockets is shown. On the bottom, a Schwann cell tongue (arrowhead) has grown to describe three and three quarters turns around the bundle of collagen. Osmium tetroxide immersion fixation. × 48,000. *C.* "Line drawing to show simple ensheathing by part of one Schwann cell of part of the next at a junctional zone (in 1), and (in 2) interdigitation of one cell with the next along unmyelinated axons." (*C* from Eames, R. A., and Gamble, H. J.: Schwann cell relationships in normal human cutaneous nerves. J. Anat., *106*:417, 1970. Reprinted by permission of Cambridge University Press.)

appear to be an exclusive feature of unmyelinated fibers. They appear to be commonplace in mature nerves as they also occur in cat, guinea pig, baboon, rabbit, and mouse. In man they are not present before the eighteenth week of fetal life, but it is not known at what age they become prominent (Ochoa, 1971). Although collagen pockets are numerous in aging and in neuropathies, the view that they may result from the degeneration of unmyelinated axons requires substantiation, and this author is skeptical. Gamble (1964) regarded collagen pockets as the consequence of active engulfing by Schwann cells of suitably oriented elongated structures.

That the Schwann cells of unmyelinated fibers are not syncytial was clear to Elfvin (1958), who rejected the erroneous concept and emphasized that the Schwann sheath was built up of a series of cells. What then is the surface relation of axons and Schwann cells at the cell junctions? Eames and Gamble (1970) have illustrated these junctions from reconstructions of longitudinal sections of nerves in man (Fig. 7–5C). The axons are not exposed at any point along their course, as the adjacent Schwann cells overlap. The cytoplasm of the ensheathed Schwann cell tip may be darker than normal, which may be a useful aid in the interpretation of unusual configurations in transverse sections.

Cytoplasmic Features of Schwann Cells Associated With Unmyelinated Axons

These cells have elongated bacilliform nuclei, in line with the main axis of the fibers (see Fig. 7–1B). In transverse sections the nuclear contour is generally smooth, but some plasticity of shape is apparent from the way the nucleus occasionally adapts to the shape of adjacent axons (Figs. 7–6A and 7–7A).

The granular contents of the nucleus are often more or less evenly distributed, with some emphasis near the periphery (see Fig. 7–4). Peripheral clumping of chromatin may be marked (Fig. 7–6A). Mitotic figures are not normally seen in mature nerves, but these Schwann cells are clearly capable of division following nerve injury.

The cytoplasm remote from the nuclear region is rather featureless, and microtubules, microfilaments, and mitochondria are usually the only visible contents. When stretched into

tenuous extensions, Schwann cell processes may be indistinguishable from axons (see Fig. 7–8C). The perinuclear cytoplasm, which is richer in organelles, contains mitochondria, sparse granular endoplasmic reticulum, and a Golgi complex in addition to microtubules and filaments (Fig. 7–7B). One or more centrioles aligned parallel to the nucleus may be present in the sections (Fig. 7–6B). Dense bodies and lysosomes may be prominent and appear to increase with age (Fig. 7–6C). Weller and Herzog (1970) have studied some aspects of enzyme histochemistry of lysosomes in the Schwann cells of unmyelinated fibers in man. Distinguishing some of these normal organelles from dead intracellular mycobacteria may be difficult, as the latter lose their distinctive features (Rees and Valentine, 1962).

In some species the cytoplasm of the Schwann cells is more electron dense than the axoplasm by virtue of a higher concentration of filaments. It may also occur in man that away from a Schwann cell junction some of the Schwann cell processes in unmyelinated fibers exhibit marked electron density. In normal human nerves fixed in osmium tetroxide such deviations were not recorded by Ochoa and Mair (1969a, 1969b), but in abnormal nerves fixed in glutaraldehyde, dark Schwann cell processes were interpreted as being necrotic by Carlsen and his associates (1969). Similar appearances have been termed "mosaic Schwann cells" by Appenzeller and Kornfeld (1972). The meaning of these dark cell processes is not entirely clear. Superficially similar electron density may occur as a result of soaking nerves in hypertonic solutions prior to fixation (Elfvin, 1962).

Apart from the absence of π granules in Schwann cells of unmyelinated fibers, the general features of these cells are on the whole similar to those of Schwann cells of myelinated fibers. This is in keeping with the concept that these cells belong to the same type; there is evidence that Schwann cells from unmyelinated fibers may myelinate regenerating axons from myelinated nerves after cross anastomosis (Simpson and Young, 1945; Hillarp and Olivecrona, 1946).

Axoplasm of Unmyelinated Axons

Within the amorphous matrix of the axoplasmic gel there are suspended microfila-

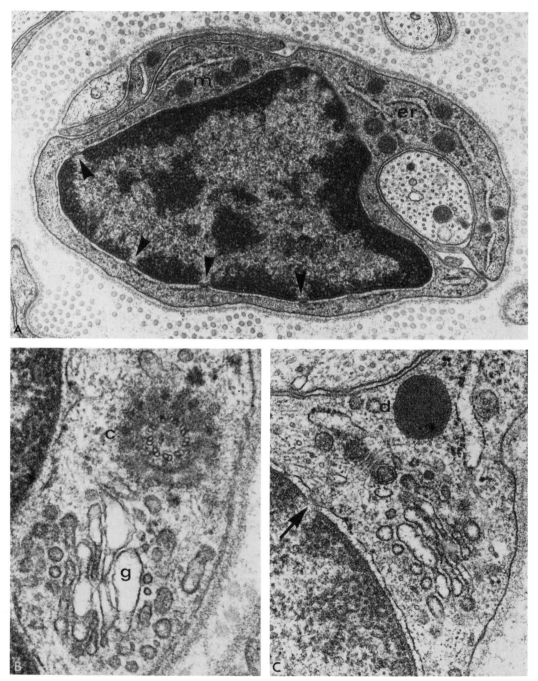

Figure 7–6   *A*. Unmyelinated axon in an unusually active Schwann cell cut through the nucleus. Notice nuclear pores (arrowheads), granular endoplasmic reticulum (er) and mitochondria (m). Glutaraldehyde immersion fixation, osmium tetroxide. × 27,200. *B*. Schwann cell of an unmyelinated fiber cut through the nucleus, showing Golgi complex (g) and a centriole (c). Note that the subunits of the centriole are duplets and not triplets. × 58,000. *C*. Section through nucleus, showing nuclear pore (arrow), Golgi complex, and membrane-bound dense body (d). × 51,000.

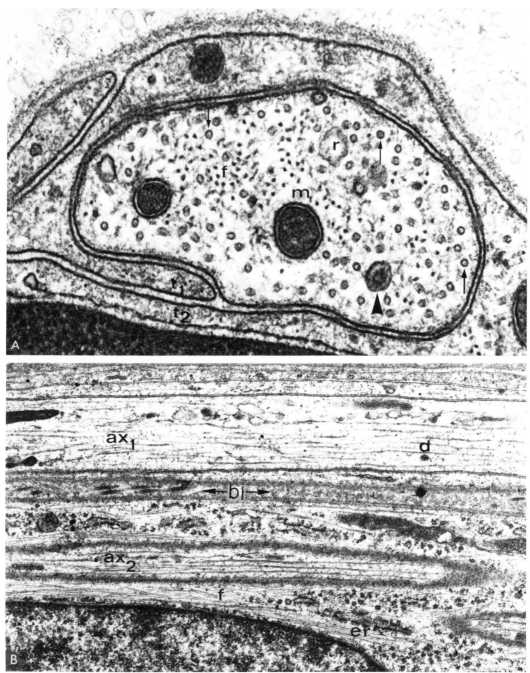

Figure 7–7 *A*. Transverse section of a somewhat flattened axon cut through the nuclear region of the fiber from the sural nerve of a child aged nine. The ingrowing Schwann cell tongue (t_1) separates axon from t_2, defining a relatively long mesaxon. The axoplasm contains mitochondria (m), microtubules, some of them dense-cored (arrows), microfilaments (f), and agranular endoplasmic reticulum (r). A dense-cored vesicle (arrowhead) is also present. Glutaraldehyde immersion fixation, osmium tetroxide. × 75,000. *B*. Section from the medial popliteal nerve of a normal baboon. The axon on the top (ax_1), cut longitudinally, shows a uniform caliber and contains an assortment of organelles (d), dense-cored vesicle). Another axon (ax_2) is cut longitudinally as it changes into a different plane; it is limited by a coarse line corresponding to the surface membranes of axon and Schwann cell cut obliquely. Endoneurial collagen intervenes between the basal laminae. Schwann cell cytoplasm with filaments (f), sparse microtubules, granular endoplasmic reticulum (er), and mitochondria occur near the nucleus. Glutaraldehyde perfusion fixation, osmium tetroxide. × 19,600.

ments and microtubules (Fig. 7–7A). The latter became obvious with the advent of aldehyde fixation for electron microscopy, although in nerves fixed with osmium tetroxide they were roughly described as "tubules" by Whitear (1960) in unmyelinated axons in the mouse cornea, and as "thick filaments" by Elfvin (1961) in unmyelinated axons from the cat splenic nerve. Technical refinement has made it possible to visualize the subunit organization of microtubules and microfilaments in various cell processes and the roles of these fibrous proteins in nonrandom movement of particles within the cytoplasm are becoming understood (Palay et al., 1962; Porter, 1966; Rodríguez-Echandía et al., 1968; Schmitt, 1968; Wuerker and Kirkpatrick, 1972). Aspects of axoplasmic transport of organelles and monoamine storage vesicles in autonomic unmyelinated axons have been studied by fluorescence microscopy and by electron microscopy (Dahlström, 1965, 1971; Mayor and Kapeller, 1967; Rodríguez-Echandía et al., 1970; Banks et al., 1971). The caliber of the microtubules is very regular as they are made up of a constant number of subunits of fixed size. What are sometimes mistaken for "dilated microtubules" are in fact elements of the agranular endoplasmic reticulum, limited by unit membrane, which occur sparsely in the axoplasm (Fig. 7–7A).

Elongated mitochondria oriented longitudinally are present on an average of one per unmyelinated axon in cross sections of the medial popliteal nerve of the baboon. In the sural nerve of man, Dyck and Lambert (1969) reported from none up to four mitochondria per cross section of unmyelinated axon.

Dense-cored vesicles are not abundant in unmyelinated axons in somatic nerves, but they do occur here and there along the course of most axons (Figs. 7–7A and B; see also Fig. 7–6A). This must mean that such vesicles occur in somatic as well as in autonomic axons, which is hardly surprising in view of their presence in some sensory nerve endings (Landon, 1972). Since the pioneer studies by von Euler and Hillarp (1956) in autonomic nerves, dense cored vesicles have been believed to contain catecholamines. The composition and significance of such vesicles in somatic nerve fibers is unknown.

Ribosomes and glycogen granules are not normally present in axons. On the whole, the features of unmyelinated axons are qualitatively similar to those of myelinated axons and also to those of immature axons.

Changes in Unmyelinated Fibers Due to Aging

After full differentiation of the structural features of unmyelinated fibers in man, regressive changes become noticeable in the third or fourth decade of life and increase with aging (Ochoa and Mair, 1969b). The regressive character of these changes is clear not only from the loss of axons involved but also from the fact that an exaggerated picture featuring identical changes is common in a number of neuropathies (Ochoa, 1970a; 1970c). An early change appears to be the budding of the Schwann cell processes into a number of flattened tongues (Fig. 7–8A). Ultimately loss of axons becomes obvious, this being best appreciated from the presence of typical budded Schwann cell bands devoid of axons (Fig. 7–8B). Such denervated bands outlive the axons, are often rounded or ovoid in shape, and usually occur in groups like the fibers of origin. They are quite different from those Schwann cell bands remaining after degeneration of myelinated fibers.

Miniature profiles, rounded in cross section and enveloped by Schwann cells, become prominent with age in unmyelinated fibers (Fig. 7–8C). They bear the same spatial relationship to Schwann cells as the unmyelinated axons and resemble closely the terminal branches of cutaneous nerve fibers (Cauna, 1968). They were identified as axon sprouts, probably produced by collateral regeneration, in the sural nerve in man, by Ochoa and Mair (1969b). These profiles may be as small as $0.2 \mu m$ in diameter, although most are in the region of 0.4 to $0.8 \mu m$, which is quite close in size to the population of the smallest developing axons in the sural nerve in the human fetus (Ochoa, 1971). They may be abundant in some neuropathies in which they may distort the frequency curves of axon diameter distribution, causing bimodality (see Fig. 7–10B). These profiles did not occur in affected unmyelinated nerves of rats that had been treated with nerve growth factor antiserum (Aguayo et al., 1972).

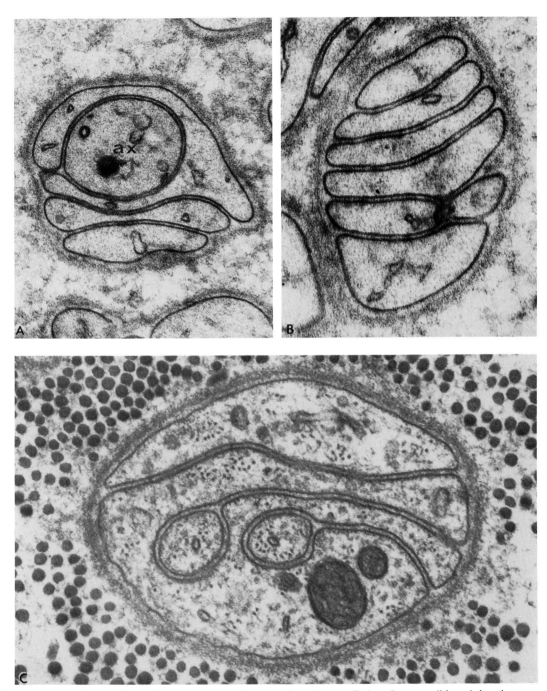

Figure 7–8 *A.* Section from the sural nerve of an adult patient suffering from a mild peripheral neuropathy. Unmyelinated axon (ax) contained in a budded Schwann cell band. Fixation enhances cell membranes but fails to preserve organelles. Potassium-permanganate immersion fixation, osmium tetroxide. × 51,000. *B.* Budded unmyelinated Schwann cell band devoid of axons. Source and preparation as in *A.* × 58,500. *C.* Section from the sural nerve of a healthy man aged 59. Unmyelinated Schwann cell band contains two miniature rounded profiles handled as axons by Schwann cell processes. The cytoplasm of the rounded profiles and Schwann cells appears similar. Notice the absence of microtubules. Osmium tetroxide immersion fixation. × 63,000.

Effects of Chemical Fixation on Fine Structure of Unmyelinated Fibers

The natural shape, volume, and composition of tissues become distorted after preparation for conventional electron microscopy, fixation being an all-important stage in the procedure. The choice of fixative may result in preferential preservation of some of the subcellular components and loss of others. The fibers shown in Figures 7–7A and 7–8A and C provide examples of some effects of primary fixation with glutaraldehyde, potassium permanganate, and osmium tetroxide on the structure of axons and Schwann cells. The osmolality of the fixative may have profound effects on shape and volume of cells. When studying the effect of treating nerves with solutions of different compositions before and during fixation, Elfvin (1962) noted striking changes in both Schwann cells and axons of unmyelinated fibers (Fig. 7–9). The change in volume did not necessarily affect axons

and Schwann cells to the same extent, and in one instance there was paradoxical swelling of Schwann cells and shrinkage of axons. Electron density of the Schwann cell cytoplasm became selectively increased when the nerves were treated with hypertonic solutions.

It appears likely that nearly circular axonal profiles (as shown in Figures 7–3A, 7–4B and C, and 7–5A) correspond more closely to the natural shape of the axons than do irregular profiles. Preparation procedures generally reputed to cause minimal distortion of shape, such as freeze-etching, result in unmyelinated axons of circular or oval shape (Bischoff, 1970; Devine et al., 1971). Volume changes in axons following fixation should be borne in mind when measuring axon size.

NUMBERS AND CALIBER OF UNMYELINATED FIBERS

Counting and measuring slices of nerve fibers has been a habit of meticulous neuro-

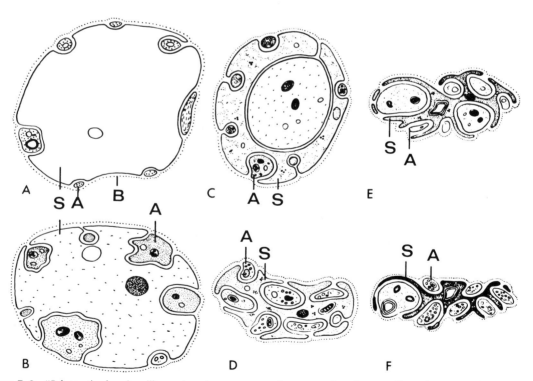

Figure 7–9 "Schematic drawing illustrating the structure of cross sectioned unmyelinated nerve fibers which have been exposed to hypotonic or hypertonic milieu for two hours before fixation with osmium tetroxide. The soaking fluids were (A) distilled water; (B) Tyrode's solution without NaCl; (C) NaCl Tyrode; (D) 2 NaCl Tyrode; (E) 5 NaCl Tyrode; (F) 10 NaCl Tyrode. A, axon; S, Schwann cell; B, basement membrane." (From Elfvin, L. G.: Electron microscopic studies on the effect of anisotonic solutions on the structure of unmyelinated splenic nerve fibers of the cat. J. Ultrastruct. Res., 7:1, 1962. Reprinted by permission.)

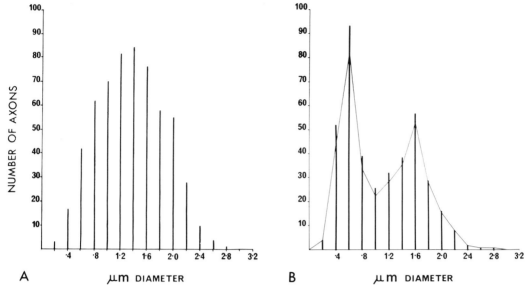

Figure 7–10 Frequency distribution of unmyelinated axon diameters in the sural nerve. *A.* The nerve, from a boy aged 15, was fixed in osmium tetroxide and measurements were made by semiautomatic means. (From Ochoa, J., and Mair, W. G. P.: The normal sural nerve in man. I. Ultrastructure and numbers of fibres and cells. Acta Neuropathol., *13*:197, 1969. Reprinted by permission.) *B.* From an adult patient suffering from isoniazid neuropathy. Below the continuous line are the genuine unmyelinated axons; above, are sprouts as yet not myelinated. (From Ochoa, J.: Isoniazid neuropathy in man: quantitative electron microscope study. Brain, *93*:831, 1970. Reprinted by permission.)

anatomists since the inception of conventional histologic study of tissue sections. At the turn of the century, Ingbert (1903) undertook the colossal enterprise of counting all myelinated nerve fibers in all the dorsal nerve roots on one side in man; he reached an estimated total of about 650,000. Ranson and his colleagues (1935) were the first to perform thorough counts of unmyelinated axons by light microscopy, and paid particular attention to the nerves of man. They showed that the highest numbers occurred in cutaneous nerves, and although their silver stains appear bound to underestimate the number of unmyelinated axons (see Fig. 7–2), their average ratio of more than three unmyelinated to one myelinated fiber is close to the figure that Ochoa and Mair (1969a), using the electron microscope, calculated for the normal sural nerve in man. Unexpected agreement can be explained if the particular arrangement of unmyelinated fibers in cutaneous nerves is considered; axons are held in separate Schwann cell cords, probably allowing axonal individuality to be discriminated even when their profile is only roughly outlined by silver stains (cf. Figure 7–4*C*).

Gasser (1950) also counted unmyelinated axons stained with silver, but he went further and undertook to measure their diameters

after strict control of the optical problem and correction for shrinkage. In the saphenous nerve of the cat he reported a size range of 0.4 to 1.25 μm and a unimodal distribution of diameters. A similar distribution and a range of 0.25 to 1.4 μm was later reported in the sural nerve of the cat by Gasser (1955) using the electron microscope.

Counts and measurements of unmyelinated axons in normal human nerves have been made by several authors from electronmicrographs. Weller (1967) reported histograms of diameters of unmyelinated axons in control sural nerves of a child of six months of age and of an adult. Axon diameters ranged from 0.5 to 3.5 μm and were distributed in unimodal curves. The peak in the adult was about 1.5 μm, as was the peak in the control of Aguayo, Nair, and Bray (1971). Similar unimodal curves with peaks in the region of 1.4 to 1.6 μm were consistently found by Ochoa and Mair (1969a) in a group of normal individuals under the age of 25 years. Over 700 axons were counted in each case. Sizes ranged from 0.2 to 3.0 μm, but axons over 2.8 μm in diameter were rarely seen (Fig. 7–10*A*). Dyck and Lambert (1969) measured about 100 axons in each of two adult control sural nerves and reported a diameter range of 0.3 to 1.5 μm. Subsequently Dyck, Lambert, and Nichols (1971) reported on further estimations on sural nerves from nine controls, for which they used a Zeiss particle analyzer. Axon diameters ranged from 0.2 to 2.0 μm and were not always distributed in unimodal curves. Peaks were at 0.6 to 0.8 μm. Lack of complete agreement of the various figures reported can be explained by different degrees of volume change following preparation of the nerves for electron microscopy. In the medial popliteal nerve of the baboon, fixed by perfusion with glutaraldehyde, Fowler and Ochoa (unpublished data) consistently found unimodal distribution curves with peaks in the region of 1 μm. Similar results have been found by Marotte (1972) in the median nerve of the guinea pig. Bimodal curves due to the presence of an additional population of immature axons, presumably regenerated, were reported in aging by Ochoa and Mair (1969b) and in neuropathies by Ochoa (1970a, 1970b, 1970c). An example is given in Figure 7–10B, in which spurious unmyelinated axons (immature sprouts from myelinated fibers) were also included and then discounted. Distinction was possible because of the characteristic arrangement of genuine unmyelinated fibers in cutaneous nerves in man. Abnormal bimodality of histograms of diameters of unmyelinated axons has also been found in damaged nerves in baboons (Fowler and Ochoa, unpublished data).

With regard to the number of unmyelinated axons in cutaneous nerves in man, Dyck, Lambert and Nichols (1971) have made available calculated figures for total numbers of unmyelinated axons in six sural nerves from healthy adults. Numbers ranged from 17,309 to 53,000. Values per unit area could be predicted to vary individually and also with the volume change caused by different preparation procedures; Dyck and his co-workers (1971) reported 19,447 to 68,813 per square millimeter, whereas Ochoa and Mair (1969a) found 21,755 to 33,859 per square millimeter.

References

Aguayo, A. J., Martin, J. B., and Bray, G. M.: Effects of nerve growth factor antiserum on peripheral unmyelinated nerve fibers. Acta Neuropathol. (Berl.), *20*:288, 1972.

Aguayo, A. J., Nair, C. P. V., and Bray, G. M.: Peripheral nerve abnormalities in the Riley-Day syndrome. Arch. Neurol., *24*:106, 1971.

Allt, G.: Ultrastructural features of the immature peripheral nerve. J. Anat., *105*:283, 1969.

Appenzeller, O., and Kornfeld, M.: Indifference to pain. A chronic peripheral neuropathy with mosaic Schwann cells. Arch. Neurol., *27*:322, 1972.

Banks, P., Mayor, D., Mitchell, M., and Tomlinson, D.: Studies on the translocation of noradrenaline-containing vesicles in post-ganglionic sympathetic neurones in vitro. Inhibition of movement by colchicine and vinblastine and evidence for the involvement of axonal microtubules. J. Physiol. (Lond.), *216*:625, 1971.

Bischoff, A.: *in* Babel, J., Bischoff, A., and Spoendlin, H. (eds.): Ultrastructure of the Peripheral Nervous System and Sense Organs. London, J. & A. Churchill, 1970.

Bishop, G. H., Heinbecker, P., and O'Leary, J. L.: The function of the non-myelinated fibers of the dorsal roots. Am. J. Physiol., *106*:647, 1933.

Bondareff, W.: An intercellular substance in rat cerebral cortex: submicroscopic distribution of ruthenium red. Anat. Rec., *157*:527, 1967.

Boughton, T. H.: The increase in the number and size of the medullated fibers in the oculomotor nerve of the white rat and of the cat at different ages. J. Comp. Neurol. Psychol., *16*:153, 1906.

Bruce, A. N.: Über die Beziehung der sensiblen Nervendigungen zum Entzündungsvorgang. Arch. Exp. Pathol. Pharmakol., *63*:424, 1910.

Carlsen, F., Knappeis, G. G., and Schmalbruch, H.: Schwann cell "necrosis" in unmyelinated nerve fibres of patients with polyneuropathy. Virchows Arch., Pathol. Anat., *348*:306, 1969.

Cauna, N.: Light and electron microscopal structure of sensory end-organs. *In* Kenshalo, D. R. (ed.): The Skin Senses. Springfield, Ill. Charles C Thomas, 1968.

Celander, O., and Folkow, B.: The nature and the distribution of afferent fibres provided with the axon reflex arrangement. Acta Physiol. Scand., *29*:359, 1953.

Cravioto, H.: The role of Schwann cells in the development of human peripheral nerves. An electron microscopic study. J. Ultrastruct. Res., *12*:634, 1965.

Dahlström, A.: Observations on the accumulation of noradrenaline in the proximal and distal parts of peripheral adrenergic nerves after compression. J. Anat., *99*:677, 1965.

Dahlström, A.: Effects of vinblastine and colchicine on monoamine containing neurons of the rat, with special regard to the axoplasmic transport of amine granules. Acta Neuropathol. (Berl.), Suppl. 5:226, 1971.

Davenport, H. A., and Bothe, R. T.: Cells and fibers in spinal nerves. II. A study of C2, C6, T4, T9, L3, S2, and S5 in man. J. Comp. Neurol., *59*:167, 1934.

Devine, C. E., Simpson, F. O., and Bertaud, W. S.: Freeze-etch studies on the innervation of mesenteric arteries and vas deferens. J. Cell Sci., *9*:411, 1971.

Doggenweiler, C. F., and Frenk, S.: Staining properties of lanthanum on cell membranes. Proc. Natl. Acad. Sci. U.S.A., *53*:425, 1965.

Dyck, P. J., and Lambert, E. H.: Dissociated sensation in amyloidosis. Compound action potential, quantitative histologic and teased-fiber, and electron microscopic studies of sural nerve biopsies. Arch. Neurol., *20*:490, 1969.

Dyck, P. J., Lambert, E. H., and Nichols, P. C.: Quantitative measurement of sensation related to compound action potential and number and sizes of myelinated and unmyelinated fibers of sural nerve in health, Friedreich's ataxia, hereditary sensory neuropathy, and tabes dorsalis. *In* Handbook of Electroencephalography and Clinical Neurophysiology. Vol. 9. Amsterdam, Elsevier Publishing Co., 1971, pp. 9–83.

Eames, R. A., and Gamble, H. J.: Schwann cell relationships in normal human cutaneous nerves. J. Anat., *106*:417, 1970.

Elfvin, L. G.: The ultrastructure of unmyelinated fibers in the splenic nerve of the cat. J. Ultrastruct. Res., *1*:428, 1958.

Elfvin, L. G.: Electron-microscopic investigation of filament structures in unmyelinated fibers of cat splenic nerve. J. Ultrastruct. Res., 5:51, 1961.

Elfvin, L. G.: Electron microscopic studies on the effect of anisotonic solutions on the structure of unmyelinated nerve fibers of the cat. J. Ultrastruct. Res., 7:1, 1962.

von Euler, U. S., and Hillarp, N. Å.: Evidence for the presence of noradrenaline in submicroscopic structures of adrenergic axons. Nature (Lond.), *177*:44, 1956.

Evans, D. H. L., and Murray, J. G.: Regeneration of non-medullated nerve fibres. J. Anat., 88:465, 1954.

Fernández-Morán, H.: The submicroscopic organization of vertebrate nerve fibers. An electron microscope study of myelinated and unmyelinated nerve fibers. Exp. Cell Res., 3:282, 1952.

Friede, R. L., and Samorajski, T.: Myelin formation in the sciatic nerve of the rat. A quantitative electron microscopic, histochemical and radioautographic study. J. Neuropathol. Exp. Neurol., 27:546, 1968.

Fontana, F.: Traité sur le Vénin de la Vipère sur les Poisons Américains. Firenze, Italy, 1781.

Gamble, H. J.: Comparative electron-microscopic observations on the connective tissues of a peripheral nerve and a spinal nerve root in the rat. J. Anat., 98:17, 1964.

Gamble, H. J.: Further electron microscope studies of human foetal peripheral nerves. J. Anat., *100*:487, 1966.

Gamble, H. J., and Eames, R. A.: An electron microscope study of the connective tissues of human peripheral nerve. J. Anat., *98*:655, 1964.

Gasser, H. S.: Unmedullated fibers originating in dorsal root ganglia. J. Gen. Physiol., *33*:651, 1950.

Gasser, H. S.: *In* Discussion *of* The Hypothesis of Saltatory Conduction. Cold Spring Harbor Symp. Quant. Biol. *17*:32, 1952.

Gasser, H. S.: Properties of dorsal root unmedullated fibers on the two sides of the ganglion. J. Gen. Physiol., *38*:709, 1955.

Geren, B. B.: The formation from the Schwann cell surface of myelin in the peripheral nerves of chick embryos. Exp. Cell Res., 7:558, 1954.

Guttmann, L.: Topographic studies on disturbances of sweat secretion after complete lesions of peripheral nerves. J. Neurol. Psychiatry, *3*:197, 1940.

Hall, S. M., and Williams, P. L.: The distribution of electron-dense tracers in peripheral nerve fibres. J. Cell Sci., 8:541, 1971.

Hallin, R. G., and Torebjörk, H. E.: Afferent and efferent C units recorded from human skin nerves in situ. Acta Soc. Med. Ups., *75*:277, 1971.

Hess, A., and Lansing, A. I.: The fine structure of peripheral nerve fibers. Anat. Rec., *117*:175, 1953.

Hillarp, N., and Olivecrona, H.: The role played by the axon and the Schwann cells in the degree of myelination of the peripheral nerve fibre. Acta Anat. 2:17, 1946.

Ingbert, C.: An enumeration of the medullated nerve fibers in the dorsal roots of the spinal nerves of man. J. Comp. Neurol., *13*:53, 1903.

Katz, B., and Schmitt, O. H.: Electric interaction between two adjacent nerve fibers. J. Physiol. (Lond.), *97*:471, 1940.

King, R. H. M., and Thomas, P. K.: Electron microscope observations on aberrant regeneration of unmyelinated axons in the vagus nerve of the rabbit. Acta Neuropathol. (Berl.), *18*:150, 1971.

Landon, D. N.: The fine structure of the equatorial regions of developing muscle spindles in the rat. J. Neurocytol., *1*:189, 1972.

Lewis, T.: The Blood Vessels of the Human Skin and Their Responses. London, Shaw & Sons, 1927.

Lewis, T., and Landis, E. M.: Some physiological effects of sympathetic ganglionectomy in the human being and its effect in a case of Raynaud's malady. Heart, 15:151, 1929.

Luft, J. H.: Ruthenium red and violet. Anat. Rec., 171: 369, 1971.

Marotte, L.: Personal communication, 1972.

Mayor, D., and Kapeller, K.: Fluorescence microscopy and electron microscopy of adrenergic nerves after constriction at two points. J. R. Microscop. Soc., 87: 277, 1967.

Moberg, E.: Objective methods for determining the functional value of sensibility in the hand. J. Bone Joint Surg., *40B*:454, 1958.

Münzer, F. T.: The discovery of the *cell of Schwann* in 1839. Q. Rev. Biol., *14*:387, 1939.

Nageotte, J.: L'Organisation de la Matière dans ses Rapports avec la Vie. Paris, Felix Alcan, 1922.

Ochoa, J.: The structure of developing and adult sural nerve in man and the changes which occur in some diseases. A light and electron microscopic study. University of London, Ph.D. Thesis, 1970a.

Ochoa, J.: Isoniazid neuropathy in man: quantitative electron microscope study. Brain, *93*:831, 1970b.

Ochoa, J.: Electron microscope observations on unmyelinated fibres in normal and pathological human nerves. Proceedings VI International Congress of Neuropathology. Paris, Masson, 1970c.

Ochoa, J.: The sural nerve of the human foetus: electron microscope observations and counts of axons. J. Anat., *108*:231, 1971.

Ochoa, J., and Mair, W. G. P.: The normal sural nerve in man. I. Ultrastructure and numbers of fibres and cells. Acta Neuropathol. (Berl.), *13*:197, 1969a.

Ochoa, J. and Mair, W. G. P.: The normal sural nerve in man. II. Changes in the axons and Schwann cells due to ageing. Acta Neuropathol. (Berl.), *13*:217, 1969b.

Palay, S. L., McGee-Russell, S. M., Gordon, S., Jr., and Grillo, M. A.: Fixation of neural tissues for electron microscopy by perfusion with solutions of osmium tetroxide. J. Cell Biol., *12*:385, 1962.

Peters, A., and Muir, A. R.: The relationship between axons and Schwann cells during development of peripheral nerves in the rat. Q. J. Exp. Physiol. *44*:117, 1959.

Porter, K. R.: Cytoplasmic microtubules and their functions. *In* Wolstenholme, G. E. W., and O'Connor, M. (eds.): Ciba Foundation Symposium on Principles of Biomolecular Organization. Boston, Little, Brown & Co., 1966, p. 308.

Ranson, S. W.: Non-medullated nerve fibers in the spinal nerves. Am. J. Anat., *12*:67, 1911.

Ranson, S. W.: The structure of the spinal ganglia and of the spinal nerves. J. Comp. Neurol., *22*:159, 1912.

Ranson, S. W.: Unmyelinated nerve-fibres as conductors of protopathic sensation. Brain, *38*:381, 1915.

Ranson, S. W., Droegemueller, W. H., Davenport, H. K., and Fisher, C.: Number, size and myelination of the sensory fibers in the cerebrospinal nerves. Res. Publ. Assoc. Res. Nerv. Ment. Dis., *15*:3, 1935.

Rees, R. J. W., and Valentine, R. C.: The appearance of dead leprosy bacilli by light and electron microscopy. Int. J. Lepr., *30*:1, 1962.

Remak, R.: Weitere mikroskopische Beobachtungen über Primitivfasern des Nervensystems der Wirbeltiere. Frorieps Neue Notizen, *3*:35, 1837.

Remak, R.: Observationes anatomicae et microscopicae de systematis nervosi structura. Berlin, Sumptibus et Formis Reimerianis, 1838.

Revel, J. P., and Ito, S.: The surface components of cells. *In* Davis, B. D., and Warren, L. (eds.): The Specificity of Cell Surfaces. Englewood Cliffs, N.J., Prentice-Hall, 1967.

Rodríguez-Echandía, E. L., Piezzi, R. S., and Rodríguez, E. M.: Dense-core microtubules in neurons and gliocytes of the toad *Bufo arenarum* Hensel. Am. J. Anat., *122*:157, 1968.

Rodríguez-Echandía, E. L., Zamora, A., and Piezzi, R. S.: Organelle transport in constricted nerve fibers of the toad *Bufo arenarum* Hensel. Z. Zellforsch. Mikrosk. Anat., *104*:419, 1970.

Rothman, S., and Coon, J. M.: Axon reflex responses to acetylcholine in the skin. J. Invest. Dermatol., *3*:79, 1940.

Schmitt, F. O.: The molecular biology of neuronal fibrous proteins. *In* Neuronal Fibrous Proteins. Neurosci. Res., *6*:119, 1968.

Schmitt, F. O., and Samson, F. E.: Brain cell microenvironment. Neurosci. Res., *7*:281, 1969.

Schröder, M.: Die Hyperneurotisation Büngnerscher Bänder bei der experimentellen Isoniazid-Neuropathie: Phasenkontrast- und elektronenmikroskopische Untersuchungen. Virchows Arch., Zellpathol. *1*: 131, 1968.

Schwann, T.: Mikroskopische Untersuchungen über die Uebereinstimmung in der Struktur und dem Wachstum der Tiere und Pflanzen. Berlin, Sander, 1839.

Simpson, S. A., and Young, J. Z.: Regeneration of fibre diameter after cross-unions of visceral and somatic nerves. J. Anat., *79*:48, 1945.

Spencer, P. S.: Light and electron microscopic observations on localised peripheral nerve injuries. University of London, Ph.D. Thesis, 1971.

Thomas, P. K.: The effect of repeated regenerative activity on the structure of peripheral nerve. *In* Research Committee of the Muscular Dystrophy Group (ed.): Research in Muscular Dystrophy. London, Pitman, 1968.

Torebjörk, H. E., and Hallin, R. G.: C-fibre units recorded from human sensory nerve fascicles in situ. A preliminary report. Acta Soc. Med. Ups., *75*:81, 1970.

Tuckett, I. L.: On the structure and degeneration of non-medullated nerve fibres. J. Physiol. (Lond.), *19*:267, 1895.

Webster, H. de F.: The geometry of peripheral myelin sheaths during their formation and growth in rat sciatic nerves. J. Cell Biol., *48*:348, 1971.

Weddell, G.: The pattern of cutaneous innervation in relation to cutaneous sensibility. J. Anat., *75*:346, 1941.

Weddell, G.: The relationship between pain sensibility and peripheral nerve fibres. *In* Knighton, R. S., and Dumke, P. R.: Pain. Boston, Little, Brown & Co., 1966.

Weddell, G., Pallie, W., and Palmer, E.: The morphology of peripheral nerve terminations in the skin. Q. J. Microsc. Sci., *95*:483, 1954.

Weller, R. O.: An electron microscopic study of hypertrophic neuropathy of Dejerine and Sottas. J. Neurol. Neurosurg. Psychiatry, *30*:111, 1967.

Weller, R. O., and Herzog, I.: Schwann cell lysosomes in hypertrophic neuropathy and in normal human nerves. Brain, *93*:347, 1970.

Whitear, M.: An electron microscope study of the cornea in mice, with special reference to the innervation. J. Anat., *94*:387, 1960.

Wuerker, R. B., and Kirkpatrick, J. B.: Neuronal microtubules, neurofilaments, and microfilaments. Int. Rev. Cytol., *33*:45, 1972.

Chapter 8

THE MUSCLE SPINDLE

Richard S. Smith

The muscle spindle has three main components: a bundle of specialized muscle fibers, motor nerves, and sensory nerves. The muscle fibers, called intrafusal muscle fibers, are innervated by fusimotor (or "gamma") nerve fibers and also possess a sensory innervation that lies in the central or equatorial region of the muscle fibers. Enclosing the equatorial region is an epithelial–connective tissue capsule that gives the muscle spindle its characteristic shape and from which its name is derived. It is the primary aim of this chapter to describe what is known of the morphologic and functional relationships among its three main components. The development of muscle spindles and pathologic changes occurring in them are also treated briefly, but very little is said about their functional significance in the control of movement, since this would necessitate a detailed consideration of the functions of the central nervous system.

Muscle spindles were described by a number of histologists in the second half of the nineteenth century. Owing to the small diameter of the intrafusal muscle fibers and to the unusual arrangement of nuclei within them, some workers thought that they represented either pathologic structures or foci of growth. The great neurohistologist Golgi (1880) described them as "a bundle of incompletely developed muscle fibers surrounded by a special sheath and to be found in muscles at every period of their growth." Others considered the spindle to be a sense organ, and by the end of the century, largely through the work of Sherrington and Ruffini, there was good evidence to support this view. Ruffini (1898) separated the sensory endings into two categories, the primary (annulospiral) endings, which lie on the central regions of the intrafusal fibers, and secondary (flower spray) endings, which lie more laterally. Substantial evidence for the presence of motor endings on the intrafusal muscle fibers was not produced for another 30 years, when it was established through degeneration experiments that nerve endings toward the ends, or poles, of the intrafusal fibers were of ventral root origin. Thus, by 1933 when Matthews ushered in a new experimental approach to the muscle spindle by electronically recording its sensory discharge in response to elongation of the muscle, the spindle was known to be a stretch receptor that received a motor nerve supply.

The impetus behind the continuing investigation of the muscle spindle is the belief that its function is to play a role in the unconscious control of motor activity. Since muscle spindles are equally numerous in flexor and in extensor muscles, the basic role of the spindle is not likely to be maintenance of posture through stretch reflexes (Liddell and Sherrington, 1924, 1925) involving the antigravity muscles. Merton's (1953) idea that the spindle is a part of a servo-system whose function is to control the length of muscle is very elegant and has offered great drive to the more recent investigation of spindle function. The basic simplicity of the idea, however, is to a large extent overwhelmed by the complexity of the muscle spindle as it is now understood. It must be admitted then that while the idea that the muscle spindle is important for the control of skeletal muscle is both useful in guiding experimental work and basically correct, nevertheless the actual significance of the muscle spindle still eludes us. Those who wish to explore the complex inter-

151

relationship between the concepts underlying experimental work on the muscle spindle and the results of these experiments are directed to general reviews of the field (Matthews, 1964; Granit, 1970; Matthews, 1972). The function of stretch receptors in muscle has been reviewed briefly and authoritatively by Jansen (1966), the motor innervation of muscle spindles has been reviewed by Barker and associates (1972), the structure and function of intrafusal muscle fibers by Smith and Ovalle (1972), and a comprehensive bibliography of work on the muscle spindle has been published by Eldred and co-workers (1967). Much that is treated in this chapter will be more clearly understood if the reader has the opportunity to view the excellent commercially available motion pictures of living muscle spindles produced by Professor Ian Boyd.

DEVELOPMENT OF THE SPINDLE

The first easily definable stage in the histogenesis of vertebrate skeletal muscle is the differentiation of mononucleated myoblasts from their precursor mesenchymal cells. The myoblasts continue to divide, producing several generations of daughter cells. By a mechanism that is still not understood, the individual myoblasts fuse to form multinucleated muscle fibers. The newly formed muscle fibers, called myotubes, have centrally placed nuclei that are surrounded by a peripheral rim of myofibrils. Further development may follow either of two courses. Most of the myotubes develop into ordinary extrafusal muscle fibers. During this process the proliferation of myofibrils is accompanied by migration of the nuclei so that they come to lie beneath the sarcolemma. Details of this developmental sequence are discussed in a recent review and a symposium (Holtzer, 1970; Banker et al., 1972).

The second developmental course leads to the formation of intrafusal muscle fibers. Since by definition the muscle spindle is an association of neural and muscular elements, the first recognizable stage occurs when sensory nerve endings become associated with myotube fibers. At this stage, which in man is about 12 to 14 weeks in utero (Cuajunco, 1940), a thin equatorial capsule is present around the sensory nerve terminals and myotube fibers. The developmental sequence from this stage to the adult spindle is not completely understood, but it is clear from an examination of the structure of adult intrafusal fibers that the process is different in detail from that occurring in extrafusal fibers.

Animal studies indicate that the full adult complement of intrafusal fibers is not present in the very early stages of development. In the rat, in which spindles are recognizable only a few days before birth, the spindle at birth contains only two intrafusal muscle fibers; one nuclear bag and one nuclear chain fiber. The normal number of intrafusal fibers in the rat, two nuclear bag fibers and two nuclear chain fibers, may be reached by longitudinal splitting of the original pair of fibers (Bravo-Rey et al., 1969; Marchand and Eldred, 1969). In the process of longitudinal splitting, the equatorial nuclei do not divide but are merely shared among the daughter fibers. Longitudinal splitting of the kind postulated could, if the process did not go through to completion, result in the branched form that has been described for some intrafusal fibers. (One also notes that a propensity to split longitudinally might bear some relationship to the abnormal number of small intrafusal fibers reported in cases of myotonia dystrophica [Daniel and Strich, 1964]). It should be kept in mind, however, that ordinary skeletal muscle fibers were once thought to multiply through a process of longitudinal division. There is now no good evidence for, and much against (e.g., Kelly and Zachs, 1969), this mode of multiplication in embryonic extrafusal muscle fibers. Thus, if intrafusal muscle fibers do proliferate by longitudinal division, this represents a unique process in developing muscle.

Intrafusal muscle fibers are notably different from extrafusal muscle fibers in that they receive a sensory innervation. The sensory nerves are believed to be the first nerve fibers to reach the developing muscle spindle. Hence it is not surprising that researchers have suspected that intrafusal fibers are trophically dependent on their sensory innervation. Zelena and her associates have investigated this dependence in a series of studies (Zelena and Hnik, 1963; Zelena, 1964). They found that if muscle spindles were deprived of their sensory innervation either before or when spindles were first detectable, then spindles either failed to develop or disappeared from the denervated muscle. Reinnervation of the muscle following the period when the spindles normally matured failed to cause typical muscle spindles to appear. Once spindles had matured they were relatively insensitive to denervation. Hyperinnervation of muscles by nerve branches from a crushed nerve caused, if the muscle were innervated during the critical period of spindle development, more than the normal number of spindles to appear. These experiments indicate that for a short time while the muscle fibers are in the myotube stage, the development of muscle spindles is critically dependent on their sensory innervation. Once this period of time has passed muscle fibers can no longer respond to the trophic influence of sensory nerves to become intrafusal muscle fibers. The effect of removing the motor supply to the spindle at any stage, or of removing the sensory innervation after the "critical period," is merely to cause a slow atrophy of the intrafusal fibers.

THE ADULT MUSCLE SPINDLE

The Capsule

In the central or equatorial zone of the spindle the intrafusal muscle fibers and sensory nerve endings are surrounded by a cellular and connective tissue capsule. Figure 8–1 is a low-power electron micrograph of a cross section of a muscle spindle from a rat showing the capsular layers at one end of the capsule. It is apparent that the capsule is composed of several cellular layers of which some, called the outer capsule, enclose the entire spindle while others, called the inner capsule, may invest groups of, or individual, intrafusal muscle fibers and sensory nerve endings very closely. The outer capsule is continuous with the perineurium of the sensory nerves that enter it and is made up largely of flat epithelial cells connected by tight junctions. These cells contain a large number of vesicles that are believed to be pinocytotic in origin. Numerous collagen fibrils are found on the outer surface of the capsule and between all the capsular layers. The number of cell layers in the capsule diminishes as the capsule narrows toward its poles. At the two ends of the capsule its lumen is said to communicate freely with the extra-cellular space.

Small blood vessels are commonly found within the layers of the outer capsule (Fig. 8–1). The close association of these vessels with the spindle may be presumed to be of functional importance since it is known that the muscle spindle is very sensitive to lack of oxygen (Matthews, 1933).

The capsule, or parts of it, is generally supposed to be filled with lymph (Sherrington, 1894) although this supposition has been contested (Brzezinski, 1961a, 1961b). Observation of isolated mammalian spindles in this laboratory suggests that the majority of the intracapsular space is tightly filled with a gelatinous material that is not freely exchangeable with the extracellular space.

Intrafusal Muscle Fibers

When one considers the very large number of light microscopic studies on mammalian spindles it is surprising that the two forms of intrafusal muscle fibers, the nuclear bag and the nuclear chain fibers, were recognized only recently. The nuclear chain fiber was described both in man and in the cat in the early 1960's (Cooper and Daniel, 1963; Boyd, 1962). The two types of fiber were distinguished by their size and by the arrangement of nuclei at the equatorial region (Figs. 8–2 and 8–3). Nuclear bag fibers generally are longer and have a greater diameter than the nuclear chain fibers. In the equatorial region the nuclear bag fibers contain many tightly packed rounded nuclei; this is the "nuclear bag" after which the fibers are named. Flanking this accumulation of nuclei are the myotube regions—named after their resemblance to embryonic muscle cells—containing a single row of centrally placed nuclei. The equatorial regions of nuclear chain fibers contain a single row of centrally placed oval nuclei surrounded by a peripheral layer of myofibrils. The polar regions of both kinds of intrafusal muscle fibers contain myofibrils and peripherally placed nuclei. Nuclear bag fibers usually extend well beyond the spindle capsule, inserting into the perimysium adjacent to extrafusal muscle fibers. Nuclear chain fibers, on the other hand, usually terminate inside the capsule by inserting on adjacent nuclear bag fibers or onto the capsule wall. Occasionally nuclear bag fibers continue through one spindle capsule and extend into a second capsule. Such a pair of capsules, each complete

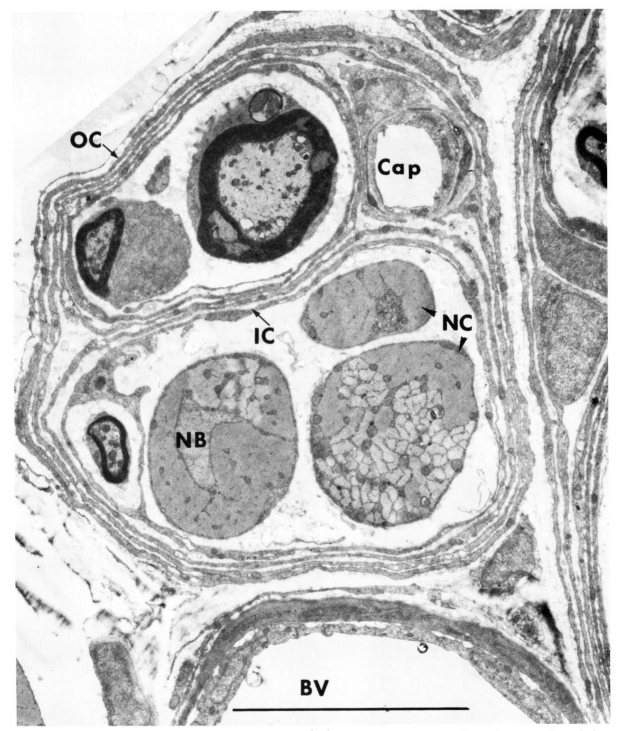

Figure 8–1 An electron micrograph of a cross section of a muscle spindle from a rat. The section passes through the region of the capsule but not through any sensory terminals. OC, outer capsule. IC, inner capsule.

A capillary (Cap) is enclosed in the layers of the outer capsule, and myelinated nerve fibers are present. Three intrafusal muscle fibers are enclosed in the inner capsule, two nuclear chain fibers (NC) and one nuclear bag fiber (NB). The spindle is situated very close to an intramuscular blood vessel, BV. Scale bar, 10 μm.

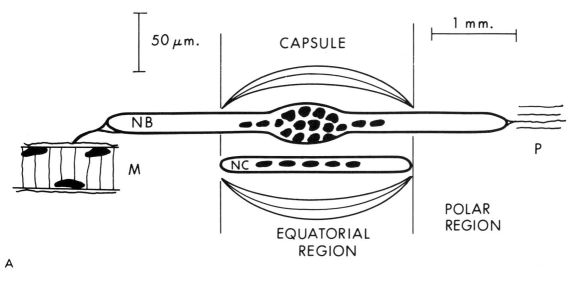

A

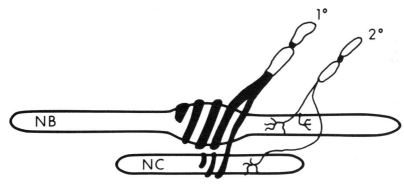

B

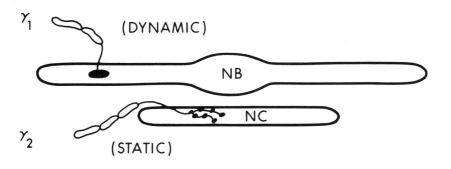

C

Figure 8–2 Diagrams of the structure and innervation of the muscle spindle. *A.* Nuclear bag (NB) and nuclear chain (NC) muscle fibers are encapsulated about their equatorial region. Nuclear bag fibers pass out of the capsule and attach to perimysial connective tissue, P, or to endomysium around the extrafusal muscle fibers. The vertical and horizontal scale bars indicate typical dimensions. *B.* Primary (1°) endings are situated on the central nucleated regions of both nuclear bag and nuclear chain muscle fibers. The secondary (2°) endings are lateral to the primary endings. *C.* In one interpretation of the histologic findings on the motor innervation of spindles, the nuclear bag and nuclear chain fibers are separately innervated. γ_1 (dynamic) fusimotor axons innervate nuclear bag fibers while γ_2 (static) fusimotor axons innervate nuclear chain fibers. (See note added at end of summary.)

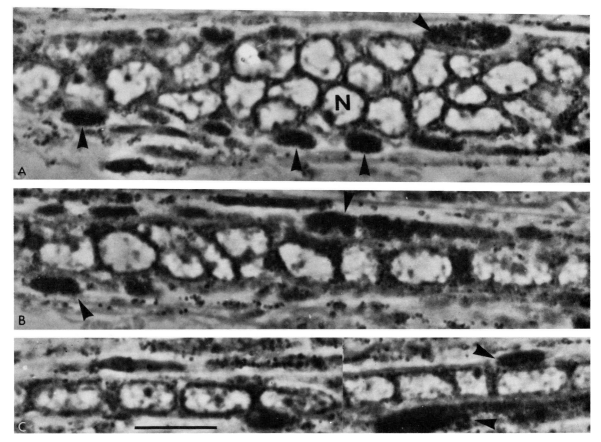

Figure 8–3   Light micrographs of thin sections taken longitudinally through the nucleated region of intrafusal muscle fibers of a cat spindle. The tissue has been treated to reveal the presence of succinic dehydrogenase (and hence mitochondria), which is stained darkly. *A.* The section passes through the center of the nuclear bag region. Round closely packed nuclei (N) are seen with mitochondria showing as dark particles between them. At the edge of the muscle fiber sections of the spirally wound primary ending are seen (arrows). The sensory endings are packed with mitochondria. *B.* The section passes from the heavily nucleated region of the nuclear bag fiber at the left to the myotube region at the right. The nuclei become elongated in the myotube region and the spaces between nuclei contain many mitochondria. Sensory endings are present at the edges of the fiber (arrows). *C.* The section passes through the nucleated region of a nuclear chain fiber (cf. *A*). The nuclei are elongated and are arranged in single file. Mitochondria occur between the nuclei and in sensory endings (arrows). Scale bar, 10 μm.

with sensory innervation and linked together by nuclear bag fibers is called a tandem muscle spindle.

The number of nuclear bag and nuclear chain fibers in a muscle spindle varies according to the muscle and the animal species. In man the lumbrical muscles contain spindles with one or two nuclear bag fibers and no, or few, nuclear chain fibers. The same muscles may also contain, as do the neck muscles, more complicated spindles with up to 14 intrafusal muscle fibers; three or four of these are typically nuclear bag fibers while the rest are nuclear chain fibers.

Only recently has the electron microscope been used to advantage in the study of the structure of the muscle spindle (see Smith and

Ovalle, 1972). In general the results support the classification of intrafusal muscle fibers into the two categories, nuclear bag fibers and nuclear chain fibers. Table 8–1 summarizes the major features of each of the two kinds of fibers. Myofibrils in the nuclear bag fiber are more closely packed and less distinct than in the nuclear chain fiber. The pattern of striation is slightly different in the two kinds of fiber; nuclear bag fibers have a thicker Z line and a less prominent M line than do nuclear chain fibers. Nuclear bag fibers also have a much less well-developed sarcotubular system (sarcoplasmic reticulum and transverse tubules) than do nuclear chain fibers. The sarcotubular system of the nuclear chain fiber is in fact surprisingly complex. In these fibers

TABLE 8–1 STRUCTURAL CHARACTERISTICS OF NUCLEAR BAG AND NUCLEAR CHAIN MUSCLE FIBERS

	Nuclear Bag Fibers	**Nuclear Chain Fibers**
Equatorial nuclei	Rounded, tightly packed, more than one abreast	Elongated nuclei in centrally placed row
Length	The longest fibers extending beyond the capsule	Shortest fibers often ending within the capsule
Diameter	Largest	Smallest
Myofibrils	Tightly packed Little interfibrillar sarcoplasm	Separated by abundant sarcoplasm
Striations	Atypical M line Thick Z line	Typical M line Thin Z line
Sarcotubular system	Poorly developed, few triads	Complex Numerous diads, triads and pentads Terminal cisternae of sarcoplasmic reticulum dilated
Sarcoplasmic contents	Mitochondria few and short Little glycogen	Many large mitochondria Glycogen abundant

junctions between the T tubes and the dilated terminal cisternae of the sarcoplasmic reticulum occur frequently, not only as the familiar triads of extrafusal muscle fibers but also as diads and pentads. Elements of the T system may also form side-to-side junctions with the sarcolemma in nuclear chain fibers.

Mitochondria in both the nuclear chain and nuclear bag fibers are oriented longitudinally between the myofibrils in contrast to their radial arrangement in extrafusal fibers. The mitochondria in the nuclear chain fibers are, however, more numerous and larger than in nuclear bag fibers.

The differences in myofibril arrangement, striation pattern, sarcotubular complexity, and sarcoplasmic contents are all in line with the idea that structurally the nuclear bag fiber resembles the slow type of extrafusal fiber while the nuclear chain fiber resembles a fast muscle fiber (Hess, 1970).

In the equatorial regions both types of fibers contain a central core of nuclei and a complex conglomeration of mitochondria, vesicles, rough and smooth sarcoplasmic reticulum, and glycogen granules. Surrounding the central core is a rim of myofibrils in which leptomeres or "microladders" may be found (Katz, 1961). The microladders are structures with alternating light- and dark-staining bands having a period of approximately 200 nm; they are closely associated with myofibrils, but their function is unknown.

Several workers have reported very close side-to-side apposition of nuclear chain fibers. The width of the gap between the cells is only about 20 nm and is devoid of basement membrane. These contacts are of interest for two reasons; they might give rise in the light microscope to the appearance of fibers that are splitting (see the section on development of the spindle), and it is possible that they may play a role in the contraction of nuclear chain fibers, which are reported to contract in synchrony.

One important idea relating to the function of intrafusal muscle fibers is that their mechanical properties are directly responsible for the dynamic features of the sensory discharge. Since most of the evidence for this idea comes not from the observation of the intrafusal fibers but from records of the sensory discharge, this idea is considered later in the discussion of the sensory endings.

Evidence gained from the direct observation of living isolated muscle spindles indicates that nuclear bag fibers when excited, whether directly by electrical stimulation or indirectly via fusimotor axons, shorten more slowly and develop tension less rapidly than do nuclear chain fibers. No direct evidence has been obtained, however, that either type of muscle fiber produces a propagated mechanical response. On the other hand, examination of the electrical properties of intrafusal muscle fibers does indicate that one type of intrafusal fiber, probably the nuclear chain fiber, can propagate an electrical impulse (Eyzaguirre, 1960; Bessou and Laporte, 1965; Bessou and Pages, 1969). While the available evidence suffers from a number of uncertainties, it does at least agree with the interpretation of the ultrastructural features of the two kinds of muscle fibers: the nuclear bag fiber resembles a slow fiber while the nuclear chain fiber resembles a twitch fiber.

The evidence that intrafusal muscle fibers in mammalian muscle spindles may be divided into two clear categories—nuclear bag fibers and nuclear chain fibers—is sufficiently abundant that counterevidence is in danger of being ignored. The counterevidence is as follows. Cuajunco (1927) divided intrafusal muscle fibers into three classes on the basis of their diameters. Later Barker formed the opinion that intrafusal fibers could be classified as nuclear bag, nuclear chain, and intermediate (Barker and Gidumal, 1961; Barker, 1962).

The intermediate fiber resembled a nuclear bag fiber, but was shorter and narrower and had a less prominent collection of equatorial nuclei than did the average nuclear bag fiber. More recently Barker and Stacey (1970) reported the existence of three kinds of intrafusal fibers in rabbit muscle. The "intermediate" fiber in this case resembled a nuclear bag fiber in its arrangement of equatorial nuclei, but resembled the nuclear chain fiber in details of its ultrastructure. Since the morphologic description of muscle spindles in the rabbit has never agreed too well with that of other mammalian spindles (Barker and Hunt, 1964), Ovalle and Smith (1972) examined spindles in the lumbrical muscles of the cat and the monkey by using serially sectioned muscles stained for the enzyme myosin ATPase. Again, three types of intrafusal muscle fibers could be distinguished. Two enzymatically different types of nuclear bag fibers were found, while the nuclear chain

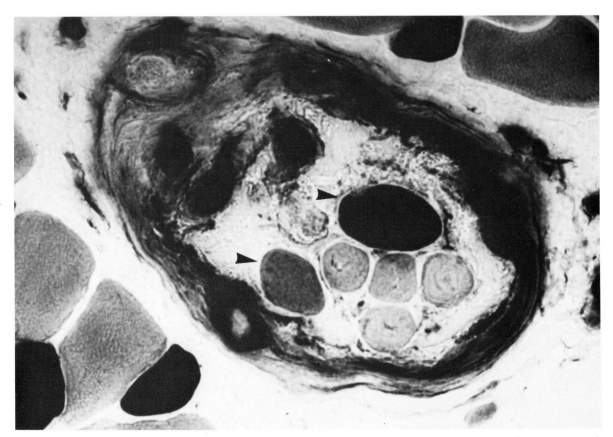

Figure 8–4   A light micrograph of a transverse frozen section of a monkey spindle. Two nuclear bag fibers are present (arrows) together with four smaller-diameter nuclear chain fibers. The group of intrafusal fibers is enclosed by a thick capsule. The section has been treated to reveal acid-stable myosin ATPase. Each of the nuclear bag fibers shows a different staining reaction while the nuclear chain fibers are histochemically homogeneous. Note also the extrafusal muscle fibers.

fibers were homogeneous in their reaction (Fig. 8–4). These findings do not correlate with any functional studies that have been performed to date, hence their meaning is obscure. Such findings, however, should be sufficient to dispel any equanimity one might feel about the completeness of our understanding of intrafusal muscle fibers.

The Sensory Endings

Since Ruffini (1898) described two kinds of sensory endings in the cat there has been a general agreement that there are two types of sensory receptors in most mammalian spindles. The primary (annulospiral) ending is always present, as shown in Figure 8–2, spirally wound on the central region of the nuclear bag muscle fibers. Small branches of the primary ending may innervate the central nucleated region of the nuclear chain muscle fibers. Secondary (flower spray) endings lie lateral to the primary endings and mainly innervate the nuclear chain fibers although, again, branches of this ending may be found on the myotube regions of the nuclear bag fibers. While most spindles contain one primary ending, the numbers of secondary endings may vary from none to five. Primary endings are connected to large diameter group I nerve fibers while secondary endings are connected to the smaller group II nerve fibers.

Electron microscopy has revealed no essential fine structural differences between the two types of endings. Both types are packed with mitochondria, vesicles, granules, and tubules whose function is not known. The sensory terminals lie in close apposition to the muscle fibers; the intercellular gap of only 15 to 35 nm contains no basement membrane, and no Schwann cell covers the endings. Both these latter features clearly distinguish sensory terminals from motor endings in the electron microscope. Some sensory endings, particularly the spirals of the primary endings, are deeply invaginated into the surface of the muscle fibers while others merely appose themselves to the muscle fiber. It is possible that specialized areas of contact exist between all sensory endings and the muscle surface since close junctions of the zonula adherens variety have been described by some workers.

In 1933 B. H. C. Matthews, using electrophysiologic techniques, discovered two types of stretch receptors in mammalian skeletal muscle. The discharge of what he called the A endings ceased during a muscle twitch, while the discharge of his B endings increased. Matthews interpreted these findings in the following way: the A endings were thought to represent muscle spindle endings that, because the spindles were in parallel with the extrafusal fibers, shortened when the muscle contracted. B endings on the other hand, because they were excited during muscle contraction, were thought to be Golgi tendon organs, which are known to be in series with extrafusal muscle. Practically all investigators have subsequently agreed with Matthews, and the pause of the sensory discharge during contraction of the muscle is still used to identify spindle receptors in physiologic experiments (Fig. 8–5B). Matthews also described one other important property of the spindle receptors; their discharge was not only sensitive to the steady length of the muscle, but also responded to the rate of extension of the muscle. If a muscle spindle is suddenly lengthened the sensory discharge often shows an initial transient burst of activity (the dynamic phase of the discharge) whose magnitude is related to the rate of elongation (Fig. 8–5C). The dynamic discharge decays to a steady level (static discharge) on attainment of a new steady length.

It was not until much later that attempts were made to study the differences in the properties of primary and secondary endings by classifying the properties of the endings according to the conduction velocity of the axons that served them. The assumption was made that in the cat, on which most of the work has been performed, a distinction between the two kinds of endings could be made by assuming that primary endings are attached to nerve fibers with conduction velocities above 72 m per second (at 37° C). This is equivalent to axons of 12 μm diameter or larger. Secondary endings are supposed to be served by axons smaller than 12 μm in diameter. (For a discussion of the origins and possible objections to these assumptions see P. B. C. Matthews [1964]). Cooper (1959, 1961) discovered that secondary endings had much less sensitivity to the rate of stretching of the muscle than did the primary endings (see Fig. 8–8). Other differences were subsequently found in the discharge of the two types of endings: the discharge from the primary ending is more erratic than that from

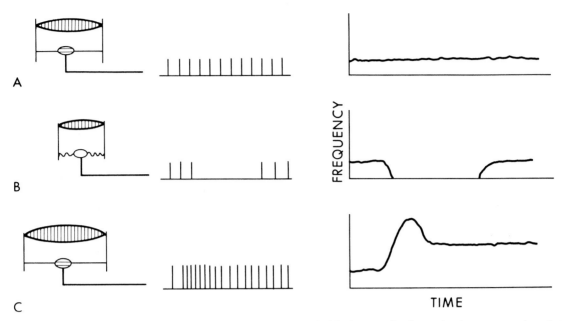

Figure 8–5 *A.* At the left the muscle spindle is shown in parallel with the extrafusal muscle. At a constant length the primary ending discharges a steady train of nerve impulses. On the right is a diagrammatic version of a plot of the frequency of the impulses against time. *B.* If the extrafusal muscle is stimulated it shortens; this also shortens the spindle. A pause in the train of sensory impulses results; this is shown on the right as a sudden decrease in frequency of the discharge. *C.* If the muscle is stretched the spindle is also stretched. The primary endings show a transient high rate of discharge (the dynamic discharge), which declines to a new steady (static) discharge.

the secondary ending and it has a very great sensitivity to very small extensions that is absent in secondary endings (Stein and Matthews, 1965; Matthews and Stein, 1968). For large but physiologic extensions, however, the mean frequency of nerve impulses in the axons leading from each kind of receptor increases linearly by roughly the same amount with increasing muscle length.

The most striking difference between the discharges originating in the primary and secondary endings is the rate, or velocity, sensitivity of the primary ending and its absence in the secondary ending. As early as 1933 B. H. C. Matthews suggested that the rate sensitivity of the spindle discharge might reflect the mechanical properties of the intra-

fusal muscle fibers. The properties of intrafusal muscle fibers must, of necessity, influence the way in which the sensory endings are excited. Figure 8–6 shows the flow of events between the input to the muscle spindle, either a change in length or excitation of the intrafusal fibers, and the final output of the receptor. The form of the extension of the muscle is modified by the mechanical properties of the intrafusal muscle fibers. The resulting deformation of the central region of the muscle fibers causes in turn a deformation of the sensory endings. Mechanoelectric transduction then takes place producing an electrical current—the generator current—which excites the nerve to produce a train of action potentials (Katz, 1950; Lippold et al.,

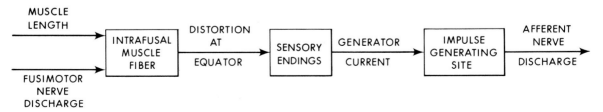

Figure 8–6 A flow diagram illustrating the sequence of events taking place between the input to the muscle spindle, change in muscle length or fusimotor activity, and the output of the spindle, a train of impulses in the sensory nerves.

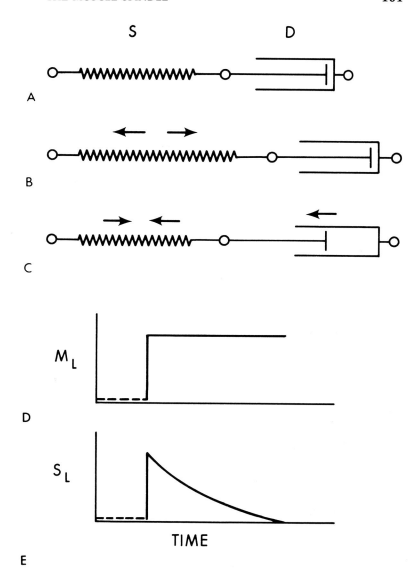

Figure 8–7 A mechanical analogy to explain the sensitivity of primary spindle endings to the rate of change of length of the muscle. *A.* The nuclear bag fiber is supposed to consist of an elastic portion (S), which is the nucleated region, and a viscous portion (D), which is each pole of the fiber. *B.* If the spindle is suddenly extended then the viscous portion remains the same length because it cannot flow rapidly, so the elastic portion is forced to extend. *C.* If held at the new length the viscous portion gradually extends allowing the elastic portion to shorten. *D.* The steplike change in muscle length (M_L). *E.* The ensuing changes in length of the elastic portion of the fiber (S_L).

1960). The mechanical hypothesis of the origin of the rate sensitivity of primary endings supposes that the central nucleated region of the nuclear bag fiber has elastic properties but is not very viscous. The poles of the nuclear bag fiber on the other hand are postulated to have appreciable viscosity. A very simple model of such a muscle fiber is shown in Figure 8–7. On rapid extension the viscous portion of the fiber (D) does not alter in length while the spring (S) extends. When the fiber is held at the new length the viscous portion will slowly extend, allowing the spring to decrease in length. If the primary ending is sensitive to the length of the nuclear bag (the spring) then it will behave in a rate-sensitive fashion. More sophisticated versions of this scheme have been proposed with the result that the actual form of the discharge of the primary ending can be modeled very closely. The lack of rate sensitivity in the secondary endings is explained by the lack of any such dramatic change in mechanical properties along the length of the nuclear chain fiber. It is apparent from the flow diagram of Figure 8–6 that other processes, such as mechano-electric transduction, could be rate sensitive. A certain amount of direct evidence exists in support of the mechanical hypothesis (Boyd, 1966; Smith, 1966). More important, however, for the interpretation of fusimotor influences on the sensory discharge is the idea that the rate-sensitive response originates in the nuclear bag fiber.

Fusimotor Innervation

While it had been known for some time that intrafusal muscle fibers received a motor supply from small-diameter myelinated nerve fibers, and while it had also been suggested that these fibers were specific to intrafusal fibers (Leksell, 1945), it remained for Hunt and associates (1951) to establish the fact. The latter workers showed that in the cat stimulation of motor nerve fibers with conduction velocities of less than 45 μm per second (diameters of 7 μm and less) would increase the discharge in sensory nerves from spindles, but would not cause any measurable contraction in the muscle containing the receptors. Following this work it was thought for some years that the fusimotor (gamma) axons were all of the same functional type. New morphologic studies by Boyd and by Barker, however, completely transformed thinking on the nature of fusimotor innervation.

It should be said at the outset of any morphologic description of the fusimotor innervation of muscle spindles that the evidence is extremely controversial. Boyd's (1962) description remains the most appealing to the physiologist since it can be made to fit much of the functional behavior of spindles. Boyd described a separate motor supply for the nuclear bag and nuclear chain muscle fibers. He found platelike endings (γ_1 endings) at the polar ends of nuclear bag fibers while diffuse motor endings (γ_2 endings) were located more centrally on the nuclear chain fibers, the type of motor innervation illustrated in Figure 8–2. Barker's group have contrary evidence that neither the motor nerve supply nor the type of motor ending is specific to either type of intrafusal muscle fiber; they state in fact that the innervation of the two kinds of muscle fibers may overlap. The disagreement is perhaps not so surprising when one examines Boyd's (1962) reconstruction of a typical muscle spindle. In this reconstruction five γ_1 motor fibers of about 3 μm diameter form endings on two nuclear bag fibers while seven γ_2 fibers of about 1 μm diameter innervate four nuclear chain fibers. It is possible that the morphologic relationships of such a complex array of fine nerve terminals cannot be determined with any high degree of certainty by conventional light microscopic techniques. In any case, the two sets of evidence are sufficiently contradictory that no decision can be made on morphologic grounds as to which

scheme represents the true pattern of innervation. Functional studies, however, do supply an independent line of evidence that tends to support Boyd's hypothesis.

More recently, Barker's group has described, in addition to the γ_2 or "gamma trail" endings, two forms of the plate endings; these are termed "P_1 plates" and "P_2 plates" (Barker et al., 1972). The P_2 plates and the trail endings are supplied by pure fusimotor axons while the P_1 plates, which closely resemble extrafusal endplates, are supplied by branches of axons to the extrafusal skeletal muscle. The latter type of innervation, termed skeletofusimotor or β innervation, appears to be a common feature of distally placed limb muscles, but its particular significance is not understood.

Electron microscopic studies cannot, by their nature, resolve the problem of how the intrafusal muscle fibers are connected to their many fusimotor axons. Such studies have, however, provided evidence that there are at least two structural varieties of motor terminals that differ mainly in the arrangement of the postsynaptic side of the junction. The sarcolemma beneath plate endings is folded, and the subneural sarcoplasm is filled with a variety of organelles, including a sole plate nucleus. Beneath trail endings the sarcolemma is not folded, and the sarcoplasm there does not contain as marked an accumulation of organelles.

Functionally, fusimotor axons have been divided into two types: dynamic and static. These were first differentiated by their effect on the stretch response of the primary endings (Matthews, 1962; Jansen and Matthews, 1962; Crowe and Matthews, 1964). Repetitive stimulation of single fusimotor axons of the dynamic type caused the dynamic component of the stretch-response of the primary endings to be increased (Fig. 8–8). Stimulation of static fusimotor axons either had no effect on the dynamic sensitivity of primary endings or decreased this sensitivity slightly. Later, Appelberg, Bessou, and Laporte (1966) reported that stimulation of dynamic fusimotor axons usually had no effect on the discharge of secondary endings while stimulation of static fusimotor axons did increase the discharge from these endings.

The simplest interpretation of these findings can be made in terms of Figures 8–2 and 8–7. If it is supposed that dynamic fusimotor axons innervate nuclear bag fibers alone, then

PASSIVE   DYNAMIC   STATIC

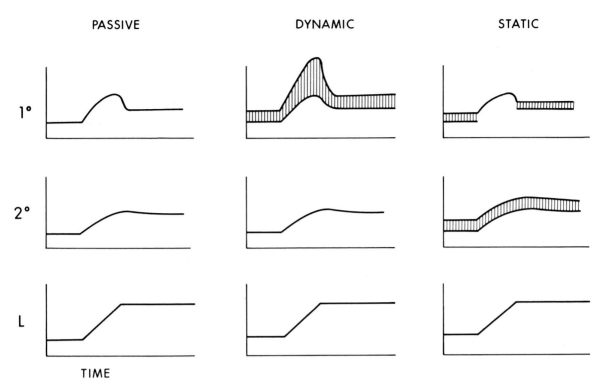

TIME

Figure 8–8 Diagram to show the effect of stretching the muscle spindle on the frequency of discharge of primary and secondary sensory endings with and without fusimotor stimulation. The bottom row of graphs shows the change of length of the spindle with time. In each case the extension is ramplike, i.e., a constant velocity length change is imposed on the spindle, and this terminates in a new, increased, length. The first column illustrates the response of primary (1°) and secondary (2°) endings to the increase in length in the absence of fusimotor stimulation. The primary ending exhibits a marked rate sensitivity while the secondary ending shows only a very small sensitivity to the rate of extension. In the second column the extension takes place in the presence of repetitive stimulation of dynamic fusimotor axons. The steady discharge and the dynamic discharge of the primary ending are increased by the amount shown by the hatching. The discharge of the secondary endings shows no change. In the third column the extension takes place in the presence of stimulation of static fusimotor axons. The static discharge of primary endings is increased while the dynamic phase is unaffected or even decreased. The response of secondary endings is uniformly increased.

contraction of the poles of the fiber would alter their mechanical properties. The altered mechanical properties of the nuclear bag fiber could then explain the increased sensitivity of the primary ending to the velocity of extension. In addition, it is assumed that a separate fusimotor innervation to the nuclear bag and nuclear chain fibers can best explain the unique effect of dynamic fusimotor axons on the discharge of primary endings and the strong effect of stimulation of static axons on the discharge of secondary endings. Proponents of this hypothesis are among the first to admit the difficulties attendant to it (Matthews, 1964; Jansen, 1966). Since the chain of events occurring in the excitation of sensory endings shown in Figure 8–6 is not fully understood, and since the contribution of branches of the sensory endings on each kind of intrafusal muscle fiber to the final discharge

is unknown, any explanation of fusimotor effects must remain tentative. Alternative views of the fusimotor innervation, particularly those that postulate a completely functional, completely overlapping innervation are less satisfactory still. In order to explain the differential effects of static and dynamic axons on the two types of sensory endings this latter type of hypothesis must include further assumptions for which there is no evidence (see Jansen, 1966). As evidence accumulates (e.g., Brown et al., 1969), it seems likely that the scheme represented in Figure 8–2 will prove to be at least functionally correct.

Sympathetic nerve fibers to the spindle are considered briefly here in this discussion of motor innervation since not only do they serve the blood vessels of the capsule, but they may also be demonstrated to have an effect on the spindle discharge. Hunt (1960) and

Eldred, Schnitzlein, and Buchwald (1960) showed that stimulation of the sympathetic trunk would cause, after approximately a 20 second delay, an increased spindle discharge. The increase in sensory discharge was later followed by a period in which the discharge was depressed. Similar effects could be caused by intraarterial injection of adrenaline. Since Hunt's work demonstrated the sympathetic nervous effect in muscles devoid of blood supply, it is impossible to ascribe the results totally to an alteration of blood flow. At the present time, however, it is also difficult to accept the alternate view that sympathetic nerves have some kind of direct motor influence on the muscle spindle.

PATHOLOGIC CHANGES

The early work of Sherrington (1894) and Batten (1897) led to the commonly accepted opinion that the intrafusal muscle fibers do not atrophy following nerve section. This view can still be found in the literature (Patel et al., 1968) although Tower (1932) had shown marked atrophy and degeneration in intrafusal muscle fibers of the cat's hind limb following denervation. Tower showed that dorsal root ganglionectomy resulted in degenerative changes in the equatorial regions of the intrafusal muscle fibers while ventral root section caused atrophy of the polar regions. Boyd (1962) confirmed Tower's findings and showed that sectioning the ventral roots caused nuclear chain fibers to atrophy more rapidly than the nuclear bag fibers. Thus, the experimental work is entirely in line with what is known of the development of the spindle: the spindle is structurally dependent both on the sensory and the motor nerve supply. In addition, Boyd's (1962) results are consistent with the view that the nuclear chain and nuclear bag fibers represent two different types of muscle fibers. The failure to detect a change of diameter among the intrafusal fibers in clinical cases of denervation (Patel et al., 1968) probably reflects the fact that these changes do not occur as early as they do in extrafusal muscle. Intrafusal muscle fibers do not undergo complete disintegration following denervation; they have been shown to persist in an atrophied state for as long as two years following nerve section (Gutmann and Zelena, 1962). In addition, tenotomy, which causes a marked atrophy of extrafusal muscle fibers, does not

produce great changes in the intrafusal fibers (Yellin and Eldred, 1970; Zelena, 1964).

Changes in the structure of the muscle spindle concurrent with disease states have been described. Among the more recent of these reports are the following. Holmes et al. (1960) described glycogen deposits in spindles in a case of glycogen storage disease. Banker and Victor (1966) reported intracapsular inflammatory cells in a case of childhood dermatomyositis. Daniel and Strich (1964) described five cases of myotonic dystrophy in which the numbers of intrafusal muscle fibers were greatly increased while the diameters of the fibers were decreased. The intrafusal fibers also contained pyknotic nuclei and foci of necrosis, and the fibers were surrounded by an abnormal amount of reticulin and connective tissue. Lindsey and co-workers (1966) showed splitting or fragmentation of infrafusal muscle fibers in nemaline myopathy while Gonatas and associates (1966) reported nemaline bodies in intrafusal fibers in the same condition.

Several surveys of biopsy material have been carried out. Lapresle and Milhaud (1964) found 150 spindles in 1200 biopsies; they selected 52 spindles for study and found 38 that were abnormal. The abnormalities reported were capsular thickening and atrophy and degeneration of intrafusal fibers in muscular dystrophy. In polymyositis some spindles were found with round cell infiltration. In cases of neurogenic atrophy of muscle, spindles were found with atrophic intrafusal fibers, increased muscle nuclei, degenerative changes in the nerve endings, and proliferation of connective tissue. Patel et al. (1968) studied 257 spindles found in 1000 biopsies from normal muscle and muscle showing changes due to denervation atrophy, nonspecific atrophy, muscular dystrophy, myotonia dystrophica, and chronic polymyositis. These workers conclude that "no specific histopathological change in the spindle or the intrafusal fibers could be detected in any of these cases." They did, however, note what appeared to be increases in the number of nuclei and pyknotic nuclei in intrafusal fibers as well as connective tissue changes in some cases. In a similar extensive survey Cazzato and Walton (1968) concluded that the extent of structural alteration in a variety of neuromuscular disorders was related to the time of onset and the stage of the disease.

One cannot agree with the opinion that

muscle spindles are disease resistant. Obviously, some changes do take place; the fact that they may take place at a rate different from those affecting extrafusal muscle need not lessen the disruptive effect of the disease on so complicated a structure. Specific changes in the structure of muscle spindles due to disease states probably will not be described until ultrastructural studies are undertaken.

Many of the pathologic conditions in which muscle spindles are involved are more subtle than those just described. These are likely to be disturbances of function that are not reflected in structural alterations but only in patterns of activity. The possible role of the muscle spindle in spasticity and rigidity has been discussed by a number of authors (Hoffman, 1962; Jansen, 1962; Landau et al., 1960; Rushworth, 1960; Steg, 1962). These discussions are not pursued here, partly because they are concerned with pathologic conditions of the central nervous system that do not fall within the scope of this volume, and partly because the role of the muscle spindle in the control of normal movement is not understood (Matthews, 1964). In general one can say that the definition of the role of the muscle spindle in pathologic conditions awaits a better understanding of both its normal structure and function.

SUMMARY

The contemporary view of the muscle spindle is changing rapidly. This fact makes it important to emphasize that any summary of the present state of knowledge represents a hypothetical position. While areas of controversy have been indicated here, the details of controversial issues have been avoided so that a reasonably coherent picture of the muscle spindle could be presented. This picture of the muscle spindle is of a system containing three pairs of components: two kinds of intrafusal muscle fibers are innervated by two kinds of fusimotor nerve fibers, while sensory information to the spinal cord originates in two kinds of sensory endings. The two kinds of intrafusal muscle fibers, the nuclear bag and nuclear chain fibers, may be distinguished by their structure both at the light microscopic and ultrastructural levels. The details of their ultrastructure are in line with what is known of their function; the nuclear bag fiber contracts slowly and does not propagate an impulse, while the nuclear chain fiber contracts rapidly and may, under normal conditions, propagate an impulse. It is likely that the two kinds of intrafusal muscle fibers receive separate motor innervation via dynamic (to nuclear bag fibers) and static (to nuclear chain fibers) fusimotor axons. Of the two kinds of sensory endings the primary endings, which mainly innervate the nuclear bag fibers, show a marked sensitivity to the rate of extension of the muscle. This rate sensitivity is thought to have its origin in the mechanical properties of the nuclear bag muscle fiber. The secondary endings, which mainly innervate the nuclear chain fibers, do not show this marked rate sensitivity. Stimulation of dynamic fusimotor axons enhances the rate sensitivity of the primary endings and also increases their static discharge. Dynamic fusimotor axons have no effect on the discharge of secondary endings. Stimulation of static fusimotor axons increases the static discharge of primary sensory endings but either has no effect on, or decreases, their rate sensitivity. Activity of static fusimotor axons also increases the static discharge of secondary endings. While these relationships and effects must be significant to the role which the spindle plays in the function of the animal, it is unfortunately true that this general role is not understood. Hence, the meaning of the detailed function of the muscle spindle remains obscure.

The muscle spindle is a complex organ that is sensitive to many influences. Its long-term integrity and development are probably under the trophic control of both motor and sensory axons, and its normal function is very sensitive to changes in blood supply. Nevertheless few specific changes in spindle morphology have yet been reported in disease states.

Note Added.   Since this chapter was written further attempts have been made to resolve the controversy over the motor innervation of intrafusal muscle fibers. Workers in Britain and France have produced preliminary reports that indicate that the innervation may be represented by a combination of the schemes originally espoused by Boyd and Barker (Brown and Butler, 1973; Laporte, 1973). Static fusimotor axons may innervate both nuclear bag and nuclear chain fibers while dynamic fusimotor fibers may innervate nuclear bag fibers alone. Thus, in Figure 8–2*B* a branch of the static axon may lead to the nuclear bag fiber. Reference to Figure

8–8 will show that this scheme would be compatible with the physiologic findings.

Acknowledgments: The author is grateful to Dr. W. K. Ovalle, who supplied the photograph for Figure 8–1. The author's own work is supported by the Muscular Dystrophy Association of Canada and the Medical Research Council of Canada.

REFERENCES

Appelberg, B., Bessou, P., and Laporte, Y.: Action of static and dynamic fusimotor fibers on secondary endings of cat's spindles. J. Physiol. (Lond.), *185*: 160, 1966.

Banker, B. Q., and Victor, M.: Dermatomyositis (systemic angiopathy) of childhood. Medicine, *45*:261, 1966.

Banker, B. Q. R., Przybylski, J., Van der Meulen, J. P., and Victor, M.: Research in Muscle Development and the Muscle Spindle. Amsterdam, Excerpta Medica, 1972.

Barker, D.: The structure and distribution of muscle receptors. *In* Barker, D. (ed.): Symposium on Muscle Receptors. Hong Kong, Hong Kong University Press, 1962.

Barker, D., and Gidumal, J. L.: The morphology of intrafusal muscle fibres in the cat. J. Physiol. (Lond.), *157*:513, 1961.

Barker, D., and Hunt, J. P.: Mammalian intrafusal muscle fibres. Nature, *203*:1193, 1964.

Barker, D., Harker, D., Stacey, M. J., and Smith, C. R.: Fusimotor innervation. *In* Banker, B. Q., et al. (eds.): Research in Muscle Development and the Muscle Spindle. Amsterdam, Excerpta Medica, 1972.

Barker, D., and Stacey, M. J.: Rabbit intrafusal muscle fibres. J. Physiol. (Lond.), *210*:70, 1970.

Batten, F.: The muscle spindle under pathological conditions. Brain, *20*:138, 1897.

Bessou, P., and Laporte, Y.: Potentials fusoraeux provoqués par la stimulation des fibres fusimotrices chez le chat. C. R. Acad. Sci. (Paris), *260*:4827, 1965.

Bessou, P., and Pages, B.: Intracellular recording from spindle muscle fibres of potentials elicited by static fusimotor axons in the cat. Life Sci., *8*:417, 1969.

Boyd, I. A.: The structure and innervation of the nuclear bag muscle fibre system and the nuclear chain muscle fibre system in mammalian muscle spindles. Philos. Trans. R. Soc. Lond. [Biol. Sci.], *245*:81, 1962.

Boyd, I. A.: The mechanical properties of mammalian intrafusal muscle fibres. J. Physiol. (Lond.), *187*:10, 1966.

Bravo-Rey, M. C., Yamaski, J. N., Eldred, E., and Maier, A.: Ionizing irradiation on development on the muscle spindle. Exp. Neurol., *25*:595, 1969.

Brown, M. C., and Butler, R. G.: Depletion of intrafusal muscle fibre glycogen by stimulation of fusimotor fibres. J. Physiol. (Lond.), *229*:25P, 1973.

Brown, M. C., Goodwin, G. M., and Matthews, P. B. C.: After-effects of fusimotor stimulation on the response of muscle spindle primary afferent endings. J. Physiol. (Lond.), *205*:677, 1969.

Brzezinski, D. K. von.: Unrersuchungen zur Histochemie der Muskelspindeln. I. Mitteilüng: Topochemie der Polysaccharide. Acta Histochem., *12*:75, 1961a.

Brzezinski, D. K. von.: Untersuchungen zur Histochemie der Muskelspindeln. II. Mitteilüng: Zur Topochemie und Funktion des Spindelraumes und der Spindelkapsel. Acta Histochem., *12*:277, 1961b.

Cazzato, G., and Walton, J. N.: The pathology of the muscle spindle. A study of biopsy material in various muscular and neuro-muscular diseases. J. Neurol. Sci., *7*:15, 1968.

Cooper, S.: The secondary endings of muscle spindle. J. Physiol. *149*:27P, 1959.

Cooper, S.: The responses of the primary and secondary endings of muscle spindles with intact motor innervation during applied stretch. Q. J. Exp. Physiol., *46*:389, 1961.

Cooper, S., and Daniel, P. M.: Muscle spindles in man; their morphology in the lumbricals and the deep muscles of the neck. Brain, *86*:563, 1963.

Crowe, A., and Matthews, P. B. C.: Further studies of static and dynamic fusimotor fibres. J. Physiol. (Lond.), *174*:132, 1964.

Cuajunco, F.: Embryology of the neuromuscular spindles. Contrib. Embryol. Carnegie Inst., *19*:1927.

Cuajunco, F.: Development of the neuromuscular spindle in human fetuses. Contrib. Embryol. Carnegie Inst., *28*:95, 1940.

Daniel, P. M., and Strich, S. J.: Abnormalities in the muscle spindles in dystrophia myotonica. Neurology (Minneap.), *14*:310, 1964.

Eldred, E., Yellin, H., Gabbois, L., and Sweeney, S.: Bibliography on muscle receptors; their morphology, pathology, and physiology. Exp. Neurol., Suppl. 3, 1967.

Eldred, E., Schnitzlein, H. N., and Buchwald, J.: Response of muscle spindles to stimulation of the sympathetic trunk. Exp. Neurol., *2*:13, 1960.

Eyzaguirre, C.: The electrical activity of mammalian intrafusal fibres. J. Physiol. (Lond.), *150*:169, 1960.

Golgi, C.: Annotazioni intorno all'istologia normale e patologica dei muscoli voloutari. Arch. Sci. Med., *5*:194, 1880.

Gonatas, N. K., Shy, G. M., and Godfrey, E. H.: Nemaline myopathy. N. Engl. J. Med., *274*:535, 1966.

Granit, R.: The Basis of Motor Control. Integrating the Activity of Muscles, Alpha and Gamma Motoneurons and their Leading Control Systems. New York, Academic Press, 1970.

Gutmann, E., and Zelena, J.: Morphological changes in the denervated muscle. *In* Gutmann, E. (ed.): The Denervated Muscle. Prague, Publishing House of the Czechoslovak Academy of Sciences, 1962, p. 57.

Hess, A.: Vertebrate slow muscle fibres. Physiol. Rev., *50*:40, 1970.

Hoffmann, W. W.: Observations on peripheral servo mechanisms in Parkinsonian rigidity. J. Neurol. Neurosurg. Psychiatry, *25*:203, 1962.

Holmes, J. M., Houghton, C. R., and Woolf, A. L.: A myopathy presenting in adult life with features suggestive of glycogen storage disease. J. Neurol. Neurosurg. Psychiatry, *23*:302, 1960.

Holtzer, H.: Myogenesis. *In* Scheide, O. A., and de Vellis, J.: Cell Differentiation. New York, Van Nostrand Reinhold Co., 1970.

Hunt, C. C.: The effect of sympathetic stimulation on mammalian muscle spindles. J. Physiol. (Lond.), *151*:332, 1960.

Hunt, C. C., and Kuffler, S. W.: Further study of efferent small-nerve fibres to mammalian muscle spindles.

Muscle spindle innervation and activity during contraction. J. Physiol. (Lond.), *113*:283, 1951.

Jansen, J. K. S.: Spasticity-functional aspects. Acta Neurol. Scand., *38*:Suppl. 3:41, 1962.

Jansen, J. K. S.: On the functional properties of stretch receptors of mammalian skeletal muscles. *In* de Renck, A. V. S., and Knight, J. (eds.): Ciba Foundation Symposium on Myotatic, Kinesthetic and Vestibular Mechanisms. London, J. & A. Churchill, Ltd., 1966.

Jansen, J. K. S., and Matthews, P. B. C.: The central control of the dynamic response of muscle spindle receptors. J. Physiol. (Lond.), *161*:357, 1962.

Katz, B.: Depolarization of sensory terminals and the initiation of impulses in the muscle spindle. J. Physiol. (Lond.), *111*:248, 1950.

Katz, B.: The terminations of the afferent nerve fibre in the muscle spindle of the frog. Proc. R. Soc. Lond. B., *243*:221, 1961.

Kelly, A. M., and Zacks, S. I.: The histogenesis of rat intercostal muscle. J. Cell. Biol., *42*:135, 1969.

Landau, W. M., Weaver, R. A., and Hornbein, R. F.: Fusimotor nerve function in man. Arch. Neurol., *3*:10, 1960.

Laporte, Y.: Evidence for common innervation of bag and chain muscle fibres in cat spindles. *In* Stein, R. B., Pearson, K. G., Smith, R. S., and Redford, J. B. (eds.): Control of Posture and Locomotion. New York, Plenum Press, 1973.

Lapresle, J., and M. Milhaud: Pathologie du fuseau neuromusculaire. Rev. Neurol. (Paris), *110*:97, 1964.

Leksell, L.: The action potential and excitatory effects of the small ventral root fibres to skeletal muscle. Acta Physiol. Scand., *10*:Suppl. 31, 1945.

Liddell, E. G. T., and Sherrington, C.: Reflexes in response to stretch (myotatic reflexes). Proc. R. Soc. Lond. B, *96*:212, 1924.

Liddell, E. G. T., and Sherrington, C.: Further observations on myotatic reflexes. Proc. R. Soc. Lond. B., *97*:267, 1925.

Lindsey, J. R., Hopkins, I. J., and Clark, D. B.: Pathology of nemaline myopathy. Bull. Johns Hopkins Hosp., *119*:378, 1966.

Lippold, O. C. J., Nicholls, J. G., and Redfearn, J. W. T.: Electrical and mechanical factors in the adaptation of a mammalian muscle spindle. J. Physiol. (Lond.), *153*:209, 1960.

Marchand, E. R., and Eldred, E.: Postnatal increase of intrafusal fibres in the rat muscle spindle. Exp. Neurol., *25*:655, 1969.

Matthews, B. H. C.: Nerve endings in mammalian muscle. J. Physiol. (Lond.), *78*:1, 1933.

Matthews, P. B. C.: The differentiation of two types of fusimotor fiber by their effects on the dynamic response of muscle spindle primary endings. Q. J. Exp. Physiol., *47*:324, 1962.

Matthews, P. B. C.: Muscle spindles and their motor control. Physiol. Rev., *44*:220, 1964.

Matthews, P. B. C.: Mammalian muscle receptors and their central actions. Monograph 23 of the Physiological Society. London, Edward Arnold Ltd., 1972.

Matthews, P. B. C., and Stein, R. B.: The sensitivity of muscle afferents to small sinusoidal changes of length. J. Physiol. (Lond.), *200*:723, 1968.

Merton, P. A.: Speculations on the servo control of movement. *In* Malcolm, J. L., Gray, J. A. B., and Freeman, J. S. (eds.): The Spinal Cord. Ciba Symposium. London, J. & A. Churchill, Ltd., 1953, p. 247.

Ovalle, W. K., and Smith, R. S.: Histochemical identification of three types of intrafusal muscle fibers in the cat and monkey based on the myosin ATPase reaction. Can. J. Physiol. Pharmacol., *50*:195, 1972.

Patel, A. N., Lalitha, V. S., and Dastur, D. K.: The spindle in normal and pathological muscle: an assessment of the histological changes. Brain, *91*:737, 1968.

Ruffini, A.: On the minute anatomy of the neuromuscular spindles of the cat, and on their physiological significance. J. Physiol., *23*:190, 1898.

Rushworth, G.: Spasticity and rigidity: an experimental study and review. J. Neurol. Neurosurg. Psychiatry, *23*:99, 1960.

Sherrington, C. S.: On the anatomical constitution of nerves of skeletal muscles; with remarks on recurrent fibres in the ventral spinal nerve-root. J. Physiol. (Lond.), *17*:211, 1894.

Smith, R. S.: Properties of intrafusal muscle fibres. *In* Granit, R. (ed.): Muscular Afferents and Motor Control. Nobel Symposium I. Stockholm, Alqvist and Wiksell, 1966, p. 69.

Smith, R. S., and Ovalle, W. K.: The structure and function of intrafusal muscle fibers. *In* Cassens, R. G. (ed.): Muscle Biology. Vol. 1. New York, Marcel Dekker Inc., 1972.

Steg, G.: The function of muscle spindles in spasticity and rigidity. Acta Neurol. Scand., *38*:Suppl. 3:53, 1962.

Stein, R. B., and Matthews, P. B. C.: Differences in variability of discharge frequency between primary and secondary muscle spindle afferent endings of the cat. Nature (Lond.), *208*:1217, 1965.

Tower, S.: Atrophy and degeneration in the muscle spindle. Brain, *55*:77, 1932.

Yellin, H., and Eldred, E.: Spindle activity of the tenotomized gastrocnemius muscle in the cat. Exp. Neurol., *29*:513, 1970.

Zelena, J.: Development, degeneration, and regeneration of receptor organs. *In* Singer, M., and Schade, J. P. (eds.): Mechanisms of Neural Regeneration. Prog. Brain Res., *13*:175, 1964.

Zelena, J., and Hnik, P.: Effect of innervation on the development of muscle receptors. *In* Gutmann, E., and Hnik, P. (eds.): The Effect of Use and Disuse on Neuromuscular Functions. Prague, Publishing House of the Czechoslovak Academy of Sciences, 1963, p. 95.

Chapter 9

MICROSCOPIC ANATOMY AND FUNCTION OF THE CONNECTIVE TISSUE COMPONENTS OF PERIPHERAL NERVE

P. K. Thomas *and* Yngve Olsson

The attention given to the study of the structure and activity of the conducting elements in peripheral nerve has tended to divert interest from the connective tissue components. Investigations in recent years have emphasized the considerable importance of these supporting structures both in the normal functioning of peripheral nerves and in disease states.

The classic observations by Key and Retzius (1876) and Ranvier (1878) laid the foundations for all subsequent studies. Key and Retzius suggested a subdivision into epineurium, perineurium, and endoneurium, which correspond respectively to the perifascicular tissue, the lamellated sheath, and the intrafascicular tissue of Ranvier (Fig. 9–1). The terminology introduced by Key and Retzius was generally adopted and, although various modifications have subsequently been advocated, still remains the most satisfactory. As is discussed later, there are morphologic grounds for believing that the perineurium should not be considered as typical connective tissue, but should be regarded as part of the membranous covering that invests the whole of the nervous system, both central and peripheral.

MORPHOLOGIC ASPECTS

The structural arrangements in the nerve trunks and their peripheral terminations differ considerably from those in the nerve roots and are therefore considered separately.

Peripheral Nerve Trunks

EPINEURIUM

The epineurium consists of a condensation of areolar connective tissue that surrounds the perineurial ensheathment of the fascicles of uni- and multifascicular nerves. Although continuous with the surrounding connective tissues, the attachment is loose, so that nerve trunks are relatively mobile except where tethered by entering vessels or by branches. Greater amounts of connective tissue are present where nerves cross joints (Sunderland, 1965). In human nerve trunks, Sunderland and Bradley (1949) found that the epineurium usually constitutes anything from 30 to 75 per cent of the cross sectional area with extremes of 22 and 88 per cent. In general, the more numerous the fascicles, the greater is the quantity of epineurium.

The collagen bundles are oriented predominantly in the axis of the nerve trunk. By electron microscopy, the diameter of the fibrils has been found to average 80 nm in the rat and rabbit nerve trunks (Schmitt et al., 1942; Thomas and Jones, 1967), 80 to 110 nm around the nodose ganglion of the rat and

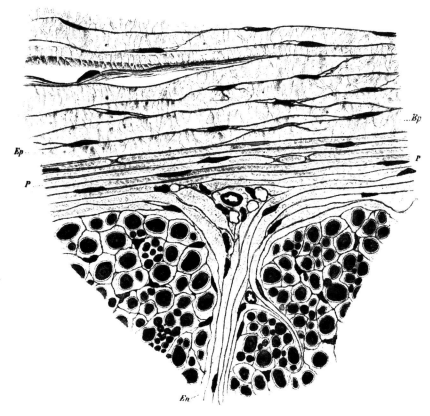

Figure 9–1   Portion of transverse section through part of brachial plexus of rabbit, showing disposition of epineurium (Ep), perineurium (p) and endoneurium (En). The structure labeled endoneurium is an intrafascicular perineurial "partition" (see text for explanation). (From Key, A., and Retzius, G.: Studien in der Anatomie des Nervensystems und des Bindegewebes. Stockholm, Samson & Wallin, 1876.)

rabbit vagus nerve (Lieberman, 1968), and 60 to 110 nm in human nerve trunks (Gamble and Eames, 1964). Elastic fibers have been identified by light microscopy and electron microscopy, particularly adjacent to the perineurium (Ranvier, 1878; Thomas, 1963a). They are again mainly oriented longitudinally.

Apart from fibroblasts, the epineurium may contain mast cells, there being considerable species differences in the numbers present (Olsson, 1968). This is discussed later in greater detail in relation to the cellular content of the endoneurium. Variable quantities of fat are also present, particularly in the larger nerve trunks.

The vasa nervorum enter the epineurium where they communicate with a longitudinal anastomotic network of arterioles and venules (see Chapter 10). The epineurium also contains lymphatic vessels, which are not present within the fascicles. The literature on the lymph drainage of nerves was collected by Sunderland (1965). He concluded that there

is a lymphatic capillary network in the epineurium that is drained by lymphatic channels that accompany the arteries of the nerve trunk and pass into the regional lymph nodes.

PERINEURIUM

It is in relation to the perineurium that there has been the greatest amount of disaccord in the literature. Key and Retzius (1876) were quick to recognize that its essential component is a lamellated arrangement of flattened cells. The disagreement has centered on the embryologic origin of these cells and whether a separate connective tissue layer is definable external to the lamellated cellular layer that can be distinguished from the epineurium.

The perineurium provides an ensheathment for both the somatic and peripheral autonomic nerves and their ganglia (Shantha and Bourne, 1968). Its cellular lamellae are

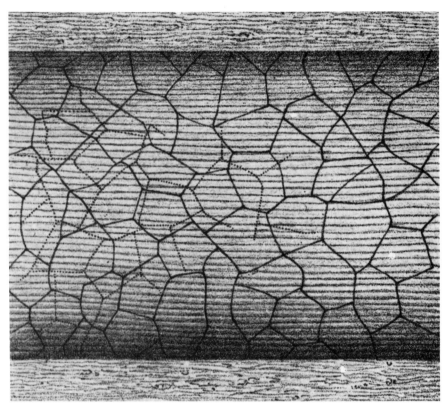

Figure 9–2   Surface view of forelimb nerve of dog, showing mosaic of flattened perineurial cells. (From Key, A., and Retzius, G.: Studien in der Anatomie des Nervensystems und des Bindegewebes. Stockholm, Sanson & Wallin, 1876.)

composed of concentric sleeves of flattened polygonal cells (Lehman, 1957; Shantha-veerappa and Bourne, 1962) and were well illustrated by Key and Retzius (1876) in their original descriptions (Fig. 9–2). The number of lamellae varies, mainly depending upon the diameter of the fascicle; the larger the fascicle the greater is the number of lamellae. Up to 15 layers are present around the fascicles of mammalian nerve trunks.

Electron microscopy confirms the flattened lamellar arrangement of the perineurial cells (Fig. 9–3*A*) (Röhlich and Knoop, 1961; Shanthaveerappa et al., 1963; Thomas, 1963a). They are bounded on both sides by basal lamina (basement membrane), although this may be deficient over short lengths. The basal lamina is sometimes of substantial thickness, particularly in human nerves, where it may reach a width of as much as 0.5 μm (Gamble and Eames, 1964). The cytoplasm, except in the perinuclear region, is not voluminous, the total width of the cytoplasm sometimes being reduced to 10 nm. Endoplasmic reticulum and mitochondria are chiefly concentrated near

the nucleus, and glycogen particles are often numerous. A prominent feature is the occurrence of multiple pinocytotic vesicles shown in Figure 9–3*B*, with caveolae opening on both internal and external aspects of the cell (Gamble and Eames, 1964; Waggener et al., 1965; Cravioto, 1966).

Ross and Reith (1969) drew attention to the presence of bundles of closely aggregated filaments, similar in appearance to the myofilaments of smooth muscle. Associated with the filaments are localized electron-opaque regions adjacent to the cell membrane which resemble the "attachment devices" of smooth muscle (Pease and Molinari, 1960); they had been interpreted as hemidesmosomes by Thomas and Jones (1967). These structural specializations led Ross and Reith to propose a contractile function for perineurial cells. They commented on their resemblance to the sheathlike contractile cells of the rat and mouse testis (Clermont, 1958; Ross, 1967). Direct verification of perineurial contractility has not yet been obtained.

Thomas (1963a) and Cravioto (1966) noted

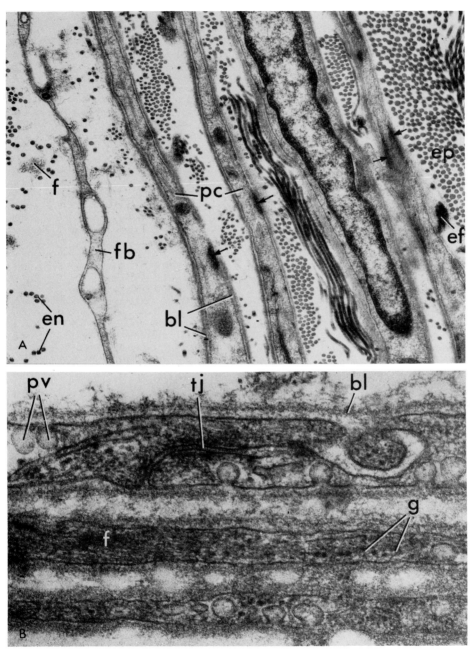

Figure 9–3 *A.* Transverse section through perineurium of sural nerve of rat. The flattened perineurial cells (pc) are bounded on either side by basal lamina (bl). Electron-dense regions (arrows) are visible in these cells, which may represent "attachment devices" for contractile filaments. ep, Epineurium; en, endoneurial collagen; ef, elastic fiber; f, endoneurial fibrils; fb, fibroblast process. Note difference in caliber between the collagen fibrils of the epineurium and those of the perineurium and endoneurium. × 21,000. *B.* Transverse section through perineurium of nerve of guinea pig. In the upper part of the figure, two overlapping perineurial cells are linked by a "tight junction" (tj). The cells contain multiple pinocytotic vesicles (pv), bundles of filaments (f), and groups of glycogen granules (g). They are surrounded on either side by a basal lamina (bl). × 60,000.

that contiguous perineurial cells either over-lapped or interdigitated with one another. Basal lamina is not interposed between their adjacent membranes. In places, contiguous cells are linked by "tight junctions," where the extracellular space is obliterated and the surface membranes are separated by a gap of 9 nm (see Fig. 9–3B) (Thomas and Jones, 1967). As is discussed later, the existence of such cell contacts can be related to the diffusion barrier property of the perineurium, and the presence of multiple endocytotic vesicles to a possible transport system across the cells. Histochemical studies by Shanthaveerappa and Bourne (1962) demonstrated that the perineurial cells possess a wide range of phosphorylating enzymes and have a high level of ATPase and creatine phosphatase activity. They are therefore equipped to act as a metabolically active diffusion barrier. These authors suggested the term "perineural epithelium" for the perineurial cells in the belief that they are of neural crest origin. Yet it is clear that they do not have the morphologic features of a true epithelium, and this term is therefore inappropriate.

The perineurial cell lamellae are separated by clefts, although the cells may branch and give rise to processes that cross the spaces and contribute to adjacent lamellae, and clefts occasionally become obliterated by fusion of the basal laminae of adjoining lamellae. The clefts contain collagen fibrils that are oriented in a lattice-like arrangement in which there are circular, longitudinal, and obliquely disposed bundles. The diameter of the collagen fibrils is substantially less than in the epineurium, averaging 52 nm in the rat sural nerve (Thomas, 1963a; Thomas and Jones, 1967). The same difference is apparent in human nerves, where a range of 40 to 65 nm was recorded (Gamble and Eames, 1964). The perineurial clefts also contain elastic fibers, often closely associated with the basal laminae, and very occasional cells not bounded by a basal lamina that are probably fibroblasts (Burkel, 1967; Thomas and Jones, 1967). Bundles of fibrous long spacing collagen may be present, particularly in the older subject.

A number of observers have claimed that there is a condensation of collagenous connective tissue surrounding the perineurial lamellae that should be designated the perineurium (Röhlich and Weiss, 1955; Clara and Özer, 1959), the cellular lamellae being referred to as "perilemma" by Röhlich and Weiss (1955), "neurothelium" by Lehman (1957), "perineural epithelium" by Shanthaveerappa and Bourne (1962), and "perineurothelium" by Cravioto (1966). It is difficult to detect any demarcation between the collagen immediately external to the outermost cellular lamella of the perineurium and the epineurium. Moreover, there is an abrupt change in the diameter of the collagen fibrils and in the staining properties of the collagen at the outermost perineurial lamella (Thomas and Jones, 1967; Denny-Brown, 1946). It therefore seems more satisfactory to categorize all the connective tissue external to the outermost lamella as epineurium.

Sunderland (1965) claimed that concentric lamellae of collagen fibrils in the perineurium are separated from one another by interlamellar clefts lined by mesothelial cells, the "perineurial spaces," which are possibly in communication centrally with the subdural and subarachnoid spaces. The innermost portion was believed to be made up of a smooth membrane composed of flattened mesothelial cells. This interpretation has not been borne out by the electron microscope studies: there is nothing to suggest "perineurial spaces" as such. The clefts between alternate lamellae are filled with collagen fibrils and other connective tissue elements.

The perineurium is traversed by blood vessels linking the longitudinal anastomotic network of arterioles and venules in the epineurium with the longitudinally oriented intrafascicular capillary network. The vessels carry in with them a perineurial "sleeve" for some distance (Thomas, 1963a; Burkel, 1967). These perineurial sleeves do not come into close opposition with the vascular walls, and the termination of the sleeves therefore provides a communication between the endoneurial and epineurial connective tissue spaces (Burkel, 1967).

When a fascicle is about to branch, this is anticipated by the formation of an intrafascicular perineurial partition. Compartmentation by perineurial lamellae has also been described within the nodose ganglion and may be related to a somatotopic organization of cells within the ganglion (Lieberman, 1968). A perineurial ensheathment follows the branches out to the periphery, where the smallest subdivisions may be surrounded by a single layer of perineurial cells (the sheath of Henle). It becomes continuous with the capsules of the muscle spindles and the encapsulated end organs (Shanthaveerappa and Bourne, 1963). At unencapsulated endings, and at the neuromuscular junction, the ensheathment terminates with an open end (Burkel, 1967). Saito and Zacks (1969) showed that at the neuromuscular junction, the perineurial cell processes form a bell-shaped covering that does not make direct contact with the fiber. A gap of 1 to 1.5 μm exists between the termination of the perineurial sheath and the basal lamina covering the muscle fiber. This therefore provides a point of communication between the endoneurial space and the exterior.

The perineurium of the dental nerves is also "open-ended" and its manner of termination is of considerable interest (Obst, 1971). As the nerves enter the tooth pulp, the perineurial cells first lose the basal lamina from their external aspects and subsequently from their internal surfaces. Finally, their close association with each other is lost, so that the nerve bundles become surrounded by cells that are indistinguishable from fibroblasts.

ENDONEURIUM

The endoneurium comprises the intrafascicular connective tissue. Reference to the original illustrations of Key and Retzius (1876) indicates that these authors used the term to describe intrafascicular perineurial partitions (see Fig. 9–1). The endoneurial collagen fibrils are of similar diameter to those of the perineurium, this also being true of human nerves (Thomas, 1963a; Thomas and Jones, 1967; Gamble and Eames, 1964). It is mainly oriented longitudinally and shows condensations around the nerve fibers and capillaries.

There are substantial intrafascicular spaces containing a finely granular or fibrillar material that is not readily resolvable in electron microscope preparations. In particular, a space regularly exists immediately internal to the perineurium, and there is also a tendency for the nerve fibers to be grouped into small bundles with intervening clefts.

The nature of the connective tissue ensheathment of the nerve fibers has been debated, part of the problem being related to confusion over terminology. By light microscopy, Young (1942) defined a thin sheath immediately external to the Schwann cell that

is inflected at the nodes of Ranvier. This referred to as the neurilemma, although the term has been used by other writers in different senses. It is probably equivalent to the sheath of Plenk and Laidlaw or inner endoneurial sheath (Plenk, 1927, 1934; Laidlaw, 1930). External to this is a layer of longitudinal collagen fibrils that is not inflected at the nodes, constituting the outer endoneurial sheath or sheath of Key and Retzius. The situation was analyzed by electron microscopy by Thomas (1963a). The myelinated nerve fibers are invested by a basal lamina that turns in at the nodes and is continuous across them, surrounding the Schwann cell nodal processes and the intervening "gap substance" (Landon and Williams, 1963). External to this, around the larger myelinated nerve fibers, is a narrow zone of collagen fibrils with a circular and oblique orientation. It is difficult to demonstrate in ultrathin sections, and is best seen in somewhat thicker sections. It is likely that the inner endoneurial sheath seen by light microscopy corresponds to these collagen fibrils together with the basal lamina. External to this are the longitudinal collagen fibrils of the outer endoneurial sheath. No separation into inner and outer endoneurial sheaths is visible around the smaller myelinated and unmyelinated fibers, the collagen fibrils there being less numerous and oriented longitudinally.

"Collagen pockets" are seen in relation to Schwann cells associated with unmyelinated axons (Gamble and Eames, 1964). They consist of small bundles of collagen fibrils that indent the cells or are surrounded by mesaxon-like arrangements (see Chapter 7). Gamble and Eames suggested that the Schwann cells actively envelop the collagen fibrils and believed that such collagen pockets could have a skeletal function. There are, however, indications that many are the consequence of the degeneration of unmyelinated axons, the site of the axon being replaced by collagen fibrils (Thomas, 1973). Collagen pockets are more numerous in chronic neuropathies.

Nageotte (1932) described fine elastic fibers within the endoneurium. By electron microscopy, no elastic fibers have been identified, but bundles of unbranched fibrils 10 to 12.5 nm in diameter are conspicuous in all species that have been examined including man (Thomas, 1963a; Gamble, 1964; Lieberman, 1968). These are similar in appearance to the fibrils related to elastic fibers, but are not associated with the amorphous component. They have an axial periodicity of approximately 17.5 nm (Lieberman, 1968).

The nature of the cellular content of the endoneurium has given rise to discussion. Light microscopists spoke about "endoneurial cells" that were presumably fibroblasts, and such cells were identified in the quantitative studies undertaken by Abercrombie and Johnson (1946a) and Thomas (1948). In an early electron microscope study, Causey and Barton (1959) claimed that there was an insignificant number of intrafascicular fibroblasts, this leading them to the conclusion that the endoneurial collagen was likely to be of Schwann cell origin. It was subsequently shown that appreciable numbers of endoneurial fibroblasts are present, although their precise proportion to other intrafascicular cells depends upon whether the subperineurial fibroblasts are also included and upon the fiber composition of the nerve (Thomas, 1963a). Nerves containing a large proportion of small myelinated fibers and many unmyelinated fibers will possess a relatively greater proportion of Schwann cells than nerves to muscle in which there are many large myelinated fibers and few unmyelinated fibers. The proportions of intrafascicular cells has been assessed in the human sural nerve by Ochoa and Mair (1969). Lieberman (1968) found that the free cells in the endoneurium of the nodose ganglion of the rat, rabbit, and guinea pig were almost all fibroblasts. These cells give rise to extremely elongated processes that ramify within the fascicle. Occasional cells with the cytologic features of macrophages are also seen in normal animals. Mast cells may be present, their numbers displaying considerable species variation, being numerous in the rat, but rare in the rabbit and guinea pig and uncommon in man (Torp, 1961; Olsson, 1968, 1971).

Renaut (1881) described structures, usually referred to as the corpuscles of Renaut, that are detectable in the endoneurium of normal human nerves and in various other species. They consist of elongated torpedo-shaped bodies and are usually observed immediately internal to the perineurium. They are composed of irregular concentric lamellae of fine filamentous material and contain occasional cells. Their manner of origin is uncertain. A more extensive description is to be found in Chapter 15.

Spinal Roots

The cellular elements of the endoneurium in the spinal roots resemble those of peripheral nerve. The quantity of collagen is substantially less and is not organized into sheaths around the nerve fibers (Gamble, 1964). The region of attachment of the spinal roots to the cord is characterized by an irregular but sharply defined transition from peripheral nerve to central nervous tissue, the Obersteiner-Redlich zone. The glial portion of the root may extend for a short distance outside the cord. Light microscope studies established that the nerve fibers pass through a double lamina cribrosa formed on the peripheral side by connective tissue and on the central side by a dense layer of glial fibers (Tarlov, 1937). At this point, Schwann cells are replaced by oligodendrocytes. Electron microscopy has established the details of this transitional zone (Maxwell et al., 1969; Steer, 1971). The Schwann cells give place abruptly to oligodendrocytes at nodes of Ranvier without the occurrence of transitional cells, as Tarlov had claimed. The central portion of the root is limited at its periphery by marginal glia, composed of astrocytes rather than oligodendroglia, as believed by Tarlov, which is covered by a basal lamina. The basal lamina becomes reflected to ensheath the nerve fibers in the peripheral portion of the root and to surround the outer limits of the endoneurium. Collagen fibrils are restricted to the peripheral side of the junctional zone.

The nature of the ensheathment of the spinal roots and the details of the transition between the meninges and the coverings of the peripheral nerves have been recurrent topics of morphologic speculation. Although the subject has not yet been fully clarified, recent electron microscope studies, in particular by Andres (1967), Waggener and Beggs (1967), McCabe and Low (1969), Haller and Low (1971) and Himango and Low (1971), have gone a long way toward establishing the structural arrangements that exist. The spinal roots traverse the subarachnoid space covered by a multicellular root sheath and penetrate the dura at the subarachnoid angle (Fig. 9–4). External to the subarachnoid angle, the nerve roots possess epineurium, perineurium, and endoneurium as in the peripheral nerve trunks. The epineurium becomes continuous with the dura and the endoneurium persists

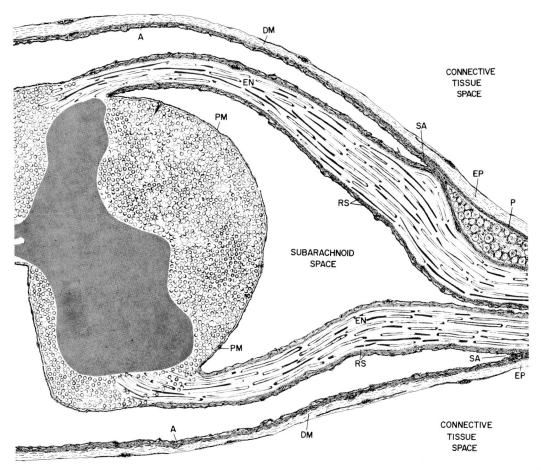

Figure 9–4 Diagram illustrating relationships of the peripheral nerve sheaths to the meningeal ensheathment of the spinal cord. The epineurium (EP) is in continuity with the dura mater (DM). The endoneurium (EN) persists from the peripheral nerves through the spinal roots to their junction with the spinal cord. At the subarachnoid angle (SA) the greater portion of the perineurium (P) passes between the dura and the arachnoid (A), but a few layers appear to continue over the roots as the inner layer of the root sheath (RS). The arachnoid is reflected over the roots at the subarachnoid angle and becomes continuous with the outer layers of the root sheath. At the junction with the spinal cord, the outer layers become continuous with the pia mater (PM). (From Haller, F. R., and Low, F. N.: The fine structure of the peripheral nerve root sheath in the subarachnoid space in the rat and other laboratory animals. Am. J. Anat., *131*:1, 1971. Reprinted by permission.)

without interruption as far as the junction of the roots with central nervous tissue. It is the fate of the perineurium that has given rise to the greatest difficulty, but it is evident that the outer layers of the perineurium separate from the nerve and pass between the dura and the arachnoid to form the "dural mesothelium" (Pease and Schultz, 1958); the inner layers merge with the root sheath.

Haller and Low (1971) demonstrated that the root sheath is composed of cellular and fibrous lamellae that can be divided into two layers. The outer consists of loosely associated cells with substantial intervening spaces that

are in continuity with the subarachnoid space and contain extracellular connective tissue components. It resembles the lining of the subarachnoid space elsewhere, that is, the pia and arachnoid, and the coverings of the arachnoid trabeculae and vascular adventitia. Where the roots become attached to the cord, the cells of the outer layer of the root sheath become continuous with the pia. At the subarachnoid angle, the outer layer probably becomes reflected to join the pia or is attached to it by punctate cell junctions (McCabe and Low, 1969). The inner layer consists of much more flattened cells that are closely associated with each other and are intermittently invested with a basal lamina. They contain multiple pinocytotic vesicles and more nearly resemble the perineurium, but are not readily classifiable as perineurial cells. It is this layer of the root sheath that becomes continuous with the perineurium peripherally. It overlies a basal lamina that encloses the endoneurium of the root and terminates at or lateral to the junction of the nerve root with the cord (Gamble, 1972). The perineurium is therefore also "open-ended" at this site.

Himango and Low (1971) drew attention to the structural arrangements at the junction of the dorsal and ventral roots. They observed that the subarachnoid space opens into a "lateral recess" that extends between the dorsal and ventral roots and that may constitute a communication between the subarachnoid and endoneurial spaces. It has long been suspected that such a communication exists, but no convincing demonstration of its location has been produced.

Ontogenesis

The embryologic origin of the coverings of peripheral nerves remains in question. It is accepted that the epineurium is of mesodermal origin. Masson (1942), from observations on the human fetus, concluded that the perineurium and the endoneurium, along with the Schwann cells, are derived from the neural crest, but there is no experimental verification of this suggestion in any species. Shanthaveerappa and Bourne (1962) argued that the perineurium is of ectodermal origin since it was supposed that it is continuous with the leptomeninges, which are themselves possibly of neural crest origin. In amphibia, there is good evidence that the meninges are mainly derived from the neural crest (Hörstadius, 1950). However, the observations of Haller and Low (1971) on the nerve root sheath indicate that the perineurium is not continuous with the pia-arachnoid, and the basis for this argument is therefore removed.

Electron microscope observations made on the human fetus by Gamble and Breathnach (1965) demonstrated that the perineurium is derived from cells having the morphologic features of fibroblasts, and the same is true during regeneration across gaps in nerves (Thomas and Jones, 1967). Moreover, the peritubular cells of the testis, which closely resemble perineurial cells, also appear to arise during development by the transformation of fibroblasts (Ross, 1967). Yet the cellular lamellae of the mature perineurium cannot be considered as "connective tissue" (see Ross and Reith, 1969). Low (1961) introduced the concept that the basal laminae or "boundary membranes" of cells defined the limits of the connective tissue space. This space contains formed elements such as connective tissue fibers and free cells including fibroblasts, mast cells, and histiocytes, all of which lack basal laminae. Thomas (1963a) applied this concept to peripheral nerve, in which the Schwann cells, capillary endothelial cells and pericytes, and perineurial cells all possess basal laminae and are thus outside the connective tissue space. The concept was applied by Fredrickson and Haller (1970) to the subarachnoid space, which they envisage as a "cleared out" connective tissue space. The cells of the outer layer of the root sheath, which forms part of the lining of this space, do not possess basal laminae, and the intercellular spaces between them, which connect with the subarachnoid space, contain fibrous connective tissue elements. The cells of the inner layer are partly ensheathed by basal laminae and rest on a basal lamina that surrounds the endoneurial connective tissue space of the root.

Nervi Nervorum

The occurrence of pain and tenderness related to nerve trauma, such as with compressive lesions of the ulnar nerve at the elbow, or pain in acute lesions of the cranial nerves of presumed vascular origin in diabetic subjects (see Chapter 47), attests to the local innervation of the connective tissues of nerve trunks. This is a field that has received little systematic attention. Hromada (1963) reviewed the somewhat meager literature and made observations on nerve trunks, spinal roots, and spinal and sympathetic ganglia of human fetuses and various laboratory animals. In addition to vasomotor innervation by way of perivascular plexuses, free endings are present in the epineurium, perineurium, and endoneurium, and encapsulated endings in the epineurium, derived from fibers in the nerve trunk (Fig. 9–5).

Bacsich (1969) has commented upon the occurrence of Timofeew's corpuscles, which

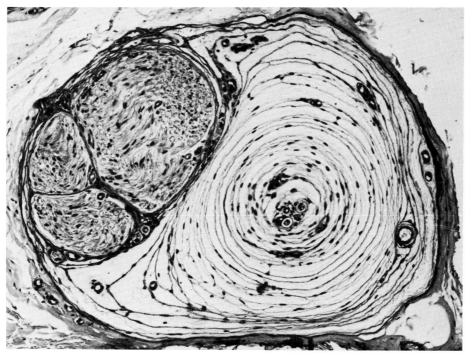

Figure 9–5 Transverse section through pacinian corpuscle within perineurium of a fascicle in human sural nerve. Periodic acid-Schiff stain. × 140.

are an encapsulated sensory organ similar to the pacinian corpuscle but smaller in size, in close relationship to the pelvic autonomic nerves and ganglia. Curiously, these sensory corpuscles have an ephemeral existence restricted to late fetal and early postnatal life.

FUNCTIONAL ASPECTS

Mechanical Properties

Peripheral nerve trunks, in common with other biologic tissues, possess viscoelastic properties, the elasticity predominantly residing in the epineurial connective tissues (Haftek, 1970). They possess considerable tensile strength: the human medial popliteal nerve will withstand longitudinal loads of up to 33 kg and the median nerve up to 22 kg (Sunderland and Bradley, 1961a). The tensile strength of nerve roots is substantially less, being of the order of 2 to 3 kg (Sunderland and Bradley, 1961b); this can be related to their lesser collagen content.

Under normal circumstances, the nerve fibers pursue a zigzag course within the fascicles. When the nerve is elongated, the fibers become straightened and, in a multi-fascicular nerve, the branching fascicular plexuses become taut. If a nerve in a slack condition is examined macroscopically, particularly with oblique incident illumination, the fasciculi show a light and dark banding in an apparently spiral arrangement. These "spiral bands of Fontana" disappear when the nerve is in an elongated state. The bands were attributed by Sunderland (1968) to undulations in the fascicles, but they have recently been shown by Clarke and Bearn (1972) to be an optical effect related to the zigzag course of the nerve fibers within the fascicles, as had been the initial interpretation placed on this phenomenon by Fontana (1781). After limited elongation of this degree the nerve, by its elastic properties, is able to return to its former length. Whether the contractile properties of the perineurium postulated by Ross and Reith (1969) play any part in these adjustments has yet to be established. Estimates of the degree of elongation possible before damage results have varied considerably. This probably partly depends upon whether the author has included the initial lengthening related to straightening of the fibers and fascicles.

The contents of the fascicles, which are bounded by the impervious perineurial cellular layer, are under pressure, bulging out if the perineurium is slit (Shanes, 1953). The collagen of the perineurium forms a lattice of longitudinal, circular, and oblique bundles (Thomas, 1963a). It is possible that this arrangement protects against kinking of the nerve when it is bent.

Sunderland (1945) investigated the distribution of fat in human nerves and commented upon its predominance in the sciatic nerve in the buttock and thigh. He suggested that it had a protective function in cushioning the fascicles against damage by compression. When generalized wasting occurs, the epineurial fat appears to behave in the same way as the general fatty tissue elsewhere in the body, and its loss may be one of the factors predisposing to the occurrence of pressure palsies in wasted, bedridden patients. The susceptibility to compression injury is likely to be less in multifascicular nerves with considerable quantities of epineurium than in unifascicular nerves (Sunderland, 1968).

Connective Tissues in Nerve Injury

STRETCH INJURY

Analyses of the events that occur when a nerve is stretched beyond physiologic limits have not yielded consistent descriptions. Sunderland and Bradley (1961a) reviewed the previous literature and recorded observations of their own. The subject has recently been reinvestigated by Haftek (1970).

The results obtained by Haftek for gradual straightening of the tibial nerve of the rabbit are shown in Figure 9–6. The initial portion of the graph, A to B, represents elongation of the epineurium and the straightening of the nerve fibers and fascicles. The second portion, B to C, is a straight line. Here there is a linear relationship between load and extension in which the nerve behaves as an elastic material and obeys Hooke's law. Beyond the elastic limit, C, extension is no longer proportional to load and the nerve does not return to its original length when the load is removed. Following this, further elongation continues (D to E) with a steadily increasing load in which the nerve behaves as a viscous material until complete rupture occurs at E. Haftek found that the first structure to rupture is the epineurium; this occurs when the elastic limit of the nerve is reached. Up to this stage, the caliber of the fascicles diminishes, with obliteration of the endoneurial spaces together with axonal narrowing and myelin disruption. During the lengthening after the elastic limit of the nerve has been reached, the next event is rupture of the perineurial sheaths, followed, after further elongation, by interruption of nerve fibers within the fascicles and finally by complete severance of the nerve. The endoneurial sheaths never become divided before the perineurium or the peri-

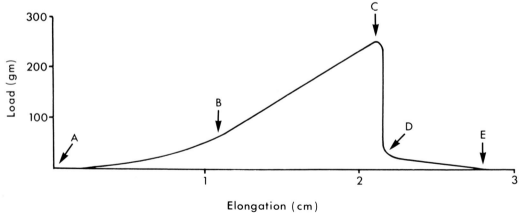

Elongation (cm)

Figure 9–6 Relationship between load and elongation during gradual stretching of the rabbit tibial nerve to the point of complete rupture. Between A and B the fascicles and nerve fibers are straightened and the epineurium is extended. Between B and C, the nerve is progressively stretched; the relationship between load and elongation is linear and the nerve behaves as an elastic material. At C, the limit of elasticity is reached and the load decreases abruptly. Between D and E there is further elongation with a steadily decreasing load until at E complete rupture of the nerve takes place. (From Haftek, J.: Stretch injury of peripheral nerve. Acute effects of stretching on rabbit peripheral nerve. J. Bone Joint Surg., 52B:354, 1970. Reprinted by permission.)

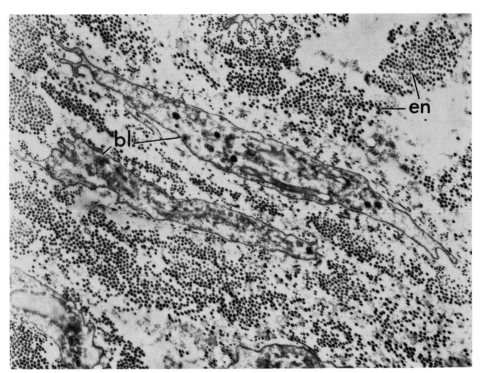

Figure 9–7 Transverse section through rat sural nerve two hours after a localized crush injury. The crushed nerve fibers are represented by flattened basal laminal tubes (bl) containing cellular debris. en, Endoneurial collagen. × 13,000.

neurium before the epineurium. The longitudinal extent of damage is considerable and is not confined to a single localized region, being observed over a length of 3 to 5 cm. The alterations in the nerve fibers resulting from elongation and compression within the narrowed perineurial sleeves are seen throughout the nerve. Haftek found that the pattern of damage is essentially the same for gradual and sudden stretching.

CRUSH INJURY

The effects of compression on nerve fibers induced by a pneumatic cuff are described in Chapter 34. Here the disruption caused by more severe compressive injuries that interrupt axonal continuity is considered.

Experimental procedures designed to interrupt axonal continuity without tearing the connective tissue components of the nerves have usually involved the use of smooth-tipped forceps or constricting ligatures. Early experiments employing light microscopy by Calugareanu (1901) and later amplified by Causey and Palmer (1952) demonstrated that mixed axoplasm and myelin is displaced to either side of the compressed region where it distends the endoneurial connective tissue sheaths but remains within them. Once the compression is released, the displaced material rapidly flows back into the compressed region. These events indicate that the endoneurial sheaths possess a high degree of elasticity (Lubińska, 1952).

Employing electron microscopy, Haftek and Thomas (1968) analyzed the changes produced by compression of rat nerves by smooth-tipped forceps. They showed that in the region of the compression, the basal laminal tubes that ensheath the nerve fibers persist (Fig. 9–7). The displaced axoplasm, myelin, and Schwann cell cytoplasm produce substantial distention of the basal laminal tubes to either side of the compressed region, but the displaced material usually remains within these tubes, confirming Lubińska's light microscope observations. Immediately adjacent to the compressed region, where extreme distention of the tubes is evident, confluence between adjacent tubes sometimes takes place by rupture of adjoining portions of basal lamina. The displaced material then flows back into the tubes in the crushed region.

It is known that functional recovery after

localized crush injuries of this type is much superior to recovery after nerve transection. Light microscopy showed that this is attributable to the persistence of the endoneurial connective tissue sheaths in the crushed region (Young, 1949). The regenerating axons cross the injured region within their own sheaths and thus return to their former terminations at the periphery. The electron microscope studies of Haftek and Thomas (1968) demonstrated that the regenerating axons and their accompanying Schwann cells traverse the injured region within the persisting basal laminal tubes, and it is therefore these that maintain the continuity required for the guidance of the axons to their previous peripheral connections.

NERVE TRANSECTION

When a nerve is sectioned, the ends rapidly draw apart. Ross and Reith (1969) attributed this to active perineurial contractility, and certainly this retraction can be shown to reside in the epineurium or perineurium and not within the nerve fascicles (Jacobovits and Thomas, 1972). Outgrowths occur from both cut ends. That from the distal stump takes place more rapidly and constitutes an important part of the process by which the gap is bridged. This outgrowth was considered by Nageotte (1932) and Masson (1932) to be composed of Schwann cells and their view was supported by later workers (Young et al., 1940; Rexed, 1942), although Holmes and Young (1942) found that at times a large outgrowth is found to be composed almost entirely of fibrous connective tissue. A different view was taken by Denny-Brown (1946), who considered that the cells that emerge from the distal stump are a specialized type of fibroblast that grows out from the endoneurium and perineurium. He believed that Schwann cells only appear in the outgrowth when it becomes invaded by axons and considered that they accompany the regenerating axons as they emerge from the proximal stump of the nerve. Since differentiation between Schwann cells and fibroblasts is difficult by light microscopy, the situation was examined by electron microscopy by Thomas (1966). He confirmed, in experiments on transected rat and rabbit nerves, that anastomosing columns of Schwann cells extend out from the Büngner bands in the distal stump and that these are embedded in a connective tissue framework, probably mainly of endoneurial and perineurial origin.

When regeneration across the gap in the nerve takes place, groups of regenerating axons and associated Schwann cells become surrounded by perineurial cells so that the junctional region comes to consist of numerous small fascicles (Masson, 1932; Nageotte, 1932). The origin of these perineurial cells was investigated by electron microscopy by Thomas and Jones (1967). They observed that the bundles of regenerating nerve fibers become surrounded by cells having the morphologic features of fibroblasts, which later assume the appearance of perineurial cells, including the acquisition of a basal laminal ensheathment.

CHANGES DURING NERVE DEGENERATION

During wallerian degeneration, the basal laminal tubes ensheathing the myelinated nerve fibers persist, either expanding around the myelin ovoids, some of which are of greater diameter than the normal fibers, or collapsing between the ovoids to form crenations. With removal of the degenerating axon and myelin, the accompanying Schwann cell proliferation takes place within the confines of these tubes leading to longitudinally continuous columns of cells, the bands of Büngner (Nathaniel and Pease, 1963a; Thomas, 1963b, 1964a). Light microscope studies clearly showed that the endoneurial connective tissue sheaths remain as definable structures throughout wallerian degeneration (Holmes and Young, 1942). After expanding during the initial stages of degeneration, the endoneurial tubes progressively diminish in size if they remain denervated, this taking place mainly during the initial three months after injury. The magnitude of the reduction is considerable and amounts to an 80 to 90 per cent diminution in size of the endoneurial tubes of the largest myelinated nerve fibers, this being associated with a reduction in the cross sectional area of the fascicles (Sunderland and Bradley, 1950a, 1950b).

It is known that the quantity of endoneurial and perineurial collagen in denervated peripheral stumps doubles by 200 days after nerve transection (Abercrombie and Johnson, 1946b). This appears to be a process initiated by wallerian degeneration and is unaffected by reinnervation (Abercrombie and Johnson, 1947).

In ultrathin sections, the endoneurial collagenous sheaths are less impressive structures than when seen by light microscopy, but Thomas (1963b, 1964a) was able to show that additional collagen fibrils with a longitudinal orientation are laid down within the inner endoneurial sheath and immediately external to the basal laminal tubes that had ensheathed the intact nerve fibers. Despite the endoneurial tube shrinkage and collagenization, denervated distal stumps are able to accept regenerating axons for very long periods, certainly for several years after injury, although maturation of the fibers may be reduced (Young, 1949).

The mechanical properties of degenerated peripheral nerve trunks were investigated by Sunderland and Bradley (1961c). They showed that the denervated distal stump of forelimb nerves of the cat had similar elastic properties and was able to carry the same load as the normal proximal stump. The experiment was, however, performed at three weeks after operation, and the effect of later changes in the connective tissues in denervated nerve is not known.

The source of the intrafascicular collagen in peripheral nerve has given rise to some discussion. In quantitative studies by light microscopy, Thomas (1948) found an appreciable increase in the numbers of cells identified as fibroblasts in degenerating nerve. Although not yet assessed quantitatively at the ultrastructural level, where the identification of cells is more certain, fibroblasts are often encountered in electron microscope preparations of degenerating nerve and appear to be increased in number (Thomas, 1964a). Yet there have been claims that Schwann cells are responsible for collagen production (Masson, 1932; Causey and Barton, 1959; Nathaniel and Pease, 1963b). Attempts to confirm this by isotopically labeling collagen precursors have not so far yielded convincing results. It is possible, however, that Schwann cells may be partly responsible for determining the site of deposition of the collagen fibrils (Thomas, 1964b).

The appearances in the perineurium during wallerian degeneration were examined by Shanthaveerappa and Bourne (1964). In transected rat and cat nerves, excluding the immediate site of injury, the perineurium in the proximal and distal stumps showed no histologic or structural changes when examined by light microscopy. There is also little change in the epineurium (Sunderland, 1968).

Perineurium as a Perifascicular Diffusion Barrier

As has already been emphasized, an important property of the perineurium is its capacity to act as a perifascicular diffusion barrier. This has been demonstrated for numerous substances (see reviews by Martin, 1964; Shantha and Bourne, 1968; Olsson et al., 1971). It implies that such substances, if present in the extracellular spaces around the nerves, are unable to diffuse into the endoneurium of the fascicles or do so only at a greatly reduced speed. The perineurium is therefore involved in the homeostasis of the nerve by being able to regulate the composition of the endoneurial fluid. This function is performed not only by the perineurium, but also by the endoneurial blood vessels which are equipped with specialized permeability properties (see Chapter 10).

THE PERINEURIAL DIFFUSION BARRIER UNDER NORMAL CONDITIONS

The existence of a perifascicular diffusion barrier in peripheral nerves can be demonstrated by both morphologic and neurophysiologic methods. In the typical morphologic experiment, a substance is injected around a nerve. After an appropriate delay and fixation of the tissue, the distribution of the substance in the nerve is determined by microscopic methods. Neurophysiologically, a diffusion barrier can be shown in the following way. An agent with the capacity to reduce either the action potentials or the resting potential is applied to the surface of a nerve. By comparing the time required to block these potentials in normal and in desheathed nerves, a conclusion can be drawn about the barrier function of the nerve sheaths (Martin, 1964). Obviously this type of experiment is restricted to the demonstration of certain slowly diffusible substances for which the nerve sheaths reduce but do not totally abolish their diffusion into the endoneurium.

A perifascicular diffusion barrier has been shown to exist in normal large peripheral nerves of various animals for many but not all substances. Martin (1964), in reviewing the literature, listed previously tested substances with regard to their ability to pass into the endoneurium from the surface of a peripheral nerve trunk. For one group of agents, the nerve sheaths act as a complete diffusion barrier, so that the substances cannot be demonstrated in the endoneurium of the fascicles but only in the perifascicular tissue. This group of substances comprises various dyes such as lithium carmine (Weiss and Röhlich, 1954), trypan blue (Emiroglu, 1955; Clara and Özer, 1960), Evans blue (Olsson and Reese, 1971), Congo red (Emiroglu, 1955), methyl blue and methylene blue (Martin, 1964). In addition, India ink behaves in the same way (Weiss and Röhlich, 1954; Kristensson and Olsson, 1971), as do several protein tracers, i.e., ferritin (Waggener et al., 1965), fluorochrome labeled serum proteins (Olsson, 1966; Olsson and Reese, 1971; Kristensson and Olsson, 1971) and horseradish peroxidase (Olsson and Reese, 1969, 1971; Klemm, 1970; Kristensson and Olsson, 1971).

For another group of substances, diffusion through the nerve sheath is only partially restricted. These substances can therefore reach the endoneurium after a certain delay. According to Martin (1964), the molecular weight of such substances is lower than that of those in the first group. This class of agents includes several ionic species such as potassium, barium and calcium chloride, choline chloride, glucose, and many other substances (Feng and Liu, 1949; Crescitelli, 1951; Crescitelli and Geissman, 1951; Krnjević, 1954a). Finally, a group of substances with low molecular weight can diffuse into the endoneurium without any significant restriction (oxygen, carbon dioxide, ethanol) (Huxley and Stämpfli, 1951; Krnjević, 1954a).

There is thus a perifascicular diffusion barrier in normal adult nerves to numerous substances of widely differing chemical composition and molecular weight. In the past, the morphologic identity of this barrier has been extensively discussed. Some of the earliest studies, for instance that of Feng and Gerard (1930), did not attempt to localize the barrier function more specifically, but related it to the peripheral nerve connective tissue sheaths in general (epineurium and perineurium). Other investigators using neurophysiologic or light microscopic methods came to the conclusion that the perineurium or the epineurium alone exerted the barrier function of the nerve sheaths (Krnjević,

1954b; Martin, 1964; Crescitelli, 1951; Causey and Palmer, 1953). The site of the barrier can now be elucidated with much greater accuracy since several "permeability tracers" are available that can be localized by fluorescence or electron microscopy such as fluorochrome-labeled serum proteins, ferritin, and horseradish peroxidase (Steinwall and Klatzo, 1966; Kerr and Muir, 1960; Waggener et al., 1965; Graham and Karnovsky, 1966). If such methods are applied, information can be obtained regarding the site and mechanism of the perifascicular diffusion barrier to macromolecular protein tracers, but it should be remembered that the chemical differences between the substances, which range from inorganic ions to macromolecules, are so great that it is unlikely that their passage into the endoneurium is impeded by exactly the same mechanisms.

Fluorochrome-labeled albumin that has been injected around the sciatic nerves of mice, rats, and rabbits spreads easily in the epineurium, but even after long application times no albumin can be observed in the endoneurium of the nerve fascicles (Olsson and Reese, 1971; Kristensson and Olsson, 1971). Usually a bright fluorescent zone indicating a high concentration of albumin can be seen in the perineurium, which is distinctly delineated from the nonfluorescent endoneurium (Fig. 9–8A). This type of experiment shows that the epineurium is not the site of the barrier and that the perifascicular diffusion barrier to albumin is located in the perineurium. The limitation in resolving power of the fluorescence microscopic technique makes it impossible to relate the barrier function to any particular cell layers within this structure. The application of horseradish peroxidase as a permeability tracer has added more detailed information on the site and mechanism of the perifascicular diffusion barrier, since this protein can be localized both by light and electron microscopy (Graham and Karnovsky, 1966). By light microscopy, peroxidase can be seen to fill the spaces between the outermost perineurial cell layers in both mouse and rat sciatic nerves (Fig. 9–9A) (Olsson and Reese, 1969, 1971; Klemm, 1970). In the mouse nerve, there is only one of a limited number of concentric layers of perineurial cells that completely surrounds the fascicles; the other layers show occasional gaps between perineurial cells. Peroxidase stops abruptly at the level of the outermost complete concentric layer although

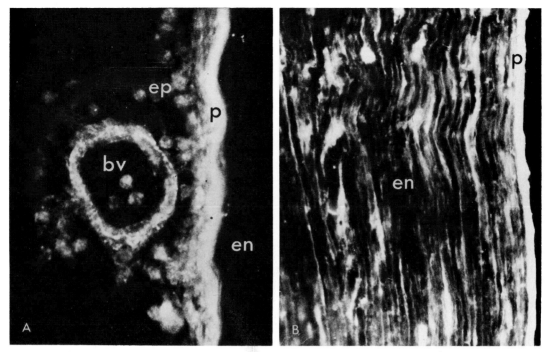

Figure 9–8 *A.* Normal adult mouse sciatic nerve. The fluorescent tracer Evans blue–labeled albumin (white areas) was injected around the nerve. The tracer has spread extensively in the epineurium (ep), but is efficiently prevented from diffusing into the endoneurium (en) by the perineurium (p). bv, Blood vessel. *B.* Same experiment, but with a seven day old mouse. The tracer has now passed through the perineurium (p) and has diffused widely into the endoneurium (en). The same pattern of endoneurial penetration is also observed in various pathologic conditions including trauma and long-lasting ischemia.

a small amount reaches the next layer (Olsson and Reese, 1971).

The relationship between the peroxidase tracer and the perineurial cell surfaces appears to be the same in sciatic nerves of both the mouse and the rat (Olsson and Reese, 1971; Klemm, 1970). In both species the tracer passes into the covering basal lamina and is seen in numerous pits and vesicles of the perineurial cells. To what extent pinocytosis of peroxidase actually occurs is open to question because lanthanum injected after fixation also fills many of the vesicles and invaginations (Olsson and Reese, 1971). As in the cerebral vascular endothelium, the basis of the impermeability to peroxidase appears to be a lack of significant transport of the tracer by pinocytosis across the perineurial cell cytoplasm (Reese and Karnovsky, 1967). Furthermore, intercellular diffusion between adjacent cells of the complete layers of perineurium is totally restricted by the tight junctions connecting these cells (Olsson and Reese, 1969, 1971; Klemm, 1970). Basically similar findings have also been made in the rat sciatic nerve by Waggener et al., (1965) employing ferritin as an electron microscopic

marker, and it therefore seems justified to assume that the location of the barrier is in the same perineurial cell layers for other protein tracers such as fluorochrome-labeled albumin.

The vast majority of studies on the structure and permeability of the perineurium has been performed on large nerves of adult animals. The permeability of the perineurium of immature individuals is only incompletely known. Recently a study was made on the perineurial permeability to fluorochrome-labeled albumin and to peroxidase in newborn mice, rats, and guinea pigs (Kristensson and Olsson, 1971). In young mice and rats, the perineurium did not act as a diffusion barrier; the protein tracers easily passed into the endoneurium of the sciatic nerves, apparently by diffusion between adjacent perineurial cells, which in the immature animals are not everywhere closed by extensive tight junctions (Figs. 9–8B and 9–9B) (Gamble and Breathnach, 1965). The permeability gained its mature character in these species around three weeks postnatally. Guinea pigs, on the other hand, were equipped from birth with a perineurium of mature character, at least as far as permeability is concerned.

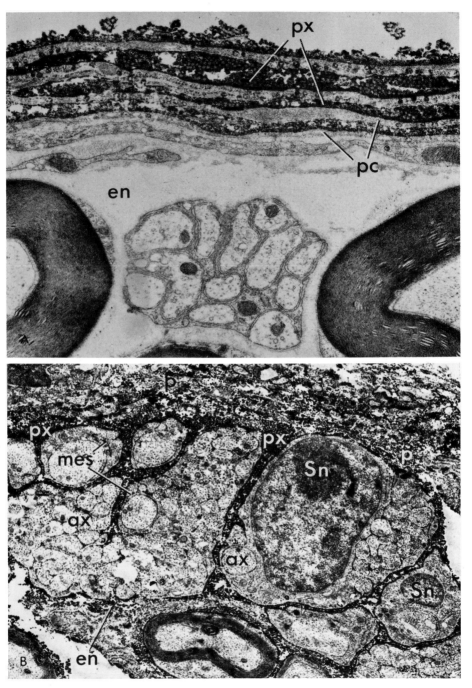

Figure 9–9   *A.* Normal adult sciatic nerve of mouse. Peroxidase (px), showing as dark areas between the perineurial cellular lamellae (pc), was injected around the nerve and its distribution studied by electron microscopy. The tracer is prevented from reaching the endoneurial spaces (en) by an inner perinurial cell layer. *B.* Same experiment, but with a seven day old mouse. Peroxidase (px) has passed into the endoneurium (en) where it fills spaces around the Schwann cells. Sn, Schwann cell nuclei. Note also penetration along mesaxons (mes) of unmyelinated fibers. ax, Axons.

The deficient barrier function of the perineurium in immature mice and rats may have implications for the development of some pathologic lesions of peripheral nerves occurring in young animals (Kristensson and Olsson, 1971). It can be anticipated that the penetration of toxic and infectious agents into the nerves of such animals will occur more readily than in adult animals. In fact, the mitotic inhibitors, colchicine and vinblastine, and the histamine liberator, compound 48/80, can induce toxic effects in newborn mice and rats that are not seen in adult animals (Kristensson et al., 1971; Hansson et al., 1971). A deficient barrier function of the perineurium may be one factor facilitating the transfer of certain viruses into the fascicles, from which site transport to the central nervous system may follow (Kristensson and Olsson, 1971).

There are still several parts of the peripheral nervous system such as peripheral ganglia and autonomic and cranial nerves that have not yet been analyzed with regard to the barrier function of the perineurium. A complete mapping of the perineurial permeability also appears to be a fruitful field of study since there is some reason to believe that the diffusion barrier is not equally efficient in all areas of the peripheral nervous system. For instance, the sheaths covering the spinal nerve roots are permeable from the subarachnoid space both for fluorochrome-labeled serum proteins and for ferritin (Klatzo et al., 1964; Waggener et al., 1965). The perineurial barrier at neuromuscular junctions also appears to be deficient since horseradish peroxidase injected intramuscularly can diffuse in and reach the terminal axons in this area (Zacks and Saito, 1969).

THE PERINEURIAL DIFFUSION BARRIER UNDER PATHOLOGIC CONDITIONS

To summarize the findings in normal nerves, large peripheral nerve trunks are equipped with perifascicular diffusion barriers that are probably engaged in the regulation of the internal milieu of the fascicles. The perineurium, by acting as a barrier to macromolecular substances, is likely to protect the nerve fibers from various disease promoting agents. Certain toxins, antigens, and viruses can be cited as examples of pathogenic macromolecules of this nature (Waggener et al., 1965). It therefore appears important to know whether pathologic condi-

tions are associated with permeability changes in the perineurium. Reduced perineurial permeability would facilitate the diffusion of such agents into the nerve parenchyma, and the composition of the endoneurial fluid would be influenced by the fluid compartments around the nerves. As a first step in the analysis of this question, a series of investigations was undertaken to study the effect of various pathologic conditions on the barrier function of the perineurium to protein tracers (Kristensson and Olsson, 1971; Söderfeldt, 1972; Olsson and Kristensson, 1973; Lundborg et al., 1973). Direct injury to a peripheral nerve readily increases the perineurial permeability. For instance, crushing mouse sciatic nerves with a jeweler's forceps induces an abnormal permeability at the site of the lesion (Olsson and Kristensson, 1973). The increased perineurial permeability has an early onset and a duration of several weeks. Protein tracers such as fluorescent albumin and peroxidase can then diffuse into the endoneurium at the site of the lesion and spread in endoneurial spaces along the nerve. On the other hand, the permeability of the perineurium distal to the immediate lesion, where the nerve is undergoing wallerian degeneration, appears to be unchanged (Olsson and Kristensson, 1973).

The permeability of the perineurium to protein tracers therefore seems to be rapidly influenced by trauma, but the vulnerability of this function is quite different with regard to ischemic injury. Protein tracers injected around peripheral nerves of mice and rabbits even 24 hours after complete ischemia do not penetrate the perineurium (Kristensson and Olsson, 1971; Lundborg et al., 1972). This phenomenon makes it possible to use fresh autopsy material for studies on the permeability of the human perineurium (Söderfeldt et al., 1973).

The permeability of the perineurium to proteins also appears to be remarkably resistant to certain mediators of the inflammatory response (Söderfeldt, 1972). Even though histamine has no appreciable effect on the perineurial permeability in otherwise normal nerves some change in this function may occur in experimental allergic neuritis (Allt, 1972). In an electron microscopic study, he observed extravasated serum protein both in the endoneurial spaces and between the perineurial cell layers and proposed the possibility of a macropinocytotic transport of proteins from the endoneurium across the perineurial cells. If confirmed, such a mechanism would be of great importance, since the perineurium could then be actively involved in the restoration of the composition of the endoneurial fluid, for instance in edematous conditions of peripheral nerves. A further striking observation is that the perineurium may be seen to provide a barrier to the entry of pus cells into the fascicles (Denny-Brown, 1946). A nerve that is related to an abscess may be surrounded by large numbers of pus cells, and yet these often do not penetrate the perineurium.

There is thus some information on the permeability of the perineurium to macromolecular substances in certain pathologic conditions of adult peripheral nerves, but much remains to be investigated. For example, a pathologic process influencing a nerve during maturation may interfere with the structural organization of the perineurium at a time when the tight junctions are formed. In fact, it has recently been shown in the rat that severe protein malnutrition during such a period causes a long-lasting deficiency in the barrier function of the perineurium (Sima, 1972). A reasonable explanation for this phenomenon is that the malnutrition in some way interferes with the formation of cellular contacts in the perineurium, allowing extracellular diffusion of protein tracers through the perineurium into the endoneurium.

Intrafascicular Diffusion Pathways

The interior of the peripheral nerve fascicles can therefore be regarded as a compartment isolated under normal conditions from its surroundings by the perineurium, which has the capacity to influence the composition of the endoneurial fluid. However, the actual composition of this fluid is currently unknown and its physiologic significance is therefore poorly understood. More is known about the movements of this fluid and its diffusion pathways inside the fascicles. Substances injected into the endoneurium readily spread in both directions along the nerve. On the basis of their experimental findings, Weiss et al. (1945) also proposed that there is normally a flow of endoneurial fluid directed distally. The initial edema occurring at the site of trauma to a nerve also spreads in this direction (Olsson, 1966; Mellick and Cavanagh, 1967a).

Chemical and, as discussed earlier, ultra-structural investigations, have shown that there is a substantial extracellular space inside peripheral nerve fascicles (Manery and Hastings, 1939; Krnjević, 1955; Mellick and Cavanagh, 1967b). Electron microscopy has also recently been used to outline possible diffusion pathways inside the fascicles by following the distribution of horseradish peroxidase that was introduced into the endoneurium (Klemm, 1970; Böck and Hanak, 1971; Olsson and Reese, 1971; Kristensson and Olsson, 1971). This protein spreads extensively in the intercellular spaces around the nerve fibers and in subperineurial spaces. Peroxidase is frequently found immediately outside the Schwann cells, infiltrating between the connective tissue fibers and invading the basal lamina of these cells. It also passes into the outer mesaxon of myelinated axons. In unmyelinated fibers, the mesaxon is filled and the peroxidase is also seen in cytoplasmic vesicles of several types of cells including Schwann cells, the innermost perineurial cells, and the pericytes of the vessel walls.

It has generally been assumed that axons of peripheral neurons show a slight uptake of exogenous proteins under normal conditions. It has, however, recently been demonstrated that fluorochrome-labeled albumin and peroxidase injected into a muscle in mice and rats normally accumulate in lysosomal organelles of the corresponding motor nerve cells in the spinal cord (gastrocnemius muscle) or the brain stem (tongue). This accumulation of foreign protein in the neurons is most probably the result of axonal uptake in the peripheral nerve branches (Zacks and Saito, 1969), followed by a retrograde axonal transport of the protein to the nerve cell perikaryon (Kristensson and Olsson, 1973). This interesting and not yet fully explored phenomenon deserves further investigation since it may be one route by which neurovirulent and toxic agents reach the central nervous system.

CONCLUSIONS

The observations brought together in this chapter make it clear that the tissues ensheathing the peripheral nerves and nerve roots are of considerable structural and functional complexity. The endoneurial connective tissues provide support for the nerve fibers and are of importance for the guidance of axons during regeneration. The tensile strength and elastic properties of nerve trunks appear largely to reside in the epineurium. The perineurium has been shown to act as a perifascicular diffusion barrier, and it has been postulated that this is related to a homeostatic effect on the endoneurial connective tissue fluid environment of the nerve fibers. The large content of micropinocytotic vesicles in the perineurial cells possibly indicates a transcellular transport system, but it remains to be discovered whether the transport is unidirectional or bidirectional, and what categories of substance are translocated. Finally, if it is established that the perineurium has contractile properties, it may be involved in adjustments of nerve length such as in the neighborhood of joints.

References

Abercrombie, M., and Johnson, M. L.: Quantitative histology of Wallerian degeneration. I. Nuclear population in rabbit sciatic nerve. J. Anat., *80*:37, 1946a.

Abercrombie, M., and Johnson, M. L.: Collagen content of rabbit sciatic nerve during Wallerian degeneration. J. Neurol. Neurosurg. Psychiatry, *9*:113, 1946b.

Abercrombie, M., and Johnson, M. L.: The effect of reinnervation on collagen formation in degenerating sciatic nerves of rabbits. J. Neurol. Neurosurg. Psychiatry, *10*:89, 1947.

Allt, G.: Involvement of the perineurium in experimental allergic neuritis: Electron microscopic observations. Acta Neuropathol., *20*:139, 1972.

Andres, K. H.: Über die Feinstruktur der Arachnoidea und Dura Mater von Mammalia. Z. Zellforsch. Mikrosk. Anat., *79*:272, 1967.

Bacsich, P.: On the presence of Timofeew's sensory corpuscles in the autonomic plexuses of the human prostate and seminal vesicles. J. Anat., *104*:182, 1969.

Böck, P., and Hanak, H.: Die Verteilung exogener Peroxydase im Endoneuralraum. Histochemie, *25*:361, 1971.

Burkel, W. E.: The histological fine structure of perineurium. Anat. Rec., *158*:177, 1967.

Calugareanu, D.: Recherches sur les modifications histologiques dans les nerfs comprimés. J. Physiol. Pathol. Gén., *3*:413, 1901.

Causey, G., and Barton, A. A.: The cellular content of the endoneurium of peripheral nerve. Brain, *82*:594, 1959.

Causey, G., and Palmer, E.: Early changes in degenerating mammalian nerves. Proc. R. Soc., B, *139*:597, 1952.

Causey, G., and Palmer, E.: The epineural sheath of a nerve as a barrier to the diffusion of phosphate ions. J. Anat., *87*:30, 1953.

Clara, M., and Özer, N.: Untersuchungen über die sogenannte Nervenscheide. Acta Neuroveg., *20*:1, 1960.

Clarke, E., and Bearn, J. G.: The spiral nerve bands of Fontana. Brain, *95*:1, 1972.

Clermont, Y.: Contractile elements in the limiting membrane of the seminiferous tubules. Exp. Cell Res., *15*:438, 1958.

Cravioto, H.: The perineurium as a diffusion barrier—ultrastructural correlates. Bull. Los Angeles Neurol. Soc., *31*:196, 1966.

Crescitelli, F.: Nerve sheath as a barrier to the action of certain substances. Am. J. Physiol., *166*:229, 1951.

Crescitelli, F., and Geissman, T. A.: Certain effects of antihistamines and related compounds on frog nerve fibers. Am. J. Physiol., *164*:509, 1951.

Denny-Brown, D.: Importance of neural fibroblasts in the regeneration of nerve. Arch. Neurol. Psychiatry, *55*:171, 1946.

Emiroglu, F.: The permeability of the peripheral nerve sheath in frogs. Arch. Int. Physiol. Biochim., *63*:161, 1955.

Feng, T. P., and Gerard, R. W.: Mechanism of nerve asphyxiation: with a note on the nerve sheath as a diffusion barrier. Proc. Soc. Exp. Biol. Med., *27*:1073, 1930.

Feng, T. P., and Liu, Y. M.: The connective tissue sheath of the nerve as effective diffusion barrier. J. Cell. Comp. Physiol., *34*:1, 1949.

Fontana, F.: Traité sur le vénin de la vipère sur les poisons américains. Florence, 1781 (cited by Clarke and Bearn, 1972).

Fredrickson, R. G., and Haller, F. R.: The subarachnoid space interpreted as a special portion of the connective tissue space. Proc. N. Dak. Acad. Sci., *24*:142, 1970.

Gamble, H. J.: Comparative electron-microscopic observations on the connective tissue of a peripheral nerve and a spinal nerve root in the rat. J. Anat., *98*:17, 1964.

Gamble, H. J.: Personal communication, 1972.

Gamble, H. J., and Breathnach, A. S.: An electron-microscope study of human foetal peripheral nerves. J. Anat., *99*:573, 1965.

Gamble, H. J., and Eames, R. A.: An electron microscope study of the connective tissues of human peripheral nerve. J. Anat., *98*:655, 1964.

Graham, R. C., and Karnovsky, M. J.: The early stages of absorption of injected horseradish peroxidase in the proximal tubules of mouse: ultrastructural cytochemistry by a new technique. J. Histochem. Cytochem., *14*:291, 1966.

Haftek, J.: Stretch injury of peripheral nerve. Acute effects of stretching on rabbit peripheral nerve. J. Bone Joint Surg., *52B*:354, 1970.

Haftek, J., and Thomas, P. K.: Electron-microscope observations on the effects of localized crush injuries on the connective tissues of peripheral nerve. J. Anat., *103*:233, 1968.

Haller, F. R., and Low, F. N.: The fine structure of the peripheral nerve root sheath in the subarachnoid space in the rat and other laboratory animals. Am. J. Anat., *131*:1, 1971.

Hansson, G., Kristensson, K., Olsson, Y., and Sjöstrand, J.: Embryonal and postnatal development of mast cells in rat peripheral nerve. Acta Neuropathol., *17*:139, 1971.

Himango, W. A., and Low, F. N.: The fine structure of a lateral recess of the subarachnoid space in the rat. Anat. Rec., *171*:1, 1971.

Holmes, W., and Young, J. Z.: Nerve regeneration after immediate and delayed suture. J. Anat., *77*:63, 1942.

Hörstadius, S.: The neural crest. London, Oxford University Press, 1950.

Hromada, J.: On the nerve supply of the connective tissue of some peripheral nervous system components. Acta Anat., *55*:343, 1963.

Huxley, A. F., and Stämpfli, R.: Effect of potassium and

sodium on resting and action potentials of single myelinated nerve fibers. J. Physiol. (Lond.), *112*:496, 1951.

Jacobovits, J., and Thomas, P. K.: Unpublished observations, 1972.

Kerr, D. N., and Muir, A. R.: A demonstration of the structure of disposition of ferritin in human liver cell. J. Ultrastruct. Res., *3*:313, 1960.

Key, A., and Retzius, G.: Studien in der Anatomie des Nervensystems und des Bindegewebes. Stockholm, Samson & Wallin, 1876.

Klatzo, I., Miguel, J., Ferris, P. J., Prokop, J. D., and Smith, D. E.: Observations on the passage of the fluorescein labelled serum proteins (FLSP) from the cerebro-spinal fluid. J. Neuropath. Exp. Neurol., *23*:18, 1964.

Klemm, H.: Das Perineurium als Diffusionsbarriere gegenüber Peroxydase bei epi- und endoneuraler Applikation. Z. Zellforsch. Mikrosk. Anat., *108*:431, 1970.

Kristensson, K., and Olsson, Y.: The perineurium as a diffusion barrier to protein tracers. Differences between mature and immature animals. Acta Neuropathol., *17*:127, 1971.

Kristensson, K., and Olsson, Y.: Diffusion pathways and retrograde axonal transport of protein tracers in peripheral nerves. Prog. Neurobiol., *1*:85, 1973.

Kristensson, K., Lycke, E., and Sjöstrand, J.: Spread of herpes simplex virus in peripheral nerves. Acta Neuropathol., *17*:44, 1971.

Krnjević, K.: Some observations on perfused frog sciatic nerves. J. Physiol. (Lond.), *123*:338, 1954a.

Krnjević, K.: The connective tissue of the frog sciatic nerve. Q. J. Exp. Physiol., *39*:55, 1954b.

Krnjević, K.: The distribution of Na and K in cat nerves. J. Physiol. (Lond.), *128*:473, 1955.

Laidlaw, G. F.: Silver staining of the endoneurial fibers of the cerebrospinal nerves. Am. J. Pathol., *6*:435, 1930.

Landon, D. N., and Williams, P. L.: Ultrastructure of the node of Ranvier. Nature (Lond.), *199*:575, 1963.

Lehman, H. J.: Über Struktur und Funktion der perineuralen Diffusionsbarriere. Z. Zellforsch. Mikrosk. Anat., *46*:232, 1957.

Lieberman, A. R.: The connective tissue elements of the mammalian nodose ganglion. An electron microscope study. Z. Zellforsch. Mikrosk. Anat., *89*:95, 1968.

Low, F. N.: The extra-cellular portion of the human blood-air barrier and its relation to tissue space. Anat. Rec., *139*:105, 1961.

Lubińska, L.: Elasticity and distensibility of nerve tubes. Acta Biol. Exp. (Warsz.), *16*:73, 1952.

Lundberg, G., Nordborg, C., Rydevik, B., and Olsson, Y.: The effect of ischemia on the permeability of the perineurium to protein tracers in rabbit tibial nerve. Acta Neurol. Scand., *49*:287, 1973.

Manery, J. F., and Hastings, A. B.: The distribution of electrolytes in mammalian tissues. J. Biol. Chem., *127*:657, 1939.

Martin, K. H.: Untersuchungen über die perineurale Diffusionsbarriere an gefriergetrockneten Nerven. Z. Zellforsch. Mikrosk. Anat., *64*:404, 1964.

Masson, P.: Experimental and spontaneous Schwannomas (peripheral gliomas), part 1. Am. J. Pathol., *8*:367, 1932.

Masson, P.: Tumeurs encapsulées et benignes des nerfs. Rev. Can. Biol., *1*:209, 1942.

Maxwell, D. S., Kruger, L., and Pineda, A.: The trigeminal

nerve root with special reference to the central-peripheral transition zone: an electron microscope study in the Macaque. Anat. Rec., *164*:113, 1969.

McCabe, J. S., and Low, F. N.: The subarachnoid angle: an area of transition in peripheral nerve. Anat. Rec., *164*:15, 1969.

Mellick, R., and Cavanagh, J. B.: Longitudinal movement of radioiodinated albumin within extravascular spaces of peripheral nerves following three systems of experimental trauma. J. Neurol. Neurosurg. Psychiatry, *30*:458, 1967a.

Mellick, R., and Cavanagh, J. B.: Extracellular space of normal peripheral nerve and normal skin as measured by radioactive sulfate in the chicken. Exp. Neurol., *18*:224, 1967b.

Nageotte, J.: Sheaths of the peripheral nerves. Nerve degeneration and regeneration. *In* Penfield, W. (ed.): Cytology and Cellular Pathology of the Nervous System. New York, Hoeber, 1932, p. 189.

Nathaniel, E. J. H., and Pease, D. C.: Degenerative changes in rat dorsal roots during Wallerian degeneration. J. Ultrastruct. Res., *9*:511, 1963a.

Nathaniel, E. J. H., and Pease, D. C.: Collagen and basement membrane formation by Schwann cells during nerve regeneration. J. Ultrastruct. Res., *9*:550, 1963b.

Obst, T.: Über das Endgebiet des Perineuriums an den Zahnnerven der Ratte. Z. Zellforsch. Mikrosk. Anat., *114*:515, 1971.

Ochoa, J., and Mair, W. G. P.: The normal sural nerve in man. I. Ultrastructure and numbers of fibres and cells. Acta Neuropathol., *13*:197, 1969.

Olsson, Y.: Studies on vascular permeability in peripheral nerves. I. Distribution of circulating fluorescent serum albumin in normal, crushed and sectioned rat sciatic nerve. Acta Neuropathol., *7*:1, 1966.

Olsson, Y.: Mast cells in the nervous system. Int. Rev. Cytol., *24*:27, 1968.

Olsson, Y.: Mast cells in human peripheral nerve. Acta Neurol. Scand., *47*:357, 1971.

Olsson, Y., and Kristensson, K.: The perineurium as a diffusion barrier to protein tracers following trauma to nerves. Acta Neuropathol., *23*:105, 1973.

Olsson, Y., and Reese, T. S.: Inaccessibility of the endoneurium of mouse sciatic nerve to exogenous proteins. Anat. Rec., *163*:318, 1969.

Olsson, Y., and Reese, T. S.: Permeability vasa nervorum and perineurium in mouse sciatic nerve studied by fluorescence and electron microscopy. J. Neuropathol., Exp. Neurol., *30*:105, 1971.

Olsson, Y., Kristensson, K., and Klatzo, J.: Permeability of blood vessels and connective tissue sheaths in the peripheral nervous system to exogenous proteins. Acta Neuropathol., Suppl. 5, 61, 1971.

Pease, D. C., and Molinari, S.: Electron microscopy of muscular arteries; pial vessels of the cat and monkey. J. Ultrastruct. Res., *3*:447, 1960.

Pease, D. C., and Schultz, R. L.: Electron microscopy of rat cranial meninges. Am. J. Anat., *102*:301, 1958.

·Plenk, H.: Über argyrophile Fasern (Gitterfasern) und ihre Bildungszellen. Ergeb. Anat. Entwicklungsgesch., *27*:302, 1927.

Plenk, H.: Die Schwannsche Scheide der markhaltigen Nervenfasern. Z. Mikrosk. Anat. Forsch., *36*:191, 1934.

Ranvier, L.: Leçons sur l'histologie du système nerveux. Paris, F. Savy, 1878.

Reese, T. S., and Karnovsky, M. J.: Fine structural localization of a blood-brain barrier to exogenous peroxidase. J. Cell Biol., *34*:207, 1967.

Renaut, J.: Recherches sur quelques points particuliers de l'histologie des nerfs. 1. La gaine lamelleuse et la système hyalin intravaginal. Arch. Physiol. Norm. Pathol. (Paris), 8:161, 1881.

Rexed, B.: Über die Aktivität der Schwannschen Zellen bei der Nervenregeneration. I. Die Überbrückung neuritloser Nervenlücken. Z. Mikrosk. Anat. Forsch., 51:177, 1942.

Röhlich, P., and Knoop, A.: Elektronenmikroskopische Untersuchungen an den Hüllen des N. Ischiadicus der Ratte. Z. Zellforsch. Mikrosk. Anat., 53:299, 1961.

Röhlich, P., and Weiss, M.: Studies on the histology and permeability of the peripheral nervous barrier. Acta Morphol. Acad. Sci. Hung., 5:335, 1955.

Ross, M. H.: The fine structure and development of the peritubular contractile cell component in the seminiferous tubules of the mouse. Am. J. Anat., 121:523, 1967.

Ross, M. H., and Reith, E. J.: Perineurium: evidence for contractile elements. Science, 165:604, 1969.

Saito, A., and Zacks, S. I.: Ultrastructure of Schwann and perineurial sheaths at the mouse neuromuscular junction. Anat. Rec., 164:379, 1969.

Schmitt, F. O., Hall, C. E., and Jakus, M. A.: Electron microscope investigations of the structure of collagen. J. Cell. Comp. Physiol., 20:11, 1942.

Shanes, A. M.: Effects of sheath removal on bullfrog nerve. J. Cell. Comp. Physiol., 41:305, 1953.

Shantha, T. R., and Bourne, G. H.: The perineural epithelium—a new concept. In Bourne, G. H. (ed.): The Structure and Function of Nervous Tissue, Vol. 1. New York and London, Academic Press, 1968, p. 379.

Shanthaveerappa, T. R., and Bourne, G. H.: The "perineural epithelium," a metabolically active, continuous, protoplasmic cell barrier surrounding peripheral nerve fasciculi. J. Anat., 96:527, 1962.

Shanthaveerappa, T. R., and Bourne, G. H.: New observations on the structure of the Pacinian corpuscle and its relation to the perineural epithelium of peripheral nerves. Am. J. Anat., 112:97, 1963.

Shanthaveerappa, T. R., and Bourne, G. H.: The effects of transection of the nerve trunk on the perineural epithelium with special reference to its role in nerve degeneration and regeneration. Anat. Rec., 150:35, 1964.

Shanthaveerappa, T. R., Hope, J., and Bourne, G. H.: Electron microscope demonstration of the perineural epithelium in rat peripheral nerve. Acta Anat. (Basel), 52:193, 1963.

Sima, A.: Personal communication, 1972.

Söderfeldt, B.: Personal communication, 1972.

Söderfeldt, B., Olsson, Y., and Kristensson, K.: The perineurium as a diffusion barrier to protein tracers in human peripheral nerve. Acta Neuropathol., 25:120, 1973.

Steer, J. M.: Some observations on the fine structure of rat dorsal spinal nerve roots. J. Anat., 109:467, 1971.

Steinwall, O., and Klatzo, I.: Selective vulnerability of blood-brain barrier in chemically induced lesions. J. Neuropathol. Exp. Neurol., 25:542, 1966.

Sunderland, S.: The adipose tissue of peripheral nerve. Brain, 68:118, 1945.

Sunderland, S.: The connective tissues of peripheral nerves. Brain, 88:841, 1965.

Sunderland, S.: Nerves and Nerve Injury. Edinburgh and London, E. & S. Livingstone, 1968.

Sunderland, S., and Bradley, K. C.: The cross-sectional area of peripheral nerve trunks devoted to nerve fibres. Brain, 72:428, 1949.

Sunderland, S., and Bradley, K. C.: Endoneurial tube shrinkage in the distal segment of a severed nerve. J. Comp. Neurol., 93:411, 1950a.

Sunderland, S., and Bradley, K. C.: Denervation atrophy of the distal stump of a severed nerve. J. Comp. Neurol., 93:401, 1950b.

Sunderland, S., and Bradley, K. C.: Stress-strain phenomena in human peripheral nerve trunks. Brain, 84:102, 1961a.

Sunderland, S., and Bradley, K. C.: Stress-strain phenomena in human spinal nerve roots. Brain, 84:120, 1961b.

Sunderland, S., and Bradley, K. C.: Stress-strain phenomena in denervated peripheral nerve trunks. Brain, 84:125, 1961c.

Tarlov, I. M.: Structure of the nerve root. I. Nature of the junction between the central and the peripheral nervous system. Arch. Neurol. Psychiatry, 37:555, 1937.

Thomas, G. A.: Quantitative histology of Wallerian degeneration. II. Nuclear population in two nerves of different fibre spectrum. J. Anat., 82:135, 1948.

Thomas, P. K.: The connective tissue of peripheral nerve: an electron microscope study. J. Anat., 97:35, 1963a.

Thomas, P. K.: The fate of the endoneurial tube during Wallerian degeneration. J. Anat., 97:476, 1963b.

Thomas, P. K.: Changes in the endoneurial sheaths of peripheral myelinated nerve fibres during Wallerian degeneration. J. Anat., 98:175, 1964a.

Thomas, P. K.: The deposition of collagen in relation to Schwann cell basement membrane during Wallerian degeneration. J. Cell Biol., 23:375, 1964b.

Thomas, P. K.: The cellular response to nerve injury. 1. The cellular outgrowth from the distal stump of transected nerve. J. Anat., 100:287, 1966.

Thomas, P. K.: The ultrastructural pathology of unmyelinated nerve fibres. In Desmedt, J. E. (ed.): New Developments in Electromyography and Clinical Neurophysiology. Vol. 2. Karger, Basel, 1973, p. 227.

Thomas, P. K., and Jones, D. G.: The cellular response to nerve injury. 2. Regeneration of the perineurium after nerve section. J. Anat., 101:45, 1967.

Torp, A.: Histamine and mast cells in nerves. Med. Exp., 4:180, 1961.

Waggener, J. P., and Beggs, J.: The membranous coverings of neural tissues: an electron microscope study. J. Neuropathol. Exp. Neurol., 26:412, 1967.

Waggener, J. P., Bunn, S. M., and Beggs, J.: The diffusion of ferritin within the peripheral nerve sheath: an electron microscopy study. J. Neuropathol. Exp. Neurol., 24:430, 1965.

Weiss, M., and Röhlich, P.: Significance of the interstice of the peripheral nerve. Acta Morphol. Acad. Sci. Hung., 4:309, 1954.

Weiss, P., Wang, H., Taylor, A. C., and Edds, M. V.: Proximo-distal fluid convection in the endoneurial spaces of peripheral nerves, demonstrated by color and radioactive (isotope) tracers. Am. J. Physiol., 143:521, 1945.

Young, J. Z.: The functional repair of nervous tissue. Physiol. Rev., 22:318, 1942.

Young, J. Z.: Factors influencing the regeneration of nerves. Adv. Surg., 1:165, 1949.

Young, J. Z., Holmes, W., and Sanders, F. K.: Nerve regeneration. Importance of the peripheral stump and the value of nerve grafts. Lancet, 2:128, 1940.

Zacks, S. J., and Saito, A.: Uptake of exogenous horseradish peroxidase by coated vesicles in mouse neuromuscular junctions. J. Histochem. Cytochem., 17:161, 1969.

Chapter 10

VASCULAR PERMEABILITY IN THE PERIPHERAL NERVOUS SYSTEM

Yngve Olsson

The blood vessels play an important role in providing adequate nutritional supplies to various parts of the peripheral nervous system (see Adams, 1942; Sunderland, 1968; Lundborg and Brånemark, 1968; Olsson, 1972). As is well known, the transfer of substances (nutrients and metabolites) between the blood and the nerve parenchyma occurs across the vascular walls, where the permeability properties of the endothelial lining appear to be of particular significance. The special permeability properties of blood vessels in the peripheral nervous system also appear to influence the distribution and character of the tissue damage in a large variety of pathologic conditions of peripheral nerves, roots, and ganglia (Waksman, 1961; Olsson, 1972). Our current knowledge of the permeability properties of the blood vessels under normal and pathologic conditions and the vascularization of the peripheral nervous system are considered here, since both histologic and ultrastructural data about the vessels are necessary for understanding their permeability properties.

VASCULAR MORPHOLOGY

The vascularization of peripheral nerve trunks has been reviewed repeatedly (Adams, 1942; Sunderland, 1968; Lundborg and Brånemark, 1968; Olsson, 1972). Cardinal features of these vessels are the richness of anastomoses and the presence of microvascular networks or plexuses (Fig. 10–1). Nutrient arteries from adjacent large vessels give

off many small branches, which by anastomoses form the epineurial and perineurial vascular plexuses. Numerous vessels also pierce the perineurium to join the endoneurial vascular network. This is composed mainly of capillaries running longitudinally along the nerves. Occasionally such vessels pass obliquely or perpendicularly to the main axis of the nerve.

The blood supply to each dorsal root

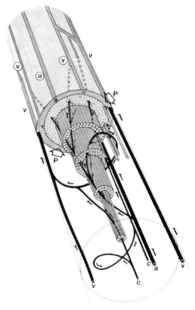

Figure 10–1 Schematic drawing illustrating the vascularization of a normal peripheral nerve trunk. Veins (v) and arteries (a) penetrate the perineurium (P) and form an endoneurial vascular plexus mainly composed of capillaries (c). Note the capillary loops surrounding the nerve fibers. (From Lundborg, G.: Ischemic nerve injury. Scand. J. Plast. Reconstruct. Surg., Suppl. 6, 1970. Reprinted by permission.)

190

ganglion originates from the spinal branch of the corresponding segmental artery (Adamkiewicz, 1886; Bergmann and Alexander, 1941; Brierley, 1955). The capillary network is particularly abundant in the gray matter of the ganglia where capillary loops surround each neuron. The ganglia also contain small venules, and the ganglionic vessels communicate with vessels in the adjacent parts of the roots and peripheral nerve (Waksman, 1961; Adamkiewicz, 1886).

The intraneural pattern of veins is basically similar to the arterial arrangement (Quénu and Lejars, 1892, 1894), although according to Waksman (1961) there are species differences with regard to the presence of small veins in the endoneurium. For instance, the sciatic nerve of the guinea pig contains an appreciable number of small veins and venules, whereas the rabbit nerve possesses a true capillary network.

The small vessels in the peripheral nervous system are surrounded by connective tissue with large extracellular spaces (Olsson, 1972). Otherwise, the vessel wall is composed of the same structural components as blood vessels of other tissues, that is, basal laminae (basement membranes), pericytes, endothelial cells, and also, in certain vessels, smooth muscle cells (see Fig. 10–8). As is discussed later, particular ultrastructural features of the endothelial cell layer are of crucial importance for the permeability properties of the blood vessels in the peripheral nervous system.

VASCULAR PERMEABILITY IN NORMAL PERIPHERAL NERVE

The term "vascular permeability" refers to the exchange of all kinds of substances between blood and a tissue. It is well known that such factors as the chemical nature, size, and electrical charge are of great importance in such a transfer of substances and that the passage across the vascular walls may occur in quite different ways. In contrast to the numerous studies of the central nervous system, there are few in which the permeability of different substances in blood vessels of the peripheral nervous system has been compared (Waksman, 1961; Olsson, 1971; Welch and Davson, 1972). Such experimental studies have most often examined the permeability to various protein tracers; most of the infor-

mation presented here concerns the microvascular permeability in this restricted sense.

Permeability to Protein Tracers

Originally, basic research on vascular permeability in the central nervous system was performed using acid dyes with great affinity for serum albumin such as trypan blue and Evans blue (see Broman, 1949). More recently, albumin labeled with a fluorescent or radioactive marker has been the tracer of choice (Steinwall and Klatzo, 1966; Brightman et al., 1970). Following intravenous injection in the early studies the dyes were localized grossly by their blue color or microscopically in thick frozen sections. These tracers can now also be identified in formalin-fixed tissue sections by fluorescence microscopy, allowing their detailed cellular localization (Steinwall and Klatzo, 1966).

The fine structural localization of an exogenous protein tracer can be determined with great accuracy if the peroxidase technique described by Graham and Karnovsky (1966) is

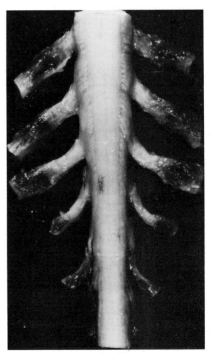

Figure 10–2 Spinal cord with roots and ganglia from a chimpanzee that had been injected with Evans blue intravenously 48 hours before sacrifice. The dorsal root ganglia are stained, whereas the cord remains unstained.

applied. Horseradish peroxidase is then used as a protein tracer, which after fixation with a glutaraldehyde-paraformaldehyde mixture and appropriate incubation, can be localized both by light and by electron microscopy. These methods have all been applied in studies on vascular permeability to proteins in peripheral nerve (see Waksman, 1961; Olsson, 1966a, 1972).

Numerous studies on the blood-brain barrier have shown that trypan blue and Evans blue injected intravenously cause a blue staining of all parenchymatous organs except the brain and spinal cord (Fig. 10–2) (Broman, 1949, Brightman et al., 1970). The distribution of the dye in the peripheral nervous system, however, differs from that in the brain and is influenced by a number of factors such as the topographical site, the area within the nerve (epineurium, endoneurium), and the animal species. For instance, the dorsal root ganglia and the epineurium are intensely stained, whereas the endoneurium is either completely unstained or shows only a slight bluish coloration (Figs. 10–2 and 10–3) (Doinikow, 1913; Tschetschujeva, 1929; Waksman, 1961; Olsson, 1968a, 1971).

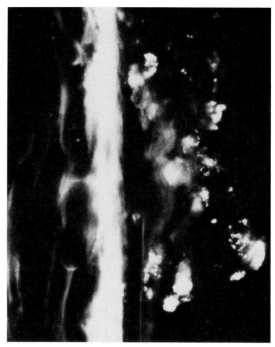

Figure 10–4 Guinea pig peripheral nerve after intravenous injection of fluorescent labeled albumin. The tracer has leaked out of epineurial vessels and has diffused widely in the epineurium and the perineurium. There is also uptake of the tracer in the cytoplasm of several cells.

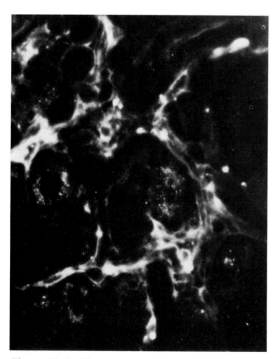

Figure 10–3 Fluorescence micrograph from a dorsal root ganglion of a guinea pig that had been injected with Evans blue before sacrifice. The tracer has passed out of the ganglionic vessels and surrounds neurons.

Observations by fluorescence microscopy have provided further information on vascular permeability in peripheral nerve. After the intravenous injection of albumin or gamma globulin labeled with the fluorescent marker Evans blue or fluorescein isothiocyanate, these proteins can be traced to the lumen of epineurial blood vessels almost immediately, and appear later in the connective tissue around the vessels (Olsson, 1966a, 1968a, 1971). The proteins in the extracellular spaces can migrate to the innermost parts of the perineurium, but their further diffusion into the endoneurium is prevented by the barrier function of the perineurium (Olsson, 1966a, 1971; see also Chapter 9). This pattern of spread, shown in Figure 10–4, has been observed in all species thus far examined, and a similar extravasation has also been described for other protein tracers such as iodine-131–labeled albumin, ferritin, and horseradish peroxidase (Waksman, 1961; Boddingius et al., 1972; Olsson and Reese, 1971).

The epineurial blood vessels thus share with many other blood vessels in the body the ability to allow the passage of serum proteins across their walls (cf. Mancini, 1963). In such tissues, there is normally a slow flow of serum proteins from the blood vessels to the extracellular spaces. The extravascular proteins are then resorbed into lymphatics and later conveyed back to the blood. In this connection it should be recalled that lymphatics are present in the epineurium, but are absent from the endoneurium of nerve fascicles (Sunderland, 1968).

The routes by which protein tracers leak out of epineurial vessels have been elucidated with the peroxidase method (Olsson and Reese, 1971). Horseradish peroxidase injected intravenously passed out of these vessels by diffusion between adjacent endothelial cells where the junctions are of the open variety (Fig. 10–5; see also Fig. 10–9*B*). These junctions are similar to those found in some other permeable vessels such as in cardiac and skeletal muscle, lung, and liver (Karnovsky, 1967; Schneeberger-Keeley and Karnovsky, 1968; Papadimitriou and Walters, 1968). A few fenestrated vessels are also present in the epineurium, and the possibility therefore exists that the proteins may, in part, escape from the circulation through such pores (Olsson and Reese, 1971). The same

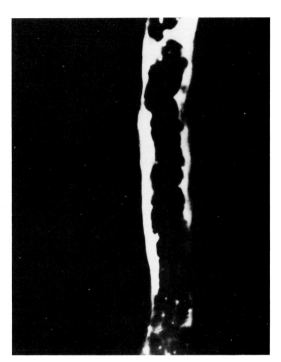

Figure 10–6 Endoneurial blood vessel from a rat sciatic nerve showing intravenously injected fluorescent tracer only in the lumen of the vessel.

holds true for pinocytotic transfer of the proteins through the endothelial cells. Following passage through the endothelium, protein tracers can easily penetrate the vascular basal laminae and then freely diffuse in the extracellular spaces of the epineurium (Olsson and Reese, 1971).

The amount of extravasated tracer in the endoneurium is usually considerably smaller than that in the epineurium, and in certain species such as the mouse and rat no tracer is seen outside the lumen of endoneurial capillaries (Fig. 10–6) (Olsson, 1966a, 1971; Olsson and Reese, 1971). In many other vertebrates (e.g., guinea pig, rabbit, cat, monkey), however, passage of intravenously injected protein tracers into the endoneurium can be observed, but the amount of extravasated tracer is usually small and varies considerably between various individuals and between various fascicles in multifascicular nerves (Fig. 10–7) (Waksman, 1961; Olsson, 1967, 1971). For instance, some of the fascicles in the sciatic nerve of the rabbit and the guinea pig contain extravasated tracer, whereas other fascicles in the same animals do not show any signs of tracer outside the vessels (Olsson, 1971).

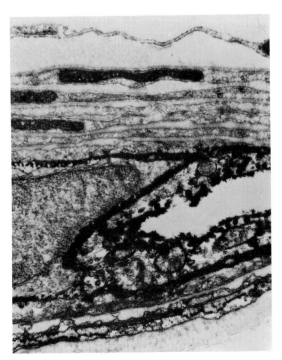

Figure 10–5 Blood vessel in a mouse sciatic nerve at the border between the epineurium and the perineurium. The dark tracer has passed between endothelial cells and then in the vascular basal lamina (basement membrane).

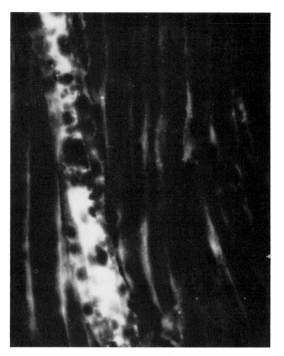

Figure 10–7 Endoneurial blood vessel from a guinea pig sciatic nerve showing passage of the fluorescent tracer out of the vascular lumen. The tracer is present in perivascular spaces and in the interstices between nerve fibers.

Some conflicting opinions appear to exist concerning the permeability of endoneurial vessels in the rabbit, which is probably due to differences in the methods applied. Thus Doinikow (1913) noticed that only minimal amounts of trypan blue could pass into the rabbit nerve parenchyma. Waksman (1961) also was of the opinion that the parenchyma of the rabbit sciatic nerve remained completely unstained by parenterally administered trypan blue and did not contain radio-labeled albumin or diphtheria toxin or toxoid after intravenous injection. In these experiments the presence of extravasated tracer was judged macroscopically, light microscopically, or by radioautography. Using the sensitive fluorescence microscope technique, Lundborg (1970) and Olsson (1967, 1971) managed to detect extravasated fluorochrome-labeled albumin in the endoneurium of rabbit sciatic and tibial nerves, thus proving that the "barrier" function of the endoneurial vessels to proteins in this species is not absolutely efficient.

Applying the peroxidase technique, Olsson and Reese (1971) studied the morphologic basis for the impermeability of endoneurial vessels in mouse sciatic nerve. Intravenously injected horseradish peroxidase remained in the lumen of the vessels, and the extracellular diffusion of this protein tracer was prevented by tight junctions between the endothelial cells (Figs. 10–8 and 10–9A). These junctions were similar to those in the brain parenchyma, where they are considered to be of major importance for the blood-brain barrier phenomenon to this protein tracer (Reese and Karnovsky, 1967). The endoneurial endothelial cells of the mouse sciatic nerve also lacked fenestrae, and protein transport by pinocytosis across the endothelial lining appeared to be insignificant since the covering basal lamina did not contain peroxidase.

The ultrastructural basis for the passage of protein tracers from the blood into the endoneurium of the peripheral nerves of certain other species has not yet been elucidated. Presumably differences in their endothelium as compared with the mouse account for this phenomenon. For instance, some junctions may be open or fenestrae may be present.

The dorsal root ganglia and presumably the spinal roots contain blood vessels of the permeable variety (Tschetschujeva, 1929;

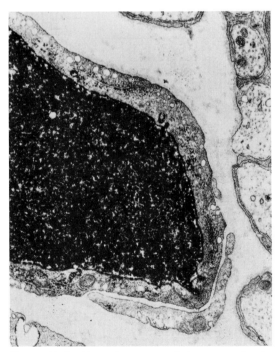

Figure 10–8 Normal mouse sciatic nerve showing intravenously injected peroxidase remaining in the lumen of an endoneurial capillary. The dark tracer does not penetrate through the tight junctions joining adjacent endothelial cells, and there is therefore no tracer in the perivascular spaces.

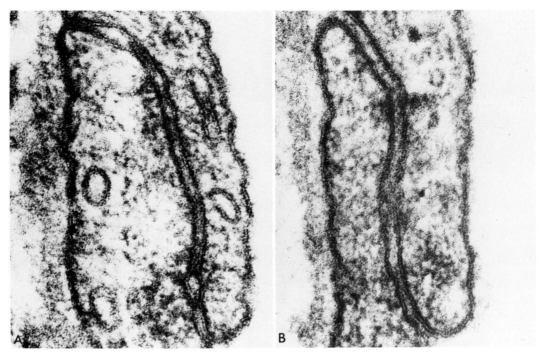

Figure 10–9   *A.* Apposition between adjacent endothelial cells in a mouse endoneurial capillary. Note that the adjacent plasma membranes come very close together at several points. Compare with Figure 10–10. *B.* Apposition between adjacent endothelial cells in a mouse epineurial capillary. Along the line of apposition the adjacent plasma membranes are separated by a gap that can be followed from the lumen to the basement membrane.

Waksman, 1961; Olsson, 1968a, 1971). Intravenously injected dyes such as trypan blue or Evans blue stain these areas, whereas adjacent parts of the cord remain unstained (see Fig. 10–2). This phenomenon occurs in all animal species thus far examined, including higher vertebrates, and is not restricted to these dyes (Olsson, 1971). Fluorochrome-labeled serum proteins, ferritin, and peroxidase are equally distributed (Rosenbluth and Wissig, 1964; Olsson, 1968a, 1971).

Permeability to Nonproteinaceous Substances

The endoneurial blood vessels in the sciatic nerve of rabbits, mice, and guinea pigs have been found to be impermeable to silver nitrate given in drinking water over several months (Waksman, 1961). Several investigators have also observed that different radio-labeled ions such as sodium-24, chlorine-36, and sulfur-35 thiourea do not penetrate as rapidly into peripheral nerves as into other soft tissues (Manery and Bale, 1941; Dainty and Krnjević, 1955; Welch and Davson, 1972). All these

observations are therefore in line with the results from experiments with protein tracers, which generally show a low rate of penetration into the endoneurium of the peripheral nerves.

More recently, Aker (1972) presented most interesting data on the hematic barriers in peripheral nerves in which a fluorescent diaminoacridine dye of low molecular weight (259.7) was used as a permeability tracer. His observations indicated that the endothelial lining of endoneurial vessels also acted as an efficient diffusion barrier to a substance of this low molecular weight.

VASCULAR PERMEABILITY IN PATHOLOGIC CONDITIONS

Two different aspects of the vascular permeability are of interest with regard to the mechanisms of pathologic processes of the peripheral nervous system. First of all, variations in the normal vascular permeability in various parts of the system may influence the localization of lesions caused by blood-borne agents. Second, various pathologic processes may induce an increased vascular permeability leading to extravasation of serum constituents and to the formation of edema.

Vasa Nervorum as Diffusion Barrier to Disease-Promoting Agents

Waksman (1961) presented an extensive investigation of the possible role of endoneurial vessels in preventing noxious agents from gaining access to the parenchyma in peripheral nerves from the blood. Clinical and histologic observations on the distribution of lesions in diphtheritic and allergic neuritis had previously demonstrated that rabbit peripheral nerves were remarkably resistant to these diseases, whereas those of the guinea pig became heavily damaged (Waksman and Adams, 1956). Waksman therefore studied the distribution in the peripheral nervous system of intravenously injected dyes, proteins, and diphtheria toxin and toxoid. He showed that the diphtheria toxin and toxoid could pass freely into the nerves of the guinea pig but not into the rabbit nerve parenchyma. He therefore proposed that the differential susceptibility of the rabbit and guinea pig to diphtheritic polyneuritis was due to species differences in the normal permeability of vasa nervorum.

The concept that the vasa nervorum may have the capacity to prevent certain circulating noxious agents from exerting their effects in nerve is also supported by some other observations with the histamine liberator: Compound 48/80 (Olsson, 1966c, 1968c). This compound, after systemic injection, causes histamine release and degranulation of mast cells in most tissues of rats, although mast cells in the endoneurium of the sciatic nerve resist the effect of this substance (Olsson, 1966c). This effect has been attributed to the inability of the compound to enter the endoneurium from the endoneurial blood vessels and to the capacity of the perineurium to act as a diffusion barrier, thereby preventing diffusion of the compound from the surrounding tissues into the endoneurium.

Increased Permeability of Vasa Nervorum in Edema

It is well known that increased vascular permeability occurs in numerous pathologic processes in other organs. The altered permeability causes an increased rate of flow of plasma from the blood into the tissues, and consequently exudates accumulate. Since the plasma proteins form an important part of exudates, the permeability of the blood vessels to these and similar proteins is of especial interest.

In other parts of the body, exudates are most frequently encountered in inflammatory diseases of infectious or allergic origin, and the same is probably true also for the peripheral nervous system (cf. Boddingius et al., 1972). In fact, histologic studies have repeatedly revealed edematous separation of nerve fibers in such conditions, for instance in herpes zoster infection and the Guillain-Barré syndrome (Krücke, 1955; Sigwald and Nonailhat, 1970). Other well-known examples of gross or histologic edema in peripheral nerve include vaccinogenic and serogenic neuropathies in which the neural edema is considered to play a crucial pathogenetic role (Gathier and Bruyn, 1970a, 1970b).

For obvious reasons, it is hard to make morphologic studies on capillary permeability in human peripheral nerves under edematous conditions. Furthermore, minor degrees of edema probably escape attention in histologic preparations, and it is therefore necessary to apply experimental methods on laboratory animals, for instance with protein tracing techniques or electron microscopy, to reveal the origin, spread, and detailed localization of edema in peripheral nerves.

With regard to inflammatory exudates of allergic origin, there are several electron microscopic reports of the presence of endoneurial edema in experimental allergic neuritis (Lampert, 1969; Schröder and Krücke, 1970; Allt, 1972). Of particular interest is Lampert's observation (1969) that proteinaceous exudates were most marked in the areas that contained extravasated mononuclear cells, but the actual route and time course in relation to the cellular infiltration in this experimental disease remain to be established.

Experimental studies on extravasation of protein tracers in infectious diseases of peripheral nerves are extremely few. Recently Boddingius et al. (1972) reported marked exudation of intravenously injected trypan blue and ferritin in mice with leprous neuropathy. The protein-containing exudates were particularly marked in areas with the most severe lesions, and ultrastructural abnormalities were noticed in endoneurial capillaries (Boddingius et al., 1972; Boddingius, 1972).

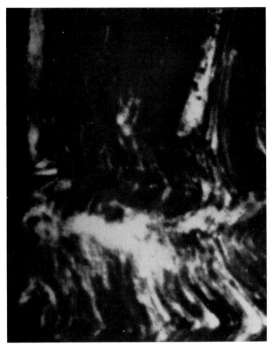

Figure 10–10 A crush lesion of a rat sciatic nerve is followed by leakage of intravenously injected protein tracer into the endoneurium. The tracer then spreads in the spaces between cords of Schwann cells, forming fluorescent lines running longitudinally along the nerve.

The permeability of the vasa nervorum has also been studied with protein-tracing techniques after nerve injury produced in various laboratory animals. Mechanical lesions, transection, and ligature of peripheral nerves are followed by an almost immediate exudation of circulating albumin at the site of the lesion, and during the following hours the extravasated albumin rapidly spreads distally into the endoneurium (Fig. 10–10) (Olsson, 1966; Mellick and Cavanagh, 1967, 1968). This leakage is most marked during the first day after injury and is confined to blood vessels in the immediate vicinity of the lesion. In the more distal segments, there is usually a delay of more than 24 hours before there is evidence of increased vascular permeability.

In addition to the early changes in vascular permeability in traumatized nerves there is a second wave of increased permeability that usually peaks at about two weeks after the injury (Olsson, 1966; Mellick and Cavanagh, 1968). In contradistinction to the early response, this delayed change in permeability probably involves blood vessels throughout the nerve distal to the lesion. The delayed permeability change is not restricted to

traumatic neuropathies but is also present in various other disorders of peripheral nerve (Olsson, 1968; Seneviratne, 1972).

Besides mechanical injuries, various toxic and metabolic conditions are common causes of peripheral nerve disease. Recently a report appeared claiming that increased permeability of endoneurial vessels occurs in diabetic neuropathy induced by alloxan (Seneviratne, 1972), and the same phenomenon is known to occur in neuropathy caused by the drug isonicotinic acid hydrazide (Fig. 10–11) (Olsson, 1968b). In such conditions extravasation of intravenously injected labeled albumin can be detected by fluorescence microscopy in areas with histologically demonstrable demyelination and axonal damage (Olsson, 1968b). In addition, Lampert et al. (1970) found electron microscopic evidence of endoneurial edema in tellurium-induced neuropathy of newborn rats.

The delayed type of increased vascular permeability to protein tracers also follows radiation injury under certain conditions. Lundborg and Schildt (1971) exposed rabbits to whole body radiation of 1100 rads corre-

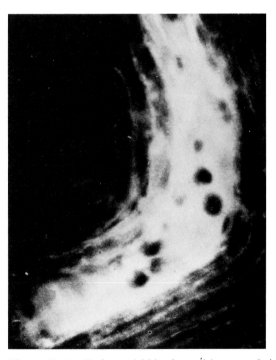

Figure 10–11 Endoneurial blood vessel in a rat sciatic nerve containing intravenously injected fluorescent protein tracer. A peripheral neuropathy was induced with isonicotinic acid hydrazide, and the tracer has now passed out of the vascular lumen and spreads in the intercellular spaces.

sponding to the median lethal dose. Increased vascular permeability was not evident until the nerve had been exposed to a slight ischemic injury before irradiation. Signs of increased permeability began on the fourth day and reached a maximum around the eighth day.

The effect of acute transient ischemia on the permeability of the vasa nervorum in rabbit peripheral nerve has recently been studied by Lundborg (1970). A controlled temporary ischemia was produced in the hind limb by a pneumatic cuff, and Evans blue was injected intravenously to indicate disturbances in the vascular permeability. Not even six hours of ischemia caused extravasation in the endoneurium in the tibial nerve, but after eight hours there was a slight, and after 10 hours a prominent, endoneurial edema containing extravasated tracer. It is also interesting to note that extravasation began in the epineurium at a time when no exudation was seen in the endoneurium, indicating that the endoneurial vessels may be more resistant to this type of injury than the epineurial vessels.

Rather little is known about the mechanisms by which the increased vascular permeability in experimental peripheral neuropathies is initiated and maintained. The early response in traumatic neuropathies is probably a consequence of the direct trauma to the blood vessels, but the liberation of endogenous chemical mediators may also be involved (Olsson, 1966). Such mediators may well include amines released from mast cells that are disrupted as a result of trauma (Olsson, 1966b, 1968c). The delayed response is obviously not exclusively an effect of the direct trauma since similar permeability changes can be induced by nontraumatic peripheral nerve lesions such as that produced by isonicotinic acid hydrazide and alloxan (Olsson, 1968; Seneviratne, 1972). It may well be that other chemical mediators are formed in the degenerating nerves that have the capacity to maintain the delayed response. In addition, the formation of new blood vessels may occur, and these vessels may not have the same functional properties as their mature counterparts (Olsson, 1966a, 1968c).

CONCLUDING REMARKS

Available information clearly shows the importance of vascular permeability for both the normal integrity of the peripheral nervous system and its role in numerous pathologic conditions. The regulation of the internal milieu of the endoneurium in the peripheral nervous system is achieved by the endoneurial blood vessels and by the perineurium (see Chapters 9 and 10). These vessels are impermeable or only slightly permeable to proteins in most parts of the system except for dorsal root ganglia and spinal nerve roots. Variations in permeability between such areas and between different animal species are presumably important for the distribution of lesions caused by various blood-borne agents of a toxic and infectious nature. In such states the pathologic alterations are most severe in areas with permeable vessels, whereas areas with impermeable vessels are usually unaffected by the disease.

The other important aspect of vascular permeability in the peripheral nervous system concerns its role in the genesis of edema in various pathologic conditions. The experimental data have shown that a protein-rich endoneurial edema of that origin occurs in a large variety of conditions such as wallerian degeneration, toxic and metabolic neuropathies, leprous neuropathy, and long-lasting ischemia. In clinical practice, increased permeability of endoneurial vessels therefore most probably occurs in similar conditions. On the basis of general pathologic experience, one can then expect the most severe edema to occur in the acute phases of the peripheral nerve diseases and in infectious and allergic neuritis. In this connection it should be recalled that edematous separation of nerve fibers is frequently a prominent manifestation in early cases of the Guillain-Barré syndrome, and fibrin-containing exudates have certainly been described in the endoneurium of rabbit sciatic nerves following the induction of allergic neuritis (Schröder and Krücke, 1970).

The peripheral nerve fascicles have particular anatomical features that probably make the resorption of endoneurial edema more difficult than that of edema elsewhere. In other tissues, an edematous condition implies that there is an increased rate of flow of serum constituents from the vessels to the extracellular spaces from which resorption occurs partly into lymphatic vessels. The interior of the nerve fascicles lacks lymphatic drainage, and the presence of the impermeable perineurium probably restricts the diffusion of edema out of the fascicles. It therefore seems reasonable to assume that nerve lesions with increased vascular permeability are associated with chronic edema and that this type of edema may induce secondary changes inside the fascicles. It could well be that such an edema is a stimulating factor in fibrosis and perhaps has an influence on the nerve fibers themselves. Further experimental studies should be directed to elucidate this interesting aspect of the pathogenesis of peripheral nerve lesions.

REFERENCES

Adamkiewicz, A.: Der Blutkreislauf der Ganglienzelle. Berlin, 1886. Cited by Adams, W. E., 1942.

Adams, W. E.: The blood supply of nerves. I. Historical review. J. Anat. (Lond.), 76:323, 1942.

Aker, F. D.: A study of hematic barriers in peripheral nerves of albino rabbits. Anat. Rec., 174:21, 1972.

Allt, G.: Involvement of the perineurium in experimental allergic neuritis: electron microscopic observations. Acta Neuropathol. (Berl.), 20:139, 1972.

Bergmann, L., and Alexander, L.: Vascular supply of the spinal ganglia. Arch. Neurol. Psychiatry, 46:761, 1941.

Boddingius, J., Rees, R. J. W., and Weddell, A. G. H.: Defects in the blood-nerve barrier in mice with leprosy neuropathy. Nature [New Biol.], 237:190, 1972.

Boddingius, J.: Ultrastructural changes in peripheral nerves in leprosy. J. Anat., 111:516, 1972.

Brierley, J. B.: Sensory ganglia: recent anatomical physiological and pathological contributions. Acta Psychiatr. Neurol. Scand., 30:553, 1955.

Brightman, M., Klatzo, I., Olsson, Y., and Reese, T. S.: The blood-brain barrier to proteins under normal and pathological conditions. J. Neurol. Sci., 10:215, 1970.

Broman, T.: The permeability of the cerebrospinal vessels in normal and pathological conditions. Copenhagen, Ejnar Munksgaard 1949.

Dainty, J., and Krnjević, K.: The rate of exchange of Na^{24} in cat nerves. J. Physiol. (Lond.), 128:489, 1955.

Doinikow, B.: Histologische und histopathologische Untersuchungen am peripheren Nervensystem mittels vitaler Färbung. Folia Neurobiol. (Leipzig), 7:731, 1913.

Gathier, J. C., and Bruyn, G. W.: The vaccinogenic peripheral neuropathies. In Vinken, P. J., and Bruyn, G. W. (eds.): Handbook of Clinical Neurology. Vol. 8. Amsterdam, North Holland Publishing Company, 1970a, p. 86.

Gathier, J. C., and Bruyn, G. W.: The serogenetic peripheral neuropathies. In Vinken, P. J., and Bruyn, G. W. (eds.): Handbook of Clinical Neurology. Vol. 8. Amsterdam, North Holland Publishing Company, 1970b, p. 95.

Graham, R. C., and Karnovsky, M. J.: The early stages of absorption of injected horseradish peroxidase in the proximal tubules of mouse kidney: ultrastructural cytochemistry by a new technique. J. Histochem. Cytochem., 14:391, 1966.

Karnovsky, M. J.: The ultrastructural basis of capillary permeability studied with peroxidase as a tracer. J. Cell. Biol., 35:213, 1967.

Krücke, W.: Erkrankungen der peripheren Nerven. In Döring, G., Herzog, E., Krücke, W., and Orthner, H. (eds.): Handbuch der speziellen patologischen Anatomie und Histologie. XIII/5. Berlin, Göttingen, Heidelberg, Springer Verlag, 1955, pp. 1–203.

Lampert, P. W.: Mechanism of demyelination in experimental allergic neuritis. Lab. Invest., 20:127, 1969.

Lampert, P. W., Garro, F., and Pentschew, A.: Tellurium neuropathy. Acta Neuropathol. (Berl.), 15:308, 1970.

Lundborg, G.: Ischemic nerve injury. Scand. J. Plast. Reconstr. Surg., Suppl. 6, 1970.

Lundborg, G., and Brånemark, P. J.: Microvascular structure and function of peripheral nerves. Adv. Microcirc., 1:66, 1968.

Lundborg, G., and Schildt, B.: Microvascular permeability in irradiated rabbits. Acta Radiol. (Stockh.), 10:311, 1971.

Manery, J. F., and Bale, W. F.: The penetration of radioactive sodium and phosphorus into the extra- and intracellular phases of tissues. Am. J. Physiol., 132:215, 1941.

Mancini, R. E.: Connective tissue and serum proteins. Int. Rev. Cytol., 14:193, 1963.

Mellick, R. S., and Cavanagh, J. B.: Longitudinal movement of radioiodinated albumin within extravascular spaces of peripheral nerves following three systems of experimental trauma. J. Neurosurg. Psychiatr., 30:458, 1967.

Mellick, R. S., and Cavanagh, J. B.: Changes in blood vessel permeability during degeneration and regeneration in peripheral nerves. Brain, 41:141, 1968.

Olsson, Y.: Studies on vascular permeability in peripheral nerves. 1. Distribution of circulating fluorescent serum albumin in normal, crushed and sectioned rat sciatic nerve. Acta Neuropathol. (Berl.), 7:1, 1966a.

Olsson, Y.: Studies on vascular permeability in peripheral nerves. II. Distribution of circulating fluorescent serum albumin in rat sciatic nerve after local injection of histamine, 5-hydroxytryptamine and Compound 48/80. Acta Physiol. Scand. 69: Suppl., 284, 1966b.

Olsson, Y.: The effect of the histamine liberator Compound 48/80 on mast cells in peripheral nerve. Acta Pathol. Microbiol. Scand., 68:563, 1966c.

Olsson, Y.: Phytogenetic variations in the vascular permeability of peripheral nerves to serum albumin. Acta Pathol. Microbiol. Scand., 69:621, 1967.

Olsson, Y.: Topographical differences in the vascular permeability of the peripheral nervous system. Acta Neuropathol. (Berl.), 10:26, 1968a.

Olsson, Y.: Studies on vascular permeability in peripheral nerves. 3. Permeability changes of vasa nervorum and exudation of serum albumin in INH-induced neuropathy of the rat. Acta Neuropathol. (Berl.), 11:103, 1968b.

Olsson, Y.: Mast cells in the nervous system. Int. Rev. Cytol., 24:27, 1968c.

Olsson, Y.: Studies on vascular permeability in peripheral nerves. IV. Distribution of intravenously injected protein tracers in the peripheral nervous system of various species. Acta Neuropathol. (Berl.), 17:114, 1971.

Olsson, Y., and Reese, T. S.: Permeability of vasa nervorum and perineurium in mouse sciatic nerve studied by fluorescence and electron microscopy. J. Neuropathol. Exp. Neurol., 30:105, 1971.

Olsson, Y.: The involvement of vasa nervorum in diseases of peripheral nerves. *In* Vinken, P. J., and Bruyn, G. E. (eds.): Handbook of Clinical Neurology. Vol. 12. Amsterdam, North Holland Publishing Co., 1972, p. 644.

Papadimitriou, J. M., and Walters, M. N. I.: Fluid flow in the liver demonstrated with horseradish peroxidase. Am. J. Anat., *123*:475, 1968.

Quénu, J., and Lejars, F., 1892, 1894. Cited by Adams, W. E., 1942.

Reese, T. S., and Karnovsky, M. J.: Fine structural localization of a blood-brain barrier to exogenous peroxidase. J. Cell Biol., *34*:207, 1967.

Rosenbluth, J., and Wissig, S. L.: The distribution of exogenous ferritin in toad spinal ganglia and the mechanism of its uptake by neurons. J. Cell Biol., *23*:307, 1964.

Schneeberger-Keeley, E. E., and Karnovsky, M. J.: The ultrastructural basis of alveolar-capillary membrane permeability to peroxidase used as a tracer. J. Cell Biol., *37*:781, 1968.

Schröder, J. M., and Krücke, W.: Zur Feinstruktur der experimentell-allergischen Neuritis beim Kaninchen. Acta Neuropathol. (Berl.), *14*:261, 1970.

Seneviratne, K. N.: Permeability of blood nerve barriers in the diabetic rat. J. Neurol. Neurosurg. Psychiatry, *55*:156, 1972.

Sigwald, J., and Nonailhat, F.: The Guillain-Barré syndrome. *In* Vinken, P. J., and Bruyn, G. W. (eds.): Handbook of Clinical Neurology. Vol. 7. Amsterdam, North Holland Publishing Co., 1970, p. 495.

Steinwall, O., and Klatzo, I.: Selective vulnerability of the blood-brain barrier in chemically induced lesions. J. Neuropathol. Exp. Neurol., *25*:542, 1966.

Sunderland, S.: Nerve and nerve injuries. Edinburgh and London, E. & S. Livingstone Ltd., 1968.

Tschetschujeva, T.: Uber die Speicherung von Trypanblue in Ganglien des Nervensystems. Z. Gesamte Exp. Med., *69*:208, 1929.

Waksman, B. H.: Experimental study of diphtheric polyneuritis in the rabbit and guinea pig. III. The blood-nerve barrier in the rabbit. J. Neuropathol. Exp. Neurol., *20*:35, 1961.

Waksman, B. H., and Adams, R. D.: A comparative study of experimental allergic neuritis in the rabbit, guinea-pig and mouse. J. Neuropathol. Exp. Neurol., *15*:293, 1956.

Welch, K., and Davson, H.: The permeability of capillaries of the sciatic nerve of the rabbit to several materials. J. Neurosurg., *36*:21–26, 1972.

Chapter 11

THE BIOLOGY OF SCHWANN CELLS

Arthur K. Asbury

The biologic behavior of the Schwann cell has attracted the interest of investigators for over 100 years. In this chapter, selected aspects of Schwann cell activity are considered, with emphasis on their role in pathologic states. The terms "neurilemma cell" and "sheath cell" as used by other authors are here taken to be synonymous with "Schwann cell." Some ultrastructural features of Schwann cells are illustrated in Figure 11–1.

ORIGIN OF SCHWANN CELLS

Although most authorities agree that Schwann cells are of neurectodermal origin, considerable difference of opinion has been voiced as to whether they are derived principally from the neural crest or from the neural tube itself. Harrison (1924) concluded, in summarizing his extensive embryologic investigations, that most Schwann cells originated in the neural crest from whence they migrated early in embryonic life. Kuntz (1922), who used techniques similar to those employed by Harrison, had suggested that many of the Schwann cells in motor nerves arise in the ventral portion of the neural tube and migrate via the ventral roots. Later, Raven (1937) found that a large portion of sheath cells (taken to be synonymous with Schwann cells for our purposes) originate in the ventral neural tube, as demonstrated by his ingenious experiments using xenoplastic grafts. This technique exploits the measureable differences in nuclear sizes between two genera of amphibians, thus making it possible

to determine the cellular contribution of either neural crest or neural tube embryo grafts. In a more recent radioautographic study of chick embryo in which grafts labeled with tritiated thymidine were utilized, Weston (1963) also found that a large proportion of Schwann cells took origin in the neural tube and migrated ventrally in company with motor nerve fibers. The present weight of evidence derived from embryologic studies favors the view that Schwann cells are neurectodermal in origin, but some doubt remains concerning the relative contributions of the neural crest and the neural tube. For more detailed exploration of this subject, the reader should consult the reviews of Hörstadius (1950), Causey (1960), and Weston (1970).

Not all authors have agreed that the Schwann cell derives from neurectoderm. Cajal (1960) believed Schwann cells were recruited by neurites from primitive pluripotential cells in the adjacent mesenchyme, and Yntema (1943) agreed in part with this opinion. More recently, Feigin (1969) and Feigin and Ogata (1971) have argued, on the basis of study of pathologic material by conventional light microscopic techniques, that the Schwann cell is a mesenchymal element. Their argument is based on the observation that peripheral myelin and Schwann cells are on occasion found within plaques of multiple sclerosis in the central nervous system and have no apparent connection with any peripheral nerve structure, such as perivascular plexuses, from which they might have arisen. The peripheral myelin in this instance is said to ensheath central axons that have been

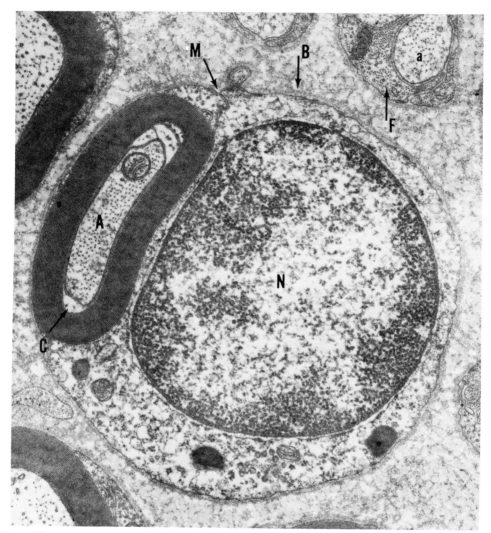

Figure 11–1 Electron micrograph of a Schwann cell with a normal myelinated axon from rabbit trigeminal nerve. The myelin sheath and axon are sectioned transversely at the level of the nucleus (N). The outer mesaxon originates at the Schwann cell surface at M. A thin layer of adaxonal Schwann cell cytoplasm (C) is seen at the top and the bottom of the axon (A). The entire Schwann cell is covered by basement membrane (B). Parts of two other myelinated axons are seen at top left and bottom left. Schwann cell cytoplasm with an invaginated unmyelinated axon (a) is seen at top right. Many small fibrils (F) are present in the Schwann cell cytoplasm, in addition to microtubules. × 24,000. (Electron micrograph by courtesy of Dr. J. R. Baringer.)

previously demyelinated. To explain their observations, Feigin and Ogata suggested that the Schwann cell is a mesenchymal element that, in plaques of multiple sclerosis, derives from primitive central nervous system cells. As further evidence, they cite the capacity of Schwann cells to make collagen and to transform into macrophages. These latter two arguments are controversial at best, and the observed "isolation" of Schwann cells and peripheral myelin in plaques of multiple sclerosis is fraught with possibilities for error.

Thus one must at present consider the case for mesenchymal derivation of the Schwann cell as unproved.

PROLIFERATION OF SCHWANN CELLS

During the development of peripheral nerve, intense proliferation of Schwann cells is prominent. This phenomenon has been most completely studied in rodents in which myelination of peripheral nerve is just beginning at the time of birth. Peters and Muir (1959), in their classic description of the events leading to myelination of nerve fibers by Schwann cells, showed that the numbers of Schwann cells in rat phrenic nerve increased by twentyfold in the final three embryonic days and that as many as 5 per cent of the Schwann cell nuclei were in mitosis at any single point during this period. They saw no Schwann cells in mitosis postnatally in rat phrenic nerve, but Diner (1965), using the electron microscope, found Schwann cells in mitosis in rat sciatic nerve throughout the first postnatal week. Schwann cells in which mitosis was taking place contained bundles of immature axons embedded in their cytoplasm. Apparently, once a Schwann cell has reduced its complement of enfolded axons to a single one and myelination is initiated, no further divisions of the Schwann cell take place unless some pathologic state supervenes.

Proliferation of Schwann cells in developing mouse sciatic nerve has been studied more quantitatively by radioautography and by adapting methods of determining the kinetics of cell proliferation (Asbury, 1967). It was found in two day old mouse sciatic nerve that about three quarters of the Schwann cells had ceased to divide; of these many presumably were initiating the sequence of myelin formation. The remaining one quarter of Schwann cells that were proliferating continued to divide at intervals of approximately 24 hours, with some ceasing to divide with each successive generation. This is best seen by examining the labeling index (proportion of cells incorporating tritiated thymidine injected an hour prior to sacrifice) on successive postnatal days. The labeling index drops from 16 per cent of all Schwann cells on the day of birth to 5 per cent by the fifth day and finally to 1 per cent by the ninth postnatal day (Asbury, unpublished observation). These observations are roughly comparable to those of Friede and Samorajski (1968) in the neonatal rat when one allows for differences in technique.

The duration of synthesis phase (that portion of interphase during which the cell nucleus takes up thymidine prefatory to the next division) in Schwann cells in two day old mouse sciatic nerve is approximately 8 to 10 hours, as determined by two different labeling methods (Asbury, 1967; Bradley and Asbury,

1970a). It is of interest that, in adult mouse sciatic nerve, Schwann cells that are proliferating in response to proximal transection of the nerve similarly exhibit an 8 to 10 hour synthesis phase (Bradley and Asbury, 1970a). These observations suggest a constancy of synthesis phase in Schwann cells whenever they proliferate. It remains to be seen whether constancy of generation time also obtains in dividing Schwann cells.

In the fully developed adult nerve there is a linear relationship between the size of myelinated axons and the length of their internodes (distance from one node of Ranvier to the next). The smallest myelinated fibers have the shortest internodes, approximately 0.4 mm, and the largest fibers have the longest internodes, approximately 1.4 mm. In order to achieve this arrangement in adult nerve, Schwann cells must space themselves along developing axons in an exact manner so that in the mature nerve the relation between axonal diameter and internodal length is maintained. Thus Schwann cell proliferation and the order in which division ceases would be controlled by a precise mechanism. One might speculate that proliferation would cease first in those Schwann cells associated with axons destined to be the largest, and the cells that continue to proliferate the longest would be those associated with the smallest myelinated axons or perhaps unmyelinated fibers. In this way, longitudinal growth of nerve that occurs during the period between the first and the last Schwann cell divisions would allow for the appropriate spacing of Schwann cells and account for the linear relationship between axonal size and internodal length. This possibility is supported by the oft-repeated observation that the largest fibers begin to myelinate first (see Skoglund and Romero, 1965, for references).

Another way can be postulated in which the linear relationship between axonal size and internodal length may come about in mature nerve. Friede and Samorajski (1968) suggest that myelination in all nerve fibers so destined begins more or less simultaneously in rat sciatic nerve. Berthold and Skoglund (1968) in studying ventral root maturation in the kitten found numbers of unusual short internodes measuring from 10 to 50 μm in length after myelination was well-advanced in the larger fibers. These short intercalated internodes showed extreme buckling, bulging, and redundancy of the myelin sheath and degenerating myelin in some. It appeared as though the foreshortened, accordion-folded internodes were compressed by adjacent internodes that were extending in length, and eventually the short ones were squeezed away from the axon. In an attempt to synthesize the observations just described, one might postulate that early in development all myelinated fibers have short internodes, but in later stages, the larger fibers attain longer internodes by a process of elongation of certain internodes and elimination of others.

As recorded in several electron microscope studies, the sequence of events in developing peripheral nerve in the human fetus appears to be similar to that in rodents, but the timing is different (Gamble and Breathnach, 1965; Cravioto, 1965; Gamble, 1966; Ochoa, 1971). In human nerve, Schwann cell proliferation is complete and myelination itself is well-advanced by the end of the second trimester of pregnancy, but in rodent nerve this process takes place on the last embryonic day or so and first two weeks postnatally (Friede and Samorajski, 1968; Webster, 1971).

MORPHOLOGIC FEATURES OF SCHWANN CELLS

Within the peripheral nervous system, Schwann cells ensheath every axon, whether myelinated or unmyelinated, from the root entry and exit zones to the distal axonal terminations. Their characteristic morphologic features are described fully in Chapters 6 and 7 and need not be repeated here except to emphasize a few salient aspects. First of all, peripheral myelin is derived from Schwann cell surface membrane by a complex process of infolding and compaction to form the characteristic lamellated myelin pattern. Second, a single Schwann cell forms each internode of myelin in its entirety, and a single Schwann cell never associates itself with more than one myelinated axon. In contrast, with unmyelinated fibers, up to 30 or so small axons lie in troughlike invaginations of a single Schwann cell surface. Third, all Schwann cells are coated by basement membrane, a feature that allows their clear distinction from fibroblasts, macrophages, and mast cells, but not from pericytes, which also have basement membrane. Basement membrane forms a continuous tubelike covering across nodes of

Ranvier, the latter representing the junction between two adjacent Schwann cells.

SCHWANN CELL RELATIONSHIP TO AXONS

Schwann cells and axons manifest an intimate and interdependent relationship with one another. Except in special instances, the ability of an axon to conduct normally probably depends upon Schwann cell investment, and conversely the structural integrity of myelin sheath depends upon its containing an intact axon. Nevertheless, the axon seems to play a controlling role in this relationship, a point of view illustrated by the seldom cited cross union experiments of Simpson and Young (1945). In rabbits, they transected neighboring nerve trunks, one with a full complement of heavily myelinated fibers and the other with only a few lightly myelinated fibers, and sutured the proximal stump of the heavily myelinated nerve trunk to the distal stump of the lightly myelinated one. After several months they noted that regeneration had taken place and that there were now many myelinated fibers in the distal stump that had previously contained only unmyelinated fibers and a few lightly myelinated ones. In light of what has been learned about myelination and remyelination in the past two decades, it must be concluded that the Schwann cells in the distal stump, which had originally made little or no myelin, were now induced to spin thick myelin sheaths. The only other possibility would have the Schwann cells in the proximal stump proliferating to a massive extent and migrating into the distal stump ahead of the regenerating axons to take up their former duties in a new location. This seems highly unlikely because little proliferation and outgrowth of Schwann cells from the proximal stump is observed (Thomas, 1966). From this evidence, we are led to the conclusion that Schwann cells are multipotential with respect to their ability to make myelin, and whether a given Schwann cell makes myelin or not during development depends upon the type of axon or axons with which it becomes associated.

Beyond their role in myelin formation and maintenance, Schwann cells also seem to have a nutritive function with respect to the axon. It is well known that severe local ischemia of nerve trunk produces axonal damage as well as injury to other elements of the nerve trunk. Pertinent examples may be seen in the peripheral nerve lesions encountered in periarteritis nodosa, and other ischemic neuropathies (for further discussion see Asbury, 1970b). This observation implies that the axon depends in some measure upon locally derived metabolites for its sustenance. Direct evidence is provided by the experiments of Singer and Salpeter (1966), who found by serial radioautographic analyses that tritiated 1-histidine is transported from the lumen of endoneurial capillaries through Schwann cell and myelin sheath into the axon.

SCHWANN CELLS IN WALLERIAN DEGENERATION

Many of the early events in wallerian degeneration are axonal, such as transient focal accumulation of organelles in paranodal axoplasm (Webster, 1962b) and the appearance within hours of abundant acid phosphatase activity within axoplasm in the distal stump (Gould and Holt, 1961). Schwann cells also are involved intimately in the process of wallerian degeneration from the earliest stages, as well as playing a major and determining role in the success of subsequent regeneration.

In wallerian degeneration one of the first changes in Schwann cells is seen in the Schmidt-Lanterman incisures, which are best seen in longitudinal section as periodic oblique discontinuities in the myelin sheath. Ultrastructurally the incisure, or cleft, is formed by splitting of the major dense line of each myelin lamella to enclose a small collar of Schwann cell cytoplasm (Robertson, 1958). Each collar overlaps the neighboring one in a telescoping fashion to produce the characteristic oblique interruption of the myelin sheath seen by light microscopy. Clefts are thought to provide a pathway connecting the perikaryal Schwann cell cytoplasm to the thin inner rim of adaxonal cytoplasm. Clefts have been observed to open and close at intervals (Singer and Bryant, 1969), a phenomenon said to produce flow of cytoplasm into the adaxonal layer. During wallerian degeneration, Webster (1965) has claimed, the number of clefts per internode increases in the first 12 to 24 hours, with a disproportionate number of new clefts forming paranodally. Segmentation of myelin

into ovoids begins paranodally, the boundaries of each ovoid being formed by clefts.

Concomitant with segmentation of myelin and formation of degenerating ovoids, striking increases of Schwann cell lysosomal activity take place (Holtzman and Novikoff, 1965). Myelin ovoids are encased in an envelope of Schwann cell cytoplasm and are progressively subdivided into smaller digestive vacuoles. Thus the early stages of myelin degradation occur in an autophagic manner within the same Schwann cells that originally produced the myelin sheath. According to Holtzman and Novikoff (1965), later digestion of myelin occurs in "transformed" Schwann cells, which exhibit intense lysosomal activity and otherwise have all the structural characteristics of macrophages. Whether Schwann cells are actually transformed into typical appearing macrophages is a matter of considerable controversy and is reviewed in more detail in the section on Schwann cells as phagocytes.

As for destruction of the axon, most observers have agreed that it degenerates and fragments in a relatively autochthonous fashion. Recently Singer and Steinberg (1972) challenged this view and suggested a much more active role for Schwann cells in mediating the destruction of the axon. In their electron microscopic studies of wallerian degeneration and colchicine intoxication in the newt, they found early swelling of Schwann cell cytoplasm in the adaxonal layer and Schmidt-Lanterman clefts, followed by lysis and erosion of both the inner Schwann cell limiting membrane and the axolemma with invasion of axoplasm by Schwann cell organelles. Most axoplasmic elements disappeared quickly except neurofilaments, which became compressed into a core at the center of the axon to be digested later. According to the view of Singer and Steinberg, once the axon is deprived of "trophic" factors by interruption of axoplasmic flow because of proximal transection, then the Schwann cell quickly turns upon its own myelin sheath and the axon and destroys both.

Proliferation of Schwann cells is a regular feature of wallerian degeneration. Early studies of the phenomenon by light microscopy were hampered by the inability to identify with assurance the nature of all the cells participating in the reaction. The result was that estimates of intrinsic cell proliferation were somewhat falsely high (Abercrombie and Johnson, 1946; Thomas, 1948). With

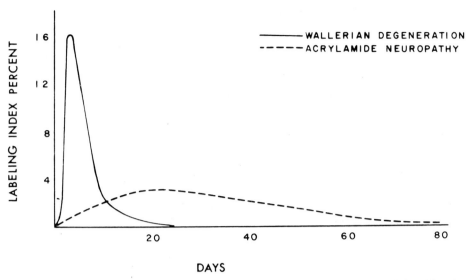

Figure 11–2   Proliferation of Schwann cells as determined by the incorporation of tritiated thymidine in two types of experimental neuropathy. The proportion of all Schwann cells taking up label is indicated on the ordinate, and the days after nerve transection in the case of wallerian degeneration and the days after the first signs of axonal breakdown in the case of acrylamide neuropathy are indicated on the abscissa. In wallerian degeneration there is a brief wave of Schwann cell proliferative activity, but in acrylamide polyneuropathy proliferation is more prolonged and less intense.

the advent of newer techniques, confirmation of Schwann cell proliferation was obtained, and uncertainties about Schwann cell identification, even by light microscopy when the preparations were technically critical, diminished. In well-myelinated nerves, a two to three fold increase in Schwann cells occurs in the distal nerve in response to a single crush, the proliferating Schwann cells tending to line up in columns to form the "bands of Büngner" within Schwann tubes (Holmes and Young, 1942). Schwann tubes have been shown by Thomas (1964) to consist of the original basement membrane and adjacent collagen fibers. If the nerve is crushed a second time, a further increase in Schwann cells occurs (Abercrombie and Santler, 1957). Indeed this ability of Schwann cells to proliferate in response to wallerian degeneration persists even if the nerve is crushed up to nine times (Thomas, 1970).

When proliferation of Schwann cells in mouse sciatic nerve is studied radioautographically using tritiated thymidine, a·brief wave of divisions takes place and rapidly subsides (Fig. 11–2) (Bradley and Asbury, 1970a). Friede and Johnstone (1967) have also studied Schwann cell proliferation by histologic radioautography in rat sciatic nerve during wallerian degeneration, and found a somewhat later and more prolonged response

than in the mouse. The vigorous wave of proliferation in wallerian degeneration contrasts with the indolent but sustained proliferation of Schwann cells in experimental polyneuropathy produced by acrylamide in the mouse as shown in Figure 11–2 (Bradley and Asbury, 1970b). The difference in these two patterns of Schwann cell proliferation is probably accounted for by the differing rates of axonal breakdown, rapid and simultaneous in wallerian degeneration and protracted in acrylamide neuropathy. Yet a third pattern is seen in experimental allergic neuritis, a primarily demyelinative neuropathy, in which Schwann cell proliferation occurs as a secondary wave 10 days following invasion of the nerve by intensely proliferating inflammatory cells (Asbury and Arnason, 1968).

SCHWANN CELLS AS PHAGOCYTES

The concept that Schwann cells might manifest phagocytic capability was first broached by Weiss (1944) and Weiss and Wang (1945) and was based on their tissue culture observations of nerve explants. In a more recent review, Guth (1956) states that "proliferated neurilemma cells are phagocytic and account for the bulk of the phagocytic activity in degeneration." Palmer, Rees, and Weddell (1961) injected either carbon particles or colloidal gold into degenerating nerve and also into the severance gap, and found that the inert material was phagocytized. They claimed that the cells that had taken up the foreign material were derived from Schwann cells, although the observed cells were indistinguishable from macrophages in any locus and had numerous processes and no basement membrane. Holtzman and Novikoff (1965) similarly suggested that macrophages they observed in degenerating rat sciatic nerve were "transformed" Schwann cells. Although this point of view has been often repeated, Schwann cell transformation into macrophage has not been documented rigorously. On the contrary there is a substantial body of evidence to suggest that macrophages in degenerating nerve are of hematogenous origin.

In recent years, extensive experimental analysis of the origins of macrophages in a wide range of pathologic reactions indicates that macrophages derive from monocytes that take origin in bone marrow and circulate in peripheral blood (Konigsmark and Sidman, 1963; Volkman and Gowans, 1965; Spector et al., 1965; Van Furth and Cohn, 1968; Roser, 1970). With these data in mind, one would suspect that reactions calling forth macrophages in peripheral nerve are not different from phagocytic responses in other tissues. Olsson and Sjöstrand (1969) tentatively concluded from their radioautographic study in the mouse that part of the macrophage population in degenerating peripheral nerve was hematogenous. Using a different radioautographic approach, Asbury (1970a) adduced evidence that virtually all macrophages in wallerian degeneration were hematogenous in origin.

This experiment (Asbury, 1970a) is described in more detail because it takes advantage of an approach that allows a clearer interpretation than is possible with the usual maneuver of injecting a labeling substance and making an experimental lesion shortly thereafter. Multiple daily doses of tritiated thymidine were given to mice in the neonatal period, and the mice were allowed subsequently to grow to maturity. In this way, Schwann cells and endothelial cells in peripheral nerve remained permanently labeled, but normally renewing cell populations, such as bone marrow– and lymph node–derived circulating leukocytes, became unlabeled through repeated division. After several months, over 60 per cent of Schwann cells were still labeled, but only a rare circulating lymphocyte (Table 11–1). When wallerian degeneration was studied at 5, 10, and 15 days following transection of the nerve, virtually none of the macrophages contained any tritium label (Fig. 11–3). The finding that the macrophage population was completely unlabeled at all time points, including five days following nerve transection, strongly suggests that they could not be derived from Schwann cells, a highly labeled population. Because the circulating leukocytes were entirely unlabeled, it was concluded that phagocytes in degenerating mouse sciatic nerve were most likely of hematogenous origin.

TABLE 11–1 CELL COUNTS AND LABELING INDICES IN TRANSECTED ADULT MOUSE SCIATIC NERVE*

Cell Type	5 Days		10 Days		15 Days	
	Number	*Per Cent Labeled*	*Number*	*Per Cent Labeled*	*Number*	*Per Cent Labeled*
Schwann	362	40	360	24	384	11
Phagocyte	37	0	86	0	73	1
Endothelial	31	39	7	28	14	7
Polymorphonuclear	28	0	24	0	9	0
Mononuclear	28	0	19	0	12	0
Mast cell	3	0	1	0	1	0
Unclassified	11	0	3	0	7	28
Total	500		500		500	

*Nerves were transected 5, 10, and 15 days previously. Mice received daily thymidine–^{3}H injections for the first 10 postnatal days, and were sacrificed five months later.

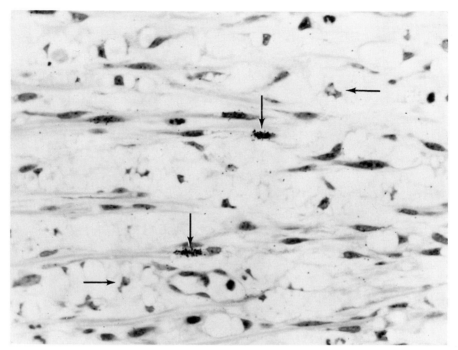

Figure 11–3 Histologic radioautogram of mouse sciatic nerve 15 days after proximal nerve transection. Schwann cell nuclei are seen as elongated spindle-shaped structures, often in columns. Several nuclei are still heavily labeled (vertical arrows). See text for explanation; also see legend for Figure 11–4. Many lipid-laden macrophages, none of which are labeled, are scattered in the interstices of the degenerating nerve (horizontal arrows).

At successive intervals following nerve transection, labeling of Schwann cells decreased progressively from a control value of 63 per cent to 11 per cent by 15 days (Fig. 11–4). This decline represents serial dilution of labeled DNA by the vigorous proliferative response known to occur in Schwann cells during wallerian degeneration. Seeking an alternate explanation for the unlabeled macrophages, one might ask whether Schwann cells could divide enough times to dilute incorporated label below threshold level prior to transformation into macrophages. This possibility is unlikely for two reasons: first, because at five days after transection too brief an interval after onset of Schwann cell proliferation had been provided for the necessary number of cell divisions to occur, and second, because the rate of decline of labeling index does not indicate a rapid enough proliferative rate to account for the observation that all macrophages were unlabeled.

Question was raised concerning the long-term effects of incorporated tritium in the Schwann cells. Could it hamper their ability to proliferate in response to nerve transection proximally? This question was explored by examining the most heavily labeled portion of the Schwann cell population, those cells with 25 silver grains or more per nucleus. The rate of proliferation in this subpopulation of Schwann cells was comparable to that for all labeled Schwann cells including the lightly labeled ones. This evidence suggests that radiation effects were negligible.

If Schwann cells begin the process of myelin degradation by forming autophagic vacuoles, and if macrophages migrate into degenerating nerve from the blood stream to complete the process of myelin breakdown, then it follows logically that Schwann cells and macrophages must interact at some stage to effect the exchange of myelin breakdown products. The exact nature of this putative event has not been clearly defined, despite a welter of electron microscopic studies of wallerian degeneration.

SCHWANN CELL SURFACES

One need only consider that peripheral myelin is specialized Schwann cell surface membrane to realize that Schwann cells possess extraordinary cell surface character-

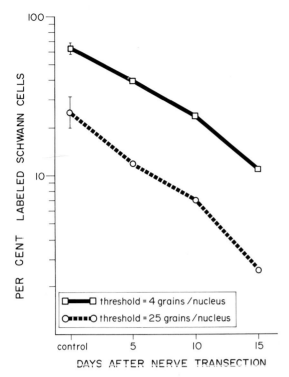

Figure 11–4 Graph of Schwann cell labeling index plotted semilogarithmically against time after nerve transection. Control values were obtained from untransected nerves. Vertical bars indicate the range from mouse to mouse. Control values represent the numbers of labeled Schwann cells in normal nerves in adult mice that had received daily injections of tritiated thymidine for the first 10 postnatal days and then were allowed to mature. Average labeling index of Schwann cells at five months of age was 63 per cent. Decreasing values of Schwann cell labeling are noted at 5, 10, and 15 days following transection because of Schwann cell proliferation in response to wallerian degeneration (solid line). Even Schwann cells with the heaviest labeling of nuclei (interrupted line) proliferated in the reaction at a rate comparable to all Schwann cells, indicating that radiation damage of Schwann cells did not occur.

istics. A single Schwann cell enclosing a large axon may produce up to 100 lamellae of compact myelin, each extending for a distance of 1.5 mm. Rough calculation shows that a single Schwann cell may lay down an expanse of membrane measuring more than 10 mm².

In neuropathic states, when axons disappear, Schwann cells thus liberated tend to produce sinuous cytoplasmic process, which intertwine and convolute with other similar processes (Fig. 11–5). Ochoa and Vial (1967) studied in detail the geometry of Schwann cell cytoplasm complexes in chronic neuropathies in humans. They postulated that Schwann cell surfaces tend to grow in contact with the surface of other Schwann cell processes to produce formations of such complexity. Schwann cell processes also encircle small bundles of collagen fibers much as they might invest an unmyelinated fiber. These collagen–Schwann cell formations have been termed collagen pockets (Gamble, 1964; Gamble and Eames, 1964). Although collagen pockets may on occasion be encountered in otherwise normal nerve, their presence in any number suggests loss of unmyelinated fibers (Ochoa and Mair, 1969; Aguayo et al., 1971). Recently Ohta and co-workers (1973) have equated complex Schwann cell cytoplasm formations and collagen pockets with regenerative nerve sprouting rather than with nerve fiber loss alone.

OTHER SCHWANN CELL CHARACTERISTICS

Brief mention should be made of several other Schwann cell qualities. They are the nerve elements most vulnerable to ischemia (Eames and Lange, 1967). Minor amounts of x-irradiation may compromise the ability of Schwann cells to proliferate during subsequent wallerian degeneration (Cavanagh, 1968). Schwann cells appear to provide a haven for *Mycobacterium leprae* bacilli in lepromatous leprosy (Lumsden, 1964; Job, 1970). In some systemic storage diseases involving primarily the central nervous system, Schwann cells may also participate in the cytoplasmic accumulation of storage product, for example in Krabbe's disease (Bischoff and Ulrich, 1969) and metachromatic leukodystrophy (Webster, 1962a), giving rise to a demyelinative neuropathy.

Endoneurial collagen fiber production by Schwann cells has been postulated. Nathaniel and Pease (1963) ascribed to Schwann cells the production of endoneurial collagen in regenerating dorsal roots in the rat because, in their view, too few fibroblasts were present to account for the amount of collagen deposition they observed. The question of Schwann cell production of collagen is somewhat complicated by the fact that basement membrane is also a form of collagen, although basement membrane collagen is formed from a different combination and configuration of polypeptide chains than interstitial collagen and also has a different polysaccharide matrix (see review of Grant and Prockop, 1972). Schwann

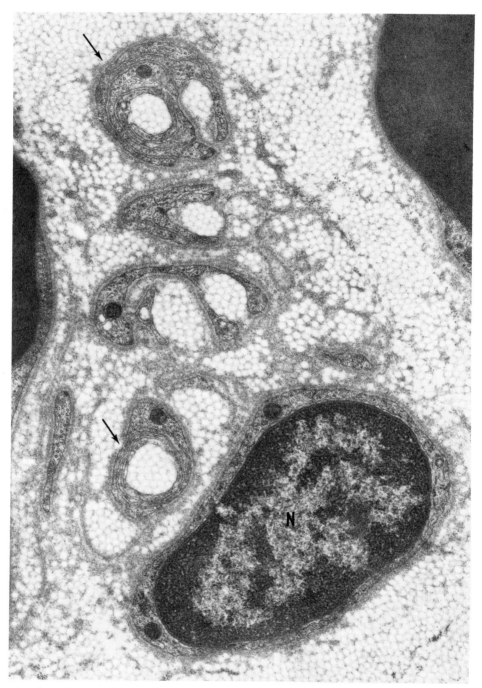

Figure 11–5   Electron micrograph of a sural nerve biopsy from a patient with chronic *n*-hexane neuropathy. Note the complex Schwann cell formations (arrows) often enclosing small bundles of collagen fibers. Each formation is bounded by basement membrane. Parts of two myelin sheaths are seen at right and left, and a Schwann nucleus (N) is seen at lower right. × 17,000.

cells are lined with basement membrane, which the Schwann cell is thought to be capable of synthesizing. In vitro evidence for this point is provided by Church, Tanger, and Pfeiffer (1973), who showed that cloned cultures of neoplastic Schwann cells synthesize collagen monomer. In addition, embryonic corneal epithelium and spinal cord may also synthesize collagen (Trelstad and Coulombre, 1971; Trelstad et al., 1973). Although it is likely that Schwann cells can produce the collagen contained in their basement membrane, considerable doubt exists whether Schwann cells have a role in the production of endoneurial collagen fibers.

REFERENCES

Abercrombie, M., and Johnson, M. L.: Quantitative histology of wallerian degeneration. I. Nuclear population in rabbit sciatic nerve. J. Anat., 80:37, 1946.

Abercrombie, M., and Santler, J.: An analysis of growth in nuclear population during wallerian degeneration. J. Cell. Comp. Physiol., 50:429, 1957.

Aguayo, A. J., Nair, C. P. V., and Bray, G. M.: Peripheral nerve abnormalities in the Riley-Day syndrome. Arch. Neurol., 24:106, 1971.

Asbury, A. K.: Schwann cell proliferation in developing mouse sciatic nerve. J. Cell Biol., 34:735, 1967.

Asbury, A. K.: The histogenesis of phagocytes during wallerian degeneration. Proceedings of VIth International Congress of Neuropathology. Paris, Masson et Cie, 1970a, p. 666.

Asbury, A. K.: Ischemic disorders of peripheral nerve. In Vinken, P. J., and Bruyn, G. W. (eds.): Handbook of Clinical Neurology. Vol. 8. Amsterdam, North-Holland Publishing Co., 1970b.

Asbury, A. K., and Arnason, B. G.: Experimental allergic neuritis: a radioautographic study. J. Neuropathol. Exp. Neurol., 27:581, 1968.

Berthold, C. H., and Skoglund, S.: Postnatal development of feline paranodal myelin-sheath segments. II. Electron microscopy. Acta Med. Soc. Upsal., 73:127, 1968.

Bischoff, A., and Ulrich, J.: Peripheral neuropathy in globoid cell leukodystrophy (Krabbe's disease). Ultrastructural and histochemical findings. Brain, 92:861, 1969.

Bradley, W. G., and Asbury, A. K.: Duration of synthesis phase in neurilemma cells in mouse sciatic nerve during degeneration. Exp. Neurol., 26:275, 1970a.

Bradley, W. G., and Asbury, A. K.: Radioautographic studies of Schwann cell behavior. I. Acrylamide neuropathy in the mouse. J. Neuropathol. Exp. Neurol., 29:500, 1970b.

Cajal, S. R.: Studies on vertebrate neurogenesis. Translated by L. Guth. Springfield, Ill., Charles C Thomas, 1960.

Causey, G.: The Cell of Schwann. Baltimore, Williams and Wilkins Co., 1960.

Cavanagh, J. B.: Effects of x-irradiation on the prolif-

eration of cells in peripheral nerve during wallerian degeneration in the rat. Br. J. Radiol., 41:275, 1968.

Church, R. L., Tanzer, M. L., and Pfeiffer, S. E.: Collagen and procollagen production by a clonal line of Schwann cells. Proc. Nat. Acad. Sci. U.S.A., 70:1943, 1973.

Cravioto, H.: The role of Schwann cells in the development of human peripheral nerves. J. Ultrastruct. Res., 12:634, 1965.

Diner, O.: Les cellules de Schwann en mitose et leurs rapports avec les axones au cours du developpement du nerf sciatique chez le rat. C.R. Acad. Sci. (Paris), 261:1731, 1965.

Eames, R. A., and Lange, L. S.: Clinical and pathological study of ischaemic neuropathy. J. Neurol. Neurosurg. Psychiatry, 30:215, 1967.

Feigin, I.: Mesenchymal tissues of the nervous system. J. Neuropathol. Exp. Neurol., 28:6, 1969.

Feigin, I., and Ogata, J.: Schwann cells and peripheral myelin within human central nervous tissues: the mesenchymal character of Schwann cells. J. Neuropathol. Exp. Neurol., 30:603, 1971.

Friede, R. L., and Johnstone, M. A.: Responses of thymidine labeling of nuclei in gray matter and nerve following sciatic transection. Acta Neuropathol. (Berl.), 7:281, 1967.

Friede, R. L., and Samorajski, T.: Myelin formation in the sciatic nerve of the rat. J. Neuropathol. Exp. Neurol., 27:546, 1968.

Gamble, H. J.: Comparative electron-microscope observations on the connective tissues of a peripheral nerve and a spinal nerve root in the rat. J. Anat., 98:17, 1964.

Gamble, H. J.: Further electron microscope studies of human foetal peripheral nerves. J. Anat., 100:487, 1966.

Gamble, H. J., and Breathnach, A. S.: An electron microscope study of human foetal peripheral nerves. J. Anat., 99:573, 1965.

Gamble, H. J., and Eames, R. A.: An electron microscope study of the connective tissues of human peripheral nerve. J. Anat., 98:655, 1964.

Gould, R. P., and Holt, S. J.: Observations on acid phosphatase and esterases in the rat sciatic nerve undergoing wallerian degeneration. In Cytology of Nervous Tissue. London, Taylor & Francis, 1961, p. 45.

Grant, M. E., and Prockop, E. J.: The biosynthesis of collagen. N. Engl. J. Med., 286:194–199, 242–249, 291–300, 1972.

Guth, L.: Regeneration in the mammalian peripheral nervous system. Physiol. Rev., 36:441, 1956.

Harrison, R. G.: Neuroblast versus sheath cell in the development of peripheral nerves. J. Comp. Neurol., 37:123, 1924.

Holmes, W., and Young, J. Z.: Nerve regeneration after immediate and delayed suture. J. Anat., 77:63, 1942.

Holtzman, E., and Novikoff, A. B.: Lysosomes in the rat sciatic nerve following crush. J. Cell Biol., 27:651, 1965.

Hörstadius, S.: The Neural Crest. London, Oxford University Press, 1950.

Job, C. K.: Mycobacterium leprae in nerve lesions in lepromatous leprosy. Arch. Pathol., 89:195, 1970.

Konigsmark, B. W., and Sidman, R. L.: Origin of brain macrophages in the mouse. J. Neuropathol. Exp. Neurol., 22:643, 1963.

Kuntz, A.: Experimental studies on the histogenesis of the sympathetic nervous system. J. Comp. Neurol., 34:1, 1922.

Lumsden, C. E.: Leprosy and the Schwann cell in vivo and in vitro. *In* Cochrane, R. G., and Davey, C. T. (eds.): Leprosy in Theory and Practice. 2nd edition. Bristol, Wright & Sons, 1964.

Nathaniel, E. J. H., and Pease, D. C.: Collagen and basement membrane formation by Schwann cells during nerve regeneration. J. Ultrastruct. Res., *9*:550, 1963.

Ochoa, J.: The sural nerve of the human foetus: electron microscope observations and counts of axons. J. Anat., *108*:231, 1971.

Ochoa, J., and Mair, W. G. P.: The normal sural nerve in man. II. Changes in the axons and Schwann cells due to aging. Acta Neuropathol. (Berl.), *13*:217, 1969.

Ochoa, J., and Vial, J. D.: Behavior of peripheral nerve structures in chronic neuropathies, with special reference to the Schwann cell. J. Anat., *102*:95, 1967.

Ohta, M., Ellefson, R. D., Lambert, E. H., and Dyck, P. J.: Hereditary sensory neuropathy, type II. Arch. Neurol., *29*:23, 1973.

Olsson, Y., and Sjöstrand, J.: Origin of macrophages in wallerian degeneration of peripheral nerves demonstrated autoradiographically. Exp. Neurol., *23*:102, 1969.

Palmer, E., Rees, R. J. W., and Weddell, G.: The phagocytic activity of Schwann cells. *In* Cytology of Nervous Tissue. London, Taylor & Francis, 1961, p. 49.

Peters, A., and Muir, A. R.: The relationship between axons and Schwann cells during development of peripheral nerves in the rat. Q.J. Exp. Physiol., *44*:117, 1959.

Raven, C. P.: Experiments on the origin of the sheath cells and sympathetic neuroblasts in amphibia. J. Comp. Neurol., *67*:221, 1937.

Robertson, J. D.: The ultrastructure of Schmidt-Lanterman clefts and related shearing defects of the myelin sheath. J. Biophys. Biochem. Cytol., *4*:39, 1958.

Roser, B.: The origins, kinetics, and fate of macrophage populations. J. Reticuloendothel. Soc., *8*:139, 1970.

Simpson, S. A., and Young, J. Z.: Regeneration of fibre diameter after cross-union of visceral and somatic nerves. J. Anat., *79*:48, 1945.

Singer, M., and Bryant, S. V.: Movement in the myelin Schwann sheath of the vertebrate axon. Nature (Lond.), *221*:1148, 1969.

Singer, M., and Salpeter, M. M.: The transport of ^{3}H-1-histidine through the Schwann and myelin sheath into the axon, including a re-evaluation of myelin function. J. Morphol., *120*:281, 1966.

Singer, M., and Steinberg, M. C.: Wallerian degeneration: a re-evaluation based on transected and colchicine-poisoned nerves in the amphibian, Triturus. Am. J. Anat., *133*:51, 1972.

Skoglund, S., and Romero, C.: Postnatal growth of spinal nerves and roots. Acta Physiol. Scand., *66*:Suppl. 260, 1965.

Spector, W. G., Walters, M. N. I., and Willoughby, D. A.: The origin of the mononuclear cells in inflammatory exudates induced by fibrinogen. J. Pathol. Bacteriol., *90*:181, 1965.

Thomas, G. A.: Quantitative histology of wallerian degeneration. II. Nuclear population in two nerves of different fibre spectrum. J. Anat., *82*:135, 1948.

Thomas, P. K.: The cellular response to nerve injury. 1. The cellular outgrowth from the distal stump of transected nerve. J. Anat., *100*:287, 1966.

Thomas, P. K.: The cellular response to nerve injury. III. The effect of repeated crushes. J. Anat., *106*: 463, 1970.

Trelstad, R. L., and Coulombre, A. J.: Morphogenesis of the collagenous stroma in the chick cornea. J. Cell Biol., *50*:840, 1971.

Trelstad, R. L., Kang, A. H., Cohen, A. M., and Hay, E. D.: Collagen synthesis in vitro by embryonic spinal cord endothelium. Science, *179*:295, 1973.

Van Furth, R., and Cohn, Z. A.: The origin and kinetics of mononuclear phagocytes. J. Exp. Med., *128*:415, 1968.

Volkman, A., and Gowans, J. L.: The origin of macrophages from bone marrow in the rat. Br. J. Exp. Pathol., *46*:62, 1965.

Webster, H. deF.: Schwann cell alterations in metachromatic leukodystrophy: preliminary phase and electron microscopic observations. J. Neuropathol. Exp. Neurol., *21*:534, 1962a.

Webster, H. deF.: Transient focal accumulation of axonal mitochondria during the early stages of wallerian degeneration. J. Cell Biol., *12*:361, 1962b.

Webster, H. deF.: The relationship between Schmidt-Lanterman incisures and myelin segmentation during wallerian degeneration. Ann. N.Y. Acad. Sci., *122*:29, 1965.

Webster, H. deF.: The geometry of peripheral myelin sheaths during their formation and growth in rat sciatic nerves. J. Cell Biol., *48*:348, 1971.

Weiss, P.: In vitro transformation of spindle cells of neural origin into macrophages. Anat. Rec., *88*:205, 1944.

Weiss, P., and Wang, H.: Transformation of adult Schwann cells into macrophages. Proc. Soc. Exp. Biol. Med., *58*:273, 1945.

Weston, J. A.: A radioautographic analysis of the migration and localization of trunk neural crest cells in the chick. Dev. Biol., *6*:279, 1963.

Weston, J. A.: The migration and differentiation of neural crest cells. *In* Abercrombie, M., Brachet, J., and King, T. (eds.): Advances in Morphogenesis. Vol. 8. New York, Academic Press, 1970.

Yntema, C. L.: Deficient efferent innervation of the extremities following removal of the neural crest in Amblystoma. J. Exp. Zool., *94*:319, 1943.

Chapter 12

AXOPLASMIC TRANSPORT — A BASIS FOR NEURAL PATHOLOGY

Sidney Ochs

Our concept of neuronal function has been revolutionized in recent years by the awareness that systems of material transport exist within the nerve fibers. The neuron cell body is recognized as having a relatively high level of protein synthesis carried out in the ribosomes associated with endoplasmic reticulum, the classic Nissl bodies (Palay and Palade, 1955). The synthesized proteins and other materials are then conveyed along the length of the nerve fiber by both a slow and a fast rate of axoplasmic transport. In part, transported materials serve to maintain those processes in the nerve essential for the conduction of the nerve impulse. In accord with the view of the membrane as a lipid bilayer with globular protein placed in it (Singer, 1972), the proteins consumed in the implied turnover in the nerve membrane would be constantly replenished through axoplasmic transport. The proteins in the membrane likely confer ion selectivity upon it. The failure of membrane potential and excitability in a nerve distal to a transection, which occurs during wallerian degeneration (cf. Chapter 16), suggests the loss of some key elements, probably protein, needed for the maintenance of function.

This dependency was first inferred by Waller (1852), who found, on cutting a nerve or the ventral root, the occurrence of degeneration distal to the transection, and on cutting the dorsal root, degeneration in the dorsal root fibers proximal to the cut. Waller, therefore, inferred a "nutritive" (trophic) control of the sensory fibers by the dorsal root ganglion

and a similar "trophic" control over the motor fibers by motor neurons in the spinal cord. His conception may be appreciated from the following translation:

As long as the influence of the ganglion over the nerve fibers occurs, this equilibrium (forces of renewal as opposed to those of degeneration) is maintained, but as soon as the connection of the ganglion corpuscle with the nerve fiber is destroyed its peripheral (severed) end is eliminated (subjected to forces of degeneration) (Waller, 1852).

Such specific reference to the dependence of the nerve fiber on the cell body (corpuscle) for its viability may seem too modern a reading if we consider the present view of the neuron to have started with Waldeyer (1891). The origin of the nerve fiber from the cell body had, however, already been described by Remak, Helmholtz, and Wagner before Waller's investigations (cf. Ramon y Cajal, 1928; Van der Loos, 1967; Clarke and O'Malley, 1968). The historical development of the concept of the control exerted by the cell body over nerve fibers will be treated elsewhere.

In addition to the dependence of the nerve fiber on the cell body and transported materials, nerve terminal structures and transmission at the synapse are influenced by down-transported elements. Synaptic transmission is seen to fail some 48 or so hours after motor nerve transection. Transsynaptic effects in muscle after nerve section are shown by the changes in metabolism, twitch duration, hyperexcitability with reduced membrane potential, and the presence of new receptor protein outside the endplate region found in muscle fiber deprived of its motor nerve (Gutmann, 1964; Guth, 1968; Drachman, 1974). Similar "trophic" influences are known for the secondary cells related to the sensory endings; the classic case is the regressive changes seen in taste buds following their denervation (Zelená, 1964; Guth, 1971).

This dynamic view of the neuron can provide a rationale for a number of nerve and muscle diseases whose etiology is at present obscure. An alteration in the amount of the materials made in the cell body or a defect in the metabolic processes of axonal transport of the nerve fiber could lead to failure of nerve excitability, synaptic transmission, sensory reception or the function of innervated cells, i.e., of muscle, or in the central nervous system, of other neurons in which a similar trophic control has been invoked. Studies relating axoplasmic transport to various neuropathologic entities were described several years ago at a symposium on axonal flow (Friede and Seitlberger, 1971), and a systematic view of a variety of neuropathologic entities possibly related to axoplasmic transport is discussed in this book by Dyck (Chapter 15).

In this chapter the main properties of fast axoplasmic transport and the mechanism that has been proposed to account for it are described. Only in relatively recent years has a fast movement of materials been recognized in addition to the slow transport system first indicated by the work of Weiss and Hiscoe (1948). A satisfactory view of slow transport and a likely mechanism have been difficult to arrive at, but recent new contributions pointing toward their clarification are briefly noted. Emphasis is placed on the fast transport system because it better accounts for the rapid wallerian changes occurring a few days after transection and over long lengths of nerve than does slow transport with the rate of several millimeters per day ascribed to it. In the main, the properties of fast axoplasmic transport described in this chapter are those observed in mammalian nerve by using an isotope labeling technique. Furthermore, fast axoplasmic transport can be maintained in vitro, and this has opened the way for studies showing the close dependence of fast transport on oxidative metabolism. Those studies indicate that the supply of energy required by the underlying transport mechanism is most likely in the form of adenosine triphosphate.

The dependence of fast axoplasmic transport on metabolism explains the requirement of nerve for its vascular supply. This is discussed with respect to recent experiments on the effects of vascular stripping and compression in vivo to produce ischemia to cause a block of fast axoplasmic transport. Finally, axoplasmic transport in the central nervous system and its use to trace fiber systems are presented because of the important developments to be expected in this field. It is hoped that this brief survey and the references given will serve as a guide to what is a potentially important field of study for the clinician.

FAST AXOPLASMIC TRANSPORT

Comparative Aspects and Materials Carried

A determination of the rate of fast axoplasmic transport in the nerves of different mammalian species was recently carried out for two reasons: (1) the uniformity or lack of uniformity of the rate of fast axoplasmic transport bears on the mechanism proposed to account for it; and (2) if the same rate of fast axoplasmic transport is present in a wide range of animals, the result can be extrapolated to man (Ochs, 1972a). The immediate impetus for the study stemmed from the previously reported range of fast axoplasmic transport rates of from 50 mm per day to over 2000 mm per day (Schmitt, 1968; Dahlström, 1971). Such rate variations are likely to be due in part to the lower rates present in some invertebrate and lower vertebrate nerve fibers and in part to the different techniques used to assess the rate (Grafstein, 1969; Davison, 1970). In the accumulation method in which naturally present or labeled components pile up above a ligation, several peaks arise at different times; this in turn has suggested two or more rates of flow (Lubińska, 1964; McEwen and Grafstein, 1968; Barondes, 1969; Karlsson and Sjöstrand, 1970). The more direct evaluation of the transport rate by the outflow pattern of labeled activity within the nerve itself eliminates some of the complication of analysis inherent in the accumulation technique. A sufficiently long length of nerve is needed for direct evaluation of the pattern in the nerve, and fortunately such lengths are available in the sciatic nerve

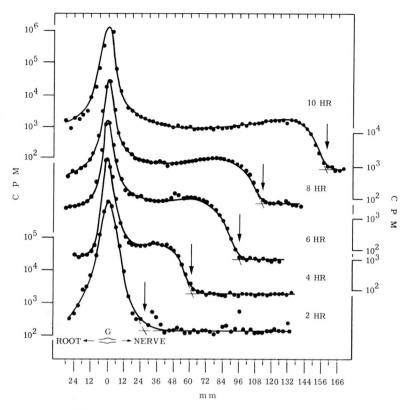

Figure 12–1 Distribution of radioactivity in the dorsal root ganglia and sciatic nerves of five cats taken between 2 and 10 hours after injecting ^{3}H-leucine into the L7 ganglia (G). The activity present in 5 mm segment of roots, ganglia, and nerves (abscissa) is given on the ordinate in logarithmic divisions. The ordinate scale for the nerve two hours after injection is given at the bottom left with divisions in counts per minute. At the top left a scale is given for the nerve taken 10 hours after injection. Only partial scales are shown at the right for the nerves taken four, six, and eight hours after injection. (From Ochs, S.: Fast transport of materials in mammalian nerve fibers. Science. *176*:252–260, 21 April, 1972. Copyright 1972 by the American Association for the Advancement of Science.

of most mammals. In these studies a labeled amino acid precursor, e.g., ^{3}H-leucine or ^{3}H-lysine, is injected into the seventh lumbar (L7) dorsal root ganglion, where it is rapidly incorporated into proteins within the neuron cell bodies, the labeled proteins then moving out in the nerve fibers. After a time determined by the rate of transport, the nerve is sectioned and the activity in each small section counted and the pattern of labeled activity plotted as a function of distance along the nerve. A characteristic crest is seen representing the earliest outflow of labeled activity in the nerve (Fig. 12–1). The position of the crest advances linearly with time at a rate, measured from the foot of the crest back to the dorsal root ganglion, of 410 ± 50 (S.D.) mm per day (Ochs, 1972a). This same rate has been found in the nerves of animals ranging in size from the goat down to the rat (Table 12–1). The plateau behind the crest represents materials exiting later from the cell bodies and some materials retained in the fibers.

The composition of labeled activity in the crest and in the plateau region behind it was determined by subcellular centrifugation and gel filtration of the soluble fraction. A wide

range of soluble proteins, polypeptides, and, as well, the particulate fraction were found to be labeled (Ochs et al., 1967; McEwen and Grafstein, 1968; Kidwai and Ochs, 1969; Sabri and Ochs, 1973). Various other com-

TABLE 12–1 RATES OF FAST AXOPLASMIC TRANSPORT—ADULT NERVES*

Nerve Type	No. of Nerves	Species	Rate
Motor (sciatic)	18	Rat	411 ± 50
	5	Monkey	400 ± 35
Sensory (sciatic)	14	Monkey	416 ± 30
	26	Cat	409 ± 50
	2	Rabbit	394 (360, 415)
	2	Goat	389 (382, 396)
	4	Dog	423 ± 15
Dorsal root	17	Monkey	428 ± 44
Corresponding sciatic nerve	18	Monkey	420 ± 28
Dorsal column spinal cord	3	Monkey	397 ± 57
	4	Cat	391 ± 59

*Rate values are given as mean and standard deviation. Measured in sensory nerves after L7 dorsal root ganglia injection with ^{3}H-leucine, in motor nerves after ^{3}H-leucine uptake by L7 motor neuron. (From Ochs, S.: Rate of fast axoplasmic transport in mammalian nerve fibers. J. Physiol., 227:627–646, 1972. Reprinted by permission.)

ponents carried down within the nerve fibers by fast axoplasmic transport include glycoproteins and glycolipids, with the full complement of fast transported components yet to be determined (McEwen et al., 1971; Elam and Agranoff, 1971).

Specific substances carried down by fast axoplasmic transport include catecholamines present in granules in autonomic nerve fibers as shown by their accumulation above a ligation (Dahlström and Häggendal, 1966) and acetylcholinesterase, which is also present in the particulate fraction (Lubińska and Niemierko, 1970). In our laboratory, using a double-ligation technique, we found the rate of fast transport for acetylcholinesterase to be 431 mm per day, a value sufficiently close to the 410 mm per day rate found with isotope techniques to indicate that the double-ligation technique gives the same measure of rate (Ranish and Ochs, 1972).

The similarity of the rate of transport found for materials with a wide range of molecular weights extending from small molecules to particles of comparatively large size is of great theoretical interest. It indicates, as is discussed in a later section, that a common "conveyor belt" system is involved in the mechanism of fast transport. In contrast, the slow transport system has different properties. As shown by isotope studies, a greater preponderance of high molecular weight soluble proteins and a lesser amount of labeled particles are carried by the slow than by the fast transport system (Kidwai and Ochs, 1969; McEwen and Grafstein, 1968).

Rate of Transport During Maturation and Aging

In some studies in which the accumulation technique was used variations in the rate of fast transport within the first month after birth were reported (Hendrickson and Cowan, 1971; Marchisio and Sjöstrand, 1971). A direct comparison of rates using the crest technique in adult cats and newborn kittens was therefore initiated (Ochs, 1973a). For this, sufficiently long lengths of sciatic nerve are needed, and fortunately these are available in kittens two weeks old. The whole of the characteristic crest could be displayed and thus the rate of fast axoplasmic transport measured (Ochs, 1973a). The L7 dorsal root ganglia were injected with ³H-leucine, and

TABLE 12–2 RATES OF FAST AXOPLASMIC TRANSPORT—NEWBORN AND AGED ANIMALS*

Animal	Age	No. of Nerves	Rate
Kitten	2 weeks	27	389±29
Kitten	3 weeks	31	397±32
Kitten	4 weeks	10	397±40
Kitten	6 weeks	10	426±26
Cat	8–20 years	8	430±27
Dog	8–12 years	15	469±47
Dog	Young adult	5	439±34

*Apparently faster rate in aged dogs may be due to a systematic error. Control values also high. Difference between any of these groups and the 410 ± 50 (S.D.) mm per day of all controls not statistically different by Student's t test. (From Ochs, S.: Effect of maturation and aging on the rate of fast axoplasmic transport in mammalian nerve. Progr. Brain Res., 40:349–362, 1973. Reprinted by permission.)

after periods of downflow of usually three hours, the rate found for the two week old kitten was 395 mm per day (Table 12–2). The difference between this value and the 410 mm per day adult rate was not statistically significant as indicated by Student's t test. At the other end of the age scale, cats and dogs older than eight years were studied. Some apparently had faster rates, but statistically, the variations in rate seen did not differ from those of young adults. Therefore, the rate in animals ranging in age from kittens two weeks old to animals up to 20 years of age (a very old age for the cat) is remarkably constant, a finding in accord with a uniform mechanism underlying the fast axoplasmic transport system.

Invariance of Rate in Different Nerve Fiber Types

When ³H-leucine is injected into the ventral horn region of the L7 segment of the cord, the motor neuron cell bodies take up the precursor and a similar crest of labeled proteins is seen to move out into the motor fibers of the sciatic nerve. Comparison with the crest position found in sensory fibers after L7 ganglion injection shows that the same fast rate is present in motor and sensory fibers (Ochs and Ranish, 1969; Ochs, 1972a).

The rate of fast axoplasmic transport is also independent of nerve fiber diameter. This was shown by injecting the L7 dorsal root ganglia of cats with ^{3}H-leucine and later removing and preparing small lengths of sciatic nerve taken from the front of the crest for radioautography (Ochs, 1966). In cross sections of the nerve, myelinated fibers with diameters ranging from 3 to 23 μm were all found to have grains of radioactivity located over their axonal region (Ochs, 1972a). The conclusion was that the rate of fast axoplasmic transport is the same in fibers of all diameters because, if the rate were slower in the smaller fibers, no grains would be present in them, and similarly, if faster, only those fibers would contain grains. The same procedure modified for electron microscope radioautography was used and the tracer was found in the non-myelinated as well as the myelinated fibers at the forward part of the crest (Ochs and Jersild, 1974). This indicated a similar fast rate of axoplasmic transport in the nonmye-linated fibers, i.e., one close to 410 mm per day. Byers and co-workers (1973) had earlier reported a fast rate of axoplasmic transport in the nonmyelinated fibers of vagus nerve, and a fast rate was reported for the non-myelinated nerve fibers of the garfish olfac-tory nerve (Gross and Beidler, 1973). When corrected for a temperature of 37°C, the rate in the garfish fibers was 403 mm per day (Gross, 1973). The evidence, therefore, is that the rate of fast axoplasmic transport present over the whole range of myelinated nerve fiber diameters, and also in nonmyelinated fibers, shows a remarkable uniformity indica-tive of a single underlying mechanism of transport.

Mechanism of Fast Axoplasmic Transport

In order to account for the known charac-teristics of fast axoplasmic transport, a hypothesis was proposed in analogy to the sliding filament theory of muscle (Ochs, 1971a, 1972b). A "transport filament" binds the materials transported and it moves along the microtubules or neurofilaments of the axon by means of cross bridges (Fig. 12–2). By this means the heterogeneous labeled components known to be transported are carried down the axon at the same fast rate. This applies also to the plateau portion of the outflow curve characteristic of fast transport as shown by comparing the composition of labeled com-ponents in the crest and plateau regions (Sabri and Ochs, 1973).

The microtubules appear to be the station-ary element along which the transport fila-ment moves. This is suggested by the electron micrographs taken by Smith, Järlfors, and Beránek (1970) of a lamprey nerve fiber near a synapse. While possibly in this case the association of vesicles and microtubules may be related to only synaptic transmission,

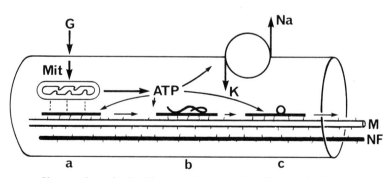

Figure 12–2 Transport filament hypothesis. Glucose (G) enters the fiber, and after glycolysis and oxidative phos-phorylation in the mitochondrion (Mit), the adenosine triphosphate (ATP) produced supplies energy to the sodium pump shown controlling the level of sodium (Na) and potassium (K) ions in the fiber and to the "transport filaments" as well. These are shown as black bars to which various components are bound and so carried down the fiber: the mitochondria (a) temporarily attaching as indicated by dashed lines to both forward and retrograde moving transport filaments and thus giving rise to a fast to-and-fro movement (though with a slow net forward movement), soluble protein (b) shown as a folded or globular configuration, and polypeptides and small particulate elements (c) as well. Simpler molecules are also bound to transport filaments. Thus, a wide range of components is carried along the fiber at the same fast rate. Cross bridges between the transport filament and the microtubules (M) or neurofilaments (NF) or both effect the movement in a fasion similar to that of the sliding filament theory of muscle, the required energy being supplied by adenosine triphos-phate. The cross bridges are shown arising from both microtubules as such spurs or side arms are seen in high-resolution electron micrographs (see Chapter 5).

electron micrographs of mammalian nerve further removed from the synapse show spurlike projections at the periphery of microtubules that have an appearance suggestive of the postulated cross bridges, as described by Tennyson in Chapter 5.

As in the sliding filament theory of muscle in which adenosine triphosphate is required to supply energy for cross bridge action and the relative movement of actin and myosin filaments sliding past one another, energy would be required for cross bridge action in the nerve. A close dependence of fast axoplasmic transport on oxidative metabolism was found (Ochs and Hollingsworth, 1971; Ochs and Smith, 1971; Ochs, 1974a). Fast axoplasmic transport requires oxygen, and as shown in in vitro studies, after anoxia was initiated by switching over to a nitrogen environment, fast axoplasmic transport became blocked within approximately 15 minutes. At the time when fast transport failed, the level of high-energy phosphate (the combined amount of adenosine triphosphate and phosphocreatine), which normally was found to have a concentration of approximately 1.2 uM per gram, fell to about half its control value (Sabri and Ochs, 1973). This appears to be below a critical level of adenosine triphosphate needed to sustain fast axoplasmic transport. Further evidence for such a critical level has recently been reviewed (Ochs, 1974a). A correlation of the block of fast axoplasmic transport with high-energy phosphate levels was seen after various metabolic blocking agents were used to stop transport and metabolism at different times. Additional support for the utilization of adenosine triphosphate by the fast axoplasmic transport mechanism is the presence of magnesium and calcium–activated adenosinetriphosphatase in myelinated nerve (Khan and Ochs, 1972). This enzyme appears to have many of the actomyosin-like properties previously shown in brain preparations by Berl and Puszkin (1970), and on the hypothesis presented, would be required for adenosine triphosphate utilization by the postulated cross bridges (Khan and Ochs, 1974).

Oxidative phosphorylation supplying adenosine triphosphate exists all along the length of the nerve. This was shown by making a short region of the nerve in advance of the downflowing crest of activity anoxic by covering it with narrow strips of plastic coated with petrolatum in order to prevent the entry of oxygen at that site (Ochs, 1971b). The resulting anoxia caused a block of fast axoplasmic transport as shown by the damming of activity just above the anoxic region and lack of penetration of labeled components into it (Fig. 12–3). On the basis of such studies the conclusion was reached that the adenosine triphosphate present in the oxygenated length of the fiber cannot diffuse into the anoxic region to sustain transport, nor can the labeled components diffuse very far once their supply of adenosine triphosphate fails (Ochs, 1971b).

The reversibility of the block of fast transport after a period of local anoxia was studied by removing the plastic strips covering the nerve and allowing a further period of time for in vitro transport. When the strips were removed after approximately one hour of local anoxia, complete reversibility was found. After one and three quarters hours an apparently complete block of transport was seen. A more extended study of reversibility indicated, however, that the block of fast transport was in fact only a partial defect. When more time was allowed for recovery a full return of the pattern and rate of fast axoplasmic transport was seen (Leone and Ochs, 1973). In those studies nerves were placed in chambers so that maximal action potential could be recorded while fast axoplasmic transport could afterward be measured. As in earlier such in vitro studies, electrical responses and fast axoplasmic transport were both found to fail within approximately 15 minutes (a range of from 10 to 30 minutes) of the onset of initiation of nitrogen anoxia (cf. Ochs et al., 1970; Ochs, 1974b). The close correlation in the time of block of these two nerve functions is in accord with the concept of a common pool of adenosine triphosphate supplying energy to the sodium pump controlling ionic asymmetry across the axonal membrane and thus excitability, and as well, to the fast transport mechanism (see Fig. 12–2). The recovery of these two functions after replacing nitrogen with 95 per cent oxygen and 5 per cent carbon dioxide was found to be good after approximately an hour and a half of anoxia. After longer times of anoxia, one and three quarters to two and a half hours, there was only partial return of fast axoplasmic transport with a changed slope and slower rate while electrical responses showed a good recovery. This differential effect of anoxia was shown to be due to a delayed recovery of fast axoplasmic transport.

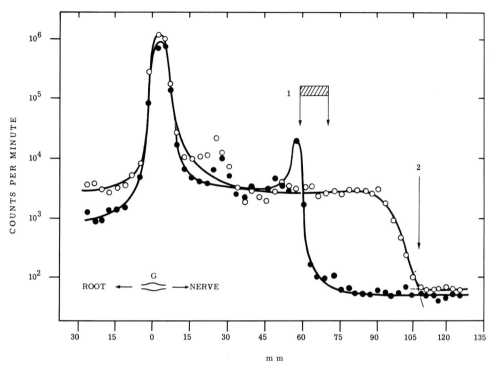

Figure 12–3 Local anoxic block of downflow shown after injection of the L7 dorsal root ganglion with ^{3}H-leucine. The nerve from one side (•) was removed after two hours of downflow in the animal and placed in a chamber containing 95 per cent oxygen and 5 per cent carbon dioxide for three hours of downflow in vitro. A short length of the nerve (arrow 1 and hatched bar) was covered with petrolatum. Damming occurred with the peak of radioactivity at the proximal edge of the anoxic region with a fall to the baseline a short distance inside the covered region. The control nerve (○ and arrow 2) shows the usual fast transport in vitro. (From Ochs, S.: Local supply of energy to the fast axoplasmic transport mechanism. Proc. Natl. Acad. Sci. U.S.A., *68*:1279–1282, 1971. Reprinted by permission.)

Because the time required for recovery was limited in in vitro studies, limb compression was used in vivo to produce ischemia and anoxia, and fast axoplasmic transport was tested at later times as is described in a subsequent section.

Vascular Supply and Ischemic Block of Fast Transport

As noted earlier, fast axoplasmic transport is closely dependent for its maintenance on oxidative metabolism although some in vivo observations might suggest otherwise. For example, in the preparation of a transected nerve for suturing, rather long lengths of nerve can be mobilized, and in the process of freeing the nerve from the surrounding tissue, the small blood vessels that enter and supply the nerve along its length are torn or cut away. The relative impunity with which this can be done without resulting wallerian degeneration attests not to the limited metabolic require-

ment of nerve, but rather to the extensive collateral circulation present in nerve trunks (Adams, 1942; Lundborg and Brånemark, 1968; Sunderland, 1968). The supply vessels that enter the nerve at intervals along its length, the arteriae nutriae, divide into ascending and descending rami; these course in the epineurium as perifascicular vascular plexuses and enter the nerve to anastomose in intrafascicular plexuses. As a result, the stripping of the smaller supply vessels may not give rise to a defect in the nerve because of the extensive collateral supply present. If in addition, however, a major arterial supply vessel is also eliminated, the nerve fails. According to Okada (1905), when only the major blood supply of the sciatic nerve branching from the inferior gluteal artery is ligated, wallerian degeneration ensues. This was not corroborated by Adams (1942), who has pointed out that there are marked variations in the pattern of vascular supply of the sciatic nerve. The difference in results found may depend on the time required for collateral supply

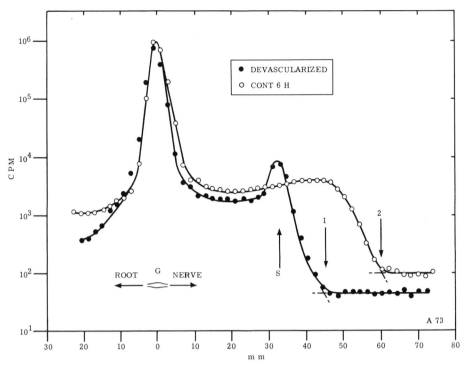

Figure 12–4 Devascularization of sciatic nerve (•) accomplished by stripping small vessels from sciatic nerve and clamping supply from inferior gluteal artery at sciatic notch. Downflow blocked with damming above stripped (S) area. Arrow 1 indicates blocked and arrow 2 indicates control (O) downflows.

to be established when a major supply is eliminated. In any case, the dependence of nerve function on vascular supply may be clearly shown when only a single vessel is left available to supply a nerve. This was arranged for by ligations of the popliteal nerve and elimination of all supply vessels but one. Then, when that one blood vessel was clamped off, nerve excitability was lost within 10 to 26 minutes as shown by the failure of muscle contractions in response to nerve stimulation (Porter and Wharton, 1949). This is the same period of time seen in in vitro studies of mammalian nerves in which excitability and transport fail after oxygen is replaced with nitrogen (Lehmann, 1937; Wright, 1946; Ochs, 1972b).

The dependence of fast axoplasmic transport on vascular supply in sciatic nerves was studied by stripping of their local blood vessels and, as well, by clamping off the major supply vessel arising from the inferior gluteal artery (Ochs, Ranish, and Maroon, unpublished experiments). The capability of fast axoplasmic transport into the devascularized region was studied by injecting the ganglia with ³H-leucine and determining the pattern

of downflow. A block of transport into the devascularized nerve was revealed by the damming of activity above the stripped region and failure of penetration of labeled components into it (Fig. 12–4). When only the smaller supply vessels to the sciatic nerve were stripped away without ligating the major vascular supply from the inferior gluteal artery, a normal downflow pattern was seen within the stripped regions. Such studies, therefore, confirm the importance of collateral circulation and further show the dependence of fast axoplasmic transport on vascular supply needed to maintain an adequate oxidative metabolism.

Pressure Ischemia and Fast Axoplasmic Transport

Anoxia may be produced in the nerve of a limb by stopping the circulation with blood pressure cuffs raised to pressures above systolic blood pressure. In the human, Lewis, Pickering and Rothschild (1931) describe a centripetal loss of motor and sensory functions in the arms beginning at about 15 minutes after the onset of ischemia produced by pressure cuffs. The effects were attributed to the ischemia of the nerve fibers rather than to pressure per se acting on the nerve fibers. The sensation of touch, of passive movement, of heat and cold, and of fast-conducted pain were lost before that of slow-conducted pain (Lewis and Pochin, 1938). The latter observation suggests that the non-myelinated nerve fibers may be somewhat more resistant to anoxia. This was noted in electrical studies of action potentials in which C fiber responses persisted longer than the alpha and beta responses of the A group after initiation of anoxia (Grundfest, 1940).

The production of ischemia by cuff compression is less easily done in the hind limb of the cat than in man, in part because of the truncated pyramidal shape of the cat hind limb and in part because of the protection afforded by the bony structures to the nerves, which was also suggested as a protecting factor in the direct compression studies of nerve by Denny-Brown and Brenner (1944). Bentley and Schlapp (1943a) found that compression of the lower leg of the cat might not block nerve conduction for times up to two hours,

but when applied higher on the limb caused the nerve to become inactive within 30 minutes. This apparently was due to the need for higher cuff pressures in the latter instance rather than to a diffusion of oxygen from surrounding tissue in the former case as was considered at the time. In a following paper, higher pressures of up to 250 mm of mercury were used, and a block of nerve conduction within 30 minutes was reported (Bentley and Schlapp, 1943b). An examination of the survival times of action potentials by Frankenhaeuser (1949) also showed a block of conduction in 25 to 30 minutes when the upper thigh was compressed. Pressures as high as 700 mm of mercury were considered necessary to effect a conduction block with pressure cuffs according to Lundborg (1970), who measured the actual resulting lower pressures within the limb with a probe.

The technique of cuff compression of the hind limb in cats to make the nerve ischemic was studied for its effect on fast axoplasmic transport (Ochs, Ranish, and Maroon, unpublished data; Leone and Ochs, 1973). The cuff was placed as high on the thigh as possible, and enough time was allowed for downflow

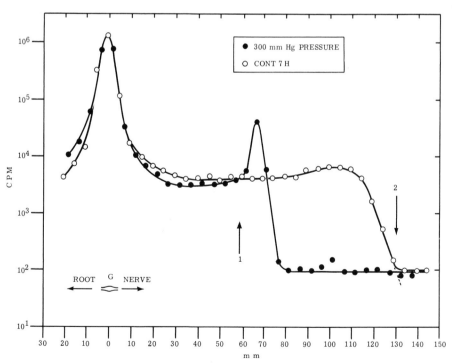

Figure 12–5 Pressure cuff applied to one leg (•) as high on thigh as possible. Arrow 1 shows edge of cuff; effective pressure to make nerve ischemic below this at site just distal to damming. There is no entry of activity into ischemic region. Arrow 2 shows downflow of control nerve (O).

after injecting the L7 dorsal root ganglion so that the activity would have normally moved down to the region of compression. Pressure ischemia at cuff pressures of 300 mm of mercury blocked fast axoplasmic transport as shown by the failure of penetration of the advancing crest of activity into that region (Fig. 12–5). A damming of activity also occurs above the ischemic region, a pattern similar to that seen when local anoxia is produced in vitro by covering a region of nerve in advance of the down-moving crest or after the stripping of vessels in vivo to eliminate blood supply (see Figs. 12–3 and 12–4). The possibility exists, however, that compression may have additional effects besides ischemia. Such additional effects may be evaluated by investigating reversibility after pressure ischemia; if compression does have an added effect, we might expect a prolonged block or a failure of reversibility of fast axoplasmic transport after a prolonged period of compression.

As described in the foregoing paragraphs, fast axoplasmic transport in vitro showed an apparent dissociation from electrical responses, with a partial recovery of transport seen after periods of anoxia lasting one and three quarters to two and a half hours (Leone and Ochs, 1973). Limb compression allowed the period of recovery to be extended. Various durations of anoxia up to six hours were produced in anesthetized animals by cuff compression at pressures of 300 mm of mercury. Then, a recovery time of 16 to 20 hours was allowed before the L7 ganglia were injected with ^{3}H-leucine so that fast axoplasmic transport could then be assessed in the nerves on compressed and control sides. A complete recovery of fast axoplasmic transport was found after periods of compression ischemia lasting as long as four hours. After compression times of six hours, however, an irreversible block was seen. This limitation on the time of reversibility after anoxia found in our studies was close to the seven hour limit of reversibility found by Lundborg (1970) using electrical responses and lack of wallerian degeneration. As the pressures used by Lundborg were much higher with a similar time period of reversibility, strength is given to the conclusion that the block of transport by compression ischemia is likely due to an interruption of an adequate blood circulation and oxygen supply rather than to pressure effects per se.

Role of Microtubules and Neurofilaments in Transport

In the theory of fast axoplasmic transport the microtubules or neurofilaments or both are considered to represent the stationary element along which the transport filaments move by means of cross bridges (see Fig. 12–2). Most likely the microtubule is the element involved. Evidence for that view is the effect of the mitotic blocking agents colchicine and the vinca alkaloids on transport. These agents arrest mitosis by binding to microtubular subunits, thus causing a disaggregation of microtubules in the spindles of dividing cells and a block of mitosis. A similar binding of colchicine to the microtubular protein subunits extracted from brain cells was found (Weisenberg et al., 1968). Following this lead, it was found that colchicine locally injected under the epineurium of a nerve trunk blocks fast transport as shown by the failure of accumulation of catecholamines at a ligation distal to the injected site (Dahlström, 1968). In similar fashion a block of fast transport of acetylcholinesterase was found (Kreutzberg, 1969). However, electron microscopy of crayfish nerve fibers exposed to colchicine and vinblastine in amounts that blocked transport showed the microtubules in the fiber still intact (Fernandez et al., 1970; Samson, 1971). The evidence suggests that these agents may have a more subtle action on the transport mechanism than a disassembly of microtubules—possibly an action on the postulated cross bridges.

Colchicine and vinblastine produce different patterns of block of fast axoplasmic transport in vitro, and evidence that they act by some means other than through a disaggregation was obtained (Ochs, 1973b). In studies of the effect of low temperature, fast axoplasmic transport was found to be "cold blocked" at temperatures near 0° C (at temperatures below 11° C) and to recover its normal rate and pattern of transport rapidly when the nerves were rewarmed to 38° C (Ochs, 1973b). If, during cold block, there is a disaggregation of microtubules as was indicated for frog nerve by Echandia and Piezzi (1968), the reaggregation would have to be very rapid, and according to the hypothesis of transport, the transport filament would also have to be repositioned on the reassembled microtubules without delay. A reaggregation response quicker than that reported for heliozoal axopodia, a time of 30 to 45 minutes, would be required (Tilney and Porter, 1967). Colchicine or vinblastine when added during the period of cold block would, if the microtubules are dissociated into subunits during cold block, combine with the subunits and thus prevent their reaggregation on rewarming. These agents did not augment the block when nerves were exposed to them in the cold for up to three hours (Ochs, 1973b). This should have been sufficient time for the agents to enter the fiber and bind to the subunits. An added effect did, however, appear when colchicine was present during cold blocks that lasted 16 hours and then the nerve was rewarmed. The added effect may not, however, be due to binding and an interference with reaggregation, but rather to additional changes produced by the prolonged period of cold block, a point under present investigation.

The linearly directed elements, the microtubules or neurofilaments or both, are considered as the stationary element in transport and may serve to channel or "route" different materials into the individual branches of a neuron. Such routing might be expected in the case of the dorsal root ganglion neuron in which one class of substance moves out to supply the afferent terminals of the sensory nerve branch and another class of substance enters the branch leading into the dorsal root to supply substances to the terminals involved in synaptic transmission within the spinal cord. The rate of fast axoplasmic transport in the two branches of the L7 dorsal root ganglion neurons was assessed in monkeys in which a sufficiently long length of dorsal root is present to allow the full extent of the crest of fast transported activity to be assessed, and the rate was found to be the same in the two branches of the neuron (cf. Table 12–1 and Ochs, 1972a). One characteristic finding in those studies was that a threefold to fivefold greater amount of labeled material was transported into the peripheral nerve as compared to the centrally directed dorsal root. This marked difference in amount could be accounted for if the fiber branches on the nerve side have a greater diameter than the root fiber branches and thus more volume. Freeze-substitution was used to verify that the diameters and thus the axonal volumes of the fiber branches on the two sides were the same (Ochs and Erdman, 1974). On this ground the disparity in the amount of activity carried into the two branches of the neuron could very well be due to a routing of materials along the different sets of linearly organized microtubules or neurofilaments present in nerve and dorsal root branches of the dorsal root ganglion neuron.

Retrograde Transport and Chromatolysis

Another means of routing materials within nerve fibers is the movement of materials in the retrograde direction. This is connected with the phenomenon of chromatolysis in cell bodies seen several days after cutting their axons (cf. Chapter 14). Various hypotheses have been advanced to account for chromatolysis (Cragg, 1970). By exclusion, the "signal" for chromatolysis was determined to be the ascent (or failure of ascent) of some critical material in the interrupted nerve fiber rather than the possible action of degenerated substances that reach the cell bodies through the circulation (Ochs et al., 1961). Since there is an increased phase of protein synthesis during chromatolysis (Brattgård et al., 1958; Watson, 1965), it seems likely that the signal substance acts as part of a feedback control to change or regulate the level of cell synthesis. The speculation has been made that the signal substance is the nerve growth factor (Fuxe, 1974).

Direct evidence for a retrograde movement of material in nerve fibers was first shown by Lubińska (1964) and her colleagues by the accumulation of acetylcholinesterase just distal to a nerve ligation in an amount less than that accumulated above the ligation. Recently, Lubińska and Niemierko (1970) showed that acetylcholinesterase is carried down the nerve fibers at a fast rate. Our studies have shown a faster forward rate of 431 mm per day, a value not significantly different from the 410 mm per day rate found for other proteins. The retrograde rate seen was approximately half the forward rate, namely 220 mm per day (Ranish and Ochs, 1972). Retrograde transport is dependent on oxidative metabolism (Edström and Hanson, 1973).

Retrograde transport is also shown by the accumulation of horseradish peroxidase in neuron cell bodies after its uptake at the nerve terminals (Kristensson and Olson, 1971; LaVail and LaVail, 1972). In the older literature toxins and viruses have been reported as moving upward in nerve fibers, and no doubt such retrograde movement will be reinvestigated and related to the presently known characteristics of axoplasmic transport (cf. Kristensson et al., 1971).

During chromatolysis the rate of axoplasmic transport has been reported as increased, decreased, or unchanged (Ochs et al., 1960; Grafstein and Murray, 1969; Hendrickson and Cowan, 1971). Our more recent studies on transport in motor fibers showed no change in the rate (Ochs et al., 1962; Ochs, 1972a). This point was also investigated with respect to the sensory fibers (Ochs, unpublished experiments). At various times up to 90 days after cutting sciatic nerves at the popliteal fossa in cats, the L7 dorsal root ganglia were injected with ^{3}H-leucine and the displacement of the crest used to compare the rate in nerves on control and cut (chromatolytic) sides. No difference in the rate on the two sides was seen throughout the whole of the period of chromatolysis. This result may be stated as a general principle: namely, fast axoplasmic transport is "all-or-none" in the axon and independent of the mechanisms of synthesis present in the cell body. According to the proposed mechanism of transport, once the transport filament enters the fiber it is subjected to the local conditions present at any given point along the nerve, a principle conceptually equivalent to the all-or-none principle long recognized for the nerve action potential (Kato, 1950).

THE MECHANISM OF SLOW TRANSPORT

Weiss and Hiscoe (1948), on morphologic grounds, related the swelling and beading present in nerve fibers just above constrictions made in a nerve to the damming up within the fibers of the contents of the axoplasm moving uniformly as a whole down inside the nerve fibers at an estimated rate of 1 to 3 mm per day. Such a bulk flow of axoplasm was analogized to the flow of lava (Weiss, 1972). A full discussion of this conception of slow transport is not possible here, but some considerations that prevent acceptance of this view should be noted; a further discussion may be found elsewhere (Ochs, 1974c). The outflow pattern of labeled activity seen after nerve cell body uptake incorporation of phosphorus-32 (or-

thophosphate) or ^{3}H-leucine is a declining exponential curve, a pattern that does not fit the bulk flow concept (Ochs et al., 1962; Miani, 1963; Ochs and Johnson, 1969). Also, the shape of the fibers in the region above a cut or a constriction seen with electron microscopy is not in accord with the concept (Spencer, 1972). The fibers in such cases may show collateral branching (Perroncito, 1905; Ramon y Cajal, 1928; Shawe, 1955) as was also seen when freeze-substitution was used to better preserve the form of the nerve fibers (Ochs, unpublished observations). The rapid to-and-fro movement of the mitochondria, shown in nerve fibers by microscopic observation with Nomarski optics, is considered due to a temporary binding to the transport filaments with a net slow proximodistal movement. Such temporary binding gives rise to the slow transport of the mitochondria and other materials (Ochs, 1974c).

TRANSPORT IN CENTRAL NERVE FIBERS

Some portion of the branches of dorsal root ganglion cell fibers entering the cord ascend in the dorsal columns of the spinal cord. It was of interest to compare the rate of transport along the length in these central nervous system fibers to the rate found for the fibers descending into the sciatic nerve (Ochs, 1972a). The ganglia were injected with ^{3}H-leucine, and after a suitable period of time for fast axoplasmic transport had been allowed, the dorsal columns were removed and sectioned, and the outflow pattern in them was determined by the usual means (Fig. 12–6). The distribution of activity found in the dorsal columns was arranged in the figure so that it could be directly compared with the pattern in the sciatic nerves. And, as can be seen, the distance to which the crest had moved in the dorsal columns is closely comparable to that in the peripheral nerves. This is taken as evidence that the rate of fast axoplasmic transport in the fibers of the dorsal column and peripheral nerve is the same. When the fibers in the dorsal column were interrupted by applied pressure or by freezing at temperatures below −20° C, a failure of fast axoplasmic transport above that site was seen with a damming of activity

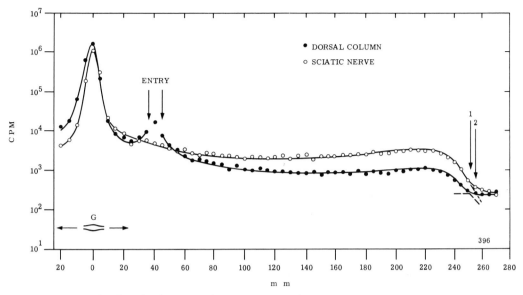

Figure 12–6   Transport in dorsal columns of the cat spinal cord after injection of ^{3}H-leucine into L7 dorsal ganglia of a large cat. Dorsal column and nerve patterns of outflow display activity similar to that shown in Figure 12–5. Both peroneal and tibial nerves were taken down to the ankle, allowing the full pattern of activity and the crests to be seen over this longer distance at 14.5 hours. This entry zone for the dorsal column curve indicates some adventitious addition of activity where fibers branch. (From Ochs, S.: Rate of fast axoplasmic transport in mammalian nerve fibres. J. Physiol., 227:627–646, 1972. Reprinted by permission.)

before it, evidence for an intraaxonal transport (Fig. 12–7).

The dorsal column studies demonstrate that the same system underlying fast axoplasmic transport is likely to be present in central fibers as well as in peripheral nerve. The generality of fast transport in the central nervous system will, however, have to be determined by similar studies in other tract systems. Such information may bear on the capability of regeneration of central nervous system tract fibers, which unfortunately is feeble compared to that of peripheral nerve (Ramon y Cajal, 1928). It is to be hoped that further studies of fast axoplasmic transport may lead to new insights whereby the capability for regeneration can be augmented.

Axoplasmic transport was used in a study of regeneration of spinal root fibers. The ventral roots of the L7 segment from one side of the spinal cord were grafted to the cut ends of the L7 dorsal roots on the other side, and the ventral roots regenerated and grew into the cord via the dorsal root (Barnes and Worrall, 1968). To show the earliest time of growth of fibers into the dorsal root, ^{3}H-leucine was injected into the ventral horn of the L7 segment of the spinal cord containing the motor neuron somas of the grafted ventral root. A regeneration of fibers into the dorsal root was

later determined by a slope of activity carried into the dorsal roots by slow transport as early as two weeks after such union (Ochs and Barnes, 1969). Corroboration of the time of ingrowth was obtained in that study of axoplasmic transport by the increased levels of acetylcholinesterase found appearing in the grafted dorsal roots two weeks after the graft had been made and later rising to levels usually present only in ventral roots (Ranish et al., 1972).

Studies of axoplasmic transport of materials related to synaptic transmission within the fiber tracts of the central nervous system have already led to significant clinical advances. The course of monoamine fiber tracts in the brain stem has been revealed by making lesions along their path and finding an increase of monoamines accumulated in the fibers proximal to the lesion, i.e., facing the cell bodies, and a depletion in the fibers distal to the lesion as would occur when the axoplasmic transport of monoamines from the nerve cell bodies to their terminals is blocked (Anden et al., 1966). The various neuronal systems revealed by this technique include dopamine fibers passing from the substantia nigra to the striatum and noradrenaline and serotonin tract fibers from brain stem nuclear regions into the hypo-

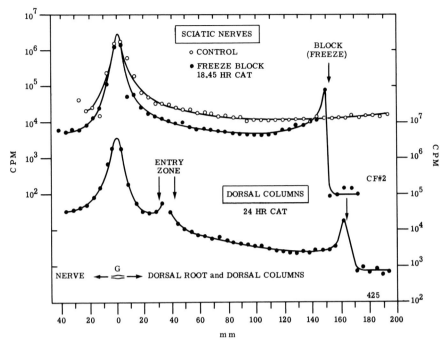

Figure 12-7 Upper curves represent outflow in the two sciatic nerves of a cat over a period of 18.45 hours. The control (○) shows only the plateau at this time; the crest would be much further distally at this time. The other nerve (●) was frozen (arrow) to produce a block, which is seen by damming above and fall of activity distal to the block. The lower curve (●) represents transport into the cord, the entry zone representing branching of fibers with cord ascent shown toward the right. At the arrow the columns had been frozen, and damming before the site and a drop after it shows block. Abscissa in millimeters, ordinate in counts per minute (CPM) on a log scale.

thalamus, thalamus, and cortex. The mapping of a number of separate monoamine pathways can be clearly shown in the smaller brain of the rat by combining such lesions with fluorescent techniques (Ungerstedt, 1971). The nigrostriatal system has been related to neural motor control mechanism; in parkinsonism patients, a reduced level of dopamine found in the striatum led to the introduction of L-dopa, a precursor of dopamine, as a successful therapeutic agent (Hornykiewicz, 1972). Changes in the amount and types of the neurotransmitter-related materials at the terminals of the dopamine, noradrenaline, and possibly serotonin fiber systems have been correlated with changes in alertness and emotional state, and provide a rationale for the action of psychotrophic agents (Phillis, 1970; Cooper et al., 1974; Kopin, 1972).

Use has been made of axoplasmic transport as a method to trace fiber pathways within the central nervous system. After injection of a labeled amino acid, e.g., ³H-leucine, near the cell bodies of a nuclear group for its uptake and incorporation, the subsequent transport of labeled proteins in the axons and course of those fiber tracts can be seen in suitable tissue sections prepared for radioautography. The advantage of this "transport radioautography" technique over the usual neuroanatomical methods in which lesions are made in nuclear groups and the ensuing degeneration in the fibers is traced by appropriate stains is that lesions often include interspersed and nearby fibers arising from other nuclear sites. These fibers, adding their degeneration to that of the intended nuclear group, make analysis difficult. In the transport radioautography technique the labeled precursor is taken up only by the cell bodies and does not enter the axon, thus making possible a discrimination between fibers arising from a given nuclear group (cell bodies) and fibers en passant (cf., Ochs and Burger, 1958).

Transport radioautography was used in a study of the central projections in the cord after injection of the ninth spinal ganglion of the toad and the L7 dorsal root ganglion of cats with ³H-leucine, and the results were compared with those of the Nauta method (Lasek et al., 1968). For the most part, the two methods were equivalent, but some projections were picked up by the transport radioautography method that were not seen in the Nauta preparations. An extra fiber group not otherwise apparent had also been found by Goldberg and Kotani (1967), who used labeled precursor injected into the eye to study the course of fiber terminations in the metamorphosing bullfrog tadpole. In addition to the expected tectal terminations, an additional projection system to the thalamus was revealed. Similarly, O'Steen and Vaughan (1968) injected ^{3}H-hydroxytryptophan into the retina of rats and found an additional optic path projection leading into the hypothalamus, presumably to transmit photic information to the pineal gland, which in this species is part of a system of neuroendocrine response to light.

Cowan and co-workers (1972) investigated the course of optic fibers in the monkey by using transport radioautography, and Edwards (1972) injected the red nucleus to determine its projections to the thalamus. As pointed out by Cowan and associates (1972), when times are kept brief, fast transport carries labeled activity mainly into the boutons termineaux and these are labeled while the fibers do not contain much activity (cf., Droz and Barondes, 1969). By this means the pattern of terminations, either axosomatic or axodendritic, or both, on the neurons to which a given nuclear group projects can be revealed. When more time is allowed for downflow by slow transport, the fibers are heavily labeled and can be traced toward their synaptic terminals. The higher level of activity seen is due to the higher concentration of labeled protein associated with slow transport as compared to fast transport (Ochs and Johnson, 1969; Grafstein, 1969). Further extensions of the technique of transport radioautography should prove useful in studies in which new patterns of connectivity due to collateral regrowth following a lesion are to be determined.

CONCLUSION

It is intriguing to observe how earlier concepts apparently completely supplanted by new ones can later return in modified form. The ancient misconceptions of animal spirits moving in nerve fibers became replaced by the modern concept of the electrical nature of the nerve impulse and chemical transmission at synapses. Virchow (1863), in contributing to the development of the cellular

theory of pathology, successfully contested the "neuralists" and their subsidiary view that diseases arise primarily from the nervous system as failures of "trophic" supply. Now that material transport in nerve fibers is known to exist, an alteration of trophic control as a result of disease is again a valuable concept. The older notion of special trophic nerve fibers has been rejected, and our present view is that control substances move down within all the nerves by axoplasmic transport. These trophic materials act within the nerve fiber, at the nerve terminal, and after crossing the terminal membrane, on muscle or glands or other neurons. The nature of such trophic materials and their modification in disease remains to be determined. If defects of supply of trophic material are referred to as *neurotrophic* diseases we may refer to the process of material transport in nerve in general as *neurophery* (Greek *pheros*—carrying) and then speak of *neuropheric* diseases, i.e., alterations in the process of axoplasmic transport with, as a special case, the failure of supply of trophic substances. It seems quite likely that a vigorous study of these processes should, before long, lead to a new understanding of nervous system diseases.

Acknowledgment: The assistance of Dr. N. Ranish, Dr. J. Maroon, John Leone, and Larry Smith in some of the experiments reported is much appreciated. This work was supported by grants from NSF GB 28664 X, PHS RO1 NS 8706–04, and The John A. Hartford Foundation, Inc.

REFERENCES

Adams, W. E.: The blood supply of nerves. II. The effects of exclusion of its regional sources of supply on the sciatic nerve of the rabbit. J. Anat., 77:243–250, 1942.

Anden, N. E., Fuxe, K., Hamberger, B., and Hökfelt, T.: A quantitative study on the nigrostriatal dopamine neuron system in rat. Acta Physiol. Scand., 67:306–312, 1966.

Barnes, C. D., and Worrall, N.: Reinnervation of spinal cord by cholinergic neurons. J. Neurophysiol., 31: 689–694, 1968.

Barondes, S. H.: Axoplasmic transport. *In* Lajtha, A. (ed.): Handbook of Neurochemistry. Vol. 2, Structural Neurochemistry. New York, Plenum Press, 1969, pp. 435–446.

Bentley, F. H., and Schlapp, W.: Experiments on the blood supply of nerves. J. Physiol., 102:62–71, 1943a.

Bentley, F. H., and Schlapp, W.: The effects of pressure on conduction in peripheral nerve. J. Physiol., 102: 72–82, 1943b.

Berl, S., and Puszkin, S.: Mg^{2+}-Ca^{2+}-activated adenosine triphosphatase system isolated from mammalian brain. Biochemistry, 9:2058–2067, 1970.

Brattgård, S.-O., Edström, J.-E., and Hydén, H.: The productive capacity of the neuron in retrograde reaction. Exp. Cell Res., Suppl. 5:185–200, 1958.

Byers, M. R., Fink, B. R., Kennedy, R. D., Middaugh, M. E., and Hendrickson, E. E.: Effects of lidocaine on axonal morphology, microtubules, and rapid transport in rabbit vagus nerve in vitro. J. Neurobiol., 4:125–143, 1973.

Clarke, E., and O'Malley, C. D.: The Human Brain and Spinal Cord. Berkeley, Calif., University of California Press, 1968.

Cooper, J. R., Bloom, F. E., and Roth, R. H.: The Biochemical Basis of Neuropharmacology. 2nd Edition. New York, Oxford University Press, 1974.

Cowan, W., Gottlieb, D., Hendrickson, A. E., Price, J., and Woolsey, T.: The autoradiographic demonstration of axonal connections in the CNS. Brain Res., 37:21–51, 1972.

Cragg, B. G.: What is the signal for chromatolysis? Brain Res., 23:1–21, 1970.

Dahlström, A.: Effect of colchicine on transport of amine storage granules in sympathetic nerves of rat. Eur. J. Pharmacol., 5:111–113, 1968.

Dahlström, A.: Axoplasmic transport (with particular respect to adrenergic neurons). Philos. Trans. R. Soc. Lond. [Biol. Sci.], 261:325–358, 1971.

Dahlström, A., and Häggendal, J.: Some quantitative studies on the noradrenaline content in the cell bodies and terminals of a sympathetic adrenergic neuron system. Acta Physiol. Scand. 67:271–277, 1966.

Davison, P. F.: Axoplasmic transport: physical and chemical aspects. In Schmitt, F. O. (ed.): The Neurosciences: Second Study Program. New York, Rockefeller University Press, 1970, pp. 851–857.

Denny-Brown, D., and Brenner, C.: Paralysis of nerve induced by direct pressure and by tourniquet. Arch. Neurol. Psychiatry, 51:1–26, 1944.

Drachman, D. B. (ed.): Trophic function of the neuron. Ann. N.Y. Acad. Sci., 228:1–423, 1974.

Droz, B.: Accumulation de protéines nouvellement synthétisées dans l'appareil de Golgi du neurone: étude radioautographique en microscopie électronique. C. R. Acad. Sci. (Paris), 260:320–322, 1965.

Droz, B., and Barondes, S. H.: Nerve endings: rapid appearance of labeled protein shown by electron microscopic radioautography. Science, 165:1131–1133, 1969.

Echandia, R. E. L., and Piezzi, R. S.: Microtubules in the nerve fibers of the toad Bufo Arenarum Hensel. Effect of low temperature on the sciatic nerve. J. Cell Biol., 39:491–497, 1968.

Edström, A., and Hanson, M.: Retrograde axonal transport of proteins in vitro in frog sciatic nerve. Brain Res., 61:311–320, 1973.

Edwards, S. B.: The ascending and descending projections of the red nucleus in the cat: an experimental study using an autoradiographic tracing method. Brain Res., 48:45–63, 1972.

Elam, J. S., and Agranoff, B. W.: Transport of proteins and sulfated mucopolysaccharides in the goldfish visual system. J. Neurobiol., 2:379–390, 1971.

Fernandez, H. L., Huneeus, F. C., and Davison, P. F.: Studies on the mechanism of axoplasmic transport in the crayfish cord. J. Neurobiol., 1:395–409, 1970.

Frankenhaeuser, B.: Ischaemic paralysis of a uniform nerve. Acta Physiol. Scand., 18:75–98 (Suppl. 61–64), 1949.

Friede, R. L., and Seitlberger, F. (eds.): Symposium on Pathology of Axons and Axonal Flow. Acta Neuropathol. Suppl. V. New York, Springer-Verlag, 1971.

Fuxe, K.: Dynamics of degeneration and growth of neurons. A report on the Wenner-Grenn Conference. IBRO News, 2:N6–N9, 1974.

Goldberg, S., and Kotani, M.: The projection of optic nerve fibers in the frog Rana catesbiana as studied by radioautography. Anat. Rec., 158:325–331, 1967.

Grafstein, B.: Axonal transport: communication between soma and synapse. In Advances in Biochemical Psychopharmacology. Vol. 1. New York, Raven Press, 1969, pp. 11–25.

Grafstein, B., and Murray, M.: Transport of protein in goldfish optic nerve during regeneration. Exp. Neurol., 25:494–508, 1969.

Gross, G. W.: The effect of temperature on the rapid axoplasmic transport in C-fibers. Brain Res., 56:359–363, 1973.

Gross, G. W., and Beidler, L. M.: Fast axonal transport in the C-fibers of the garfish olfactory nerve. J. Neurobiol., 4:413–428, 1973.

Grundfest, H.: Bioelective potentials. Physiol. Rev., 11:213–242, 1940.

Guth, L.: "Trophic" influences of nerve on muscle. Physiol. Rev., 48:645–687, 1968.

Guth, L.: Degeneration and regeneration of taste buds. In Handbook of Sensory Physiology. Vol. 4, Chemical Senses. Part 2. Taste. (L. M. Beidler, ed.). Berlin, Springer-Verlag, 1971, pp. 63–74.

Gutmann, E.: Neurotrophic relations in the regeneration process. Progr. Brain Res., 13:72–112, 1964.

Hendrickson, A. E., and Cowan, M. N.: Changes in the rate of axoplasmic transport during postnatal development of the rabbit's optic nerve and tract. Exp. Neurol., 30:403–422, 1971.

Hornykiewicz, O.: Dopamine and extrapyramidal motor function and dysfunction. In Kopin, I. J. (ed.): Neurotransmitters. Res. Publ. Assoc. Res. Nerv. Ment. Dis., Vol. 50. Baltimore, Williams & Wilkins Co., 1972, pp. 390–415.

Karlsson, J. O., and Sjöstrand, J.: Synthesis, migration and turnover of protein in retinal ganglion cells. J. Neurochem., 18:749–767, 1970.

Karlsson, J. O., and Sjöstrand, J.: Axonal transport of proteins in retinal ganglion cells. Amino acid incorporation into rapidly transported proteins and distribution of radioactivity to the lateral geniculate body and the superior colliculus. Brain Res., 37:279–285, 1972.

Kato, G.: Microphysiology of Nerve. 2d Edition. Tokyo, Nakayama, 1950.

Khan, M. A., and Ochs, S.: Mg^{2+}-Ca^{2+} ATPase in mammalian nerves: relation to fast axoplasmic transport and block with colchicine. Am. Soc. Neurochem. Abst., 3:93, 1972.

Khan, M. A., and Ochs, S.: Magnesium or calcium activated ATPase in mammalian nerve. Brain Res., 81:413–426, 1974.

Kidwai, A. M., and Ochs, S.: Components of fast and slow phases of axoplasmic flow. J. Neurochem., 16:1105–1112, 1969.

Kopin, I. J. (ed.): Neurotransmitters. Res. Publ. Assoc. Res. Nerv. Ment. Dis., Vol. 50. Baltimore, Williams & Wilkins Co., 1972.

Kreutzberg, G. W.: Neuronal dynamics and axonal flow.

IV. Blockage of intra-axonal enzyme transport by colchicine. Proc. Natl. Acad. Sci. U.S.A., *62*:722–728, 1969.

Kristensson, K., and Olsson, Y.: Uptake and retrograde axonal transport of peroxidase in hypoglossal neurons. Electron microscopical localization in the neuronal perikaryon. Acta Neuropathol. (Berl.), *19*: 1–9, 1971.

Kristensson, K., Lycke, E., and Sjöstrand, J.: Spread of herpes simplex virus in peripheral nerves. Acta Neuropathol. (Berl.), *17*:44–53, 1971.

Lasek, R., Joseph, B. S., and Whitlock, D. G.: Evaluation of a radioautographic neuroanatomical tracing method. Brain Res., *8*:319–336, 1968.

LaVail, J. H., and LaVail, M. M.: Retrograde axonal transport in the central nervous system. Science, *176*:1416–1417, 1972.

Lehmann, J. E.: The effect of asphyxia on mammalian A nerve fibres. Am. J. Physiol., *119*:111–120, 1937.

Leone, J., and Ochs, S.: Reversibility of fast axoplasmic transport following differing durations of anoxic block in vitro and in vivo. Soc. Neurosci. (Abst.), *3*:147, 1973.

Lewis, T., and Pochin, E. E.: Effects of asphyxia and pressure on sensory nerves of man. Clin. Sci., *3*:141–155, 1938.

Lewis, T., Pickering, G. W., and Rothschild, P.: Centripetal paralysis arising out of arrested bloodflow to the limb, including notes on a form of tingling. Heart, *16*:1–32, 1931.

Lubińska, L.: Axoplasmic streaming in regenerating and in normal nerve fibres. Progr. Brain Res., *13*:1–71, 1964.

Lubińska, L., and Niemierko, S.: Velocity and intensity of bidirectional migration of acetylcholinesterase in transected nerves. Brain Res., *27*:329–342, 1970.

Lundborg, G.: Ischemic nerve injury. Scand. J. Plast. Reconstr. Surg. Suppl., *6*:3–113, 1970.

Lundborg, G., and Brånemark, P.-I.: Microvascular structure and function of peripheral nerves. Adv. Microcirc., *1*:66–88, 1968.

Marchisio, P. C., and Sjöstrand, J.: Axonal transport in the avian optic pathway during development. Brain Res., *26*:204–211, 1971.

McEwen, B. S., and Grafstein, B.: Fast and slow components in axonal transport of protein. J. Cell Biol., *38*:494–508, 1968.

McEwen, B. S., Forman, D. S., and Grafstein, B.: Components of fast and slow axonal transport in the goldfish optic nerve. J. Neurobiol., *2*:361–377, 1971.

Miani, N.: Analysis of the somato-axonal movement of phospholipids in the vagus and hypoglossal nerves. J. Neurochem., *10*:859–874, 1963.

Ochs, S.: Axoplasmic flow in neurons. *In* Garto, J. (ed.): Macromolecules and Behavior. New York, Appleton-Century-Crofts, 1966.

Ochs, S.: Characteristics and a model for fast axoplasmic transport in nerve. J. Neurobiol., *2*:331–345, 1971a.

Ochs, S.: Local supply of energy to the fast axoplasmic transport mechanism. Proc. Natl. Acad. Sci. U.S.A., *68*:1279–1282, 1971b.

Ochs, S.: Rate of fast axoplasmic transport in mammalian nerve fibres. J. Physiol., *227*:627–646, 1972a.

Ochs, S.: Fast transport of materials in mammalian nerve fibers. Science, *176*:252–260, 1972b.

Ochs, S.: Effect of maturation and aging on the rate of fast axoplasmic transport in mammalian nerve. Progr. Brain Res., *40*:349–362, 1973a.

Ochs, S.: Cold-block of fast axoplasmic transport: Re-

versibility and effects of colchicine and vinblastine. Soc. Neurosci. (Abst.), *3*:147, 1973b.

Ochs, S.: Energy metabolism and supply of nerve by axoplasmic transport. *In* Larrabee, M. (ed.): Metabolism in relation to function in ganglia and peripheral nerves of vertebrates. Fed. Proc. *33*:1049–1057, 1974a.

Ochs, S.: Fast axoplasmic transport—energy metabolism and mechanism. *In* Hubbard, J. I. (ed.): The Vertebrate Peripheral Nervous System. New York, Plenum Press, 1974b.

Ochs, S.: Systems of material transport in nerve fibers (axoplasmic transport) related to nerve function and trophic control. In: Trophic function of the neuron. Drachmann, D. B. (Ed.) Ann. N.Y. Acad. Sci., *228*: 202–223, 1974c.

Ochs, S., and Barnes, C.: Regeneration of ventral root fibers into dorsal roots shown by axoplasmic flow. Brain Res., *15*:600–603, 1969.

Ochs, S., and Burger, E.: Movement of substance proximo-distally in nerve axons as studied with spinal cord injections of radioactive phosphorus. Am. J. Physiol., *194*:499–506, 1958.

Ochs, S., and Erdman, J.: "Routing" of fast transported materials in nerve fibers. Abst. Soc. Neurosci., *4*:359, 1974.

Ochs, S., and Hollingsworth, D.: Dependence of fast axoplasmic transport in nerve on oxidative metabolism. J. Neurochem., *18*:107–114, 1971.

Ochs, S., and Jersild, R. A., Jr.: Fast axoplasmic transport in nonmyelinated nerve fibers shown by electron microscopic radioautography. J. Neurobiol., *5*:373–377, 1974.

Ochs, S., and Johnson, J.: Fast and slow phases of axoplasmic flow in ventral root nerve fibers. J. Neurochem., *16*:845–853, 1969.

Ochs, S., and Ranish, N.: Characteristics of the fast transport system in mammalian nerve fibers. J. Neurobiol., *1*:247–261, 1969.

Ochs, S., and Smith, C.: Fast axoplasmic transport in mammalian nerve in vitro after block of glycolysis with iodoacetic acid. J. Neurochem., *18*:833–844, 1971.

Ochs, S., Booker, H., and DeMyer, W. E.: Note on the signal for chromatolysis after nerve interruption. Exp. Neurol., *3*:206–208, 1961.

Ochs, S., Dalrymple, D., and Richards, G.: Axoplasmic flow in ventral root nerve fibers of the cat. Exp. Neurol., *5*:349–363, 1962.

Ochs, S., Hollingsworth, D., and Helmer, E.: Dependence of fast axoplasmic transport in mammalian nerve on metabolism and relation to excitability. Fed. Proc., *29*:264, 1970.

Ochs, S., Johnson, J., and Ng, M.-H.: Protein incorporation and axoplasmic flow in motoneuron fibers following intra-cord injection of leucine. J. Neurochem., *14*:317–331, 1967.

Ochs, S., Kachmann, R., and DeMyer, W. E.: Axoplasmic flow rates during regeneration. Exp. Neurol., *2*: 627–637, 1960.

Okada, E.: Experimentelle Untersuchungen über die vasculäre Trophik des peripheren Nervs. Arb. Neurol. Inst. Wien. Univ., *12*:59, 1905 (quoted by Adams, 1942).

O'Steen, W. K., and Vaughan, G. M.: Radioactivity in the optic pathway and hypothalamus of the rat after intraocular injection of tritiated 5-hydroxytryptophan. Brain Res., *8*:209–212, 1968.

Palay, S. L., and Palade, G. E.: The fine structure of neurons. J. Biophys. Biochem. Cytol., *1*:69–88, 1955.

Perroncito, A.: La rigenerazione delle fibre nervose. Boll. Soc. Med. Chir. Pavia, *4*:434–444, 1905.

Phillis, J. W.: The Pharmacology of Synapses. New York, Pergamon Press, 1970.

Porter, E. L., and Wharton, P. S.: Irritability of mammalian nerve following ischaemia. J. Neurophysiol., *12*:109–116, 1949.

Ramon y Cajal, S.: Degeneration and Regeneration of the Nervous System. (Trans. and ed. by R. M. May.) Cambridge, Oxford University Press, 1928.

Ranish, N., and Ochs, S.: Fast axoplasmic transport of acetylcholinesterase in mammalian nerve fibers. J. Neurochem., *19*:2641–2649, 1972.

Ranish, N., Ochs, S., and Barnes, C. D.: Regeneration of ventral root axons into dorsal roots as shown by increased acetylcholinesterase activity. J. Neurobiol., *3*:245–257, 1972.

Sabri, M. I., and Ochs, S.: Characterization of fast and slow transported proteins in dorsal root and sciatic nerve of cat. J. Neurobiol., *4*:145–165, 1973.

Samson, F. E.: Mechanism of axoplasmic transport. J. Neurobiol., *2*:347–360, 1971.

Schmitt, F. O.: Fibrous proteins—neuronal organelles. Proc. Natl. Acad. Sci. U.S.A., *60*:1092–1101, 1968.

Schultze, M.: The general characters of the structures composing the nervous system. *In* Stricker, S. (ed.): Human Comparative Histology. Vol. 1. London, New Sydenham Society, 1870.

Shawe, G. D. H.: On the number of branches formed by regenerating nerve fibres. Br. J. Surg., *42*:474–488, 1955.

Singer, S. J.: A fluid lipid-globular protein mosaic model of membrane structure. Ann. N.Y. Acad. Sci., *195*: 16–23, 1972.

Smith, S. S., Järlfors, U., and Beránek, R.: The organization of synaptic axoplasm in the lamprey (*Petromyzon marinus*) central nervous system. J. Cell Biol., *46*:199–219, 1970.

Spencer, P. S.: Reappraisal of the model for "bulk axoplasmic flow." Nature [New Biol.], *240*:283, 1972.

Sunderland, S.: Nerve and Nerve Injuries. Edinburgh and London, E. & S. Livingstone, 1968.

Tilney, L. G., and Porter, K. R.: Studies on the microtubules in *Heliozoa*. II. The effect of low temperature on these structures in the maintenance of the axopodia. J. Cell Biol., *34*:327–343, 1967.

Torrey, T. W.: The relation of taste buds to their nerve fibers. J. Comp. Neurol., *59*:203–220, 1934.

Ungerstedt, U.: Stereotaxic mapping of the monamine pathways in the rat brain. Acta Physiol. Scand. Suppl., *367*:1–48, 1971.

Van der Loos, H.: The history of the neuron. *In* Hyden, H. (ed.): The Neuron. Amsterdam, Elsevier Publishing Co., 1967.

Virchow, R.: Cellular Pathology. New York, Dover Publications, 1971. (English transl. by L. J. Rather from 2nd German edition. Philadelphia, Lippincott, 1863.)

Waldeyer, W.: Uber einige neurere Forschungen im Gebiete der Anatomie des Centralnervensystems. Dtsch. Med. Wochenschr., *17*:1213–1218, 1244–1246, 1267–1269, 1287–1289, 1331–1332, 1352–1356, 1891.

Waller, A. V.: Sur la reproduction des nerfs et sur la structure et les fonctions des ganglions spinaux. Arch. Anat. Physiol. Wissensch. Med. (Berl.), 392–401, 1852.

Watson, W. E.: An autoradiographic study of the incorporation of nucleic-acid by neurons and glia during nerve regeneration. J. Physiol., *180*:741–753, 1965.

Weisenberg, R. C., Borisy, G. G., and Taylor, E. W.: The colchicine-binding protein of mammalian brain and its relation to microtubules. Biochemistry, *7*:4466–4479, 1968.

Weiss, P.: Neuronal dynamics and axonal flow. V. The semi-solid state of the moving axonal column. Proc. Natl. Acad. Sci. U.S.A., *69*:620–623, 1972.

Weiss, P., and Hiscoe, H. B.: Experiments on the mechanism of nerve growth. J. Exp. Zool., *107*:315–395, 1948.

Wright, E. B.: A comparative study of the effect of oxygen lack on peripheral nerve. Am. J. Physiol., *147*:78–89, 1946.

Zelená, J.: Development, degeneration, and regeneration of receptor organs. Progr. Brain Res., *13*:175–213, 1964.

Chapter 13

THE STRUCTURAL PROTEINS
OF PERIPHERAL NERVE

David E. Pleasure

The structural proteins of peripheral nerve share several distinguishing features: presence in relatively high concentration; absence of known enzymatic properties; and capacity to aggregate with other molecules to form skeletal, contractile, or membranous organelles. Interstitial collagen microfibrils are polymers of collagen monomer (Grant and Prockop, 1972). Basement membrane also contains collagen as a major component, linked by covalent and noncovalent bonds to several other glycoproteins (Kefalides, 1972a, 1972c). Microtubules are aggregates of tubulin (Kirkpatrick et al., 1970; Davison and Huneeus, 1970) and participate in the movement of transmitter vesicles through the axoplasm (Thoa et al., 1972; Kopin and Silberstein, 1972), chromosomes through the cytosol during cell mitosis (Taylor, 1965), and the release of tropocollagen precursors by fibroblasts (Ehrlich and Bornstein, 1972). Neurofilaments, 6 to 10 nm in diameter, are polymers of filarin and are found only in neurons (Huneeus and Davison, 1970; Shelanski et al., 1971). Neurofilaments accumulate in axons and the perikarya of neurons when axoplasmic flow is interrupted (Smith et al., 1970). Their functions are unknown. Actin-like microfilaments, aggregates of an actin-like protein (Wessells et al., 1971), occur in fibroblasts (Yang and Perdue, 1972), perineurial cells (Ross and Reith, 1969), and the growth cones of nascent axons (Tennyson, 1970; Spooner and Wessells, 1970); they are probably contractile elements (Yamada et al., 1970; Mascarenhas and LaFountain, 1972). The major proteins of myelin, proteolipid and the basic proteins, form complexes with charged and neutral lipids (Braun and Radin, 1969; Carnegie, 1971), and are essential for the biosynthesis and stability of the myelin sheath (Pleasure et al., 1973a).

Nerve function is compromised when synthesis or transport of the structural proteins is interfered with, or when the normal balance between formation and degradation of the intracellular and extracellular organelles is lost. For example, segmental demyelination occurs when either synthesis of myelin proteolipid and basic proteins is inhibited by diphtheria toxin (Pleasure et al., 1973a), or when myelin catabolism is accelerated to a degree beyond the capacity of the Schwann cell to replace the myelin that is lost, as in exposure to hexachlorophene (Pleasure et al., 1973b). Regeneration of axons and myelin sheaths is impeded by excessive deposition of interstitial collagen in nerve (Holmes and Young, 1942; Abercrombie and Johnson, 1946, 1947; Pleasure and Towfighi, 1972). Axoplasmic flow is interrupted and axonal sprouting slowed if axonal microtubules are depolymerized by colchicine (Edstrom and Mattsson, 1972; Kopin and Silberstein, 1972), or if microtubular remodeling is prevented by deuterium oxide (Anderson, et al., 1972).

COLLAGEN

Tropocollagen, a molecule 1.5 nm in diameter and 300 nm long (Grant and Prockop, 1972), is the major constituent of two extracellular structures: interstitial collagen micro-fibrils, 30 to 120 nm in diameter in nerve (Thomas, 1963; Gamble, 1964; Gamble and Eames, 1964); and basement membrane, a meshwork of 3 to 4 nm diameter filaments set in an amorphous glycoprotein matrix (Kefalides, 1973).

Tropocollagen makes up 25 to 50 per cent of the total protein in peripheral nerves (Abercrombie and Johnson, 1946; Roberts et al., 1958). It is most abundant in small cutaneous nerve twigs and least plentiful in the nerve roots (Gamble and Eames, 1964; Morris et al., 1972). Interstitial collagen accounts for the tensile strength of nerve and also of the basement membrane that lines the lumen of vasa nervorum and surrounds perineurial cells and Schwann cells (Thomas, 1963; Shanthaveerappa and Bourne, 1966; Ross and Reith, 1969; Saito and Zacks, 1969; Gamble and Eames, 1964). Basement membrane helps to make up the blood-nerve barrier and is important in guiding nerve regeneration.

Chemistry of Interstitial Collagen

Cross striations, seen at intervals of 68 nm along interstitial collagen microfibrils, are attributable to ordered stacking of tropocollagen molecules. Tropocollagen in newly formed microfibrils is held in place only by noncovalent bonds, but mature collagen microfibrils are stabilized by covalent links between the peptide chains of neighboring tropocollagen molecules (Grant and Prockop, 1972). Each tropocollagen molecule is made up of three peptide chains, 1000 amino acids long. The peptides are coiled together to form a triple helix (Grant and Prockop, 1972). Two of the three peptides are identical (alpha$_1$ chains) while the third, though the same length, is different in amino acid sequence (alpha$_2$ chain) (Piez et al., 1963).

The unusual triple helical configuration of collagen is attributed, in part, to a recurrent amino acid sequence within the individual polypeptide chains in which glycine is followed by proline and then hydroxyproline (Fig. 13-1). The rigid pyrrolidine rings of proline and trans-4-hydroxyproline put constraints on the degree of bending permitted the peptide chain and reduce the number of intramolecular hydrogen bonds that can be formed. Instead, the glycines form hydrogen

bonds with carbonyl groups of the other two peptides in the molecule (Traub et al., 1969; Grant and Prockop, 1972). Glycine-X-lysine and glycine-X-hydroxylysine (X being any amino acid) also occur repetitively in collagen. Galactose or glucosylgalactose is covalently bound to the hydroxyl group of hydroxylysine (Butler and Cunningham, 1966). The epsilon amino groups of lysine and hydroxylysine participate in cross linking to other collagen molecules in the collagen microfibrils (see Fig. 13-2) (Siegel and Martin, 1970; Siegel et al., 1970; Grant and Prockop, 1972).

Chemistry of Basement Membrane Collagen

Basement membrane collagen resembles interstitial collagen in large content of glycine, hydroxyproline, and hydroxylysine, as well as in triple helical configuration (Kefalides, 1973). There are, however, significant differences. Basement membrane collagen contains three identical alpha chains (Kefalides, 1971, 1972b), each slightly larger than the peptides of interstitial collagen (Grant et al., 1972b). The hydroxylysine content is greater (Kefalides, 1972b, 1973), and a significant proportion of the trans-hydroxyproline is hydroxylated in the 3 rather than the 4 position on the ring (Kefalides, 1971; Grant et al., 1972a). Basement membrane collagen contains 20 times more hexose than interstitial collagen, chiefly in the form of glucosylgalactose disaccharide linked to hydroxylysine (Kefalides, 1971, 1972b). Steric hindrance by this disaccharide may explain the inability of basement membrane tropocollagen to form typical striated microfibrils (Grant and Prockop, 1972). Each alpha chain of basement membrane tropocollagen is covalently linked to a cystine-containing glycopeptide, and noncovalently bound to other glycopeptides (Kefalides, 1972a, 1973; Hudson and Spiro, 1972a, 1972b).

Biosynthesis of Tropocollagen

CELLS RESPONSIBLE FOR BIOSYNTHESIS

Most cell lines synthesize collagen in tissue culture, but fibroblasts are by far the most

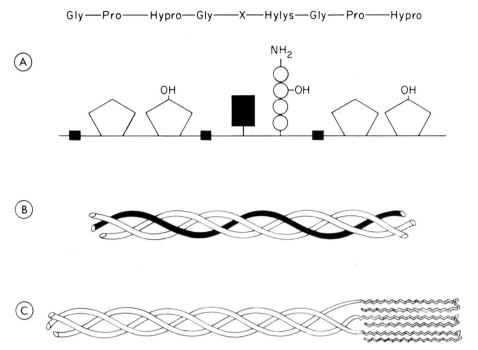

Gly—Pro——Hypro—Gly—X—Hylys—Gly—Pro——Hypro

Figure 13–1   Structure of tropocollagen. *A*. A typical nine amino acid sequence is shown. The glycine-proline-hydroxy-proline triplet (three amino acids at left and three at right ends of the sequence) is important in determining the secondary and tertiary structure of tropocollagen (see text for explanation). The hydroxyl group of hydroxylysine is the site for covalent binding of galactose or glucosylgalactose. *B*. The tropocollagen triple helix. In interstitial tropocollagen, two of the three peptides are identical alpha₁ chains (shown in white) while the third, an alpha₂ chain (shown in black), differs in amino acid sequence. *C*. Basement membrane tropocollagen. The three alpha chains of basement membrane tropo-collagen are identical. Each is covalently linked to a glycopeptide containing cystine (shown as a thin, doubled back fila-ment) and noncovalently linked to other glycopeptides (not shown). *A* modified from Grant, M. E., and Prockop, D. J.: The biosynthesis of collagen. N. Engl. J. Med., *286*:194, 242, 291, 1972. *C* modified from Kefalides, N. A.: Structure and biosynthesis of basement membranes. Int. Rev. Connect. Tissue Res., *6*:63, 1973.)

active, devoting about 15 per cent of total protein production to collagen (Green et al., 1966). Most interstitial collagen is produced by cells of mesodermal origin, but neuro-ectodermal cells secrete extracellular filaments with the characteristic cross striations of collagen microfibrils during early stages of development of the cornea and neuraxis (Cohen and Hay, 1971). "Pure cultures" of Schwann cells also synthesize material re-sembling interstitial collagen (Murray and Stout, 1940, 1942).

It is likely that epineurial interstitial col-lagen microfibrils are made by epineurial fibroblasts (Saito and Zacks, 1969). Within the endoneurium, more than 90 per cent of cell nuclei belong to Schwann cells and less than 10 per cent to fibroblasts (Thomas, 1963; Ochoa and Mair, 1969). Schwann cells often enclose collagen microfibrils within basement membrane–lined pockets, particularly in the cutaneous nerves (Gamble and Eames, 1964, 1970), suggesting that these cells are making

collagen, but it is possible that this configura-tion results, instead, from the tendency of Schwann cells to wrap around slender cylin-ders. As yet, it has not been established which cells are responsible for endoneurial inter-stitial collagen synthesis.

Schwann cell processes are surrounded by a basement membrane, usually about 25 nm thick (Gamble and Eames, 1964), and peri-neurial cells by an even thicker basement membrane (Thomas, 1963; Shanthaveerappa and Bourne, 1966; Ross and Reith, 1969; Saito and Zacks, 1969). It is uncertain whether the Schwann cells and perineurial meso-thelial cells synthesize basement membrane (Nathaniel and Pease, 1963), but both Schwann cells and perineurial cells are of neuroecto-dermal origin, as is lens capsule, which is known to synthesize basement membrane (Kefalides, 1973). Recently, Church and co-workers (1973) reported that a clonal line of rat Schwann cells synthesized collagen actively in vitro.

Processing of Collagen

Six sequential steps in collagen biosynthesis have been distinguished (Grant and Prockop, 1972). Three are intracellular: (1) synthesis of collagen polypeptide chains on the polyribosomes, (2) hydroxylation of some of the prolines and lysines in the polypeptides, and (3) glycosylation of the hydroxylysines. Intracellular processing takes approximately 20 minutes in tendon fibroblasts (Dehm and Prockop, 1971), and one hour in lens capsule basement membrane–forming cells (Grant et al., 1972a). Subsequent extracellular processing includes: (4) selective proteolysis of the polypeptide chains to remove a cystine-containing "transport piece," (5) oxidative deamination of epsilon amino groups of lysine and hydroxylysine to form aldehydes, and (6) aldehyde participation in cross linking between adjacent tropocollagen molecules by Schiff base formation or aldol condensation (see Fig. 13–2). Extracellular processing is not completed until from weeks to years after tropocollagen is synthesized (Veis et al., 1972).

INTRACELLULAR PROCESSING OF COLLAGEN

Trans-4-hydroxyproline and hydroxylysine are not incorporated directly into peptides; instead, prolines and lysines in newly synthesized protocollagen are hydroxylated by the enzymes protocollagen proline hydroxylase and protocollagen lysine hydroxylase (Kivirikko et al., 1972). The number of proline and lysine residues hydroxylated prior to collagen extrusion varies from tissue to tissue, but is greater in basement membrane than interstitial collagen. If hydroxylation is prevented, incompletely hydrolyzed collagen accumulates within the cells, is proteolyzed, and is excreted as small peptide fragments (Harsch et al., 1972; Ehrlich and Bornstein, 1972). Proline hydroxylation is inhibited by incorporation of the proline analogues, cis-4-hydroxyproline or azetidine-2-carboxylic acid into protocollagen in place of proline (Takeuchi et al., 1969; Rosenbloom and Prockop, 1970, 1971; Harsch et al., 1972). Lysine hydroxylation is inhibited by incorporation of dehydrolysine into protocollagen in place of lysine (Christner and Rosenbloom, 1971; Harsch et al., 1972). The activities of protocollagen proline hydroxylase and protocollagen lysine hydroxylase, both iron-dependent enzymes, are reduced by the chelator, alpha, alpha'-dipyridyl (Prockop and Juva, 1965). Hereditary human deficiency of protocollagen lysine hydroxylase has been described. Affected children have abnormalities of connective tissue, including lax joints and kyphoscoliosis. Muscle bulk is reduced, and motor milestones retarded (Pinnell et al., 1972; Eyre and Glimcher, 1972).

EXTRUSION AND SELECTIVE PROTEOLYSIS OF PROCOLLAGEN

Microtubules participate in the release of collagen from cells, and agents that cause depolymerization of microtubules slow the rate of collagen production by these cells (Hsie and Puck, 1971; Hsie et al., 1971; Puck et al., 1972; Ehrlich and Bornstein, 1972).

Newly extruded collagen is in a triple helix configuration, like collagen monomer, but there is an additional cystine-containing glycopeptide, 13 nm long and 2 nm wide, attached to the amino terminal of each alpha chain of the collagen molecule (Dehm et al., 1972; Grant and Prockop, 1972). This interstitial "procollagen" or "transport form" does not polymerize into normal collagen microfibrils until a proteolytic enzyme, procollagen peptidase, splits the extra segment off (Layman et al., 1971; Bellamy and Bornstein, 1971; Dehm et al., 1972). In lens capsule, a similar transition between basement membrane procollagen and collagen occurs, but the split-off "transport piece" may remain linked to the collagen by S-S or noncovalent bonds (Grant et al., 1972b). In a hereditary disease of sheep and cattle, dermatosparaxis, procollagen peptidase activity is absent, and malformed fragile collagen microfibrils containing cystine are present, particularly in the dermis (Lapiere et al., 1971).

CROSS LINKING OF COLLAGEN

Newly formed interstitial collagen microfibrils have little tensile strength and dissolve in water at high salt concentrations (Grant and Prockop, 1972). As cross links form, tensile strength increases and solubility decreases (Fig. 13–2). Interstitial collagen microfibrils remain friable and salt-soluble if cross links are prevented by the lathyrogen, beta-amino proprionitrile, which inhibits the deamination

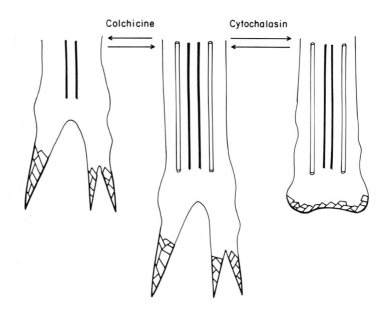

Figure 13–4 Colchicine and cytochalasin B inhibit axonal outgrowth in different ways. Microtubules (shown as hollow cylinders) and neurofilaments (shown as thick bars) do not extend into the pseudopods of axonal growth cones, where actin-like filaments (shown as thin lines) are the only organelles and appear to insert into cell membrane. Colchicine and cytochalasin B both inhibit axonal outgrowth, but colchicine does so by causing depolymerization of microtubules with consequent retraction of axonal sprouts, whereas cytochalasin B has no visible effect on microtubules, but inhibits mobility of growth cone pseudopods and changes the orientation of the actin-like microfilaments (Tennyson, 1970; Spooner and Wessells, 1970; Wessells et al., 1971).

lumen about 15 nm wide (Fig. 13–3) (Smith et al., 1970; Burton, 1970).

The microtubular subunits have been named "tubulin" (Weisenberg et al., 1968; Kirkpatrick et al., 1970). Tubulin weighs 110,000 daltons and is composed of two polypeptide chains, distinct in amino acid composition and sequence though almost identical in molecular weight. Colchicine and other agents favor the depolymerization of microtubules to tubulin (Handel, 1971); loss of microtubules causes retraction of cellular processes and prevents cell mitosis (Fig. 13–4) (Taylor, 1965; Wisniewski et al., 1968; Tilney, 1968). Agents that stabilize microtubules, such as deuterium oxide, interfere with microtubular remodeling (Anderson et al., 1972); cells retain their specialized processes in the presence of deuterium oxide, but further development ceases (Tilney and Gibbins, 1969).

Tubulin makes up from 15 to 40 per cent of total soluble protein in vertebrate brain (Shelanski, 1971; Forrest and Klevecz, 1972) and 15 per cent of squid axoplasmic protein (Davison and Huneeus, 1970). Microtubules are present in the neuronal perikaryon, dendrites, and axons, but do not extend into axonal growth cone pseudopods (see section on actin-like microfilaments). Tubulin is also present in fibroblasts, making up 2 per cent of total fibroblast protein (Nagayama and Dales, 1970), and in Schwann cells in unknown concentration (Hendelman and Bunge, 1966).

Chemistry of Microtubules

Tubulin monomer is extracted from tissue by homogenization and can be precipitated from the homogenate by ammonium sulfate, vincristine, or vinblastine (Marantz et al., 1969); further purification of tubulin can be accomplished by cation exchange chromatography (Weisenberg et al., 1968; Bryan and Wilson, 1971). Microtubules are comparatively labile organelles, but are stabilized by addition of hexylene glycol or deuterium oxide. Such stabilization permits isolation of intact microtubules from tissue homogenates by differential ultracentrifugation (Kirkpatrick et al., 1970).

Tubulin has a sedimentation rate ($S^o_{20,w}$) of 5.8, weighs 110,000 daltons, and binds 1 mole of colchicine and 2 moles of guanosine triphosphate (GTP) per mole of protein (Weisenberg et al., 1968; Davison and Huneeus, 1970). It contains 1 mole of phosphate per mole of protein, covalently bound to serine (Eipper, 1972). In the presence of a reducing agent and a protein denaturant, tubulin dissociates into two polypeptides that differ minimally in molecular weight (56,000 versus 53,000 to 54,000), but are substantially different in amino acid composition and cyanogen bromide peptides (Bryan and Wilson, 1971; Feit et al., 1971a; Fine, 1971). Each of the polypeptides contains several cystines or cysteines (Bryan and Wilson, 1971), which suggests that they may be bound together in tubulin, at least in part, by S-S bonding.

Biosynthesis and Degradation of Tubulin

Neuronal tubulin is synthesized in the perikaryon and reaches the axons by slow axoplasmic flow (Grafstein ,et al., 1970; Feit et al., 1971b). Tubulin synthesis increases to meet extraordinary demands; for example, the rapid outgrowth of autonomic neurites produced by nerve growth factor is accompanied by enhanced tubulin synthesis (Fine and Bray, 1971). The form in which tubulin is transported in the cytoplasm has not been established, but it is likely that tubulin monomer, rather than the microtubule, is the mobile species (Tilney, 1968).

In tissue cultures in which cell division is synchronized, there is a cyclic rhythm of tubulin synthesis and degradation appropriate to cellular needs. Rapid catabolism of tubulin occurs during the stage of DNA replication (Forrest and Klevecz, 1972). Neuronal tubulin is synthesized continuously, and acid and neutral proteinases in axoplasm (Orrego, 1971) may be responsible for degradation of tubulin so as to achieve a steady state.

Tubulin Pool and the Function of Microtubules

In unicellular organisms and neurons, an intracellular pool of preformed tubulin is available for microtubule polymerization, and a given tubulin molecule can pass reversibly from this pool into microtubules (see Fig. 13–3) (Tilney, 1968; Coyne and Rosenbaum, 1970; Piatigorsky et al., 1972). Microtubules are depolymerized if tubulin is removed from this pool by precipitation with vincristine (Bensch and Malawista, 1968; Nagayama and Dales, 1970). This results in loss of cell processes and inhibition of mitosis. The equilibrium between tubulin and microtubules is shifted toward microtubules in the presence of high concentrations of deuterium oxide, and there is a concurrent inhibition of remodeling of cellular processes (Tilney, 1968).

It has been suggested that a microtubule-associated adenosinetriphosphatase (Nagayama and Dales, 1970) serves as a source of energy permitting a conformational change in microtubules, and that this change in confor-

mation in some way causes the movement of transmitter vesicles and other materials through the cell (Schmitt, 1968; Smith, 1971). This theory has not yet been proved, but it has recently been shown that assembly of tubulin into microtubules in vitro requires the presence of guanosine triphosphate or adenosine triphosphate (Weisenberg, 1972; Borisy and Olmsted, 1972). A change in the equilibrium between tubulin and microtubules produced by the action of cyclic adenosine monophosphate (Gillespie, 1971; Hsie and Puck, 1971; Puck et al., 1972), which phosphorylates tubulin in the presence of a cyclic phosphodiesterase (Murray and Froscio, 1971), may be the means by which various hormones, including nerve growth factor, induce differentiation of target tissues (Roisen et al., 1972a, 1972b).

Role of Microtubules in Nerve

Microtubules in nerve are involved in axonal sprouting, axoplasmic flow, and collagen synthesis. Depolymerization of microtubules, e.g., by colchicine, causes retraction of axonal sprouts, though there is no immediate effect upon the motility of the axonal growth cone pseudopods (see Fig. 13–4). Colchicine slows the rate of regeneration of transected nerves in vivo as well as in vitro (Hoffman, 1952; Pinner-Poole and Campbell, 1969; Handel, 1971; Daniels, 1972). Either depolymerization (Edstrom and Mattsson, 1972) or abnormal stabilization of microtubules (Anderson et al., 1972) interrupts both slow and fast axoplasmic flows; there is a diminution in the rate of transport of transmitter vesicles to nerve endings (Thoa et al., 1972; Kopin and Silberstein, 1972), and neurofilaments accumulate within the nerve perikaryon and axons (Wisniewski and Terry, 1967).

Both colchicine and deuterium oxide slow the rate of transcellular movement of procollagen (transport form) from fibroblasts, suggesting that microtubules are necessary for processing of collagen precursors (Ehrlich and Bornstein, 1972). The function of microtubules in Schwann cells, other than in the mitotic spindle apparatus, is not known. Neither depolymerization of microtubules by colchicine nor stimulation of microtubule polymerization by dibutyrl cyclic adenosine monophosphate had any immediate effect upon the rate of myelin synthesis by Schwann cells in vitro (Pleasure, unpublished data).

It is possible that some of the inherited axonal neuropathies are the result of mutations affecting the synthesis of neuronal microtubules (Dyck et al., 1971). No such genetic defect has been recognized in vertebrates, but several mutations causing morphologic and functional aberrations in the microtubules of unicellular organisms have been documented (Randall, 1969; McVittie, 1969).

NEUROFILAMENTS

Axons contain two populations of filaments: 4 to 7 nm diameter actin-like microfilaments restricted to the pseudopods of axonal growth cones (discussed in the following section); and 6 to 10 nm diameter neurofilaments, running the length of axons (Wuerker, 1970) but not present in the growth cone pseudopods or in other cells in the nerve (Wessells et al., 1971). Neurofilaments are polymers of filarin; filarin does not bind colchicine, is not precipitated by vincristine, and is distinct from both tubulin and the actin-like protein in amino acid composition and antigenic properties (Huneeus and Davison, 1970; Shelanski et al., 1971; Fine and Bray, 1971).

Chemistry of Neurofilaments

Neurofilaments are made up of 3 to 3.5 nm diameter globular subunits; these are arranged in a rhomboidal pattern when the neurofilaments are viewed in cross section, and helically in longitudinal section (Wuerker and Palay, 1969; Wuerker, 1970). Neurofilaments have been purified from squid giant axons; they constitute 20 per cent of total squid axoplasmic protein (Huneeus and Davison, 1970). They have also been purified from crude myelin preparations of mammalian brain (Shelanski et al., 1971). In the presence of protein denaturants, the neurofilaments depolymerize into filarin monomer. Squid filarin weighs 70,000 to 74,000 daltons as determined by analytical ultracentrifugation (Huneeus and Davison, 1970), and mammalian brain filarin weighs 60,000 daltons by polyacrylamide gel electrophoresis in the presence of sodium dodecyl sulfate (SDS) (Shelanski et al., 1971). The amino acid composition of the two filarin preparations and the antigenic properties of squid filarin differ from tubulin and the actin-like protein (Huneeus and Davison, 1970; Shelanski et al., 1971).

Metabolism of Neurofilaments

No data are available on the site of synthesis of filarin in neurons, but it is most likely that it is synthesized in nerve cell bodies and transported by axoplasmic flow. When an axon is cut, neurofilaments in the distal stump degenerate within two days (Ballin and Thomas, 1969), but neurofilaments increase in number in the proximal stump and neuronal perikaryon, where they remain prominent for from two to eight weeks (Zelena, 1971; Price and Porter, 1972). When axoplasmic flow is interrupted—for example, by vincristine, colchicine, or acrylamide—neurofilaments increase in number in both perikaryon and axon (Wisniewski and Terry, 1967; Schochet et al., 1968; Pleasure et al., 1969; Prineas, 1969a; Hansson and Sjostrand, 1971), but there is no comparable increase in neurofilaments in toxic neuropathies in which axoplasmic flow is normal (Pleasure et al., 1969; Prineas, 1969b). Neurofilaments also accumulate in neurons in Alzheimer's disease and senile dementia (Schmitt, 1968); whether this implies an abnormality in axoplasmic flow in these conditions is unclear.

ACTIN-LIKE MICROFILAMENTS

The motile pseudopods of the growth cones of sprouting axons (Harrison, 1910) contain 5 to 8 nm microfilaments that appear to insert into the cell membrane (Tennyson, 1970; Spooner and Wessells, 1970; Yamada et al., 1970). Similar microfilaments are present in Schwann cells, perineurial mesothelial cells, and fibroblasts (Wessells et al., 1971; Ross and Reith, 1969; Yang and Perdue, 1972). These microfilaments, polymers of an actin-like protein, participate in axonal elongation (Yamada et al., 1970) and the release of neurotransmitter vesicles (Thoa et al., 1972). They also may play a role in collagen synthesis by fibroblasts (Ehrlich and Bornstein, 1972) and in Schwann cell movements during myelin synthesis (Wessells et al., 1971).

Chemistry of Actin-like Microfilaments

Actin-like microfilaments (ALM) have been isolated from unicellular organisms by Nachmias, Huxley, and Kessler (1970) and Weihing and Korn (1972), from fibroblasts by Yang and Perdue (1972), from sympathetic neurons by Fine and Bray (1971), and from brain by Puszkin and Berl (1972). They resemble actin filaments in diameter, double helical structure (Pollard, 1970), and capacity to associate with skeletal muscle heavy meromyosin in vitro to form "arrowheads" (Nachmias et al., 1970; Goldman, 1972). As a result of the association with either actin-like microfilaments or actin, heavy meromyosin adenosinetriphosphatase is activated (Berl and Puszkin, 1970; Weihing and Korn, 1972).

Actin-like monomer can be obtained by dissociating actin-like microfilaments at very low salt concentration, and will re-form filaments when the salt concentration is raised (Puszkin and Berl, 1972). The transition between monomer and polymer resembles that between G-actin and F-actin (Kawamura and Maruyama, 1972). Actin-like monomer weighs about 45,000 daltons (Morgan, 1971; Fine and Bray, 1971; Weihing and Korn, 1972), and strongly resembles actin in amino acid composition and tryptic peptide fingerprint (Fine and Bray, 1971). The unusual amino acid, 3-methylhistidine, is present in the monomer as it is in actin (Puszkin and Berl, 1972). There are, however, significant differences between actin-like monomer and actin in antigenic properties (Puszkin and Berl, 1972).

Actin-like monomer has several features in common with tubulin. There is some immunologic cross reactivity, synthesis of both proteins is stimulated in autonomic neurons by nerve growth factor (Fine and Bray, 1971), and both actin-like microfilaments and microtubules are depolymerized to monomers by increased hydrostatic pressure (Tilney and Gibbins, 1969). There are significant differences between actin-like monomer and tubulin in amino acid composition and molecular weight, and the monomer does not bind colchicine (Tilney and Gibbins, 1969; Wessells et al., 1971), though it is precipitated by vincristine (Fine and Bray, 1971).

Functions of Actin-like Microfilaments

Cytochalasin B, a mold derivative (Carter, 1967), inhibits cell movement in tissue culture (Spooner and Wessells, 1970; Wessells et al., 1971). Schwann cell movement (Wessells et al., 1971) and procollagen synthesis by fibroblasts (Ehrlich and Bornstein, 1972) are diminished by this agent, and axonal outgrowth stops (Yamada et al., 1970). Neurotransmitter vesicle release is inhibited (Thoa et al., 1972), and the configuration of the actin-like microfilaments in axonal growth cones is altered (see Fig. 13–4) (Yamada et al., 1970). Because of this alteration in organization, it has been suggested that cytochalasin B interacts with the actin-like microfilaments to inhibit cell mobility (Wessells et al., 1971).

A protein resembling myosin has been isolated in association with actin-like microfilaments from brain and renal cells, and an interaction between this myosin-like protein and the filaments might be necessary for their function in nerve (Berl and Puszkin, 1970; Rostgaard et al., 1972). It has been demonstrated that cytochalasin B competes with myosin for binding to muscle actin, though this competition does not affect muscle contraction (Spudich and Lin, 1972). It is still uncertain whether the effects of cytochalasin B on the mobility of axons and other cell processes is due to a direct interference with the interaction of the filaments with the myosin-like protein, or whether cytochalasin B has some other effect on cells, with changes in the filament configuration as a secondary manifestation. It has been demonstrated that cytochalasin inhibits membrane transport of glucose, glucosamine, and various other small molecules, and some direct membrane action of this agent might explain the diminution in cell mobility (Krishan, 1972; Sanger and Holtzer, 1972).

The roles of actin-like microfilaments in the outgrowth of axons, formation of myelin, and synthesis of collagen are worth further study. The presence of the unusual amino acid, 3-methylhistidine, and the interaction of the microfilaments with cytochalasin B may be useful tools for determining their concentration, location, and functions.

MYELIN PROTEINS

Peripheral nervous system myelin is formed by rotation of Schwann cells around axons. After several wraps, the Schwann cell cytoplasm between successive layers of membrane is no longer visible and an almost crystalline array of unit membranes is formed (Peters and Vaugn, 1970). Peripheral nerve myelin contains three major proteins, a glycoprotein and two basic proteins. The glycoprotein differs from central nervous system proteolipid in molecular weight and amino acid composition, but resembles it in ability to form water-insoluble complexes with myelin lipids (Wolfgram and Kotorii, 1968; Braun and Radin, 1969; Folch-Pi and Stoffyn, 1972; Pleasure et al., 1973a). The two myelin basic proteins resemble central nervous system basic protein in solubility in dilute acid, large content of lysine and arginine, and susceptibility to acid proteinases (Bencina et al., 1969; London, 1971; Einstein et al., 1972; Sammeck and Brady, 1972; Brostoff et al., 1972; Eylar, 1972). In addition, there are several extended homologies between the peripheral and central nervous system myelin basic proteins in amino acid sequence (Shapira et al., 1971; Brostoff et al., 1972). These shared sequences explain the capacity of peripheral nervous system basic proteins to induce experimental allergic encephalomyelitis (Bencina et al., 1969; Paty, 1971) as well as experimental allergic neuritis (Arnason et al., 1968; Brostoff et al., 1972) in susceptible species.

Purification of Peripheral Myelin

The most widely used method for isolation of myelin from peripheral nerves was developed by Norton and Autilio (Norton, 1971). Nerve is homogenized in 0.3 M sucrose in water, layered over 0.8 M sucrose, and centrifuged. Most particulate material forms a pellet at the bottom of the tube, but myelin, because of its high lipid content and consequent low density, floats at the interface between the 0.3 and 0.8 M sucrose. The myelin is rid of axonal remnants by osmotic shock in distilled water. Then sucrose density gradient ultracentrifugation and osmotic shock are repeated. The final preparation consists of sheets of myelin membrane almost devoid of mitochondrial or microsomal contamination (Mokrasch, 1971; Pleasure and Prockop, 1972).

Electrophoresis of Myelin Proteins

Freshly prepared myelin or myelin partially delipidated by extraction with cold acetone dissolves in a mixture of phenol, formic acid, water or SDS, mercaptoethanol, and water. Polyacrylamide gel electrophoresis in either solvent system shows three major protein bands, a glycoprotein and two basic

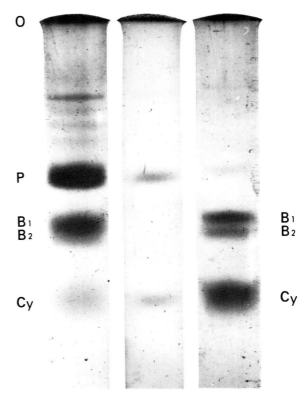

Figure 13–5 Sodium dodecyl sulfate polyacrylamide gel electrophoresis of chick peripheral nerve myelin. Whole myelin (a sample equivalent to myelin contained in one 18 day chick embryo sciatic nerve) was run on the gel on the left; a glycoprotein standard was run on the gel in the center; and basic protein standards were run on the gel on the right; the gels were stained with Coomassie blue for proteins. The molecular weight of the glycoprotein was 30,000 daltons, and of the two basic proteins, 21,000 and 19,000 daltons. *Symbols:* O, proteins remaining at origin; P, proteolipid; B₁ and B₂, basic proteins; Cy, cytochrome c standard. (From Pleasure, D. E., Feldmann, B., and Prockop, D. J.: Diphtheria toxin inhibits the synthesis of myelin proteolipid and basic proteins by peripheral nerve in vitro. J. Neurochem., *20*:81, 1973. Reproduced by permission.)

proteins, in contrast to the two major bands, a proteolipid and one basic protein, obtained with central nervous system myelin of most species (Fig. 13–5) (Mehl and Wolfgram, 1969; Eng et al., 1971; Morris et al., 1971; Pleasure et al., 1973a). If chick embryo peripheral nerve myelin is extracted with chloroform and methanol prior to gel electrophoresis, only a faint trace of the glycoprotein band is present. The two basic protein bands are not seen if the myelin preparation is extracted with dilute acid prior to electrophoresis (Pleasure, unpublished data).

Chemistry of Glycoprotein

Two groups of investigators have recently published data suggesting that the principal peripheral nervous system myelin protein contains covalently bound carbohydrate. Everly, Brady, and Quarles (1973) performed sodium dodecyl sulfate (SDS)–polyacrylamide gel electrophoresis of rat sciatic nerve myelin, and demonstrated that this protein band is periodic acid–Schiff (PAS) positive, which has been confirmed by Wood and Dawson (1973). Everly, Brady, and Quarles (1973) found, in addition, that this protein becomes radioactively labeled after intraneural administration of carbon-14 fucose.

The peripheral nervous system myelin glycoprotein resembles central nervous system proteolipid in molecular weight (about 30,000 daltons), and Pleasure, Feldmann, and Prockop (1973a) found that this peripheral nerve myelin protein, when prepared from chick embryo sciatic nerve, is partially soluble in chloroform and methanol, but adult ox peripheral nerve 30,000 dalton myelin protein is not soluble in organic solvents (Csejtey et al., 1972). Central nervous system myelin proteolipid contains covalently bound fatty acids (Folch-Pi and Stoffyn, 1972), but there have been no reports of lipid bound to the 30,000 dalton myelin glycoprotein of peripheral nerve.

In myelin, central proteolipid interacts with lipids by ionic and hydrophobic bonds (Braun and Radin, 1969), and this is probably true of the peripheral nerve 30,000 dalton myelin glycoprotein as well. When myelin is dissolved in SDS, these bonds are broken, and both neutral and anionic lipids are stripped away. Simultaneously, there is a conformational change in the protein itself, as demonstrated by the reactivity of its cysteine-sulfhydryl groups with alkylating agents. Carbon-14 iodoacetate, a reagent that selectively alkylates sulfhydryl groups at neutral pH, does not react with the cysteine-sulfhydryls in peripheral nerve myelin 30,000 dalton protein in intact peripheral nerve myelin, but does so readily when the myelin has been dissolved in SDS in water (Fig. 13–6) (Pleasure, unpublished data). Similar results have been obtained with central myelin proteolipid (Lees et al., 1971).

The peripheral nervous system 30,000 dalton myelin glycoprotein is relatively resistant to the action of proteolytic enzymes (Csejtey et al, 1972), whereas its myelin basic proteins are rapidly destroyed by exposure to such enzymes. Wolfgram and Kotorii (1968) studied the amino acid composition of that portion of peripheral nerve myelin protein that resists proteolysis and found it rich in sulfur-containing and hydrophobic amino acids, resembling the composition of central nervous system myelin proteolipid (Folch-Pi and Stoffyn, 1972). Wood and Dawson (1973), however, eluted the 30,000 dalton peripheral nerve myelin glycoprotein from SDS – polyacrylamide gels, and reported that its amino acid composition more closely resembles that of a myelin basic protein.

Chemistry of the Basic Proteins

Neural tissues are rich in acid proteinases, which are not inactivated by acetone (Deibler et al., 1972; Einstein et al., 1972). Basic proteins are excellent substrates for such proteinases, and this caused failure of early attempts at acid extraction of intact myelin basic proteins from acetone powders of whole brain or nerve (Bergstrand, 1971). Denaturation of these enzymes by preliminary homogenization of the tissue in chloroform and methanol, or reduction in enzyme concentration by purification of myelin prior to acid extraction, has been more successful. Subsequent purification of the basic proteins has been accomplished by ion exchange and gel permeation chromatography (Carnegie, 1971a; Eylar, 1972; Brostoff et al., 1972; Deibler et al., 1972).

Peripheral basic proteins are only slightly soluble in water at neutral pH, but remain in aqueous solution at acid pH. The basic proteins of peripheral nerve myelin are resolved into two bands by SDS polyacrylamide gel electrophoresis (Eng et al., 1971; Eng, 1971; Pleasure et al., 1973a). In rabbit peripheral myelin, the larger of the two basic proteins resembles central nervous system myelin basic protein in molecular weight, amino acid composition, antigenic properties, and random coil configuration in aqueous solution. The smaller of the two, molecular weight 12,000 daltons, is rich in arginine and lysine, as is central basic protein, and contains a 39 amino acid sequence identical with that of myelin basic protein of the central nervous

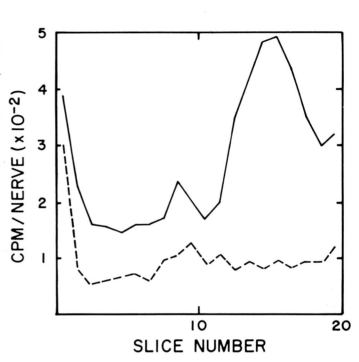

Figure 13–6 Glycoprotein cysteine in intact myelin is shielded from alkylation by iodoacetate. Intact myelin (dotted line) or myelin in 5 per cent sodium dodecyl sulfate (SDS) (solid line) was incubated for 90 minutes at 37° C with 10 μc of ^{14}C-iodoacetate (32 μc per micron). The intact myelin was washed and subsequently dissolved in SDS, and then both samples of myelin were dialyzed against SDS in water. After electrophoresis in SDS on polyacrylamide, the gels were sliced and digested, and the radioactivity in each slice was determined by liquid scintillation counting (Pleasure et al., 1973a). A parallel gel, stained for proteins with Coomassie blue, indicated the position of the protein bands (shown above the graph). No evidence for alkylation of proteolipid cysteine sulfhydryl groups in intact myelin was detected, but alkylation occurred readily in glycoprotein denatured by SDS. Basic proteins were not labeled because they contain no cysteine (Brostoff et al., 1972; Eylar, 1972).

system, including the encephalitogenic sequence around the sole tryptophan in the molecule, but differs from it in having a greater content of hydrophobic amino acids elsewhere in the molecule and a significant amount of secondary structure in aqueous solution rather than a completely random coil (Brostoff et al., 1972; Eylar, 1972).

Little or no 12,000 dalton basic protein is visible in SDS-polyacrylamide gels of human and chick peripheral nerve myelin, even when the gels are heavily loaded with myelin proteins. Instead, two basic proteins of almost identical molecular weight are seen and appear to be present in nearly equal amounts (see Fig. 13–5) (Pleasure et al., 1973a; Pleasure, unpublished data).

Location of Proteins in Myelin

Whereas membrane proteins of red blood cells and other plasma membranes can be visualized directly by freeze-etch techniques, such studies of peripheral nerve myelin show no discernible proteins on either the extracellular or intracellular aspects of the myelin membrane (Weinstein, 1969). Indirect methods for localization of myelin proteins yield conflicting results. Phosphotungstic acid and hematoxylin (PTAH) at pH 5 stains myelin basic proteins and not other myelin proteins. This histochemical method reveals the basic proteins predominantly in the major dense line (inner aspect of the Schwann cell membrane) rather than in the intraperiod line (extracellular surface of the membrane) (Adams et al., 1971). Similar results were obtained for central nerve myelin basic protein with this method (Adams et al., 1971) and also by an indirect Coombs technique, using peroxidase-labeled immunoglobulin to locate antibasic protein antibodies (Herndon et al., 1972).

If the basic proteins are located only on the inner surface of myelin membranes, it is difficult to visualize how sensitized lymphocytes detect the antigen during the development of experimental allergic encephalitis and neuritis (Levine, 1970; Kiyota and Egami,

1972). Several studies suggest that the basic proteins are present, at least in part, on the extracellular aspect of the myelin membrane. Extraction of central nervous system myelin basic protein with dilute acid causes no alteration in the appearance of the major dense line, but an increase in density of the intraperiod line (Dickinson et al., 1970). X-ray diffraction studies of peripheral nerve myelin indicate a concentration of protein on the intraperiod (extracellular) aspect of the membrane (Worthington, 1971).

Function and Synthesis of Glycoprotein and Basic Proteins

Both glycoprotein and the basic proteins form insoluble complexes with anionic lipids (Braun and Radin, 1969; Carnegie, 1971a; Pleasure and Prockop, 1972; Pleasure et al., 1973a). Experiments with diphtheria toxin, which demonstrated selective inhibition of the synthesis of glycoprotein and the basic proteins by this large-molecule protein toxin suggest the possibility that glycoprotein and the basic proteins are synthesized by polysomes located near the cell membrane (Pleasure et al., 1973a). The synthesis of peripheral nerve glycoprotein and basic proteins is particularly active during initial myelination, but continues at a slower pace throughout life (Pleasure, unpublished data). When repair of myelin is necessary after wallerian degeneration, the rate of synthesis of these proteins in adults approaches that achieved during initial myelination (Rawlins and Smith, 1971). Interference with glycoprotein and basic protein synthesis, or accelerated destruction of myelin proteins, causes loss of myelin lipid-binding capacity and segmental demyelination (Pleasure et al., 1973a; Pleasure and Parris, unpublished data).

CONCLUSIONS

Knowledge of the ways cells control the synthesis and polymerization of the structural proteins is fragmentary, but most complete with respect to collagen. Protocollagen, the collagen precursor, is synthesized and enzymatically modified within fibroblasts and probably Schwann cells, and is then extruded from the cells by a process that involves microtubules (Ehrlich and Bornstein, 1972). Once in the extracellular space, enzymatic

removal of a transport piece must occur before interstitial collagen microfibrils or basement membrane can be formed (Dehm et al., 1972; Grant et al., 1972a, 1972b). This multistep pathway offers many opportunities for control over collagen content of nerve, but which of the steps is rate-limiting and how feedback control over collagen synthesis is exerted are not known (Grant and Prockop, 1972). Feedback control is lost when a nerve is cut (Abercrombie and Johnson, 1946, 1947) or subjected to repetitive segmental demyelination (Dyck, 1969; Pleasure and Towfighi, 1972), and the consequent fibrosis has deleterious effects on axonal and myelin sheath regeneration (Holmes and Young, 1942; Pleasure and Towfighi, 1972; Miller and Levine, 1972).

Microtubules serve as intracellular cytoskeletal members; they are required for the stability of elongated cytoplasmic processes, including axons (Tilney, 1968; Davison and Huneeus, 1970). Microtubule polymerization and depolymerization are governed by alterations in the size of the intracellular tubulin pool (Tilney, 1968; Coyne and Rosenbaum, 1970), and probably by changes in the rate of flow of tubulin from site of synthesis to site of polymerization (Feit et al., 1971b). It is likely, in addition, that cells can shift the equilibrium between tubulin and microtubules as required for elongation or resorption of cellular processes, even without changes in the local or overall size of the free tubulin pool (Borisy and Olmsted, 1972; Weisenberg, 1972), but the details of this mechanism are unknown. Pharmacologic manipulation of this equilibrium by agents that stabilize microtubules or prevent tubulin polymerization has dramatic effects on a variety of cellular processes in peripheral nerve, including axonal elongation, axoplasmic flow, and collagen synthesis (Anderson et al., 1972; Thoa et al., 1972; Kopin and Silberstein, 1972; Roisen et al., 1972b; Ehrlich and Bornstein, 1972).

Neurofilaments tend to accumulate in axons and neuronal perikarya when axoplasmic flow is impeded, and this may indicate that control of the polymerization of filarin into neurofilaments is exerted at the stage of filarin synthesis and transport rather than by a rate-limiting enzymatic transformation of the monomer. Now that methods are available for the purification of filarin (Huneeus and Davison, 1970; Shelanski et al., 1971), it should be straightforward and worthwhile to study the biosynthesis and properties of this molecule further.

Actin-like microfilaments and actin-like monomer exist in equilibrium and the reversible transition between monomer and polymer permits ready remodeling of the microfilaments (Tilney and Gibbons, 1969; Puszkin and Berl, 1972). It is uncertain whether a myosin-like protein, found in association with the actin-like microfilaments in brain, in kidney, and in amebae (Puszkin and Berl, 1972; Rostgaard et al., 1972; Nachmias et al., 1970), is always present to interact with the actin-like protein in a fashion analogous to that in muscle, or whether the actin-like protein itself, by inserting on two fixed points and changing length, is capable of exerting force (Wessells et al., 1971). Cytochalasin-B may prove a useful tool for studying the role of the actin-like microfilaments in nerve (Carter, 1967; Spooner and Wessels, 1970; Wessells et al., 1971), but the independent effects of this agent on membrane transport will make interpretation difficult (Krishan, 1972; Sanger and Holtzer, 1972).

The biologically important associations that glycoprotein and the basic proteins form are with lipids. These associations govern the lipid composition and stability of myelin (Braun and Radin, 1969; Carnegie, 1971b; Pleasure et al., 1973). Schwann cells synthesize glycoprotein and the basic proteins near the myelin membrane (Pleasure et al., 1973a). The covalently linked fatty acids on central myelin proteolipid (Folch-Pi and Stoffyn, 1972) may represent enzymatic modifications of the protein that are important in governing its configuration in myelin, and it would be interesting to know if such fatty acids are also covalently bound to peripheral myelin glycoprotein.

Synthesis, transport, and assembly of the structural proteins must be tightly controlled in order to ensure proper development and function of nerve. When control is lost, because of trauma, genetic mutation, or exposure to such agents as colchicine, deuterium oxide, cytochalasin-B, or diphtheria toxin, nerve function is compromised. As our knowledge of the chemistry and function of the structural proteins advances, agents may become available that will permit acceleration of nerve regeneration after trauma or toxic injury.

Acknowledgments: Dr. L. P. Rowland, Department of Neurology, University of Pennsylvania, and Dr. N. A. Kefalides, Clinical Research Center, Philadelphia General Hospital, provided helpful criticisms.

References

Abercrombie, M., and Johnson, M. L.: Collagen content of rabbit sciatic nerve during Wallerian degeneration. J. Neurol. Neurosurg. Psychiatry, 9:113, 1946.

Abercrombie, M., and Johnson, M. L.: The effect of reinnervation on collagen formation in degenerating sciatic nerves of rabbits. J. Neurol. Neurosurg. Psychiatry, 10:89, 1947.

Adams, C. W. M., Bayliss, O. B., Hallpike, J. F., and Turner, D. R.: Histochemistry of myelin. XII. Anionic staining of myelin basic proteins for histology, electrophoresis and electron microscopy. J. Neurochem., 18:389, 1971.

Anderson, K. E., Edstrom, A., and Hanson, M.: Heavy water reversibly inhibits fast axonal transport of proteins in frog sciatic nerves. Brain Res., 43:299, 1972.

Arnason, B. G., Asbury, A. K., Astrom, K. E., and Adams, R. D.: EAN as a model for idiopathic polyneuritis. Trans. Am. Neurol. Assoc., 93:133, 1968.

Ballin, R. H. M., and Thomas, P. K.: Electron microscope observations on demyelination and remyelination in experimental allergic neuritis. Part I. Demyelination. J. Neurol. Sci., 8:1, 1968.

Ballin, R. H. M., and Thomas, P. K.: Changes at the nodes of Ranvier during Wallerian degeneration: an electron microscope study. Acta Neuropathol. (Berl.), 14:237, 1969.

Bellamy, G., and Bornstein, P.: Evidence for procollagen, a biosynthetic precursor of collagen. Proc. Natl. Acad. Sci. U.S.A., 68:1138, 1971.

Bencina, B., Carnegie, P. R., McPherson, R. A., and Robson, G.: Encephalitogenic basic protein from sciatic nerve. FEBS Letters, 4:9, 1969.

Bensch, K. G., and Malawista, S. E.: Microtubule crystals: a new biophysical phenomenon induced by vinca alkaloids. Nature (Lond.), 218:1176, 1968.

Bergstrand, H.: Isolation and partial characterization of some proteolytically and chemically derived fragments of bovine encephalitogenic protein. Eur. J. Biochem., 21:116, 1971.

Berl, S., and Puszkin, S.: Mg^{2+}-Ca^{2+}-activated adenosine triphosphatase system isolated from mammalian brain. Biochemistry, 9:2058, 1970.

Borisy, G. G., and Olmsted, J. B.: Nucleated assembly of microtubules in porcine brain extracts. Science, 177:1196, 1972.

Borisy, G. G., Olmsted, J. B., and Klugman, R. A.: In vitro aggregation of cytoplasmic microtubule subunits. Proc. Natl. Acad. Sci. U.S.A., 69:2890, 1972.

Bornstein, P.: The cross-linking of collagen and elastin and its inhibition in osteolathyrism. Is there a relation to the aging process? Am. J. Med., 49:429, 1970.

Braun, P. E., and Radin, N. S.: Interactions of lipids with a membrane structural protein from myelin. Biochemistry, 8:4310, 1969.

Brostoff, S., Burnett, P., Lampert, P., and Eylar, E. H.: Isolation and characterization of a protein from sciatic nerve myelin responsible for experimental allergic neuritis. Nature [New Biol.], 235:210, 1972.

Bryan, J., and Wilson, L.: Are cytoplasmic microtubules heteropolymers? Proc. Natl. Acad. Sci. U.S.A., 68:1762, 1971.

Burton, P. R.: Optical diffraction and translational reinforcement of microtubules having a prominent helical wall structure. J. Cell Biol., *44*:693, 1970.

Butler, W. T., and Cunningham, L. W.: Evidence for the linkage of a disaccharide to hydroxylysine in tropocollagen. J. Biol. Chem., *241*:3882, 1966.

Carnegie, P. R.: Amino acid sequence of the encephalitogenic basic protein from human myelin. Biochem. J., *123*:57, 1971a.

Carnegie, P. R.: Properties, structure and possible neuroreceptor role of the encephalitogenic protein of human brain. Nature (Lond.), *229*:25, 1971b.

Carter, S. B.: Effects of cytochalasins on mammalian cells. Nature (Lond.), *213*:261, 1967.

Christner, P. J., and Rosenbloom, J.: Effects of incorporation of trans-4,5-dehydrolysine on collagen biosynthesis and extrusion in embryonic chick tibiae. J. Biol. Chem., *246*:7551, 1971.

Church, R. L., Tanzer, M. L., and Pfeiffer, S. E.: Collagen and procollagen production by a clonal line of Schwann cells. Proc. Natl. Acad. Sci. U.S.A., *70*: 1943, 1973.

Cohen, A. M., and Hay, E. D.: Secretion of collagen by embryonic neuroepithelium at the time of spinal cord-somite interaction. Dev. Biol., *26*:578, 1971.

Cohn, R. H., Banerjee, S. D., Shelton, E. R., and Bernfeld, M. R.: Cytochalasin B: lack of effect on mucopolysaccharide synthesis and selective alterations in precursor uptake. Proc. Natl. Acad. Sci. U.S.A., *69*:2865, 1972.

Coyne, B., and Rosenbaum, J. L.: Flagellar elongation and shortening in Chlamydomonas. II. Reutilization of flagellar proteins. J. Cell Biol., *47*:777, 1970.

Csejtey, J., Hallpike, J. F., Adams, C. W. M., and Bayliss, O. B.: Histochemistry of myelin. XIV. Peripheral nerve myelin proteins: electrophoretic and histochemical correlations. J. Neurochem., *19*:1931, 1972.

Dales, S.: Concerning the universality of a microtubule antigen in animal cells. J. Cell Biol., *52*:748, 1972.

Daniels, M.: Colchicine inhibition of nerve fiber formation in vitro. J. Cell Biol., *53*:164, 1972.

Davison, P. F., and Huneeus, F. C.: Fibrillar proteins from squid axons. II. Microtubular protein. J. Mol. Biol., *52*:429, 1970.

Dehm, P., Jimenez, S. A., Olsen, B. R., and Prockop, D. J.: A transport form of collagen from embryonic tendon: electron microscopic demonstration of an NH₂-terminal extension and evidence suggesting the presence of cystine in the molecule. Proc. Natl. Acad. Sci. U.S.A., *69*:60, 1972.

Dehm, P., and Prockop, D. J.: Synthesis and extrusion of collagen by freshly isolated cells from chick embryo tendon. Biochim. Biophys. Acta, *240*:358, 1971.

Deibler, G. E., Martenson, R. E., and Kies, M. W.: Large scale preparation of myelin basic protein from central nervous tissue of several mammalian species. Prep. Biochem., *2*:139, 1972.

Deshmukh, K., and Nimni, M. E.: A defect in the intramolecular and intermolecular cross-linking of collagen caused by penicillamine. J. Biol. Chem., *244*: 1787, 1969.

Dickinson, J. P., Jones, K. M., Aparicio, S. R., and Lumsden, C. E.: Localization of encephalitogenic basic protein in the intraperiod line of lamellar myelin. Nature (Lond.), *277*:1133, 1970.

Dyck, P. J.: Experimental hypertrophic neuropathy. Pathogenesis of onion-bulb formations produced by repeated tourniquet applications. Arch. Neurol., *21*:73, 1969.

Dyck, P. J., Lambert, E. H., and Nichols, P. C.: Quantitative measurement of sensation related to compound action potential and number and sizes of myelinated and unmyelinated fibers of sural nerve in health, Friedreich's ataxia, hereditary sensory neuropathy, and tabes dorsalis. *In* Rémond, A. (ed.): Handbook of Electroencephalography and Clinical Neurophysiology. Vol. 9. Amsterdam, Elsevier Publishing Co., 1971, p. 83.

Eames, R. A., and Gamble, H. J.: Schwann cell relationships in normal human cutaneous nerves. J. Anat., *106*:417, 1970.

Edstrom, A., and Mattsson, H.: Fast axonal transport in vitro in the sciatic system of the frog. J. Neurochem., *19*:205, 1972.

Ehrlich, H. P., and Bornstein, P.: Microtubules in transcellular movement of procollagen. Nature [New Biol.], *238*:257, 1972.

Einstein, E. R., Csejtey, J., Dalal, K. B., Adams, C. W. M., Bayliss, O. B., and Hallpike, J. F.: Proteolytic activity and basic protein loss in and around multiple sclerosis plaques: combined biochemical and histochemical observations. J. Neurochem., *19*:653, 1972.

Eipper, B. A.: Rat brain microtubule protein: purification and determination of covalently bound phosphate and carbohydrate. Proc. Natl. Acad. Sci. U.S.A., *69*:2283, 1972.

Eng, L. F.: Molecular weights of the major myelin proteins. Fed. Proc., *30*:1248, 1971.

Eng, L. F., Bond, P., and Gerstl, B.: Isolation of myelin proteins from disc acrylamide gels electrophoresed in phenol-formic acid-water. Neurobiology, No. *1*: 58, 1971.

Everly, J. L., Brady, R. O., and Quarles, R. H.: Evidence that the major protein in rat sciatic nerve myelin is a glycoprotein. J. Neurochem., *21*:329, 1973.

Eylar, E. H.: The structure and immunologic properties of basic proteins of myelin. Ann. N.Y. Acad. Sci., *195*:481, 1972.

Eyre, D. D., and Glimcher, M. J.: Reducible cross links in hydroxylysine-deficient collagens of a heritable disorder of connective tissue. Proc. Natl. Acad. Sci. U.S.A., *69*:2594, 1972.

Feit, H., Slusarek, L., and Shelanski, M. L.: Heterogeneity of tubulin subunits. Proc. Natl. Acad. Sci. U.S.A., *68*:2028, 1971a.

Feit, H., Dutton, G. R., Barondes, S. H., and Shelanski, M. L.: Microtubule protein. Identification and transport to nerve endings. J. Cell Biol., *51*:138, 1971b.

Fine, R. E.: Heterogeneity of tubulin. Nature [New Biol.], *233*:283, 1971.

Fine, R. E., and Bray, D.: Actin in growing nerve cells. Nature [New Biol.], *234*:115, 1971.

Folch-Pi, J., and Stoffyn, P. J.: Proteolipids from membrane systems. Ann. N.Y. Acad. Sci., *195*:86, 1972.

Forrest, G. L., and Klevecz, R. R.: Synthesis and degradation of microtubule protein in synchronized Chinese hamster cells. J. Biol. Chem., *247*:3147, 1972.

Gagnon, J., Finch, P. R., Wood, D. D., and Moscarella, M. A.: Isolation of a highly purified myelin protein. Biochemistry, *10*:4756, 1971.

Gamble, H. J.: Comparative electron-microscopic observations on the connective tissues of a peripheral nerve and a spinal nerve root in the rat. J. Anat., *98*:17, 1964.

Gamble, H. J., and Eames, R. A.: An electron microscope study of the connective tissues of human peripheral nerve. J. Anat., *98*:655, 1964.

Gillespie, E.: Colchicine binding in tissue slices. Decrease by calcium and biphasic effect of adenosine-3',5'-monophosphate. J. Cell. Biol., *50*:544, 1971.

Goldman, R. D.: The effects of cytochalasin B on the microfilaments of baby hamster kidney (BHK-21) cells. J. Cell Biol., *52*:246, 1972.

Grafstein, B., McEwen, B. S., and Shelanski, M. L.: Axonal transport of neurotubule protein. Nature (Lond.), *227*:289, 1970.

Grant, M. E., and Prockop, D. J.: The biosynthesis of collagen. N. Engl. J. Med., *286*:194, 242, 291, 1972.

Grant, M. E., Kefalides, N. A., and Prockop, D. J.: The biosynthesis of basement membrane collagen in embryonic chick lens. I. Delay between the synthesis of polypeptide chains and the secretion of collagen by matrix-free cells. J. Biol. Chem., *247*:3539, 1972a.

Grant, M. E., Kefalides, N. A., and Prockop, D. J.: The biosynthesis of basement membrane collagen in embryonic chick lens. II. Synthesis of a precursor form by matrix-free cells and a time-dependent conversion to alpha chains in intact lens. J. Biol. Chem., *247*:3545, 1972b.

Green, H., Goldberg, B., and Todaro, G. J.: Differentiated cell types and the regulation of collagen synthesis. Nature (Lond.), *212*:631, 1966.

Handel, M. A.: Effects of experimental degradation of microtubules on the growth of cultured nerve fibers. J. Exp. Zool., *178*:523, 1971.

Hansson, H., and Sjostrand, J.: Ultrastructural effects of colchicine on the hypoglossal and dorsal vagal neurons of the rabbit. Brain Res., *35*:379, 1971.

Harrison, R. G.: The outgrowth of the nerve fibers as a mode of protoplasmic movement. J. Exp. Zool., *9*:787, 1910.

Harsch, M., Murphy, L., and Rosenbloom, J.: Metabolism by isolated fibroblasts of abnormal collagens containing analogues of proline and lysine. FEBS Letters, *26*:48, 1972.

Hendelman, W., and Bunge, M. B.: Some observations on the disposition of microtubules in relation to the myelin sheath. J. Cell Biol., *31*:46a, 1966.

Herndon, R. M., Rauch, H. C., and Einstein, E. R.: Immuno-electron microscopic location of the encephalitogenic protein in central myelin. Fed. Proc., *31*:743, 1972.

Hoffman, H.: Acceleration and retardation of the process of axon-sprouting in partially denervated muscles. Aust. J. Exp. Biol. Med. Sci., *30*:341, 1952.

Holmes, W., and Young, J. Z.: Nerve regeneration after immediate and delayed suture. J. Anat., *77*:63, 1942.

Hsie, A. W., and Puck, T. T.: Morphological transformation of Chinese hamster cells by dibutyryl adenosine cyclic 3':5'-monophosphate and testosterone. Proc. Natl. Acad. Sci., *68*:358, 1971.

Hsie, A. W., Jones, C., and Puck, T. T.: Further changes in differentiation state accompanying the conversion of chinese hamster cells to fibroblast form by dibutyryl adenosine cyclic 3':5'-monophosphate and hormones. Proc. Natl. Acad. Sci. U.S.A., *68*:1648, 1971.

Hudson, B. G., and Spiro, R. G.: Studies on the native and reduced alkylated renal glomerular basement membrane. Solubility, subunit size, and reaction with cyanogen bromide. J. Biol. Chem., *247*:4229, 1972a.

Hudson, B. G., and Spiro, R. G.: Fractionation of glycoprotein components of the reduced alkylated renal glomerular basement membrane. J. Biol. Chem., *247*:4239, 1972b.

Huneeus, F. C., and Davison, P. F.: Fibrillar proteins from squid axons. I. Neurofilament protein. J. Mol. Biol., *52*:415, 1970.

Kawamura, M., and Maruyama, K.: A further study of electron microscopic particle length of F-actin polymerized in vitro. J. Biochem., *72*:179, 1972.

Kefalides, N. A.: Isolation of a collagen from basement membranes containing three identical alpha-chains. Biochem. Biophys. Res. Commun., *45*:226, 1971.

Kefalides, N. A.: The chemistry of antigenic components isolated from glomerular basement membrane. Connect. Tissue Res., *1*:3, 1972a.

Kefalides, N. A.: Isolation and characterization of cyanogen bromide peptides from basement membrane collagen. Biochem. Biophys. Res. Comm., *47*:1151, 1972b.

Kefalides, N. A.: Structure and biosynthesis of basement membranes. Int. Rev. Connect. Tissue Res., *6*:63, 1973.

Kirkpatrick, J. B., Hyams, L., Thomas, U. L., and Howley, P. M.: Purification of intact microtubules from brain. J. Cell Biol., *47*:384, 1970.

Kivirikko, K. I., Shudo, K., Sakakibara, S., and Prockop, D. J.: Studies on protocollagen lysine hydroxylase. Hydroxylation of synthetic peptides and the stoichiometric decarboxylation of alpha-ketoglutarate. Biochemistry, *11*:122, 1972.

Kiyota, K., and Egami, S.: Electrophoretic studies of basic proteins capable of inducing experimental allergic neuritis. J. Neurochem., *19*:857, 1972.

Kopin, I. J., and Silberstein, S. D.: Axons of sympathetic neurons: transport of enzymes in vivo and properties of axonal sprouts in vitro. Pharmacol. Rev., *24*:245, 1972.

Krane, S. M., Pinnell, S. R., and Erbe, R. W.: Lysyl-procollagen hydroxylase deficiency in fibroblasts from siblings with hydroxylysine-deficient collagen. Proc. Natl. Acad. Sci. U.S.A., *69*:2899, 1972.

Krishan, A.: Cytochalasin-B: time-lapse cinematographic studies on its effects on cytokinesis. J. Cell Biol., *54*:657, 1972.

Lane, J. M., Dehm, P., and Prockop, D. J.: Effect of the proline analogue azetidine-2-carboxylic acid on collagen synthesis in vivo. I. Arrest of collagen accumulation in growing chick embryos. Biochim. Biophys. Acta, *236*:517, 1971a.

Lane, J. M., Parkes, L. J., and Prockop, D. J.: Effect of the proline analogue azetidine-2-carboxylic acid on collagen synthesis in vivo. II. Morphological and physical properties of collagen containing the analogue. Biochim. Biophys. Acta, *236*:528, 1971b.

Lapiere, C. M., Lenaers, A., and Kohn, L. D.: Procollagen peptidase: an enzyme excising the coordination peptides of procollagen. Proc. Natl. Acad. Sci. U.S.A., *68*:3054, 1971.

Layman, D. L., McGoodwin, E. B., and Martin, G. R.: The nature of the collagen synthesized by cultured human fibroblasts. Proc. Nat. Acad. Sci. U.S.A., *68*:454, 1971.

Lees, M. B.: Effect of ion removal on the solubility of rat brain proteins in chloroform-methanol mixtures. J. Neurochem., *15*:153, 1968.

Lees, M. B., Leston, J. A., and Paxman, S. A.: The heterogeneity of the trypsin-resistant protein residue from brain white matter. J. Neurochem., *18*:1791, 1971.

Levine, S.: Allergic encephalomyelitis: cellular transformation and vascular blockade. J. Neuropathol. Exp. Neurol., *29*:6, 1970.

London, Y.: Ox peripheral nerve myelin membrane. Purification and partial characterization of two basic proteins. Biochim. Biophys. Acta, *249*:188, 1971.

McEwen, B. S., Forman, D. S., and Grafstein, B.: Components of fast and slow axonal transport in the goldfish optic nerve. J. Neurobiol., 2:361, 1971.

McVittie, A.: Studies on flagella-less, stumpy, and short flagellum mutants of Chlamydomonas reinhardii. Proc. Roy. Soc. [Biol.], *173*:59, 1969.

Marantz, R., Ventilla, M., and Shelanski, M.: Vinblastine-induced precipitation of microtubule protein. Science, *165*:498, 1969.

Mascarenhas, J. P., and LaFountain, J.: Protoplasmic streaming, cytochalasin B, and growth of the pollen tube. Tissue and Cell, *4*:11, 1972.

Mehl, E., and Wolfgram, F.: Myelin types with different protein components in the same species. J. Neurochem., *16*:1091, 1969.

Miller, C., and Levine, E. M.: Neuroblastoma: syncronization of neurite outgrowth in cultures grown on collagen. Science, *177*:799, 1972.

Mokrasch, L. C.: Purification and properties of isolated myelin. Methods Neurochem. *1*:1, 1971.

Mokrasch, L. C.: Preparation and properties of animal proteins soluble in organic solvents. Prep. Biochem., *2*:1, 1972.

Morgan, J.: Microfilaments from amoeba proteins. Exp. Cell. Res., *65*:7, 1971.

Morris, J. H., Hudson, A. R., and Weddell, G.: A study of degeneration and regeneration in the divided rat sciatic nerve based on electron microscopy. I. The traumatic degeneration of myelin in the proximal stump of the divided nerve. Z. Zellforsch. Mikrosk. Anat., *124*:76, 1972a.

Morris, J. H., Hudson, A. R., and Weddell, G.: A study of degeneration and regeneration in the divided rat sciatic nerve based on electron microscopy. II. The development of the "regenerating unit." Z. Zellforsch. Anat., *124*:103, 1972b.

Morris, S. J., Louis, C. F., and Shooter, E. M.: Separation of myelin proteins on two different polyacrylamide gel systems. Neurobiology, *1*:64, 1971.

Murray, A. N., and Froscio, M.: Cyclic adenosine 3':5'-monophosphate and microtubule function: specific interaction of the phosphorylated protein subunits with a soluble brain component. Biochem. Biophys. Res. Commun., *44*:1089, 1971.

Murray, M. R., and Stout, A. P.: Schwann cell versus fibroblast as the origin of the specific nerve sheath tumor. Observations upon normal nerve sheaths and neurilemomas in vitro. Am. J. Pathol., *16*:41, 1940.

Murray, M. R., and Stout, A. P.: Demonstration of the formation of reticulin by Schwannian tumor cells in vitro. Am. J. Pathol., *15*:585, 1942.

Nachmias, V. T., Huxley, H. E., and Kessler, D.: Electron microscope observations on actomyosin and actin preparations from Physarum polycephalum, and on their interaction with heavy meromyosin subfragment I from muscle myosin. J. Mol. Biol., *50*:83, 1970.

Nagayama, A., and Dales, S.: Rapid purification and the immunological specificity of mammalian microtubular paracrystals possessing an ATPase activity. Proc. Natl. Acad. Sci. U.S.A., *66*:464, 1970.

Nathaniel, E. J. H., and Pease, D. C.: Collagen and basement membrane formation by Schwann cells during nerve regeneration. J. Ultrastruct. Res., *9*:550, 1963.

Norton, W. T.: Recent developments in the investigation of purified myelin. Adv. Exp. Med. Biol., *13*:327, 1971.

Ochoa, J., and Mair, W. G. P.: The normal sural nerve in man. I. Ultrastructure and numbers of fibres and cells. Acta Neuropathol. (Berl.), *13*:197, 1969.

Olmsted, J. B., Witman, G. B., Carlson, K., and Rosenbaum, J. L.: Comparison of the microtubule proteins of neuroblastoma cells, brain, and Chlamydomonas flagella. Proc. Natl. Acad. Sci. U.S.A., *68*:2273, 1971.

Orrego, F.: Protein degradation in squid giant axons. J. Neurochem., *18*:2249, 1971.

Paty, D. W.: An encephalitogenic basic protein from human peripheral nerve. Eur. Neurol., *5*:281, 1971.

Peters, A., and Vaugn, J. E.: Morphology and development of the myelin sheath. In Davison, A. N., and Peters, A. (eds.): Myelination. Springfield, Ill., Charles C Thomas, 1970, pp. 3–79.

Pfeiffer, S. E., and Wechsler, W.: Biochemically differentiated neoplastic clone of Schwann cells. Proc. Natl. Acad. Sci. U.S.A., *69*:2885, 1972.

Piatigorsky, J., Webster, H., and Wollberg, M.: Cell elongation in the cultured embryonic chick lens epithelium with and without protein synthesis. J. Cell Biol., *55*:82, 1972.

Piez, K. A., Eigner, E. A., and Lewis, M. S.: The chromatographic separation and amino acid composition of the subunits of several collagens. Biochemistry, *2*:58, 1963.

Pinnell, S. R., Krane, S. M., Kenzora, J. E., and Glimcher, M. J.: A heritable disorder of connective tissue. Hydroxylysine-deficient collagen disease. N. Engl. J. Med., *286*:1013, 1972.

Pinner-Poole, B., and Campbell, J. B.: Effects of low temperature and colchicine on regenerating sciatic nerve. Exp. Neurol., *25*:603, 1969.

Pleasure, D. E., and Prockop, D. J.: Myelin synthesis in peripheral nerve in vitro: sulphatide incorporation requires a transport lipoprotein. J. Neurochem., *19*:283, 1972.

Pleasure, D. E., and Towfighi, J.: Onion bulb neuropathies. Arch. Neurol., *26*:289, 1972.

Pleasure, D. E., Feldmann, B., and Prockop, D. J.: Diphtheria toxin inhibits the synthesis of myelin proteolipid and basic proteins by peripheral nerve in vitro. J. Neurochem., *20*:81, 1973a.

Pleasure, D. E., Mishler, K. C., and Engel, W. K.: Axonal transport of proteins in experimental neuropathies. Science, *166*:524, 1969.

Pleasure, D. E., Towfighi, J., Silberberg, D., and Parris, J.: Hexachlorophene disrupts central and peripheral myelin: morphological and biochemical studies. Neurology, (Minneap.), *23*:414, 1973b.

Pollard, T. D.: Shelton, E., Weihing, R. R., and Korn, E. D.: Ultrastructural characterization of F-actin isolated from Acanthamoeba castellanii and identification of cytoplasmic filaments as F-actin by reaction with rabbit heavy metomyosin. J. Mol. Biol., *50*:91, 1970.

Price, D. L., and Porter, K. R.: The response of ventral horn neurons to axonal transection. J. Cell Biol., *53*:24, 1972.

Prineas, J.: The pathogenesis of dying-back polyneuropathies. Part I. An ultrastructural study of experimental tri-ortho-cresyl phosphate intoxication in the cat. J. Neuropathol. Exp. Neurol., *28*:571, 1969a.

Prineas, J.: The pathogenesis of dying-back polyneuropathies. Part II. An ultrastructural study of experimental acrylamide intoxication in the cat. J. Neuropathol. Exp. Neurol., *28*:598, 1969b.

Prockop, D. J., and Juva, K.: Synthesis of hydroxyproline in vitro by the hydroxylation of proline in a precursor of collagen. Proc. Natl. Acad. Sci. U.S.A., *53*:661, 1965.

Puck, T. T., Waldren, C. A., and Hsie, A. W.: Membrane dynamics in the action of dibutyryl adenosine 3':5'-

cyclic monophosphate and testosterone on mammalian cells. Proc. Natl. Acad. Sci. U.S.A., *69*:1943, 1972.

Puszkin, S., and Berl, S.: Actomyosin-like protein from brain. Separation and characterization of the actin-like component. Biochim. Biophys. Acta, *256*:695, 1972.

Randall, J.: The flagellar apparatus as a model organelle for the study of growth and morphopoiesis. Proc. Roy. Soc. [Biol.], *173*:31, 1969.

Rawlins, F. A., and Smith, M. E.: Metabolism of sciatic nerve myelin in Wallerian degeneration. Neurobiology, *1*:225, 1971.

Roberts, N. R., Coelho, R. R., Lowry, O. H., and Crawford, E. J.: Enzyme activities of giant squid axoplasm and axon sheath. J. Neurochem., *3*:109, 1958.

Roisen, F. J., Murphy, R. A., and Braden, W. G.: Dibutyryl cyclic adenosine monophosphate stimulation of colcemid-inhibited axonal elongation. Science, *177*: 809, 1972a.

Roisen, F. J., Murphy, R. A., Pichichero, M. E., and Braden, W. G.: Cyclic adenosine monophosphate stimulation of axonal elongation. Science, *175*:73, 1972b.

Rosenbloom, J., and Prockop, D. J.: Incorporation of 3,4-dehydroproline into protocollagen and collagen: limited hydroxylation of proline and lysine in the same polypeptide. J. Biol. Chem., *245*:3361, 1970.

Rosenbloom, J., and Prockop, D. J.: Incorporation of cis-hydroxyproline into protocollagen and collagen. Collagen containing cis-hydroxyproline in place of proline and trans-hydroxyproline is not extruded at a normal rate. J. Biol. Chem., *246*:1549, 1971.

Ross, M. H., and Reith, E. J.: Perineurium: evidence for contractile elements. Science, *165*:604, 1969.

Rostgaard, J., Kristensen, B. I., and Nielsen, L. E.: Electron microscopy of filaments in the basal part of rat kidney tubule cells and their in situ interaction with heavy meromyosin. Z. Zellforsch. Mikrosk. Anat., *132*:497, 1972.

Saito, A., and Zacks, S. I.: Ultrastructure of Schwann and perineurial sheaths at the mouse neuromuscular junction. Anat. Rec., *164*:379, 1969.

Sammeck, R., and Brady, R. O.: Studies of the catabolism of myelin basic proteins of the rat in situ and in vitro. Brain Res., *42*:441, 1972.

Sanders, F. K., and Young, Y. Z.: The role of the peripheral stump in the control of fibre diameter in regenerating nerves. J. Physiol. (Lond.), *103*:119, 1944.

Sanger, J. W., and Holtzer, H.: Cytochalasin B: effects on cell morphology, cell adhesion, and mucopolysaccharide synthesis. Proc. Natl. Acad. Sci. U.S.A., *69*:253, 1972.

Schmitt, F. O.: Fibrous proteins-neuronal organelles. Proc. Natl. Acad. Sci. U.S.A., *60*:1092, 1968.

Schochet, S. S. Jr., Lampert, P. W., and Earle, K. M.: Neuronal changes induced by intrathecal vincristine sulfate. J. Neuropathol. Exp. Neurol., *27*:645, 1968.

Schröder, J. M.: Altered ratio between axon diameter and myelin sheath thickness in regenerated nerve fibers. Brain Res., *45*:49, 1972.

Schröder, J. M., and Krücke, W.: Zur Feinstruktur der experimentell-allergischen Neuritis beim Kaninchen. Acta Neuropathol. (Berl.), *14*:261, 1970.

Shanthaveerappa, T. R., and Bourne, G. H.: Perineurial epithelium: a new concept of its role in the integrity of the peripheral nervous system. Science, *154*: 1464, 1966.

Shapira, R., Chou, F. C. H., McKneally, S., Urban, E., and

Kibler, R. F.: Biological activity and synthesis of an encephalitogenic determinant. Science, *173*:736, 1971.

Shelanski, M. L.: Tubulin: dynamics, distribution and transport in brain. Trans. Am. Soc. Neurochem., 2:34, 1971.

Shelanski, M. L., Albert, S., DeVries, G. H., and Norton, W. T.: Isolation of filaments from brain. Science, *174*:1242, 1971.

Siegel, R. C., and Martin, G. R.: Collagen cross-linking: enzymatic synthesis of lysine-derived aldehydes and the production of cross-linked components. J. Biol. Chem., *245*:1653, 1970.

Siegel, R. C., Pinnell, S. R., and Martin, G. R.: Cross-linking of collagen and elastin: properties of lysyl oxidase. Biochemistry, *9*:4486, 1970.

Smith, D. S.: On the significance of cross-bridges between microtubules and synaptic vesicles. Philos. Trans. R. Soc. Lond. [Biol. Sci.], *261*:395, 1971.

Smith, D. S., Jarlfors, U., and Beranek, R.: The organization of synaptic axoplasm in the lamprey (Petromyzon marinus) central nervous system. J. Cell Biol., *46*:199, 1970.

Spooner, B. S., and Wessells, N. K.: Effects of cytochalasin B upon microfilaments involved in morphology of salivary epithelium. Proc. Natl. Acad. Sci. U.S.A., *66*:360, 1970.

Spudich, J. A., and Lin, S.: Cytochalasin B, its interaction with actin and actomyosin from muscle. Proc. Natl. Acad. Sci. U.S.A., *69*:442, 1972.

Takeuchi, T., Rosenbloom, J., and Prodkop, O. J.: Biosynthesis of abnormal collagens with amino acid analogues. II. Inability of cartilage cells to extrude collagen polypeptides containing L-azetidine-2-carboxylic acid or cis-4-fluoro-L-proline. Biochim. Biophys. Acta, *175*:156, 1969.

Taylor, E. W.: The mechanism of colchicine inhibition of mitosis. I. Kinetics of inhibition and the binding of H^3-colchicine. J. Cell Biol., *25*:145, 1965.

Tennyson, V. M.: The fine structure of the axon and growth cone of the dorsal root neuroblast of the rabbit embryo. J. Cell Biol., *44*:62, 1970.

Thoa, N. B., Wooten, G. F., Axelrod, J., and Kopin, I. J.: Inhibition of dopamine-beta-hydroxylase (DBH) and norepinephrine (NE) release from sympathetic nerves by colchicine, vinblastine and cytochalasin-B and its enhancement by dibutyryl cyclic-AMP. Fed. Proc., *31*:566, 1972.

Thomas, P. K.: The connective tissue of peripheral nerve: an electron microscope study. J. Anat., *97*:35, 1963.

Thomas, P. K.: The deposition of collagen in relation to Schwann cell basement membrane during peripheral nerve regeneration. J. Cell Biol., *23*:375, 1964.

Tilney, L. G.: The assembly of microtubules and their role in the development of cell form. Dev. Biol. Suppl., *2*:63, 1968.

Tilney, L. G., and Gibbins, J. R.: Microtubules and filaments in the filopodia of the secondary mesenchyme cells of Arbacia punctulata and Echinarachnius parma. J. Cell Sci., *5*:195, 1969.

Traub, W., Yonath, A., and Segal, D. M.: On the molecular structure of collagen. Nature, *221*:914, 1969.

Veis, A., Anesey, J. R., Garvin, J. E., and Dimuzio, M. T.: High molecular weight collagen: a long-lived intermediate in the biogenesis of collagen fibrils. Biochem. Biophys. Res. Commun., *48*:1404, 1972.

Weihing, R. R., and Korn, E. D.: Acanthamoeba actin. Composition of the peptide that contains 3-methylhistidine and a peptide that contains N^e-methyllysine. Biochemistry, *11*:1538, 1972.

Weinstein, R. S.: The structure of cell membranes. N. Engl. J. Med., *281*:86, 1969.

Weisenberg, R. C.: Microtubule formation in vitro in solutions containing low calcium concentrations. Science, *177*:1104, 1972.

Weisenberg, R. C., Borisy, G. G., and Taylor, E. W.: The colchicine-binding protein of mammalian brain and its relation to microtubules. Biochemistry, *7*:4466, 1968.

Wessells, N. K., Spooner, B. S., Ash, J. F., Bradley, M. O., Luduena, M. A., Taylor, E. L., Wrenn, J. T., and Yamada, K. M.: Microfilaments in cellular and developmental processes. Contractile microfilament machinery of many cell types is reversibly inhibited by cytochalasin B. Science, *171*:135, 1971.

Wisniewski, H., and Terry, R. D.: Experimental colchicine encephalopathy. I. Induction of neurofibrillary degeneration. Lab. Invest., *17*:577, 1967.

Wisniewski, H., Shelanski, M. L., and Terry, R. D.: Effects of mitotic spindle inhibitors on neurotubules and neurofilaments in anterior horn cells. J. Cell Biol., *38*:224, 1968.

Wolfgram, F., and Kotorii, K.: The composition of the myelin proteins of the peripheral nervous system. J. Neurochem., *15*:1291, 1968.

Wood, J. G., and Dawson, R. M. C.: A major myelin glycoprotein of sciatic nerve. J. Neurochem., *21*:717–719, 1973.

Worthington, C. R.: X-ray analysis of nerve myelin. *In* Adelman, W. J., Jr. (ed.): Biophysics and Physiology of Excitable Membranes. New York, Van Nostrand Reinhold, 1971, pp. 1–45.

Wuerker, R. B.: Neurofilaments and glial filaments. Tissue and Cell, *2*:1, 1970.

Wuerker, R. B., and Palay, S. L.: Neurofilaments and microtubules in anterior horn cells of the rat. Tissue and Cell, *1*:387, 1969.

Yamada, K. M., Spooner, B. S., and Wessells, N. K.: Axon growth: roles of microfilaments and microtubules. Proc. Natl. Acad. Sci. U.S.A., *66*:1206, 1970.

Yang, Y., and Perdue, J. F.: Contractile proteins of cultured cells. I. The isolation and characterization of an actin-like protein from cultured chick embryo fibroblasts. J. Biol. Chem., *247*:4503, 1972.

Zelena, J.: Neurofilaments and microtubules in sensory neurons after peripheral nerve section. Z. Zellforsch. Mikrosk. Anat., *117*:191, 1971.

SECTION III

*Pathology of the
Peripheral Nervous System*

Chapter 14

PATHOLOGY OF THE NERVE CELL BODY IN DISORDERS OF THE PERIPHERAL NERVOUS SYSTEM

John Prineas *and* Peter S. Spencer

The fact that it is necessary, in a text such as this, to provide separate accounts of the pathologic changes that affect nerve cell processes and those that affect nerve cell bodies illustrates clearly enough the largely descriptive nature of current nerve cell pathology. Morphologic studies have demonstrated a close correlation between axonal interruption or cell loss and nervous dysfunction; in terms of cell dysfunction, however, the significance of the various structural alterations that have been observed in neurons and the pathogenesis of these changes remain almost entirely unknown. It must also be emphasized that nerve cells are particularly sensitive to poor fixation and postmortem artifacts, and that the classic histologic methods have sometimes failed to distinguish such changes. Current electron microscopic techniques, and particularly the combined use of tissue culture methods and electron microscopy, have been most revealing in this regard, and it may be anticipated that the cellular pathology of the neuron will be radically revised and extended over the next few years.

METHODS OF STUDY

The common staining procedures used to study the general morphology of the nerve cell include hematoxylin and eosin preparations, which also display inclusion bodies and cellular infiltrates and blood vessel changes; reduced silver stains such as Bodian's pro-

targol and Cajal's silver method for neurofibrils and synaptic terminals; and the various modifications of the Nissl technique, which stain the nucleus and cell body and part of the dendritic system of the nerve cell. For studies involving measurements of cell size, it should be noted that with the latter technique, which is used as an all purpose cell survey stain, cell membranes and the margins of nerve cells stain poorly and appear smaller than with procedures such as the combined periodic acid–Schiff Gallocyanin–chrome alum method, which also stains the cell margin (Cammermeyer, 1961). Routine histologic examination of the spinal cord also requires myelin and glial fiber preparations, and the common histochemical procedures to detect lipid, carbohydrate, and protein-containing complexes are frequently called for. For details of these staining methods and for the techniques for sampling and fixing nervous tissue, the reader is referred to accounts by Tedeschi (1970) and Segarra (1970). One micron thick sections of epoxy-embedded material that has been fixed and prepared for electron microscopy by using standard methods are unsurpassed for fine cytologic detail. These sections, stained with toluidine blue, are ideal specimens for optical microscopy in terms of thickness and contrast, and they warrant the use of apochromatic objectives. Although used mainly in experimental studies, in which fixation can be carried out by whole body perfusion, this method will also be rewarding in examination of autopsy material fixed by

253

immersion. Quite large sections, up to several millimeters square, may be cut without difficulty with glass knives mounted in standard ultramicrotomes. In small animals, such as the cat, full cross sections of the cord and dorsal root ganglia can be prepared in this way.

Electron microscopy has been an almost routine extension of the histologic examination in experimental work, and it is used increasingly in the study of human biopsy and autopsy material. In experimental animals, adequate fixation of the brain and whole spinal cord is readily achieved by total body perfusion through the left ventricle or aorta; a large volume of fixative delivered rapidly under pressure (3 liters in 15 minutes at 150 mm of mercury in the rabbit) is necessary, and in the anesthetized animal, a delay of more than a few seconds between opening the chest and commencing the perfusion usually results in poor fixation. Further details of perfusion fixation are provided by Bohman and Maunsbach (1970), Wiśniewski, Raine, and Kay (1972), and Price and Porter (1972). Correct orientation and selection of areas for electron microscopy are particularly important when dealing with nervous tissue, and this is facilitated by embedding tissue in the form of thin slices less than 0.5 mm thick and several millimeters square. Sections for light microscopy may be cut from the surface of these slices, making it possible to trim selected areas for subsequent examination by electron microscopy. In man, the opportunity to examine adequately fixed neuronal perikarya in peripheral nervous system disorders is limited to parasympathetic neurons in the intestinal tract wall and sympathetic tissue obtained at biopsy. In general, autopsy material is not suitable for electron microscopy because of the rapid breakdown of most cell constituents that begins moments after death; however, useful information may be obtained by this method particularly when the object of the study is a stable intracellular or extracellular inclusion body, storage product, or a group of virus particles (Schochet et al., 1969; Morecki and Zimmerman, 1969).

PREPARATIVE ARTIFACTS AND POSTMORTEM CHANGES

Certain changes that occur in nerve cells at the time of or following death, or during the preparation of tissue for histologic examination, may mimic antemortem changes of

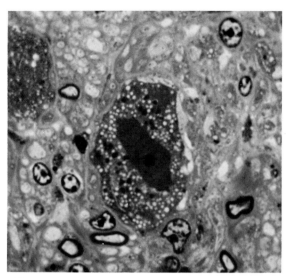

Figure 14–1 Postmortem artifact in a primate neuron. Note the shrunken, angulated outline of the neuron in the center of the field, the presence of numerous cytoplasmic vacuoles, and the dark, abnormally shaped nucleus. Monkey tissue, four hours postmortem, fixed by immersion in glutaraldehyde and postfixed in osmium tetroxide; 1 μm Epon section stained with toluidine blue. × 1200.

pathologic significance (Cammermeyer, 1961; Andres, 1963; Adams and Sidman, 1968). The most reliable evidence of neuronal disease is a loss of nerve cells and the presence of reactive changes in the surrounding tissues. The latter invariably accompany nerve cell damage of more than a few days' duration; and if these are absent, and no topographic variation appropriate to the clinical illness can be demonstrated, the possibility must be considered that any neuronal alteration present may be a nonspecific agonal change or a preparative artifact.

The most common preparative artifact is known as the dark or spiky cell change. Affected neurons appear shrunken and stain darkly; the nucleus is pyknotic, and it is difficult to distinguish the nucleolus and Nissl bodies (Fig. 14–1). Motor neurons appear spiky and angulated, and the normally round cells of the sympathetic and dorsal root ganglia become multifaceted. These cells may occur scattered among neurons of normal appearance, or all neurons in one area may be affected. Associated changes include shrinkage spaces around some neurons and pyknosis of glial cell nuclei. Autolysis, the combined effects of anoxia and autolysis, or some feature of the fixative used have all been held responsible for this appearance. The most likely explana-

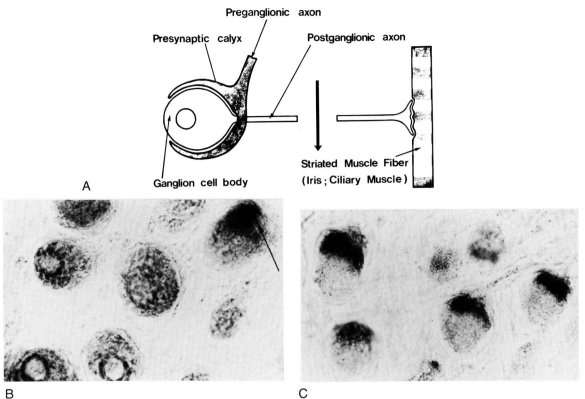

Figure 14–6   The effects of section of postganglionic nerves on the metabolism of preganglionic neurons. Section of postganglionic axons of the chicken ciliary ganglion, as indicated in the diagram (*A*), results in enhanced acetylcholines-terase activity in the preganglionic nerve endings. *B*. Intact ganglion cells. Arrow indicates normal acetylcholinesterase activity. *C*. Axonotomized ganglion cells. Koelle method was used to demonstrate acetylcholinesterase activity. × 580. (From Koenig, H. L., and Droz, B.: Effect of nerve section on protein metabolism of ganglion cells and preganglionic nerve endings. Acta Neuropathol. (Berl.), Suppl. 5:119, 1971. © Springer-Verlag, Berlin, Heidelberg, New York. Reprinted by permission.)

subacute myelo-opticoneuropathy (Shiraki, 1971) and acute idiopathic polyneuritis with conspicuous peripheral axonal degeneration (Haymaker and Kernohan, 1949; Asbury et al., 1969). Although the appearances associated with the axonal reaction are relatively specific for axonal damage, there are degenerative disorders in which similar appearances occur in neuronal perikarya prior to cell death, and it may be that in some of the neuropathies just mentioned the cell body changes are not reactive but are related to the mechanism responsible for axonal degeneration in these disorders. For example, light microscopic changes similar to those seen in the axonal reaction have been observed, albeit rarely, in Werdnig-Hoffmann disease, amyotrophic lateral sclerosis, and poliomyelitis (Einarson, 1949; Bodian, 1949), and also in subacute inclusion body encephalitis (Brain et al., 1948), in herpes simplex infected neurons (Kristensson and Haltia, 1970), in pyramidal cells of the cerebral cortex in patients dying from severe malnutrition and pellagra (Meyer, 1901), in anterior horn cells in kwashiorkor and following prolonged electrical stimulation of a peripheral nerve (Barr and Bertram, 1951; Hydén, 1950).

A number of acute axonal neuropathies have been described in which the nerve cell bodies in the spinal cord either appear normal or show minor, nonspecific changes in the presence of severe distal axonal breakdown. Cavanagh (1954) has commented on this in tri-ortho-cresyl phosphate neuropathy in the chicken, in which it was also observed that affected neurons retain their normal capacity to respond to axonal transsection. The same observation has been made in tri-ortho-cresyl phosphate neuropathy in the cat (Prineas, 1969a).

ACUTE CELL NECROSIS

Nerve cells subjected to acute irreversible metabolic or toxic injury undergo changes referred to as acute cell necrosis. The common appearance consists of a shrinkage and an increased angularity of the cell, the spiky appearance resulting from increased staining of the dendrites. Compaction or loss of Nissl bodies occurs, resulting in a cell that stains more densely or less densely than normal or one in which the cytoplasm becomes glassy and excessively eosinophilic (Fig. 14–7). Oval basophilic bodies, considered to be enlarged boutons terminaux, may appear on the surface of the cell. A further form of acute cell necrosis, resembling Nissl's acute cell disease, with swelling of the neuron has been observed in anterior horn cells following the intrathecal injection of 5-fluoro-orotic acid (Koenig, 1960).

Degenerating neurons are removed by phagocytic cells (neuronophages), which persist for a time as small clusters of microglia at

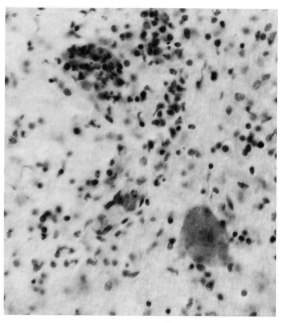

Figure 14–7 Acute necrosis of anterior horn cells in poliomyelitis. The larger collections of mononuclear cells and microglia mark sites of degenerated nerve cells. Hematoxylin and eosin. × 330.

the site of the degenerated nerve cell as shown in Figure 14–7. Whether degenerate nerve cells ever disappear in the absence of microglial phagocytic activity is not certain although it is said to occur. Rarely, degenerating nerve cells become encrusted with basophilic calcareous material sometimes incorporating iron, and these deposits may persist for years. When the necrotic process involves all tissue elements of the cord, as in acute ischemic lesions, acute radionecrosis, necrotic myelitis due to herpes zoster infection, and with trauma, the white matter undergoes spongy and lacunar degeneration, extravasation of blood may be a feature, and blood vessels may be necrotic. As the lesions resolve, the cord shrinks and may exhibit cavity formation.

Acute cell necrosis is seen in ischemic and hypoxic injury of the cord, in hypoglycemia, associated with trauma to the cord, and in virus infections. Anterior horn cells and dorsal root ganglion cells are less susceptible to the effects of anoxia and hypoglycemia than cells elsewhere in the central nervous system, and they will survive anoxic episodes that would be sufficient to cause irreversible damage to cortical neurons. Tureen (1936) described a reversible type of anoxic injury in anterior horn cells in the cat: Following 15 minutes of ischemia of the cord, Nissl bodies disappeared within 7 hours; at 36 hours the cytoplasm was deeply basophilic, but no recognizable Nissl bodies could be seen; and after 72 hours, Nissl bodies began to reappear. It has also been observed that the smaller neurons in the anterior gray matter of the cord are much more susceptible to spinal cord asphyxia than the larger motor neurons (Harreveld, 1964; Tarlov and Gelfam, 1960). This has been related to the fact that large motor neurons, which have high levels of phosphorylase activity and low levels of succinate dehydrogenase activity, may be more dependent on anaerobic glycogen metabolism and less dependent on oxidative phosphorylation than the smaller neurons (Campa and Engel, 1970). Similarly, hypoglycemia readily leads to irreversible damage to cortical neurons in the absence of changes in the spinal cord. In recurrent hypoglycemic encephalopathy due to islet cell tumors of the pancreas, however, there may be selective destruction of anterior horn cells (Richardson et al., 1959).

In acute and subacute neurotropic virus infections involving the spinal cord, neuronophagia of the degenerating nerve cells by pleomorphic mononuclear cells, and residual nodules of microglial phagocytes, are particularly prominent. In rabies, the latter are referred to as Babes nodules. Perivascular and diffuse infiltrates of lymphocytes, larger mononuclear cells, and occasionally polymorphonuclear leukocytes are conspicuous in the gray matter and in the meninges and are associated with vascular congestion and sometimes hemorrhage. If the inflammatory response is particularly vigorous, as for example in poliomyelitis, there may be more widespread necrosis and hemorrhage, following which the cord appears shrunken and its architecture disturbed, and cavities may be seen in the gray matter. The loss of nerve cells is reflected in a loss of fibers from the anterior nerve roots, and a loss of intersegmental fibers from the anterior parts of the lateral funiculi and throughout the anterior funiculi. This picture has been observed in the spinal cord in poliomyelitis, rabies, encephalitis lethargica, Russian spring-summer encephalitis, equine encephalitis, St. Louis encephalitis, and Japanese B encephalitis; in all these conditions the anterior horn cells may be involved with resulting amyotrophy if the patient survives. Similar changes have been observed in the lumbar and dorsal gray matter of the spinal cord in subjects with myoclonus affecting the legs following x-irradiation of the spinal cord, a disorder described as subacute myoclonic spinal neuronitis by Campbell and Garland (1956). In all these conditions, including poliomyelitis, nerve cell destruction involves not only large anterior horn cells but also cells of the intermediolateral columns, interneurons, and neurons in the posterior gray matter. It has been suggested that the involvement of interneurons may be responsible for the muscle spasm that may occur during the acute clinical illness in some of these disorders (Kabat and Knapp, 1944).

In herpes zoster and in rabies, affected dorsal root and cranial sensory ganglia exhibit acute cell necrosis associated with inflammatory changes similar to those just described. In zoster, the changes are usually limited to a single ganglion and the adjacent parts of the spinal nerve roots and spinal nerves. The inflammatory process may extend into the cord at the same level, however, with destruction of neurons in the anterior and posterior horns most marked on the side of the affected ganglion (Head and Campbell, 1900; Lhermitte

and Nichols, 1924; Denny-Brown et al., 1944). An extensive necrotic myelitis sometimes occurs involving all tissue elements over many segments of the cord, and it has been noted that inflammatory changes here may not be conspicuous and the lesion is essentially one of hemorrhagic necrosis, suggesting that some factor in addition to invasion of the neuraxis by virus may be involved in this disorder (Rose et al., 1964).

When viral inclusion bodies are a feature of a particular neurotropic or pantropic virus infection of the central nervous system, these may be seen in spinal cord neurons, although cord involvement is usually not prominent in subacute sclerosing panencephalitis, typical Cowdry type A inclusion bodies have been described in neurons of the anterior and posterior gray matter of the spinal cord, associated with inflammatory changes and some loss of neurons (Brain et al., 1948). In human rabies, Negri and lyssa bodies have been observed as an occasional finding in neurons of the spinal gray matter and in dorsal root and cranial sensory ganglia (Dupont and Earle, 1965).

The factors responsible for nerve cell damage in neurotropic virus infections include direct cytopathic effects of these agents, immune responses to viral antigens, and possibly immune responses directed at normal tissue components liberated or modified by the virus infection (Fenner, 1968; Bull. W.H.O., 1972). Shortly after a cell is infected with poliovirus, host cell protein and cellular ribonucleic acid synthesis are depressed owing to virus-coded protein that renders messenger ribonucleic acid incapable of attaching new ribosomes. In rabies encephalitis, on the other hand, although a variety of degenerative changes, including the formation of cytoplasmic inclusion bodies, have been observed in neurons, the significance of these with respect to cell death is disputed, and it is held that nerve cell necrosis in this infection may be determined by the inflammatory response (Dupont and Earle, 1965). In other virus infections, such as herpes simplex, there is evidence that the virus may persist in neurons in a latent form, without ultrastructural changes and with no clinical illness (Stevens and Cook, 1972).

Acute cell necrosis is not a prominent feature in the slow virus infections that involve spinal cord neurons. In these disorders, which include scrapie in the sheep and kuru and

Jakob-Creutzfeldt disease in man, there is a loss of nerve cells throughout the spinal gray matter, with the remaining nerve cells exhibiting chronic cell change discussed in the following section, chromatolysis, prominent lipofuscin deposition, and in particular, vacuolation of the neuronal cytoplasm (Bertrand et al., 1937; Klatzo et al., 1959).

CHRONIC DEGENERATIVE CHANGES AND NERVE CELL LOSS

Minor degrees of nerve cell loss are sometimes difficult to detect in the central gray matter as the supporting tissues contract and reduce the distance between the remaining nerve cells. Reactive fibrous astrogliosis is an almost invariable accompaniment of nerve

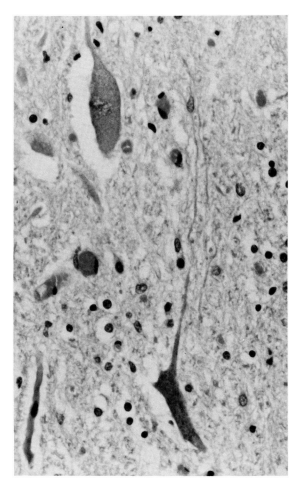

Figure 14–9 Chronic cell degeneration of anterior horn cells in familial amyotrophic lateral sclerosis. Hematoxylin and eosin. × 380. (Courtesy of Prof. J. G. McLeod.)

cell damage, and this is a useful indication of gray matter damage (Fig. 14–8). A paucity of nerve cells without fibrous gliosis is said to occur if neurons degenerate in fetal life or if there is a developmental abnormality of nerve cells (Levi-Montalcini, 1964). Microglial proliferation and spaces in the neuropil may be seen if nerve cell loss is recent.

Chronic Cell Degeneration

In certain chronic disorders in which there is a conspicuous loss of nerve cells from the central nervous system, the outstanding pathologic alteration in neurons remaining in affected areas of gray matter is a degenerative change referred to as chronic cell degeneration or atrophic change. This nonspecific appearance is seen in various metabolic and

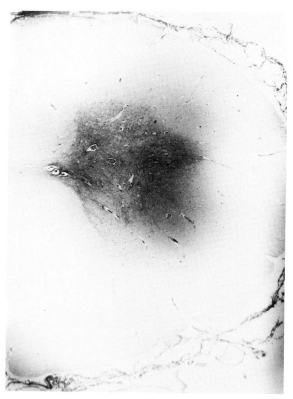

Figure 14–8 Prominent fibrillary gliosis in anterior horn of cervical spinal cord of a patient with sporadic juvenile amyotrophic lateral sclerosis. Holzer stain. Original × 8. (From Nelson, J. S., and Prensky, A. L.: Sporadic juvenile amyotrophic lateral sclerosis. A clinicopathological study of a case with neuronal cytoplasmic inclusions containing RNA. Arch. Neurol., 27:300, 1972. Copyright 1972, American Medical Association. Reprinted by permission.)

degenerative disorders that affect the spinal cord and brain stem nuclei, including amyotrophic lateral sclerosis, Werdnig-Hoffmann disease and other chronic spinal muscular atrophies, sensorimotor polyneuropathy and atypical motor neuron disease associated with carcinoma (Norris et al., 1969; Brain et al., 1968), and Jakob-Creutzfeldt disease. This is also the usual pattern of neuronal degeneration seen in Gudden's atrophy and in transsynaptic and retrograde transsynaptic degeneration. The affected cells appear shrunken, angulated, and darkly staining (Fig. 14–9). Neurofibrils are irregularly thickened, and lipofuscin is present in excessive amounts. The Nissl bodies are lost or clumped together or persist only around the nucleus, which remains central (peripheral chromatolysis). Axons may appear thickened and corkscrew-shaped, and become visible in hematoxylin and eosin preparations. Phagocytosis of the degenerating cells may be seen. The enzyme histochemistry of this type of neuronal degeneration has been investigated in Werdnig-Hoffmann disease, amyotrophic lateral sclerosis, progressive idiopathic polyneuropathy, Friedreich's ataxia, and Jakob-Creutzfeldt disease, but so far no specific change in any particular enzyme system has been detected (Huttenlocher and Cohen 1966; Engel 1968; Robinson 1966a, 1966b, 1968; Friede and DeJong, 1964; Friede 1968; Koenig 1968).

The pathologic changes in affected nerve cells differ in each of the various types of amyotrophic lateral sclerosis that are now recognized, and this has helped distinguish possibly unrelated disease entities within this group of clinically similar disorders. In classic sporadic amyotrophic lateral sclerosis the predominant cell change is chronic cell degeneration as just described, and this affects chiefly the larger nerve cells in the areas of gray matter involved in this disease (Wohlfart and Swank, 1941). Typical central chromatolysis has been described in cases of short duration, but this is rare. In the classic sporadic form of the disease, unlike the Guamanian and Kii peninsula types, neurofibrillary degeneration is not a feature: this was specifically looked for and found to be absent in the spinal cords of 87 subjects with classic amyotrophic lateral sclerosis examined by Hirano and co-workers (1968b). Argyrophilic axonal swellings up to 110 μm in diameter are not an uncommon finding in the anterior gray matter of the cord in the classic form (Wohlfart, 1959), and these have also been observed in the familial adult type of the disease (Takahashi et al., 1972). Carpenter (1968) has demonstrated that the swellings are composed largely of neurofilaments and that they arise from the proximal portion of the axon within 70 μm of the parent cell body. The nature of the rare, minute, single or multiple eosinophilic cytoplasmic inclusion bodies (Bunina bodies) occasionally observed in anterior horn cells in sporadic, familial, and Guamanian amyotrophic lateral sclerosis is not known (Fig. 14–10A) (Bunina, 1962; Hirano, 1965).

An unusual type of anterior horn cell degeneration has been observed in a number of cases of familial amyotrophic lateral sclero-

Figure 14–10 A. Bunina bodies (arrow) from a patient with sporadic amyotrophic lateral sclerosis. Hematoxylin and eosin. $\times$ 890. (From Hirano, A.: Pathology of amyotrophic lateral sclerosis. *In* Gajdusek, D. C., Gibbs, C. J., and Alpers, M. (eds.): Slow, Latent and Temperate Virus Infections. National Institute of Neurological Diseases and Blindness Monograph No. 2, 1965, p. 23. Reprinted by permission.) B. Lewy body–like cytoplasmic inclusions in an anterior horn cell of a patient with familial amyotrophic lateral sclerosis. Luxol fast blue, cresyl violet. $\times$ 560. (From Takahashi, K., Nakamura, H., and Okada, E.: Hereditary amyotrophic lateral sclerosis. Histochemical and electron microscopic study of hyaline inclusions in motor neurons. Arch. Neurol., *27*:292, 1972. Copyright 1972, American Medical Association. Reprinted by permission.)

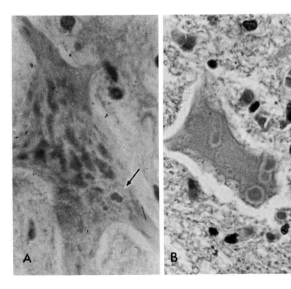

sis of the adult-onset autosomal dominant variety. In this disorder, which is also characterized by posterior column and spinocerebellar tract degeneration, Hirano (1965), Hirano, Kurland, and Sayre (1967); Metcalf and Hirano (1971), and Takahashi, Nakamura, and Okada (1972) have observed swollen anterior horn cells containing hyaline eosinophilic cytoplasmic inclusions that show some resemblance, both histochemically and ultrastructurally, to Lewy bodies (Fig. 14–10*B*). Consisting of a densely staining central core and a lightly staining peripheral zone, the inclusions contain protein and phospholipid, and are composed of radially arranged fibrils 7 to 10 nm in diameter, circular profiles 10 to 80 nm across, and a granular core.

A further type of cytoplasmic inclusion body has been observed in nerve cells in cases of juvenile sporadic amyotrophic lateral sclerosis (Wohlfart and Swank, 1941; Berry et al., 1969; Nelson and Prensky, 1972). Affected neurons are markedly swollen and contain large, irregular, single or multiple bodies with a thin basophilic rim, and a core that stains lightly in hematoxylin and eosin preparations and is intensely argyrophilic (Fig. 14–11). Histochemical studies indicate that the bodies are composed of protein and ribonucleic acid. Affected cells also contain neurofibrillary tangles.

In the chronic spinal muscular atrophies in which degenerative changes are confined to lower motor neurons in the spinal cord and brain stem, which include the infantile form (Werdnig-Hoffmann disease), the juvenile and adult-onset types, and the sex-linked and dominantly inherited forms of which scapuloperoneal amyotrophy is one, neuronal degeneration is usually of the nonspecific, chronic cell degenerative type described earlier, and this is associated with cell loss and reactive changes in the supporting tissues (Kaeser, 1965; Fenichel, 1968). In some cases of Werdnig-Hoffmann disease the cord is smaller than normal, with underdevelopment of the anterior horns. Such cases may show, in addition to areas of cell loss and gliosis, regions in which the anterior horn cells appear smaller and more numerous than usual, without gliosis or other evidence of gray matter damage. This suggests that, at least in some cases of this disease, there may be a developmental arrest of anterior horn cells (Greenfield and Stern, 1927; Byers and Banker, 1961; Malamud, 1968). Central chromatolysis, prom-

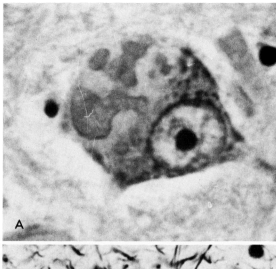
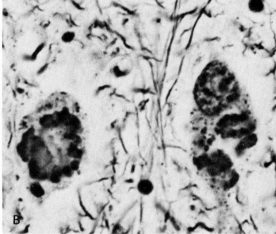

Figure 14–11 Argyrophilic inclusions in motor neurons in sporadic amyotrophic lateral sclerosis. *A*. Hematoxylin and eosin. × 480. *B*. Bodian's silver stain. × 400. (From Nelson, J. S., and Prensky, A. L.: Sporadic juvenile amyotrophic lateral sclerosis. A clinicopathological study of a case with neuronal cytoplasmic inclusions containing RNA. Arch. Neurol., 27:300, 1972. Copyright 1972, American Medical Association. Reprinted by permission.)

inent microglial proliferation, and neuronophagia have been described in rapidly progressive cases, and Engel (1968) noted the occurrence of small eosinophilic intranuclear inclusion bodies in anterior horn cells in two sporadic cases. There are also reports of neuronal degeneration in Werdnig-Hoffmann disease involving a marked accumulation of mitochondria (Chou and Fakadej, 1971) and the appearance of argyrophilic masses in the cytoplasm of affected cells (Norman, 1958). In three typical cases of Werdnig-Hoffmann disease, Chou (1971) observed a selective loss of large-diameter fibers in the anterior spinal

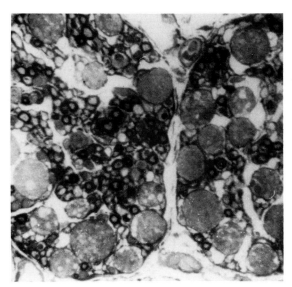

Figure 14–12 Werdnig-Hoffmann disease. Anterior root showing large amorphous bundles of glial filaments between the myelinated nerve fibers. One micron Epon section stained with Paragon. × 500. (Courtesy of Dr. S. M. Chou.)

nerve roots, associated with bundles of astroglial processes 50 to 70 μm in diameter extending up to 1.5 cm into the affected roots from the spinal cord (Fig. 14–12). Chou related these observations to the type 1 muscle fiber atrophy that occurs in this disease, and he suggested that the accompanying neuronal degeneration may be related to a primary ectopic glial hyperplasia.

At autopsy, the majority of cases of the neurogenic type of arthrogryposis multiplex congenita in man and in some animals have shown changes very similar to those seen in Werdnig-Hoffmann disease (Drachman and Banker, 1961; Drachman, 1968; Whittem, 1957). As in Werdnig-Hoffmann disease, the question has been raised concerning a possible developmental abnormality in the motor neurons in the spinal cord and brain stem nuclei in this disorder, as in some cases areas of gray matter have been observed in which neurons are depleted but reactive changes are minimal or absent (Drachman and Banker, 1961).

The fine structural changes accompanying chronic cell degeneration of spinal neurons in man have not been defined, although as already mentioned, ultrastructural features in Werdnig-Hoffmann disease and of certain intracellular inclusion bodies associated with chronic cell degeneration have been described.

Andrews and Maxwell (1968), however, have studied neuronal perikarya of motor neurons in a hereditary motor neuron disease in mice (wobbler mice) described by Duchen and Strich (1968), in which motor neurons of the spinal cord and brain stem nuclei exhibit, on routine histologic examination, chronic cell degeneration, swollen chromatolytic cells with eccentric nuclei, and a loss of nerve cells from the anterior horns of the spinal cord and from the motor nuclei in the brain stem. These workers observed an unusual vacuolar degeneration of neuronal cytoplasm, involving enlargement of the Golgi cisternae and dilatation of the granular endoplasmic reticulum. The vacuoles were multiple and sometimes almost completely replaced the neuronal cytoplasm. Other intracellular organelles maintained a relatively normal appearance (Fig. 14–13). Attention was drawn to the fact that in paraffin sections the vacuoles were difficult to define and the appearances were very similar to those seen in the axonal reaction.

Neuronal Storage Disorders

In the group of familial systemic lipidoses there is a genetic error in the metabolism of a complex class of lipids known as the sphingolipids (Suzuki and Suzuki, 1973). In general, the sphingolipidoses are neuronal degenerative disorders characterized by an excessive accumulation of partially degraded sphingolipids in many types of cell, including neurons, throughout the central and peripheral nervous systems. In these conditions, which include Niemann-Pick disease, Gaucher's disease, Fabry's disease, metachromatic leukodystrophy, and the gangliosidoses, affected nerve cells are swollen by an accumulation in the cytoplasm of faintly eosinophilic, PAS-positive, lipid-containing granules (Fig. 14–14). Usually, some loss of neurons is evident and reactive gliosis and macrophages containing some of the abnormal storage product may be seen.

Niemann-Pick disease includes a heterogeneous group of disorders characterized by abnormally high levels of phospholipids and an enormous accumulation of sphingomyelin in many tissues. In the infantile neuropathic form of this disease, there is widespread and severe neuronal ballooning, and in Purkinje cells, Wallace, Schneck, Kaplan, and Volk (1965) have demonstrated numerous 1 to 2 μm membrane-bound cytoplasmic vacuoles containing loosely arranged lamellar structures.

Lesions of peripheral and autonomic neurons do not appear to have been recorded in Gaucher's disease, another group of systemic

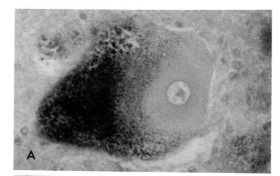
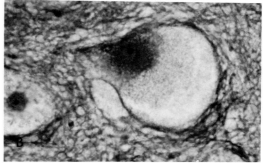

Figure 14–14 Swollen anterior horn cells each displaying an eccentrically-placed nucleus and cytoplasm filled with a finely granular, PAS-positive material. *A.* G_{M1} gangliosidosis. *B.* Tay-Sachs disease. Both × 320. (Courtesy of Dr. Kinuko Suzuki.)

sphingolipidoses in which there appears to be a genetic block of glucocerebroside degradation.

Peripheral neuropathy and autonomic dysfunction are features of Fabry's disease, which is a generalized sphingolipidosis associated with a deficiency of the enzyme ceramide trihexosidase that is associated with an accumulation of ceramide trihexoside in various tissues, including nervous tissues and the walls of blood vessels. These glycolipid granules, which are about 1 μm in diameter and consist of concentrically arranged lamellae with a periodicity of approximately 4 nm, accumulate

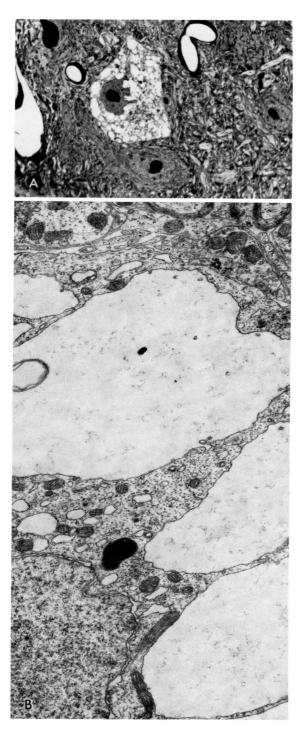

Figure 14–13 Wobbler mouse ventral horn cells. *A.* Degenerate neuron illustrating severe cystic change. Epoxy-embedded section stained with Giemsa stain. × 950. *B.* Membrane-bound intracellular vacuoles occupy much of the cytoplasm. Other cell constituents appear normal. Tissue fixed by perfusion with glutaraldehyde and formaldehyde and postfixed with osmium tetroxide. × 25,700. (From Andrews, J. M., and Maxwell, D. S.: Motor neuron diseases in animals. *In* Norris, F. H., Jr., and Kurland, L. T. (eds.): Motor Neuron Diseases: Research on Amyotrophic Lateral Sclerosis and Related Disorders. New York, Grune & Stratton, 1968. Reprinted by permission.)

in nerve cells in Meissner's and Auerbach's plexuses, sympathetic ganglia, and spinal cord, particularly in the intermediolateral cell columns (Rahman and Lindenberg, 1963). Whether the peripheral axonal degeneration in this disease is related to the enzyme deficiency and abnormal storage of glycolipid in neurons, or to the blood vessel changes and ischemia, has not been determined (Kocen and Thomas, 1970).

In metachromatic leukodystrophy there is a deficiency of arylsulfatase, and in this disorder peripheral neuropathy is associated with an abnormal accumulation of glycolipid within neurons and more especially within glia. The storage product, cerebroside sulphatide, which possesses specific staining properties, is seen in the kidney, liver, leukocytes, and peripheral nerves, and it also occurs in quite large quantities in anterior horn cells, in brain stem motor neurons, and in dorsal root ganglion cells. The fine structure of the accumulations is variable; small inclusions may be granular while larger ones are lamellar with a repeat period of 4 to 9 nm (Suzuki et al., 1967).

At the present time, at least five enzymatically distinct ganglioside storage diseases are known; they fall into two families, the G_{M1} and G_{M2} gangliosidoses. Classic Tay-Sachs disease with hexosaminidase A deficiency is one of four known G_{M2} gangliosidoses. It cannot be distinguished by light microscopy from G_{M1} gangliosidosis, since most neurons in both types of disease are swollen and filled with a finely granular PAS-positive material associated with an eccentrically placed nucleus. In Tay-Sachs disease, swollen neurons are filled with membranous cytoplasmic inclusion bodies about 1 μm in diameter composed of regularly ordered, concentrically arranged membranes with a 5 to 7 nm periodicity (Terry and Weiss, 1963). The granules are associated with acid phosphatase activity, suggesting a relationship to lysosomes (Wallace et al., 1964). The pattern of neuronal inclusion bodies varies in other gangliosidoses; in juvenile G_{M2} gangliosidosis, numerous abnormal bodies of various sizes and structures are seen, including lamellar types, lipofuscin, membranovesicular bodies, and large conglomerates of all these types of inclusions (Menkes et al., 1971).

In the acute and subacute forms of Gaucher's disease, which probably results from a genetically determined deficiency of tissue glycosyl ceramide hydrolase, anterior horn cells and autonomic ganglion cells may be slightly distended and occasionally vaculoated.

Three other neuronal storage diseases may be mentioned, all unrelated to each other and to the sphingolipidoses: the juvenile form of amaurotic familial idiocy or Batten's disease, Pompe's disease, and Hurler's syndrome (gargoylism). In the juvenile type of amaurotic familial idiocy, not to be confused with juvenile type G_{M2} gangliosidosis, the cytoplasmic bodies are granular and multiloculated, resemble lipofuscin granules, and are thought to be derived from lysosomes (Zeman and Donahue, 1963; Gonatas et al., 1963). In the generalized glycogen storage diseases, and particularly in type 2 glycogenosis with acid maltase deficiency (Pompe's disease), large confluent masses of glycogen occur in neuronal cytoplasm throughout the brain stem as well as in autonomic ganglia, glial cells, and Schwann cells (Mancall et al., 1965). In gargoylism, a type of mucupolysaccharidosis, neuronal inclusion granules, known as Zebra bodies, are found and consist of transversely arranged lamellae (Aleu et al., 1965).

Lafora Bodies

The large round basophilic bodies known as Lafora bodies, which occur singly or in groups in the cytoplasm of neurons in the

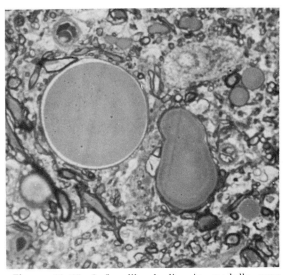

Figure 14–15 Lafora-like bodies in medulla near cuneate nucleus of a patient with presenile dementia, motor neuron disease, and sensory abnormalities. Toluidine blue stain. × 750. (From Suzuki, K., David, E., and Kutschman, B.: Presenile dementia with "Lafora-like" intraneuronal inclusions. Arch. Neurol., 25:69, 1969. Copyright 1969, American Medical Association. Reprinted by permission.)

dentate nucleus and elsewhere in the central nervous system in familial myoclonic epilepsy, have also been observed in this disease within nerve cell processes in the anterior gray matter of the spinal cord and in axons of spinal nerve roots. Chromatolysis of anterior horn cells has also been noted in such cases (Schwarz and Yanoff, 1965). Although clinical evidence of peripheral nervous dysfunction is usually lacking in Lafora's disease, this has been described in a late-onset case reported by Suzuki, David, and Kutschman (1971). In this patient is was noted that, in addition to typical acid mucopolysaccharide–containing Lafora bodies in nerve cell processes in the anterior gray matter of the spinal cord and in other regions, there was also a loss of anterior horn cells (Fig. 14–15).

Chediak-Higashi Granules

In Chediak-Higashi disease, a hereditary disorder that may be associated with polyneuropathy seen in man, Aleutian mink, a strain of Hereford cattle, and the beige mouse, the lysosome-like granules characteristically seen in leukocytes are also found in Schwann cells and in neurons of the spinal cord and autonomic ganglia (Fig. 14–16) (Lockman et al., 1967; Kritzler et al., 1964). In an ultrastructural study of dorsal root ganglion cells in Aleutian mink of different ages, Sung and Okada (1970) observed that, as in other tissues, the granules resembled lysosomes in younger animals, but with increasing age the granules appeared more like lipofuscin granules except that they were larger, tended to fuse together, and had a more conspicuous lamellar substructure. In the beige mouse the enlarged lysosomes may possibly arise from within the Golgi-related specialized smooth endoplasmic reticulum, suggesting that there exists in this disease an alteration in the normal function of this cytoplasmic organelle (Essner, 1972).

Neurofibrillary Degeneration

The appearance of thick argyrophilic strands in the cytoplasm of degenerating nerve cells is referred to as neurofibrillary degeneration and is classically associated with cortical neuronal degeneration in Alzheimer's disease, postencephalitic parkinsonism, and in senescence. Certain peripheral nervous disorders are also characterized by this type of neuronal degeneration. In affected cells, the normally fine argyrophilic neurofibrils are replaced by thick tangles of fibrillar argyrophilic material arranged in circular or flame-shaped masses that may be large enough to displace other cytoplasmic constituents and the cell nucleus to one side. These neurofibrillary tangles may persist after the death and disappearance of the cell. In some types of experimentally induced neurofibrillary degeneration, tangle formation is reversible, and the cell may revert to a normal appearance. Electron microscope studies have revealed different types of argyrophilic material in different disorders:

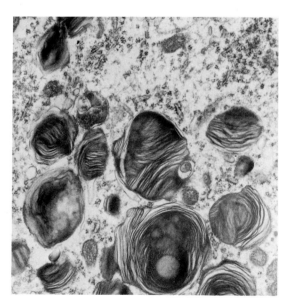

Figure 14–16 Perikaryon of anterior horn cell in spinal cord of Aleutian mink with Chediak-Higashi disease. Dense laminated structures, essentially similar to membranous cytoplasmic bodies as seen in human Tay-Sachs disease, are prominent. Tissue fixed by perfusion with glutaraldehyde and postfixed with osmium tetroxide. × 27,500. (From Hirano, A.: Electron microscopy in neuropathology. *In* Zimmerman, H. M. (ed.): Progress in Neuropathology. Vol. 1. New York, Grune & Stratton, 1971. Reprinted by permission.)

TEN NANOMETER NEUROFILAMENTS

An accumulation of what appear to be normal 10 nm (range 6 to 14 nm) thick neurofilaments occurs in anterior horn cells and dorsal root ganglion cells as part of the axonal reaction, and in the lizard, 6 to 7 nm filamentous tangle formation may be seen as a

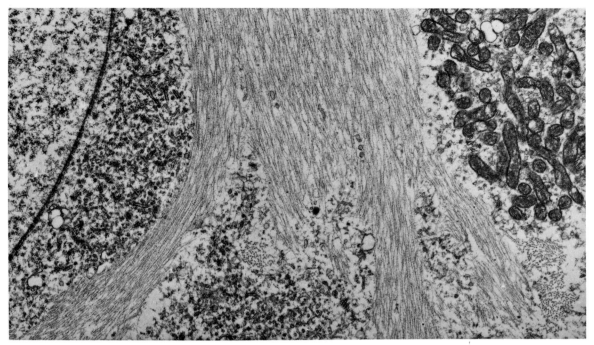

Figure 14–17   Anterior horn cell of a rabbit treated with intrathecal vincristine. Dense bundles of neurofilaments are seen in the cytoplasm. Tissue fixed by intracardiac perfusion with paraformaldehyde and glutaraldehyde and post-fixed in osmium tetroxide. × 10,000. (From Shelanski, M. L., and Wiśniewski, H.: Neurofibrillary degeneration induced by vincristine therapy. Arch. Neurol., *20*:199, 1969. Copyright 1969, American Medical Association. Reprinted by permission.)

transient stage late after the onset of chromatolysis (Pannese, 1963). A similar increase in apparently normal neurofilaments is seen in anterior horn cells in tri-ortho-cresyl phosphate neuropathy in the cat and in spinal neurons in copper-deficient sheep (swayback) (Prineas, 1969a, Cancilla and Barlow, 1966). Schochet and co-workers (1969) have reported the occurrence of large aggregates of approximately 10 nm filaments that distended the cell and displaced the cell nucleus in anterior horn cells and motor neurons of the brain stem in a patient with late-onset chronic spinal muscular atrophy.

Drugs that inhibit spindle formation during mitosis have been found to cause a marked neuronal accumulation of about 10 nm thick filaments that resemble normal neurofilaments. These spindle inhibitors include colchicine, podophyllotoxin, vincristine, and vinblastine. The latter two are alkaloids from the periwinkle plant, *Vinca rosea*, and are used in the treatment of leukemia. Intrathecal injection of these compounds in experimental animals produces a rapid accumulation of approximately 10 nm filaments in neurons of the spinal cord and brain stem, and at the

same time a loss of normal approximately 24 nm thick neurotubules (Fig. 14–17) (Wiśniewski and Terry, 1967; Wiśniewski et al., 1968; Schochet et al., 1968a). Within a few days of the injection, neurotubules reappear and neurofilaments decrease in number. Similar changes have been demonstrated in tissue cultures of spinal cord and dorsal root ganglion cells treated with these spindle inhibitors (Fig. 14–18) (Seil and Lampert, 1968; Peterson and Bornstein, 1968; Peterson, 1969). Large aggregates of 10 nm filaments have been observed in anterior horn cells, dorsal root ganglion cells, and motor neurons in the brain stem in children with leukemia treated with vincristine (Shelanski and Wiśniewski, 1969). An accumulation of neurofilaments (10 to 14 nm across) associated with a loss of neurotubules has also been observed in spinal cord neurons following intrathecal injections of aluminum compounds in certain animal species (Terry and Peña, 1965). Several mechanisms have been proposed to account for the accumulation of perikaryal filamentous material in experimental neurofibrillary degeneration. It has been suggested that the protein subunits of neurofilaments and neurotubules are similar and that depolymerization of neurotubular protein by mitotic spindle inhibitors might release these subunits to form filaments. Embree, Hamberger, and Sjöstrand (1967), on the other hand, observed that the neurofibrillary tangles induced by aluminum phosphate incorporate labeled leucine, suggesting active synthesis of the filaments. In contrast to this finding is the observation of Masurovsky, Bunge, and Bunge (1967), who demonstrated neurofibrillary tangles in dorsal root ganglion cells in vitro following x-irradiation of sufficient strength to disrupt severely the machinery necessary for protein synthesis (Fig. 14–19).

TWISTED 20 NM TUBULES

In Alzheimer's disease, neurofibrillary tangles in cortical neurons contain aggregates of 20 nm thick tubules with a periodic narrowing to 10 nm every 80 nm (Terry, 1963; Kidd, 1964). As normal neurotubules are about 24 nm thick with a lumen approximately 15 nm wide and are probably not argentophilic, it is considered that the abnormal tubules in Alzheimer's disease are more likely to be related to neurofilaments. Spinal cord neurons in Alzheimer's disease do not exhibit neurofibrillary degeneration (McMenemey,

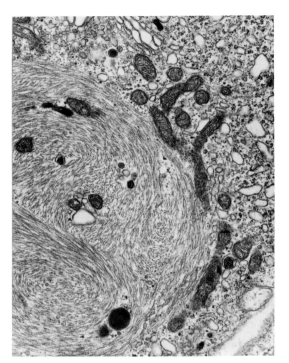

Figure 14–19 Tangle of approximately 9 to 12 nm filaments containing entrapped organelles in the cytoplasm of a cultured rat dorsal root ganglion neuron eight days after x-irradiation. Tissue fixed in osmium tetroxide. (Courtesy of Drs. E. B. Masurovsky, M. B. Bunge, and R. P. Bunge.)

1963). Spinal cord neurons in familial Alzheimer's disease may, however, exhibit neurofibrillary degeneration, but whether or not these tangles are composed of twisted tubules has not been determined (Feldman et al., 1962). In the Guamanian amyotrophic lateral sclerosis–parkinsonism–dementia complex, twisted tubules have been observed in degenerating neurons in Sommer's sector, as shown in Figure 14–20, and it may be that twisted tubules are also a feature of the neurofibrillary degeneration of neurons in the intermediolateral cell columns and in the anterior horns of the spinal cord, which is a common finding in this disease (Hirano et al., 1961, 1968a). Characteristic Alzheimer-type twisted tubules have been observed only in man and have not been produced experimentally.

HIRANO BODIES

Eosinophilic rod-shaped bodies with an affinity for silver stains, present in cortical neurons exhibiting neurofibrillary degenera-

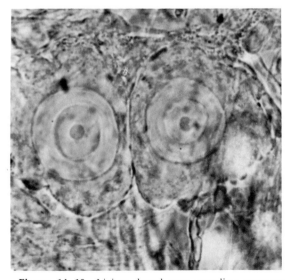

Figure 14–18 Living dorsal root ganglion neurons, exposed in vitro to 0.5 μg per milliliter vinblastine for three days. Neurofilaments have accumulated in the form of prominent perinuclear inclusions. × 660. (Courtesy of Ms. E. R. Peterson.)

tion and granulovacuolar bodies in patients with the Guamanian amyotrophic lateral sclerosis–parkinsonism–dementia complex, Alzheimer's disease, or Pick's disease, have a fine structure of aggregates of sheetlike material incorporating regularly arranged beaded filaments (Fig. 14–21) occurring in association with Alzheimer-type twisted tubules (Hirano et al., 1968a; Schochet et al., 1968b). Similar beaded filaments have been observed in association with aggregates of approximately 10 nm filaments in spinal and brain stem motor neurons in a late-onset case of chronic spinal muscular atrophy (Fig. 14–22) (Schochet et al., 1969).

Neurofibrillary degeneration of anterior horn cells is also seen in postencephalitic parkinsonism and in amyotrophic lateral sclerosis endemic to the Kii peninsula region of Japan (McMenemey et al., 1967; Tatetsu, 1958; Shiraki, 1969). Tangle formation has been described in the intermediolateral cell columns in progressive supranuclear palsy (Steele et al., 1964). The fine structure of altered spinal neurons in these conditions has not been determined.

The relationship between neurofibrillary degeneration of the cell body and axonal breakdown is not understood. Terry and

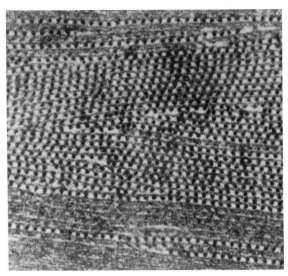

Figure 14–21   Hirano body in pyramidal cell in Sommer's sector of a Guamanian patient with amyotrophic lateral sclerosis. Tissue fixed by immersion in glutaraldehyde and postfixed in osmium tetroxide. × 124,000. (From Hirano, A.: Pathology of amyotrophic lateral sclerosis. *In* Gajdusek, D. C., Gibbs, C. J., and Alpers, M. (eds.): Virus Infections. National Institute of Neurological Diseases and Blindness Monograph No. 2, 1965, p. 23. Reprinted by permission.)

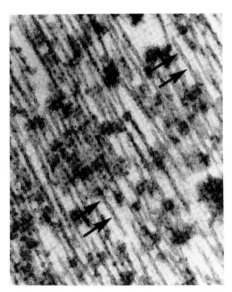

Figure 14–20   Twisted tubules in a pyramidal cell in Ammon's horn of a Guamanian patient who died of parkinsonism-dementia complex. The constrictions are indicated by the arrows. × 64,000. (From Wiśniewski, H., Terry, R. D., and Hirano, A.: Neurofibrillary pathology. J. Neuropathol. Exp. Neurol., *29*:163, 1970. Reprinted by permission.)

Wiśniewski (1970) and Lampert (1971) have suggested that neurofibrillary tangles in cortical neurons may mechanically impede axoplasmic flow, leading to degeneration of the terminal arborizations of axons and dendrites and formation of a neuritic (senile) plaque. Recently, however, doubt has been cast on this explanation since neurofibrillary degeneration and plaque formation are not always concomitant pathologic changes (Wiśniewski et al., 1973). In the case of the mitotic spindle inhibitors, the loss of neurotubules has been singled out by most authors as possibly the important factor leading to axonal degeneration, and the suggestion that this may interfere with normal axonal transport is supported by the observation that when colchicine and vinblastine are applied locally to lumbar sympathetic ganglia, there is a marked accumulation of noradrenaline, and an increase in the number of dense-core vesicles (storage granules) in the neuronal perikarya (Dahlström, 1971; Hökfelt and Dahlström, 1970). Also the local application of spindle inhibitors has been shown to cause a local rearrangement of neurotubules and distal fiber degeneration plus a proximal axonal reaction in the corresponding neuron

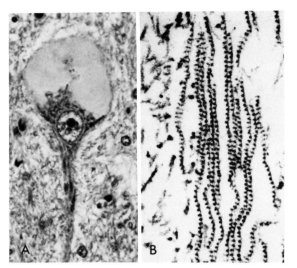

Figure 14–22 Anterior horn cell degeneration associated with neurofibrillary degeneration and beaded filament formation in a subject with late-onset chronic spinal muscular atrophy. *A.* Large hyaline inclusions distend the perikaryon. Hematoxylin and eosin. × 400. *B.* Beaded filaments observed at the periphery of the inclusions. Tissue fixed in formaldehyde and postfixed in osmium tetroxide. × 91,000. (From Schochet, S. S., Jr., Hardman, J. M., Ladewig, P. P., and Earle, K. M.: Intraneuronal conglomerates in sporadic motor neuron disease. Arch. Neurol., *20*:548, 1969. Armed Forces Institute of Pathology Photograph Neg. 68–7615; Neg. 68–8628–2. Copyright 1969, American Medical Association. Reprinted by permission.)

(Dahlström, 1971; Schlaepfer, 1971; Pilmar and Landmesser, 1972). Bradley (1970) has stressed the fact that axonal degeneration in vincristine neuropathy in the guinea pig equally affects distal and proximal segments of peripheral nerves, and that the mechanism underlying this type of axonal degeneration is probably different from that responsible for axonal degeneration of the dying back type.

NEURONAL PERIKARYA IN AXONAL NEUROPATHIES

The most remarkable feature of the pathology of the nerve cell body in polyneuropathies characterized by primary axonal degeneration is the fact that nerve cells giving rise to degenerating axons frequently appear normal or show changes that appear to be reactive rather than degenerative in nature, even in the presence of widespread axonal breakdown, which in some instances extends into the spinal nerve roots. Axonal neuropathies in which the nerve cells in the spinal cord have been

reported to appear normal on routine light microscopy include acrylamide neuropathy in the mouse and in the cat (Bradley and Asbury, 1970; Prineas, 1969b), cases of vincristine neuropathy in man (Bradley et al., 1970), vincristine neuropathy in the guinea pig (Bradley, 1970), isoniazid neuropathy in man and rats (Zbinden and Studer, 1955; Cavanagh, 1967), carnosinase deficiency neuropathy (Terplan and Cares, 1972) and thallium neuropathy in vitro (Spencer et al., 1973b). The axonal neuropathies in which nerve cells in the cervical and lumbar enlargements of the spinal cord exhibit appearances similar to those seen in the axon reaction have been mentioned earlier. Other changes have been noted under the light microscope: indentation of anterior horn cells by axonal spheroids in infantile neuroaxonal dystrophy and in β-β-iminodipropionitrile (IDPN) intoxication in rats has been reported by Chou and Hartmann (1964). Some loss of anterior horn cells has been reported in dominantly inherited sensorimotor polyneuropathies by Hughes and Brownell (1972), England and Denny-Brown (1952), Brodal, Boyesen, and Frövig (1953), and Wohlfahrt (1926); in hereditary spinocerebellar degenerations by Boller and Segarra (1969); in hereditary polyneuropathy by Dejerine and Sottas (1893); in the neuropathy associated with the malabsorption syndrome by Smith (1955); and in infantile neuroaxonal dystrophy by Haberland, Brunngraber, and Whitting (1972). The predominantly sensory axonal polyneuropathies in which it has been reported that dorsal root ganglion cells appear normal or show changes resembling those seen in the axonal reaction include subacute myelo-opticoneuropathy (Shiraki, 1971), some cases of diabetic neuropathy (Greenbaum et al., 1964), hereditary sensory neuropathy in mice, and organic mercury poisoning in rats (Cavanagh, 1968).

Ultrastructural studies have revealed no significant pathologic alterations in randomly sampled lumbar anterior horn cells and dorsal root ganglion cells in thiamine deficiency polyneuropathy in rats (Prineas, 1970), in anterior horn cells in β-β-iminodipropionitrile neuropathy in rats, and in dorsal root ganglion cells in hereditary sensory neuropathy in mice (Janota, 1972). In acrylamide neuropathy in the cat, anterior horn cells and dorsal root ganglion cells supplying the foot muscles reveal a mild dispersion of the granular endoplasmic reticulum with some dissociation of polyribosomes and single ribosomes (Prineas, 1969b). In rodents, both acrylamide and mercury intoxication lowers the rate of labeled amino acid incorporation into anterior horn and dorsal root ganglion cells prior to the onset of axonal alterations (Cavanagh, 1968; Asbury et al., 1973). The only axonal neuropathies in which distinctive fine structural changes have been observed in the nerve cell bodies are vincristine neuropathy, which has been discussed earlier, thallium neuropathy studied in vitro, tri-ortho-cresyl phosphate in cats and chickens, and infantile neuroaxonal dystrophy. In the latter, Kamoshita, Neustein, and Landing (1968) and also Toga, Bérard-Badier, and Gambarelli-Dubois (1970) noted conspicuous mitochondrial alterations in neuronal perikarya and in dendrites. In tri-ortho-cresyl phosphate neuropathy in cats during the stage of progressive axonal breakdown, anterior horn cells and dorsal root ganglion cells supplying the foot muscles show an increase in the amount of smooth endoplasmic reticulum and the appearance of membrane-bound cisternae in the peripheral cytoplasm, some dispersion of the granular endoplasmic reticulum with freeing of polyribosomes and individual ribosomes into the cytoplasm, and an increase in the number of neurofilaments and neurotubules present comparable to that seen in the axonal reaction (Fig. 14–23) (Prineas, 1969a). Similar peripheral cisternae have been observed in spinal neurons of chickens with tri-ortho-cresyl phosphate neuropathy (Bischoff, 1970). Le Vay, Meier, and Glees (1971) distinguished between the reaction of small, dark spinal ganglion cells in which the endoplasmic reticulum proliferated and of larger cells that underwent a cytoplasmic filamentous proliferation in response to tri-ortho-cresyl phosphate. Thallium neuropathy has been investigated using an organotypic tissue culture model of the peripheral nervous system (Spencer et al., 1973b). In this ultrastructural study, thallium salts selectively disrupted neuronal mitochondria, the effect being most marked in the axon, where the normal axoplasm was replaced by a series of vacuoles derived from swollen mitochondria (Fig. 14–24) (the reader is referred to Bunge's account in Chapter 18 for a discussion of pathologic changes in peripheral neurons in vitro).

Neuropathies in which axons degenerate and break down without an intermediate

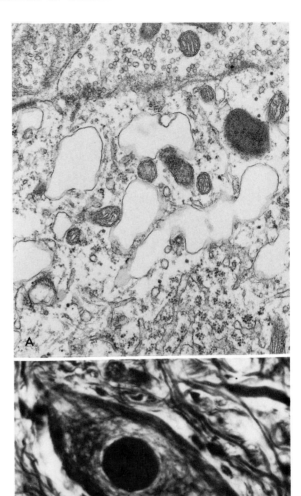

Figure 14–23 Anterior horn cells in tri-ortho-cresyl phosphate neuropathy in cats. *A.* Membrane-bound cisternae in the peripheral cytoplasm. × 12,000. *B.* There is an excessive amount of neurofibrillary material, particularly around the periphery of the cell. Bodian stain. × 375. Tissue fixed by intraaortic perfusion with paraformaldehyde and glutaraldehyde and postfixed in osmium tetroxide. (From Prineas, J.: The pathogenesis of dying-back polyneuropathies. 1. An ultrastructural study of experimental tri-ortho-cresyl phosphate intoxication in the cat. J. Neuropathol. Exp. Neurol., *28*:571, 1969. Reprinted by permission.)

stage of axonal swelling, referred to as "atrophying dystrophies" by Seitelberger (1971), include both dying back neuropathies in which degeneration of the axons begins distally and affects the longest axons first (Cavanagh, 1964), and those in which axonal breakdown is equally apparent in the proxi-

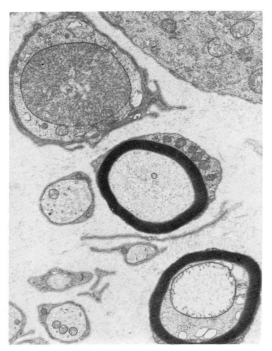

Figure 14–24 Dorsal root fibers and portions of a ganglion cell exposed in vitro to 5 μg per milliliter (10^{-5}M) thallium sulfate. Note the enormously enlarged perikaryal mitochondrion and the vacuolated axonal mitochondrion. Tissue fixed by immersion in glutaraldehyde and postfixed with osmium tetroxide. × 7000.

mal and distal segments of peripheral nerves. Ultrastructural studies have revealed different axoplasmic alterations in different dying back polyneuropathies without implicating any particular system of subcellular organelles in axonal degeneration of this type (Prineas, 1970). This, together with the fact that nerve fibers of different size and function are involved in different neuropathies, indicates that there is probably a variety of subcellular mechanisms that may lead to axonal degeneration with preservation of the perikaryon. The pathogenesis of axonal degeneration in neuropathies associated with the formation of discontinuous axonal swellings (axonal spheroids or Axonschollen) has been the subject of rather more detailed speculations. Referred to as neuroaxonal dystrophies by Seitelberger (1971) and Jellinger and Jirásek (1971), these disorders include some in which pathologic changes have been recognized only in the central nervous system and others in which changes have been described in both the peripheral and the central nervous systems. The latter include infantile neuroaxonal dystrophy (Seitelberger's disease) (Bérard-

Badier et al., 1971; Haberland et al., 1972); iminodipropionitrile neuropathy (Chou and Hartmann, 1964), acrylamide neuropathy (Prineas, 1969b), hereditary sensory neuropathy in mice (Janota, 1972), carnosinase deficiency in man (Terplan and Cares, 1972), and p-bromophenylacetylurea neuropathy in rats (Blakemore and Cavanagh, 1969). The axonal spheroids most commonly appear on the preterminal parts of axons and presynaptic terminals ("axoterminal neuroaxonal dystrophy"). In some conditions, however, they are located on axons close to the nerve cell body. They are composed of accumulations of altered axoplasmic organelles and are different in appearance from reactive and regenerating axons (Lampert, 1967). In the conditions already mentioned, and in those neuroaxonal dystrophies that at present are regarded as purely central nervous system disorders, such as natural and experimental vitamin E deficiency, Wilson's disease, Hallervorden-Spatz disease, and senile neuroaxonal dystrophy, spheroids consistently occur in the dorsal funiculi of the cord and in the gracile nucleus. As axoterminal neuroaxonal dystrophy may be regarded as a type of dying back degeneration, it would not be surprising if future studies reveal peripheral axonal spheroid formation in all conditions associated with spheroid formation in the posterior funiculi and in the gracile nucleus. Chou and Hartmann (1964) introduced the idea of "axostasis" or stagnation of flow of axoplasm to account for spheroid formation in iminopropionitrile neuropathy in rats. Following a single injection of this chemical, an acute "waltzing syndrome" develops that is permanent. Earlier histologic studies revealed what were thought to be necrotic "ghost cells" in the anterior gray matter of the cord. Chou and Hartmann noted that these large amorphous bodies were composed of thick neurofilaments (40 nm in diameter) and mitochondria, and that they were in fact axonal swellings that arose close to the parent cell body (Fig. 14–25). They developed from uniformly swollen anterior horn cell axons, and by six weeks were twice as large as the adjacent nerve cell. Similar changes were observed in nerve fibers in the dorsal root ganglia, and at a later stage, in the spinal nerve roots and in the sciatic nerves. Axons remained in continuity with the spheroids and were not observed to break down. These authors refer to the accumulation of neurofilaments and mitochondria that

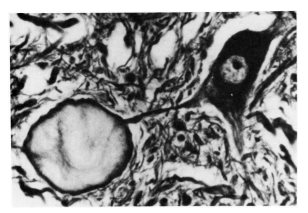

Figure 14–25 Lumbar anterior horn cell in a β-β-iminodipropionitrile-treated rat. A large axonal spheroid is seen arising from the axon a short distance from the cell body. Tissue fixed by perfusion with formalin. Luxol fast blue and Bodian stain. × 620. (From Chou, S. M., and Klein, R. A.: Autoradiographic studies of protein turnover in motoneurons of IDPN-treated rats. Acta Neuropathol. (Berl.), *22*:183, 1972. © Springer-Verlag, Heidelberg, New York, Reprinted by permission.)

occurs in axons proximal to points of constriction, and they suggested that spheroid formation may be due to slowing of axoplasmic flow (the concept of bulk axoplasmic flow is now in question—cf. Spencer, 1972, and Chapter 12). Blakemore and Cavanagh (1969), on the other hand, have suggested that axonal spheroid formation may be due to frustrated axonal regeneration: In *p*-bromophenylacetylurea neuropathy in rats, these workers observed that axonal spheroids increased in number and in size in the dorsal columns pari passu both in the intact ends of damaged axons along the dorsal columns and at the termination of the dorsal columns, and this occurred during the recovery stage of the neuropathy when the peripheral axons were regenerating. Spheroid formation was not observed in the peripheral nervous system, and it was suggested that the different local environment of peripheral regenerating axons might account for this. In contrast to iminodipropionitrile neuropathy and acrylamide neuropathy and hereditary sensory neuropathy in mice, in which axonal spheroids are composed largely of neurofilaments, the major component of the spheroids in *p*-bromophenylacetylurea neuropathy was found to be an anastomosing tubular membrane system similar to that seen in degenerating axoplasm in tri-ortho-cresyl phosphate neuropathy, in infantile neuroaxonal dystrophy (Bischoff 1967; Herman et al., 1969) and in spheroids in the gracile nucleus of aged rats (Spencer, personal ob-

servation). A number of investigators have also been impressed by the mitochondrial changes seen at an early stage in the development of spheroids in several types of neuroaxonal dystrophy. Schochet (1971) has stressed the fact that diverse mitochondrial abnormalities are a particularly conspicuous feature of dystrophic axons in experimental vitamin E deficiency in rats; the mitochondria are larger, pleomorphic and contain more

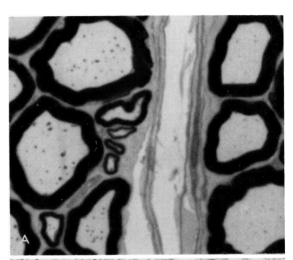

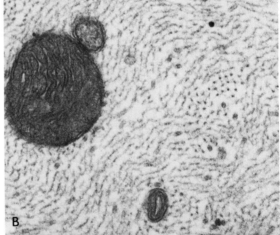

Figure 14–26 First sacral spinal nerve roots of a cat with acrylamide neuropathy. *A.* Adjacent anterior (*right*) and posterior (*left*) nerve roots. Note the enlarged mitochondria in the dorsal root fibers. Toluidine blue. × 1600. *B.* Posterior root. One axoplasmic mitochondrion is markedly enlarged and the neurofilaments are more densely packed than normal. × 35,000. Tissue fixed with paraformaldehyde and glutaraldehyde and postfixed with osmium tetroxide. (From Prineas, J.: The pathogenesis of dying-back neuropathies. 2. An ultrastructural study of experimental acrylamide intoxication in the cat. J. Neuropathol. Exp. Neurol., *28*:598, 1969. Reprinted by permission.)

cristae than normal mitochondria, and degenerate forms proceeding to nonautophagic dissolution are also a feature. Koenig (1971) also noted prominent changes in mitochondria in axons and nerve cell bodies in the neuroaxonal dystrophy produced by intrathecal injections of substances that inhibit cell respiration. And in acrylamide neuropathy, in which distal axonal degeneration is associated with the formation of small neurofilament-rich spheroids at the extremities of long central and peripheral axons, similar mitochondrial alterations associated with an increase in the number of neurofilaments is a prominent finding in the larger myelinated axons in the posterior spinal nerve roots (Fig. 14–26) (Prineas, 1969b; Spencer and Schaumburg, 1974).

DORSAL ROOT GANGLIA

Polyneuropathies in which axonal degeneration extends into the spinal nerve roots are sometimes referred to as radiculoneuropathies, and when there is a loss of ganglion cells, as ganglioneuropathies or ganglioradiculoneuropathies. In many dying back neuropathies involving first sensory neurons, degeneration of the terminal portion of the centrally directed axon in the posterior columns and in the gracile and cuneate nuclei is a feature. It is interesting to note that in a number of demyelinating neuropathies associated with some axonal loss, posterior column changes have not been described; if these are in fact absent, axonal loss in such disorders may depend on factors other than a primary neuronal disturbance (see Dyck's discussion of posterior column degeneration in Chapter 15).

Interstitial and Demyelinating Neuropathies

In neuropathies in which the primary pathologic changes affect the connective tissue and blood vessels of the nerve, and in the demyelinating neuropathies, the dorsal root ganglia and the cranial sensory ganglia may exhibit alterations similar to those seen in the peripheral nerves, and may be visibly enlarged in the various types of hypertrophic neuropathy such as sporadic hypertrophic

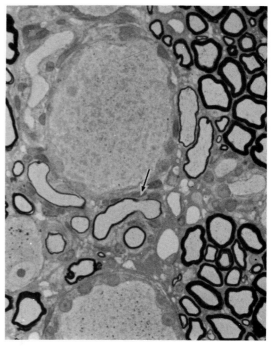

Figure 14–27 Feline dorsal root ganglion. This micrograph illustrates the normal appearance of a sensory neuron and the nonmyelinated and thinly myelinated portions of the initial complex that comprises the glomerulus, the initial segment, and the length of axon proximal to the bifurcation. The appearance of adjacent internodes with disproportionately thin myelin sheaths (arrow) resembles the picture seen during local fiber remyelination. Tissue fixed by perfusion with paraformaldehyde and glutaraldehyde and postfixed with osmium tetroxide; 1 μm Epon section stained with toluidine blue. × 480.

polyneuropathy with onion bulb formation (Green et al., 1965). Nerve cell loss is usually slight or absent, although this may occur and lead to a loss of fibers from the posterior columns. It should be noted that the initial segments of large axons in normal ganglia are thinly myelinated, an appearance that could be confused with remyelination following demyelination (Fig. 14–27) (Spencer et al., 1973a). In sporadic generalized primary amyloidosis and in the Andrade and Indiana types of familial amyloid neuropathy, deposits of amyloid similar to those seen in the peripheral nerves commonly occur in the sensory ganglia (Navasquez and Treble, 1938; Andrade, 1952; Mahloudji et al., 1969) and may be more prominent here than elsewhere in the peripheral nervous system (Krücke, 1959). The deposits are found in the capsule of the ganglion, around blood vessels in the epineurium, as small stellate and floccular perivascular deposits in the endoneurium, and in the adventitia and media and occasionally in the intima of endoneurial blood vessels, where they may be associated with disappearance of the internal elastic lamina and narrowing of the blood vessel lumen Lampert, 1968). When a loss of nerve cells has been observed, this has been ascribed to the compressive effects of the deposits or to interference with the blood supply. Deposits of amyloid have also been observed in gasserian ganglia removed from patients with trigeminal neuralgia who, at the time of operation, showed no other sign of amyloidosis (Daly et al., 1957). Human amyloid deposits are found almost exclusively in extracellular locations. When deposits are stained with Congo red they exhibit characteristic green birefringence when examined in polarized light. The deposits are composed of either aggregates of 7.5 nm filaments (type 1) or 10 nm rods divided into segments at 4 nm intervals (type 2). It has been suggested that a possible mechanism for amyloid formation may be an intracellular lysosomal catheptic digestion of light polypeptide chains of immunoglobulins, the products being liberated by the cell to form extracellular (amyloid) deposits (Glenner et al., 1971).

The inflammatory interstitial polyneuropathies, including acute idiopathic polyneuritis (Asbury et al., 1969), recurrent idiopathic polyneuropathy (Goto et al., 1969; Thomas et al., 1969; Borit and Altrocchi, 1971), and in certain animal species, experimental allergic encephalomyelitis and neuritis frequently involve the sensory ganglia, usually without much evidence of nerve cell destruction. Some loss of nerve cells with proliferation of satellite cells and secondary degeneration of axons in the posterior columns has been observed in acute idiopathic polyneuritis, however (Haymaker and Kernohan, 1949). In other conditions associated with invasion of the dorsal root ganglia and cranial sensory ganglia by inflammatory and neoplastic cells, such as Marek's disease in chickens, the Chédiak-Higashi syndrome (Kritzler et al., 1964), leukemia, Hodgkin's disease, sarcoidosis, and facial herpes simplex infection (Richter, 1944; Howard, 1905), destruction of nerve cells is variable and may be absent. Nerve cell destruction is a constant accompaniment, however, of the inflammatory response in rabies and in herpes zoster infections. Degenerative changes in ganglion cells in herpes zoster appear to

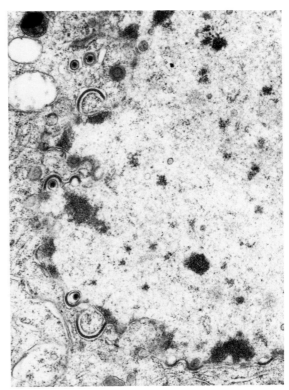

Figure 14–28   Zosteriform herpes simplex in the mouse. The nucleus of a dorsal root ganglion cell exhibits focal reduplication and increased density of the inner nuclear membrane with budding of virus particles into the cytoplasm. Tissue fixed by immersion in glutaraldehyde and postfixed in osmium tetroxide. × 21,000. (From Dillard, S. H., Cheatham, W. J., and Moses, H. L.: Electron microscopy of zosteriform herpes simplex in the cat. Lab. Invest., 26:391, 1972. Reprinted by permission.)

be at least partly due to a direct effect of the virus infection. In an ultrastructural study of a herpes zoster–like disorder in mice infected with a neurotropic strain of herpes simplex, Dillard, Cheatham, and Moses (1972) observed, in dorsal root ganglion cells innervating infected dermatomes, the typical changes of herpesvirus infection, including dissolution of nucleoli, clumping and peripheral condensation of chromatin, intranuclear hollow and core-containing capsids, and focal budding of the nuclear membrane with envelopment of viral nucleocapsids (Fig. 14–28). Similar changes were also observed in sympathetic ganglia and in ganglion cells in the bowel wall. Schwann cells associated with unmyelinated axons, satellite cells, and perineurial and endoneurial cells contained only immature virus particles. These observations suggest that cell to cell spread is an unlikely mechanism of neural spread of herpesvirus and support other evidence that herpesvirus travels along axons, possibly in a form not recognizable electron microscopically, to produce a primary infection of neurons. (Baringer and Griffith, 1970).

The selective involvement of the dorsal root ganglia in certain interstitial and demyelinating polyneuropathies may be related to the fact that, in some animal species, the endoneurial capillaries in the dorsal root ganglia and in the dorsal and ventral spinal nerve roots are more permeable to large molecules than endoneurial capillaries elsewhere in the peripheral nerves. In adult animals in most of the mammalian species examined, tracers such as albumin labeled with Evan's blue or fluorescein readily leave the vessels in the dorsal root ganglia and can be seen in the spaces around the nerve cells (Waksman, 1961; Olsson, 1967). In the peripheral nerves, however, the permeability of endoneurial vessels varies in different species: in rats and mice, proteins do not penetrate the endoneurial vessel barrier; in rabbits and guinea pigs there is a leakage of protein, especially in the latter species (Olsson, 1971). A correlation has been made between this differential permeability and the restriction of experimental allergic neuritic and diphtheritic lesions to the dorsal root ganglia and spinal nerve roots in the rabbit, and the more widespread distribution of lesions in these two neuropathies in the guinea pig (Waksman et al., 1957; Waksman, 1961).

Ganglioneuropathies

Much the same histologic picture is observed in the dorsal root ganglia in different chronic degenerative disorders that result in a marked loss of ganglion cells. These include Friedreich's ataxia (Hughes et al., 1968; Castaigne et al., 1970), some cases of diabetic neuropathy (Greenbaum et al., 1964), carcinomatous sensory neuropathy (Denny-Brown, 1948; Henson et al., 1954; Croft et al., 1965), some cases of dominantly inherited sensorimotor polyneuropathy (Hughes and Brownell, 1972), familial dysautonomia (Pearson et al., 1971), hereditary sensory radicular neuropathy (Denny-Brown, 1951; Campbell and Hoffman, 1964; Castaigne et al., 1970), and globoid cell leukodystrophy (Sourander and Olsson, 1968). The outstanding pathologic alteration in each of these disorders is a loss of ganglion cells, which may be accompanied by some reduction in the size of the ganglia. Nonspecific changes observed in the remaining nerve cells include shrinkage and darkening of the cell with the appearance of a surrounding "shrinkage space," chromatolysis, cytoplasmic vacuolization, and necrosis with neuronophagia. Proliferation of satellite cells appears to be a constant accompaniment of ganglion cell degeneration; this may occur at an early stage in the degenerative process and even before structural changes are apparent in the nerve cell body. The single layer of spindle-shaped satellite cells around the nerve cell body, shown in Figure 14–29, is replaced by concentrically

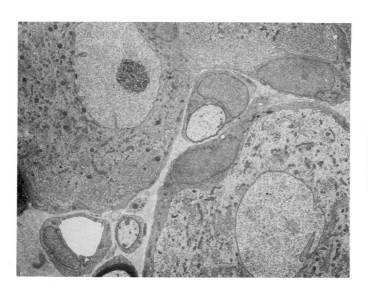

Figure 14–29 Dorsal root ganglion neurons from a newborn kitten, illustrating their normal fine structure. Each neuron is bordered by a thin layer of satellite cell cytoplasm. Fixed by intraaortic perfusion with formaldehyde and glutaraldehyde and postfixed in osmium tetroxide. × 3500.

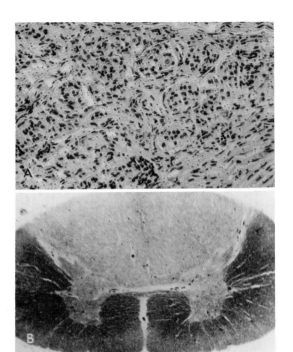

Figure 14–30 *A*. Dorsal root ganglion from a patient with carcinomatous sensory neuropathy showing proliferation of satellite cells to form nodules of Nageotte and an almost total loss of neurons. Hematoxylin and eosin. × 120. *B*. Section of the lumbar cord stained for myelin, showing extensive degeneration in the posterior columns in a patient with carcinomatous neuropathy. × 10. (Courtesy of Dr. H. Schaumburg.)

arranged layers of satellite cells, and with the disappearance of the nerve cell body, these form compact groups of cells (nodules of Nageotte or residualknötchen") (Fig. 14–30). Myelinated fibers are lost from affected ganglia, and the remaining axons may exhibit irregular beading and clublike terminations (retraction bulbs). Also common is the appearance of groups of very fine axons in isolated tangles or related to apparently normal or degenerating nerve cells. In the latter situation these have been referred to as basket fibers; they are thought to represent regenerating fibers comparable to collateral sprouts seen in partially damaged peripheral nerves. Tangles of fine unmyelinated or myelinated axons forming small neuromas related to blood vessels in the vicinity of the spinal cord or within the substance of the spinal cord have been reported in most ganglioneuropathies. Similar whorls of myelinated or unmyelinated nerve fibers related to blood vessels within or near the spinal cord are particularly common in diabetic subjects with and without overt

diabetic neuropathy (Adelman and Aronson, 1972). They are also seen in other disorders associated with damage to the spinal nerve roots or spinal cord, such as prolapsed intervertebral disk, trauma, neurofibromatosis, and syringomyelia (van Bogaert, 1953). The origin of the neuromas is discussed by Koeppen, Ordinario, and Barron (1968), and Adelman and Aronson (1972): it has variously been suggested that they arise from perivascular nerves or represent regenerating posterior root, anterior horn cell, or central axon. Schlesinger (1895) first observed that myelin in the neuromas stains brown with the Weigert-Pal method, suggesting that the myelin is peripheral rather than central myelin, which stains black by this method. This has been confirmed by using the combined luxol fast blue–periodic acid–Schiff technique of Feigin and Cravioto (1961). Also Lampert and Cressman (1964), in an electron microscope study, observed that posterior funiculotomy in rats leads to a growth of neurites with peripheral-type myelin and Schwann cells from the posterior roots near the necrotic zone into the damaged region of the cord.

Both distally and proximally directed axons disappear with degeneration and loss of the ganglion cells, leading to a reduction in the number of nerve fibers in the posterior nerve roots and in the posterior columns (see Fig. 14–30). It has been suggested that the degeneration of secondary sensory neurons present in some of these conditions, such as the degeneration of the mesial fillet in Friedreich's ataxia, may be due to transneuronal degeneration (Greenfield and Meyer, 1963).

Thickening and hyalinization of the walls of small arteries in the dorsal root ganglia is said to be a feature of diabetic neuropathy, but the significance of this has not been established (Greenbaum et al., 1964). Lymphocytic infiltrates have been observed in the dorsal root ganglia in carcinomatous sensory neuropathy, suggesting a possible viral or autoimmune pathogenesis in this disorder (Henson et al., 1954; Croft et al., 1965). Horwich, Porro, and Posner (in press) examined five dorsal root ganglion biopsies by light and electron microscopy. They found pronounced neuronal loss in the presence of numerous inflammatory cells, but detected no evidence of virus particles. Denny-Brown (1951) and van Bogaert (1953) noted, in the dorsal root ganglia in cases of hereditary sensory neuropathy, the presence of eosinophilic hyaline material, associated with cells with large pale nuclei, in the capsule, in the endoneurial space around surviving nerve cells, and in the perineurium and ensheathing nerve fibers in the spinal nerve roots. It is likely that this material, which was absent in the otherwise typical cases studied by Campbell and Hoffman (1964) and Castaigne, Escourolle, and ReCondo (1970), is similar in nature to the material observed by Schoene and co-workers (1970) in the endoneurial space in sural nerve biopsies obtained from two patients with hereditary sensory neuropathy: the subperineurial space was widened and, in this region and throughout the endoneurial space, there was an accumulation of a granular ground substance associated with large cells containing prominent cytoplasmic vacuoles and long ramifying cytoplasmic processes. Electon microscopy suggested that these cells were fibroblasts and revealed that the ground substance was composed of amorphous material and 8 to 10 nm thick filaments.

An acute hemorrhagic ganglioneuropathy has been described in intoxication with cadmium compounds in various species (Gabbiani et al., 1967). This has been studied in organotypic cultures of rat sensory ganglia by Tischner and Schröder (1972), who observed degeneration of ganglion cells associated with the appearance of large aggregates of glycogen and voluminous whorls of 10 to 12 nm neurofilaments within the cytoplasm of affected cells.

Dissociated Sensory Loss

In a number of sensory polyneuropathies and ganglioneuropathies, some forms of sensation are more severely affected than others. It has been suggested that this may be due to selective involvement of particular types of nerve cells in the dorsal root ganglia. In hereditary amyloid neuropathy and in familial dysautonomia, in which there is a selective loss of pain and temperature sensation and autonomic dysfunction, sural nerve biopsies have revealed a disproportionate reduction in the number of unmyelinated fibers. Dyck and Lambert (1969) felt it necessary to postulate a proximally situated lesion, perhaps in the dorsal root ganglia, to account for the loss of unmyelinated fibers in amyloid neuropathy, because experimental studies

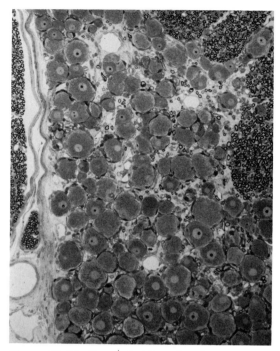

Figure 14–31 Postnatal feline dorsal root ganglion illustrating the range of size of neurons. Tissue fixed by perfusion with paraformaldehyde and glutaraldehyde and postfixed with osmium tetroxide; 1 μm Epon section stained with toluidine blue. × 120.

have shown that large myelinated fibers are affected more than unmyelinated fibers by compression and ischemia. Aguayo and colleagues (1971) noted, in a sural nerve biopsy from a patient with familial dysautonomia, that in addition to a reduction in the number of unmyelinated fibers there was a paucity of Schwann cells unassociated with unmyelinated fibers, suggesting agenesis rather than degeneration of unmyelinated nerve fibers. These investigators proposed that in this disorder there may be a failure of migration of small neurons from the neural crest into the dorsal root ganglia and autonomic ganglia (Fig. 14–31). In Friedreich's ataxia, vibration and position sense are more severely affected than pain and temperature sense, and histologic studies have revealed a striking loss of large myelinated fibers with preservation of fine myelinated fibers and unmyelinated fibers in peripheral sensory nerves, posterior spinal nerve roots, and Flechsig's middle root zone of the dorsal columns (Mott, 1907; Dyck and Lambert, 1966; McLeod, 1971). This contrasts with the changes observed in hereditary sensory radicular neuropathy, in which an early selective loss of pain and temperature sensibility is associated with an almost total loss of large myelinated fibers with relative preservation of unmyelinated fibers in cutaneous sensory nerves (Schoene et al., 1970) and degeneration affecting chiefly Flechsig's posterior root zones in the dorsal columns (Denny-Brown, 1951). The significance of middle root zone degeneration in Friedreich's ataxia and other ataxic diseases such as tabes dorsalis, and posterior root zone degeneration in disorders associated with a gross loss of superficial modalities of sensation has been discussed by Greenfield (1954), who concluded that these different patterns of posterior column degeneration, quite apart from the alterations in the peripheral nerves, support the view that different types of dorsal root ganglion cells are involved in these disorders. The condition described by Swanson, Buchan, and Alvord (1965) seems to be the sole example among the ganglioneuropathies with dissociated sensory loss in which a selective loss of a particular type of nerve cell has been reported. The patient studied had a familial disorder with insensitivity to pain and anhydrosis, and at autopsy was found to have absence of Lissauer's tracts, a loss of small axons in the dorsal roots, and smaller than usual dorsal root ganglia in which the neurons were of uniformly large size. It was suggested that there might have been a developmental lack of small neurons. The spinal dura was thickened and there were extensive leptomeningeal adhesions, however, and it is possible that the changes observed were due in part to a diffuse radiculopathy secondary to the meningeal lesion.

One experimental study in which pathologic changes have been confined to a particular cell type in the dorsal root ganglia is that reported by Joó, Szolcsányi, and Jancsó-Gabor (1969): capsaicin, a pain-producing substance found in the red pepper that produces a persistent impairment of sensitivity to chemically induced pain, was injected subcutaneously into rats; electron microscopy of dorsal root ganglia supplying the treated area of skin revealed mitochondrial changes in the small dark nerve cells but not in the large light nerve cells.

AUTONOMIC GANGLIA

The sympathetic ganglia, like the dorsal root ganglia, may be involved in various types of interstitial neuropathy, including amyloid neuropathy, acute idiopathic polyneuritis and recurrent idiopathic polyneuropathy (Schlesinger et al., 1962; Haymaker and Kernohan, 1949; Asbury et al., 1969; Borit and Altrocchi, 1971). Infiltrates of chronic inflammatory cells have been observed in sympathetic ganglia in rabbits following intradermal injections of human sympathetic ganglia mixed with Freund's adjuvant, a condition termed experimental autonomic neuropathy by Appenzeller, Arnason, and Adams (1965). In degenerative disorders associated with nerve cell loss, changes similar to those that accompany cell loss in the dorsal root ganglia may be seen, including proliferation of satellite cells with the formation of residual nodules, the presence of skeins of fine regenerating axons related to the surviving nerve cells or forming small isolated neuromas in the ganglia and in the gray rami, and increased prominence of fibrous tissue septa (Döring et al., 1955). This picture has been observed in diabetic and alcoholic polyneuropathy by Olsson and Sourander (1968), Budzilovich (1970), and Appenzeller and Richardson (1966), in familial dysautonomia by Pearson, Budzilovich and Finegold (1971), in subacute myelo-optico-neuropathy by Shiraki (1971), and in Refsum's syndrome by Cammermeyer (1956). Similar changes have been observed, however, in other conditions in the absence of overt autonomic dysfunction (Döring et al., 1955; Appenzeller, 1969), and the functional significance and specificity of such changes has yet to be established. Appenzeller and Richardson (1966) noted unusually large nerve cells in the thoracic sympathetic ganglia in patients with diabetic polyneuropathy. These giant neurons were said to exhibit various degenerative changes including displacement and pyknosis of the nucleus, and an accumulation of PAS-positive refractile eosinophilic material that did not stain with fat stains. Similar degenerating giant neurons were observed in the sympathetic ganglia in patients with alcoholic polyneuropathy, but they were absent in ganglia from diabetic and alcoholic subjects without clinical evidence of polyneuropathy. It was suggested that this finding may be related to the occurrence of autonomic disturbances, particularly orthostatic hypotension, in these two types of polyneuropathy. Hensley and Soergel (1968) reported similar findings in subjects with diabetic diarrhea and polyneuropathy, and also noted the occur-

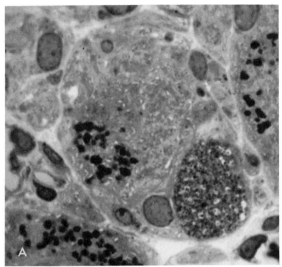

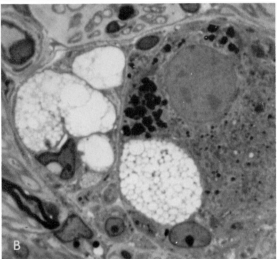

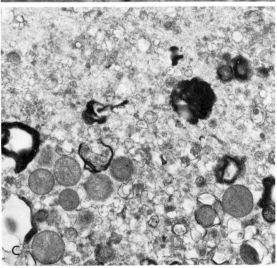

rence of swollen nerve cell processes in the dendritic tracts and dendritic glomeruli in prevertebral ganglia in these patients. Similar lesions were absent in diabetic subjects without neuropathy, in patients with alcoholic polyneuropathy, and in patients with various other disorders. It was considered that these observations correlate with the results of physiologic studies that point to impaired afferent sympathetic pathways, rather than sympathetic denervation of the small bowel, in diabetic diarrhea (Whalen et al., 1969). The significance of these findings in diabetics has been questioned by Spencer and Schaumburg (in press), who examined biopsies of sympathetic ganglia from 17 diabetic subjects with peripheral neuropathy and 5 without neuropathy, and from 5 age-matched atherosclerotic subjects without diabetes. Material was fixed for electron microscopy and compared with normal monkey ganglia fixed by perfusion. As reported by Olsson and Sourander (1968), no giant neurons were found and abnormal neurons were rarely detected in a few of the ganglia examined (Fig. 14–32). Spencer and Schaumburg felt that, apart from the vascular changes shown in Figure 14–33, which were more conspicuous in the diabetic material, and an equivocal loss of neurites, the diabetic ganglia revealed no specific abnormal features. It was also noted that sympathetic neurons are very susceptible to artifactual change and that a deliberate delay in fixation induced cytoplasmic vacuolation and enlargement.

Morphologic studies of the submucosal and myenteric plexuses by Vinnik, Kern, and Struthers (1962), Drewes and Olsen (1965), Berge, Sprague, and Bennett (1956), Hensley and Soergel (1968), and of the thoracolumbar sympathetic and presacral nerves by Vinnik and co-workers (1962) and Malins and French (1957) in patients with diabetic diarrhea have for the most part been normal.

Figure 14–32 Sympathetic ganglion neurons from a diabetic patient, aged 77, with peripheral neuropathy but without autonomic neuropathy. Biopsy material fixed by immersion in glutaraldehyde and postfixed in osmium tetroxide. *A.* In addition to the normal neuromelanin granules, a mass of abnormal granular material is seen associated with the central neuron. One micron Epon section stained with toluidine blue. × 1200. *B.* Abnormal foamy material is associated with the neuronal perikaryon. One micron Epon section stained with toluidine blue. × 1200. *C.* The fine structure of the abnormal granular material illustrated in *A.* Vesicular and filamentous profiles and altered mitochondria are prominent. × 15,000.

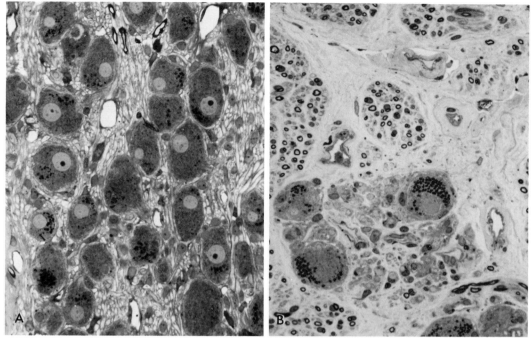

Figure 14–33 *A.* Normal primate sympathetic ganglion. Monkey tissue fixed by perfusion with paraformaldehyde and glutaraldehyde and postfixed with osmium tetroxide. × 300. *B.* Sympathetic ganglion from a diabetic patient with peripheral neuropathy but without autonomic neuropathy (age 77 years). Note the markedly thickened walls of the blood vessels. Biopsy tissue fixed by immersion in glutaraldehyde and postfixed in osmium tetroxide. × 300. One micron Epon sections stained with toluidine blue.

Lewy Bodies

The spherical hyaline eosinophilic bodies found in the cytoplasm of neurons in the pigmented nuclei of the brain stem in Parkinson's disease, described by Lewy in 1912, also occur in this disease in neurons of the sympathetic ganglia and in the intermediolateral cell columns and posterior horns of the spinal gray matter (Hartog Jager and Bethlem, 1960). The bodies are usually concentrically laminated with a deeply staining central core. They stain light blue with Nissl stains and are PAS-negative (Greenfield and Bosanquet, 1953). Ultrastructural studies have shown that they are typically composed of a core of radially arranged 7 to 8 nm thick filaments associated with circular profiles 50 nm in diameter and more irregular filaments, and a granular core 7.5 to 20 nm across (Duffy and Tennyson, 1965).

Lewy bodies have been a prominent finding in the sympathetic ganglia and in pigmented neurons in the brain stem of some patients with idiopathic orthostatic hypotension but without other neurologic signs (Johnson et al., 1966), and in subjects with orthostatic

hypotension associated with a loss of pain and temperature sensation (Roessmann et al., 1971) or with pyramidal and extrapyramidal deficits and amyotrophy. In the latter syndrome, some loss of neurons from the sympathetic ganglia has been observed, and vascular hypersensitivity to levarterenol, consistent with sympathetic denervation, has been demonstrated (Fig. 14–34) (Vanderhaeghen et al., 1970). Frequently associated with Lewy body formation in sympathetic ganglia are round or irregular eosinophilic hyaline bodies lying between the nerve cells. These have been regarded as extracellular Lewy bodies, but Roessmann, van der Noort, and McFarland (1971), in an electron microscope study, noted that at least some of these structures were swollen axons containing fibrillar or osmiophilic granular material, and it was suggested that they may represent degenerating preganglionic nerve terminals.

A further group of patients with orthostatic hypotension and evidence of a diffuse central nervous system disorder has been reported in whom Lewy body formation or other histologic evidence of Parkinson's disease has been lacking. Extrapyramidal, pyramidal,

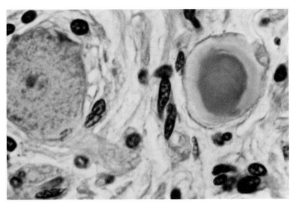

Figure 14–34 Stellate sympathetic ganglion from a patient with idiopathic orthostatic hypotension. Circular concentric hyaline formation (Lewy body) adjacent to a ganglion cell. Hematoxylin and eosin. (From Vanderhaeghen, J.-J., Périer, O., and Sternon, J. E.: Pathological findings in idiopathic orthostatic hypotension. Arch. Neurol., 22:207, 1970. Copyright 1970, American Medical Association. Reprinted by permission.)

cerebellar, and lower motor neuron deficits, and urinary and fecal incontinence have been present during life, and postmortem examination has revealed a loss of nerve cells with gliosis in the intermediolateral cell columns, the inferior olivary nuclei, the cerebellum, and certain other areas in the central nervous system (Shy and Drager, 1960; Johnson et al., 1966; Schwarz, 1967; Graham and Oppenheimer, 1969; Hughes et al., 1970). When changes have also been observed in the sympathetic ganglia, these have been mild and nonspecific. Roessmann, van der Noort, and McFarland (1971) and Thapedi, Ashenhurst, and Rozdilsky (1971) have reviewed the autopsy findings reported in cases of idiopathic orthostatic hypotension with and without Lewy body formation and have noted that whereas changes in the peripheral autonomic ganglia were inconstant and frequently absent, a loss of cells from the intermediolateral cell columns was observed in virtually every case studied, and that this may be the important although not exclusive determinant of autonomic dysfunction in this group of diseases. There have been recent reports of patients with the clinical and histologic features of the Shy-Drager syndrome in whom Lewy body formation has also been a feature, and it is now suggested that idiopathic orthostatic hypotension of the Shy-Drager type and idiopathic orthostatic hypotension associated with Lewy body formation and other histologic features of Parkinson's disease may be differ-

ent expressions of the same progressive multisystem degenerative disease (Thapedi et al., 1971; Graham and Oppenheimer, 1969).

In familial dysautonomia, described by Riley and co-workers (1949) and further studied by Solitaire and Cohen (1965), and the clinically related autonomic disorders described by Vassela and co-workers (1968) and Easterly and co-workers (1968), a number of studies have failed to reveal pathologic changes in the peripheral autonomic nervous system or in the dorsal root ganglia, and it has been proposed that the underlying biochemical alterations in these disorders may be unaccompanied by morphologic alterations (Yatsu and Zussman, 1964). Pearson, Budzilovich, and Finegold (1971) noted, however, in one patient with the Riley-Day syndrome, a marked reduction in the number of nerve cells in the sympathetic ganglia, shown in Figure 14–35, and dorsal root ganglia, together with a loss of submucosal axons in the tongue and some loss of large-diameter fiber axons in the dorsal roots; and Aguayo, Nair, and Bray

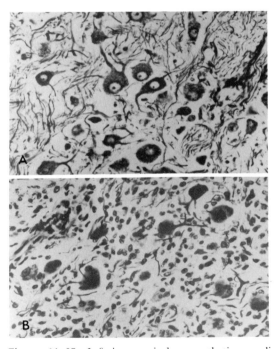

Figure 14–35 Inferior cervical sympathetic ganglia from one year old children. *A.* That of normal child shows large neurons, well-developed dendritic processes, and many axons. *B.* In a child with familial dysautonomia the ganglion shows a few small, darkly staining neurons, poorly developed dendritic processes, and few axons. Many small cells are distributed throughout the section. Silver stain. × 200. (Courtesy of Dr. J. Pearson.)

(1971) have reported a striking reduction of unmyelinated nerve fibers in the peripheral sensory nerves in this disorder.

Nerve Growth Factor

Nerve growth factor is a protein, found in snake venom and mouse salivary gland, that stimulates the growth and differentiation of developing sensory and autonomic neurons. It has been detected by bioassay in sympathetic ganglia in chick embryos and in human plasma and spinal fluid (see Levi-Montalcini and Angeletti, 1968). It acts maximally during late embryonic development and early postnatal life, and injected into newborn mice, causes hypertrophy and hyperplasia of the sympathetic ganglia (Zaimis, 1971). Weiss (1971) has reported that its action in the sensory ganglia in chick embryos is restricted to the medio-dorsal nerve cells and spares the ventrolateral cells. Nerve growth factor antiserum injected shortly after birth in a number of animal species results in destruction of neurons in sympathetic ganglia; referred to as immuno-sympathectomy, this has been observed in the mouse to result in a 98 per cent reduction in the number of neurons in the superior cervical ganglion (Levi-Montalcini and Angeletti, 1966). Electron microscopy of affected ganglion cells has been reported by Sabatini and co-workers (1965): within a few hours of the injection the cells display infolding of the nuclear membrane, condensation of nuclear chromatin, swelling of the nucleus and mitochondria, and lysis of the cell. In a quantitative electron microscope study of immuno-sympathectomized rats, Aguayo, Martin, and Bray (1972) noted a 76 per cent reduction in the number of unmyelinated cervical pre- and postganglionic sympathetic nerve fibers with no evidence of regenerative activity six weeks after an early postnatal injection of antiserum. In view of the selective involvement of sympathetic and dorsal root ganglion cells in immunosympathectomized animals, it has been suggested that a lack of nerve growth factor may be the mechanism underlying autonomic and sensory dysfunction in familial dysautonomia (Dancis and Smith, 1966; Aguayo et al., 1971).

The extent and nature of parasympathetic involvement in peripheral nervous system disorders is largely unknown. Most attention has been given to disorders that affect gastro-intestinal tract motility: A loss of parasympathetic neurons from the wall of the gastrointestinal tract has been reported in patients with Hirschsprung's disease by Bodian, Stephens and Ward (1949), with Chagas' disease by Okumura and Correa Neto (1961), with achalasia of the esophagus by Rake (1927), and with familial dysautonomia by Solitaire and Cohen (1965) and by Pearson, Axelrod, and Dancis (1974). The myenteric and the submucosal plexuses are particularly well developed in the rectum, and rectal biopsy has become a routine procedure in the diagnosis of disorders that affect nerve cell bodies throughout the peripheral and central nervous systems such as the lipidoses. The characteristic lesions of metachromatic leukodystrophy and infantile neuroaxonal dystrophy have also been observed in the nerve plexuses in the wall of the rectum (Nakai and Landing, 1960; Kamoshita et al., 1968).

REFERENCES

Adams, R. D., and Sidman, R. L.: Introduction to Neuropathology. New York, McGraw-Hill Book Co., 1968.

Adelman, L. S., and Aronson, S. M.: Intramedullary nerve fiber and Schwann cell proliferation within the spinal cord (schwannosis). Neurology (Minneap.), 22:726, 1972.

Aguayo, A., Martin, J. B., and Bray, G. M.: Effects of nerve growth factor antiserum on peripheral unmyelinated nerve fibers. Acta Neuropathol. (Berl.), 20:288, 1972.

Aguayo, A., Cherunada, P. V., Nair, C. P. U., and Bray, G. M.: Peripheral nerve abnormalities in the Riley-Day syndrome. Arch. Neurol., 24:106, 1971.

Aleu, F. P., Terry, R. D., and Zellweger, H.: Electron microscopy of two cerebral biopsies in gargoylism. J. Neuropathol. Exp. Neurol., 24:304, 1965.

Andrade, C.: A peculiar form of peripheral neuropathy. Familiar atypical generalized amyloidosis with special involvement of the peripheral nerves. Brain, 75:408, 1952.

Andres, K. H.: Untersuchungen über morphologische Veränderungen in Spinalganglien während der retrograden Degeneration. Z. Zellforsch. Mikrosk. Anat. 55:49, 1961.

Andres, K. H.: Electron microscopy studies on preparation related and postmortem structural changes in spinal ganglia cells. Z. Zellforsch. Mikrosk. Anat., 59:78, 1963.

Andrews, J. M., and Maxwell, D. S.: Motor neuron diseases in animals. In Norris, F. H., Jr., and Kurland, L. T. (eds.): Motor Neuron Diseases: Research on Amyotrophic Lateral Sclerosis and Related Disorders. New York and London, Grune & Stratton, 1968.

Appenzeller, O.: The vegetative nervous system. In Vinken, P. J., and Bruyn, G. W. (eds.): Handbook of Clinical Neurology. Vol. 1. Amsterdam, North Holland Publishing Co., 1969.

Appenzeller, O., and Richardson, E. P., Jr.: The sympathetic chain in patients with diabetic and alcoholic polyneuropathy. Neurology (Minneap.), *16*:1205, 1966.

Appenzeller, O., Arnason, B. G., and Adams, R. D.: Experimental autonomic neuropathy: an immunologically induced disorder of reflex vasomotor function. J. Neurol. Neurosurg. Psychiatry, *28*:510, 1965.

Asbury, A. K., Arnason, B. G., and Adams, R. D.: The inflammatory lesion in idiopathic polyneuritis. Its role in pathogenesis. Medicine (Baltimore), *48*:173, 1969.

Asbury, A. K., Cox, S. C., and Kanada, D.: ³H leucine incorporation in acrylamide neuropathy in the mouse. Proc. Am. Acad. Neurol., April, 1973.

Asbury, A. K., Victor, M., and Adams, R. D.: Uremic polyneuropathy. Arch. Neurol., *8*:413, 1963.

Bailey, A. A.: Changes with age in the spinal cord. A.M.A. Arch. Neurol. Psychiatry, *70*:299, 1953.

Baringer, J. R., and Griffith, J. F.: Experimental herpes simplex encephalitis: early neuropathologic changes. J. Neuropathol. Exp. Neurol., *29*:89, 1970.

Barr, M. L., and Bertram, E. G.: The behaviour of the nuclear structures during depletion and restoration of Nissl material in motor neurons. J. Anat., *85*:171, 1951.

Barr, M. L., and Hamilton, J. D.: A quantitative study of certain morphological changes in spinal motor neurons during axon reaction. J. Comp. Neurol., *89*: 93, 1948.

Barron, K. D.: Enzyme histochemistry of the central nervous system. *In* Minckler, J. (ed.): Pathology of the Nervous System, Vol. 1. New York, McGraw-Hill Book Co., 1968.

Barron, K. D., and Doolin, P. F.: Neuronal responses to axon injury. *In* Norris, F. H., Jr., and Kurland, L. T. (eds.): Motor Neuron Diseases: Research on Amyotrophic Lateral Sclerosis and Related Disorders. New York and London, Grune & Stratton, 1968.

Barron, K. D., and Sklar, S.: Response of lysosomes of bulbospinal motoneurons to axon section. Neurology (Minneap.), *11*:866, 1961.

Barron, K. D., and Tuncbay, T. O.: Phosphatase in cuneate nuclei after brachial plexectomy. Arch. Neurol., *7*:203, 1962.

Bérard-Badier, M., Gambarelli, D., Pinsard, N., Hassoun, J., and Toga, M.: Infantile neuroaxonal dystrophy or Seitelberger's disease. 2. Peripheral nerve involvement: electron microscopic study in one case. Acta Neuropathol. (Berl.), Suppl. 5:30, 1971.

Berge, K. G., Sprague, R. G., and Bennett, W. A.: The intestinal tract in diabetic diarrhoea. A pathologic study. Diabetes, *5*:289, 1956.

Berry, R. G., Chambers, R. A., Duckett, S., et al.: Clinicopathological study of juvenile amyotrophic lateral sclerosis. Neurology (Minneap.), *19*:312, 1969.

Bertrand, I., Carré, H., and Lucam, F.: La "tremblante" du mouton. Ann. Anat. Pathol. (Paris), *14*:565, 1937.

Bielschowsky, M.: Allgemeine Histologie ünd Histopathologie des Nervensystems. *In* Bumke, O., and Foerster, O. (eds.): Handbuch der Neurologie. Vol. 1. Berlin, Julius Springer, 1935.

Bischoff, A.: The ultrastructure of tri-ortho-cresyl phosphate poisoning. 1. Studies on myelin and axonal alterations in the sciatic nerve. Acta Neuropathol. (Berl.), *9*:158, 1967.

Bischoff, A.: Ultrastructure of tri-ortho-cresyl phosphate poisoning in the chicken. 2. Studies on spinal cord alterations. Acta Neuropathol. (Berl.), *15*:142, 1970.

Blakemore, W. F., and Cavanagh, J. B.: "Neuroaxonal dystrophy" occurring in an experimental "dying-back" process in the rat. Brain, *92*:789, 1969.

Bodian, D.: Poliomyelitis. London, Pitman Medical Publishing Co., 1949.

Bodian, D., and Mellors, R. C.: The regenerative cycle of motor neurons, with special reference to phosphatase activity. J. Exp. Med., *81*:469, 1945.

Bodian, M., Stephens, F. D., and Ward, B. C. H.: Hirschsprung's disease and idiopathic megacolon. Lancet, *1*:6, 1949.

Bogaert, L. van: Etude histopathologique d'une observation d'arthropathie mutilante symétrique familiare (famille de B); sa non-appartenance à la syringomyélie, ses rapports avec la neuropathie radiculaire sensorielle héréditaire (Hicks et Denny-Brown). Acta Neurol. Belg., *53*:37, 1953.

Bohman, S.-O., and Maunsbach, A. B.: Effects on tissue structure of variations in colloid osmotic pressure of glutaraldehyde fixatives. J. Ultrastruct. Res., *30*:195, 1970.

Boller, F., and Segarra, J. M.: Spino-pontine degeneration. Europ. Neurol., *2*:356, 1969.

Borit, A., and Altrocchi, P. H.: Recurrent polyneuropathy and neurolymphomatosis. Arch. Neurol., *24*:40, 1971.

Bots, G. T. A. M.: Pathology of nerves. *In* Vinken, P. J., and Bruyn, G. W. (eds.): Handbook of Clinical Neurology. Vol. 7. Amsterdam, North-Holland Publishing Co., 1970.

Bradley, W. G.: The neuromyopathy of vincristine in the guinea pig. An electrophysiological and pathological study. J. Neurol. Sci., *10*:133, 1970.

Bradley, W. G., and Asbury, A. K.: Radioautographic studies of Schwann cell behaviour. 1. Acrylamide neuropathy in the mouse. J. Neuropathol. Exp. Neurol., *24*:500, 1970.

Bradley, W. G., Lassman, L. P., Pearle, G. W., and Walton, J. N.: The neuromyopathy of vincristine in man. Clinical, electrophysiological and pathological studies. J. Neurol. Sci., *10*:107, 1970.

Brain, W. R., Croft, P., and Wilkinson, M.: The course and outcome of motor neuron disease. *In* Norris, F. H., Jr., and Kurland, L. T. (eds.): Motor Neuron Diseases: Research on Amyotrophic Lateral Sclerosis and Related Disorders. New York and London, Grune & Stratton, 1968.

Brain, W. R., Greenfield, J. G., and Russell, D. S.: Subacute inclusion encephalitis (Dawson type). Brain, *71*:365, 1948.

Brodal, A. S., Boyesen, S., and Frövig, A. G.: Progressive neuropathic (peroneal) muscular atrophy (Charcot-Marie-Tooth disease). Arch. Neurol., *70*:1, 1953.

Budzilovich, G. N.: Peripheral sympathetic nervous system in diabetes mellitus. *In* Proceedings of the Sixth International Congress of Neuropathology. Paris, Masson & Cie, 725, 1970.

Bull. W.H.O.: Virus-associated immunopathology: animal models and implications for human disease. *47*:257, 1972.

Bunina, T. L.: On intracellular inclusions in familial amyotrophic lateral sclerosis. Zh. Neuropatol. Psikhiatr. *62*:1293, 1962.

Byers, R. K., and Banker, B. Q.: Infantile muscular atrophy. Arch. Neurol., *5*:140, 1961.

Cammermeyer, J.: Neuropathological changes in hereditary neuropathies: manifestation of the syndrome heredopathia atactica polyneuritiformis in the presence of interstitial hypertrophic polyneuropathy. J. Neuropathol. Exp. Neurol., *15*:340, 1956.

Cammermeyer, J.: The importance of avoiding "dark" neurons in experimental neuropathology. Acta Neuropathol. (Berl.), *1*:245, 1961.

Cammermeyer, J.: Peripheral chromatolysis after transection of mouse facial nerve. Acta Neuropathol (Berl.), 2:213, 1963.

Campa, J. F., and Engel, W. K.: Histochemistry of motor neurons and interneurons in the cat lumbar spinal cord. Neurology (Minneap.), 20:559, 1970.

Campa, J. F., and Engel, W. K.: Histochemical and functional correlations in anterior horn neurons of the cat spinal cord. Science, 171:198, 1971.

Campbell, A. M. G., and Garland, H.: Subacute myoclonic spinal neuronitis. J. Neurol. Neurosurg. Psychiatry, 19:268, 1956.

Campbell, A. M. G., and Hoffman, H. L.: Sensory radicular neuropathy associated with muscle wasting in two cases. Brain, 87:67, 1964.

Cancilla, P. A., and Barlow, R. M.: Structural changes of the central nervous system in swayback (enzootic ataxia) of lambs. 2. Electron microscopy of the lower motor neuron. Acta Neuropathol. (Berl.), 6:251, 1966.

Carpenter, S.: Proximal axonal enlargement in motor neuron disease. Neurology (Minneap.), 18:841, 1968.

Castaigne, P., Escourolle, R., and ReCondo, J. de: Lésions des ganglions spinaux dans les hérédo-dégénérescences. *In* Proceedings of Sixth International Congress of Neuropathology. Paris, Masson & Cie, 1970, p. 717.

Cavanagh, J. B.: The toxic effects of tri-ortho-cresyl phosphate on the nervous system. J. Neurol. Neurosurg. Psychiatry, 17:163, 1954.

Cavanagh, J. B.: The significance of the "dying-back" process in experimental and human neuronal disease. Int. Rev. Exp. Pathol., 3:219, 1964.

Cavanagh, J. B.: On the pattern of change in peripheral nerves produced by isoniazid intoxication in rats. J. Neurol. Neurosurg. Psychiatry, 30:26, 1967.

Cavanagh, J. B.: Organo-phosphorus neurotoxicity and the "dying back" process. *In* Norris, F. H., Jr., and Kurland, L. T. (eds.): Motor Neuron Diseases: Research on Amyotrophic Lateral Sclerosis and Related Disorders. New York and London, Grune & Stratton, 1968.

Cavanagh, J. B., and Mellick, R. S.: On the nature of the peripheral nerve lesions associated with acute intermittent porphyria. J. Neurol. Neurosurg. Psychiatry, 28:320, 1965.

Cavanagh, M. W.: Quantitative effects of the peripheral innervation area of nerves and spinal ganglion cells. J. Comp. Neurol., 94:181, 1951.

Chou, S. M.: Infantile spinal muscular atrophy: correlation between alterations in anterior spinal roots and muscle fiber atrophy. Second International Congress on Muscle Disease. Excerpta Medica International Congress Series No. 237, 1971, p. 44.

Chou, S. M., and Fakadej, A. V.: Ultrastructure of chromatolytic motoneurons and anterior spinal roots in a case of Werdnig-Hoffmann disease. J. Neuropath. Exp. Neurol., 30:368, 1971.

Chou, S. M., and Hartmann, H. A.: Axonal lesions and waltzing syndrome after IDPN administration in rats. With a concept—"axostasis." Acta Neuropathol. (Berl.), 3:428, 1964.

Chou, S. S., and Klein, R. A.: Autoradiographic studies of protein turnover in motoneurons of IDPN-treated rats. Acta Neuropathol. (Berl.), 22:183, 1972.

Corbin, K. B., and Gardner, E. D.: Decrease in the number of myelinated fibers in human spinal roots with age. Anat. Rec., 68:63, 1937.

Cragg, B. G.: What is the signal for chromatolysis? Brain Res., 23:1, 1970.

Croft, P. B., Henson, R. A., Urich, H., and Wilkinson, P. C.: Sensory neuropathy with bronchial carcinoma: a study of four cases showing serological abnormalities. Brain, 88:501, 1965.

Dahlström, A.: Effects of vinblastine and colchicine on monoamine containing neurons of the rat. With special regard to the axoplasmic transport of amine granules. Acta Neuropathol. (Berl.), Suppl. 5:226, 1971.

Daly, D. D., Love, J. G., and Docherty, M. B.: Amyloid tumour of gasserian ganglion. J. Neurosurg., 14: 347, 1957.

Dancis, J., and Smith, A. A.: Familial dysautonomia. N. Engl. J. Med., 274:207, 1966.

Déjérine, J., and Sottas, J.: Sur la névrite interstitielle, hypertrophique et progressive de l'enfance. C.R. Soc. Biol. (Paris) 45:63, 1893.

Denny-Brown, D.: Primary sensory neuropathy with muscular changes associated with carcinoma. J. Neurol. Neurosurg. Psychiatry, 11:73, 1948.

Denny-Brown, D.: Hereditary sensory radicular neuropathy. J. Neurol. Neurosurg. Psychiatry, 14:237, 1951.

Denny-Brown, D., and Sciarra, D.: Changes in the nervous system in acute porphyria. Brain, 68:1, 1945.

Denny-Brown, D., Adams, R. D., and Fitzgerald, P. J.: Pathologic features of herpes zoster. Arch. Neurol. Psychiatry, 51:216, 1944.

Dillard, S. H., Cheatham, W. J., and Moses, H. L.: Electron microscopy of zosteriform herpes simplex infection in the mouse. Lab. Invest., 26:391, 1972.

Döring, G. von, Herzog, E., Krücke, W., and Orthner, H.: Erkrankungen des peripheren Nervensystems, Erkrankungen des vegetativen Nervensystems. *In* Lubarsch, O., Henke, F., and Rössle, R. (eds.): Handbuch der speziellen pathologischen Anatomie und Histologie. Vol. 13, Part 5. Berlin, Springer Verlag, 1955.

Drachman, D. B.: Congenital deformities produced by neuromuscular disorders of the developing embryo. *In* Norris, F. H., Jr., and Kurland, L. T. (eds.): Motor Neuron Diseases: Research on Amyotrophic Lateral Sclerosis and Related Disorders. New York and London, Grune & Stratton, 1968.

Drachman, D. B., and Banker, B. Q.: Arthrogryposis multiplex congenita. Arch. Neurol., 5:77, 1961.

Drewes, V. M., and Olsen, S.: Histological changes in the small bowel in diabetes mellitus. A study of peroral biopsy specimens. Acta Pathol. Microbiol. Scand., 63:478, 1965.

Duchen, L. W., and Strich, S. J.: An hereditary motor neurone disease with progressive denervation of muscle in the mouse. J. Neurol. Neurosurg. Psychiatry, 31:535, 1968.

Duffy, P. E., and Tennyson, V. M.: Phase and electron microscopic observations of Lewy bodies and melanin granules in the substantia nigra and locus caeruleus in Parkinson's disease. J. Neuropathol. Exp. Neurol., 24:398, 1965.

Dupont, J. R., and Earle, K. M.: Human rabies encephalitis. A study of forty-nine fatal cases with a review of the literature. Neurology (Minneap.), 15:1023, 1965.

Dyck, P. J., and Lambert, E. H.: Numbers and diameters of nerve fibers and compound action potential of sural nerves: controls and hereditary neuromuscular disorders. Trans. Am. Neurol. Assoc., 91:214, 1966.

Dyck, P. J., and Lambert, E. H.: Dissociated sensation in amyloidosis. Compound action potential, quantitative histologic and teased-fiber, and electron micro-scopic studies of sural nerve biopsies. Arch. Neurol., 20:490, 1969.

Easterly, N. B., Cantolino, S. J., Alter, B. P., et al.: Pupillotonia, hyporeflexia and segmental hypohydrosis: autonomic dysfunction in a child. J. Pediatr., 73:852, 1968.

Einarson, L.: On internal structure of motor cells of anterior horns and its changes in poliomyelitis. Acta Orthop. Scand., 19:27, 1949.

Embree, L. J., Hamberger, J. A., and Sjöstrand, J.: Quantitative cytochemical studies and histochemistry in experimental neurofibrillary degeneration. J. Neuropathol. Exp. Neurol., 26:427, 1967.

Engel, W. K.: Motor neuron histochemistry in ALS and infantile spinal muscular atrophy. In Norris, F. H., Jr., and Kurland, L. T. (eds.): Motor Neuron Diseases: Research on Amyotrophic Lateral Sclerosis and Related Disorders. New York and London, Grune & Stratton, 1968.

England, A. C., and Denny-Brown, D.: Severe sensory changes, and trophic disorder, in peroneal muscular atrophy (Charcot-Marie-Tooth type). A.M.A. Arch. Neurol. Psychiatry, 67:1, 1952.

Essner, E.: Personal communication, 1972.

Essner, E., and Novikoff, A. B.: Human hepatocellular pigments and lysosomes. J. Ultrastruct. Res., 3:374, 1960.

Evans, D. H. L., and Gray, E. G.: In Anatomical Society of Great Britain and Ireland: Cytology of the Nervous Tissue. London, Taylor & Francis Ltd., 1961.

Feigin, I., and Cravioto, H.: A histochemical study of myelin: a difference in the solubility of the glycolipid components in the central and peripheral nervous system. J. Neuropathol. Exp. Neurol., 20: 245, 1961.

Feldman, R. G., Chandler, K. A., Levy, L. L., and Glaser, G. H.: Familial Alzheimer's disease. Neurology (Minneap.), 12:603, 1962.

Fenichel, G. M.: The spinal muscular atrophies. In Norris, F. H., Jr., and Kurland, L. T. (eds.): Motor Neuron Diseases: Research on Amyotrophic Lateral Sclerosis and Related Disorders. New York and London, Grune & Stratton, 1968.

Fenner, F.: The Biology of Animal Viruses. Vol. 1. New York, Academic Press, 1968.

Friede, R. L.: Enzyme histochemical observations in amyotrophic lateral sclerosis. In Norris, F. H., Jr., and Kurland, L. T. (eds.): Motor Neuron Diseases: Research on Amyotrophic Lateral Sclerosis and Related Disorders. New York and London, Grune & Stratton, 1968.

Friede, R. L., and De Jong, R. N.: Neuronal enzymatic failure in Creutzfeldt-Jakob disease. Arch. Neurol., 10:181, 1964.

Friede, R. L., and Johnstone, M. A.: Responses of thymidine labeling of nuclei in gray matter and nerve following sciatic transection. Acta Neuropathol. (Berl.), 218:231, 1967.

Gabbiani, G., Gregory, A., and Baic, D.: Cadmium induced selective lesions of sensory ganglia. J. Neuropathol. Exp. Neurol., 26:498, 1967.

Glenner, G. G., Ein, D., Eanes, E. D., Bladen, H. A., Terry, W., and Page, D. L.: Creation of "amyloid" fibrils from Bence Jones proteins in vitro. Science, 174:712, 1971.

Gonatas, N. K., Terry, R. D., Winkler, R., Korey, S. R., Gomez, C. J., and Stein, A.: A case of juvenile lipidosis: electron microscopic and biochemical observation of a cerebral biopsy. J. Neuropathol. Exp. Neurol., 22:557, 1963.

Goto, Y., Hamaguchi, K., Hirai, S., Matsuyam, H., and Kameya, T.: Chronic polyneuritis with repeated remissions and exacerbations—report of a case with autopsy findings. Clin. Neurol., 9:239, 1969.

Graham, J. G., and Oppenheimer, D. R.: Orthostatic hypotension and nicotine sensitivity in a case of multiple system atrophy. J. Neurol. Neurosurg. Psychiatry, 32:28, 1969.

Green, L. N., Herzog, I., and Aberfeld, D.: A case of hypertrophic interstitial neuritis coexisting with dementia and cerebellar degeneration. J. Neuropathol. Exp. Neurol., 24:682, 1965.

Greenbaum, D., Richardson, P. C., Salmon, M. V., and Urich, H.: Pathological observations on six cases of diabetic neuropathy. Brain, 87:201, 1964.

Greenfield, J. G.: The Spinocerebellar Degenerations. Oxford, Blackwell Scientific Publications, 1954.

Greenfield, J. G.: Infectious diseases of the central nervous system. In Blackwood, W., et al. (eds.): Greenfield's Neuropathology. 2nd edition. London, Edward Arnold Ltd., 1963.

Greenfield, J. G., and Bosanquet, F. D.: The brain stem lesions in parkinsonism. J. Neurol. Neurosurg. Psychiatry, 16:213, 1953.

Greenfield, J. G., and Meyer, A.: General pathology of the nerve cell and neuroglia. In Blackwood, W., et al. (eds.): Greenfield's Neuropathology. 2nd edition. London, Edward Arnold Ltd., 1963.

Greenfield, J. G., and Stern, R. O.: The anatomical identity of the Werdnig-Hoffmann and Oppenheim forms of infantile muscular atrophy. Brain, 50:652, 1927.

Haberland, C., Brunngraber, E. G., and Whitting, L. A.: Infantile neuroaxonal dystrophy. Neuropathological and biochemical study of a case. Arch. Neurol., 26:391, 1972.

Hare, W. K., and Hinsey, J. C.: Reaction of dorsal root ganglion cells to section of peripheral and central processes. J. Comp. Neurol., 73:489, 1940.

Harreveld, A. van: Effect of spinal cord asphyxiation. Progr. Brain Res., 12:280, 1964.

Hartog Jager, W. A. den, and Bethlem, J.: The distribution of Lewy bodies in the central and autonomic nervous system in idiopathic paralysis agitans. J. Neurol. Neurosurg. Psychiatry, 23:283, 1960.

Haymaker, W., and Kernohan, J. W.: The Landry-Guillain-Barré syndrome. A clinicopathologic report of fifty fatal cases and a critique of the literature. Medicine (Baltimore), 28:59, 1949.

Head, H., and Campbell, A. W.: The pathology of herpes zoster and its bearing on sensory localisation. Brain, 23:353, 1900.

Hensley, G. T., and Soergel, K. H.: Neuropathologic findings in diabetic diarrhea. Arch. Pathol. 85:587, 1968.

Henson, R. A., Russell, D. S., and Wilkinson, M.: Carcinomatous neuropathy and myopathy, a clinical and pathological study. Brain, 77:82, 1954.

Herman, M. M., Huttenlocher, P. R., and Bensch, K. G.: Electron microscopic observations in infantile neuroaxonal dystrophy. Report of a cortical biopsy and review of the recent literature. Arch. Neurol., 20:19, 1969.

Hillarp, N.: Peripheral autonomic mechanisms. In Field, J. (ed.): Handbook of Physiology. Vol. 2. Washington, The American Physiological Society, 1960.

Hirano, A.: Pathology of amyotrophic lateral sclerosis. *In* Gajdusek, D. C., Gibbs, C. J., and Alpers, M. (eds.): Slow, Latent and Temperate Virus Infections. National Institute of Neurological Diseases and Blindness Monograph No. 2, 1965.

Hirano, A.: Electron microscopy in neuropathology. *In* Zimmerman, H. M. (ed.): Progress in Neuropathology. Vol. 1. New York, Grune & Stratton, 1971.

Hirano, A., Kurland, L. T., and Sayre, G. P.: Familial amyotrophic lateral sclerosis. Arch. Neurol., *16*: 232, 1967.

Hirano, A., Malamud, N., and Kurland, L. T.: Parkinsonism-dementia complex, and endemic disease on the island of Guam. 2. Pathological features. Brain, *84*:662, 1961.

Hirano, A., Dembitzer, H. M., Kurland, L. T., and Zimmerman, N. M.: The fine structure of some intraganglionic alterations. J. Neuropathol. Exp. Neurol., *27*:167, 1968a.

Hirano, A., Malamud, N., Kurland, L. T., and Zimmerman, H. M.: A review of the pathologic findings in amyotrophic lateral sclerosis. *In* Norris, F. H., Jr., and Kurland, L. T. (eds.): Motor Neuron Disease. New York and London, Grune & Stratton, 1968b.

Hökfelt, T., and Dahlström, A.: Electronmicroscopical observations on the distribution and transport of noradrenaline storage particles after local treatment with mitosis inhibitors. Acta Physiol. Scand., Suppl. *357*:10, 1970.

Horwich, M., Porro, R., and Posner, J.: The subacute sensory neuropathy "ganglioradiculitis" associated with cancer. Neurology, in press.

Howard, W. T.: Further observations on the relation of lesions of the gasserian and posterior root ganglia to herpes occurring in pneumonia and cerebrospinal meningitis. Am. J. Med. Sci., *130*:1012, 1905.

Hudson, G., Lazarow, A., and Hartmann, J. F.: A quantitative electron microscopic study of mitochondria in motor neurons following axonal section. Exp. Cell Res., *24*:440, 1961.

Hughes, J. T., and Brownell, B.: Spinal cord ischemia due to arteriosclerosis. Arch. Neurol., *15*:189, 1966.

Hughes, J. T., and Brownell, B.: Pathology of peroneal muscular atrophy (Charcot-Marie-Tooth disease). J. Neurol. Neurosurg. Psychiatry, *35*:648, 1972.

Hughes, J. T., Brownell, B., and Hewer, R. L.: The peripheral sensory pathway in Friedreich's ataxia. An examination by light and electron microscopy of the posterior nerve roots, posterior root ganglia and peripheral sensory nerves in cases of Friedreich's ataxia. Brain, *91*:803, 1968.

Hughes, R. C., Cartlidge, N. E. F., and Millac, P.: Primary Neurogenic orthostatic hypotension. J. Neurol. Neurosurg. Psychiatry, *33*:363, 1970.

Huttenlocher, P. R., and Cohen, R. B.: Oxidative enzymes in spinal motor neurons in Werdnig-Hoffmann disease. Neurology (Minneap.), *16*:398, 1966.

Hydén, H.: *In* Weiss, P. (ed.): Genetic Neurology. Chicago, University of Chicago Press, 1950.

Hydén, H.: The neurone. *In* Brachet, J., and Mirsky, A. (eds.): The Cell: Biochemistry, Physiology, Morphology. Vol. 4. New York, Academic Press, 1960.

Hydén, H.: Cytophysiological aspects of the nucleic acids and proteins of nervous tissue. *In* Elliot, K. A. C., Page, I. H., and Quastrel, J. H. (eds.): Neurochemistry. Springfield, Ill., Charles C Thomas, 1962.

Jakob, H.: Sekundäre, retrograde und transynaptische Degeneration. *In* Henke, F., and Lubarsch, O. (eds.): Handbuch der speziellen pathologischen Anatomie und Histologie. Vol. 13, Part 1. Berlin, Springer Verlag, 1957.

Janota, I.: Ultrastructural studies of an hereditary sensory neuropathy in mice (dystonia musculorum). Brain, *95* Pt. 3:529, 1972.

Jellinger, K., and Jirásek, A.: Neuroaxonal dystrophy in man: character and natural history. Acta Neuropathol. (Berl.), Suppl. *5*:3, 1971.

Jellinger, K., and Neumayer, E.: Myélopathie progressive d'origine vasculaire: contribution anatomoclinique aux syndromes d'une hypovascularisation chronique de la moelle. Acta Neurol. Psychiatr. Belg., *62*:944, 1962.

Johnson, R. H., Lee, G. de J., Oppenheimer, D. R., et al.: Autonomic failure with orthostatic hypotension due to intermediolateral column degeneration. A report of two cases with autopsies. Q. J. Med., *35*:276, 1966.

Joó, F., Szolcsányi, J., and Jancsó-Gábor, A.: Mitochondrial alterations in the spinal ganglion cells of the rat accompanying the long-lasting disturbance induced by capsaicin. Life Sci., *8*:621, 1969.

Kabat, H., and Knapp, M. E.: The mechanism of muscle spasm in poliomyelitis. J. Pediatr., *24*:123, 1944.

Kaeser, H. E.: Scapuloperoneal muscular atrophy. Brain, *88*:407, 1965.

Kamoshita, S., Neustein, H. B., Landing, B. H.: Infantile neuroaxonal dystrophy with neonatal onset. Neuropathologic and electron microscopic observation. J. Neuropathol. Exp. Neurol., *27*:300, 1968.

Kidd, M.: Alzheimer's disease. An electron microscopical study. Brain, *87*:307, 1964.

Klatzo, I., Gajdusek, D. C., and Zigas, V.: Pathology of kuru. Lab. Invest., *8*:799, 1959.

Kocen, R. S., and Thomas, P. K.: Peripheral nerve involvement in Fabry's disease. Arch. Neurol., *22*:81, 1970.

Koenig, H.: Experimental myelopathy produced with a pyrimidine analogue. Arch. Neurol., *2*:463, 1960.

Koenig, H. L.: Relations entre la distribution de l'activité acétylcholinestérasique et celle de l'ergastoplasme dans les neurons du ganglion ciliaire du poulet. Arch. Anat. Microsc. Morphol. Exp., *54*:937, 1965.

Koenig, H.: Histochemical clues to metabolic abnormalities in nerve cells. *In* Norris, F. H., Jr., and Kurland, L. T. (eds.): Motor Neuron Diseases: Research on Amyotrophic Lateral Sclerosis and Related Disorders. New York and London, Grune & Stratton, 1968.

Koenig, H.: Some observations on the experimental production of acute neuroaxonal and synaptosomal dystrophy. Acta Neuropathol. (Berl.), Suppl. *5*:126, 1971.

Koenig, H. L., and Droz, B.: Effect of nerve section on protein metabolism of ganglion cells and preganglionic nerve endings. Acta Neuropathol. (Berl.), Suppl. *5*:119, 1971.

Koeppen, A. H., Ordinario, A. T., and Barron, K. D.: Aberrant intramedullary peripheral nerve fibers. Arch. Neurol., *18*:567, 1968.

Kristensson, K., and Haltia, M.: Ultrastructural and cytochemical studies of chromatolysis in neurons. *In* Proceedings of the Sixth International Congress of Neuropathology. Paris, Masson & Cie, 1970, p. 1015.

Kristensson, K., and Olsson, Y.: Diffusion pathways and retrograde axonal transport of protein tracers in peripheral nerves. Progr. Neurobiol., *1*:87, 1973.

Kritzler, R. A., Tener, J. Y., Lindenbaum, J., et al.: Chediak-Higashi syndrome: cytologic and serum lipid observations in a case and family. Am. J. Med., *36*:583, 1964.

Krücke, W.: Die paramyloidose. Ergeb. Inn. Med. Kinderheilkd., *11*:299, 1959.

Lampert, P.: A comparative electron microscopic study of reactive, degenerating, regenerating and dystrophic axons. J. Neuropathol. Exp. Neurol., *26*:345, 1967.

Lampert, P. W.: Amyloid and amyloid-like deposits. *In* Minckler, J. (ed.): Pathology of the Nervous System. Vol. 1. New York, McGraw-Hill Book Co., 1968.

Lampert, P.: Fine structural changes of neurites in Alzheimer's disease. Acta Neuropathol. (Berl.), Suppl. *5*:49, 1971.

Lampert, P., and Cressman, M.: Axonal regeneration in the dorsal columns of the spinal cord of adult rats: an electron microscopic study. Lab. Invest., *13*:825, 1964.

La Velle, A., and La Velle, F. W.: Neuronal reaction to injury during development. Exp. Neurol., *1*:82, 1959.

Leech, R. W.: Changes in satellite cells of rat dorsal root ganglia during central chromatolysis. An electron microscope study. Neurology (Minneap.), *17*:349, 1967.

Le Vay, S., Meier, C., and Glees, P.: Effects of tri-ortho-cresyl-phosphate on spinal ganglia and peripheral nerves of chicken. Acta Neuropathol. (Berl.), *17*:103, 1971.

Levi-Montalcini, R.: Events in the developing nervous system. *In* Purpura, D., and Schadé, J. P. (eds.): Growth and Maturation of the Brain. Progress in Brain Research. Vol. 4. New York, American Elsevier Publishing Co., 1964.

Levi-Montalcini, R., and Angeletti, P. U.: Immuno-sympathectomy. Pharmacol. Rev., *18*:619, 1966.

Levi-Montalcini, R., and Angeletti, P. U.: Nerve growth factor. Physiol. Rev., *48*:534, 1968.

Lewy, F. H.: Paralysis Agitans: pathologische anatomie. *In* Lewandowsky, F. D. (ed.): Handbuch der Neurologie. Berlin, Julius Springer, 1912.

Lhermitte, J. A., and Nichols, M.: Les lésions spinales du zona. La myélite zostérienne. Rev. Neurol. (Paris), *1*:361, 1924.

Lieberman, A. R.: The axon reaction: A review of the principal features of perikaryl responses to axon injury. Int. Rev. Exp. Pathol., *14*:49, 1971.

Lockman, L. A., Kennedy, W. R., and White, J. G.: The Chediak-Higashi syndrome. Electrophysiological and electron microscopic observations on the peripheral neuropathy. J. Pediatr., *70*:942, 1967.

Luse, S. A.: The neuron. *In* Minckler, J. (ed.): Pathology of the Nervous System. Vol. 1. New York, McGraw-Hill Book Co., 1968.

Mahloudji, M. Teasdall, R. D., Adamkiewicz, J. J., Hartmann, W. H., Lambird, P. A., and McKusick, V. A.: The genetic amyloidoses. With particular reference to hereditary neuropathic amyloidosis, type II (Indiana or Rukavina type). Medicine (Baltimore), *48*:1, 1969.

Malamud, N.: Neuromuscular system disease. *In* Minckler, J. (ed.): Pathology of the Nervous System. Vol. 1. New York, McGraw-Hill Book Co., 1968.

Malins, J. M., and French, J. J.: Diabetic diarrhoea. Q.J. Med., *26*:467, 1957.

Mancall, E. L., Aponte, G. E., and Berry, R. G.: Pompe's disease (diffuse glycogenosis) with neuronal storage. J. Neuropathol. Exp. Neurol., *24*:85, 1965.

Mannen, T.: Studies on vascular lesions in the spinal cord in the aged: clinicopathological study. Acta Gerontol. Jap., *37*:17, 1963.

Marinesco, G.: Über Veränderung der Nerven und des Rückenmarks nach Amputationen. Neurol. Zentralbl. (Leipzig) *11*:463, 1892.

Masurovsky, E. B., Bunge, M. B., and Bunge, R. P.: Cytological studies of organotypic cultures following x-irradiation in vitro. I Changes in neurons and satellite cells. J. Cell Biol., *32*:467, 1967.

McLeod, J. G.: An electrophysiological and pathological study of peripheral nerves in Friedreich's ataxia. J. Neurol. Sci., *12*:333, 1971.

McMenemey, W. H.: The dementias and progressive diseases of the basal ganglia. *In* Blackwood, W., McMenemey, W. H., Meyer, A., Norman, R. M., and Russell, D. S. (eds.): Greenfield's Neuropathology. 2nd edition. London, Edward Arnold Ltd., 1963.

McMenemey, W. H., Barnard, R. O., and Jellinek, E. H.: A late sequel of epidemic encephalitis (von Economo). Rev. Roum. Neurol., *4*:251, 1967.

Menkes, J. H., O'Brien, S., Okada, S., Grippo, J., Andrews, J. M., and Cancilla, P. A.: Juvenile G_{M2} gangliosidosis. Biochemical and ultrastructual studies on a new variant of Tay-Sachs disease. Arch. Neurol., *25*:14, 1971.

Metcalf, C. W., and Hirano, A.: Clinico-pathological studies of a family with amyotrophic lateral sclerosis. Arch. Neurol., *24*:518, 1971.

Meyer, A.: On parenchymatous systemic degenerations mainly in the central nervous system. Brain, *24*:47, 1901.

Morecki, R., and Zimmerman, H. M.: Human rabies encephalitis. Fine structure study of cytoplasmic inclusions. Arch. Neurol., *20*:599, 1969.

Mott, F. W.: A case of Friedreich's disease with autopsy. Arch. Neurol. (London), *3*:180, 1907.

Nakai, H., and Landing, B. H.: Suggested use of rectal biopsy in the diagnosis of neural lipidoses. Pediatrics, *26*:225, 1960.

Nandy, K.: Histologic and histochemical study of motor neurons with special reference to experimental degeneration, aging and drug actions. *In* Norris, F. H., Jr., and Kurland, L. T. (eds.): Motor Neuron Diseases: Research on Amyotrophic Lateral Sclerosis and Related Disorders. New York and London, Grune & Stratton, 1968.

Navesquez, S. de, and Treble, H. A.: A case of primary generalized amyloid disease with involvement of the nerves. Brain, *61*:116, 1938.

Nelson, J. S., and Prensky, A. L.: Sporadic juvenile amytrophic lateral sclerosis. A clinicopathological study of a case with neuronal cytoplasmic inclusions containing RNA. Arch. Neurol., *27*:300, 1972.

Newberne, J. W., Robinson, V. B., Estill, L., and Brinkman, D. C.: Granular structures in brains of apparently normal dogs. Am. J. Vet. Res., *21*:782, 1960.

Nissl, F.: Über die Veränderungen der Ganglienzellen am facialiskern des Kaninchens nach Ausreibung der nerven. Allg. Z. Psychiatr., *48*:197, 1891.

Norman, R. M.: Malformations of the nervous system, birth injury and diseases and early life. *In* Greenfield, J. G., Blackwood, W., McMenemey, W. H., et al. (eds.): Neuropathology. London, Edward Arnold, 1958.

Norris, F. H., McMenemey, W. H., and Barnard, R. O.: Anterior horn cell pathology in carcinomatous neuromyopathy compared with other forms of motor neuron disease. *In* Norris, F. H., Jr., and Kurland, L. T. (eds.): Motor Neuron Diseases: Research on Amyotrophic Lateral Sclerosis and Related Disorders. New York and London, Grune & Stratton, 1968.

Okumura, M., and Correa Neto, A.: Producas experimental de "megas" em enimais inoculados com Trypanosoma cruzi, Rev. Hosp. Clín. Fac. Med. São Paulo, *16*:338, 1961.

Olsson, Y.: Phylogenetic variations in the vascular permeability of peripheral nerves to serum albumin. Acta Microbiol. Scand., *69*:621, 1967.

Olsson, Y.: Studies on vascular permeability in peripheral nerves. IV. Distribution of intravenously injected protein tracers in the peripheral nervous system of various species. Acta Neuropathól. (Berl.), *17*:114, 1971.

Olsson, Y., and Sourander, P.: Changes in sympathetic nervous system in diabetes mellitus. J. Neurovisc. Relat., *31*:86, 1968.

Pannese, E.: Investigations on the ultrastructural changes of the spinal ganglion neurons in the course of axon regeneration and cell hypertrophy. 2. Changes during cell hypertrophy and comparison between the ultrastructure of nerve cells of the same type under different functional conditions. Z. Zellforsch. Mikrosk. Anat., *61*:561, 1963.

Pant, S. S., Asbury, A. K., and Richardson, E. P., Jr.: The myelopathy of pernicious anemia. A neuropathological reappraisal. Acta Neurol. Scand., *44*:Suppl. 5, 1968.

Pearse, A. G. E.: Histochemistry. 2nd edition. London, J. & A. Churchill, 1960.

Pearson, J., Budzilovich, G., and Finegold, M. J.: Sensory motor and autonomic dysfunction: the nervous system in familial dysautonomia. Neurology (Minneap.), *21*:486, 1971.

Pearson, J., Axelrod, F., and Dancis, J.: Familial dysautonomia. Current concepts of dysautonomia: neuropathological defects. Ann. N.Y. Acad. Sci., *228*:288, 1974.

Penfield, W. G.: Alterations of the golgi apparatus in nerve cells. Brain, *43*:290, 1920.

Peterson, E. R.: Neurofibrillar alterations in cord-ganglion cultures exposed to spindle inhibitors. J. Neuropathol. Exp. Neurol., *28*:168, 1969.

Peterson, E. R., and Bornstein, M. B.: The neurotoxic effects of colchicine on tissue cultures of cord-ganglia. J. Neuropathol. Exp. Neurol., *27*:121, 1968.

Pilmar, G., and Landmesser, L.: Axotomy mimicked by localised colchicine application. Science, *177*:1116, 1972.

Price, D. L., and Porter, K. R.: The response of ventral horn neurons to axonal transection. J. Cell Biol., *53*:24, 1972.

Prineas, J.: The pathogenesis of dying-back polyneuropathies. 1. An ultrastructural study of experimental tri-ortho-cresyl phosphate intoxication in the cat. J. Neuropathol. Exp. Neurol., *28*:571, 1969a.

Prineas, J.: The pathogenesis of dying-back polyneuropathies. 2. An ultrastructural study of experimental acrylamide intoxication in the cat. J. Neuropathol. Exp. Neurol., *28*:598, 1969b.

Prineas, J.: Peripheral nerve changes in thiamine-deficient rats. Arch. Neurol., *23*:541, 1970.

Rahman, A. N., and Lindenberg, R.: The neuropathology of hereditary dystrophic lipidosis. Arch. Neurol., *9*:373, 1963.

Rake, G. W.: Pathology of achalasia of cardia. Guy's Hosp. Rep., *77*:141, 1927.

Ramón y Cajal, S.: Variaciones morfológicas normales y patológicas del reticulo neurofibrilar. Trab. Lab. Invest. Biol. Univ. Madrid, 3, 1904.

Ramón y Cajal, S.: Die Neuronenlehre. *In* Bumke, O.,

and Foerster, O. (eds.): Handbuch der Neurologie. Vol. 1. Berlin, Julius Springer, 1935.

Richardson, J. C., Chambers, R. A., and Heywood, P. M.: Encephalopathies of anoxia and hypoglycemia. Arch. Neurol., *1*:178, 1959.

Richter, R.: Observations bearing on presence of latent herpes simplex virus in human Gasserian ganglion. J. Nerv. Ment. Dis., *99*:356, 1944.

Riley, C. M., Day, R. L., Greeley, D. M., et al.: Central autonomic dysfunction with defective lacrimation. 1. Report of five cases. Pediatrics, *3*:468, 1949.

Robinson, N.: A histochemical study of motor neurone disease. Acta Neuropathol. (Berl.), *7*:101, 1966a.

Robinson, N.: Friedreich's ataxia. A histochemical and biochemical study. Part 1.: Enzymes of carbohydrate metabolism. Part 2. Hydrolytic enzymes. Acta Neuropathol. (Berl.), *6*:25, 1966b.

Robinson, N.: Peroneal muscular atrophy. A histochemical study. Acta Neuropathol. (Berl.), *11*:301, 1968.

Roessman, U., van der Noort, S., and McFarland, D. E.: Idiopathic orthostatic hypotension. Arch. Neurol., *24*:503, 1971.

Rose, F. C., Brett, E. M., and Burston, J.: Zoster encephalomyelitis. Arch. Neurol., *11*:155, 1964.

Sabatini, M. T., Pellegrino de Iraldi, A., and de Robertis, E.: Early effects of antiserum against the nerve growth factor on fine structure of sympathetic neurons. Exp. Neurol., *12*:370, 1965.

Schlaepfer, W. W.: Vincristine-induced axonal alterations in rat peripheral nerve. J. Neuropathol. Exp. Neurol., *30*:488, 1971.

Schlesinger, A. S., Duggins, V. A., and Masucci, E. F.: Peripheral neuropathy in familial primary amyloidosis. Brain, *85*:357, 1962.

Schlesinger, H.: Ueber das wahre Neurom des Rueckenmarkes. Arb. Inst. Anat. Physiol. Centralnervens. Vol. 3. Vienna and Leipzig, F. Deuticke, 1895.

Schochet, S. S.: Mitochondrial changes in axonal dystrophy produced by vitamin E deficiency. Acta Neuropathol. (Berl.) Suppl., *5*:54, 1971.

Schochet, S. S., Jr., Lampert, P. W., and Earle, K. M.: Neuronal changes induced by intrathecal vincristine sulfate. J. Neuropathol. Exp. Neurol., *27*:645, 1968a.

Schochet, S. S., Lampert, P. W., and Lindenberg, R.: Fine structure of the Pick and Hirano bodies in a case of Pick's disease. Acta Neuropathol. (Berl.), *11*:330, 1968b.

Schochet, S. S., Jr., Hardman, J. M., Ladewig, P. P., and Earle, K. M.: Intraneuronal conglomerates in sporadic motor neuron disease. Arch. Neurol., *20*:548, 1969.

Schoene, W. C., Asbury, A. K., Åström, K. E., and Masters, R.: Hereditary sensory neuropathy. A clinical and ultrastructural study. J. Neurol. Sci., *11*:463, 1970.

Schwarz, G. A.: The orthostatic hypotension syndrome of Shy-Drager: A clinicopathologic report. Arch. Neurol., *16*:123, 1967.

Schwarz, G. A., and Yanoff, M.: Lafora's disease. Arch. Neurol., *12*:172, 1965.

Segarra, J. M.: Histological and histochemical staining methods: a selection. *In* Tedeschi, C. G. (ed.): Neuropathology, Methods and Diagnosis. Boston, Little, Brown, & Co., 1970.

Seil, F. J., and Lampert, P. W.: Neurofibrillary tangles induced by vincristine and vinblastine sulphate in central and peripheral neurones in vitro. Exp. Neurol., *21*:219, 1968.

Seitelberger, F.: Neuropathological conditions related to neuroaxonal dystrophy. Acta Neuropathol. (Berl.), Suppl. *5*:17, 1971.

Shelanski, M. L., and Wiśniewski, H.: Neurofibrillary degeneration induced by vincristine therapy. Arch. Neurol., 20:199, 1969.

Shiraki, H.: The neuropathology of amyotrophic lateral sclerosis (ALS) in the Kii Peninsula and other areas of Japan. In Norris, F. H., Jr., and Kurland, L. T. (eds.): Motor Neuron Diseases. New York and London, Grune & Stratton, 1969.

Shiraki, H.: Neuropathology of subacute myelo-optico-neuropathy "SMON." Jap. J. Med. Sci. Biol., 24:217, 1971.

Shy, G. M., and Drager, G. A.: A neurological syndrome associated with orthostatic hypotension. Arch. Neurol., 2:511, 1960.

Sjöstrand, J.: Proliferative changes in glial cells during nerve regeneration. Z. Zellforsch. Mikrosk. Anat., 68:481, 1965.

Sjöstrand, J.: Glial cells in the hypoglossal nucleus of the rabbit during nerve regeneration. Acta Physiol. Scand., 67:Suppl. 270, 1966.

Smith, K. R.: The fine structure of neurons of dorsal root ganglia after stimulating or cutting sciatic nerve. J. Comp. Neurol., 116:103, 1961.

Smith, W. T.: Neuropathologic changes associated with steatorrhoea. Excerpta Med. Amst. (Section 8) 860, 1955.

Solitaire, G. B., and Cohen, G. S.: Peripheral autonomic nervous system in congenital or familial dysautonomia: Riley-Day syndrome. Neurology (Minneap.), 15:321, 1965.

Sourander, P., and Olsson, Y.: Peripheral neuropathy in globoid cell leukodystrophy (morbus Krabbe). Acta Neuropathol. (Berl.), 11:69, 1968.

Spencer, P. S.: Light and electron microscope observations on localised peripheral nerve injuries (2 vols.). Thesis. London, 1971.

Spencer, P. S.: Reappraisal of the model for "bulk axoplasmic flow." Nature [New Biol.], 240:282, 1972.

Spencer, P. S., and Schaumburg, H. H.: Acrylamide neurotoxicity—a review. Can. J. Neurol. Sci., in press.

Spencer, P. S., and Schaumburg, H. H.: Unpublished observations.

Spencer, P. S., Raine, C. S., and Wiśniewski, H.: Axon diameter and myelin sheath thickness—unusual relationships in dorsal root ganglia. Anat. Rec., 176:225, 1973a.

Spencer, P. S., Peterson, E. R., Madrid, A. R., and Raine, C. S.: Effects of thallium on neuronal mitochondria in organotypic cord-ganglia-muscle combination cultures. J. Cell Biol., 58:79, 1973b.

Steele, J. C., Richardson, J. C., and Olszewski, J.: Progressive supranuclear palsy. Arch Neurol., 10:333, 1964.

Stevens, J. G., and Cook, M. L.: Latent herpes simplex virus in neural tissue. In Wolfgram, F., Ellison, G. W., Stevens, J. G., and Andrews, J. M. (eds.): Multiple Sclerosis. New York, Academic Press, 1972.

Sulkin, N. M., and Sulkin, D. F.: Age differences in response to chronic hypoxia on the fine structure of cardiac muscle and autonomic ganglion cells. J. Gerontol., 22:485, 1967.

Sung, J. H.: Neuroaxonal dystrophy in mucoviscidosis. J. Neuropathol. Exp. Neurol., 23:567, 1964.

Sung, J. H., and Okada, K.: Alterations of lysosomes in neurons in Chediak-Higashi disease in man and mink. In Proceedings of the Sixth International Congress of Neuropathology. Paris, Masson & Cie., 1970, p. 1007.

Suzuki, K., and Suzuki, K.: Disorders of sphingolipid metabolism. In Goull, G. E. (ed.): Biology of Brain Dysfunction. New York, Plenum Press, 1973.

Suzuki, K., David E., and Kutschman, B.: Presenile dementia with "Lafora-like" intraneuronal inclusions. Arch. Neurol., 25:69, 1971.

Suzuki, K., Suzuki, K., and Chen, G. C.: Isolation and chemical characterization of metachromatic granules from a brain with metachromatic leukodystrophy. J. Neuropathol. Exp. Neurol., 26:537, 1967.

Swanson, A. G., Buchan, G. C., and Alvord, E. C., Jr.: Anatomic changes in congenital insensitivity to pain. Absence of small primary sensory neurons in ganglia, roots and Lissauer's tract. Arch. Neurol., 12:12, 1965.

Takahashi, K., Nakamura, H., and Okada, E.: Hereditary amyotrophic lateral sclerosis. Histochemical and electron microscopic study of hyaline inclusions in motor neurons. Arch. Neurol., 27:292, 1972.

Takano, I.: Electron microscopic studies on retrograde chromatolysis in the hypoglossal nucleus and changes in the hypoglossal nerve following its severance and ligation. Okajimas Folia Anat. Jap., 4:1, 1964.

Tarlov, I. M., and Gelfam, S.: Rigidity from spinal interneuron destruction. Histologic study. Trans. Am. Neurol. Assoc., 85:120, 1960.

Tatetsu, S.: Neuropathological changes found in cases with lesion of substantia nigra, especially regarding the changes of the nerve fibers from substantia nigra. Rec. Adv. Res. Nerv. System (Tokyo), 3:135, 1958.

Tedeschi, C. G.: Fixation and selection of blocks for microscopic study. In Tedeschi, C. G. (ed.): Neuropathology, Methods and Diagnosis. Boston, Little, Brown & Co., 1970.

Terplan, K. L., and Cares, H. L.: Histopathology of the nervous system in carnosinase enzyme deficiency with mental retardation. Neurology (Minneap.), 22:644, 1972.

Terry, R. D.: The fine structure of neurofibrillary tangles in Alzheimer's disease. J. Neuropathol. Exp. Neurol., 22:629, 1963.

Terry, R. D., and Peña, C.: Experimental production of neurofibrillary degeneration. 2. Electron microscopy, phosphatase histochemistry and electron probe analysis. J. Neuropathol. Exp. Neurol., 24:200, 1965.

Terry, R. D., and Weiss, M.: Studies in Tay-Sachs disease. 2. Ultrastructure of the cerebrum. J. Neuropathol. Exp. Neurol., 22:18, 1963.

Terry, R. D., and Wiśniewski, H.: The ultrastructure of the neurofibrillary tangle and the senile plaque. In Wolstenholme, G. W. W., and O'Connor, M. (eds.): CIBA Foundation Symposium on Alzheimer's Disease and Related Conditions. London, J. & A. Churchill, 1970, p. 143.

Thapedi, I. M., Ashenhurst, E. M., and Rozdilsky, B.: Shy-Drager syndrome. Report of an autopsied case. Neurology (Minneap.), 21:26, 1971.

Thomas, P. K., Lascelles, R. G., Hallpike, J. F., and Hewer, R. L.: Recurrent and chronic relapsing Guillain-Barré polyneuritis. Brain, 92:589, 1969.

Tischner, K. H., and Schröder, J. M.: The effects of cadmium chloride on organotypic cultures of rat sensory ganglia. A light and electron microscope study. J. Neurol. Sci., 16:383, 1972.

Toga, M., Bérard-Badier, M., Gambarelli-Dubois, D.: La dystrophie neuroaxonale infantile ou maladie de Sietelberger. Étude clinique, histologique et ultrastructurale de deux observations. Acta Neuropathol. (Berl.), 15:327, 1970.

Torvik, A., and Heding, A.: Histological studies on the

effect of actinomycin on retrograde nerve cell reaction in the facial nucleus of mice. Acta Neuropathol. (Berl.), *9*:146, 1967.

Tureen, L. L.: Effect of experimental temporary vascular occlusion of the spinal cord. Arch. Neurol. Psychiatry, *35*:789, 1936.

Vanderhaeghen, J.-J., Périer, O., and Sternon, J. E.: Pathological findings in idiopathic orthostatic hypotension. Arch. Neurol., *22*:207, 1970.

Vassela, F., Emrich, H. M., Krans-Rupert, R., et al.: Congenital sensory neuropathy with anhydrosis. Arch. Dis. Child., *43*:124, 1968.

Vinnik, I. E., Kern, F., Jr., and Struthers, J. E., Jr.: Malabsorption and the diarrhoea of diabetes mellitus. Gastroenterology, *43*:507, 1962.

Waksman, B. H.: Experimental study of diphtheritic polyneuritis in the rabbit and guinea pig. 3. The blood nerve barrier in the rabbit. J. Neuropathol. Exp. Neurol., *20*:35, 1961.

Waksman, B. H., Adams, R. D., and Mansmann, H. C.: Experimental study of diphtheritic polyneuritis in the rabbit and guinea pig. J. Exp. Med., *105*:591, 1957.

Walberg, F.: The fine structure of the cuneate nucleus in normal cats and following interruption of afferent fibers. An electron microscopic study with particular reference to findings made in Glees and Nauta sections. Exp. Brain Res., *2*:107, 1966.

Wallace, B. J., Volk, B. W., and Lazarus, S. S.: Fine structural localization of acid phosphatase acting in neurons of Tay-Sach's disease. J. Neuropathol. Exp. Neurol., *23*:676, 1964.

Wallace, B. J., Schneck, L., Kaplan, H., and Volk, B. W.: Fine structure of the cerebellum of children with lipidoses. Arch. Pathol., *80*:466, 1965.

Weiss, P.: The in vitro effect of the nerve growth factor on chicken embryo spinal ganglia: an electron microscopic evaluation. J. Comp. Neurol., *141*:117, 1971.

Whalen, G. E., Soergel, K. H., and Greenen, J. E.: Diabetic diarrhea. A clinical and pathophysiological study. Gastroenterology, *56*:1021, 1969.

Whittem, J. H.: Congenital abnormalities in calves. Arthrogryposis and hydranencephaly. J. Pathol. Bacteriol., *73*:375, 1957.

Wiśniewski, H., and Terry, R. D.: Experimental colchicine encephalopathy. 1. Induction of neurofibrillary degeneration. Lab. Invest., *17*:577, 1967.

Wiśniewski, H., Ghetti, B., and Terry, R. D.: Neuritic (senile) plaques and filamentous changes in aged Rhesus monkeys. J. Neuropathol. Exp. Neurol., *32*:566, 1973.

Wiśniewski, H., Raine, C. S., and Kay, W. J.: Observations on viral demyelinating encephalomyelitis. Canine distemper. Lab. Invest., *26*:589, 1972.

Wiśniewski, H., Shelanski, M. L., and Terry, R. D.: Effects of mitotic spindle inhibitors on neurotubules and neurofilaments of anterior horn cells. J. Cell Biol., *38*:224, 1968.

Wohlfart, G.: Degenerative and regenerative changes in the ventral horns, brainstem and cerebral cortex in amyotrophic lateral sclerosis. Acta Univ. Lundensis (new series 2), *56*:1, 1959.

Wohlfart, G., and Swank, R. L.: Pathology of amyotrophic lateral sclerosis: fiber analysis of the ventral roots and pyramidal tracts of the spinal cord. Arch. Neurol. Psychiatry, *46*:783, 1941.

Wohlfahrt, S.: De l'amyotrophie progressive à type Charcot-Marie. Acta Med. Scand., *63*:195, 1926.

Yatsu, F., and Zussman, W.: Familial dysautonomia (Riley-Day syndrome). Case report with postmortem findings of a patient at age 31. Arch. Neurol., *10*:459, 1964.

Zaimis, E.: Nerve growth factor: the target cells. *In* Zaimis, E., and Knight, J. (eds.): Nerve Growth Factor and its Antiserum. London, Athlone Press, 1972.

Zbinden, G., and Studer, A.: Zur Wirkung von Vitaminen der B-Gruppe auf die experimentelle Isoniazid-'Neuritis.' Schweiz. Z. Pathol., *18*:1198, 1955.

Zeman, W., and Donahue, S.: Fine structure of the lipid bodies in juvenile amaurotic idiocy. Acta Neuropathol. (Berl.), *3*:144, 1963.

Chapter 15

PATHOLOGIC ALTERATIONS OF THE PERIPHERAL NERVOUS SYSTEM OF MAN

Peter James Dyck

The emphasis in this chapter is on general aspects of the pathology of peripheral nerve. Specific pathologic changes are discussed in Section V, Diseases of the Peripheral Nervous System. This chapter should be read in conjunction with the other chapters in Pathology of the Peripheral Nervous System.

ANATOMICAL FACTORS AND PATHOLOGIC CHANGE

The unusual structure of the peripheral nervous system makes it difficult to study and classify pathologic changes. This fiber network is made up of cytoplasmic processes of cell bodies that lie in the spinal cord and in spinal and autonomic ganglia. Lower motor neurons arise in the ventral horn of the spinal cord, extend through the subarachnoid and ganglionic regions of the nerve root, the segmental nerve, the plexus, and the peripheral nerve, and ramify and end on muscle fibers. Spinal ganglion neurons arise in cutaneous receptors and make a variety of connections within the spinal cord. These nerve cells have most unusual shapes compared to other cells in the body. For example, large peripheral sensory neurons may be 1.8 m long and for most of their length be only 0.00001 m in diameter.

Because the peripheral nervous system ramifies widely throughout the body and because it has extensions into the central nervous system, it is not possible to perform a complete examination of this system at biopsy or even at autopsy. It is particularly difficult to evaluate the pathologic changes in three dimensions. Usually, only a portion of the brachial, lumbar, and sacral plexuses and a portion of an occasional limb nerve are taken. To get a satisfactory sample for pathologic examination it is necessary to obtain tissue from the spinal cord, subarachnoid and ganglionic portions of roots, segmental nerve and plexus, and peripheral nerve at various levels, including terminal ramifications. Even with extensive sampling, the essential lesion may be missed. In some cases it may be necessary to take out entire nerve trunks and branches so that serial tissue blocks can be prepared to discover focal pathologic lesions.

Because of the great length of nerve cells, their symbiosis with Schwann cells, and the great variability in the diameter of these cells (from 18 μm to 0.2 μm), a diversity of techniques is necessary to understand the three-dimensional morphologic alterations. These techniques include light microscopy using myelin and axis cylinder stains and specialized stains, phase contrast microscopy, electron microscopy, teased-fiber preparations, and histometric evaluation of light and electron micrographs and of teased-fiber preparations.

A significant problem in interpretation of pathologic alterations in nerves is the inability to identify the functional and physiologic types of a fiber from its appearance. It is not possible to distinguish, on morphologic grounds, motor from sensory fibers or unmyelinated dorsal root C fibers from post-ganglionic sympathetic unmyelinated fibers. Furthermore, it is impossible to recognize specific fibers from mechanoreceptors or from warm, cold, or pain receptors. Fibers from receptors in skin cannot be distinguished, by their morphologic features, from fibers subserving deep structures.

In the interpretation of pathologic change it also must be recognized that not all the changes that are seen, even though abnormal, come directly from the disease process in question. Anatomical factors may be involved. If a portion of the neuron is damaged, it may affect other portions of the neuron quite far removed from the site of the injury, as is discussed later in this chapter. Cachectic persons may have compression of their peroneal and ulnar nerves at the knee and elbow merely from lying in bed. As shown by Hopkins and Morgan-Hughes (1967), guinea pigs poisoned with diphtheria toxin are more likely to develop degenerative changes in the plantar nerves if they are allowed to walk in wire cages or in cages with solid floors than if suspended by a harness so that pressure on the plantar nerves is avoided. In amyloid neuropathy, deposits in the carpal ligament may cause compression of the median nerve and damage to its fibers. The effect of tumor, hemorrhage, or edema about a nerve is largely dependent on whether the nerve is enclosed within a bony or rigid fascial compartment or is lying in loose tissue. In the skull and vertebral canal, nerves at foramina of exit are likely to be damaged because they can be easily compressed here.

The nature of the microscopic anatomy plays a role in pathologic states. Necrotizing angiopathy of nerves is largely confined to arterioles with diameters between 75 and 300 μm. Such arterioles are only rarely seen in nerve roots and in spinal ganglia, and it appears that this is the reason why these regions are seldom affected by this disorder (Dyck et al., 1972). Furthermore, these arterioles are commonplace in the epineurium, but are seldom if ever seen in the perineurium or endoneurium. For this reason, the pathologic alterations of necrotizing angiopathy are seen in the vessels between fascicles rather than within fascicles.

Although its role is poorly understood, the perineurium undoubtedly plays a significant part in maintaining the proper environment for nerve tissue. A peripheral nerve trunk may be flooded by pus and inflammatory cells throughout the epineurium but with none passing through the perineurium into the endoneurial area. As discussed by Olsson in a preceding chapter, the endothelium of capillaries and of precapillaries probably also plays an important role in maintaining the proper environment of nerves.

HISTOLOGIC METHODS

The choice of nerve, the technique, the usefulness, and the sequelae of biopsy of peripheral nerve are discussed in the chapter by Stevens and coauthors.

The first consideration in using nerve tissue from autopsy material is to obtain it as soon as possible after death and to preserve it adequately. It is most desirable to obtain the tissue within one hour of death; if at all possible, it should be obtained within four hours. In those cases of peripheral neuropathy that merit an extensive evaluation of the peripheral nervous system, it may be necessary to obtain additional consent to remove limb nerves. It is important to consider the clinical conduction velocity and electromyographic characteristics so that tissue can be taken from appropriate anatomical sites. It is necessary also to remember the peculiar elongated structure of nerve cells of the peripheral nervous system and their central nervous system extensions so that sampling represents the various levels of the cells.

In cases of inherited neuropathy, portions of peripheral nerve, of brain, and of parenchymatous organs should be obtained quickly after death and preserved in liquid nitrogen for later biochemical studies. Even with postmortem material, tissue should be obtained for teased-fiber preparations. For this purpose, the nerve selected should be one affected by the disorder and one for which normative histometric measurements are available. (Such measurements are available for sural nerve at ankle and midcalf levels, cutaneous fascicles of the superficial peroneal nerve, nerve to the peroneus brevis, and lateral fascicles of the deep peroneal nerve.) Histometric evaluations of the number and sizes of neurons of S1 ganglia from persons of various ages are also available (Ohta et al., 1974).

The many histologic methods that are used

for peripheral nerve tissue can be found in such books as the one by Romeis (1948) and in the manual of the Armed Forces Institute of Pathology (Luna, 1968). A few histologic procedures that are especially helpful are described here.

FIXATION

Generally, peripheral nerve tissue either is fixed initially in an aldehyde or is stored in liquid nitrogen. Fresh nerve stored in bulk for biochemical studies or affixed to cryostat chucks for histochemical studies is stored in liquid nitrogen. For most postmortem studies, fixation in 10 per cent formalin in phosphate buffer is used. Although expensive, additional fixation of selected small blocks or of thin slices of large blocks in 1 per cent osmium tetroxide in phosphate buffer results in good sections from which to judge myelinated fiber density and abnormality. Extensive histometric evaluations have been based on nerves fixed with Flemming's fixative and stained with the Kulschitsky-Pal modification of Weigert's method. This also produces good profiles of the myelin sheath in transverse section at somewhat less expense. In most of our own histometric evaluations of both biopsy and postmortem material, we have prepared the tissue so that the same routine could be used for paraffin and epoxy sections and for preparation of teased fibers. The same fixation schedule permits evaluation by light, phase contrast, and electron microscopy.

In our fixation routine, 2 per cent glutaraldehyde in 0.1M cacodylate buffer at pH 7.35 to 7.4 is used. The duration of fixation depends on the size of the tissue sample. When whole sural nerves are fixed, the portion to be used for teased fibers is removed in 45 minutes, while the portion to be used for histologic sections is removed in three to four hours. For fascicular biopsy specimens, fixation is for 20 minutes and one and a half hours, respectively. In both cases, after a wash for 30 to 60 minutes in the same buffer to which 3 per cent sucrose has been added, the nerve is cut into appropriate blocks or divided into fascicles and additionally fixed in 1 per cent osmium tetroxide in the same buffer for one and one half to three hours, depending on the size of the fascicle. The doubly fixed fascicles are embedded in epoxy for thick and thin sections for phase contrast and electron

microscopy. Other parts of the fascicles are placed in 66 per cent glycerin for 48 hours and in 100 per cent glycerin for 24 hours for teased-fiber preparation.

Silver stains have been widely used for selective staining of axis cylinders, but because of lack of specificity, vagaries in staining, the uncertainty of staining all unmyelinated fibers, and the better resolution of the electron microscope, these methods are now used less frequently.

Fixation of peripheral nerves for electron microscopy is not entirely satisfactory. Fixation with aldehydes results in much better preservation of the contents of the axis cylinders than does osmium tetroxide fixation alone, but it appears also to be associated with shrinkage of the axis cylinder and with distortion of the myelin sheath. The ideal length of time in the glutaraldehyde fixative appears to be critically dependent on the volume of the tissue. With the use of osmium tetroxide alone, the myelin sheath assumes a rounded profile that is assumed from cryostat studies to be the in vivo shape. The preservation of microtubules and neurofilaments, however, is disappointingly poor. The factors that make for good preservation of microtubules are not entirely understood. Low temperature and various fixatives and ions in the fixative solutions are reported to have a deleterious effect on microtubules (Porter and Tilney, 1965; Ohnishi and Dyck, unpublished data; Schultz and Case, 1968).

TEASED-FIBER PREPARATION

Evaluation of teased fibers begins with adequate preparation. Optimal fixation with aldehyde is a prerequisite to the preparation of good teased fibers. Our method of preparing teased fibers is illustrated in Figure 15–1. With curved, pointed forceps, epineurium and perineurium are stripped off on lightly glycerinated glass slides under a dissecting microscope. Fascicles are separated, and from each, small strands of nerve fibers are torn from the bundle of fibers. From these strands, single fibers or bundles of only a few fibers are torn away by holding the proximal end of the parent strand with one forceps and pulling the proximal end of the other strand with the other forceps. For a right-handed person, the left forceps remains motionless while the right one traces an inverted

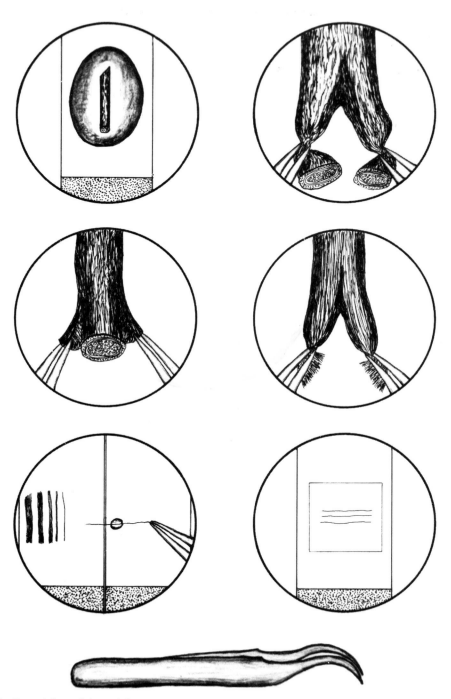

Figure 15–1   From left to right and from top to bottom, consecutive steps in fiber teasing: a fascicle of nerve, fixed in glutaraldehyde and osmium tetroxide, lying in pool of glycerin on glass slide; proximal ends are grasped and fascicles are pulled apart; epineurium and perineurium are stripped off; strands of fibers are pulled apart; from separated strands of nerve, a single teased fiber is slid onto an adjacent slide as described in the text; teased fibers in place under cover slip.

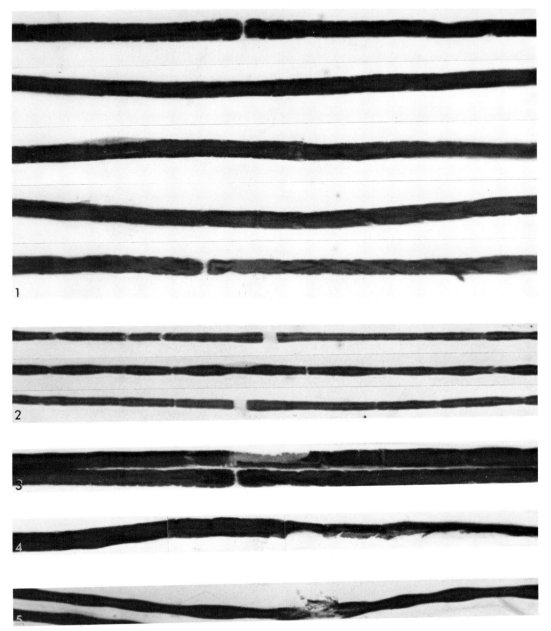

Figure 15–2 Teased-fiber preparations showing, from top down (× 380): (1) Five consecutive portions along the length of a teased fiber. Nodes of Ranvier are seen in first and fifth strips. Unstained Schwann cell nucleus is seen in third strip. (2) Three consecutive portions along the length of a teased fiber, showing excessive separation at nodes of Ranvier (top and bottom strips), separation at Schmidt-Lanterman incisures, and undulating thickness of fiber, all due to improper fixation (osmium tetroxide alone) for this method of teasing. (3) Two adjacent teased fibers with the upper showing patchy loss of myelin, an artifact encountered during teasing when excessive hardening has occurred with glutaraldehyde fixation. (4) A more severe artifact in which the lower right half of the fiber has been split and pulled away during teasing from tissue that is excessively hard. (5) Artifact in middle of strip of fiber due to grasping with forceps. These artifacts are inevitable in this method and should be ignored. This fiber also shows the effect of excessive stretching; the undulating appearance comes from excessive stretching before adequate fixation.

U-shaped pathway. The tip of the forceps is always kept in contact with the glass slide to prevent the fiber from curling up around it. Teasing is always performed from the proximal end of the fascicle so that branches are not torn off.

A clean slide is laid on the right side of the slide on which the teasing is done. With the forceps, the proximal end of each separate fiber is grasped and slid onto the clean slide through a minute drop of glycerine — again, the tip of the forceps kept constantly touching the glass. As the middle of the new slide is reached, the points of the forceps are allowed to spread apart. The friction of the fiber on the glass will straighten the fiber and will cause it to pull loose from the tips of the forceps. Three or four teased fibers are placed in the center of the glass slide. If proper technique is used, the proximal ends of the fibers will always be oriented in the same way, the fibers will be straight, and there will be a minimum of glycerin with them (Fig. 15–2).

A drop of mounting medium is applied to the cover slip, under observation under the dissecting microscope so that the apex of this drop is at the center of the fiber, and the cover slip is dropped onto the slide. As the drop spreads outward it will carry most of the glycerin at its moving front, displacing it to the edges of the cover slip. The cover slip edges may be sealed with nail polish.

Using these methods on suitably prepared tissue, an experienced, diligent person can prepare 150 to 300 teased fibers per day.

ARTIFACTS

It is important to recognize the artifacts, shown in Figure 15–2, that can be produced by the method described here. Excessive stretching of the nerve during biopsy or of the fiber during teasing when the tissue is inadequately fixed produces separation at nodes of Ranvier and at Schmidt-Lanterman incisures. In addition the fiber may assume a varicose appearance that mistakenly may be assumed to be due to pathologic abnormality. Separation at nodes and at Schmidt-Lanterman incisures is particularly common when this method of teasing is used on tissue fixed with osmium tetroxide alone; with correct aldehyde fixation, it is not seen. The morphologic changes at the ends of teased fibers

should be ignored since these may represent damage by the forceps.

The optimal time of glutaraldehyde fixation for nerve to be embedded in epoxy may be too long for nerve that is to be teased. Excessive fixation leads to separation of bits of myelin from the teased fiber or an actual splitting.

In properly fixed material, this method of teasing does not produce artifacts even at the electron microscope level. For electron microscopy, teasing is done in freshly prepared epoxy rather than in glycerin (Dyck and Lais, 1970; Spencer and Thomas, 1970). Figure 15–3 shows electron micrographs, at low and high power, of transverse sections of different parts along the length of one teased fiber of the sural nerve of a child with hypertrophic neuropathy of the Charcot-Marie-Tooth type. The preservation of structures is not unlike that with the usually prepared nerve.

HISTOMETRIC EVALUATION

Histometric evaluation of various structures of spinal cord, spinal ganglia, and peripheral nerve has two purposes. The first is descriptive. Questions to be answered are: What are the normal numbers and size distributions, at various ages and at various levels, of fibers of afferent tracts of spinal cord that contain central processes of spinal ganglia neurons? What are the normal numbers and size distributions, at various ages and at various levels, of anterior horn cells, of spinal ganglia neurons, and of fibers of mixed, muscle, and cutaneous nerves? What is the normal relationship, at various ages, of length of internode to diameter of myelinated fibers at various sites and levels of peripheral nerves and of afferent spinal cord tracts? What is the normal relationship of the number of lamellae of myelin to the perimeter of axis cylinders in central and peripheral processes of lower motor and primary sensory neurons? In nerve fibers of various types, what are the densities of microtubules, neurofilaments, endoplasmic reticulum, and mitochondria? How are these measurements affected by various disorders of the peripheral nervous system?

The second purpose is investigative. A variety of measurements have been made on nerves during development and with advancing age to elucidate how nerve fibers

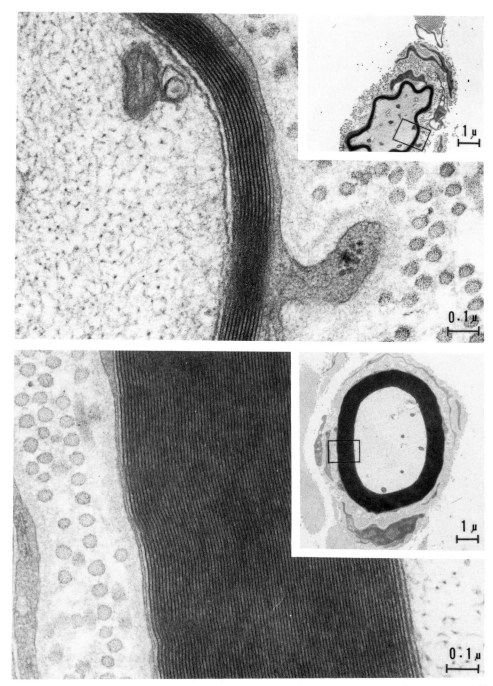

Figure 15–3   Transverse sections at the same magnification (× 79,050) from two sites on the same teased fiber from a child with hypertrophic neuropathy of the Charcot-Marie-Tooth type. In insets, both at the same low magnification (× 5,088), rectangles show area reproduced at higher magnification. These pictures illustrate that good electron microscopic preservation is possible by the method of teasing described in the text. (From Dyck, P. J., and Lais, A. C.: Electron microscopy of teased nerve fibers: method permitting examination of repeating structures of same fiber. Brain Res., *23*:418, 1970. Reprinted by permission of the Elsevier Publishing Co.)

develop and how they later degenerate. On transverse sections of nerves, the numbers and diameters of myelinated and unmyelinated fibers have been determined in infancy and with increasing age and in various peripheral neuropathies. In Chapter 3, Webster discusses the spatial changes of Schwann cell membrane as it forms in a spiral fashion around the axolemma. On electron micrographs, measurements have been made of the number of lamellae of myelin and of the perimeter of the axis cylinder. These relationships are being studied to understand the change that occurs with development and with old age.

Extensive studies have been made on the relationship of the length of internodes to the diameters of myelinated fibers for sural nerve and for muscle nerves of man at various ages (Dyck et al., 1973; Stevens et al., 1973). Such measurements are being used in studies of nerves of patients with peripheral neuropathy to provide information regarding previous degeneration and regeneration or previous segmental demyelination and remyelination. Measurement of the numbers and sizes, at various levels, of afferent spinal cord tracts, anterior horn and spinal ganglion neurons, and mixed, muscle, and cutaneous nerves might provide information on the occurrence, nature, and pathogenic mechanism of such processes as neuronal degeneration, neuronal atrophy, axonal regeneration, and segmental demyelination and remyelination.

At present, methods and normative values for various levels and ages are not available for anterior horn cells or for afferent spinal cord tracts of man.

NUMBER AND SIZE OF CYTONS OF SPINAL GANGLIA

Values for the normal volume of the first sacral ganglion and the numbers and sizes of its neurons at various ages have been published (Ohta et al., 1974). For histometric evaluation, this ganglion should be removed within a few hours of death. Transverse serial sections (usually 1000 to 2000 8-μm sections) are made. The sections that mark the beginning and end of the ganglion have to be identified.

The first and last sections and a sampling of sections in between are photographed at two magnifications. The low-power photographs are used to determine the area of the sections. From this and the number of sections between the samples, the volume can be determined. The photographs at the higher magnification are used for counts of nerve cells and of their size distribution. It should be recognized that corrections of these counts are necessary because the cell or its nucleus or nucleolus (whichever is used for counting) appears in more than one section. A second correction is necessary because of the tendency to overcount large cells or their particles. The frequency distribution is based on measurements of the diameter of nerve cells cut through the nucleolus, thus ensuring that the measurement is made at the equator of the cell. The exact methods of fixation, counting, sizing, and computation may be obtained from the studies by Offord and co-workers (1974) and by Ohta and co-workers (1974). Representative histograms of cytons (cell bodies) of the first sacral ganglion of man at various ages are shown in Figure 15–4.

NUMBER AND SIZE OF FIBERS

Histometric measurements of myelinated and unmyelinated fibers in transverse sections and teased fibers from healthy nerves of man have been made on cutaneous nerves (sural nerve at midcalf and ankle level, and superficial peroneal at ankle level) and muscle nerves (lateral fascicle of deep peroneal nerve and nerve to peroneus brevis) (Dyck et al., 1965; Swallow, 1966; Ochoa and Mair, 1969a, 1969b; Dyck et al., 1973; Stevens et al., 1973). Typical histograms of the diameters of myelinated and unmyelinated fibers of sural nerve are shown in Figure 15–5, and of diameters of myelinated fibers of the nerve to peroneus brevis in Figure 15–6.

To determine the numbers and frequency distributions of diameters of myelinated and unmyelinated fibers per nerve and per square millimeter of fascicular area, three sets of photographic enlargements of transverse sections of the nerve are required: (1) at a low power to measure the size of the nerve; (2) at a higher power to measure the diameters of myelinated fibers; and (3) at a much higher power, under the electron microscope, to measure the diameter of unmyelinated fibers. A suitable histologic preparation is obtained

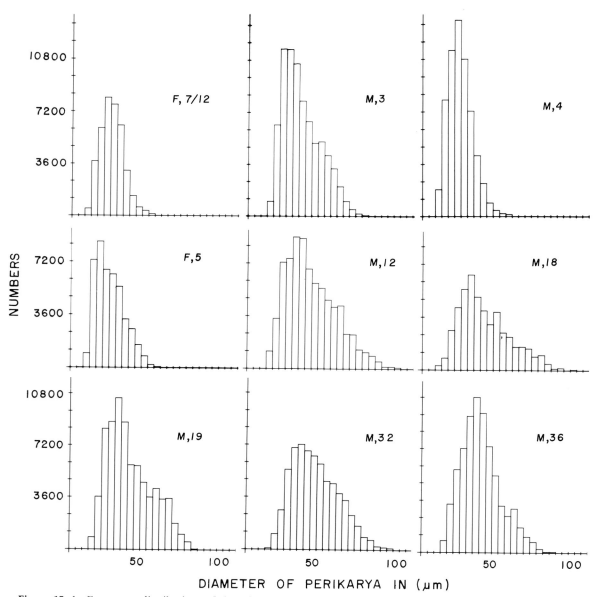

Figure 15-4 Frequency distributions of size of neurons of representative first sacral ganglia of man at various ages. (From Ohta, M., Offord, K., and Dyck, P. J.: Morphometric evaluation of first sacral ganglion of man. J. Neurol. Sci., *22*:73–82, 1974. Reprinted by permission of Elsevier Publishing Co.)

by fixation in glutaraldehyde and osmium tetraoxide followed by embedding in epoxy. Some blocks will contain the entire nerve (paraffin sections may be used) and others will contain only whole fascicles.

Enlargements at the lowest magnification are made of sections of the whole nerve, for measurement of the transverse fascicular area. This measurement is made with a planimeter or a digitizer attachment and a programmable calculator or computer. We trace the outline of the outer border of the endoneurial area of fascicles.

Photographs at the middle magnification (× 1500) are made of random areas (corresponding to an area greater than 0.2 mm²) of fascicles or of transverse sections of the nerve, through a phase contrast microscope, for use in determining the frequency distribution of the diameters of the fibers. A photographic enlargement of a reticle is used for accurate measurement of the magnification. We use a Zeiss TGZ 3 particle size analyzer set for standard range and exponential and frequency distribution. The analyzer light spot is approximated to the size of the myelin

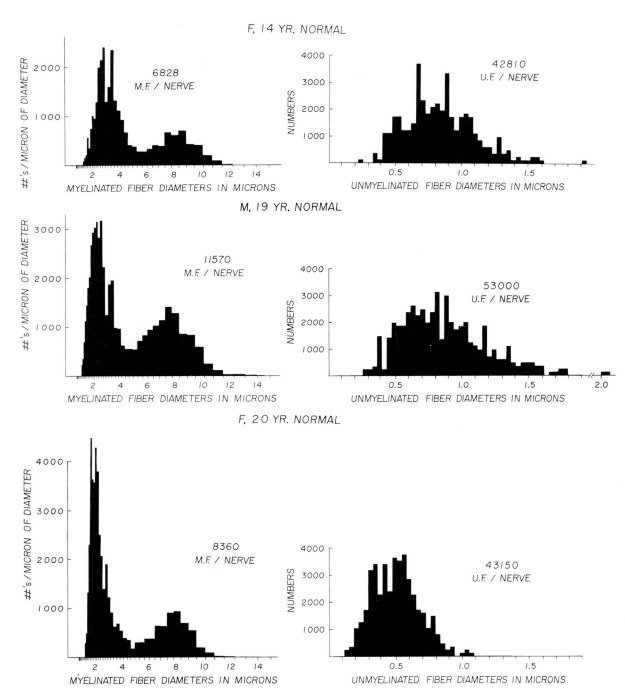

Figure 15–5 Frequency distributions of myelinated (*left*) and unmyelinated (*right*) fibers of sural nerve of man at various ages. (From Dyck, P. J., Lambert, E. H., and Nichols, P. C.: Quantitative measurement of sensation related to compound action potential and number and sizes of myelinated and unmyelinated fibers of sural nerve in health, Friedreich's ataxia, hereditary sensory neuropathy, and tabes dorsalis. *In* Rémond, A. (ed.): Handbook of Electroencephalography and Clinical Neurophysiology. Vol. 9. Amsterdam, Elsevier Publishing Co., 1971, p. 83. Reprinted by permission.)

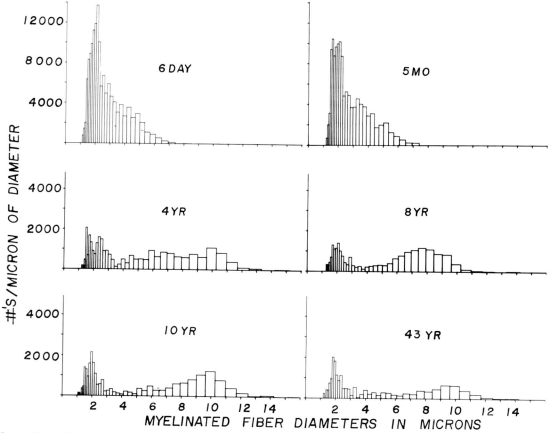

Figure 15–6 Frequency distribution of myelinated fibers of nerve to peroneus brevis muscle in man at various ages. (From Stevens, J. C., Lofgren, E. P., and Dyck, P. J.: Histometric evaluation of branches of peroneal nerve: Technique for combined biopsy of muscle nerve and cutaneous nerve. Brain Res., 52:37–59, 1973. Reprinted by permission of the Elsevier Publishing Co.)

sheath profile on the photograph, and the foot switch is depressed, thereby perforating the paper and identifying the measured fiber. Fibers that have an oval profile are considered to be cut obliquely; in these, the lesser axis is assumed to be the correct diameter. The diameter of the fiber is tallied for size in the appropriate counter and also in a counter for the total. A separate tally is made of myelinated fibers that touch the left and lower borders of the photograph and of distorted fibers whose diameters have not been measured. A programmable calculator and plotter are used to derive the transverse fascicular area, the number of myelinated fibers per nerve and per square millimeter of fascicular area, and an exponential plot of the number of fibers per micron of diameter. The exponential plot and the small-diameter categories used give a more precise definition of the small-fiber peak, compared to the linear plots often used.

For determination of the numbers and sizes of unmyelinated fibers, the highest magnification, electron micrographs at enlargements of approximately × 15,000, is used. The numbers and size distribution of diameters are obtained in the same way as for myelinated fibers with the exception that the Zeiss TGZ 3 counter is utilized in the standard range and linear and frequency distribution modes.

MORPHOMETRY OF TEASED FIBERS

Teased myelinated fibers to be evaluated histometrically should be obtained without preselection. They are identified serially as they are obtained. Next, they are graded according to their condition as outlined in the next section. Then measurements are made, with a light microscope and an ocular grid, of the internode length (IL), of the length of demyelinated regions, and, at regular intervals, of the diameter of the fibers. Only fibers classified as condition A, B, C, or D can be evaluated.

The mean (mean of IL), standard deviation, and coefficient of variation of internode length (CV of IL) and the length of demyelinated regions of a fiber are determined. We usually obtain such measurements on 100 teased fibers of a nerve. Mean values for the mean IL and mean CV of IL of 100 fibers are then derived to obtain the mean IL and the mean CV of IL of the nerve. Demyelinated regions are not included in the measurement of IL. Since small and large fibers may not be selected in the correct ratio as found from evaluation of transverse sections and since the CV of IL is somewhat greater for small fibers than for large fibers, an adjustment of these mean values for the nerve is made.

The teased fibers are grouped into small fibers and large fibers according to their mean IL (as an example, for the sural nerve, a value of 625 μm or larger is used to designate large fibers). The mean of IL and of CV of IL of small fibers (designated mean IL_s and CV of IL_s) and of large fibers (designated mean IL_l and CV of IL_l are determined separately. From the ratio between small and large fibers, the adjusted mean IL of nerve and the adjusted CV of IL of nerve can be determined. If 60 per cent of the fibers are small and 40 per cent are large, the adjusted mean IL of nerve equals 0.6 (mean IL_s) plus 0.4 (mean IL_l) and the adjusted CV of IL of nerve equals 0.6 (mean CV of IL_s) plus 0.4 (mean CV of IL_l).

In practice, we use a programmable calculator to obtain these indices from the following entered data: number of fibers, condition of fiber, correction factor to convert divisions of ocular micrometers to microns, serial entry of IL in divisions of ocular micrometer, and serial entry of diameter of fiber at regular intervals along its length.

Histometric data from teased fibers of a normal cutaneous nerve, the sural nerve, are shown in Table 15–1; the data for a normal muscle nerve, the lateral fascicle of the deep peroneal nerve, are shown in Table 15–2. Values of mean IL of nerve and of CV of IL of nerve may be strikingly abnormal in disease.

RATIO OF LAMELLAE OF MYELIN TO PERIMETER

To determine the number of lamellae of myelin per micron of perimeter of axis cylinder, (abbreviated, lamellae/1 μm of P), we developed a program for a digitizer

TABLE 15–1 INTERNODE LENGTH (IL) OF TEASED MYELINATED FIBERS OF HEALTHY SURAL NERVES*

Nerve	Age (yr), Sex	Mean IL of Nerve			
		Midcalf		Ankle	
		Small	Large	Small	Large
96–71	10, M	324	943	293	906
73–71	11, M	339	897	353	854
62–71	14, M	333	951	330	849
25–71	20, F	364	977	305	940
23–71	23, M	337	1017	313	936
24–71	26, M	294	979	356	1003
70–71	31, M	325	1187	345	850
79–71	37, M	266	919	317	881
26–71	44, M	287	947	286	1035
113–71	46, M	258	1055	281	941
56–71	52, M	393	860	354	799
108–71	59, M	265	991	302	794
74–71	70, F	277	961	308	911
Mean IL, all nerves		312.5	975.7	318.7	899.9
SD		41.6	80.8	26.5	72.2

*From Dyck, P. J., Schultz, P. W., and Lais, A. C.: Mensuration and histologic typing of teased myelinated fibers of healthy sural nerve of man. *In* Kakulas, B. K. (ed.): Clinical Studies in Myology. Excerpta Medica International Congress Series. Amsterdam, Excerpta Medica, 1973. Reprinted by permission.

TABLE 15-2 INTERNODE LENGTH (IL) OF TEASED MYELINATED FIBERS OF HEALTHY LATERAL FASCICLES OF DEEP PERONEAL NERVE*

| | | | Small Fibers | | | Large Fibers | | | Small and Large Fibers | |
| | | | | | | | | | Adjusted | Adjusted |
Nerve	Age (yr)	Num-ber†	Mean IL (μm)	SD (μm)	Mean CV of IL	Mean IL (μm)	SD (μm)	Mean CV of IL	Mean IL of Nerve (μm)	CV of IL of Nerve
71-71	2	6.1	257	84	9.7	495	72	9.1	390	9.5
96-71	10	6.4	368	125	8.7	838	114	10.5	716	10.0
75-71	18	6.3	380	139	17.1	1198	245	10.5	716	14.4
78-71	18	5.5	405	131	19.4	930	115	9.9	668	14.6
115-71	21	6.4	312	145	16.1	1015	162	11.3	628	13.9
54-71	30	6.5	393	138	13.7	968	164	9.6	646	11.7
70-71	31	6.7	274	148	15.8	941	160	11.4	674	13.1
44-71	33	5.9	329	112	14.4	894	111	9.5	595	12.1
79-71	37	6.1	371	133	14.2	937	154	11.7	660	12.9
113-71	46	6.4	322	119	14.9	1135	188	10.1	598	13.2
51-71	58	5.6	361	146	19.2	1002	166	12.4	637	16.3
108-71	59	6.7	279	125	13.3	910	163	15.8	450	14.0
1-72	67	6.2	323	111	15.9	837	126	11.2	487	14.4
74-71	70	6.7	301	143	18.1	774	86	9.7	467	15.2

*From Stevens, J. C., Lofgren, E. P., and Dyck, P. J.: Histometric evaluation of branches of peroneal nerve: technique for combined biopsy of muscle nerve and cutaneous nerve. Brain Res., 52:37-59, 1973. Reprinted by permission of the Elsevier Publishing Co.

†Mean number of internodes per teased fiber.

and a programmable calculator. Electron micrographs of myelinated fibers are prepared at known magnifications. The number of major dense lines is counted under a dissecting microscope and the axolemma is traced with the cursor of the digitizer. These measurements are made on 80 to 200 fibers. The evaluated fibers can be divided into "small" and "large" categories, depending on the number of lamellae of myelin or the perimeter of the axis cylinder. For sural nerves of persons 10 years old and older, we have determined that large fibers have a myelin sheath thickness of 52 lamellae or more and an axis cylinder perimeter of 10 μm or more. Ratios of lamellae per micron of perimeter can be determined for small (lamellae/1 μm of P_s) and for large (lamellae/1 μm of P_l) fibers, and from the ratio of large and small fibers in the nerve an adjustment can be made for incorrect sampling of large and small fibers as just discussed.

In addition, because two criteria (thickness of myelin sheath and size of axon) can be used to designate large and small fibers, the ratio may be different, depending on which criterion is used. In abnormal nerves, such as sural nerves in Friedreich's ataxia, if the criterion of myelin sheath thickness is used, "old internodes" of large fibers can be shown to have an abnormally high lamellae/1 μm of

P value, indicating a decrease in volume of axis cylinder rather than an increase in volume of myelin (Dyck and Lais, 1973).

HISTOLOGIC STRUCTURES WITH POSSIBLE PATHOLOGIC SIGNIFICANCE

The incidence of fiber degeneration and regeneration is low in nerves of healthy persons of all ages, but increases with age. This includes fibers that have degenerated into linear rows of myelin ovoids, fibers with intercalated internodes, fibers with excessive variability of internode length and diameter, fibers with irregularity of the myelin sheath of some internodes, fibers with segmental demyelination and remyelination, and fibers that have uniformly short internodes relative to their diameters. These changes are discussed in greater detail later.

A histologic structure referred to as "Renault's corpuscle" was first described in the nerves of man, horse, dog, and ass by Renaut (1881a, 1881b) (Figure 15-7A). Subsequently they have been seen in nerves of persons with various disorders. They have been extensively studied and reported in the German and

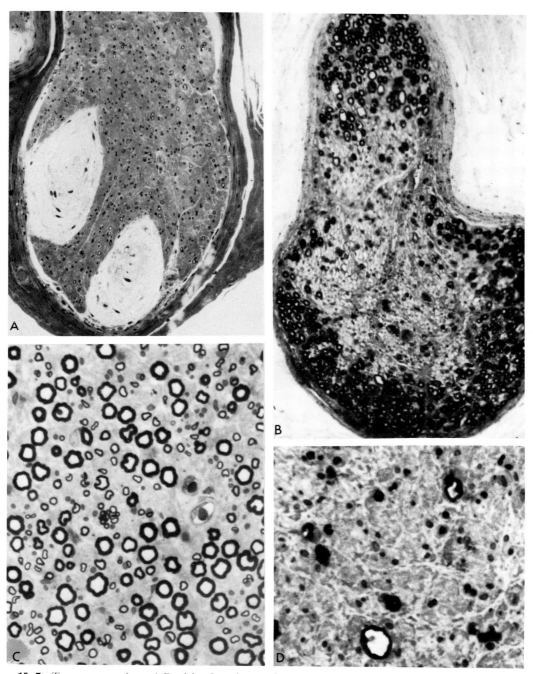

Figure 15–7 Transverse sections. *A.* Fascicle of sural nerve from patient with hypertrophic neuropathy of the Charcot-Marie-Tooth type, with two large Renault's corpuscles seen as two oval light areas touching the perineurium. × 150. These also are seen in healthy nerves. *B.* Fascicle of median nerve of patient with rheumatoid arthritis and necrotizing angiopathic neuropathy. Note central fascicular degeneration of myelinated fibers. × 150. *C.* Intrafascicular area, showing normal density of myelinated fibers. × 500. *D.* Intrafascicular area of nerve from patient with necrotizing angiopathic neuropathy, showing markedly decreased density of myelinated fibers. Only degenerating myelin ovoids and myelin balls are seen. × 500.

French literature (Krücke, 1955; Dyck et al., 1970). In the English literature they usually have been described as infarcts (Kernohan and Woltman, 1938). The corpuscles usually are found on the inside of the perineurium and protrude into the endoneurial space. In longitudinal profile they taper at both ends and merge with the perineurium. In transverse sections they consist of concentric lamellae of filamentous strands. Oval, plump, pale nuclei—cellules godronnées of Renaut—are associated with filamentous strands. At the center of the corpuscle there usually are three or four plump nuclei similar to those noted in mucoid degeneration. The lamellae stain light pink with hematoxylin and eosin, pale green with trichrome, not at all with methyl violet, and strongly blue with alcian blue at pH 2.5. The staining reaction suggests that they contain acid mucopolysaccharides. They are seen in the nerves of healthy persons, in greater frequency with increasing age, and according to Asbury and co-workers (1972), especially adjacent to limb joints. The consensus is that Renaut's corpuscles are not specific for a particular disease and certainly are not infarcts of nerve (Okada, 1903).

Schwann cell inclusions occur particularly at polar regions of the nuclei of Schwann cells and near nodes of Ranvier. One of these is the π granule of Reich (Fig. 15–8). In paraffin or thick epoxy sections stained with thionine, toluidine blue, or methylene blue, these metachromatic granules are seen. Usually they are rod-shaped and approximately 1 μm long. They are directed radially or circumferentially to the direction of the fiber. In the electron microscope they undoubtedly correspond to Schwann cell cytoplasmic lamellar bodies, also called zebra bodies. They have a periodicity of approximately 4.8 nm, may be surrounded by a double membrane, and may occur singly or in clusters. They have been described by Thomas and Slatford (1964) in nerve of the rabbit, by Evans and co-workers (1965) in nerves of patients with various neuromuscular disorders, by Gonatas (1967) in nerves of a patient with a disorder resembling Refsum's disease, and by us (Dyck and Lambert, 1970) in a series of nerves from healthy persons and nerves from patients with hypothyroid neuropathy. Although they probably are a result of a degeneration phenomenon, they do not appear to be specific for a disease.

Another Schwann cell inclusion is the Elzholz body (μ granule of Reich). These myelin-like droplets in the cytoplasm of Schwann cells are Marchi-positive and are often seen adjacent to Schwann cell nuclei and in Schwann cells near nodes of Ranvier as well as in teased fibers, where they may be mistaken for myelin ovoids. Under the electron microscope, osmiophilic bodies of two kinds are seen. The first is a myelin whorl without axis cylinder contents; it may lie outside the myelin sheath or between the sheath and the axolemma. The other is a homogeneous oil droplet.

Glycogen granules abound in perineurial and blood vessel cells. Small clumps of glycogen granules also are seen in Schwann cell cytoplasm at polar ends of the nuclei and near nodes of Ranvier (Fig. 15–8D and E). At both sites they often are associated with mitochondria. An occasional glycogen granule is seen in axis cylinders. Their presence in electron micrographs is markedly enhanced with adequate aldehyde fixation.

FIBER DEGENERATION

Abnormalities Seen in Transverse and Longitudinal Sections

In human disorders of the peripheral nervous system there usually is an admixture of degenerative and regenerative changes. For this reason they are discussed together. The changes to be described are largely those affecting myelinated fibers; for unmyelinated fibers the nature of the degenerative changes is probably simpler, but they are less well understood.

In transverse frozen or embedded sections of nerve, the following histologic abnormalities may be recognized: a decrease in number of myelinated or unmyelinated fiber profiles (see Fig. 15–7), excessive dilatation of myelin sheath profile (ballooning), single myelin balls or clusters of balls, and sudanophilic material near myelin ovoids or at the sites of former myelinated fibers.

Improper fixation and cutting sometimes may produce an artifact that has a superficial resemblance to myelin ovoids and balls. Sections taken from the site of the razor blade cut of inadequately fixed nerve may show what appear to be abnormal myelin sheaths (Fig. 15–9). Such an artifact is recognized by the thickened, split myelin encroaching on the

(Text continued on page 314.)

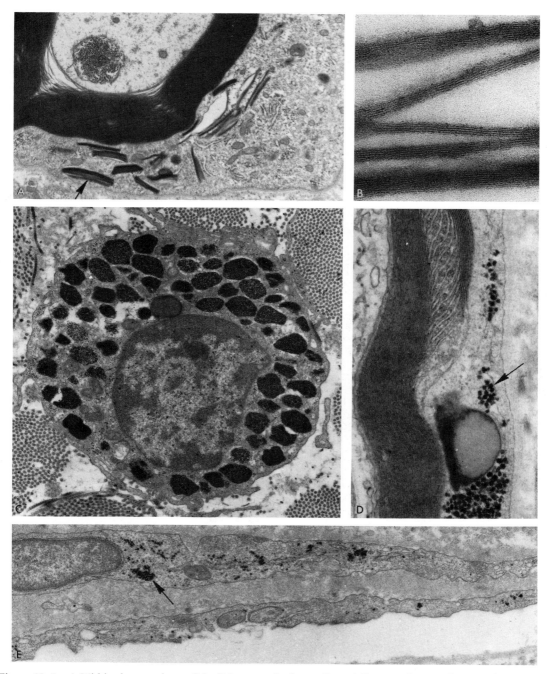

Figure 15–8   *A.* Within the cytoplasm of the Schwann cell of a myelinated fiber are clusters of π granules (arrow) (also called Schwann cell cytoplasmic lamellar bodies or zebra bodies). $\times$ 8480. *B.* Higher magnification of π granule cluster. *C.* Electron micrograph of mast cell from nerve. The metachromatic staining properties of this cell may be confused with the metachromasia of metachromatic leukodystrophy disease granules or with deposits of amyloid. $\times$ 11,280. *D.* Portion of longitudinal section through a Schmidt-Lanterman incisure, showing deposit of glycogen (arrow). $\times$ 39,480. *E.* Perineurial cell with glycogen (arrow). $\times$ 20,800.

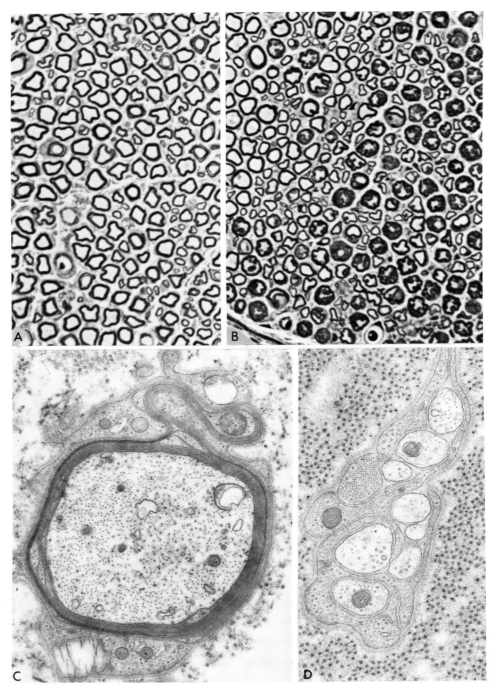

Figure 15–9   *A* and *B*. Transverse sections of peroneal nerve of rat, showing no artifact (*A*) and, in approximately half the fibers, an artifact of myelin (*B*) that was produced by cutting the nerve prior to fixation in glutaraldehyde and osmium tetroxide and making a histologic section near this cut. × 500. *C*. Transverse section of remyelinated internode, showing characteristic thin myelin sheath and lack of compaction of myelin lamellae. × 19,000. *D*. Unmyelinated axonal sprouts with myelin ovoids and myelin balls. × 25,200.

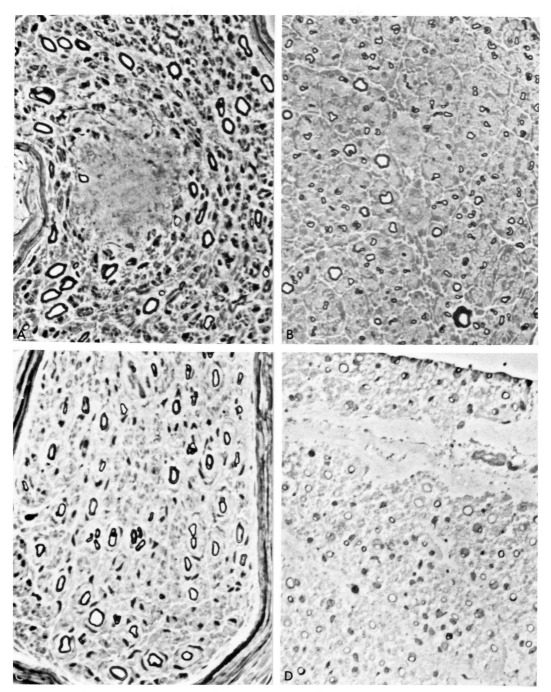

Figure 15–10   Transverse sections of sural nerve of man at the same magnification (× 500), showing differences in size distribution of fibers in: *A*, dominantly inherited amyloidosis; *B*, Friedreich's ataxia; *C*, dominantly inherited hypertrophic neuropathy; and *D*, recessively inherited hypertrophic neuropathy. See text for further explanation.

axis cylinder, the absence of homogeneous myelin balls, and the absence of hyperplasia of the Schwann cell cytoplasm. The damaged myelin sheaths occur in islands. With deeper sections the abnormality lessens.

The size distribution of the fibers may be suggestive of various disorders. In Figure 15–10, photograph *A*, of sural nerve, shows the central plaque of amyloidosis surrounded predominantly by large fibers, a finding typical of dominantly inherited amyloidosis. In photograph *B*, of nerve from a patient with Friedreich's ataxia, most of the myelinated fibers are small. The lower two photographs of nerve are from patients with hypertrophic neuropathy. *C*, from a patient with a dominantly inherited variety, shows a relatively normal thickness of myelin sheath; *D*, from a patient with a recessively inherited variety, shows very thin myelin sheaths.

In longitudinal sections, the abnormalities may consist of linear rows of myelid ovoids or balls within nerve strands. They may be at various stages of fiber degeneration. A superficial section of a fiber with irregularity of myelin may spuriously suggest linear rows of myelin balls. Sections of nerve stained with silver may show varicosities of the axis cylinders or discontinuity. Combined myelin and axis cylinder stains may show discontinuity of myelin in the presence of intact axis cylinders. Special stains may reveal the presence of abnormal lipids.

Longitudinal thick sections have limited value for recognizing mild abnormality. Irregularity of the myelin sheath may be interpreted falsely as myelin ovoids in linear rows. It is not possible to recognize variation in thickness of myelin sheath and variation of the diameter of axis cylinder or other pathologic abnormality of the fiber over the length of more than a few internodes of the same fiber in longitudinal sections.

Teased-Fiber Studies

A much more illuminating view of the morphology of nerve fiber degeneration comes from a careful evaluation of teased myelinated fibers. Such teased-fiber studies were used by Remak, Kolliker, Gombault, and Cajal. In our examination of teased myelinated fibers in various experimental neuropathies and in a variety of neuropathies in man, we have utilized a grading system to designate the histologic condition of the fibers (Dyck

et al., 1971a). In using it, it is important that the nerve fibers be obtained without preselection. To accomplish this we often divide the portion to be teased into 10 equal parts and then deliberately take an equal number of fibers from each of these 10 parts. The person doing the teasing tries to take the fibers without attention to whether they are abnormal. On the average, teased fibers should be longer than 4 mm and should be free of preparatory artifacts except at their extremities where they have been grasped. All histologic abnormalities at the ends of the fiber therefore are ignored.

The following classification describes the histologic condition of teased fibers:

A. Teased fiber of normal appearance ignoring criteria of internode length and of internode diameter. Myelin is regular except in paranodal regions. Thickness of myelin of the internode with the thinnest myelin is 50 per cent or more of that of the internode with the thickest myelin. No paranodal or internodal segmental demyelination is seen (Fig. 15–11).

B. Teased fiber with excessive irregularity, wrinkling, and folding of myelin that is not due to preparatory artifact. In other respects it has the features of condition A (Fig. 15–12).

C. Teased fiber with region or regions of paranodal or internodal segmental demyelination with or without myelin ovoids or balls in cytoplasm of the associated Schwann cells.* Thickness of myelin of the internode with the thinnest myelin is 50 per cent or more of that of the internode with the thickest myelin. Myelin may be regular or irregular (Fig. 15–13).

D. Teased fiber with region or regions of paranodal or internodal segmental demyelination with or without myelin ovoids or balls in cytoplasm of the associated Schwann cells. Thickness of myelin of the internode with the thinnest myelin is less than 50 per cent of that of the internode with the thickest myelin. Myelin of internodes may be regular or irregular (Fig. 15–14).

E. Teased strand of nerve tissue with linear rows of myelin ovoids and balls at the same stage of degeneration (Fig. 15–15).

F. Teased fiber without region or regions of segmental demyelination but with excessive variabil-

---

*In demyelination, as judged by the high-dry objective of the light microscope, no myelin can be recognized. From our previous evaluation of teased fibers under the electron microscope, four lamellae of myelin can be recognized as a thin dark line under the light microscope except when there is excessive tissue around the fiber. By paranodal demyelination it is implied that the site of the node of Ranvier is recognized and that the nodal gap is increased beyond that seen in normal fibers. In internodal demyelination a part or the entire former internode is demyelinated.

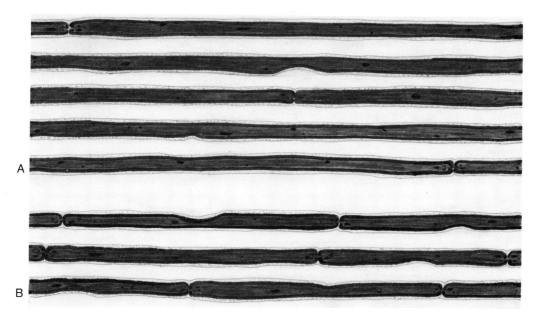

Figure 15–11 Drawings of consecutive lengths, from top to bottom, of teased myelinated fibers. *A.* A fiber in condition A as described in text. *B.* Also condition A, but note that the internode lengths (IL) are short as compared to fiber shown above. This may be a regenerated fiber; however, because of the considerable variability in mean internode lengths between fibers of a given diameter even in healthy nerve, it is not possible with certainty to designate this fiber as being regenerated.

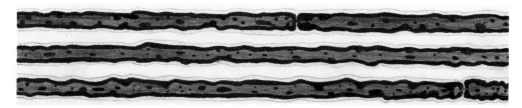

Figure 15–12 Drawing of consecutive lengths, from top to bottom, of a teased myelinated fiber in condition B as described in text.

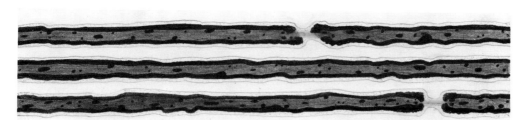

Figure 15–13 Drawing of consecutive lengths, from top to bottom of a teased myelinated fiber in condition C as described in text. Note that the myelin thickness is not as variable as it is in condition D.

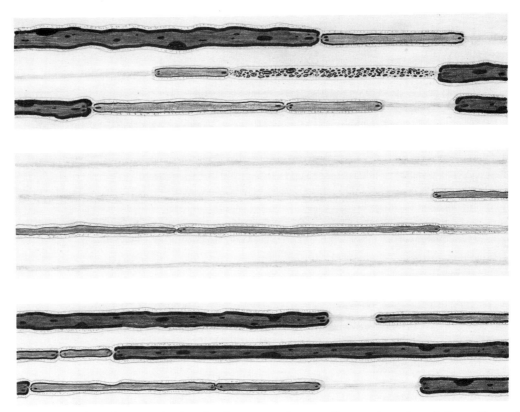

Figure 15–14 Drawing of consecutive lengths, from top to bottom of a teased myelinated fiber with condition D as described in text. Note that the ovoids of the internode in which the myelin has degenerated are much smaller in diameter than the large ovoids that form initially in condition E. Note also regions of segmental demyelination and the considerable variability of myelin thickness due to the presence of "old" and "new" internodes.

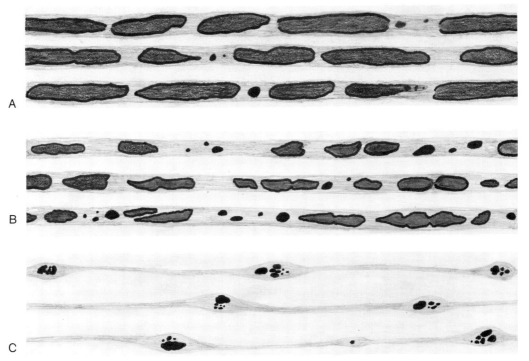

Figure 15–15 Drawings of consecutive lengths, from top to bottom of a teased myelinated fiber with condition E as described in text. *A.* Segmentation into large ovoids. *B.* Mixture of myelin ovoids and balls of intermediate size. *C.* Clusters of small myelin balls occurring at widely separated points.

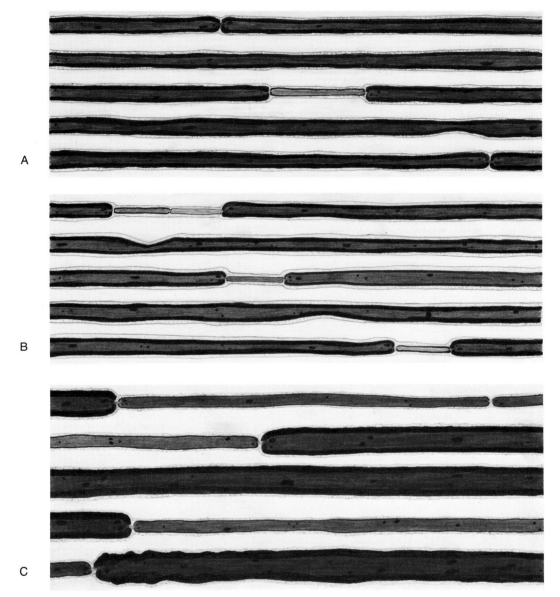

Figure 15–16   Drawings of consecutive lengths, from top to bottom, of three teased myelinated fibers in condition F as described in text. The teased fiber in *A* shows a single intercalated internode, a not uncommon finding in fibers from healthy nerve.

ity of myelin thickness between internodes. Thickness of myelin of the internodes with the thinnest myelin is less than 50 per cent of that of the internode with the thickest myelin. Myelin of internodes may be regular or irregular (Fig. 15–16).

G. Teased fiber without region or regions of segmental demyelination but with excessive variability of myelin thickness within internodes to form "globules" or "sausages" (Fig. 15–17).*

*Although the myelin thickness in the regions of the "globule" (Dayan et al., 1968) or "sausage" (Behse et al., 1972) is greater, it probably merely represents a process of infolding and reduplication of myelin rather than excessive production of myelin.

H. Teased fiber of normal appearance as described in A, but in which there are myelin ovoids or balls contiguous to two or more internodes (Fig. 15–18).

I. Teased fiber having several proximal internodes or parts of internodes with or without paranodal or internodal segmental demyelination and, distal to these, a linear row of myelin ovoids or balls (Fig. 15–19).

The classification is descriptive and only criteria are used that have a small "between observers" difference. Teased fibers are classified on the basis of a "by eye" assessment under the microscope and without measure-

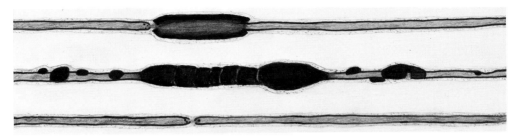

Figure 15–17 Drawings of consecutive lengths, from top to bottom, of a teased myelinated fiber in condition G as described in text.

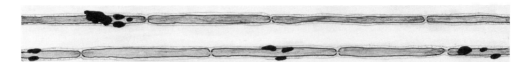

Figure 15–18 Drawings of consecutive lengths, from top to bottom, of a teased myelinated fiber in condition H as described in text. This condition clearly implies regeneration of a myelinated fiber. This condition is not to be confused with that of the teased fiber that has a single osmiophilic droplet in Schwann cell cytoplasm outside of myelin, which is discussed subsequently as the Elholtz body (μ granule of Reich).

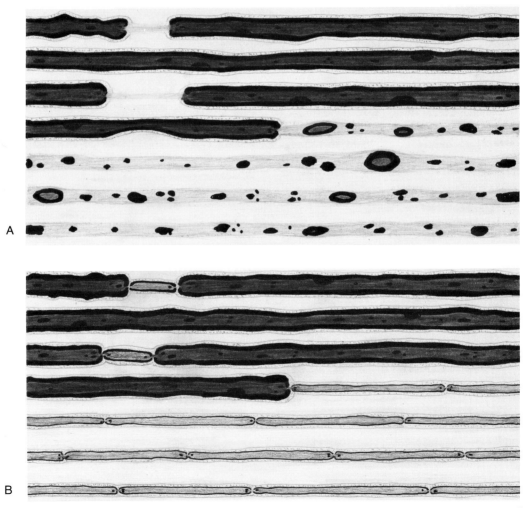

Figure 15–19 *A.* Drawing of consecutive lengths, from top to bottom, of a teased myelinated fiber in condition I as described in text. This type of fiber change is seen typically several days after and at the site of crush. *B.* The same fiber as shown above after repair has occurred—this would be graded as condition F.

TABLE 15–3   DISTRIBUTION OF 100 TEASED MYELINATED FIBERS OF NORMAL SURAL NERVE AT ANKLE LEVEL

Nerve	Age (yr), Sex	Type of Myelinated Fiber (per cent)*							
		A + B	C	D	E	F	G	H	I
96–71	10, M	100							
73–71	11, M	94			1	4			1
62–71	14, M	96				4			
25–71	20, F	97				3			
23–71	23, M	96			3	1			
24–71	26, M	96	1			3			
70–71	31, M	98				2			
79–71	37, M	93				4	3		
26–71	44, M	97				3			
113–71	46, M	96		1	1	2			
56–71	52, M	93			1	6			
108–71	59, M	97				3			
74–71	70, F	93			2	4	1		

*Teased fibers evaluated according to the new classification described in the text: A, normal appearance; B, excessive irregularity of myelin not due to preparative artifacts; C and D, segmental demyelination and thickness of myelin (that of internodes with thinnest myelin compared with that of internodes with thickest myelin; C, 50 per cent or more; D, less than 50 per cent); E, linear rows of myelin ovoids; F, 50 per cent or more difference in myelin thickness between internodes; G, thickening or reduplication of myelin to form "globules" within internodes; H, consecutive "new-appearing" internodes with adjacent myelin ovoids; I, proximally, "old-appearing" internodes, and distally, "new-appearing" internodes plus other features.

ment. Internode length and diameter are not used as criteria since these can be done better by making measurements, e.g., mean IL of fiber, and CV of IL of fiber. There is no category of "regenerated fibers" for those fibers with multiple internodes that are short considering their diameter. Such fibers would be classified as condition A. In our opinion it is usually not possible to say with certainty whether such fibers are variants of normal, regenerated fibers, or portions of fibers undergoing slow axonal atrophy that have been remyelinated. Teased fibers with regions of intercalated internodes are placed in F. Subclassification under each category is possible, e.g., condition E could have three subdivisions: (1) segmentation into large ovoids, (2) mixture of myelin ovoids and balls of intermediate size, and (3) clusters of small myelin balls occurring at widely separated points along the length of the strand of nerve tissue. The various conditions of teased fibers are not meant to correspond directly to types of fiber degeneration, e.g., wallerian degeneration, axonal degeneration, or axonal atrophy.

The frequency of occurrence of these various histologic conditions of teased myelinated fibers in healthy nerve from persons of various ages is known for the sural nerve, cutaneous branches of the superficial peroneal nerve, and the lateral fascicle of the deep peroneal nerve. Tables 15–3 and 15–4 present the summarized data for these nerves (Dyck et al., 1973;

Stevens et al., 1973). The incidence of various abnormalities increases in older persons. In peripheral neuropathy there is a striking increase in the incidence of fiber types other than A. To illustrate this change from the normal, two examples might be cited. In a typical case of necrotizing angiopathy, all or most of the myelinated fibers in an affected nerve may be condition E. In hypertrophic neuropathy of the Charcot-Marie-Tooth type, most of the fibers may be condition D. The determination of the histologic condition of fibers, especially when combined with histometric evaluation of sections and of teased fibers in a questionable case of neuropathy provides definite evidence of normality or abnormality and documents the degree and kind of abnormalities.

Electron Microscopic Correlation With Teased-Fiber Abnormality

Electron microscopic evaluation along the length of singly embedded fibers, in regard to the eight conditions just described, has not been undertaken extensively.

In conditions B and C, the axis cylinder is preserved. Abnormalities of the axis cylinder that have been described include a decrease in volume of the axis cylinder, accumulations of mitochondria and dense bodies, and pos-

TABLE 15–4 DISTRIBUTION OF TEASED MYELINATED FIBERS OF LATERAL FASCICLES OF DEEP PERONEAL NERVE

Nerve	Age (yr)	Type of Myelinated Fiber (per cent)*							
		$A + B$	C	D	E	F	G	H	I
71–71	2	100							
96–71	10	99		1					
75–71	18	94	1		1	4			
78–71	18	96			1	3			
115–71	21	95	2			3			
54–71	30	92			1	7			
70–71	31	92		1	2	5			
44–71	33	91			1	8			
79–71	37	94			2	4			
113–71	46	87	2		5	6			
51–71	58	93			1	6			
108–71	59	95			1	4			

*Teased fibers evaluated according to the new classification described in the text: A, normal appearance; B, excessive irregularity of myelin not due to preparation artifacts; C and D, segmental demyelination and thickness of myelin (that of internodes with thinnest myelin compared with that of internodes with thickest myelin; C, 50 per cent or more; D, less than 50 per cent); E, linear rows of myelin ovoids; F, 50 per cent or more difference in myelin thickness between internodes; G, thickening or reduplication of myelin to form "globules" within internodes; H, consecutive "new-appearing" internodes with adjacent myelin ovoids; I, proximally, "old-appearing" internodes, and distally, "new-appearing" internodes plus other features.

sibly abnormal clustering of neurofilaments. The ratio of the number of lamellae of myelin to the perimeter of the axis cylinder in nerves with many fibers in condition B or C has been shown to be increased, suggesting that the volume of the axis cylinder is smaller than normal since the thickness of the myelin was not found to be different from normal.

The electron microscopic features of singly embedded fibers of condition D have not been studied in enough detail to allow conclusions to be drawn. Several observations can be made, however. Myelin breakup in condition D (segmental demyelination) is into small balls (see Fig. 15–13) and not into large myelin ovoids (cf. Fig. 15–15) as in condition E (axonal degeneration). These small myelin balls degenerate into lipid droplets in autophagic vacuoles. Paranodal regions usually are affected first but not necessarily to the same degree at opposite ends of an internode. A new node of Ranvier can form at the site of a partially damaged internode. When viewed under the electron microscope, demyelinated axis cylinders are always surrounded by Schwann cell cytoplasm. In nerve showing segmental demyelination there usually is abundant evidence of remyelination. Early remyelinated internodes are short and of small diameter and have a small number of

lamellae of myelin per micron of perimeter of axis cylinder (Schröder, 1970; Dyck et al., 1973). Fibers in condition D usually also show varying degrees of onion bulb formation.

The electron microscopic features of condition E of myelinated fibers are not well known. The condition is seen in a variety of disorders affecting peripheral neurons. The presence of linear rows of myelin ovoids or myelin balls that are at the same stage of degeneration over the whole length of the teased fiber always is associated with discontinuity of the axis cylinder. Axis cylinder remnants show varying combinations of rarefaction, of clumping or dissolution of microtubules, neurofilaments, mitochondria, and dense bodies, and of dissolution of axolemma. Abnormal organelles also have been described. Myelin ovoids with an undisturbed lamellar pattern may be in autophagic vacuoles in Schwann cell cytoplasm or in macrophages. Subsequently, homogeneous lipid replaces formed myelin.

Types of Fiber Degeneration in Neuropathy

Fiber degeneration in various neuropathies usually is reported either as wallerian degeneration or as segmental demyelination. On considering the diverse mechanisms producing neuropathy and the various conditions of teased fibers, it seems unlikely that there are only two types of fiber degeneration. Recognition of other types of fiber degeneration is reflected by the use of other terms in the literature such as "axonal degeneration," "axonal atrophy," "simple atrophy," "axonal dystrophy," "primary and secondary segmental demyelination," and "hypomyelination." Because of insufficient knowledge of the three-dimensional pathologic alterations in neurons and of pathogenic mechanisms of fiber degeneration, classifications of fiber degeneration, such as proposed here, are tentative.

The type of fiber degeneration that is seen depends in part on whether the pathologic process is interstitial (between or outside of nerve cells—necrotizing angiopathy) or is parenchymatous (metabolic derangement within cells). If the process is interstitial, focal damage within nerve trunks and affecting all types of fibers is produced. If the process is parenchymatous, the damage is more diffuse and tends to affect various populations of neurons more selectively. Wallerian degeneration and several varieties of segmental demyelination are seen if the process is interstitial. Axonal degeneration, axonal atrophy, and probably a different variety of segmental demyelination from that seen in the first group usually are seen if the process is parenchymatous.

WALLERIAN DEGENERATION

Wallerian degeneration and regeneration are discussed in detail by Schröder in a subsequent chapter. In neuropathy, this type of fiber degeneration is seen especially in disorders with focal abnormalities in nerve (interstitial neuropathies). The term "wallerian degeneration" is used in the restricted sense to refer to the histologic sequence of events consequent to transection of fibers. It does not refer to other processes in which fibers may not be transected but that also result in linear rows of myelin ovoids and myelin balls and discontinuity of the axis cylinder. Therefore, it may not always be possible to ascertain from one portion of nerve whether the process is wallerian degeneration or axonal degeneration. Only with electron microscopic study and with infor-

mation regarding the pathogenesis of the fiber degeneration is this distinction possible.

In neuropathy, nerve fibers may be transected by mechanical section, compression, traction, ischemia, or thermal, electric, or radiation injury.

Compression of nerve sufficient to produce segmental demyelination at the site of constriction usually also produces wallerian degeneration of some of the fibers. There is a long-standing divergence of opinion regarding the mechanism of damage produced by tourniquet—mechanical damage versus ischemic damage. Whatever the mechanism, compression of nerve is important in human neuropathy. Acute paralysis is seen in tourniquet paralysis, in crossed-leg palsy, and in bridegroom's palsy. It also is seen in repetitive damage to nerves in a variety of entrapment syndromes, as is discussed in the chapter by Aguayo. Compression of nerve tissue also occurs from tumor, from disk material, from osteophytes, and from an inflammatory response at sites of nerve that are bounded by a bony wall (for example, foramina of exit in cranium and spinal column).

Ischemia may damage peripheral nerve tissue and cause wallerian degeneration. Ischemic damage of nerve fibers may be caused by occlusion of a major artery to a limb. It also can be caused by necrotizing angiopathy, septic or other emboli to nerve, and possibly compression. As is discussed in more detail in the section on neuropathy due to ischemia and physical agents, ischemia presumably causes transection of fibers with resultant wallerian degeneration. The site of fiber damage most likely is at watershed zones of poor perfusion and not at the occluded vessel or vessels. Differential susceptibility of tissue to anoxia results in a greater damage to nerve fibers than to other cells.

Several pathogenic factors may be important in fiber degeneration in amyloidosis. Kernohan and Woltman (1942) stated that amyloid produced its effect by either compression or ischemia. In teased fibers we have seen that amyloid nodules lying adjacent to myelinated fibers cause large saccular dilatation, probably a prewallerian phase (Dyck and Lambert, 1969). At other sites, remyelinated internodes lie adjacent to such nodules—evidence that the integrity of the axis cylinder has been maintained. The selective and almost complete degeneration of unmyelinated fibers of the nerves of the lower limbs in the dominantly inherited variety and the observed deposition of amyloid in autonomic and spinal ganglia suggest that factors other than ischemia or compression within peripheral nerve are in operation. It may be that there is a selective deposition near the perikaryon of these cells.

An inflammatory response within nerve tissue may result in sufficient damage to nerve fibers to transect them, so that they undergo wallerian degeneration. Cellular hyperimmunity probably underlies this damage. These hyperimmune macrophages initially damage the Schwann cells, but the axis cylinders commonly are affected also. A perivascular inflammatory response has been demonstrated in acute inflammatory polyradiculoneuropathy (Guillain-Barré-Strohl syndrome) and in subacute, chronic, and relapsing varieties of inflammatory polyradiculoneuropathy. The inflammatory response may be found widely distributed in roots, plexuses, and nerves and sometimes also in spinal cord. Although inadequately studied, a similar inflammatory hyperimmune reaction may underlie brachial plexus neuropathy and lumbar and sacral plexus neuropathies.

Intrinsic or extrinsic nerve tumors may transect nerve fibers. The mechanism by which this occurs is poorly understood.

AXONAL DEGENERATION

This term is used here to indicate the histologic sequence of events, in myelinated fibers, associated with degeneration of the entire neuron (neuronal degeneration) or with degeneration of the distal processes of neurons (distal axonal degeneration or dying back). As in wallerian degeneration, linear rows of myelin ovoids and myelin balls are formed (condition E). In addition, there usually are fibers in conditions B and C, which is not typical for wallerian degeneration. In disorders with axonal degeneration the fibers of nerves often show abnormalities within axis cylinders that differ from those seen in wallerian degeneration. Furthermore, there tends to be a selective involvement of populations of neurons in axonal degeneration and in axonal atrophy. In wallerian degeneration, all fibers are affected. (Actually, this point is hard to substantiate because one usually is looking at nerve distal to the site of damage — at a point where normal and abnormal fibers mix.) An important distinction from wallerian

degeneration is that, in axonal degeneration, transection of fibers cannot be demonstrated. The distinction of axonal degeneration from axonal atrophy may be only one of chronicity; it may be that axonal degeneration is associated with a more rapid process than is axonal atrophy.

NEURONAL DEGENERATION WITH AXONAL DEGENERATION

In disorders with neuronal degeneration affecting only peripheral motor neurons (also called anterior horn cell diseases), numbers of anterior horn cells and of motor fibers to muscle are decreased. Since adequate normative histometric data on the anterior horn cells in spinal cords of man at various ages are not available, it is difficult to recognize decreased numbers of cells unless the decrease is marked. Also, since muscle nerves contain many afferent fibers, recognition of loss of motor fibers may be problematic unless one has reliable normative data. Therefore, identification of degenerating nerve cells and fibers in muscle nerves becomes important. An abnormal incidence of conditions B, C, and especially E in teased fibers in muscle nerves, without abnormality in cutaneous nerves, is typical of a neuronal degeneration of peripheral motor neurons.

Stevens and co-workers (1973) have described techniques for the study of muscle and cutaneous nerves obtained by biopsy through one incision. The lateral fascicle of the deep peroneal nerve and the cutaneous fascicle of superficial peroneal nerve above the ankle were found to have a low incidence of degenerative change and consistent values of mean internode length of large and of small fibers and of their coefficients of variation.

In disorders with neuronal degeneration selectively affecting peripheral sensory neurons (also called sensory radicular neuropathies), numbers of fibers in afferent spinal cord tracts, or perikarya in spinal ganglia, and of afferent fibers in peripheral nerves are decreased. As in peripheral motor neuron degeneration, a decrease in number of fibers in spinal cord tracts and in spinal ganglia has to be severe to be recognized. Teased-fiber studies of posterior columns, although technically difficult, can now be done (Harrison et al., 1970; McDonald and Ohlrich, 1971), but as yet, adequate spinal cord data for man are not available. The numbers and sizes of perikarya, of first sacral spinal ganglia and of myelinated and unmyelinated fibers of sural nerve of man at various ages are available, as mentioned earlier in this chapter. Recognition of degenerating cells or fibers and documenting their occurrence may be most helpful in demonstrating the presence and the characteristics of a disorder. To do this, the conditions of 100 teased fibers taken at random from the sural nerve are graded as previously outlined.

The disorders with neuronal degeneration affecting peripheral motor neurons include poliomyelitis, amyotrophic lateral sclerosis, and Werdnig-Hoffmann disease. Typical examples of neuronal degeneration affecting spinal ganglia are herpes zoster, sensory neuropathy of carcinoma, and some vitamin B deficiencies such as of B_{12}.

Little is known of the pathogenic mechanism of axonal degeneration. In the case of poliomyelitis and herpes zoster, the virus invades the perikaryon and damages the nerve cell by unknown mechanisms. The nature of the mechanism of neuronal degeneration in motor neuron diseases, in the sensory neuropathy of carcinoma, and in some deficiency disease is unknown.

DISTAL AXONAL DEGENERATION

The disorders with distal axonal degeneration are different from those with neuronal degeneration in that the distal aspect of the central and peripheral cell processes degenerates to form linear rows of myelin ovoids, sparing the perikaryon. A rigid separation of the processes of neuronal degeneration and of distal axonal degeneration is not possible because of lack of sufficient information regarding the numbers and sizes of fibers in afferent spinal cord tracts, of peripheral motor and sensory cell bodies, and of motor and sensory fibers of peripheral nerve in various disorders of peripheral neurons. It is commonly stated that there is dying back in neuronal degeneration and, conversely, that loss of some neurons probably occurs in disorders with distal axonal degeneration.

Metabolic Factors. An important question to be resolved is whether the distal axonal degeneration results from failure of the metabolic apparatus of the perikaryon or from a local abnormality in the distal axon. The present view is that the perikaryon is the meta-bolic center of the nerve cell and the major site for synthesizing proteins such as enzymes. Such enzymes have to be transported to the cell's extremities. Local factors, e.g., oxygen and glucose supply, may be necessary for this transport.

That many peripheral neuropathies with distal axonal degeneration may result from disordered metabolism of the perikaryon of the nerve cell is not a new concept. The trophic influence of the anterior horn cells on peripheral nerve and on muscle was known from the effect of sectioning of a nerve. Charcot and Joffroy (1869) referred to the lack of a trophic influence on nerve and muscle in amyotrophic lateral sclerosis. Erb (1883), discussing multiple degenerative neuritis and referring to Strümpell's (1883) cases of neuropathy without inflammation, wrote that he was dealing with a neural atrophy whose origin was in the trophic central apparatus and that the absence of histologic abnormality in the spinal cord in no way proved that he was dealing exclusively with a peripheral affection. Discussing cases of amyotrophic lateral sclerosis, Mott (1895) commented,

As a rule, the more remote a part is from its seat of nutrition, the more likely is it to undergo degeneration, and we could thus explain the gradual "creeping up" of the degenerative process.

From studies of thiamine deficiency, Swank (1940) stated that,

When a neuron is subjected to a slow depletion of thiamin . . . its axis cylinder degenerates at a point most distant from its trophic cell body.

The existence of an explanation for degeneration of the central processes of spinal ganglion neurons, in peripheral neuropathies with distal axonal degeneration, is largely overlooked except in the literature on neuropathology. There have been many studies showing degeneration and decreases in numbers of fibers of the posterior columns and of peripheral nerve in the presence of normal numbers of anterior horn and spinal ganglia perikarya. These anatomical changes have been noted both in experimental neuropathy and in neuropathies of man, such as thiamine deficiency (Gudden, 1896; Swank, 1940; Prineas, 1970), diabetes mellitus (Williamson, 1904; Bosanquet and Henson, 1957; Greenbaum et al., 1964), pellagra (Aring et al., 1941), vitamin B_{12} deficiency (Greenfield and Carmichael, 1935), pantothenic acid deficiency (Swank and Adams, 1948), multiple myeloma (Victor et al., 1958; Aguayo et al., 1964), vitamin E deficiency (Pentschew and Schwarz, 1962), acrylamide intoxication (Prineas, 1969b), and tri-ortho-cresyl phosphate (TOCP) intoxication (Prineas, 1969a).

Several possible reasons for the degenerative changes and decreased number of fibers in posterior column come to mind.

1. The metabolic apparatus of the perikaryon of peripheral sensory neurons may be disordered as a result of various causes, so that the amount of proteins, enzymes, or other constituents is small or their rate of synthesis is abnormal and the integrity of the distal processes of the cells cannot be maintained.

2. Proteins, enzymes, and other constituents are synthesized normally, but a defect in axonal transport prevents their becoming available to distal processes.

3. Axonal degeneration of the central process is a secondary histologic event after damage to the peripheral process.

4. There is a local abnormality in the proximal process coincident with the abnormality in the peripheral process.

It is unlikely that axonal degeneration of the central process is secondary to damage of the peripheral process. In the pathologic studies cited, the changes in posterior columns consisted of marked loss of fibers, degeneration of fibers, and sclerosis. Such marked degrees of posterior tract change have not been seen resulting from focal pathologic change of nerve in which the majority of fibers were transected, as may occur in necrotizing vasculopathy. Well-studied postmortem cases of necrotizing vasculopathy, such as the ones of Eichhorst (1877) and Leyden (1880) in which there was extensive damage of peripheral nerve, have not shown demyelination and sclerosis of posterior tracts of spinal cord. Experimental section of the large nerve trunks with disarticulation of the hind limb at the hip in dogs by Homen (1888) showed atrophy of the ipsilateral posterior tracts. This was of greater magnitude if nerve section had been done when the dog was immature, although some atrophy could be seen after some time even in adult dogs. Sudanophilia and sclerosis were not features of this secondary effect on the posterior tracts. The marked degree of degeneration and sclerosis of posterior and other afferent spinal cord tracts seen in many cases of neuropathy is therefore probably not secondary to transection or damage of the peripheral processes

of spinal ganglia neurons. Transection of peripheral nerves, particularly near the perikaryon of the neuron, does produce pathologic alterations known as retrograde degeneration or chromatolysis, but it is thought that for the most part this is reversible (see review by Döring, 1955).

There is some evidence that a failure of axonal flow may precede at least one variety of neuropathy with distal axonal degeneration. In experimental acrylamide neuropathy, Pleasure and co-workers (1969) have shown that the normal transport of the labeled protein was blocked near the perikaryon.

Segmental Demyelination in Axonal Degeneration. The mechanism of the paranodal segmental demyelination in axonal degeneration is also poorly understood. That it occurs in conditons in which the predominant alterations of teased myelinated fibers are linear rows of myelin ovoids and myelin balls was recognized by Gombault (1880–1881, 1886) in lead neuropathy of guinea pigs, in alcoholic neuropathy, and in amyotrophic lateral sclerosis of man. Segmental demyelination in the presence of evidence of axonal degeneration was noted by Meyer (1881) in diphtheritic neuropathy, by Dreschfeld and by Karsalsoff and Serbski in alcoholic neuropathy, by Pitres and Vaillard in nerves of a gangrenous upper limb, and by Fiese and Pagenstecher in lead neuropathy (see review by Stransky, 1902). Gombault considered segmental demyelination to be a prewallerian degeneration phase. Inflammatory cells destroyed the myelin sheath first. If the process was severe, the axis cylinder was destroyed next.

Collins and co-workers (1964) postulated a different mechanism for segmental demyelination in alcoholic neuropathy — focal demyelination possibly due to a decrease in volume of the axon. Such a hypothesis would explain Krücke's (1961), Hopkins's (1970), and Hopkins and Gilliatt's (1971) observation of discontinuity of myelin in proximal nerve fibers and linear rows of myelin ovoids and myelin balls in distal fibers in some varieties of neuropathy.

In a study of uremic neuropathy, Dyck and co-workers (1971a) came to the conclusion that the myelin irregularities and the paranodal and segmental demyelination were probably secondary to axonal degeneration. This view was based on the following observations.

1. There was unequivocal degeneration of myelinated and of unmyelinated fibers, and this was most severe in distal segments of the nerves studied—approximately 5 per cent of myelinated fibers at the midcalf level and more than 50 per cent at the ankle level were seen as linear rows of myelin ovoids and balls.

2. The paranodal and segmental demyelination was not randomly distributed but occurred especially in certain fibers.

3. The regression lines for the relationship of lamellae of myelin to circumference of axis cylinder for nerves from patients with uremic neuropathy could best be explained by a selective decrease in volume of axis cylinders.

4. Unequivocal electron microscopic abnormalities were observed in preserved axis cylinders.

From these observations it was postulated that this paranodal and segmental demyelination was at least in part the result of a decrease in volume of the axis cylinder. It was also postulated that the axon does not necessarily degenerate and that a series of intercalated internodes on a single teased fiber probably was due to a previous axonal abnormality.

Ultrastructural Alterations. Several electron microscopic alterations have been seen in axonal degeneration. Since degeneration and regeneration may be occurring concomitantly, the changes described as follows may represent stages of degeneration or abortive regeneration. In tri-*o*-cresyl phosphate poisoning, aggregation of neurofilaments and neurotubules and proliferation of endoplasmic reticulum were observed in myelinated fibers of nerves by Bischoff (1967) and by Prineas (1969a). Collins and co-workers (1964) described redundant projections of membranes in the axoplasm in thiamine-deficient and chronically starved rats; within the axis cylinder they noted paranodal collections of vesicles and mitochondria. In the same disorder, Prineas (1970) noted flattened, irregular sacs around degenerating mitochondria in many fibers. Aggregation of neurofilaments and microtubules, proliferation of endoplasmic reticulum, and abnormal organelles were reported by Schröder (1968) in experimental isoniazid neuropathy. In uremic neuropathy, Dyck and co-workers (1971a) noted clumping of microtubules and neurofilaments and accumulations of abnormal mitochondria and other abnormal organelles. In acrylamide neuropathy, Prineas (1969b) found a marked increase in the number of

neurofilaments with a relative decrease in microtubules. In polyneuropathy associated with hypothyroidism, Dyck and Lambert (1970) found an increase in glycogen granules in axis cylinders of myelinated and of unmyelinated fibers and mitochondrial abnormalities. In this condition, segmental demyelination was also seen, but whether this was secondary to axis cylinder change or was due to concomitant metabolic abnormality of Schwann cells or both was not known.

The emphasis so far has been largely on axonal degeneration and not on regeneration. In many conditions in which axonal degeneration is seen, the fate of the neuron is not necessarily sealed. In various metabolic, deficiency, and toxic disorders, when the abnormality improves, it is probable that some of the neurons will recover functionally. Too little is known regarding the morphologic changes of such recovery. Axonal regrowth or sprouting most likely would occur at the degenerated tips of neurons, as shown by Schröder (1968) in isoniazid neuropathy. One would expect to find a shorter mean internode length of nerve (Fullerton et al., 1965) and an increase in the mean coefficient of variation of internode length of nerve as a result of the development of intercalated internodes at regions of previous paranodal and segmental demyelination. Such an axonal degeneration and regeneration may be the reason for the shorter internode lengths of myelinated fibers of the nerves of the elderly (Vizoso, 1950; Dyck and Lais, 1973; Stevens et al., 1973).

In the classification at the end of this chapter, there is a brief list of the conditions in which axonal degeneration is seen.

AXONAL ATROPHY

Axonal atrophy is found in chronic disorders that are probably progressive over many years. The disorders usually are inherited and are assumed to be due to an inborn error of metabolism. Characteristically, fibers disappear insidiously without the occurrence, except very occasionally, of linear rows of myelin ovoids. The effect of axonal atrophy is a gradual loss of fibers. Affected neurons shrink and the axis cylinder volume decreases. Possibly as a result of axonal shrinkage, myelin is discontinuous with paranodal and segmental demyelination, as discussed under Axonal Degeneration. In progressive disorders the affected neurons degenerate. Because of the chronicity and repeated segmental demyelination and remyelination, onion bulbs may be formed.

The concept of axonal atrophy or simple atrophy arose historically with the views on "progressive muscular atrophy" and "systematic atrophy or system degeneration." An early pathologic account of the type of fiber alteration discussed here was published by Virchow (1855) and described the postmortem examination in a case of inherited progressive muscular atrophy. He noted that the nerves were thickened, that there were fewer than normal numbers of myelinated fibers, and that there was a loss of posterior column fibers. Linear rows of myelin ovoids and myelin balls were not seen. An increase in number of nuclei and amount of connective tissue was also noted. This case now might be called neural progressive muscular atrophy or peroneal muscular atrophy or the hypertrophic variety of Charcot-Marie-Tooth disease.

In an early case of progressive muscular atrophy of long duration, described by Friedreich (1873), nerve fibers were thin and myelin was atrophic at various points along the length of fibers and especially at the distal ends of fibers. Here also the fibers were surrounded by rich connective tissue with increased numbers of nuclei and of hyperplastic neurilemma (onion bulbs).

Discussing spinocerebellar degeneration, Gowers (1893) coined the word "abiotrophy" to include all diseases with primary neuronal atrophy that affected groups of neurons with similar functions. By "primary neuronal atrophy," he meant a disturbance of metabolism of the neuron, which led gradually to its death. The observation that groups of neurons with similar functions (a system) might be selectively affected by an atrophic degenerative process had been recognized and called "systematic atrophy" by Joffroy (according to Strümpell, 1883). A striking example of such a system atrophy was recorded by Mott (1907) in a case of Friedreich's ataxia; in this case there had been a symmetrical fallout of coarse fibers in the posterior roots and in peripheral nerves.

Spatz (1938) defined the characteristics of the system atrophies: the hallmarks of acute breakdown of fibers are absent; affected centers do not show degeneration; decrease in numbers of fibers can be shown but not the stages of breakdown; the nerve cells and fibers eventually disappear, their place being taken by glia; one or two functional systems are affected; and it is different from degenerative conditions that show degeneration products. In discussing "system degeneration," Greenfield and co-workers (1958) noted that, in spinocerebellar degeneration, long and large neurons in tracts were affected first and at their periphery and that the perikarya shrank and showed chromatolysis.

It is evident from these historical views that precise pathologic definitions have not been possible. Although there may be subtypes within the axonal atrophies, exact classification of these is difficult. Differences are based on which types of neurons are involved, on the age at onset of the disorder, on the rapidity of degeneration of the neurons, and on whether there is atrophy of the entire neuron or only of distal processes.

NEURONAL DEGENERATION WITH AXONAL ATROPHY

This type of fiber degeneration is well illustrated by the events that occur in Friedreich's ataxia (the restricted definition given in Chapter 40 by Dyck and Ohta. There is some evidence that the peripheral motor or sensory neurons are normal in infancy and early childhood. We have shown that the density of myelinated nerve fibers in the sural nerve is moderately decreased in mild cases and markedly decreased in advanced cases.

From quantitative studies of sensation, recordings of the compound action potential of the sural nerve in vitro, and histometric evaluation of sural nerves from patients with Friedreich's ataxia (Dyck et al., 1971b) it is known that the Aα peripheral sensory neurons are affected first and predominantly. Postmortem examination has shown decreased numbers and atrophic cytons within spinal ganglia and demyelination with sclerosis of afferent tracts in the spinal cord (Friedreich, 1863; Mott, 1907; Hughes et al., 1968), suggesting that the cyton atrophies and disappears.

Recognition of the atrophic process in the peripheral fibers of cutaneous nerves of patients with Friedreich's ataxia came from study of teased fibers (Dyck et al., 1973). Most teased fibers had a normal appearance. Internode length (IL) and coefficients of variation (CV) of IL per fiber and per nerve as previously discussed, however, even in fibers classed as condition A, were abnormal. Because of the marked paucity of large fibers, the uncorrected mean IL of nerve was less than normal. If the remaining fibers were normal, one would expect the adjusted IL of nerve and the adjusted CV of IL of nerve to be normal. Actually, our measurements showed that the mean IL for small fibers and the mean IL for large fibers both were significantly less than normal. The mean CV of IL for small fibers was significantly greater than normal (there were too few large fibers to estimate this value for them).

An explanation for this observation came from study of large numbers of teased fibers. Occasional fibers were seen with multiple sites of paranodal and segmental demyelination; one teased fiber had 18 such sites. Occasional other teased fibers had multiple intercalated internodes. The paranodal and segmental demyelination was not occurring at random but was strikingly clustered (P values were between 2.6×10^{-5} and 5.3×10^{-11} for four samples evaluated). In fibers with multiple intercalated internodes, "old" internodes had an abnormally high value for the number of lamellae of myelin per micron of perimeter while intercalated internodes had an abnormally low value.

From these observations, a reasonable hypothesis to explain the degeneration of the Aα neurons might be as follows. An inborn error of metabolism exists in or affects Aα neurons more than other neurons. Affected cells shrink, and this probably is most severe in the peripheral axis cylinder. As the fiber shrinks, a rearrangement of internodes of myelin becomes necessary. "Old" internodes are recognized by their irregular, wrinkled myelin sheath and an abnormally high number of lamellae per micron of perimeter. During the course of degeneration, some teased fibers probably only have regions that are remyelinated and these have a small or normal number of lamellae per micron of perimeter and a normal appearance; however, they have somewhat shorter internodes than do normal fibers. The inclusion of such fibers would explain the decrease in the mean internode length of small fibers that was found. The final stage is an atrophic fiber without myelin or with multiple regions devoid of myelin. Although rare nerve strands are seen with myelin balls, these usually are very small, indicating that this probably is a final event in the process of atrophy.

From these histologic observations it also is possible to understand the sensory abnormality and the abnormality in the characteristics of the compound action potential. The cutaneous touch-pressure threshold is increased while the temperature and pain thresholds remain normal, at least early in the course of Friedreich's ataxia. These findings suggest that the fibers from low-threshold mechanoreceptors are particularly affected. From the characteristics of the compound action potential of the nerve in vitro and from the histometric evaluation, the affected fibers are probably those of Aα neurons. In early Friedreich's ataxia, the amplitude of the muscle action potential and the conduction velocity of motor fibers of limb nerves are within the range of normal. Nerve action potentials of sensory fibers, however, usually are not detectable. The compound action potential of a cutaneous nerve recorded in vitro shows a very small Aα potential compared to normal. The conduction velocity of these fibers is within or at the lower border of the range of normal values. The amplitude and conduction velocity of Aδ and C fibers are within the values of control nerves. These results correlate well with our teased-fiber studies. There is a marked decrease in number of large fibers, but enough of the remaining fibers conduct normally.

A similar type of fiber degeneration—although not necessarily of the same population of neurons—is thought to occur in peripheral sensory neurons in other varieties of spinocerebellar degenerations and in several varieties of hereditary sensory neuropathy. Although less well studied, axonal atrophy also affects the peripheral motor cells in such disorders as the progressive muscular atrophy form of Charcot-Marie-Tooth disease. In such disorders as the neuronal variety of Charcot-Marie-Tooth disease, both the peripheral sensory and the peripheral motor neurons show axonal atrophy.

DISTAL AXONAL ATROPHY

This type of fiber degeneration, with or without abnormalities of myelination and with or without hypertrophic neuropathy, is seen in chronic disorders that are usually inherited and that affect both the peripheral motor and the sensory neurons. Here also there may be atrophy and, to a lesser extent, degeneration of the perikaryon, and there are demyelination and sclerosis of afferent spinal cord tracts.

In these disorders, although the clinical symptoms are those of a peroneal muscular atrophy or of a symmetrical mixed distal neuropathy, the involvement of peripheral neurons is ubiquitous. Limb nerves, however, especially in the peroneal distribution, are affected most. In limb nerves there usually is a decrease in number of myelinated fibers per nerve and per unit of fascicular area. The frequency distribution of the diameter of myelinated fibers is abnormal. Particularly in the nerves of more severely affected persons, there is only one peak instead of the usual two peaks. The largest fibers of such nerves are considerably smaller than the largest fibers of reference nerves. Especially in long-standing disorders with axonal atrophy, varying degrees of hypertrophic neuropathy are seen. Onion bulbs occur in relationship to myelinated fibers, demyelinated regions of myelinated fibers, or former sites of myelinated fibers. The lamellae of onion bulbs are made up of circumferentially directed Schwann cells and their processes. These are separated and surrounded by longitudinally directed collagen fibrils. In disorders such as the hypertrophic neuropathy of Dejerine-Sottas, the myelin sheath is abnormally thin and this is not related to the size of the axis cylinder.

In the teased-fiber preparations of cutaneous nerves, a marked abnormality of all fibers is apparent. There is an excessive variability of internode length and diameter. From internode to internode of teased fibers there is a great variation in myelin sheath thickness. In some nerves every teased fiber (approximately 4 to 6 mm long) has regions devoid of a myelin sheath. The unadjusted mean IL of nerve for such disorders as the hypertrophic neuropathy of the Charcot-Marie-Tooth type is much less than normal. The CV of IL for such nerves is increased severalfold. In such severe disorders as Dejerine-Sottas hypertrophic neuropathy, myelinated fibers are without a myelin sheath for most of their length.

In these disorders, an abnormality of peripheral neurons can be demonstrated. In addition, however, there is an abnormality of myelination. Whether this represents a concomitant metabolic abnormality of Schwann cells is not known. In metachromatic leuko-

dystrophy, in Refsum's disease, and probably in Dejerine-Sottas hypertrophic neuropathy also, a lipid abnormality has been demonstrated (Dyck and co-workers, 1970).

SEGMENTAL DEMYELINATION

The term "segmental demyelination" is used to indicate that the myelin sheath is absent for a segment of the length of fiber but that the axis cylinder is intact. As conventionally used, the term also suggests that myelin was previously present at the demyelinated segment but has degenerated. Breakdown of myelin results not in the large myelin ovoids seen in wallerian degeneration or in axonal degeneration but in smaller ovoids and fatty droplets. As has already been implied, there may be several types of segmental demyelination.

INTERCALATED NODES

From his observations on teased fibers of nerves of healthy small mammals, Mayer (1881), incorrectly it is generally agreed, concluded that all nerve fibers undergo a constant cycle of degeneration and regeneration. His description and beautiful drawings demonstrate that he recognized a segmental granular breakdown of myelin and the characteristics of remyelinated internodes, which he called Schaltstucke (inserted or intercalated segment). Similar observations of short, small-diameter, thinly myelinated segments between long, large-diameter, thickly myelinated internodes of fibers of nerves of healthy animals were made by Renaut (1881a), who also called them "intercalated" segments.

Gombault (1880–1881) described the process of névrite periaxialis segmentaire in guinea pigs poisoned with lead. He noted discontinuity of the myelin sheath with preservation of the axis cylinder. Additionally he noted that, in regions where the myelin sheath was deficient, it was "emulsified"—a marked difference from the initial large myelin ovoids seen in wallerian degeneration. According to his view, inflammatory cells initiated the damage to myelin. If the process was severe enough, it might cause damage also of the axis cylinder and, in so doing, produce wallerian degeneration. Segmental demyelination was considered by him to be a prewallerian degeneration stage. Degeneration was not irreversible since repair could occur with the development of short, small-diameter internodes with thin myelin—evidence of remyelination. He also believed that a greater proliferation of nuclei occurred in this condition than in wallerian degeneration. He described segmental demyelination in nerves taken at autopsy in several disorders, including the condition of alcoholic neuropathy. Here he found that linear rows of myelin ovoids and myelin balls were common.

Fundamental observations were made that were important for an understanding of the process of segmental demyelination and remyelination. These included Speidel's (1932) observation of the development of internodes of myelin from individual Schwann cells, Schmitt and Bear's (1937) demonstration of the periodicity of myelin by x-ray diffraction, Fernández-Morán's (1950) unequivocal electron microscopic confirmation of the foregoing, and Geren's (1954) demonstration of the spiral lamellar growth of myelin lamellae in embryogenesis.

New insight regarding the formation of intercalated segments came from studies by Lubińska (1958a, 1958b, 1959, 1961). After a discrete crush of nerve, with enough time allowed for regeneration, the most distal preserved internodes were longer than half the length of the preserved proximal internodes of the same teased fiber. She also noted that the last preserved internode usually had irregularities, wrinkles, and invaginations of the myelin sheath and that paranodal demyelination occurred with the highest frequency at the first node above the crush, with a lower frequency at the second node, and only seldom at the third node. These results indicated to her that the myelin internode may survive if the damage occurs in its distal half—that is, the nucleus of the Schwann cell, which is at the center of the internode, is necessary for the maintenance of an internode of myelin. Since the last preserved internode had a wrinkled myelin sheath and no myelin breakdown was seen at widened nodes of Ranvier, she argued that the myelin loops at nodes of Ranvier had been loosened and displaced. In other studies, she showed that partial demye-

lination of an internode resulted in the formation of short (50 to 150 μm) internodes, whereas if an entire internode was demyelinated, the intercalated internodes that formed were longer (300 to 500 μm).

Plotting the relationship of internode length to internode diameter in nerves of man at autopsy, Vizoso (1950) found that in later life there was ". . . a multiplication of nodes, presumably due to degeneration and reformation." This suggested to him that there were two populations of internodes: those that remain with the individual through life and others that formed after the growth period was over and therefore remain close to the minimal length.

Fullerton and co-workers (1965) showed that measurement of internode lengths of teased fibers provided information about the previous history of fiber degeneration and regeneration. In grown animals, nerve fibers that had regenerated after crush had short internodes of approximately the same length. After administration of diphtheritic toxin, teased fibers contained a mixture of short and long internodes.

The greater variability of internode length (expressed as CV of IL) in teased fibers of nerves of older persons probably is caused by the formation of intercalated internodes with age (Vizoso, 1950; Dyck et al., 1973; Stevens et al., 1973). The development of such internodes may also explain why the length of internodes has not been found to continue to increase to the time of maximal lengthening of the nerve during growth of the limb in which it is situated. Several mechanisms may be involved in naturally occurring segmental demyelination and remyelination. Compression or bruising of limb nerves is a possibility. Ischemia from atherosclerosis may be a factor. In our opinion the process of aging of neurons may be important. Several observations on nerves at various ages suggest such a mechanism: there is a decrease in number of nerve fibers with age (Corbin and Gardner, 1937); there is accumulation of lipochrome in perikarya of neurons with age; and preliminary data suggest that the number of lamellae per micron of perimeter increases with age (Dyck et al., 1973), which suggests atrophy of axis cylinders. Such neurons may undergo an insidious, naturally occurring neuronal atrophy with secondary segmental demyelination and remyelination.

TYPES OF SEGMENTAL DEMYELINATION

In experimental and in naturally occurring neuropathy, segmental demyelination and remyelination are common. Probably without exception in nerves with segmental demyelination, abnormalities of the axis cylinder also can be demonstrated. In true wallerian degeneration, segmental demyelination is not seen. In the nerve just proximal to a cut or crush, paranodal demyelination occurs. In axonal degeneration from degeneration of the neuron or of only the distal axon, segmental demyelination is seen. Our impression is that, when the process is abrupt, this segmental demyelination is seen infrequently, but if the process is more chronic, it may be seen more frequently. In the process of axonal atrophy, segmental demyelination occurs commonly. We have suggested previously (Dyck et al., 1971a, 1971c) that there are two different varieties of segmental demyelination.

In the primary type there is a selective abnormality in the development or maintenance of myelin. Because of the metabolic abnormality affecting Schwann cells, myelin may be deficient in amount, improperly constituted, or prematurely degraded. This does not preclude the possibility that the same metabolic defect also may affect the structure of the axis cylinder. One of these mechanisms probably accounts for the widespread segmental demyelination and remyelination seen in metachromatic leukodystrophy (Webster, 1962; Suzuki et al., 1967; Austin et al., 1968), in Krabbe's disease (Austin, 1963; Bischoff and Ulrich, 1968), in Refsum's disease (Kahlke, 1963; Klenk and Kahlke, 1963), and in hypertrophic neuropathy of the Dejerine-Sottas type (Dyck et al., 1970, 1971c). Schwann cells and myelin also may be selectively damaged by toxins such as diphtheria (Fisher and Adams, 1956; Waksman et al., 1957; Jacobs et al., 1966), by mononuclear cells as occurs in experimental allergic encephalitis and in experimental allergic neuritis (see Chapter 56 by Arnason), probably in acute, chronic, and relapsing inflammatory segmentally demyelinating polyradiculopathy, and possibly in vaccinogenic and various plexus neuropathies.

In the secondary type of segmental demyelination, the primary abnormality is in the axis cylinder. This type of segmental demyelination may occur in axonal degeneration and in axonal atrophy as discussed earlier. A deformation of the axis cylinder by compression, as by a tourniquet, may underlie the ensuing segmental demyelination (Ochoa et al., 1971).

PATHOLOGIC CHANGES OF INTERSTITIAL TISSUE

An important distinction that can be made in the pathologic alterations of the peripheral nervous system is whether the process is interstitial or parenchymatous. In the former, the abnormality is extrinsic to nerve fibers, whereas in the latter, the disorder is within them. For the most part, interstitial processes are focal. Because foci may arise at different times and at different anatomical locations, the patient may present with the clinical picture of a mononeuropathy or of a mononeuropathy multiplex. More rarely, however, multiple small foci may result in a clinical picture of a diffuse neuropathy. The interstitial pathologic alterations may be grouped under the headings of infections, inflammations, vascular disturbances, infiltrations (for example, with amyloid), and neoplasms. The specific pathologic changes are described under Diseases of the Peripheral Nervous System.

There are other interstitial changes that probably result as a reaction to the events of fiber degeneration or regeneration. As is discussed in greater detail by Schröder in Chapter 16, sectioning or crushing a nerve results in a marked increase in Schwann cells and macrophages, especially in the distal portion of the nerve. Segmental demyelination also appears to act as a stimulus for proliferation of Schwann cells. In all varieties of peripheral neuropathy in man there is an increase of nuclei in affected nerves. Schwann cells, macrophages, fibroblasts, and mast cells all have been shown to increase in number. With peripheral neuropathy there also is a nonspecific increase in collagen.

ONION BULBS

An important histologic reaction to repeated events affecting myelinated and unmyelinated fibers is the development of onion bulbs. The light microscopic features and ideas about pathogenesis were reviewed by Wolf and coworkers (1932). The electron microscopic features of onion bulbs in human neuropathy have been described by several workers (Gruner, 1960; Dyck and Lambert, 1966; Garcin et al., 1966; Thomas and Jones, 1967; Webster et al., 1967; Weller, 1967).

Onion bulbs are now thought not to be specific for a single disease. They usually are situated around myelinated fibers or probable sites of former myelinated fibers. The leaflets of the onion bulb are made up of Schwann cell processes that surround the core in a circumferential fashion. These are known to be Schwann cells because they often contain unmyelinated fibers and have basement membranes. Outer leaflets of onion bulbs may be fibroblasts. Between the leaflets are longitudinally directed collagen fibrils. In teased-fiber preparations of fibers surrounded by onion bulbs, the following abnormalities are noted: internode length is abnormally short, segmental demyelination and remyelination are seen, and there is a much greater variability of both internode length and diameter than in normal fibers. Rarely, internodes of myelin undergo a granular degeneration. Linear rows of myelin ovoids are not seen.

According to Dejerine and co-workers (1893, 1896, 1906) the hypertrophied "connective tissue" whorl was primary and compressed the nerve tube. Bielschowsky (1922) considered the disorder to be a blastomatous affection of Schwann cells, like neurofibromatosis. Krücke (1941, 1942) proposed that hypertrophic neuropathy developed from an abnormal permeability of blood vessels, transudation of protein-rich serum, and mobilization of mucoid substances from connective tissue and degenerating myelin. Creutzfeldt and co-workers (1951) and Thomas (1969) suggested, correctly we think, that onion bulbs develop as a reparative hyperplasia of the Schwann cells in response to demyelination.

Experimentally it has been possible to produce small onion bulbs by intraneural injection of 9,10-dimethyl-1,2-benzanthracene (Weller and Das Gupta, 1968), by repeated applications of a tourniquet (Dyck, 1969), and by lead intoxication (Lampert and Carpenter, 1965). From our studies, it appears that the histologic events in the formation of onion bulbs include the following: (1) partial or complete demyelination of an internode; (2) mitosis of the Schwann cell associated with the demyelinated internode; (3) capture of the demyelinated internode by one of the two newly formed Schwann cells, with outward displacement of the other; (4) circumferential

orientation (influenced by the second-order basement membrane) and further mitosis of the displaced Schwann cell; and (5) successive outward displacement of layers of basement membranes and Schwann cells with repeated segmental demyelination and remyelination (Dyck, 1971). Additional Schwann cells may be attracted to the demyelinating internode from other regions.

Austin (1956) regarded the formation of the onion bulb as a secondary tissue reaction accompanying myelin and axonal degeneration. According to Webster and co-workers (1967), the processes of fiber degeneration and of faulty regeneration of myelinated and unmyelinated fibers were involved. Schwann cells that had lost axons became arranged around a core. An extension of this view came from the work of King and Thomas (1971). After crush of the vagus nerve, some regenerated unmyelinated fibers became diverted into the recurrent laryngeal nerve and here formed small onion bulbs around large myelinated fibers. The finding of what appeared to be small unmyelinated fibers in the lamellae of onion bulbs does suggest that regeneration of fibers is involved (see Wolf et al., 1932). Earlier workers had assumed these to be sprouts from the regenerating axon, while Zacks and co-workers (1968) and Ochoa and Mair (1969b) suggested that they could be regenerated unmyelinated axons.

Several studies have shown that repeated wallerian degeneration does not produce onion bulbs (Dyck, 1969; Thomas, 1969). Probably repeated segmental demyelination and remyelination and axonal regeneration and sprouting are involved in the formation.

CLASSIFICATION OF PATHOLOGY OF PERIPHERAL NERVOUS SYSTEM

This classification of the pathology of the peripheral nervous system is based on the following criteria: single or multiple nerve trunk; interstitial or parenchymatous; type of fiber degeneration; population of neurons affected; type of histologic reaction to fiber degeneration; and specific etiologic agent, biochemical derangement, or association with disease. The classification is neither perfect nor exhaustive.

Mononeuropathy
  Congenital absence of cranial nerve nuclei
  Mechanical transection, contusion, compression, entrapment, abrasion, and stretch
  Thermal damage—burns and frostbite
  Electrical burns, lightning, and damage by other forms of physical energy
  Compression
    Entrapment syndromes—acute radial, ulnar, peroneal, and other nerve palsies
    Tourniquet paralysis—anterior leg compartment syndrome
    Abnormal deposition in fascial bands with metabolic disease states
  Infections—herpes zoster, syphilis, leprosy
  Mononeuropathy of ischemia—artery occlusion from atherosclerosis, thrombosis, embolism, necrotizing angiopathy, Volkmann's ischemic paralysis, tight compartment syndrome, tight plaster cast, hemorrhagic diathesis, and others
  Tumor
Multiple Neuropathy
  Interstitial
    Infections—leprosy, syphilis
    Cellular immunity
      Acute inflammatory segmentally demyelinating polyradiculoneuropathy
      Chronic and relapsing inflammatory segmentally demyelinating polyradiculoneuropathy with or without hypertrophic neuropathy
      Vaccinogenic neuropathy
      ?Postexanthematous neuropathy
      ?Brachial plexus neuropathy
      ?Lumbar and sacral plexus neuropathy (also called femoral neuropathy)
    Ischemia
      Necrotizing angiopathy—periarteritis nodosa, rheumatoid arthritis, systemic lupus erythematosus, Wegener's granulomatosis, Churg-Strauss syndrome, and others
      Peripheral vascular disease
      Embolic, from acute and subacute bacterial endocarditis
      Hemorrhage secondary to bleeding diathesis
    Amyloidosis
      Primary without inheritance
      Dominantly inherited
        Portuguese type
        Indiana type

Tumor
  Primary
  Metastatic
Parenchymatous
  Axonal degeneration with or without segmental demyelination
    Neuronal degeneration with axonal degeneration
      Anterior horn cell—amyotrophic lateral sclerosis, Werdnig-Hoffmann disease, poliomyelitis
      Primary sensory neurons—carcinomatous sensory radicular neuropathy, ?inflammatory sensory radicular neuropathy, herpes zoster
      Both anterior horn cell and primary sensory neuron
    Distal axonal degeneration of peripheral motor, sensory, and autonomic neurons
      Vitamin deficiency states—alcoholism, malnutrition, malabsorption, pellagra, and pernicious anemia
      Remote effects of malignant neoplasms
      Diabetes mellitus, hypothyroidism, and acromegaly
      Drugs—vinca alkaloids, nitrofurantoin, and others
      Toxins and poisons—TOCP, acrylamide, and others
      Heavy metals—arsenic, mercury, lead, thallium, bismuth, and others
      Associated with uremia
      Acute intermittent and variegate porphyria and hereditary coproporphyria
      Hypothyroidism
  Axonal atrophy with or without segmental demyelination and with or without hypertrophic neuropathy
    Neuronal degeneration with axonal atrophy
      Anterior horn cell—progressive muscular atrophy form of peroneal muscular atrophy (Charcot-Marie-Tooth) and ?proximal muscular atrophy (Kugelberg and Welander)
      Primary sensory neuron—Friedreich's ataxia, spinocerebellar degeneration, dominantly inherited sensory neuropathy (type 1), recessively inherited sensory neuropathy (type 2), recessively in-

herited sensory neuropathy (type 3, Riley-Day), and recessively inherited sensory neuropathy (type 4, Swanson-Buchanan-Alvord)
Distal axonal atrophy with or without abnormality of myelination and with or without hypertrophic neuropathy
Without clinically apparent hypertrophic neuropathy—neuronal type of peroneal muscular atrophy (Charcot-Marie-Tooth), spastic paraplegia and peroneal atrophy, ?Fabry's disease, and α and β lipoprotein deficiency
With hypertrophic neuropathy—dominantly inherited hypertrophic neuropathy form of peroneal muscular atrophy (Charcot-Marie-Tooth, Roussy-Lévy, Pierre Marie types), recessively inherited hypertrophic neuropathy form of peroneal muscular atrophy of infancy (Dejerine-Sottas type), and recessively inherited hypertrophic neuropathy with phytanic acid excess (Refsum's disease)
Segmental demyelination
Primary
Metabolic abnormality of myelin (abnormalities of myelin synthesis, myelin constituents, and degradation)—metachromatic leukodystrophy, Krabbe's disease, Refsum's disease, ?Niemann-Pick disease, and ?Fabry's disease
Toxins—diphtheria
Cellular immunity (as already listed)
Secondary
Axonal degeneration (as already listed)
Axonal atrophy (as already listed)

REFERENCES

Aguayo, A., Thompson, D. W., and Humphrey, J. G.: Multiple myeloma with polyneuropathy and osteosclerotic lesions. J. Neurol. Neurosurg. Psychiatry, n.s. 27:562, 1964.

Aring, C. D., Bean, W. B., Roseman, E., Rosenbaum, M., and Spies, T. D.: The peripheral nerves in cases of nutritional deficiency. Arch. Neurol. Psychiatry, 45:772, 1941.

Asbury, A. K., Baringer, J. R., and Cox, S. C.: Renaut bodies—an ultrastructural study. Read at the American Association of Neuropathologists annual meeting, June 9 to 11, 1972.

Austin, J., Armstrong, D., Fouch, S., Mitchell, C., Stumpf, D., Shearer, L., and Briner, O.: Metachromatic leukodystrophy (MLD) 8: MLD in adults; diagnosis and pathogenesis. Arch. Neurol., 18:225, 1968.

Austin, J. H.: Observations on the syndrome of hypertrophic neuritis (the hypertrophic interstitial radiculoneuropathies). Medicine (Baltimore), 35:187, 1956.

Austin, J. H.: Studies in globoid (Krabbe) leukodystrophy. II. Controlled thin-layer chromatographic studies of globoid body fractions in seven patients. J. Neurochem., 10:921, 1963.

Behse, F., Buchtal, F., Carlsen, F., and Knappeis, G. G.: Hereditary neuropathy with liability to pressure palsies. Brain, 95:777–794, 1972.

Bielschowsky, M.: Familiäre hypertrophische Neuritis und Neurofibromatose. J. Psychol. Neurol. (Leipzig), 29:182, 1922.

Bischoff, A.: The ultrastructure of tri-ortho-cresyl phosphate-poisoning. I. Studies on myelin and axonal alterations in the sciatic nerve. Acta Neuropathol. (Berl.), 9:158, 1967.

Bischoff, A., and Ulrich, J.: Peripheral neuropathy in globoid cell leukodystrophy (Krabbe's disease): ultrastructural and histochemical findings. Brain, 92:861, 1968.

Bosanquet, F. D., and Henson, R. A.: Sensory neuropathy in diabetes mellitus. Folia Psychiatr. Neurol. Jap., 60:107, 1957.

Charcot, J.-M., and Joffroy, A.: Deux cas d'atrophie musculaire progressive avec lésions de la substance grise et des faisceaux antéro-latéraux de la moelle épinière. Arch. Physiol. Norm. Pathol., 2(Ser. I):354;744, 1869.

Collins, G. H., Webster, H. deF., and Victor, M.: The ultrastructure of myelin and axonal alterations in sciatic nerves of thiamine deficient and chronically starved rats. Acta Neuropathol. (Berl.), 3:511, 1964.

Corbin, K. B., and Gardner, E. D.: Decrease in number of myelinated fibers in human spinal roots with age. Anat. Rec., 68:63, 1937.

Creutzfeldt, H. G., Curtius, F., and Krüger, K. H.: Zur Klinik, Histologie und Genealogie dur Déjérine-Sottasschen Krankheit. Arch. Psychiatr. Nervenkr., 186:341, 1951.

Dayan, A. D., Graveson, G. S., Robinson, P. K., et al.: Globular neuropathy. A disorder of axons and Schwann cells. J. Neurol. Neurosurg. Psychiatry, 31:552–560, 1968.

Dejerine, J.: Contribution à l'étude de la névrite interstitielle hypertrophique et progressive de l'enfance. Rev. Méd. (Paris), 16:881, 1896.

Dejerine, J., and André-Thomas: Sur la névrite interstitielle hypertrophique et progressive de l'enfance. Nouv. Iconog. Salpêtrière, 19:477, 1906.

Dejerine, J., and Sottas, J.: Sur la névrite interstitielle, hypertrophique et progressive de l'enfance. C. R. Soc. Biol. (Paris), 45:63, 1893.

Döring, G.: Pathologische Anatomie der Spinal- und Hirnnervenganglien, einschliesslich der Wurzelnerven. In Henke, F., Lubarsch, O., and Rössle, R. (eds.): Handbuch der speziellen pathologischen Anatomie und Histologie. Vol. 13, Part 5. Berlin, Springer-Verlag KG, 1955, p. 249.

Dyck, P. J.: Experimental hypertrophic neuropathy:

pathogenesis of onion-bulb formations produced by repeated tourniquet applications. Arch. Neurol., 21:73, 1969.

Dyck, P. J.: A brief review of inherited hypertrophic neuropathy. Birth Defects: Original Article Series, VII:2:66, Feb., 1971.

Dyck, P. J., and Lais, A. C.: Electron microscopy of teased nerve fibers: method permitting examination of repeating structures of same fiber. Brain Res., 23:418, 1970.

Dyck, P. J., and Lais, A. C.: Evidence for segmental demyelination secondary to axonal degeneration in Friedreich's ataxia. In Kakulas, B. K. (ed.): Clinical Studies in Myology. Int. Congr. Series. Amsterdam, Excerpta Medica, 1973, pp. 253–263.

Dyck, P. J., and Lambert, E. H.: Numbers and diameters of nerve fibers and compound action potential of sural nerve: controls and hereditary neuromuscular disorders. Trans. Am. Neurol. Assoc., 91:214, 1966.

Dyck, P. J., and Lambert, E. H.: Dissociated sensation in amyloidosis: compound action potential, quantitative histologic and teased-fiber, and electron microscopic studies of sural nerve biopsies. Arch. Neurol., 20:490, 1969.

Dyck, P. J., and Lambert, E. H.: Polyneuropathy associated with hypothyroidism. J. Neuropathol. Exp. Neurol., 29:631, 1970.

Dyck, P. J., Beahrs, O. H., and Miller, R. H.: Peripheral nerves in hereditary neural atrophies: number and diameters of myelinated fibers. Read at the Sixth International Congress of Electroencephalography and Clinical Neurophysiology, Vienna, September 5 to 10, 1965.

Dyck, P. J., Conn, D. L., and Okazaki, H.: Necrotizing angiopathic neuropathy: three-dimensional morphology of fiber degeneration related to sites of occluded vessels. Mayo Clin. Proc., 47:461, 1972.

Dyck, P. J., Lambert, E. H., and Nichols, P. C.: Quantitative measurement of sensation related to compound action potential and number and sizes of myelinated and unmyelinated fibers of sural nerve in health, Friedreich's ataxia, hereditary sensory neuropathy, and tabes dorsalis. In Rémond, A. (ed.): Handbook of Electroencephalography and Clinical Neurophysiology. Vol. 9. Amsterdam, Elsevier Publishing Co., 1971b, p. 83.

Dyck, P. J., Schultz, P. W., and Lais, A. C.: Mensuration and histologic typing of teased myelinated fibers of healthy sural nerve of man. In Kakulas, B. K. (ed.): Clinical Studies in Myology. Int. Congr. Series. Amsterdam, Excerpta Medica, 1973, pp. 246–252.

Dyck, P. J., Johnson, W. J., Lambert, E. H., and O'Brien, P. C.: Segmental demyelination secondary to axonal degeneration in uremic neuropathy. Mayo Clin. Proc., 46:400, 1971a.

Dyck, P. J., Lambert, E. H., Sanders, K., and O'Brien, P. C.: Severe hypomyelination and marked abnormality of conduction in Dejerine-Sottas hypertrophic neuropathy: myelin thickness and compound action potential of sural nerve in vitro. Mayo Clin. Proc., 46:432, 1971c.

Dyck, P. J., Ellefson, R. D., Lais, A. C., Smith, R. C., Taylor, W. F., and Van Dyke, R. A.: Histologic and lipid studies of sural nerves in inherited hypertrophic neuropathy: preliminary report of a lipid abnormality in nerve and liver in Dejerine-Sottas disease. Mayo Clin. Proc., 45:286, 1970.

Eichhorst, H.: Neuritis acuta progressiva. Virchows Arch. [Pathol. Anat.], 69:265, 1877.

Erb, W.: Bemerkungen über gewisse Formen der neurotischen Atrophie (sog. multiple degenerative Neuritis). Neurol. Centralbl., 2:481, 1883.

Evans, M. J., Finean, J. B., and Woolf, A. L.: Ultrastructural studies of human cutaneous nerve with special reference to lamellated cell inclusions and vacuole-containing cells. J. Clin. Pathol., 18:188, 1965.

Fernández-Morán, H.: Sheath and axon structures in the internode portion of vertebrate myelinated nerve fibres: an electron microscope study of rat and frog sciatic nerves. Exp. Cell Res., 1:309, 1950.

Fisher, C. M., and Adams, R. D.: Diphtheritic polyneuritis: a pathological study. J. Neuropathol. Exp. Neurol., 15:243, 1956.

Friedreich, N.: Ueber degenerative Atrophie der spinalen Hinterstränge. Virchows Arch. [Pathol. Anat.], 27:1, 1863.

Friedreich, N.: Ueber progressive Muskelatrophie, über wahre und falsche Muskelhypertrophie. Berlin, A. Hirschwald, 1873.

Fullerton, P. M., Gilliatt, R. W., Lascelles, R. G., and Morgan-Hughes, J. A.: The relation between fibre diameter and internodal length in chronic neuropathy (abstract). J. Physiol. (Lond.), 178:26P, 1965.

Garcin, R., Lapresle, J., Fardeau, M., and de Recondo, J.: Étude au microscope électronique du nerf périphérique prélevé par biopsie dans quatre cas de névrite hypertrophique de Déjérine-Sottas. Rev. Neurol. (Paris), 115:917, 1966.

Geren, B. B.: The formation from the Schwann cell surface of myelin in the peripheral nerves of chick embryos. Exp. Cell Res., 7:558, 1954.

Gombault, M.: Contribution a l'étude anatomique de la névrite parenchymateuse subaiguë et chronique: névrite segmentaire péri-axile. Arch. Neurol. (Paris), 1:11, 1880–1881.

Gombault, M.: Sur les lésions de la névrite alcoolique. C. R. Acad. Sci. [D] (Paris), 102:439, 1886.

Gonatas, N. K.: A generalized disorder of nervous system, skeletal muscle and heart resembling Refsum's disease and Hurler's syndrome. II. Ultrastructure. Am. J. Med., 42:169, 1967.

Gowers, W. R.: A Manual of Diseases of the Nervous System. 2nd Edition. Vol. 1. Philadelphia, P. Blakiston, Son & Co., 1893.

Greenbaum, D., Richardson, P. C., Salmon, M. V., and Urich, H.: Pathological observations on six cases of diabetic neuropathy. Brain, 87:201, 1964.

Greenfield, J. G., Blackwood, W., McMenemey, W. H., Meyer, A., and Norman, R. M.: Neuropathology. London, Edward Arnold, Ltd., 1958, p. 529.

Greenfield, J. G., and Carmichael, E. A.: The peripheral nerves in cases of subacute combined degeneration of the cord. Brain, 58:483, 1935.

Gruner, J. E.: La biopsie nerveuse en microscopie électronique. C. R. Soc. Biol. (Paris), 154:1632, 1960.

Gudden, H.: Klinische und anatomische Beiträge zur Kenntniss der multiplen Alkoholneuritis nebst Bemerkungen über die Regenerationsvorgänge im peripheren Nervensystem. Arch. Psychiatr. Nervenkr., 28:643, 1896.

Harrison, B. M., McDonald, W. I., Ochoa, J., and Sears, T. A.: Electron microscopic observations on a focal experimental demyelinating lesion in the cat spinal cord. J. Neurol. Sci., 10:409, 1970.

Homen, E. A.: 1. Die histologischen Veränderungen in den peripherischen Nerven, den Spinalganglien und dem Rückenmarke in Folge von Amputation. Neurol. Centralbl., 7:66, 1888.

Hopkins, A.: The effect of acrylamide on the peripheral nervous system of the baboon. J. Neurol. Neurosurg., Psychiatry, *33*:805, 1970.

Hopkins, A. P., and Gilliatt, R. W.: Motor and sensory nerve conduction velocity in the baboon: normal values and changes during acrylamide neuropathy. J. Neurol. Neurosurg. Psychiatry, n.s. *34*:415, 1971.

Hopkins, A. P., and Morgan-Hughes, J. A.: The effect of local pressure in diphtheritic neuropathy (abstract). J. Physiol. (Lond.), *189*:81P, 1967.

Hughes, J. T., Brownell, B., and Hewer, R. L.: The peripheral sensory pathway in Friedreich's ataxia: an examination by light and electron microscopy of the posterior nerve roots, posterior root ganglia, and peripheral sensory nerves in cases of Friedreich's ataxia. Brain, *91*:803, 1968.

Jacobs, J. M., Cavanagh, J. B., and Mellick, R. S.: Intraneural injection of diphtheria toxin. Br. J. Exp. Pathol., *47*:507, 1966.

Kahlke, W.: Über das Vorkommen von 3, 7, 11, 15-Tetramethyl-Hexadecansäure im Blutserum bei *Refsum*-Syndrom. Klin. Wochenschr., *41*:783, 1963.

Kernohan, J. W., and Woltman, H. W.: Periarteritis nodosa: a clinicopathologic study with special reference to the nervous system. Arch. Neurol. Psychiatry, *39*:655, 1938.

Kernohan, J. W., and Woltman, H. W.: Amyloid neuritis. Arch. Neurol. Psychiatry, *47*:132, 1942.

King, R. H., and Thomas, P. K.: Electron microscope observations on aberrant regeneration of unmyelinated axons in the vagus nerve of the rabbit. Acta Neuropathol. (Berl.), *18*:150, 1971.

Klenk, E., and Kahlke, W.: Über das Vorkommen der 3, 7, 11, 15-Tetramethyl-hexadecansäure (Phytansäure) in den Cholesterinestern und anderen Lipoidfraktionen der Organe bei einem Krankheitsfall unbekannter Genese (Verdacht auf Heredopathia atactica polyneuritiformis [Refsum-Syndrom]). Hoppe Seylers Z. Physiol. Chem., *333*:133, 1963.

Krücke, W.: Ödem und seröse Entzündung im peripheren Nerven. Virchows Arch. [Pathol. Anat.], *308*:1, 1941.

Krücke, W.: Zur Histopathologie der neuralen Muskelatrophie, der hypertrophischen Neuritis und Neurofibromatose. Arch. Psychiatr. Nervenkr., *115*:180, 1942.

Krücke, W.: Erkrankungen der peripheren Nerven. *In* Henke, F., Lubarsch, O., and Rössle, R. (eds.): Handbuch der speziellen pathologischen Anatomie und Histologie. Vol. 13, Part 5. Berlin, Springer-Verlag KG, 1955, p. 1.

Krücke, W.: Die Erkrankungen der peripheren Nerven. *In* Kaufmann, E., and Staemmler, M. (eds.): Lehrbuch der speziellen pathologischen Anatomie. Vol. 3, Part 2. Berlin, Walter de Gruyter & Co., 1961, pp. 750–752.

Lampert, P., and Carpenter, S.: Electron microscopic studies on the vascular permeability and the mechanism of demyelination in experimental allergic encephalomyelitis. J. Neuropathol. Exp. Neurol., *24*:11, 1965.

Leyden, E.: Ueber Poliomyelitis und Neuritis. Z. Klin. Med., *1*:387, 1880.

Lubinska, L.: "Intercalated" internodes in nerve fibres. Nature (Lond.), *181*:957, 1958a.

Lubińska, L.: Short internodes "intercalated" in nerve fibers. Acta Biol. Exp., *18*:117, 1958b.

Lubińska, L.: Region of transition between preserved and regenerating parts of myelinated nerve fibers. J. Comp. Neurol., *113*:315, 1959.

Lubińska, L.: Demyelination and remyelination in the proximal parts of regenerating nerve fibers. J. Comp. Neurol., *117*:275, 1961.

Luna, L. G.: Manual of Histologic Staining Methods of the Armed Forces Institute of Pathology. 3rd Edition. New York, McGraw-Hill Book Co., 1968.

Mayer, S.: Ueber Vorgänge der Degeneration und Regeneration im unversehrten peripherischen Nervensystem: eine biologische Studie. Z. Heilk., *2*:154, 1881.

McDonald, W. I., and Ohlrich, G. D.: Quantitative anatomical measurements on single isolated fibres from the cat spinal cord. J. Anat., *110*:191, 1971.

Meyer, P.: Anatomische Untersuchungen über diphtheritische Lähmung. Virchows Arch. [Pathol. Anat.], *85*:181, 1881.

Mott, F. W.: A case of amyotrophic lateral sclerosis with degeneration of the motor path from the cortex to the periphery. Brain, *18*:21, 1895.

Mott, F. W.: Case of Friedreich's disease, with autopsy and systematic microscopical examination of the nervous system. Arch. Neurol. Pathol. Lab. (Lond.), *3*:180, 1907.

Ochoa, J., Danta, G., Fowler, T. J., and Gilliatt, R. W.: Nature of the nerve lesion caused by a pneumatic tourniquet. Nature (Lond.), *233*:265, 1971.

Ochoa, J., and Mair, W. G. P.: The normal sural nerve in man. I. Ultrastructure and numbers of fibers and cells. Acta Neuropathol. (Berl.), *13*:197, 1969a.

Ochoa, J., and Mair, W. G. P.: The normal sural nerve in man. II. Changes in the axons and Schwann cells due to ageing. Acta Neuropathol. (Berl.), *13*:217, 1969b.

Offord, K., Ohta, M., and Dyck, P. J.: Method of morphometric evaluation of spinal and autonomic ganglia. J. Neurol. Sci., *22*:65–71, 1974.

Ohnishi, A., and Dyck, P. J.: Unpublished data.

Ohta, M., Offord, K., and Dyck, P. J.: Morphometric evaluation of first sacral ganglion of man. J. Neurol. Sci., *22*:73–82, 1974.

Okada, E.: Ueber Zwiebelartige Gebilde im peripherischen Nerven (Renaut'sche Körperchen) bei einem Fall von Kakke (Beriberi). Tokyo Imperial Univ. Coll. Med., *6*:93, 1903.

Pentschew, A., and Schwarz, K.: Systemic axonal dystrophy in vitamin E deficient adult rats: with implication in human neuropathology. Acta Neuropathol. (Berl.), *1*:313, 1962.

Pleasure, D. E., Mishler, K. C., and Engel, W. K.: Axonal transport of proteins in experimental neuropathies. Science, *166*:524, 1969.

Porter, K. R., and Tilney, L. G.: Microtubules and intracellular motility (abstract). Science, *150*:382, 1965.

Prineas, J.: The pathogenesis of dying-back polyneuropathies. I. An ultrastructural study of experimental tri-ortho-cresyl phosphate intoxication in the cat. J. Neuropathol. Exp. Neurol., *28*:571, 1969a.

Prineas, J.: The pathogenesis of dying-back polyneuropathies. II. An ultrastructural study of experimental acrylamide intoxication in the cat. J. Neuropathol. Exp. Neurol., *28*:598, 1969b.

Prineas, J.: Peripheral nerve changes in thiamine-deficient rats: an electron microscope study. Arch. Neurol., *23*:541, 1970.

Renaut, J.: Recherches sur quelques points particuliers de l'histologie des nerfs. I. La gaine lamelleuse et le système hyalin intravaginal. Arch. Physiol. Norm. Pathol., *8* (Ser. 2):161, 1881a.

Renaut, J.: Système hyalin de soutènement des centres nerveux et de quelques organes des sens. Arch. Physiol. Norm. Pathol., *8* (Ser. 2):845, 1881b.

Romeis, B.: Mikroskopische Technik. Vol. 15. München, Leibniz, 1948.

Schmitt, F. O., and Bear, R. S.: The optical properties of vertebrate nerve axons as related to fiber size. J. Cell. Comp. Physiol. *9*:261, 1937.

Schröder, J. M.: Überzählige Schwannzellen bei der Remyelinisation regenerierter und segmental demyelinisierter Axone im peripheren Nerven. Verh. Dtsch. Ges. Pathol., *52*:222, 1968.

Schröder, J. M.: Zur feinstruktur und quantitativen auswertung regenerierter peripherer Nervenfasern. *In* VIth International Congress of Neuropathology. Paris, Masson et Cie, 1970, pp. 628–646.

Schultz, R. L., and Case, N. M.: Microtubule loss with acrolein and bicarbonate-containing fixatives. J. Cell Biol., *38*:633, 1968.

Spatz, H.: Die "systematischen Atrophien": Eine wohlgekennzeichnete Gruppe der Erbkrankheiten des Nervensystems. Arch. Psychiatr. Nervenkr., *108*:1, 1938.

Speidel, C. C.: Studies of living nerves. I. The movements of individual sheath cells and nerve sprouts correlated with the process of myelin-sheath formation in amphibian larvae. J. Exp. Zool., *61*:279, 1932.

Spencer, P. S., and Thomas, P. K.: The examination of isolated nerve fibres by light and electron microscopy, with observations on demyelination proximal to neuromas. Acta Neuropathol. (Berl.), *16*:177, 1970.

Stevens, J. C., Lofgren, E. P., and Dyck, P. J.: Histometric evaluation of branches of peroneal nerve: technique for combined biopsy of muscle nerve and cutaneous nerve. Brain Res., *52*:37–59, 1973.

Stransky, E.: Über discontinuierliche Zerfallsprozesse an der peripheren Nervenfaser. J. Psychol. Neurol. (Leipzig), *1*:167, 1902.

Strümpell, A.: Zur Kenntniss der multiplen degenerativen Neuritis. Arch. Psychiatr. Nervenkr., *14*:339, 1883.

Suzuki, K., Suzuki, K., and Chen, G. C.: Isolation and chemical characterization of metachromatic granules from a brain with metachromatic leukodystrophy. J. Neuropathol. Exp. Neurol., *26*:537, 1967.

Swallow, M.: Fibre size and content of the anterior tibial nerve of the foot. J. Neurol. Neurosurg. Psychiatry, n.s. *29*:205, 1966.

Swank, R. L.: Avian thiamin deficiency: a correlation of the pathology and clinical behavior. J. Exp. Med., *71*:683, 1940.

Swank, R. L., and Adams, R. D.: Pyridoxine and pantothenic acid deficiency in swine. J. Neuropathol. Exp. Neurol., *7*:274, 1948.

Thomas, P. K.: Schwann-cell proliferation in chronic neuropathies. J. Anat., *105*:212, 1969.

Thomas, P. K., and Jones, D. G.: The cellular response to nerve injury. 2. Regeneration of the perineurium after nerve section. J. Anat., *101*:45, 1967.

Thomas, P. K., and Slatford, J.: Lamellar bodies in the cytoplasm of Schwann cells. Proc. Anat. Soc. Great Britain and Ireland, *98*:691, 1964.

Victor, M., Banker, B. Q., and Adams, R. D.: The neuropathy of multiple myeloma. J. Neurol. Neurosurg. Psychiatry, n.s. *21*:73, 1958.

Virchow, R.: Ein Fall von progressiver Muskelatrophie. Virchows Arch. [Pathol. Anat.], *8*:537, 1855.

Vizoso, A. D.: The relationship between internodal length and growth in human nerves. J. Anat., *84*:342, 1950.

Waksman, B. H., Adams, R. D., and Mansmann, H. C., Jr.: Experimental study of diphtheritic polyneuritis in the rabbit and guinea pig. I. Immunologic and histopathologic observations. J. Exp. Med., *105*:591, 1957.

Webster, H. deF.: Schwann cell alterations in metachromatic leukodystrophy: preliminary phase and electron microscopic observations. J. Neuropathol. Exp. Neurol., *21*:534, 1962.

Webster, H. deF., Schröder, J. M., Asbury, A. K., and Adams, R. D.: The role of Schwann cells in the formation of "onion bulbs" found in chronic neuropathies. J. Neuropathol. Exp. Neurol., *26*:276, 1967.

Weller, R. O.: An electron microscopic study of hypertrophic neuropathy of Déjérine and Sottas. J. Neurol. Neurosurg. Psychiatry, n.s. *30*:111, 1967.

Weller, R. O., and Das Gupta, T. K.: Experimental hypertrophic neuropathy: an electron microscope study. J. Neurol. Neurosurg. Psychiatry, n.s. *31*:34, 1968.

Williamson, R. T.: Changes in the spinal cord in diabetes mellitus. Br. Med. J., *1*:122, 1904.

Wolf, A., Rubinowitz, A. H., and Burchell, S. C.: Interstitial hypertrophic neuritis of Dejerine and Scottas: a report of three cases. Bull. Neurol. Inst. N.Y., *2*:373, 1932.

Zacks, S. I., Lipshutz, H., and Elliott, F.: Histochemical and electron microscopic observations on "onion bulb" formations in a case of hypertrophic neuritis of 25 years duration with onset in childhood. Acta Neuropathol. (Berl.), *11*:157, 1968.

Chapter 16

DEGENERATION AND REGENERATION OF MYELINATED NERVE FIBERS IN EXPERIMENTAL NEUROPATHIES

J. Michael Schröder

The axon of the peripheral neuron and the myelin sheath of the Schwann cell may undergo varying morphologic changes depending on the degree of physical or chemical damage. Before definite axon or myelin damage occurs, there appear to be fine structural changes with selective involvement of organelles that subdivide the two main types of peripheral neuropathy, the neuronal or the demyelinating, into various subtypes.

Although neurons (axons) and Schwann cells (myelin sheaths) can be affected separately, their close functional and structural relationship frequently results in secondary myelin change from axonal alterations or, on the other hand, axonal lesions from primary myelin or Schwann cell damage.

Depending on the type of lesion, there are different forms of nerve fiber repair showing numerous fine structural alterations. Although there is a striking capacity of the peripheral nerve fiber to regenerate and of the Schwann cell to remyelinate demyelinated or regenerated nerve fibers, complete structural restoration apparently does not occur. Abnormal sprouts of regenerating axons, alterations of the shape, thickness, and length of the newly formed myelin sheaths, and an excess of proliferated Schwann cells constitute some of the characteristic features of regenerated and remyelinated nerve fibers. In most neuropathies, degenerative and regenerative phenomena are closely related and occur in a complex mixture (cf. Chapter 15). A great deal of our knowledge about the general pathology of degenerating and regenerating myelinated nerve fibers in the peripheral nervous system is based on experimental studies. Only a brief account of these can be given.

MORPHOLOGIC ALTERATION IN FIBER DEGENERATION AND REGENERATION

Before describing "specific" or characteristic alterations in particular neuropathies one needs to know the many different fine structural aspects of wallerian degeneration. If interruption of axonal continuity occurs at any level of the peripheral nerve, the distal part of the interrupted nerve fiber will show the typical features of wallerian degeneration. Thus characteristic alterations of wallerian degeneration and its sequelae occur in many neuropathies (Fig. 16–1).

Wallerian Degeneration

In his classic paper Waller (1850) showed that nerve fibers of the distal stump of a transected nerve degenerated in a characteristic manner. The fibers of the proximal stump survived and were capable of regenerative

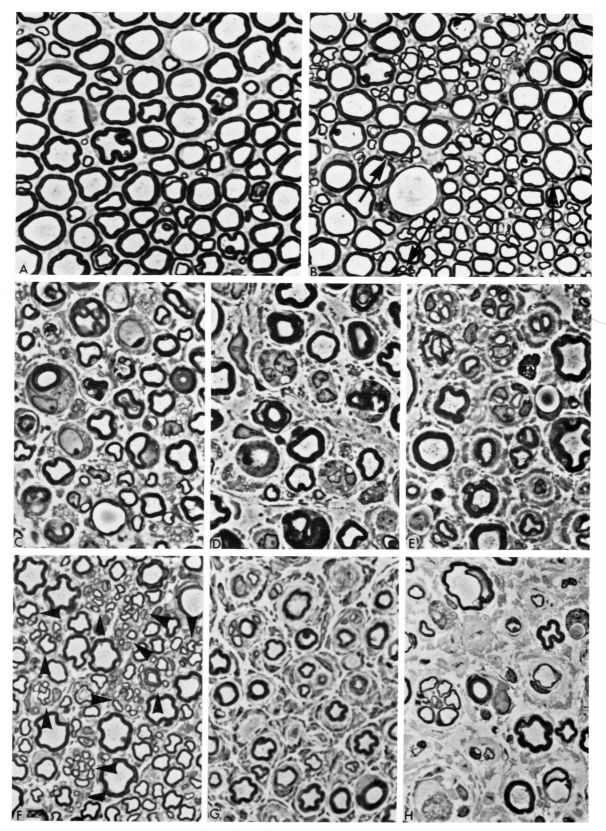

Figure 16–1   See opposite page for legend.

outgrowth. Wallerian degeneration is seen in its most developed form following complete transection of a nerve, but it occurs distal to any lesion severe enough to cause interruption of axonal continuity. The structural changes are quite similar in unmyelinated and in myelinated axons. The axonal alterations are, however, closely associated with Schwann cell changes, and these are far more complicated in myelinated than in unmyelinated nerve fibers.

The morphology of the degenerating myelinated nerve fiber varies considerably, depending on the time interval after the lesion, the distance from the lesion, and the area of the internode studied (cf. Krücke, 1955, 1961; Lehmann, 1959; Hager, 1968). It is not yet clear whether the more proximal parts of the distal stump of an interrupted nerve fiber degenerate prior to more peripheral parts. There is also some controversy whether the proximodistal advance of degeneration is faster in thin fibers than in thick ones. The time to conduction failure distal to nerve section differs remarkably in various species (cf. Gilliatt and Hjorth, 1972). The earliest and most significant physiologic changes occur at the terminal parts of the intramuscular nerve fibers (Fukami and Ridge, 1971; Gilliatt and Hjorth, 1972). In the nerve trunk the appearance of many axons of the same size and at the same distance from the area of transection varies considerably. Some axons in a plane of section may have a normal content of microtubules and neurofilaments even 48 hours after the lesion, while others are completely disintegrated.

The initial change appears to be an accumulation of organelles at the proximal and distal stumps of the fibers near the site of transection (Webster, 1962; Kreutzberg and Wechsler, 1963; Holtzman and Novikoff, 1965; Zelená et al., 1968; Donat and Wiśniewski, 1973). Apart from this focal accumulation of intra-axonal organelles, degeneration of the distal part of the axon is accompanied by a series of structural changes that finally lead to fragmentation and dissolution of axons. Thirty-six to ninety-six hours after the nerve crush, there are numerous discontinuities in the axolemma, focal swelling or condensation of axons with dilatation of the axoplasmic reticulum, dissolution of neurofilaments and microtubules, and zones of increased density and granularity (Webster, 1962.)

Axonal alterations are closely associated with secondary myelin or Schwann cell changes. Retraction of the myelin loops at the node of Ranvier (cf. Ballin and Thomas, 1968) and folding, contraction, and extension of the myelin sheath (Friede and Martinez, 1970a, 1970b) coincide with fragmentation at the Schmidt-Lanterman incisures. The occurrence of incisures at sites of axonal narrowing and at the margins of myelin segments was emphasized by Ramón y Cajal (1928), and it is of interest that Ranvier thought incisures were sites at which Schwann cell protoplasm invaded the myelin sheath, a view further advanced by Webster (1965) and by Singer and Steinberg (1972). In later stages of degeneration myelin breaks up into ovoids, and progressive removal of myelin becomes apparent (cf. Dyck, 1973; Krücke, 1974).

The basement membranes surrounding the Schwann cells persist during wallerian degeneration and form tubes (called Schwann tubes by Holmes and Young, 1942) within which the Schwann cells proliferate to give rise to longitudinal columns (bands of Büngner) as the myelin and axon remnants are removed (Nathaniel and Pease, 1963; P. K. Thomas, 1964). The fine structural changes during the formation of the bands of Büngner have been studied rather carefully since these bands provide optimal pathways for regenerating axons to reach their terminations (Bielschowsky and Unger, 1917; Ramon y Cajal, 1928; Nageotte,

---

Figure 16–1 Degeneration and regeneration of myelinated fibers in sciatic nerves of rats. *A.* Control nerve. *B.* Reinnervated contralateral nerve 12 months after a crush lesion. The largest regenerated nerve fibers show disproportionately thin myelin sheaths, whereas some of the axon diameters approach normal values. Some regenerated fibers appear to be atrophic (arrows). Myelin remnants are still seen in the perivascular space. *C* to *G.* Severe isoniazid (INH) neuropathy after four days (*C*), three weeks (*D*), seven weeks (*E*), three months (*F*), and two years (*G*). In *F* and *G* large amounts of INH were given for the first two weeks, the nerve being allowed to regenerate for the rest of the time. The bands of Büngner show initial proliferation of Schwann cells (*C* and *D*), becoming reinnervated by multiple axonal sprouts within seven weeks (*E*). Nerve fibers regenerated in small bundles (arrowheads) are most numerous after three months and have largely disappeared within two years (*G*). *H.* Sciatic nerve of a male control rat at the age of three and a half years showing all types of spontaneous nerve fiber change (degeneration and regeneration, demyelination and remyelination) as well as a great increase in the endoneurial connective tissue. Epon embedded semithin sections; *A, B, F,* and *G,* × 720; *C, D,* and *E,* × 1000; *H,* × 690.

1932; Masson, 1932; Haftek and Thomas, 1968; Schröder, 1968a; P. K. Thomas, 1970; Gonzenbach, 1972; Morris et al., 1972. See also Honjin et al., 1959; Terry and Harkin, 1959; Glimstedt and Wohlfahrt, 1960; Ohmi, 1961; Wechsler and Hager, 1962; Blümcke, 1963; Lee, 1963, and others). The cells inside the Schwann tubes account for most of the increase in number of cells that accompanies wallerian degeneration. Nuclei increase in number about 13 times during the first 25 days of degeneration. By 225 days their number has fallen again to about half of peak values (Abercrombie and Johnson, 1946; Seiler and Schröder, 1970; Bradley and Asbury, 1970). The stimulus for the cell proliferation apparently is the chemical decomposition of the myelin sheath. The chemical sequence of events switching on the proliferative process remains obscure, however, although quantitative changes of ratios of polyamines to nucleic acids may play a role (Seiler and Schröder, 1970).

In cross sections of bands of Büngner, up to 45 closely packed Schwann cell processes have been counted containing various forms of myelin remnants, homogenous lipid droplets, vacuoles, smooth and granular endoplasmic reticulum, Golgi complexes, microtubules and filaments, which are increased in number, and glycogen. If the bands of Büngner do not become reinnervated, filaments and glycogen granules are particularly numerous several weeks or months following wallerian degeneration. Round or oval Schwann cell processes, about 0.2 to 1 μm (or more) in diameter, containing microtubules and filaments only, without any other organelles in a particular plane of section, have been frequently mistaken for regenerating but not yet myelinated (unmyelinated) axons. The axon surface membrane is usually thicker and shows greater electron density than the Schwann cell surface membrane (Elfvin, 1961; Schröder, 1970a). This then may be the only feature that distinguishes regenerating axons from thin Schwann cell processes.

Experimental Neuropathy With Predominating Neuronal or Axonal Degeneration

A number of drugs and chemicals and deficiency states cause relatively selective lesions of peripheral neurons. In most of these a clear-cut nucleodistal predominance of nerve fiber degeneration (the "dying back" phenomenon) has been demonstrated. To some extent, these experimental neuropathies may serve as models of the process of degeneration of the axon and nerve cell seen in the systemic atrophies and degenerations of human neuropathology (Spatz, 1938; Greenfield, 1954; cf. Krücke, 1955, 1961; see also Chapter 15). The analogy must not, however, be carried too far, since in toxic neuropathies the degenerative processes proceed at a much faster rate than in the human systemic atrophies.

Some of the most extensively studied experimental neuropathies with distal predominance include isoniazid (INH), tri-ortho-cresyl phosphate (TOCP), vinca alkaloid, and acrylamide neuropathy. In none of these nor in other experimental neuropathies have the sites of the lesions of the complex system degenerations been studied comparatively at various time intervals, under different dosages, and in several species. Thus the observations pertaining to the time of onset of the first or later lesions and to which neuronal system is most severely affected remain controversial.

TOPOGRAPHICAL PATTERN OF INVOLVEMENT

The topographical pattern of involvement of particular neuronal systems in experimental neuropathies of the neuronal or axonal type appears to depend not only on the structural and functional characteristics of the neuronal system affected, but also on its neuronal connections and on its lymphatic and vascular supply. To illustrate, following administration of streptomycin sulfate or dihydrostreptomycin or other antibiotics (e.g., kanamycin, neomycin) a seemingly selective affection of the statoacoustic nerve occurs. It is not clear, however, whether the seventh or eighth nerve lesions are due to a selective toxic effect of the drug on the nerve, or, more likely, to an accumulation of the drug in the perilymph, or to secondary degeneration following primary damage of the neuroepithelial cells (cf. Stupp et al., 1965; Wagner et al., 1971; Gonzales, 1972).

In acute cadmium intoxication there is selective damage of spinal sensory ganglia. In organotypic cultures of rat sensory ganglia poisoned with cadmium, a series of fine structural changes have been observed in perikarya and axons. These include striking accumulations of glycogen granules, of homogenous lipid droplets, and of whorls of filaments (Tischner and Schröder, 1972). The predominant lesion from cadmium in vivo, however, appears to be endothelial change leading to severe hemorrhages, not primary affection of the ganglion cells and axons themselves (Gabbiani, 1966; Gabbiani et al., 1967; Schlaepfer, 1971b). The selectivity seen in cadmium damage, therefore, is not due to a primary sensitivity or vulnerability of a particular neuronal system, but rather to selective vulnerability of the capillaries and venules that renders the cranial and spinal sensory ganglia more exposed to the toxic effects of cadmium.

Following organomercury intoxication with methyl mercuric compounds, sensory fibers and ascending pathways in the spinal cord appeared to be predominantly involved, whereas motor fibers showed changes only rarely if at all (Hunter et al., 1940; Hunter and Russell, 1954; Cavanagh, 1968; Cavanagh and Chen, 1971a, 1971b; Miyakawa et al., 1970; Herman et al., 1973). Quantitative analysis and autoradiographic studies of peripheral nervous system structures and spinal cord revealed that the greatest uptake of labeled mercury (^{203}Hg) occurred in spinal ganglia. The selective damage of sensory nerve fibers seemed to be closely related to differential uptake of mercury by their parent cell bodies (Herman et al., 1973). Whether the selectivity of the lesions could, as in cadmium intoxication, be due to the particular structure and vulnerability of the blood vessels in the spinal ganglia has not been proved thus far (Gabbiani and Majno, 1969).

In isoniazid neuropathy, in which a distal predominance of the nerve lesion was clearly shown by Klinghardt (1965), Cavanagh (1967; 1968) noted that motor fibers selectively die back to the spinal roots, and in the spinal cord only the gracile tracts were altered. Further experimental studies in rats revealed a nonselective involvement of motor as well as sensory fibers in isoniazid neuropathy (Schröder, 1970b, 1970c). Unfortunately there are no quantitative morphologic studies available comparing motor and sensory system involvement in any neuronal or axonal neuropathy.

Another interesting disease characterized by a distinct topographical pattern of lesions is subacute myelo-opticoneuropathy (SMON).

This syndrome is characterized by sensory disturbances and motor paralyses starting in a distal portion of the lower limbs, by disturbances of autonomic function, and by loss of visual acuity (cf. Kono, 1971). Autopsy studies revealed systemic degeneration of the long tracts of the spinal cord, starting in a distal portion of Goll's and the corticospinal tracts, and degeneration of the spinal root ganglia, peripheral nerves, and optic nerves (Matsuyama, 1965; Shiraki and Oda, 1969; Shiraki, 1971). Pathologic changes of subacute myelo-opticoneuropathy similar to those in humans have been produced in cats, dogs, and monkeys following application of clioquinol (Tateishi et al., 1971, 1973). A coincidence of autoradiographic accumulation of ^{131}I-clioquinol and the site of the lesions has been discussed by Tateishi and co-workers (1972); however, further studies are needed for a better understanding of the topographical pattern in this particular neuropathy.

INTRANEURONAL SITE OF INITIAL LESION

Several lines of evidence lead to the assumption that, for example, in isoniazid neuropathy the primary lesion of affected neurons was in the axon and not in the perikaryon: (1) the incidence of lesions: many more axons than perikarya showed alterations; (2) the intensity of the lesions: axons disintegrated completely, whereas the perikarya showed, in general, only reversible changes or none at all; (3) the type of lesion: characteristic lesions occurred within axons only; within the perikarya nonspecific retrograde changes were apparent that could be secondary to axonal damage; (4) the time sequence of the lesions: there were simultaneous alterations in many axons and in some perikarya, but no perikaryal lesions preceded axonal damage; and (5) the undisturbed regenerative capacity of the neuron: there was terminal regeneration of multiple axons moving down the bands of Büngner of the degenerated nerve fibers despite continued isoniazid intoxication (Schröder, 1968a, 1970b).

Similarly, there were no specific or even characteristic alterations within the perikarya of the affected neurons in tri-ortho-cresyl phosphate and acrylamide neuropathy, (Prineas, 1969a, 1969b; cf. Chapter 15). Of the two, it was in acrylamide neuropathy that an abnormality of the slow axoplasmic flow as the possible underlying pathomechanism causing neuropathy could be demonstrated (Pleasure et al., 1969). Controversial results were, however, reported by Bradley and Williams (1973). These authors studied the waves of "fast" and "slow" axoplasmic flow of radioactivity following the injection of ^{3}H-leucine into the L7 dorsal root ganglion of cats with vincristine, acrylamide, or tri-ortho-cresyl phosphate neuropathies. There was no decrease in the amount of the axoplasmic flow of protein, since the heights of these waves in the intoxicated animals were normal. The rate of movement of the crests, however, of the "fast" waves, but not of the fronts, was reduced in all experimental groups. The velocity of the "slow" wave was reduced only in tri-ortho-cresyl phosphate neuropathy.

In contrast to the findings in neuropathies with distal axonal degeneration, in chloroquine neuropathy (or "myoneuropathy"), numerous membranous cytoplasmic bodies were observed in spinal ganglion cells (Gleiser et al., 1968; Read and Bay, 1971) as well as in some axons of dorsal root nerves and terminal nerves (Klinghardt, 1974). Possibly, chloroquine myoneuropathy may turn out to represent a "neuronal type of neuropathy" in a strict sense (the "neuronal degeneration" of P. J. Dyck, Chapter 15, or the "parenchymal process" of Krücke, 1959) showing characteristic lesions of the central and terminal parts of the affected neurons, whereas isoniazid and tri-ortho-cresyl phosphate and acrylamide neuropathies may represent different forms of an "axonal type of neuropathy" (the "axonal degeneration" of P. J. Dyck or the "neuronal degeneration with nucleodistal beginning" of Krücke, 1955) showing primary lesions within axons and secondary changes of the perikarya only.

Both the neuronal and the axonal types of neuropathy, which can develop from different causes and by different pathogenic mechanisms, may be associated with a distally accentuated ("dying back") neuropathy. It is obvious that several pathogenic mechanisms may cause a distal neuropathy. Most frequently it is argued that impairment of axoplasmic flow underlies some of the distally accentuated neuropathies (cf. Chapter 12). But it is not clear whether axoplasmic flow is altered by (1) a direct effect on the slow or fast transport mechanisms, (2) an effect on the local metabolic supporting systems for the axonal transport mechanisms, (3) a decreased supply of the transported substances from the perikaryon, or (4) an increased demand in the periphery. Also, (5) a discrepancy between the metabolic demand of the axons and the supply of essential substances from the endoneurial vessels could cause an axonal neuropathy. Thus far, it is not known whether the distal accentuation of fiber lesions in neuronal or axonal neuropathies results from a numerical accumulation of degenerating nerve fibers damaged focally at many levels throughout the length of a nerve or, more likely, whether it results from the more generalized "neuropathic" effect throughout the length of an axon. At the present time, no definite conclusions can be drawn about the many possible pathogenetic subtypes of neuronal or axonal degeneration.

NUCLEODISTAL ACCENTUATION OF NERVE FIBER DEGENERATION

In comparing the number of nerve fibers damaged at given proximal and distal levels of a nerve, it is important to use the ratios of normal to damaged fibers. If one simply counts the damaged nerve fibers per area, the usual decreased fiber density in the distal, swollen part of the nerve will not be taken into account. Even then only a single population of nerve fibers should be likened; a mixed nerve should not be compared with its cutaneous or its motor branches.

Most severe degrees of neuropathy were seen in rats tolerating a large daily dosage of isoniazid for about two weeks. At this stage, 30 to 40 times as many nerve fibers were damaged in the sciatic nerve at the lower level of the thigh as at the level of the lumbar nerve roots contributing to the sciatic nerve (Schröder, 1970b).

There are no quantitative data concerning the proximodistal ratio of the nerve fiber lesions in other experimental neuropathies of the neuronal or axonal type; it appears, however, that a similar pattern occurs (cf. Hopkins, 1970; Bradley, 1970).

LESIONS OF INTRAAXONAL ORGANELLES

Efforts have been made to define by electron microscopy which organelle constitutes the primary site of the "neuropathic" action of a substance. However, none of the fine structural changes seen in etiologically and pathogenetically different neuropathies, although characteristic, appears to be specific.

Axonal Microtubules and Neurofilaments. Dissolution of microtubules and neurofilaments within axons or their replacement by an amorphous material of low electron density appears to be one of the initial changes in isoniazid neuropathy (Schlaepfer and Hager, 1964a; Schröder, 1970a, 1970b). Similar changes are seen in wallerian degeneration following nerve section and in many other conditions. Low temperature, pressure, alterations of the pH value, and other physical or chemical lesions may lead to disruption of microtubules (cf. Tilney and Porter, 1967; Echandia and Piezzi, 1968). Microtubules and neurofilaments appear to be extremely fragile. Since they are probably involved in axoplasmic transport, any damage to them may finally lead to wallerian-type degeneration of the nerve fiber (cf. Chapter 12). It appears most likely that microtubules and neurofilaments, in fact, constitute the sites of primary attack in vinca alkaloid neuropathy and in acrylamide neuropathy (Fullerton and Barnes, 1966; Uy et al., 1967; Schochet et al., 1968; Gottschalk et al., 1968; Wiśniewski et al., 1968; Prineas, 1969b; Bradley, 1970). One line of evidence for this viewpoint is the striking accumulation of neurofilaments in central, peripheral, and terminal axons seen with the electron microscope in these neuropathies. Some regenerating axons in isoniazid neuropathy, however, were also filled with neurofilaments (Schröder, 1968a); and accumulation of neurofilaments was regularly seen in sprouting axons early after nerve crushing, together with many other accumulated organelles near the tip of the interrupted axons (Blümcke and Niedorf, 1965; Zelená et al., 1968; Donat and Wiśniewski, 1973).

Thirty minutes after endoneurial injection of vincristine sulfate, transient clustering of microtubules in the axoplasm of myelinated fibers was apparent; after 60 minutes, formation of "microtubular crystals" within axons was observed, some of which showed continuity with neurofilaments (Schlaepfer, 1971a). At this time disruption of microtubules was complete. An in vitro study of isolated interganglionic segments of crayfish ventral nerve cord revealed formation of "macrotubules" varying in diameter between 38 and 48 nm or

"C-shaped filaments" after incubation in a medium containing halothane (Hinkley and Samson, 1972). If vinblastine was added after the induction of macrotubules by halothane, discrete crystalloid forms developed in the axoplasm rather than the large arrays of paracrystalline material seen after one hour of incubation in 0.2 mM vinblastine. Macrotubule formation was inhibited by pretreatment with colchicine. Since microtubules disappear as enlarged tubules form, the enlarged tubular structures were thought to represent abnormal polymerization of microtubular elements (Tilney and Porter, 1967; Hinkley and Samson, 1972).

An interesting increase in the proportion of microtubules relative to the axon caliber and to the number of neurofilaments was described by Friede (1971). He applied a snug ligature around the sciatic nerve of rats on the fourteenth postnatal day, allowing the nerve to compress itself by its subsequent growth ("hypoplasia" of nerve fibers).

Axoplasmic Reticulum. A striking accumulation of abnormal membrane-bound vesicles and tubules within otherwise normal axoplasm was revealed by electron microscopy in tri-o-cresyl phosphate poisoning before changes became evident by light microscopy (Bischoff, 1967; Prineas, 1969a). A similar proliferation of agranular endoplasmic reticulum was also seen in myelinated nerve fibers of the spinal gray matter and in thiamine-deficient rats (Prineas, 1969a, 1970; Bischoff, 1970). Blakemore and Cavanagh (1969) studying rats poisoned with p-bromophenylacetylurea noted large central axon swellings ("neuroaxonal dystrophy") containing masses of smooth endoplasmic reticulum of a similar fine structural appearance; these masses developed long after the acute phase of poisoning had passed. The authors concluded that such changes occurred in a wide variety of natural and experimental states indicating "continued frustration of the regeneration process in damaged central axons and their terminals." In the central nervous system of apparently normal adult rats such findings among others were interpreted as a possible sign of "axonal remodeling" (Sotelo and Palay, 1971). In fact, proliferation of an agranular endoplasmic reticulum was also seen in occasional regenerating peripheral axons in isoniazid neuropathy whereas in the acute stage of the intoxication no such changes occurred (Schröder, 1968a). Zelená, Lubińska, and Gutmann (1968) have shown accumulations of a similar axoplasmic reticulum in the distal stump of crushed peripheral nerve fibers. Since proliferation of an agranular axoplasmic reticulum develops or accumulates under various conditions, it is regarded as a nonspecific sign of axonal reactivity rather than as proof of axon regeneration.

Axonal Mitochondria. Enlarged axoplasmic mitochondria with increased numbers of cristae in posterior root fibers were a prominent finding in acrylamide neuropathy (Prineas, 1969b). In addition a mitochondrion containing a paracrystalline inclusion was seen in the tibial nerve 49 days after acrylamide intoxication.

A conspicuous increase in the density and number of mitochondrial matrix granules was observed in some myelinated and a few unmyelinated axons in early isoniazid neuropathy (Schröder, 1970a). This change was not observed, however, in mitochondria of the spinal ganglia or in anterior horn cells of the spinal cord or in intrafusal nerve terminals. In the latter, numerous mitochondria included foci of an amorphous, electron-dense material similar to that seen in mitochondria of central axons following vitamin E deficiency (Schochet, 1971). Other mitochondria showed an overall increase in electron density. Both reactions are nonspecific and seen also in mitochondria in other cells and tissues (Reimer et al., 1972).

Unlike mitochondrial enlargement in which there is an increase in structural components, swelling, as frequently seen in wallerian degeneration, is due to an altered membrane permeability and imbibition of water. This is a ubiquitous change that can accompany almost any type of cell injury (Trump and Ericson, 1965). The various alterations in the structure of the cristae, such as disorderly arrangement, fragmentation, and vesiculation, seen in axon terminals in isoniazid neuropathy (Schröder, 1970c), are also found in many types of cellular injury and must be considered a nonspecific reaction. The myelin figures

occasionally present in mitochondria are thought to be derived from the phospholipids of the membranes in response to various stimuli (cf. Le Beux et al., 1969).

Axonal Lysosomes. Lysosomes, among other particles containing enzymes, are known to increase in number in the stumps of sectioned nerve fibers (Kreutzberg and Wechsler, 1963; cf. Holtzman and Novikoff, 1965, and E. Thomas, 1969). Their role and significance in toxic or metabolic neuropathies is not known. In atrophic regenerated axons, however, electron-dense lysosome-like bodies were occasionally seen to be increased in number in certain planes of sections (Schröder, 1968a; Schröder and Krücke, 1970).

Following chloroquine poisoning, numerous membranous bodies were seen within the perikarya of affected dorsal root ganglia and within a few peripheral axons (Gleiser et al., 1968; Read and Bay, 1971; Tischner, 1972; Klinghardt, 1974). Their relation to lysosomes and their pathogenetic role in initiating axonal lesions remains obscure.

The Axolemma. Discontinuities of the axolemma were frequently seen 36 to 96 hours following nerve crushing (Webster, 1962) and in various neuropathies at a time when axonal degeneration proceeds by wallerian degeneration. An increased density and thickness of the axolemma was often observed in isoniazid neuropathy (Schröder, 1970a). Thickening of membranes is, however, a widespread nonspecific reaction occurring under various conditions in a large number of surface membranes. More specific changes of the axolemma have not been analyzed in detail.

MYELIN AND SCHWANN CELL IN NEURONAL AND AXONAL NEUROPATHIES

The myelin changes seen in various neuronal and axonal neuropathies resemble those in wallerian degeneration (Fig. 16–2A to C). A few of the changes within the bands of

Figure 16–2 Myelin changes in isoniazid neuropathy 4 days after onset of isoniazid application (A through C) and experimental allergic neuritis 20 days following a second injection of an antigen emulsion (D and E). A. Disintegration of myelin ovoids within a Schwann cell showing splitting and dissolution of single and multiple myelin lamellae. × 15,000. B. Delamination of a few myelin lamellae from a compact degenerating myelin sheath with formation of small myelin ovoids between them. × 14,000. C. Formation of homogeneous lipid droplets in conjunction with a degenerating myelin sheath and numerous lamellae of a smooth endoplasmic reticulum. × 14,000. D. Vesicular and bulbous swellings of disintegrating myelin lamellae adjacent to the surface of an invading mononuclear cell in a focus of perivascular demyelination in experimental allergic neuritis. × 60,000. E. Another plane of section of the same cell as shown in D reveals penetration of the Schwann cell's basement membrane at the arrow. Part of the Schwann cell is pushed aside, and the myelin sheath is focally destroyed by the invading cell, which includes several small myelin ovoids. × 18,000.

Büngner and in Schwann cells of degenerating and regenerating nerve fibers probably were present only in experimental toxic neuropathies.

Frequently within early bands of Büngner developing in isoniazid neuropathy, there were large extracellular spaces containing finely dispersed floccular material lying between the multiple Schwann cell processes (Schlaepfer and Hager, 1964c).

In isoniazid neuropathy profiles of "empty" paracrystalline needles were observed situated both intracellularly and extracellularly within reinnervated bands of Büngner (Fig. 16–3B) (Schröder, 1970b). Crystals of a shape similar to those in the upper part of Figure 16–3B, although much larger (up to 50 μm in length), were also seen in endoneurial macrophages adjacent to spontaneously degenerated nerve fibers in a three year old control rat (Schröder, unpublished observations). It is likely that Doinikow had already noted similar structures in 1911. He observed, usually 60 to 90 days after transection of nerves, "rather thin, long needles" staining green with thionine, yellow to orange with Sudan red, and bright red with Nile blue sulphate. The intracellular needles illustrated in the lower part of Figure 16–3B have a somewhat different appearance. Similar needle-shaped or prismatic profiles projecting into a "moderately electron-dense ground substance," but occurring much more numerously, were shown by Bischoff and Ulrich (1969) in Schwann cells and histiocytes in cases of Krabbe's disease. Although some of the needle-like profiles resemble cholesterol crystals, the exact chemical composition of the various "empty" intra- and extracellular clefts of needle-like or prismoid shape remains to be defined.

Occasionally in chronic isoniazid neuropathy, corpuscles presumably corresponding to the π ("protagon-like") granules of Reich (1903; 1907) shown in Figure 16–3F, and the μ ("myelin-like") granules of Reich, named "Elzholz bodies" after Elzholz (1898) and shown in Figure 16–3E, were observed in Schwann cells of regenerated and remyelinated nerve fibers (Schröder, 1970b). Although it is difficult to relate the Schwann cell corpuscles, carefully described and depicted by Reich and Elzholz, to the structures seen with the electron microscope, it appears likely that the elongated, comma-shaped structures, largely composed of straight parallel lamellae with a periodicity of about 4 to 5 nm and most frequently seen at the polar ends of Schwann cell nuclei, correspond to Reich's "protagon-like (π) granules," which in histochemical preparations stain metachromatically with thionine and basic aniline dyes (cf. Doinikow, 1911; Schnabel and Sir, 1962; Thomas and Slatford, 1964; Evans et al., 1965; Tomonaga and Sluga, 1970; Dyck and Lambert, 1970).

Myelin-like (Elzholz) bodies, referred to as μ granules by Reich (1907), were often seen near the node of Ranvier and at other sites of the segment of normal Schwann cells and most frequently in the proximal stump of distally degenerating nerves (Elzholz, 1898). Elzholz reported that Key and Retzius (1873) as well as Stroebe (1893) and Koester (1893) had previously seen similar spherical myelin bodies staining black or dark brown to gray with osmic acid and the Marchi method. With the electron microscope a large number of myelin-like bodies have been described in various nerves and neuropathies (e.g., Webster and Spiro, 1960; Collins et al., 1964). It is not clear, however, whether all myelin-like bodies represent myelin debris, or whether they may also form as a sign of "focal degradation" indicating a nonspecific cell reaction as it is seen in many other cells and tissues (Swift and Hruban, 1964). If the periodicity of the myelin sheath with alternating major and minor dense lines is still somewhat retained within such myelin-like bodies, and if the myelin structure appears merely "collapsed"

Figure 16–3   Schwann cell inclusions. *A.* Enlarged lysosome-like bodies in a severely altered cell with multiple thin projections at the surface surrounded by the shriveled basement membrane of a degenerated nerve fiber at nine days of isoniazid neuropathy. × 13,000. *B.* Needle-like or prismatoid structures lying intracellularly in the cytoplasm of a Schwann cell or extracellularly between Schwann cell processes and regenerating axons of a band of Büngner after four weeks of isoniazid neuropathy. × 17,000. *C.* Cross striated fibrils originating at the same area but diverging in different directions in a proliferated Schwann cell following experimental allergic neuritis. × 28,000. *D.* Higher magnification of a cross striated fibril; two minor striations are apparent between the major cross striations. × 55,000. *E.* Myelin-like granule (Elzholz body) in the cytoplasm of a Schwann cell of a regenerated and remyelinated nerve fiber at three months of isoniazid neuropathy. × 24,000. *F.* Another Schwann cell of a regenerated nerve fiber in the same nerve as in *E* shows, adjacent to the nucleus, a comma-shaped lamellated inclusion that corresponds to the π granule of Reich. × 19,000.

as it is seen in Figure 16–3*E*, preceding disintegration of the myelin sheath may be assumed.

In rare instance cross striated fibrils were observed in Schwann cells following crush injuries in rats, experimental allergic neuritis in rabbits (Fig. 16–3*C* and *D*), and hypertrophic neuropathy in man (Schröder et al., 1970). These usually spindle-shaped fibrils resembled rootlet fibrils of cilia or "leptomere myofibrils" in muscle fibers (Ruska and Edwards, 1957; cf. Fawcett, 1961). They measure up to 1.23 μm in length, and up to 0.5 μm in width. The distance between the major cross striations is in the range of 110 to 200 μm (as in leptomere myofibrils). Their significance in Schwann cells is not known; however, recent serial sections in one such structure revealed a close connection with a centriole (Schröder and Šantel, unpublished observations).

Other well-defined Schwann cell inclusions consisted of tubular arrays seen in wallerian degeneration (Thomas and Sheldon, 1964), and crystalloid bodies that appeared to be characteristic for the induced inhibition of cholesterol biosynthesis (Rawlins and Uzman, 1970; Hedley-Whyte, 1973).

Regeneration of Myelinated Nerve Fibers

The capacity of the peripheral nervous system to regenerate is striking (Figs. 16–1*B* and 16–4). There are, however, limitations to nerve regeneration. The degree of recovery is determined by: type of lesion (cf. Gutmann and Sanders, 1943), reestablishment of adequate function (Weiss and Taylor, 1944; Weiss et al., 1945; Sanders and Young, 1944, 1946; Simpson and Young, 1945; Aitken et al., 1947), site of lesion in relation to the perikaryon (Ramón y Cajal, 1928; cf. Sunderland, 1968), time after the lesion (Holmes and Young, 1942), age of the individual (Moyer

et al., 1953), species (Kline et al., 1964), temperature (Deineka, 1908; Lubińska, 1952), and other factors.

Usually, in neuronal and axonal neuropathies, conditions for the outgrowth of regenerating nerve fibers and for the nerve terminals to find an appropriate end organ appear to be optimal since the endoneurial and perineurial connective tissue of the nerve remains largely intact and the bands of Büngner provide optimal pathways guiding the regenerating axons to their original site of destination. Nerve fiber restitution, occurring in an experimental toxic neuropathy, has been studied in rat sciatic nerves at periods of from 1 to 24 months following both transient and long-term intoxication with isoniazid (Schröder, 1968a, 1968b, 1970d; see also Suzuki and Pfaff, 1973). In cross sections bundles of 4 or 5 (2 to 13) small myelinating and nonmyelinating regenerating nerve fibers appeared within three to four weeks after onset of isoniazid application. One of the fibers usually tended to become larger than the others (see Fig. 16–1*D* to *H*). Apparently it is the basement membrane that causes the proliferating Schwann cells of the degenerating nerve fibers within the bands of Büngner to retain their longitudinal orientation and that confines the regenerating axons to small round or oval groups during their longitudinal outgrowth along the original proximodistal course of the damaged nerve fiber. The site of the outgrowth and the mode of branching of a nerve fiber damaged somewhere along the course of the nerve in an experimental toxic neuropathy has not been analyzed by electron microscopy. It is possible that axonal sprouting in a neuropathy proceeds in a way similar to that seen proximal to focal nerve injuries (Ramón y Cajal, 1928; Zelená et al., 1968; O'Daly and Imaeda, 1967), or as it does during development or in tissue culture (cf. Chapters 3 and 21). This type of sprouting is usually referred to as terminal regeneration

Figure 16–4 Regenerating nerve fibers in isoniazid neuropathy. Teased-fiber preparations of regenerating nerve fibers at six weeks of isoniazid neuropathy show: *A*, large mass of myelin degradation products adjacent to a thin myelinated fiber; *B*, numerous Schwann cell nuclei (arrowheads) and a μ granule (arrow) in a band of Büngner reinnervated by a small myelinated fiber with short internodes; and, *C*, a bundle of twisted thin regenerated fibers adjacent to a fiber with incompletely remyelinated internodes (arrowheads). × 620. *D*. Bundle of seven regenerating nerve fibers numbered 1 to 7) in a band of Büngner at three months of continuous isoniazid application. The largest axon (1) became remyelinated, but thus far shows two compacted myelin lamellae only. Two other axons (5 and 7) contain numerous vesicular structures and several mitochondria. The arrow indicates two further processes thought to represent degenerate axon sprouts. The Schwann cell processes contain an increased number of filaments and microtubules as well as lipid droplets, the content of which became partially extracted during embedding of the specimen. The collagen filaments are thinner between the reinnervated Schwann cells than in the surrounding endoneurium. × 17,000.

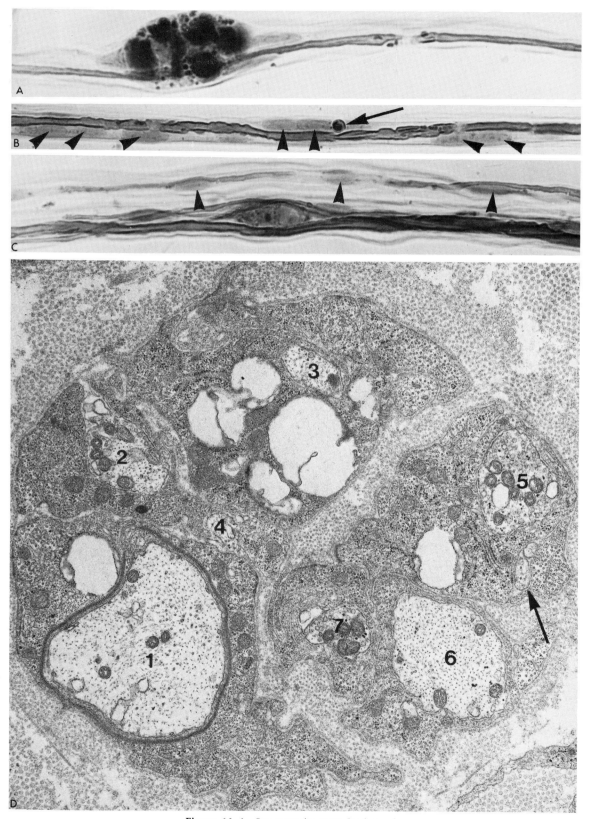

Figure 16–4 See opposite page for legend.

and occurs at or near the end of an interrupted nerve fiber (for additional information about collateral regeneration and its diverse definitions see Ramón y Cajal, 1928; Coërs and Woolf, 1959).

"Terminal axonic neoformation" was seen by Ramón y Cajal (1928) to proceed by dichotomy eventually leading to 10 to 15 branches of small nerve fibers. O'Daly and Imaeda (1967), on the other hand, observed a more fingerlike mode of branching with some four or five axons originating at the same level.

The analysis of regenerated nerve fibers in toxic experimental neuropathies is limited since it is often impossible to distinguish with certainty between a regenerated fiber and a preexisting one in transverse sections. More insight into the structural peculiarities of regenerated nerve fibers came from experimental studies of nerve section or crush injury. It is generally agreed that, following nerve section and suture, normal fiber spectra are never regained (Gutmann and Sanders, 1943). Following crush injuries, however, normal frequency distributions of diameters were reported by Gutmann and Sanders, but not by Cragg and Thomas (1964.) An analysis of the ratio between the axon diameter and the myelin sheath thickness of regenerated nerve fibers 6 and 12 months after focal crush injuries of sciatic nerves of rats revealed, contrary to the findings of Sanders (1948), a disproportionate reduction of the myelin sheath thickness of the largest regenerated nerve fibers with relatively normal axon diameters (see Fig. 16–1A and B) (Schröder, 1972). These alterations were even more prominent 6, 12, 18, and 24 months following nerve grafting in dogs (Schröder, 1970d, 1972; Schröder and Seiffert, 1972). On the other hand, there was a proportion of very thin, "atrophic" myelinated fibers with extraordinarily thick myelin sheaths. A large number of medium-sized myelinated fibers, however, showed a normal relationship between the axon caliber and the myelin sheath thickness.

Following remyelination of segmentally demyelinated nerve fibers, an even more pronounced reduction of the myelin sheath thickness was observed (as discussed later) in fibers in which there were no changes proximally at the cell body or distally at the nerve terminal of the respective neuron. Thus it appears likely that local factors such as aging of Schwann cells or physical hindrance by endoneurial collagen fibrils cause deficient remyelination. From the theoretical calculations of Rushton (1951) (see also Pickard, 1969) it can be concluded that a decrease in thickness of the myelin sheath would reduce conduction velocity more severely than would a decrease in the axon diameter. Thus, it appears reasonable to assume that the known decrease of conduction velocity of regenerated fibers is mainly caused by a proportionate reduction of the myelin sheath thickness in the largest regenerated nerve fibers (cf. Cragg and Thomas, 1964).

Measurements of internodal lengths of normal and regenerated myelinated nerve fibers in a number of species revealed a consistent reduction of the internodal length in regenerated nerve fibers (Sanders and Whitteridge, 1946; Hiscoe, 1947; Vizoso and Young, 1948; Cragg and Thomas, 1964; Jacobs and Cavanagh, 1969). It has been assumed that the internodal length of 300 to 400 (200 to 500) μm, found in regenerated nerve fibers of adult animals, represents the basic length of the Schwann cell, that is the length of the Schwann cell at the commencement of myelination during normal development (Young, 1950). Jacobs and Cavanagh (1969), however, observed much longer regenerated internodes in chickens. The number of Schmidt-Lanterman incisures, on the other hand, increased in number in regenerated nerve fibers if myelin sheaths of equal thickness were compared in normal and regenerated nerve fibers (Hiscoe, 1947; Schröder, 1972).

Within bundles of regenerated nerve fibers, among myelinated nerve fibers of larger size, there were always thin nonmyelinated axons that in other planes of section were thickly myelinated (Schröder, 1968a; 1970d). The minimal diameter of atrophic regenerated myelinated fibers was in the range of 0.4 to 0.5 μm.

The structural abnormalities of regenerated nodes of Ranvier have not been studied in detail, but it is obvious from preliminary observations that alterations in the arrangement of the nodal Schwann cell processes can occur.

Several other fine structural changes may help to distinguish regenerated from normal nerve fibers in cross and longitudinal sections. The perinuclear and periaxonal cytoplasm of the Schwann cell may be wider in regenerated than in normal nerve fibers as seen during normal development (cf. Chapter 3). Broad periaxonal cytoplasm often also occurs at the level of unusually large Schmidt-Lanterman incisures. Both structures may contain mitochondria. Cytoplasmic inclusions were occasionally apparent in Schwann cells of regenerated myelinated nerve fibers. These consisted of myelin remnants (μ granules), π granules, rootlet fibrils of centrioles (described earlier), and severely indented nuclei with aggregated heterochromatin and a small proportion of euchromatin. Microtubules and filaments, oriented longitudinally to the axis of the nerve fiber, were frequently increased in Schwann cells of regenerated nerve fibers.

Proliferated Schwann cells that will not become reinnervated by outgrowing axons ("supernumerary" or "empty" Schwann cells) tend to arrange themselves circularly around adjacent myelinated nerve fibers (the "onion bulb" formation discussed in a following section). They were often attached to free basement membranes that became separated from the degenerated nerve fibers.

EXPERIMENTAL NEUROPATHY WITH PREDOMINATING SCHWANN CELL AND MYELIN LESIONS

In 1880 Gombault demonstrated that guinea pigs develop a peripheral neuropathy as a result of chronic lead intoxication. He observed both degenerative and regenerative changes of the myelin sheaths without damage to axons. The sheaths disintegrated in a segmental fashion beginning at the nodes of Ranvier, a type of lesion that he termed "névrite segmentaire péri-axile" and that was later designated as "segmental demyelination", by Waksman, Adams, and Mansmann (1957) or "segmental fiber disease" by Krücke (1955). The latter term has the advantage of indicating axonal involvement concurrent with demyelination.

In vivo studies of segmental demyelination in various experimental neuropathies initially revealed two basic and clearly distinguishable types of selective myelin breakdown: an inflammatory type most thoroughly studied in experimental allergic neuritis, and a noninflammatory type seen in various demye-

linating toxic or metabolic neuropathies. However, in vitro studies showed a striking multiformity of myelin changes (cf. Chapter 21), and it is supposed that more types of myelin breakdown can be separated in vivo as well.

Noninflammatory Segmental Demyelination

Some of the best-studied demyelinating neuropathies of the noninflammatory type include diphtheritic, lead, tellurium, and compression neuropathy. Segmental demyelination occurring selectively or concomitantly with axonal changes has, however, been described in a large number of other conditions.

The pathogenesis of diphtheritic neuropathy has been carefully studied by light and electron microscopy and is discussed in detail by J. W. McDonald in Chapter 64 (cf. Waksman et al., 1957; Majno et al., 1960; Webster et al., 1961; Cavanagh and Jacobs, 1964; Weller, 1965; Jacobs et al., 1966; Weller and Mellick, 1966, Jacobs, 1967). In summary, a widening of the space at the node of Ranvier with focal fragmentation of myelin appeared in scattered fibers three to six days after the injection of the toxin-antitoxin mixture. One to two weeks later, when clinical neuropathy was severe, many fibers showed breakdown of myelin into ovoids and droplets of varying size. Lesions were most numerous near the nodes of Ranvier, and frequently several foci of myelin destruction occurred in different segments of the same fiber. All sizes of fibers were affected. The percentage of fibers with lesions in a given area varied; the pattern of distribution was not related to vessels. The relative sparing of axis cylinders was a constant feature. Demyelination in diphtheritic neuropathy is not due to, or associated with, an inflammatory lesion as, for instance, in the experimental allergic neuritis described in the following section.

The changes at the nodes of Ranvier were correlated with measurements of conduction velocity indicating that the fall in velocity, at a time when one third or one half of the fibers showed widening of nodal gaps, was trivial compared with that occurring in animals in which demyelination had spread from regions immediately adjacent to the nodes, and in which complete internodal segments were involved (Cavanagh and Jacobs, 1964; Morgan-Hughes, 1965, 1968; Gilliatt, 1969).

An additional finding reported by Hopkins and Morgan-Hughes (1969) indicated that in diphtheritic neuropathy nerve fibers became unduly susceptible to pressure; apparently, demyelination by diphtheria toxin can be exacerbated by local trauma or pressure too mild to produce a detectable effect on a healthy nerve.

Chronic lead intoxication causes degeneration and proliferation of Schwann cells (Gombault, 1880; Doinikow, 1911; Fullerton, 1966; Lampert and Schochet, 1968). The segment of the myelin sheath related to an afflicted Schwann cell disintegrates. Beginning at the nodes of Ranvier and Schmidt-Lanterman clefts, the myelin lamellae separate after splitting of major and minor dense lines. The separated lamellae further disintegrate into membranous blebs. Proliferated Schwann cells project beneath the basement membrane and engulf disrupted myelin lamellae. "Macrophages" were also seen penetrating through a gap in the neurilemma participating in the removal of myelin (Lampert and Schochet, 1968).

The application of a tourniquet or a spring clip to a nerve for an optimal period of time also resulted in segmental or partial demyelination (Denny-Brown and Brenner, 1944a, 1944b; Dyck, 1969; Aguayo et al., 1971; Ochoa et al., 1971, 1972). The mechanism of demyelination in this elegant experimental model has, however, not been studied in all details. Thus far it is not known whether, in fact, mechanical alterations of axons produce the demyelinating lesion as suggested by Ochoa and his co-workers (1971) or whether the mitochondria of the Schwann cells show the first lesions as might be suggested from the hypothesis that segmental demyelination following compression of a nerve is caused by ischemia (Denny-Brown and Brenner, 1944a, 1944b; cf. Chapters 39 and 40). Additional evidence for a mechanical rather than an ischemic cause of the nerve damage in chronic entrapment neuropathies was presented by Ochoa and Marotte (1973).

Another type of segmental demyelination was observed in weanling rats fed a diet containing tellurium; the animals became paralyzed in the hind legs within a few days (Garro and Pentschew, 1964; Lampert et al., 1970; Lampert and Garrett, 1971). Segmental demyelination developed secondary to degeneration of Schwann cells. Early changes of Schwann cells consisted of a focal degradation of cytoplasm characterized by the formation of membranous whorls around the degraded cytoplasm. The following disintegration of the myelin segment showed a nonspecific sequence of changes consisting of separation, splitting, and vesicular transformation of myelin lamellae. The vesicular myelin debris and fragments of compact myelin were then removed by invading cytoplasmic tongues derived from adjacent proliferating Schwann cells and from "macrophages" that penetrated the basement membrane. The focal degradation of Schwann cell cytoplasm in tellurium neuropathy was regarded as a characteristic early change distinct from that seen in other demyelinating neuropathies (Lampert and Garrett, 1971).

Recovery from paralysis and remyelination occurred despite continued ingestion of tellurium. The findings indicated that tellurium intoxication damaged Schwann cells during a critical stage in their development, i.e., the period of most active myelogenesis (Lampert et al., 1970).

Retraction of the myelin loops at the node of Ranvier apparently is a consistent early sign of segmental demyelination in many demyelinating neuropathies. Splitting at the minor and major dense lines of the myelin lamellae and transformation into membranous blebs are also regarded as nonspecific signs of myelin disintegration. Wide separation of a portion of the myelin lamellae from the rest of the myelin sheath was seen in a number of different conditions too. Thus, only nonspecific changes of the myelin sheath have been observed in these and several other toxic experimental demyelinating neuropathies. However, the Schwann cell changes preceding segmental demyelination differ strikingly in various neuropathies.

Experimental Allergic Neuritis, Marek's Disease

Segmental demyelination confined to perivascular areas of mononuclear cell infiltrates was consistently seen in experimental allergic neuritis (EAN). This can be produced by injections of emulsified peripheral nervous tissue (Waksman and Adams, 1955, 1956). Fine structural studies revealed that lymphocytes penetrated the endoneurial vascular endothelium (Åström et al., 1968), and traversed the basement membrane of peripheral myelinated nerve fibers, pushed the Schwann cell aside, and destroyed the myelin sheath (Lampert, 1969; Wisniewski et al., 1969; Schröder and Krücke, 1970).

Wiśniewski, Prineas, and Raine (1969) distinguished two types of myelin destruction; one was characterized by focal lysis of superficial lamellae at points of contact with the invading cell, which proceeded to strip away segments of the sheath; the other consisted of a vesicular disruption of myelin lying close to the invading cell (see Fig. 16–2D and E). Participation of cellular infiltrates in the process of demyelination was not seen at the nodes where retraction of myelin loops occurred (Ballin and Thomas, 1968). A subsequent study using bovine peripheral nerve antigen in rabbits confirmed the findings of Lampert (1969), although it could not be excluded with certainty that a humoral factor might cause demyelination in fibers in which invading mononuclear cells were not seen (Schröder and Krücke, 1970). Since no antibody markers have yet been used to demonstrate participation of humoral antibodies in experimental allergic neuritis (or experimental allergic encephalitis), the currently prevailing theory of a cellular pathogenic mechanism of demyelination may be maintained despite the results of some tissue culture studies (cf. Chapters 18 and 55). A basic protein isolated from human peripheral nerve was found by Paty (1971) to produce allergic encephalomyelitis is guinea pigs with very little neuritis.

Recurrent episodes of demyelination were found in the peripheral nervous system of rabbits suffering from chronic allergic encephalomyelitis (Raine et al., 1971). This ongoing demyelinative process followed a single antigen inoculation and was clearly demonstrable only in the peripheral nervous system. It was thought that in many ways the constellation of acute and chronic changes in these peripheral nerve lesions made them analogous to a demyelinating plaque of the central nervous system.

A pattern of primary demyelination related to invading mononuclear cells and essentially similar to that seen in experimental allergic neuritis has also been described in Marek's disease, a progressive paralytic disorder of chickens caused by a group B herpesvirus (Wight, 1969; Prineas and Wright, 1972).

It has been suggested that the disorder may represent a model of a virus-induced autoimmune demyelinating disease.

Remyelination of Segmentally Demyelinated Nerve Fibers

As early as 10 to 14 days after the onset of diphtheritic neuropathy and during clinical worsening, remyelination was identified in many Schwann cells (Webster et al., 1961, Webster, 1964). In animals that were poisoned with tellurium for 13 and 18 days, remyelination was advanced and detectable even by light microscopy (Lampert et al., 1970). During remyelination the myelin sheaths may be loosely compacted (Dyck, 1969), but usually, although modified by the abundance of proliferated Schwann cells, it proceeds in a way similar to that seen during myelinogenesis.

The time at which remyelination is completed is difficult to determine. In large fibers the newly formed myelin sheath is never completely restored to full thickness. Following compression of peripheral nerves by a pressure tourniquet or a spring clip, segmental demyelination occurs (Denny-Brown and Brenner, 1944a, 1944b). Although recovery of motor conduction begins early, the restitution of the myelin defect is only slightly advanced after six to eight weeks and is still defective after six months. After experimental allergic encephalitis in the peripheral nervous system the newly formed myelin sheaths reached only 50 per cent of their normal thickness by 10 months (Raine et al., 1969); they were not further advanced within 24 months after experimental allergic neuritis in rabbits (Fig. 16–5K) (Schröder, 1970d). This reduction of the myelin sheath thickness of segmentally remyelinated fibers is similarly seen in large regenerated nerve fibers in which the axis cylinders may become relatively thick whereas the myelin sheaths remain disproportionately thin (as described earlier).

The internodal length of segmentally demyelinated and remyelinated nerve fibers was usually reduced to about one half to one third of the original length and was of the same order as in regenerated nerve fibers (cf. Jacobs and Cavanagh, 1969). In chickens internodal length tended to be related to axon diameter both following demyelination after diphtheritic neuropathy and following regen-

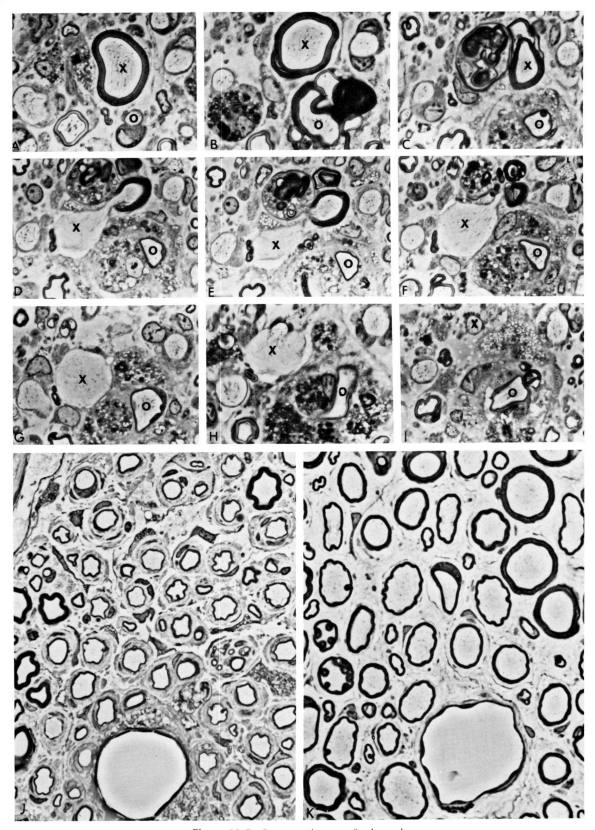

Figure 16–5 See opposite page for legend.

eration after a nerve crush. After both wallerian degeneration and diphtheritic demyelination the internodal lengths, particularly in the larger fibers, attained 1000 μm or more (Jacobs and Cavanagh, 1969), whereas in rats it reached only about 400 to 500 μm at the most.

Several abnormalities occurred at the nodes of Ranvier of some segmentally remyelinated nerve fibers (Ballin and Thomas, 1969a; Allt, 1969; Raine et al., 1969). The outer terminal myelin loops, instead of making contact with the axon, may override the Schwann cell on the opposite side of the node, a phenomenon described as "transnodal remyelination" by Dinn (1970). Most nodes, however, show a regular appearance following remyelination after segmental demyelination.

Supernumerary Schwann Cells, "Onion Bulb" Formation

During disintegration of the myelin sheaths in segmental demyelination a striking proliferation of Schwann cells occurs as it does also during wallerian degeneration. The proliferation rate has been estimated by counting the nuclei per demyelinated or remyelinated nerve fiber in semithin cross sections of epon embedded material following experimental allergic neuritis (Schröder, 1968b). The increase in the number of nuclei thus determined was on the order of 8 to 14 times, whereas in wallerian degeneration an average thirteenfold increase of the Schwann cell nuclei was observed (Abercrombie and Johnson, 1946). For comparison, in isoniazid neuropathy an increase on the order of 13 to 30 was seen (Schröder, 1968a). This was presumably due to repeated degeneration and regeneration of myelinated nerve fibers. Since in segmental demyelination only about two to four new internodes are formed instead of a single disintegrated one, there are far more

Schwann cells left over that do not participate in remyelinating the demyelinated fiber. This differs from isoniazid neuropathy in which there are multiple sprouts of regenerating nerve fibers within a single band of Büngner leading to reinnervation of most of the proliferated Schwann cells (Schröder, 1968a). Thus there are many supernumerary Schwann cells following segmental demyelination that usually become circularly arranged around remyelinating nerve fibers, as shown in Figure 16–5J, scaffolded by the persisting second-order basement membrane derived from the affected fiber (Dyck, 1969). If this sequence of demyelination and remyelination is repeated several times, "onion bulbs" may form (Lampert and Schochet, 1968; Weller and Das Gupta, 1968; Schröder, 1968b; Ballin and Thomas, 1969b; Dyck, 1969). This phenomenon is characteristically seen in chronic demyelinating neuropathies, namely hypertrophic neuropathy in which there is additional increase in the amount of intervening collagen between circularly arranged Schwann cell processes (cf. Chapter 43).

Partial Sheath Damage and Paranodal Demyelination

If a peripheral nerve was cautiously crushed and if the crush fell distal to the nucleated portion of the Schwann cell, it was shown by Lubińska (1959) that the directly affected internode could survive in a "truncated state." The nucleus of the Schwann cell, which in normal internodes was situated exactly in the middle, appeared displaced toward the periphery in the last internode, and the preserved internode was, on the average, shorter and more variable in length than other internodes, ranging from half to normal internodal length. If the lesion affected the proximal half of the internode too, the whole internode degenerated, showing that integrity of the nucleated region of the Schwann cell was

Figure 16–5   Sequelae of axon and myelin changes in experimental allergic neuritis. A to I. Serial cross sections of a number of segmentally demyelinated nerve fibers in a perivascular focus of demyelination. One axon (x) shows a prolapse-like deformation and extensive myelin changes that are even more pronounced in another fiber (o); other demyelinated axons present changes of the contour and diameter as well as of the accompanying Schwann cells. × 800. J. Perivascular area of demyelination in a sciatic nerve with numerous circularly arranged cells and cell processes around thinly remyelinated nerve fibers at 7 or 11 months following two injections of an antigen emulsion. × 650. K. Perivascular area of demyelination and remyelination in a dorsal root nerve two years after experimental allergic neuritis. The myelin sheaths remain disproportionately thin, the axon diameters appear to be reduced, and "supernumerary" Schwann cells and other cell processes surrounding the remyelinated nerve fibers are extremely thin or have disappeared. × 650.

essential for subsistence of myelin in the internode.

These observations of Lubińska's have been confirmed and extended in experimental studies of diphtheritic neuropathy (Cavanagh and Jacobs, 1964; Jacobs, 1967; Allt, 1969). Also, in nerve lesions caused by a pneumatic tourniquet, demyelination has usually been restricted to the region within 200 μm of the node of Ranvier; demyelination of whole internodal segments had been rare (Ochoa et al., 1971). Ochoa and Marotte (1973) reported a detachment and subsequent slippage of only the inner myelin lamellae occurring at the nodes of Ranvier in chronic entrapment neuropathy of guinea pigs. Apparently, the myelin sheath does not necessarily react in the all or none fashion usually seen in demyelinating neuropathies.

Following nerve crushing, paranodal demyelination, presumably by retraction of the myelin sheath at the nodes of Ranvier, was seen extending for one or two segments proximal to the level of the crush, with wallerian degeneration below this level (Lubińska, 1961). Some evidence of paranodal demyelination and remyelination has also been found in acrylamide neuropathy of baboons (Hopkins, 1970). In the latter, formation of short and thinly myelinated "intercalated" segments (Rénaut, 1881; "Schaltstücke," Mayer, 1881) was more frequently seen than loss of myelin from whole segments. In addition Lubińska (1961) noted that in occasional animals, one or two months after the crush injury, unusual appearances were seen in the last preserved internodes. The proximal portion was observed to be demyelinated; the rest of the internode, which in other fibers was simply wrinkled, displayed a series of bulbous myelin swellings interconnected by narrow necklike constrictions. It was noted that a characteristic feature of such internodes was the presence of numerous nuclei both in the demyelinated portions of the fibers and in the narrowed regions between the swellings.

Closely similar changes were observed by Spencer and Thomas (1970), who studied unusual swollen fibers with multiple "myelin bubbles" proximal to neuromas after transection of nerve in rats. These authors concluded that their findings represented "a peculiar type of demyelinating process in which the demyelination involves an already remyelinated portion of the fiber." It is of interest that Lubińska observed that fibers showing the bulbous myelin swellings invariably give rise to bundles of 8 to 15 sprouts. Apparently, paranodal demyelination and this interesting transitional zone between normal and regenerating nerve fibers deserves further fine structural investigation.

INTERDEPENDENT AXON AND MYELIN CHANGES

Demyelination results in a reduction of axonal diameter that was shown by Raine, Wisniewski, and Prineas (1969) to remain for at least 10 months and that is apparent even two years after experimental allergic neuritis (Fig. 16–5K). The density of neurofilaments and microtubules is strikingly increased within the demyelinated shrunken axis cylinders.

During the acute stage of experimental allergic neuritis an occasional prolapse-like deformation of demyelinated axons was seen in perivascular areas of demyelination (Schröder and Krücke, 1970). Serial sections revealed this to be limited to a short segment of the axon (Fig. 16–5A to I). The caliber of the demyelinated axons may vary considerably from one plane of section to another. Axoplasmic alterations consisting of an accumulation of mitochondria, membranous dense bodies, and vesicular elements known to develop in the proximal and distal stumps of severed axons were explained by Lampert (1969) as indicating that an injury severe enough to cause axonal damage had occurred along the course of the demyelinated axons. Bundles of regenerated nerve fibers after experimental allergic neuritis were also interpreted as sequelae of preceding wallerian degeneration (Fig. 16–5J) (Schröder and Krücke, 1970). A tendency of his "névrite segmentaire périaxile" to result in wallerian degeneration had already been noted by Gombault (1880).

On the other hand, axonal changes, namely, axonal atrophy, may cause secondary segmental demyelination, a type of lesion that has thus far not been analyzed experimentally, but has been observed in chronic neuropathies in man only (Dyck et al., 1971; cf. Chapters 15 and 47 through 53). Paranodal demyelination has also been considered a type of secondary myelin lesion due to primary axonal alterations. Further studies are needed, however, to elucidate the underlying pathogenic mechanism of segmental and paranodal demyelination secondary to axonal changes.

References

Abercrombie, M., and Johnson, M. L.: Quantitative histology of Wallerian degeneration. I. Nuclear population in rabbit sciatic nerve. J. Anat., *80*:37, 1946.

Aguayo, A., Nair, C. P., and Midgley, R.: Experimental progressive compression neuropathy in the rabbit. Histologic and electrophysiologic studies. Arch. Neurol., *24*:358, 1971.

Aitken, J. T., Sharman, M., and Young, J. Z.: Maturation of regenerating nerve fibers with various peripheral connections. J. Anat., *81*:1, 1947.

Allt, G.: Repair of segmental demyelination in peripheral nerves: an electron microscope study. Brain, *92*:639, 1969.

Åström, K. E., Webster, H. deF., Arnason, B. G.: The initial lesion in experimental allergic neuritis. A phase and electron microscope study. J. Exp. Med., *128*:465, 1968.

Ballin, R. H. M., and Thomas, P. K.: Electron microscopic observations on demyelination and remyelination in experimental allergic neuritis. Part 1. Demyelination. J. Neurol. Sci., *8*:1, 1968.

Ballin, R. H. M., and Thomas, P. K.: Electron microscopic observations on demyelination and remyelination in experimental allergic neuritis. Part 2. Remyelination. J. Neurol. Sci., *8*:225, 1969a.

Ballin, R. H. M., and Thomas, P. K.: Changes at the nodes of Ranvier during Wallerian degeneration: an electron microscope study. Acta Neuropathol. (Berl.), *14*:237, 1969b.

Le Beux, Y., Hetenyi, G., Jr., and Philipps, M. J.: Mitochondrial myelin-like figures: A non-specific reactive process of mitochondrial phospholipid membranes to several stimuli. Z. Zellforsch. Mikrosk. Anat., *99*:491, 1969.

Bielschowsky, M., and Unger, E.: Die Überbrückung großer Nervenlücken. Beiträge zur Kenntnis der Degeneration und Regeneration peripherischer Nerven. J. Psychol. Neurol., *22*:267, 1917.

Bischoff, A.: The ultrastructure of tri-ortho-cresyl-phosphate-poisoning. I. Studies on myelin and axonal alterations in the sciatic nerve. Acta Neuropathol. (Berl.), *9*:158, 1967.

Bischoff, A.: Ultrastructure of tri-ortho-cresyl phosphate poisoning in the chicken. II. Studies on the spinal cord alterations. Acta Neuropathol. (Berl.), *15*:142, 1970.

Bischoff, A., and Ulrich, J.: Peripheral neuropathy in globoid cell leukodystrophy (Krabbe's disease): Ultrastructural and histochemical findings. Brain, *92*:861, 1969.

Blakemore, W. F., and Cavanagh, J. B.: "Neuroaxonal dystrophy" occurring in an experimental "dying back" process in the rat. Brain, *92*:789, 1969.

Blümcke, S.: Elektronenoptische Untersuchungen an Schwannschen Zellen während der initialen Degeneration und frühen Regeneration. Beitr. Pathol. Anat., *128*:238, 1963.

Blümcke, S., and Niedorf, H. R.: Elektronenoptische Untersuchungen an Wachstumsendkolben regenerierender peripherer Nervenfasern. Virchows Arch. [Pathol. Anat.], *340*:93, 1965.

Bradley, W. G.: The neuropathy of vincristine in the guinea pig: an electrophysiological and pathological study. J. Neurol. Sci., *10*:133, 1970.

Bradley, W. G., and Asbury, A. K.: Duration of synthesis phase in neurilemma cells in mouse sciatic nerve during degeneration. Exp. Neurol., *26*:275, 1970.

Bradley, W. G., and Williams, M. H.: Axoplasmic flow in axonal neuropathies. I. Axoplasmic flow in cats with toxic neuropathies. Brain, *96*:235, 1973.

Büngner, O.: Über die Degenerations- und Regenerationsvorgänge am Nerven nach Verletzungen. Zieglers Beiträge, *10*:321, 1891.

Cavanagh, J. B.: On the pattern of changes in peripheral nerves produced by isoniazid intoxication in rats. J. Neurol. Neurosurg. Psychiatry, *30*:26, 1967.

Cavanagh, J. B.: Organo-phosphorus neurotoxicity and the "dying back" process. *In* Norris, F. H., and Kurland, L. T. (eds.): Motor Neuron Disease: Research on Amyotrophic Lateral Sclerosis and Related Disorders. New York and London, Grune & Stratton, 1968, p. 292.

Cavanagh, J. B., and Chen, F. C. K.: The effects of methyl-mercury-dicyandiamide on the peripheral nerves and spinal cord of rats. Acta Neuropathol. (Berl.), *19*:208, 1971a.

Cavanagh, J. B., and Chen, F. C. K.: Amino-acid incorporation in protein during the "silent phase" before organo-mercury and *p*-bromophenylacetylurea neuropathy in the rat. Acta Neuropathol. (Berl.), *19*:216, 1971b.

Cavanagh, J. B., and Jacobs, J. M.: Some quantitative aspects of diphtheritic neuropathy. Br. J. Exp. Pathol., *45*:309, 1964.

Cavanagh, J. B., Chen, F. C. K., Kyu, H. H., and Ridley, A.: The experimental neuropathy in rats caused by p-bromophenylacetylurea. J. Neurol. Neurosurg. Psychiatry, *31*:471, 1968.

Coërs, C., and Woolf, A. C.: The Innervation of Muscle. A Biopsy Study. Oxford, Blackwell Scientific Publications, 1959.

Collins, G. H., Webster, H. deF., and Victor, M.: The ultrastructure of myelin and axonal alterations in sciatic nerves of thiamine deficient and chronically starved rats. Acta Neuropathol. (Berl.), *3*:511, 1964.

Cragg, B. G., and Thomas, P. K.: The conduction velocity of regenerated peripheral nerve fibers. J. Physiol. (Lond.), *171*:164, 1964.

Deineka, D.: L'influence de la température ambiante sur la régénération des fibres nerveuses. Folia Neurobiol. *2*:13, 1908.

Denny-Brown, D., and Brenner, C.: Paralysis of nerve induced by direct pressure and by tourniquet. Arch. Neurol. Psychiatry, *51*:1, 1944a.

Denny-Brown, D., and Brenner, C.: Lesion in peripheral nerve resulting from compression by spring clip. Arch. Neurol. Psychiatry, *52*:1, 1944b.

Dinn, J. J.: Transnodal remyelination. J. Pathol., *102*:51, 1970.

Doinikow, B.: Beiträge zur Histologie und Histopathologie der peripheren Nerven. Histol. Arb. Großhirnrinde, *4*:445, 1911.

Donat, J. R., and Wisniewski, H. M.: The spatio-temporal pattern of Wallerian degeneration in mammalian peripheral nerves. Brain Res., *53*:41, 1973.

Dyck, P. J.: Experimental hypertrophic neuropathy. Arch. Neurol., *21*:73, 1969.

Dyck, P. J.: Ultrastructural alterations in myelinated fibers. *In* Desmedt, J. E. (ed.): New Developments in Electromyography and Clinical Neurophysiology. Vol. 2, Basel, S. Karger, 1973, pp. 192–226.

Dyck, P. J., and Lambert, E. H.: Polyneuropathy associated with hypothyroidism. J. Neuropathol. Exp. Neurol., *29*:631, 1970.

Dyck, P. J., Johnson, W. J., Lambert, E. H., and O'Brien, P. C.: Segmental demyelination secondary to axonal degeneration in uremic neuropathy. Mayo Clin. Proc., *46*:401, 1971.

Echandia, E. L. R., and Piezzi, R. S.: Microtubules in the nerve fibers of the toad Bufo arenarum Hensel. Effect of low temperature on the sciatic nerve. J. Cell Biol., *39*:491, 1968.

Elfvin, L. G.: Electron microscopic investigation of the plasma membrane and myelin sheath of autonomic nerve fibers in the cat. J. Ultrastruct. Res., *5*:388, 1961.

Elzholz, A.: Zur Kenntnis der Veränderungen im centralen Stumpf lädierter gemischter Nerven. Jb. Psychiatr., *17*:323, 1898.

Evans, M. J., Finean, J. B., and Woolf, A. L.: Ultrastructural studies of human cutaneous nerve with special reference to lamellated cell inclusions and vacuole-containing cells. J. Clin. Pathol., *18*:188, 1965.

Fawcett, D. W.: Cilia and flagella. *In* Brachet, J., and Mirsky, A. E. (eds.): The Cell. Vol. II. New York, London, Academic Press, 1961.

Friede, R. L.: Changes in microtubules and neurofilaments in constricted, hypoplastic nerve fibers. Acta Neuropathol. (Berl.), Suppl. V:216, 1971.

Friede, R. L., and Martinez, A. J.: Analysis of the process of sheath expansion in swollen nerve fibers. Brain Res., *19*:165, 1970a.

Friede, R. L., and Martinez, A. J.: Analysis of axon-sheath relations during early Wallerian degeneration. Brain Res., *19*:199, 1970b.

Fukami, Y., and Ridge, R. M. A. P.: Electrophysiological and morphological changes at extrafusal endplates in the snake following chronic denervation. Brain Res., *29*:139, 1971.

Fullerton, P. M.: Chronic peripheral neuropathy produced by lead poisoning in guinea pigs. J. Neuropathol. Exp. Neurol., *25*:214, 1966.

Fullerton, P. M., and Barnes, J. M.: Peripheral neuropathy in rats produced by acrylamide. Br. J. Ind. Med., *23*:210, 1966.

Gabbiani, G.: Action of cadmium chloride on sensory ganglia. Experientia, *22*:261, 1966.

Gabbiani, G., and Majno, G.: Endothelial microvilli in the vessels of the rat gasserian ganglion and testis. Z. Zellforsch. *97*:111, 1969.

Gabbiani, G., Gregory, A., and Baic, D.: Cadmium induced selective lesions of sensory ganglia. J. Neuropathol. Exp. Neurol., *26*:498, 1967.

Garro, F., and Pentschew, A.: Neonatal hydrocephalus in the offspring of rats fed during pregnancy non-toxic amounts of tellurium. Arch. Psychiatr. Nervenkr., *206*:272, 1964.

Gilliatt, R. W.: Experimental peripheral neuropathy. Sci. Basis Med., 203, 1969.

Gilliatt, R. W., and Hjorth, R. J.: Nerve conduction during Wallerian degeneration in the baboon. J. Neurol. Neurosurg., Psychiatry, *35*:335, 1972.

Gleiser, C. A., Bay, W. W., Dukes, T. W., Brown, R. S., Read, W. K., and Pierce, K. R.: Study of chloroquine toxicity and a drug-induced cerebrospinal lipodystrophy in swine. Am. J. Pathol., *53*:27, 1968.

Glimstedt, G., and Wohlfahrt, G.: Electron microscopic observations on Wallerian degeneration in peripheral nerves. Acta Morphol. Neerl. Scand., *3*:135, 1960.

Gombault, A.: Contribution a l'étude anatomique de la névrite parenchymateuse subaiguë ou chronique. Névrite segmentaire péri-axile (suite). Arch. Neurol. (Paris), *1*:177, 1880.

Gonzales, G.: Progressive neuro-ototoxicity of kanamycin. Ann. Otol. Rhinol. Laryngol., *81*:127, 1972.

Gonzenbach, H. R., Nickel, E., and Waser, P. G.: Elektronenmikroskopische Untersuchungen der Degeneration und Regeneration des Nervus phrenicus der weißen Ratte. Microsc. Acta, *71*:159, 1972.

Gottschalk, P. G., Dyck, P. J., and Kiely, J. M.: Vinca alkaloid neuropathy: nerve biopsy studies in rats and in man. Neurology (Minneap.), *18*:875, 1968.

Greenfield, J. G.: The Spinocerebellar Degenerations. Oxford, Blackwell Scientific Publications, 1954.

Gutmann, E., and Sanders, F. K.: Recovery of fibre numbers and diameters in the regeneration of peripheral nerves. J. Physiol. (Lond.), *101*:489, 1943.

Haftek, J., and Thomas, P. K.: Electron-microscope observations on the effects of localized crush injuries on the connective tissues of peripheral nerve. J. Anat., *103*:233, 1968.

Hager, H.: Allgemeine morphologische Pathologie des Nervengewebes. *In* Altmann, H.-W., Büchner, F., Cottier, H., Holle, G., Letterer, E., Masshoff, W., Meessen, H., Roulet, F., Seifert, G., Siebert, G., and Studer, A. (eds.): Handbuch der Allgemeinen Pathologie. Vol. 3. 1968, p. 149.

Hedley-Whyte, E. T.: Myelination of rat sciatic nerve: comparison of undernutrition and cholesterol biosynthesis inhibition. J. Neuropathol. Exp. Neurol., *32*:284, 1973.

Herman, S. P., Klein, R., Talley, F. A., and Krigman, M. R.: An ultrastructural study of methylmercury-induced primary sensory neuropathy in the rat. Lab. Invest., *28*:104, 1973.

Hinkley, R. E., and Samson, F. E.: Anesthetic-induced transformation of axonal microtubules. J. Cell Biol., *53*:258, 1972.

Hiscoe, H. B.: Distribution of nodes and incisures in normal and regenerated nerve fibers. Anat. Rec., *99*:447, 1947.

Holmes, W., and Young, J. Z.: Nerve regeneration after immediate and delayed suture. J. Anat., *77*:63, 1942.

Holtzman, E., and Novikoff, A. B.: Lysosomes in the rat sciatic nerve following crush. J. Cell Biol., *27*:651, 1965.

Honjin, R., Nakamura, T., and Imura, M.: Electron microscopy of peripheral nerve fibers. III: On the axoplasmic changes during Wallerian degeneration. Okajimas Folia Anat. Jap., *33*:131, 1959.

Hopkins, A.: The effect of acrylamide on the peripheral nervous system of the baboon. J. Neurol. Neurosurg. Psychiatry, *33*:805, 1970.

Hopkins, A. P., and Morgan-Hughes, J. A.: The effect of local pressure in diphtheritic neuropathy. J. Neurol. Neurosurg. Psychiatry, *32*:614, 1969.

Hunter, D., and Russell, D. S.: Focal cerebral and cerebellar atrophy in a human subject due to organic mercury compounds. J. Neurol. Neurosurg. Psychiatry, *17*:235, 1954.

Hunter, D., Bomford, R. R., and Russell, D. S.: Poisoning by methylmercury compounds. Q. J. Med., *9*:193, 1940.

Jacobs, J. M.: Experimental diphtheritic neuropathy in the rat. Brit. J. Exp. Pathol., *48*:204, 1967.

Jacobs, J. M., and Cavanagh, J. B.: Species differences in internode formation following two types of peripheral nerve injury. J. Anat., *105*:295, 1969.

Jacobs, J. M., Cavanagh, J. B., and Mellick, R. S.: Intraneural injection of diphtheria toxin. Br. J. Exp. Pathol., *47*:507, 1966.

Kline, D. G., Hayes, G. J., and Morse, A. S.: A comparative study of response of species to peripheral nerve injury. II. Crush and severance with primary suture. J. Neurosurg., *21*:980, 1964.

Klinghardt, G. W.: Arzneimittelschädigungen des peripheren Nervensystems unter besonderer Berücksichtigung der Polyneuropathie durch Isonicotinsäurehydrazid (experimentelle und humanpathologische Untersuchungen). Proceedings of Fifth International Congress on Neuropathology, Zürich, 1965. Amsterdam, Excerpta Medica Foundation, 1966, p. 292.

Klinghardt, G. W.: Experimentalle Untersuchungen zur Ätiologie der Polyneuropathie durch Nitrofurane und zur Histopathologie der Neuro-Myopathie durch Chlorochindiphosphat (Resochin). Beitr. Neurochir., *16*:55, 1969.

Klinghardt, G. W.: Experimentelle Schädigungen von Nervensystem und Muskulatur durch Chlorochin: Modelle einer Gangliosidose mit weiteren Speicherdystrophien. Acta Neuropathol. (Berl.) *28*:117–141, 1974.

Kono, R.: Subacute myelo-optico-neuropathy, a new neurological disease prevailing in Japan. Jap. J. Med. Sci. Biol., *24*:195, 1971.

Kreutzberg, G., and Wechsler, W.: Histochemische Untersuchungen oxydativer Enzyme am regenerierender Nervus ischiadicus der Ratte. Acta Neuropathol. (Berl.), *2*:349, 1963.

Krücke, W.: Erkrankungen der peripheren Nerven. *In* Von Lubarsch, O., Henke, F., and Rössle, R. (eds.): Handbuch der speziellen pathologischen Anatomie und Histologie. Vol. 5. Berlin, Springer Verlag, 1955, p. 1.

Krücke, W.: Die Erkrankungen der peripheren Nerven. *In* Kaufmann, E., and Staemmler, M. (eds.): Lehrbuch der speziellen pathologischen Anatomie. Vol. 3. Berlin, Walter de Gruyter, 1961, p. 750.

Krücke, W.: Pathologie der peripheren Nerven. *In* Olivecrona, H., Tönnis, W., and Krenkel, W. (eds.): Handbuch der Neurochirurgie. Vol. VII/3. Heidelberg, Springer-Verlag, 1974, pp. 1–267.

Lampert, P. W.: Mechanism of demyelination in experimental allergic neuritis. Lab. Invest., *20*:127, 1969.

Lampert, P. W., and Garrett, R. S.: Mechanism of demyelination in tellurium neuropathy. Electron microscopic observations. Lab. Invest., *25*:380, 1971.

Lampert, P. W., and Schochet, S. S.: Demyelination and remyelination in lead neuropathy. Electron microscopic studies. J. Neuropathol. Exp. Neurol., *27*:527, 1968.

Lampert, P., Garro, F., and Pentschew, A.: Tellurium neuropathy. Acta Neuropathol. (Berl.), *15*:308, 1970.

Lee, J. C.: Electron microscopy of Wallerian degeneration. J. Comp. Neurol., *120*:65, 1963.

Lehmann, H. J.: Die Nervenfaser. *In* Von Möllendorff, W., and Bargmann, W. (eds.): Handbuch der mikroskopischen Anatomie des Menschen. Vol. 4. Berlin—Göttingen—Heidelberg, Springer Verlag, 1959.

Lubińska, L.: On the arrest of regeneration of frog peripheral nerves at different temperatures. Acta Biol. Exp. (Vars.), *15*:125, 1952.

Lubińska, L.: Region of transition between preserved and regenerating parts of myelinated nerve fibers. J. Comp. Neurol., *113*:315, 1959.

Lubińska, L.: Demyelination and remyelination in the proximal parts of regenerated nerve fibers. J. Comp. Neurol., *117*:275, 1961.

Majno, G., Waksman, B. H., and Karnovsky, M. L.: Experimental study of diphtheritic neuritis in the rabbit and guinea pig. II. The effect of diphtheria toxin on lipide biosynthesis by guinea pig nerve. J. Neuropathol. Exp. Neurol., *19*:7, 1960.

Masson, P.: Experimental and spontaneous schwannomas (peripheral gliomas). Am. J. Pathol., *8*:367, 1932.

Matsuyama, H.: Autopsy cases of paralytic patients following abdominal symptoms. Jap. J. Clin. Med., *23*: 1956, 1965.

Mayer, S.: Über Vorgänge der Degeneration und Regeneration im unversehrten peripherischen Nervensystem. Z. Heilk., *2*:154, 1881.

Miyakawa, T., Deshimaru, M., Sumiyoshi, S., Teraoka, A., Udo, N., Hattoci, E., and Tatetsu, S.: Experimental organic mercury poisoning—pathologic changes in peripheral nerves. Acta Neuropathol. (Berl.), *15*:45, 1970.

Morgan-Hughes, J. A.: Changes in motor nerve conduction velocity in diphtheritic polyneuritis. Riv. Pat. Nerv. Ment., *86*:253, 1965.

Morgan-Hughes, J. A.: Experimental diphtheritic neuropathy: pathological and electrophysiological study. J. Neurol. Sci., *7*:157, 1968.

Morris, J. H., Hudson, A. R., and Weddell, G.: A study of degeneration and regeneration in the divided rat sciatic nerve based on electron microscopy. II. The development of the "regenerating unit." Z. Zellforsch. Mikrosk. Anat., *124*:103, 1972.

Moyer, E. K., Kimmel, D. L., and Winborne, L. W.: Regeneration of sensory spinal nerve roots in young and in senile rats. J. Comp. Neurol., *98*:283, 1953.

Nageotte, J.: Sheaths of the peripheral nerves. Nerve degeneration and regeneration. *In* Penfield, W. (ed.): Cytology and Cellular Pathology of the Nervous System. Vol. 1. New York, P. B. Hoeber, 1932, p. 189.

Nathaniel, E. J. H., and Pease, D. C.: Degenerative changes in rat dorsal roots during Wallerian degeneration. J. Ultrastruct. Res., *9*:511, 1963a.

Nathaniel, E. J. H., and Pease, D. C.: Regenerative changes in rat dorsal roots following Wallerian degeneration. J. Ultrastruct. Res., *9*:533, 1963b.

Nathaniel, E. J. H., and Pease, D. C.: Collagen and basement membrane formation by Schwann cells during nerve regeneration. J. Ultrastruct. Res., *9*:550, 1963c.

Ochoa, J., and Marotte, L.: The nature of the nerve lesion caused by chronic entrapment in the guinea-pig. J. Neurol. Sci., *19*:491, 1973.

Ochoa, J., Fowler, T. J., and Gilliatt, R. W.: Anatomical changes in peripheral nerves compressed by a pneumatic tourniquet. J. Anat., *113*:433, 1972.

Ochoa, J., Danta, G., Fowler, T. J., and Gilliatt, R. W.: Nature of the nerve lesion caused by a pneumatic tourniquet. Nature, *233*:265, 1971.

O'Daly, J. A., and Imaeda, T.: Electron microscopic study of Wallerian degeneration in cutaneous nerves caused by mechanical injury. Lab. Invest., *17*:744, 1967.

Ohmi, S.: Electron microscopic study on Wallerian degeneration of the peripheral nerve. Z. Zellforsch. Mikrosk. Anat., *54*:39, 1961.

Paty, D. W.: An encephalitogenic basic protein from human peripheral nerve. Eur. Neurol., *5*:281, 1971.

Pickard, W. F.: Estimating the velocity of propagation along myelinated and unmyelinated fibers. Mathematical Biosciences *5*:305, 1969.

Pleasure, D. E., Mishler, K. C., and Engel, W. K.: Axonal transport of proteins in experimental neuropathies. Science, *166*:524, 1969.

Prineas, J.: The pathogenesis of dying-back polyneuropathies. Part I. An ultrastructural study of experimental tri-ortho-cresyl phosphate intoxication in the cat. J. Neuropathol. Exp. Neurol., *28*:571, 1969a.

Prineas, J.: The pathogenesis of dying-back polyneuropathies. Part II. An ultrastructural study of experimental acrylamide intoxication in the cat. J. Neuropathol. Exp. Neurol., *28*:598, 1969b.

Prineas, J.: Peripheral nerve changes in thiamine-deficient rats. Arch. Neurol., *23*:541, 1970.

Prineas, J. W., and Wright, R. G.: The fine structure of peripheral nerve lesions in a virus-induced demyelinating disease in fowl (Marek's disease). Lab. Invest., *26*:548, 1972.

Raine, C. S., Wisniewski, H., and Prineas, J.: An ultrastructural study of experimental demyelination and remyelination. II. Chronic experimental allergic encephalomyelitis in the peripheral nervous system. Lab. Invest., *21*:316, 1969.

Raine, C. S., Wisniewski, H., Dowling, P. C., and Cook, S. D.: An ultrastructural study of experimental demyelination and remyelination. IV. Recurrent episodes and peripheral nervous system plaque formation in experimental allergic encephalomyelitis. Lab. Invest., *25*:28, 1971.

Ramón y Cajal, S.: Degeneration and Regeneration of the Nervous System. Vol. 1. London, Oxford University, 1928.

Rawlins, F. A., and Uzman, B. G.: Retardation of peripheral nerve myelination in mice treated with inhibitors of cholesterol biosynthesis. A quantitative electron microscopic study. J. Cell Biol., *46*:505, 1970.

Read, W. K., and Bay, W. W.: Basic cellular lesion in chloroquine toxicity. Lab. Invest., *24*:246, 1971.

Reich, F.: Über eine neue Granulation in den Nervenzellen. Arch. Physiol. (Leipz.), 208, 1903.

Reich, F.: Über den zelligen Aufbau der Nervenfaser auf Grund mikrohistiochemischer Untersuchungen. J. Psychol. Neurol., *8*:244, 1907.

Reimer, K. A., Ganote, C. E., and Jennings, R. B.: Alterations in renal cortex following ischemic injury. III. Ultrastructure of proximal tubules after ischemia or autolysis. Lab. Invest., *26*:347, 1972.

Rénaut, M. J.: Recherches sur quelques points particulaires de l'histologie des nerfs. Arch. Physiol., *13*:161, 1881.

Ruska, H., and Edwards, G. A.: A new cytoplasmic pattern in striated muscle fibers and its relation to growth. Growth, *21*:73, 1957.

Sanders, F. K.: The thickness of myelin sheaths of normal and regenerating peripheral nerve fibres. Proc. R. Soc. Lond. [Biol.], *135*:323, 1948.

Sanders, F. K., and Whitteridge, D.: Conduction velocity and myelin sheath thickness in regenerating nerve fibres. J. Physiol., *105*:152, 1946.

Sanders, F. K., and Young, J. Z.: The role of the peripheral stump in the control of fibre diameter in regenerating nerves. J. Physiol., *103*:119, 1944.

Sanders, F. K., and Young, J. Z.: The influence of peripheral connexion on the diameter of regenerating nerve fibres. J. Exp. Biol., *22*:203, 1946.

Schlaepfer, W. W.: Vincristine-induced axonal alterations in rat peripheral nerve. J. Neuropathol. Exp. Neurol., *30*:488, 1971a.

Schlaepfer, W. W.: Sequential study of endothelial changes in acute cadmium intoxication. Lab. Invest., *25*:556, 1971b.

Schlaepfer, W. W., and Hager, H.: Ultrastructural studies of INH-induced neuropathy in rats. I. Early axonal changes. Am. J. Pathol., *45*:209, 1964a.

Schlaepfer, W. W., and Hager, H.: Ultrastructural studies in INH-induced neuropathy in rats. II. Alteration and decomposition of myelin sheath. Am. J. Pathol., *45*:423, 1964b.

Schlaepfer, W. W., and Hager, H.: Ultrastructural studies in INH-induced neuropathy in rats. III. Repair and regeneration. Am. J. Pathol., *45*:679, 1964c.

Schnabel, R., and Sir, G.: Histochemische Untersuchungen über die π-Granula (Reich) der peripheren, markhaltigen Nervenfasern. Z. Zellforsch. Mikrosk. Anat., *56*:1, 1962.

Schochet, S. S.: Mitochondrial changes in axonal dystrophy produced by vitamin E deficiency. Acta Neuropathol. (Berl.), Suppl. V:54, 1971.

Schochet, S. S., Lampert, P. W., and Earle, K. M.: Neuronal changes induced by intrathecal vincristine sulfate. J. Neuropathol. Exp. Neurol., *27*:645, 1968.

Schröder, J. M.: Die Hyperneurotisation Büngnerscher Bänder bei der experimentellen Isoniazid-Neuropathie: Phasenkontrast- und elektronenmikroskopische Untersuchungen. Virchows Arch. [Zellpathol.], *1*:131, 1968a.

Schröder, J. M.: Überzählige Schwannzellen bei der Remyelinisation regenerierter und segmental demyelinisierter Axone im peripheren Nerven. Verh. Dtsch. Ges. Pathol., *52*:222, 1968b.

Schröder, J. M.: Die Feinstruktur markloser (Remakscher) Nervenfasern bei der Isoniazid-Neuropathie. Acta Neuropathol. (Berl.), *15*:156, 1970a.

Schröder, J. M.: Zur Pathogenese der Isoniazid-Neuropathie. I. Eine feinstrukturelle Differenzierung gegenüber der Wallerschen Degeneration. Acta neuropathol. (Berl.), *16*:301, 1970b.

Schröder, J. M.: Zur Pathogenese der Isoniazid-Neuropathie. II. Phasenkontrast- und elektronenmikroskopische Untersuchungen am Rückenmark, an den Spinalganglien und Muskelspindeln. Acta Neuropathol. (Berl.), *16*:324, 1970c.

Schröder, J. M.: Zur Feinstruktur und quantitativen Auswertung regenerierter peripherer Nervenfasern. *In* Proceedings of the Sixth International Congress of Neuropathology. Paris, Masson & Cie, 1970d, p. 628.

Schröder, J. M.: Altered ratio between axon diameter and myelin sheath thickness in regenerated nerve fibers. Brain Res., *45*:49, 1972.

Schröder, J. M.: Two-dimensional reconstruction of Schwann cell changes following remyelination of regenerated nerve fibers. *In* Hausmanowa-Petrusewicz, I. (ed.): Proceedings, Symposium on Structure and Function of Normal and Diseased Muscle and Peripheral Nerve, Kazimierz upon Vistula, Poland, 1972. In press.

Schröder, J. M., and Krücke, W.: Zur Feinstruktur der experimentellallergischen Neuritis beim Kaninchen. Acta Neuropathol. (Berl.), *14*:261, 1970.

Schröder, J. M. and Seiffert, K. E.: Untersuchungen zur homologen Nerventransplantation. Morphologische Ergebnisse. Zentralbl. Neurochir., *53*:103, 1972.

Schröder, J. M., Thomas, P. K., and Ballin, R. H. M.: Quergestreifte Fibrillen in Schwannschen Zellen. Naturwissenschaften, *57*:44, 1970.

Seiler, N., and Schröder, J. M.: Beziehungen zwischen Polyaminen und Nucleinsäuren. II. Biochemische und feinstrukturelle Untersuchungen am peripheren Nerven während der Wallerschen Degeneration. Brain Res., 22:81, 1970.

Shiraki, H.: Neuropathology of subacute myelo-optico-neuropathy, "SMON." Jap. J. Med. Sci. Biol., 24: 217, 1971.

Shiraki, H., and Oda, M.: Neuropathology of "SMON." Saishin Igaku, 24:2479, 1969.

Simpson, S. A., and Young, J. Z.: Regeneration of fibre diameter after cross-union of visceral and somatic nerves. J. Anat., 79:48, 1945.

Singer, M., and Steinberg, M. C.: Wallerian degeneration: a reevaluation based on transected and colchicine-poisoned nerves in the amphibian. Am. J. Anat., 133:51, 1972.

Sotelo, C., and Palay, S. L.: Altered axons and axon terminals in the lateral vestibular nucleus of the rat. Lab. Invest., 25:653, 1971.

Spatz, H.: Die "systematischen Atrophien." Eine wohl gekennzeichnete Gruppe der Erbkrankheiten des Nervensystems. Arch. Psychiatr., 108:1, 1938.

Spencer, P. S., and Thomas, P. K.: The examination of isolated nerve fibres by light and electron microscopy, with observations on demyelination proximal to neuromas. Acta Neuropathol. (Berl.), 16:177, 1970.

Stupp, H. F., Rauch, R., Soud, H., Lagler, F., and Brun, J. P.: Die Ursache der spezifischen Ototoxizität der basischen Streptomycesantibiotika—ein Permeabilitätsproblem. Med. et Hyg., 23:988, 1965.

Sunderland, S.: Nerves and Nerve Injury. Edinburgh and London, E. & S. Livingstone, 1968.

Suzuki, K., and La Dorna Pfaff: Acrylamide neuropathy in rats. An electron microscopic study of degeneration and regeneration. Acta. Neuropathol. (Berl.), 24:197, 1973.

Swift, H., and Hruban, Z.: Focal degradation as biological process. Fed. Proc., 23:1026, 1964.

Tateishi, J., Kuroda, S., Saito, A., and Otsuki, S.: Myelo-optic neuropathy induced by clioquinol in animals. Lancet, 2:1263, 1971.

Tateishi, J., Kuroda, S., Saito, A., and Otsuki, S.: Experimental myelo-optic neuropathy induced by clioquinol. Acta Neuropathol. (Berl.), 2:304, 1973.

Tateishi, J., Kuroda, S., Watanabe, S., Otsuki, S., and Ogata, M.: Autoradiographic distribution of ^{131}I-clioquinol in canine and feline. Folia Psychiatr. Neurol. Jap., 26:159, 1972.

Terry, R. D., and Harkin, J. C.: Wallerian degeneration and regeneration of peripheral nerves. In Korey, S. A. (ed.): Biology of Myelin. New York, Paul B. Hoeber, 1959, p. 303.

Thomas, E.: Histotopochemie und Histopathochemie des peripheren Nervensystems bei Verletzungen und Tumoren. Stuttgart, Gustav Fischer Verlag, 1969.

Thomas, P. K.: Changes in endoneurial sheaths of peripheral myelinated nerve fibers during Wallerian degeneration. J. Anat., 98:175, 1964.

Thomas, P. K.: The cellular response to nerve injury. 3. The effect of repeated crush injuries. J. Anat., 106: 463, 1970.

Thomas, P. K., and Sheldon, H.: Tubular arrays derived from myelin breakdown during Wallerian degeneration of peripheral nerve. J. Cell Biol., 22:715, 1964.

Thomas, P. K., and Slatford, J.: Lamellar bodies in the cytoplasm of Schwann cells. J. Anat., 98:691, 1964.

Tischner, K. H.: Chlorquine-induced alteration in rat sensory ganglia cultivated in vitro. A light and electron microscope study. Acta Neuropathol. (Berl.), 22:208, 1972.

Tischner, K. H., and Schröder, J. M.: The effects of cadmium chloride on organotypic cultures of rat sensory ganglia. A light and electron microscopic study. J. Neurol. Sci., 16:383, 1972.

Tilney, L. G., and Porter, K. R.: Studies on the microtubules in Heliozoa. II. The effect of low temperature on these structures in the formation and maintenance of the axopodia. J. Cell Biol., 34:327, 1967.

Tomonaga, M., and Sluga, E.: Zur Ultrastruktur der π-Granula. Acta Neuropathol. (Berl.), 15:56, 1970.

Trump, B. F., and Ericson, J. L. E.: Some ultrastructural and biochemical consequences of cell injury. In Zweifach, B. W., Grant, L. H., and McCluskey, R. T. (eds.): The Inflammatory Process. New York, Academic Press, 1965.

Uy, Q. L., Moen, T. H., Johns, R. J., and Owens, A. H.: Vincristine neurotoxicity in rodents. Johns Hopkins Med. J., 121:349, 1967.

Vizosa, A. D., and Young, J. Z.: Internodal length and fibre diameter in developing and regenerating nerves. J. Anat., 82:110, 1948.

Wagner, W. H., Chou, J. T. Y., Ilberg, C., von, Ritter, R., and Vosteen, K. H.: Untersuchungen zur Pharmakokinetik von Streptomycin. Arzneim. Forsch., 21:2006, 1971.

Waksman, B. H., and Adam, R. D.: Allergic neuritis: an experimental disease of rabbits induced by the injection of peripheral nervous tissue and adjuvants. J. Exp. Med., 102:213, 1955.

Waksman, B. H., and Adams, R. D.: A comparative study of the experimental neuritis in the rabbit, guinea-pig, and mouse. J. Neuropathol. Exp. Neurol., 15:293, 1956.

Waksman, B. H., Adams, R. D., and Mansmann, H. C.: Experimental study of diphtheritic neuritis in the rabbit and guinea pig. I. Immunologic and histopathologic observations. J. Exp. Med., 105:591, 1957.

Waller, A.: Experiments on the section of the glossopharyngeal and hypoglossal nerves of the frog, and observation on the alterations produced thereby in the structure of their primitive-fibres. Philos. Trans. R. Soc. Lond. [Biol. Sci.], 140:423, 1850.

Webster, H. deF.: Transient focal accumulations of axonal mitochondria during the early stages of Wallerian degeneration. J. Cell Biol., 12:361, 1962.

Webster, H. deF.: Some ultrastructural features of segmental demyelination and myelin regeneration in peripheral nerve. Progr. Brain Res., 13:151, 1964.

Webster, H. deF.: The relationship between Schmidt-Lantermann incisures and myelin segmentation during Wallerian degeneration. Ann. N.Y. Acad. Sci., 122:29, 1965.

Webster, H. deF., and Spiro, D.: Phase and electron microscopic studies of experimental demyelination. I. Variations in myelin sheath contour in normal guinea pig sciatic nerve. J. Neuropathol. Exp. Neurol., 19:42, 1960.

Webster, H. deF., Spiro, D., Waksman, B., and Adams, R. D.: Phase and electron microscopic studies of experimental demyelination. II. Schwann cell changes in guinea pig sciatic nerves during experimental diphtheritic neuritis. J. Neuropathol. Exp. Neurol., 20:5, 1961.

Wechsler, W., and Hager, H.: Elektronenmikroskopische Untersuchung der sekundären Wallerschen Degeneration der peripheren Säugetiernerven. Beitr. Pathol. Anat., 126:352, 1962.

Weiss, P., Edds, M. V., and Cavanaugh, M.: The effect

of terminal connections on the caliber of nerve fibers. Anat. Rec., 92:215, 1945.

Weiss, P., and Taylor, A. C.: Further experimental evidence against "neurotropism" in nerve regeneration. J. Exp. Zool., 95:233, 1944.

Weller, R. O.: Diphtheritic neuropathy in the chicken: an electron-microscope study. J. Pathol. Bacteriol., 89:591, 1965.

Weller, R. O., and Das Gupta, T. K.: Experimental hypertrophic neuropathy: an electron microscope study. J. Neurol. Neurosurg. Psychiatry, 31:34, 1968.

Weller, R. O., and Mellick, R. S.: Acid phosphatase and lysosome activity in diphtheritic neuropathy and Wallerian degeneration. Br. J. Exp. Pathol., 47:425, 1966.

Wright, P. A. L.: The ultrastructure of sciatic nerves affected by fowl paralysis (Marek's disease). J. Comp. Pathol., 79:563, 1969.

Wiśniewski, H., and Raine, C. S.: An ultrastructural study of experimental demyelination and remyelination. V. Central and peripheral nervous system lesions caused by diphtheria toxin. Lab. Invest., 25:73, 1971.

Wiśniewski, H., Prineas, J., and Raine, C. S.: An ultrastructural study of experimental demyelination and remyelination. I. Acute experimental allergic encephalomyelitis in the peripheral nervous system. Lab. Invest., 21:105, 1969.

Wiśniewski, H. Shelanski, M. L., and Terry, R. D.: Effects of mitotic spindle inhibitors on neurotubules and neurofilaments in anterior horn cells. J. Cell Biol., 38:224, 1968.

Young, J. Z.: The determination of the specific characteristics of nerve fibers. In Weis, P.: Genetic Neurology, Chicago, University of Chicago Press, 1950, p. 92.

Zelená, J., Lubińska, L., and Gutmann, E.: Accumulation of organelles at the ends of interrupted axons. Z. Zellforsch. Mikrosk. Anat., 91:200, 1968.

Chapter 17

PATHOLOGY AND PATHOPHYSIOLOGY OF UNMYELINATED NERVE FIBERS

EXPERIMENTAL PATHOLOGY

Albert J. Aguayo *and* Garth M. Bray

Unmyelinated nerve fibers are an important component of the peripheral nervous system, and their involvement in various forms of neuropathy has been documented (see Chapter 7). The clinical manifestations of such neuropathies mainly reflect disturbances of autonomic and sensory function and include postural hypotension, sweating abnormalities, impotence, and other signs of autonomic failure as well as distorted appreciation of pain and temperature sensation. Because these manifestations are common in peripheral nerve disorders it seems likely that involvement of unmyelinated fibers is of greater significance than heretofore recognized.

Evaluation of the structural and functional changes that occur in diseases affecting unmyelinated nerve fibers (Remak fibers) has been limited by the small size of their axons and the complexity of axon–Schwann cell relationships. In these fibers several axons of different origin and diameter run together through chains of longitudinally aligned Schwann cells, and there is frequent interchange of axons between adjacent Remak fibers. For these reasons, and also because unmyelinated fibers lack the distinctive staining properties of myelin, knowledge of their reactions is less advanced than that of myelinated fibers. With the development of ultramicroscopic techniques, however, it has become possible to define alterations of unmyelinated axons and Schwann cells in human peripheral nerves

(Ochoa and Mair, 1969a, 1969b; Thomas, 1970, 1973). In this chapter, experimental studies of unmyelinated nerve fibers are reviewed and the significance of their reactions to injury discussed.

NORMAL STRUCTURE AND DEVELOPMENT OF UNMYELINATED NERVE FIBERS

The concept that all nerve fibers are cylindrical structures is derived from light microscopic observations. Electron microscopy has shown that, whereas this concept applies to myelinated fibers, it is not strictly true for unmyelinated fibers in which the longitudinal arrangement is more complex. In peripheral sympathetic nerves, unmyelinated fibers are arranged in a network (Hillarp, 1959; Iwayama, 1970; Peerless and Yasargil, 1971), while in nerves with mixed fiber populations, cords of interconnecting unmyelinated fibers tend to group near myelinated ones (Gamble and Eames, 1964; Ochoa and Mair, 1969a).

Ultrastructure

The term "unmyelinated nerve fiber" as used in this chapter refers to the structure described

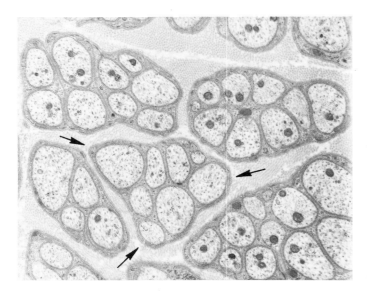

Figure 17–1 Normal unmyelinated nerve in cross section. Individual Schwann cell units are composed of axons embedded in Schwann cell cytoplasm. Each unit is surrounded by Schwann cell basal lamina. One such unit is indicated by the three arrows. Electron micrograph of adult rat cervical sympathetic trunk. × 12,000.

by Remak (1838), using light microscopy, and is not synonymous with "unmyelinated axon." Thus, individual unmyelinated fibers (Remak fibers) consist of axons embedded in Schwann cells. The exterior surface of each Schwann cell is enveloped by a basal lamina (Fig. 17–1). In cross section, structures totally enclosed by this basal lamina are designated a Schwann cell unit or complex. Although the number of axons enclosed by each Schwann cell depends on the particular nerve as well as on the species and age of the animal studied, most adult unmyelinated fibers contain 3 to 6 axons per Schwann cell unit with a range of 1 to 30 (Table 17–1). The diameter of individual axons varies little along unmyelinated nerves.

The longitudinal configuration of unmyelinated fibers is continuously varying, owing to separation and rejoining of adjacent Schwann cell units (Fig. 17–2). Consequently an individual Schwann cell unit, as defined in cross section, may represent only a portion of one Schwann cell and the axons it contains. Furthermore, the number of axons within individual Schwann cell units varies from level to level; this is primarily due to axonal interchange between Schwann cell units rather than to axonal branching (Fig. 17–3).

In unmyelinated nerve fibers, no distinct junctions can be defined between adjacent Schwann cells; rather, their processes seem to overlap and interdigitate (Eames and Gamble, 1970). An approximate estimate of the longitudinal territory occupied by individual Schwann cells can be obtained by measuring the internuclear distances of consecutive cells. These measurements are variable, but their median is approximately 90 μm for adult rat cervical sympathetic trunk, shown in Figure 17–4, and is close to 100 μm for unmyelinated fibers in rat sural nerve (Peyronnard et al., 1973, 1975).

TABLE 17–1 DIAMETERS AND PERCENTAGE DISTRIBUTION OF AXONS IN SCHWANN CELL UNITS

	Median Axonal Diameter (μm)	Mean Axonal Content	Distribution of Axons in Schwann Cell Units (%)					
			1	2	3–4	5–6	7–10	11 or More
Rat cervical sympathetic trunk (mid level, right)	0.64	4.4	20.9	12.6	18.3	14.5	18.5	15.2
Rabbit anterior mesenteric nerve (proximal level)	0.71	3.0	35.4	18.1	24.7	12.9	7.3	1.6
Mouse sural nerve (midcalf level)	0.52	5.6	16.5	9.5	22.8	16.5	21.3	13.4

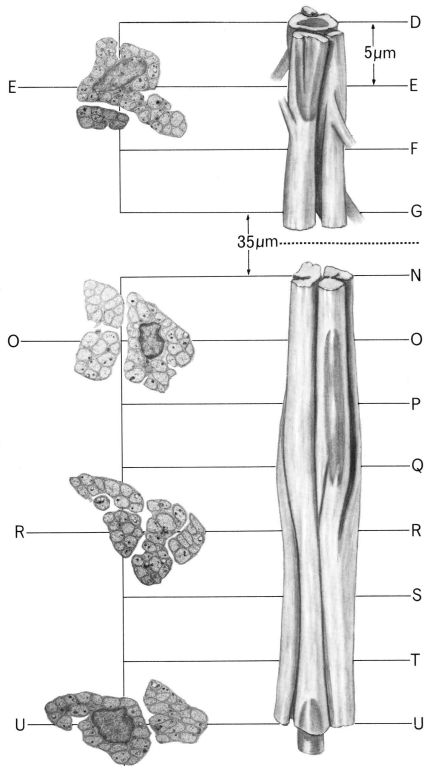

Figure 17-2   Three-dimensional reconstruction of interrelating Schwann cell units from a normal rat cervical sympathetic trunk based upon electron micrographs of serial transverse sections (D to U) cut at 5 μm intervals. Four of the electron micrographs are reproduced. The arrangement of axons within Schwann cell units varies from level to level, owing to separation and rejoining of adjacent units. Schwann cell nuclei are present at levels D, O, and U.

Normal Development

In unmyelinated nerve fibers, studied in rat cervical sympathetic trunks, early development is characterized by a complex reorganization of axon–Schwann cell relationships. Beginning prenatally and continuing during the first few days after birth, there is a marked reduction in the total number of axons and a progressive increase in Schwann cell populations (Aguayo et al., 1973a; Terry et al., 1974). Consequently, there is a decline in the number

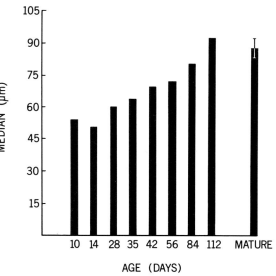

Figure 17–4 Median internuclear distances of Schwann cells in the rat cervical sympathetic trunk during various stages of development. Unmyelinated fibers were prepared by microdissection, and internuclear distances measured from approximately 400 fibers (except at 1, 10, and 14 days, when only 139, 304, and 298 fibers respectively were available); the value for mature animals was calculated from the median determined for seven different nerves and is expressed as the mean plus or minus standard deviation. (From Peyronnard, J. M., Terry, L. C., and Aguayo, A. J.: Schwann cell internuclear distances in developing rat unmyelinated nerve fibers. Arch. Neurol., 32:36, 1975. Copyright 1975, American Medical Association. Reprinted by permission.)

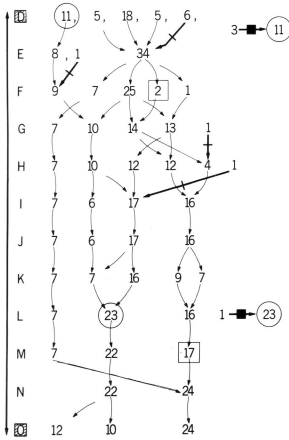

Figure 17–3 Schematic representation of the course followed by axons in the segment of unmyelinated fiber shown in Figure 17–2 that extends between two consecutive Schwann cell nuclei (D and O). At level D there are five Schwann cell units containing 11, 5, 18, 5, and 6 axons. Five microns below (level E) four units have joined in a single complex containing 34 axons. This complex divides again into four units at level F. The complexity of axon–Schwann cell relationships is demonstrated by changes at subsequent levels. Along the segment studied, nine axons have joined the fiber (←┼) from neighboring fibers while four axons have left (←■). In this study, the presence of an additional axon at levels F ② and M ⑰ could not be explained by axonal interchange from neighboring complexes.

of axons per Schwann cell unit, and at the same time the diameter of the remaining axons increases toward normal (Fig. 17–5). Because a reduction of axon–Schwann cell ratios has been observed during development in other peripheral nerves (Peters and Muir, 1959; Cravioto, 1965), it can be assumed that spontaneous axonal loss and Schwann cell multiplication are both partially responsible for this change. It is not yet known if the changes in axonal population are secondary to neuronal degeneration or to a disappearance of redundant axonal branches (Prestige, 1970; Prestige and Wilson, 1972; Reier and Hughes, 1972). The neonatal loss of unmyelinated axons may be prevented by administration of nerve growth factor (Roisen, 1972) but is accentuated by nerve growth factor antiserum (Aguayo et al., 1972b) or other procedures that decrease the number of postsynaptic neurons in the superior cervical ganglion (Black et al., 1971; Aguayo et al., 1973c). Thus, the number of preganglionic axons that mature in the cervical sympathetic trunk can be modified from the

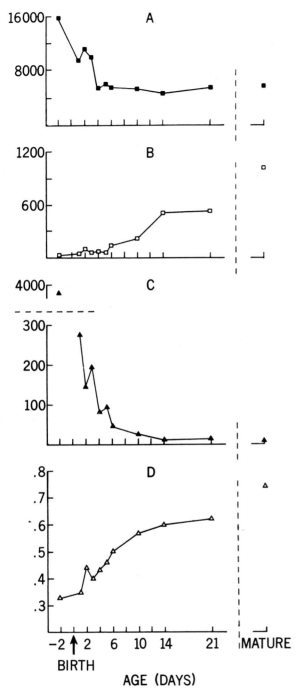

periphery, presumably by changes in the number of neurons in the superior cervical ganglion available as potential synaptic sites. The size of the axonal population, in turn, influences the extent of Schwann cell proliferation in the cervical sympathetic trunk (Aguayo et al., 1974).

In rat cervical sympathetic trunks, there are few Schwann cell units per transverse section at birth. Each unit, however, may contain more than one Schwann cell nucleus in addition to large numbers of small axons. Postnatally, Schwann cell development evolves through several stages. Schwann cell nuclei multiply intensely during the first week after birth (Terry et al., 1974). Subsequently nonproliferating Schwann cells form multiple processes. Thus, there is a rapid increase in the number of Schwann cell units per transverse section (Fig. 17–5B). In addition, Schwann cell internuclear distances gradually increase, indicating a longitudinal extension of individual Schwann cell territories during development (Fig. 17–4) (Peyronnard et al., 1975).

In general, the increase in Schwann cell plasma membrane required for the formation of cytoplasmic processes, the complete enclosure of individual axons, and the lengthening of individual Schwann cell territories along developing unmyelinated nerve fibers may be a process equivalent to that occurring in myelinated fibers during the formation of myelin sheaths.

METHODS OF STUDYING UNMYELINATED NERVE FIBERS

Several morphologic techniques and experimental models have been used to investigate unmyelinated nerves; in this section, certain of these are critically reviewed.

Morphologic Techniques

Changes in unmyelinated axons, as seen with the light microscope, have been studied with stains such as silver impregnation (Ramón y Cajal, 1903, Bielschowsky, 1904) and methylene blue (Hillarp, 1959) and by degeneration methods (Cottle and Mitchell, 1966). It is difficult, however, to assess Schwann

Figure 17–5 Quantitative data for whole transverse section of rat cervical sympathetic trunks during various stages of development. Observations from single trunks, beginning prenatally and continuing up to 21 days of age, are presented; data for mature trunks are means of four observations. Total numbers of axons and axon–Schwann cell unit ratios rapidly decline while axonal diameters and number of Schwann cell units increase. *A.* Total number of unmyelinated axons. *B.* Total number of Schwann cell units. *C.* Axon–Schwann cell unit ratios. *D.* Median axonal diameter in microns.

cell relationships with these techniques, and since the smallest unmyelinated axons are beyond the resolution of light microscopy, precise quantitative studies are not possible.

The most valuable technique used for the study of normal and altered structure of unmyelinated nerve fibers is electron microscopy. Since Gasser documented the precise relationship of unmyelinated axons and Schwann cells in 1952, electron microscopy has been used to study various reactions of these peripheral nerve fibers. Quantitative electron microscopic techniques are particularly valuable in the experimental study of unmyelinated nerve fiber responses (Dyck and Hopkins, 1972; Aguayo et al., 1972a). An important limitation of electron microscopic studies of unmyelinated nerve fibers, however, is the difficulty in obtaining satisfactory sections of any useful length for longitudinal assessment of axon–Schwann cell relationships. This difficulty can be overcome, in part at least, by the use of serial transverse sections (Gasser, 1955; Eames and Gamble, 1970; Aguayo et al., 1973c). Microdissection of unmyelinated fibers, a technique originally used by Remak (1838) and later by Tuckett (1896) and Nageotte (1932), has also proved valuable for the study of Schwann cell reactions along unmyelinated fibers (Peyronnard et al., 1973).

Other special techniques have been used to study unmyelinated nerve fibers. Adrenergic neurons and their axons have been demonstrated by fluorescence microscopy by Falck and associates (1962) and Olson (1969), and this technique has been used by Dahlström and Häggendal (1966) to assess axonal flow rates. Cholinergic fibers have been visualized by cholinesterase histochemistry (Ellison and Olander, 1972). In vivo studies of nerve fibers are possible with differential interference microscopy (Webster and Billings, 1972).

It is anticipated that scanning electron microscopy will also be used to study the surface morphology of unmyelinated fibers.

Nerves Used for Experimental Studies

Most experimental studies of unmyelinated fiber reactions have utilized autonomic nerves. Because these nerves are predominantly unmyelinated, confusion with degenerative and regenerative changes in myelinated fibers can be minimized. Autonomic nerves that have been most frequently studied by electron microscopy are the rat cervical sympathetic trunk and abdominal vagus nerve, and the rabbit anterior mesenteric nerve.

The cervical sympathetic trunk of the rat usually consists of a single fascicle between the middle and superior cervical sympathetic ganglia (Dyck and Hopkins, 1972; Aguayo et al., 1972a). In adult animals, this nerve measures approximately 20 mm in length and contains 4000 to 5000 axons, of which less than 100 are myelinated; the median diameter of unmyelinated axons is approximately 0.64 μm (see Table 17–1) (Bray and Aguayo, 1974). Quantitative parameters for this nerve, such as the total number of unmyelinated axons, the number of axon–Schwann cell units, the distribution of axonal diameters, and the ratio of axons to Schwann cells are relatively constant at different levels of the cervical sympathetic trunk.

The anterior mesenteric nerve of the rabbit is composed of 8 to 10 fascicles that arise from the anterior mesenteric ganglia and run together for approximately 10 mm before separating into divergent and tortuous branches. Median axonal diameters for this nerve are slightly larger than those of the rat cervical sympathetic trunk (Aguayo et al., 1973b); otherwise the characteristics of both nerves are similar, as shown in Table 17–1. Occasional ganglion cells are present along the course of this and most other unmyelinated nerves.

Other autonomic nerves used experimentally are the rabbit abdominal vagus nerve (Thomas et al., 1972) and the cat splenic and hypogastric nerves (Kapeller and Mayor, 1969a, 1969b). Deep petrosal nerves have been examined in mice and found to contain approximately 3000 unmyelinated axons but only one myelinated fiber (Shimozawa, 1972). The nerve to the vas deferens, studied in rats, has provided an opportunity to examine the innervation of smooth muscle by unmyelinated axons (Richardson, 1962); such studies have shown that the terminal axonal branches of this nerve are naked, lacking Schwann cell coverage.

Because most peripheral nerves contain both myelinated and unmyelinated axons, reactions of unmyelinated fibers can be studied experimentally in mixed nerves. Confusion with changes in myelinated fibers is difficult to avoid, however (Blumcke et al., 1966).

Experimental Models of Unmyelinated Nerve Fiber Reactions

Morphologic responses of unmyelinated nerve fibers have been studied in several experimental models.

Axonal Interruption. Degenerative and regenerative responses following surgical transection or crush injury have been investigated by electron microscopy (Taxi, 1959; Roth and Richardson, 1969; Iwayama, 1970; Dyck and Hopkins, 1972; Bray et al., 1972; Thomas et al., 1972; Aguayo et al., 1973b; Bray and Aguayo, 1974). Although both transection and crush injury produce axonal interruption, the Schwann cell basal lamina and connective tissue framework remain continuous after crush injury. The effects of nerve constriction have also been studied by several workers (Dahlström and Häggendal, 1966; Kapeller and Mayor, 1969a, 1969b; Geffen and Ostberg, 1969).

Toxic Agents. Changes in unmyelinated nerve fibers have been studied by fluorescence microscopy in rat cervical sympathetic trunks following administration of vinblastine (Dahlström, 1971), a drug that causes alterations in axonal tubules and filaments (Shelanski and Wiśniewski, 1969). On the other hand, resistance of unmyelinated fibers to isoniazid and acrylamide, drugs capable of causing axonal degeneration in myelinated fibers, has been suggested from physiologic studies (Hopkins and Lambert, 1972a).

Radiation Injury. Schwann cell changes in unmyelinated fibers have been observed in nerve tissue cultures exposed to x-irradiation (Masurovsky et al., 1967). Rat cervical sympathetic trunks also show predominant Schwann cell alterations and relative preservation of axons after x-irradiation (Aguayo et al., 1973c, 1975).

Chemical Sympathectomy. 6-Hydroxydopamine, a synthetic analog of dopamine, causes a long-standing depletion of catecholamines in sympathetic nerve fibers and, in mature animals, a selective but reversible degeneration of adrenergic nerve endings (Thoenen and Tranzer, 1968). The loss of axons is permanent and involves entire adrenergic neurons when larger doses of 6-hydroxydopamine are administered to newborn animals (Angeletti and Levi-Montalcini, 1970; Angeletti, 1972a). Newborn mice and rats also show pronounced changes in sympathetic ganglia after administration of guanethidine, bretyllium tosylate, or reserpine (Angeletti and Levi-Montalcini, 1972).

Immunosympathectomy. Nerve growth factor is a protein that promotes growth and differentiation of certain autonomic and sensory neurons in tissue culture and developing experimental animals. Extensive studies of this substance and its antibody have been carried out by Levi-Montalcini, Angeletti, and co-workers (Levi-Montalcini, 1972a, 1972b; Angeletti, 1972b). Administration of nerve growth factor antiserum to newborn animals leads to a loss of sympathetic neurons and their axons, most of which are unmyelinated (Levi-Montalcini and Boeker, 1960; Aguayo et al., 1972b). Destructive lesions of autonomic ganglia have followed administration of ganglionic antigens to rabbits, as described by Appenzeller, Arnason, and Adams (1965), but no detailed study of changes of unmyelinated fibers has been reported for this model.

Hereditary Sensory Neuropathy of Mice. A genetically determined disorder of dorsal root ganglion cells in mice has been shown to cause an axonal degeneration with involvement of both myelinated and unmyelinated nerve fibers (Janota, 1972; Peyronnard and Aguayo, 1972). This disorder affects the animal during the first weeks of life; it is transmitted as an autosomal recessive gene.

RESPONSES OF UNMYELINATED NERVE FIBERS TO INJURY

In this section, the ultrastructural aspects of unmyelinated nerve fiber reactions are emphasized. Observations based on other techniques are discussed as they relate to electron microscopic findings. Reactions in the three main components of unmyelinated nerves — axons, Schwann cells, and connective tissue — are described separately, even though it is recognized that they are interdependent.

Axonal Changes

Axonal interruption, whether by transection or crush, has been the most useful experimental method for understanding degenerative and regenerative responses in axons of peripheral unmyelinated nerve fibers. Therefore, particular attention is paid to responses that result from this form of injury; changes after other forms of injury are presented for comparison.

AFTER AXONAL INTERRUPTION

Degeneration. In transected or crushed unmyelinated nerves, changes vary along the length of the injured axons. Early electron microscopic reports on the degeneration of unmyelinated nerve fibers in nerves and roots that contain both myelinated and unmyelinated fibers were conflicting. Nathaniel and Pease (1963) reported that distal segments of unmyelinated fibers degenerated within 48 hours, whereas Ohmi (1962) and Lee (1963) suggested that distal stumps of such axons

had not degenerated by 35 days after transection. It has now been established in autonomic nerves that distal segments of unmyelinated axons degenerate shortly after interruption (Blumcke et al., 1968; Hamori et al., 1968; Iwayama, 1970; Dyck and Hopkins, 1972; Bray et al., 1972; Thomas et al., 1972). The difficulties in determining the exact morphologic characteristics of the degenerative process in unmyelinated nerve fibers may be explained by certain aspects of their structure. In myelinated fibers, interruption of a single axon leads to an inevitable breakdown of its myelin sheath; in contrast, several axons must be lost in unmyelinated fibers before their Schwann cell appearance is noticeably altered. Consequently, even a few interrupted myelinated axons can be recognized by the characteristic appearance of myelin debris,

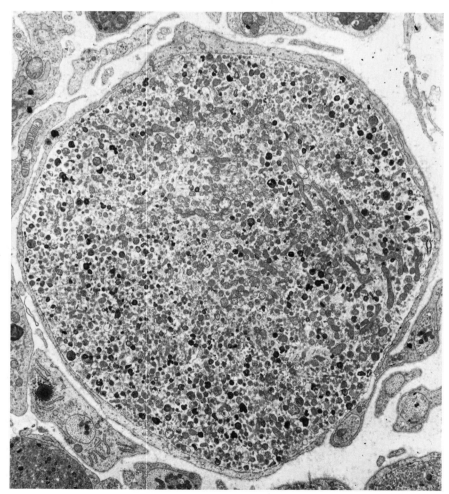

Figure 17–6 A swollen axon near the point of injury contains mitochondria and dense bodies. Schwann cell cytoplasm is stretched at the periphery of the enlarged axon. Normal appearing axons are also present. Rabbit anterior mesenteric nerve two days after transection. × 2500.

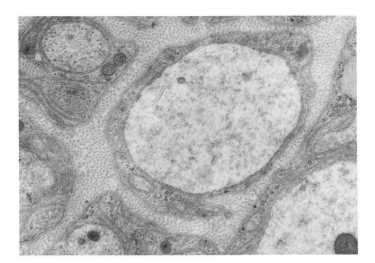

Figure 17–7 Swollen axons distal to the point of injury contain pale, amorphous material. Rat cervical sympathetic trunk one day after crush injury. × 16,000.

while degenerating unmyelinated axons may only be identified by subtle changes confined to the axon itself. The overlapping of degenerative and regenerative changes in injured unmyelinated nerves imposes additional problems in interpretation, for regenerative axonal sprouting begins while degenerative changes are still present.

Initially, after axonal interruption, large axonal swellings up to 20 times as large as the normal axonal diameter occur for the first few millimeters adjacent to the point of injury (Bray et al., 1972). These swollen axons are packed with mitochondria, vesicles, lamellar bodies, and dense amorphous structures as well as tubules and filaments in disarray (Fig. 17–6). Similar axonal changes are observed in myelinated nerve fibers after interruption (Blumcke et al., 1966; Webster, 1962). This type of reaction is more prominent in transected anterior mesenteric nerves than in crushed cervical sympathetic trunks.

Distal portions of interrupted unmyelinated axons show clear swellings during the first 24 to 48 hours after injury (Fig. 17–7). The precise fate of such axonal swellings remains obscure (Dyck and Hopkins, 1972; Thomas et al., 1972); presumably they are rapidly resorbed, for such swollen axons are transient, being rarely observed more than 48 hours after injury. Some axonal remnants may persist as dense amorphous bodies within Schwann cell cytoplasm (Iwayama, 1970). Unmyelinated axons in tissue culture also show clear swellings in response to transection, nutritional deprivation (Mire et al., 1970), and cadmium chloride poisoning (Tischner and Schröder, 1972).

Axonal swellings, also seen in constricted unmyelinated nerves, have been attributed to damming of axoplasmic flow (Kapeller and Mayor, 1969a, 1969b). In such experiments, however, it is difficult to avoid axonal interruption due to crush injury, so other mechanisms may also be involved.

As reported by Aitken and Thomas (1962) in myelinated fibers, retrograde changes also occur in unmyelinated nerves after interruption. These changes may include loss of entire neurons if axonal interruption occurs near their cell bodies. Because of the short length of unmyelinated nerves studied experimentally, retrograde changes can thus extend to the nerve cell body, causing a reduction in the number of ganglionic cells. In later stages, some axons that fail to regenerate can undergo retrograde atrophy and degeneration (Bray and Aguayo, 1974).

Regeneration. The rapidity with which unmyelinated nerve fibers regenerate has been demonstrated by functional and morphologic studies (Peebles, 1954; Murray and Thompson, 1957; Hopkins and Lambert, 1972a; Bray et al., 1972; Aguayo et al., 1973b). On the basis of these studies four phases of unmyelinated fiber regeneration have been recognized: axonal sprouting, longitudinal growth, loss of redundant sprouts, and axonal maturation.

Axonal sprouting is the initial phase of regeneration appearing one or two days after axonal interruption. Multiple axonal branches, called sprouts, are seen near the end of the proximal stump of transected nerves and in the 1 to 2 mm proximal to a nerve crush (Fig. 17–8). The axonal sprouts are similar

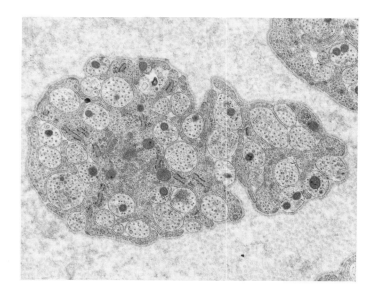

Figure 17-8 Numerous axonal sprouts are partially enclosed by Schwann cell processes in regenerating unmyelinated nerves. Electron micrograph of proximal stump of rabbit anterior mesenteric nerve. × 16,000.

in size and in their clustered appearance to those in developing nerves (Ochoa, 1971; Aguayo et al., 1973a, 1973b). In early stages following crush injury the appearance of axonal sprouts may be difficult to differentiate from that of Schwann cell processes (Dyck and Hopkins, 1972).

Several conditions seem essential for sprouting to occur: axonal interruption, neuronal preservation, synthesis of structural material for new axons, and transport of this material to the axonal tip. Various chemical and physical factors have been reported to be capable of modifying axonal sprouting in vivo and in vitro. Such factors include cyclic adenosine monophosphate (Roisen, 1972), nerve growth factor (Levi-Montalcini and Angeletti, 1968), prostaglandins (Recklies et al., 1973), a factor released from interrupted axons ("neurocletin") (Hoffman and Springell, 1951), and other substances (Yamada et al., 1971). The extent of axonal sprouting can also be influenced by various properties of the original axon, including its size (Bray et al., 1973).

Longitudinal growth of regenerating axons occurs rapidly after injury; rates of 1 to 2 mm per day for regenerating cervical sympathetic nerves were calculated by Hopkins (1970). The direction and arrangement of axonal regrowth is influenced by the type of injury. When unmyelinated axons have been interrupted by crush injury, the basal laminae of the Schwann cells remain intact and serve as guides for longitudinally oriented regrowth (Haftek and Thomas, 1968; Dyck and Hopkins, 1972). The number of axon–Schwann

cell complexes per whole transverse section of nerve is not significantly altered in such regenerating nerves (Bray et al., 1973; Bray and Aguayo, 1974). In contrast, after nerve transection, fibers extend in many directions, often following blood vessels (Evans and Murray, 1954; Bray et al., 1972; Aguayo et al., 1973b). The presence of myelinated fibers also influences the orientation of regenerating unmyelinated nerve fibers. Thus, when unmyelinated fibers regenerate in mixed nerves they tend to follow and encircle myelinated fibers (Fig. 17–9) (Evans and Murray, 1953; King and Thomas, 1971). It has been suggested that this remarkable arrangement develops because of different Schwann cell multiplication rates for myelinated fibers, reported by Abercrombie and Johnson (1946), and Romine and co-workers (1974), with regenerating unmyelinated axons tending to follow the more rapidly developing Schwann cell columns (Büngner bands) of interrupted myelinated fibers (King and Thomas, 1971).

Many regenerating axons gradually increase in diameter (maturation) while total axonal numbers progressively decline because of loss of sprouts that have failed to mature. When longitudinal regrowth and formation of synaptic connections are prevented by the isolation of regenerating proximal stumps of unmyelinated nerves within siliconized rubber tubes, all sprouts fail to mature (Aguayo et al., 1973b). Thus, as Aitken (1949) reported in myelinated fibers, the establishment of functional connections seems to be an important prerequisite for axonal diameters to increase;

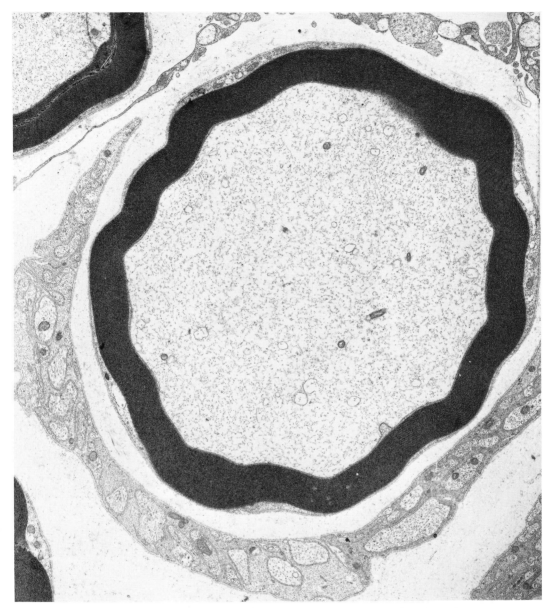

Figure 17–9   Aberrant regeneration in injured rabbit vagus nerve. A regenerating myelinated fiber appears partially encircled by a crescentic formation composed of multiple Schwann cell processes and unmyelinated axons. × 9000. (From King, R. H. M., and Thomas, P. K.: Electron microscope observations on aberrant regeneration of unmyelinated axons in the vagus nerve of the rabbit. Acta Neuropathol. (Berl.), *18*:150–159, 1971. © Springer-Verlag, Berlin, Heidelberg, New York, 1971. Reprinted by permission.)

unmyelinated axons that fail to make such connections gradually atrophy, and some disappear. The persistence of significant numbers of axons of small diameter, however, distorts the size frequency distribution for regenerating axons and influences the total number of fibers within regenerating nerves (Fig. 17–10) (Orgel et al., 1972; Dyck and Hopkins, 1972; Bray and Aguayo, 1974).

OTHER EXPERIMENTAL MODELS

Axonal swellings containing dense accumulations similar to those seen adjacent to interrupted axons are present in unmyelinated fibers of posterior roots and sensory nerves affected by the hereditary degeneration of dorsal root ganglion cells found in mice (Janota, 1972; Peyronnard and Aguayo, 1972).

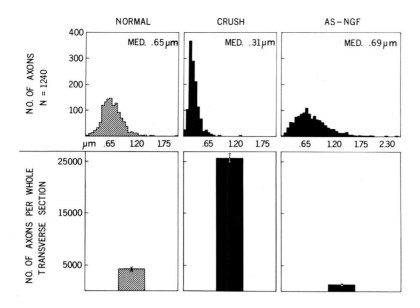

Figure 17-10 Axonal diameter histograms (*above*) and total axonal populations (*below*) in normal (cross hatched bars) and pathologic (solid bars) unmyelinated nerve fibers of rat cervical sympathetic trunks. After crush injury, there is a marked reduction in the median axonal diameters (MED.); little change in diameters follows neonatal administration of nerve growth factor antiserum (AS-NGF). Axonal populations increase fivefold two weeks after crush, but following AS-NGF, axonal counts remain only one third of normal.

These presumably represent axons degenerating as a result of a primary change in the cell body. Such axonal swellings were not, however, observed after neonatal administration of nerve growth factor antiserum, a procedure that causes a loss of sympathetic neurons and axons in rat cervical sympathetic nerves (Aguayo et al., 1972a).

Spontaneous regenerative axonal sprouting does not occur in cervical sympathetic trunks of rats treated neonatally with nerve growth factor antiserum, even though axonal populations are reduced to approximately 30 per cent of normal (Aguayo et al., 1972a). Because the surviving neurons do not sprout, it could be suggested that nerve growth factor antiserum has rendered them incapable of such a response. This hypothesis seems unlikely for they are capable of sprouting after crush injury (Bray et al., 1973). These experimental observations emphasize the effectiveness of axonal interruption as a stimulus for regenerative sprouting.

Schwann Cell Changes

The responses of Schwann cells after unmyelinated nerve fiber injury may involve changes in shape or number.

Morphologic changes in Schwann cells are present shortly after axonal interruption. Schwann cell processes are thinned and stretched by the acute axonal swellings that occur adjacent to the point of unmyelinated fiber injury (see Fig. 17-6). Some swollen axons may be covered only by Schwann cell basal lamina, suggesting that they have enlarged beyond the limits of their covering Schwann cells. Schwann cells may also be distended by clusters of regenerating axonal sprouts. Bundles of sprouts initially surrounded by Schwann cell processes are eventually segregated into smaller groups. Finally, individual axons are completely enclosed by Schwann cell cytoplasm (Dyck and Hopkins, 1972; Aguayo et al., 1973b). During regeneration, Schwann cells show evidence of increased metabolic activity, with prominent nuclei, ribosomes, and Golgi networks; dense amorphous and lamellar inclusions may also appear in their cytoplasm.

The appearance of Schwann cells is considerably different when large numbers of unmyelinated axons are lost and fail to regenerate. Following administration of nerve growth factor antiserum to newborn rats, some Schwann cells of unmyelinated fibers in the cervical sympathetic trunk have elongated processes and contain collagen pockets, although they may also enclose normal numbers of axons (Fig. 17-11). Collagen pockets within Schwann cells may result from processes wrapping around bundles of collagen. On the other hand, because many collagen pockets are similar in size to normal axons, some may be caused by collagen growing into spaces previously occupied by axons. These changes, which are present in the cervical sympathetic nerves of immunosympathectomized

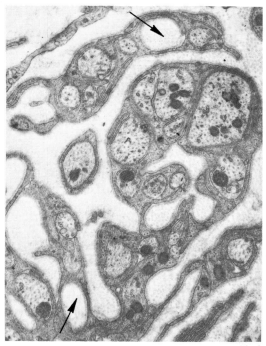

Figure 17–11 Unmyelinated nerve fibers from the cervical sympathetic nerves of a six week old rat treated neonatally with nerve growth factor antiserum. Schwann cell processes are elongated and contain numerous collagen pockets (arrows) as well as axons. × 7200.

the anterior mesenteric ganglia and observed that Schwann cell nuclei did not increase in the distal portions of these nerves. It has now been established that Schwann cell nuclei multiply in unmyelinated fibers regenerating after simple axonal interruption (Abercrombie et al., 1959; Bray et al., 1972; Peyronnard et al., 1973), although the response is less vigorous than in myelinated fibers (Abercrombie and Johnson, 1946; Romine et al., 1975).

Increased numbers of Schwann cell nuclei are apparent in cross sections of regenerating unmyelinated nerves as well as in longitudinally teased fibers (Bray et al., 1972, 1973; Peyronnard et al., 1973). Close to the site of injury, Schwann cell nuclei approximately double in number in the rat cervical sympathetic trunk following crush injury (Bray et al., 1973). The numerical increase in Schwann cells is associated with a shortening of individual Schwann cell territories, as indicated by a reduction of their median internuclear distances to approximately 50 per cent of normal (Peyronnard et al., 1973). Thus, the shortening of Schwann cell territories in regenerating unmyelinated fibers is similar to the reduction of internodal length that characterizes regenerating myelinated fibers (Fullerton et al., 1965). Short Schwann cell territories are also observed in unmyelinated as well as in myelinated nerve fibers during development (Fig. 17–12).

Schwann cell responses differ for crushed and transected unmyelinated nerves. After crush injury, Schwann cells multiply within the residual basal laminae. Thus, although their internuclear distances are reduced (Peyronnard et al., 1973). The total number of axon–Schwann cell units per whole transverse section remains relatively constant (Bray et al., 1973). After transection, however, proliferating Schwann cells accompany the regenerating axons and follow their course.

Loss of unmyelinated Schwann cells with preservation of axons has been observed after x-irradiation of nerves in tissue culture by Masurovsky, Bunge, and Bunge (1967) and after irradiation of the cervical sympathetic trunk by Aguayo and co-workers (1973c). Redundant Schwann cell basal laminae can be seen surrounding axons in such nerves and are also present in other situations in which there is shrinkage of the cross sectional area and volume of individual Schwann cell complexes (Nathaniel and Pease, 1963).

animals studied between birth and six weeks of age, as reported by Aguayo and co-workers (1972a, 1972b), are less prominent in animals studied at six to eight months of age (Bray et al., 1973). This suggests that, following axonal loss, the early changes in Schwann cells are eventually modified. Similar Schwann cell changes with elongation of processes and collagen pockets are seen in unmyelinated nerves of immature mice with hereditary dorsal root ganglion cell degeneration (Peyronnard and Aguayo, 1972). Because the axonal loss in both these instances occurs in immature animals, it is possible that immaturity may influence the configuration of the Schwann cell responses. Elongated Schwann cell processes with collagen pockets can, however, also be observed several months after axonal interruption due to crush injury of the cervical sympathetic trunk in the adult rat, suggesting that other mechanisms must also be considered (Bray and Aguayo, 1974).

It has been doubted whether Schwann cells multiply after interruption of unmyelinated axons. Joseph (1947, 1950) studied rabbit anterior mesenteric nerves after removal of

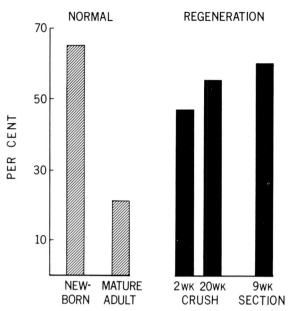

Figure 17–12 Proportion of internuclear Schwann cell distances measuring less than 60 μm. Unmyelinated nerve fibers from normal cervical sympathetic trunks of newborn and adult rats (cross hatched bars) are compared with unmyelinated fibers regenerating 2 and 20 weeks after crush injury and 9 weeks after transection (solid bars). In fibers from newborn and regenerating nerves, there are more than twice as many short internuclear distances as in normal mature nerves.

Connective Tissue Changes

In experimental lesions of unmyelinated nerves, connective tissue changes vary, depending upon the degree of perineurial and endoneurial disruption. After crush injury, the connective tissue architecture of unmyelinated nerves is relatively preserved; in this way the regenerating rat cervical sympathetic trunk retains its original unifascicular character (Dyck and Hopkins, 1972). By contrast, after transection, unmyelinated nerves regenerate in a multifascicular pattern (Aguayo et al., 1973b). During the first week after transection of rabbit anterior mesenteric nerves, spindle-shaped cells resembling endoneurial fibroblasts are present among the regenerating axonal sprouts and their associated Schwann cells. At later stages, these cells outline multiple small fascicles, many of which contain groups of unmyelinated nerve fibers. Similar changes have also been observed in transected rat cervical sympathetic trunks. It is likely that the pattern of multifasciculation that occurs after unmyelinated nerve transection prevents the degree of

axonal interchange that usually occurs between unmyelinated fibers.

PATTERNS OF UNMYELINATED NERVE FIBER RESPONSES

Although ultrastructural studies of unmyelinated nerve fibers have reemphasized the complexity of peripheral nerve histopathology, they have also suggested certain general patterns of response. In particular, two morphologic patterns distinguished by the presence or absence of regenerative activity have become apparent (Fig. 17–13) (Aguayo et al., 1973d).

Pattern A. The experimental method that best produces a regenerative appearance in unmyelinated fibers is axonal interruption. Crushed or transected unmyelinated nerves initially show reactive changes near the point of injury and rapid disappearance of distal axonal segments. The rapid onset of sprouting

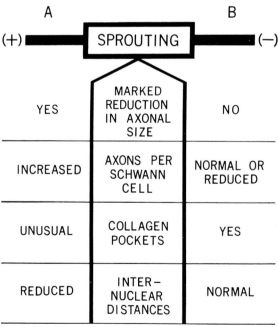

A		B
(+)	SPROUTING	(−)
YES	MARKED REDUCTION IN AXONAL SIZE	NO
INCREASED	AXONS PER SCHWANN CELL	NORMAL OR REDUCED
UNUSUAL	COLLAGEN POCKETS	YES
REDUCED	INTER-NUCLEAR DISTANCES	NORMAL

Figure 17–13 Principal changes that characterize two patterns of response in unmyelinated nerve fibers. In pattern A, regeneration follows axonal interruption; in pattern B, there is absence of regeneration following axonal loss. The presence or absence of axonal sprouting is the main factor that differentiates these two patterns by influencing the median diameter of axons and their total number. In pattern B, Schwann cells may contain collagen pockets, while in pattern A there is a shortening of Schwann cell internuclear distances.

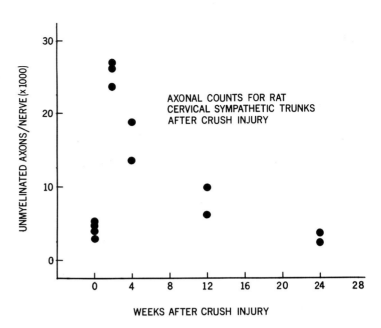

Figure 17–14 Regenerating axonal sprouts after crush injury. Rat cervical sympathetic trunks were crushed and total numbers of axons determined from each whole transverse section (●) at various times after injury. Values for control nerves are shown at zero time. Two weeks after crush there is a fivefold increase in the axonal population, which gradually declines to near normal by six months after injury.

produces a striking increase in the total number of axons and a reduction in their median diameters to approximately half of normal (see Fig. 17–10). The increase in axonal population reaches its maximum during the first few weeks after injury; during this time, axon–Schwann cell ratios are augmented and the appearance of unmyelinated nerve fibers resembles that seen during development. These changes are dynamic rather than static, for with time, there is a gradual decline in the number of sprouts and a decrease in axon–Schwann cell unit ratios (Fig. 17–14). This secondary loss presumably affects axons that have failed to complete longitudinal growth and establish terminal connections. Thus, during this phase of regeneration certain populations of axons mature while others undergo atrophy and presumably disappear. Even though total axonal populations may fall to nearly normal levels, the proportion of small axons remains increased (Bray and Aguayo, 1974).

The total number of axons that regenerate after nerve injury is also dependent upon the extent of retrograde axonal and neuronal degeneration. When injury occurs near the cell body, retrograde degeneration is more common; consequently, the population of neurons from which regenerating axons must originate is reduced. Conversely, regeneration is likely to be more complete when injury occurs remote from the cell body and close to the natural termination of the axons, as when

mixed cutaneous nerves reinnervate skin grafts (Orgel et al., 1972). Because the axonal branching that occurs in such circumstances is greater for unmyelinated than for myelinated axons, there is a persistent imbalance in the proportion of unmyelinated and myelinated fibers. Following transection or crush of unmyelinated nerve fibers, Schwann cells multiply and, as in regenerating myelinated fibers, individual Schwann cell territories become shorter than normal. The extent, duration and functional significance of this change remains to be determined.

Pattern B. A different pattern of axon and Schwann cell reactions follows axonal loss when regenerative changes are lacking. In immunosympathectomy, the experimental model that best illustrates this pattern, the loss of axons that follows neonatal administration of nerve growth factor antiserum is not accompanied by axonal sprouting from surviving nerve cells. Thus, the distribution of axonal diameters remains close to normal (see Fig. 17–10). In association with the loss of axons, some Schwann cells initially have elongated processes and contain collagen-filled pockets. These Schwann cells may redevelop normal relationships with the remaining axons. In such circumstances, quantitative analysis of the total axonal population may be the only way to differentiate these nerves from normal ones. This is particularly true if there is a proportional reduction in both unmyelinated axons and Schwann cells, as occurs when axonal loss is induced during development and thus before the full complement of Schwann cells has appeared (Aguayo et al., 1972b; Aguayo et al., 1974).

These two patterns of response in unmyelinated nerves illustrate the diversity and dynamic nature of nerve reactions to injury. Each pattern defines a particular response and does not necessarily have value in localizing the site of the primary lesion. The changes in the number, size, and arrangement of axons that result can affect conduction of nervous impulses (Hopkins and Lambert, 1972a). Dispersion of nerve impulses due to the presence of fibers with axonal diameters smaller than normal as well as to variations in the proportion of unmyelinated to myelinated fibers (pattern A) could result in functional alterations that are different from those that follow the loss of only unmyelinated axons without axonal regeneration (pattern B). For methodologic reasons, the experimental models from which these patterns emerge have mainly involved autonomic nerves. If it can be shown that these changes apply to peripheral unmyelinated fibers in general and that they occur in human neuropathies, the character and temporal sequence of certain sensory and autonomic symptoms could be better understood.

NORMAL AND ABNORMAL PHYSIOLOGY

Anthony Hopkins

Although many histologic studies were carried out on unmyelinated fibers following the discovery of the methods of silver impregnation, physiologic investigations may be said only to have begun in 1928 when Heinbecker, in Gasser's laboratory, recorded the C elevation of the compound action potential, which propagated at a velocity far slower than had previously been imagined (Bishop, 1965).

Unmyelinated fibers are found in both autonomic efferent and dorsal root afferent nerves. Studies of their physiology and pathophysiology in man are limited, and most of this section must be concerned with the results of experiments in lower mammals.

NORMAL PHYSIOLOGY

Mechanism of Conduction in Unmyelinated Fibers

Vertebrate unmyelinated axons are believed to conduct as cable structures. Because of their small size there is no possibility, at present, of recording changes in membrane potential by using intraaxonal electrodes, a technique extensively used in the exploration of the dynamics of the membrane of giant axons. It is conceivable that current may preferentially pass across the axon membrane at certain sites, but at present it is generally believed that adjacent areas of the membrane are sequentially depolarized by the approaching spike.

It is impossible to dissect out single unmyelinated axons. For single unit records, multifiber preparations are teased into bundles of small numbers of axons, of which only one is active. The diameter of the smallest myelinated fiber is about 1 μm, and such a fiber conducts at about 4.5 m per second. Very few fibers have been observed to conduct at a velocity between 3.0 and 4.5 m per second, and fibers that conduct at velocities between 2.5 and 3.0 m per second are uncommon. It is generally assumed that all axons conducting more slowly than 2.5 m per second are unmyelinated, and velocities of less than 0.7 m per second are rarely recorded. It is worth noting that if two impulses simultaneously start in two fibers conducting at 2.5 and 0.7 m per second, more than one second will separate them after they have traveled for a distance of 1 m.

DURATION AND RISE TIME OF THE SPIKE

Grundfest and Gasser (1938) gave a value of 2 milliseconds for the duration of the spike of autonomic unmyelinated axons, and Gasser (1950) found a similar value for dorsal root afferent unmyelinated axons. Paintal (1967) studied single aortic (afferent) axons. The spike duration varied between 1.2 msec for axons conducting at 2.5 m per second to about 2.8 msec for axons conducting at 1 m per second. The rise time of the spike ranged from 0.2 to 1.2 msec, varying inversely with the velocity. Paintal found practically no difference between the temporal characteristics of the fastest unmyelinated axons and those of the slowest myelinated fibers in the same nerve. Thus the rate of rise of the impulse cannot alone be responsible for the fact that conduction velocity of a myelinated fiber of 1 μm external diameter is, at 4.5 m per second, more than twice that of an unmyelinated axon of the same diameter at about 2.0 m per second. The increased velocity of the myelinated fiber must be attributed to saltatory conduction.

RELATIONSHIP BETWEEN CONDUCTION VELOCITY AND DIAMETER

The surface area of an axon of length 1 and diameter d is πdl and therefore varies linearly with diameter. If it is assumed that membrane current per square centimeter is the same in fibers of different diameters, then, as spike duration varies inversely with the diameter, the conduction velocity should tend to vary linearly with fiber diameter. Gasser (1950) observed such a relationship in dorsal root afferents, although it has also been suggested that velocity is in proportion to the square root of the diameter (Rushton, 1951). Using the light microscope to measure diameter, Gasser calculated the ratio between velocity and diameter to be 1.73. This is close to the value of 1.84 given by Dyck and Hopkins (1972) for the ratio between the fastest autonomic unmyelinated axons in the rat cervical sympathetic trunk and the diameter of the largest axons in this nerve trunk as measured by the electron microscope.

POSTSPIKE EVENTS

The chemical processes following the spike have been investigated extensively in recent years by using the rabbit sympathetic trunk in a sucrose gap (see Rang and Ritchie, 1968, for references). The sucrose gap provides an indirect way of measuring membrane potential and changes in membrane potential, although the absolute values are always a little uncertain in view of the junctional potentials arising between the sucrose and Locke's solutions.

After stimulation at 30 Hz for about five seconds, the unmyelinated axon membrane potential briefly hyperpolarizes, probably reflecting the persisting increase in potassium permeability that remains after the impulse, so that the membrane approaches the potassium equilibrium potential. This early hyperpolarization is much more prominent in dorsal root afferent unmyelinated axons than in autonomic unmyelinated axons, in which it reaches only about 3 mv (Gasser, 1958). This early phase of hyperpolarization can be exaggerated by reducing potassium ion concentration in the surrounding medium, and by cooling (Greengard and Straub, 1958).

Following this brief posttetanic hyperpolarization, there is a much longer-lasting hyperpolarization action of low amplitude. There is now good evidence that this phase is linked to the activities of the sodium pump. It is abolished by ouabain, lithium, and dinitrophenol (for references, see Rang and Ritchie, 1968). A suggestion had been put forward by Ritchie that the hyperpolarization could be accounted for in terms of depletion of potassium in the periaxonal space, as a result of its re-uptake into the nerve fiber by an electrically neutral coupled sodium-potassium pump. An electrogenic pump was subsequently suggested by other workers, however, and Rang and Ritchie (1968) have now demonstrated an electrogenic pump, although the activities of an electrically neutral coupled pump certainly contribute. Reducing the membrane conductance by replacing chloride by isethionate ion, to which the membrane is impermeable, dramatically increased the posttetanic hyperpolarization.

The initial period of hyperpolarization after repetitive stimuli may be interrupted or replaced by a period of relative depolarization, the negative afterpotential, which is believed to be due to accumulation of potassium ions in the periaxonal spaces, thereby lowering the membrane potential. It usually lasts for about 100 to 200 msec. Reducing the external potassium ion concentration reduces the negative after-potential, and, as just noted, exaggerates the early hyperpolarization. The negative after-potential is greatly increased by veratrine.

Recent investigation of sodium channels in nerve membrane have been made by using tetrodotoxin (for references, see Colquhoun et al., 1972). In low concentrations tetrodotoxin alters the sodium ionic current without altering its kinetics. Of particular interest is the resulting calculation of the number of sites of sodium channels—if they were laid in a square array there would be the surprisingly large distance of 0.2 μm between sites.

EFFECTS OF TEMPERATURE ON CONDUCTION VELOCITY

Paintal (1967) found that the temperature coefficient (Q_{10}) of three single unmyelinated axons in the cat aortic nerve was 1.3, 1.6, and 1.7 for the range between 27° and 37° C. These axons are of dorsal root origin, afferent from baroreceptors. Hopkins and Lambert (1972a) give an average Q_{10} of 1.65 for the same temperature range for autonomic C fibers, measuring the change in conduction velocity in the fastest axons of the cervical sympathetic trunk of six rats.

A Q_{10} of about 1.6 for the range from 27° to 37° C has been reported for the myelinated fibers of various species (see Paintal, 1965, for references). It is interesting to compare the delay produced by a decrease in temperature from 37° to 36° C in the transmission of an impulse in a myelinated fiber that at 37° C conducts at 75 m per second and in an unmyelinated axon that, at the same temperature, conducts at 2 m per second. Assuming a Q_{10} of 1.6 for each group, at 36° C the first axon will be conducting at 72.2 m per second and the second at 1.92 m per second. Over a length of 50 cm the first impulse will be delayed by (6.91 − 6.66) = 0.25 msec and the second by (260 − 250) = 10 msec. Thus a small change in temperature must result in a very considerable difference in the overall pattern of transmission of impulse in a mixed nerve.

Paintal (1967) and Franz and Iggo (1968) have measured the temperatures at which conduction in myelinated and unmyelinated axons is blocked. Paintal gives mean blocking temperatures of 4.3° C for 16 unmyelinated axons in the feline aortic nerve, and of 6.5° C for 16 myelinated fibers of slow conduction velocity. The figures given by the second group of workers are 2.7° and 7.2° C for feline saphenous nerve. Paintal showed a considerable overlap in the distribution of blocking temperatures of myelinated and unmyelinated axons, but Franz and Iggo found a clear distinction between the two fiber types in individual preparations. Thus investigation of, for example, the contribution of myelinated and unmyelinated axons in various

reflexes by differential block of the former by cold is valid (Paintal, 1973).

Franz and Iggo also showed that unmyelinated axons can carry trains of impulses below temperatures at which all repetitive activity in myelinated fibers had ceased (illustrated in Figure 9 of their report).

EFFECT OF AGE ON CONDUCTION VELOCITY

Hopkins and Lambert (1973) studied the cervical sympathetic trunk of growing rats. Only 1 per cent of fibers in this nerve are myelinated, even in rats aged 300 days. Conduction velocity of the fastest axons is about half the adult value 10 days after birth, and the velocity in some nerves reaches the adult range by 50 to 80 days (Fig. 17–15). This may be contrasted with the findings in myelinated fibers in the same animal (Birren and Wall, 1956). Only after about 150 days do some sciatic nerves contain myelinated axons conducting at a velocity in the range found at 300 days.

Aguayo, Terry, and Bray (1973a) have shown that the diameter of the axons in the cervical sympathetic trunk is smaller at birth than in the adult rat; it is likely that increase in diameter to the adult range is alone sufficient to account for the increase in velocity.

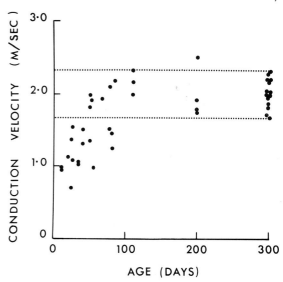

Figure 17–15 Conduction velocity of the fastest unmyelinated fibers of the cervical sympathetic trunk of rats of various ages. (From Hopkins, A. P., and Lambert, E. H.: Age changes in conduction velocity of unmyelinated fibers. J. Comp. Neurol., *147*:547–552, 1973. Reprinted by permission.)

INTRAAXONAL TRANSPORT

The intraaxonal transport of noradrenalin has recently been studied in vitro by Kirpekar, Prat, and Wakade (1972), using a fluorescent technique. Their results clearly showed that removal of the inferior mesenteric ganglion, which contains the cell bodies, has no influence on the rate of transport. Treatment with ouabain did not affect transport, but deprivation of glucose and oxygen markedly depressed transport, as did removal of sodium from the surrounding fluid. It was concluded that transport of noradrenalin depends on glycolysis or oxidative phosphorylation. This active process also requires extracellular sodium ions.

Receptors That Pass Impulses to the Cord Via Unmyelinated Axons

Müller in 1826 proposed a theory of specific nerve energies—that one nerve fiber was responsible for one particular type of sensation (cited by Collins et al., 1960). After the discovery of unmyelinated fibers, attempts were made to link these specifically to painful impulses (e.g., Ranson and Billingsley, 1916).

Bishop (1946) reviewed the earlier work, which suggested that pain was mediated by small myelinated or unmyelinated axons, based largely on a correlation of the action potential record and reflex function. He was careful to say, "What other senses this group may mediate is not known at present."

The first suggestion that unmyelinated axons could be concerned with nonnoxious stimuli came from the work of Zotterman (1939), but it was not until Douglas and Ritchie's paper (1957) that the extent of the response of unmyelinated axons to nonnoxious stimulation was realized. These workers measured the amount of receptor discharge produced by stroking the skin of the cat's leg in the distribution of the saphenous nerve. They did this by "colliding" an evoked compound action potential with the physiologic discharge. The greater the ongoing physiologic discharge, the greater is the chance that an electrically evoked impulse in any individual axon will be extinguished by an orthodromic impulse originating at the receptor; therefore the greater will be the reduction in the amplitude of whatever component of the compound action potential is

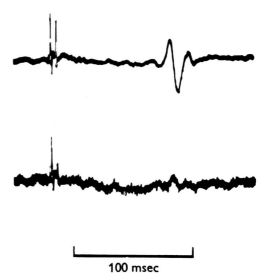

Figure 17–16 Records of the compound potential from a branch of the cat saphenous nerve. The upper control trace shows the component arising from the myelinated and the unmyelinated fibers. The lower trace shows the diminution in the amplitude of the unmyelinated component while the skin was lightly stroked with gauze. The amplitude of the myelinated component has been artificially limited by a shunt. (From Douglas, W. W., and Ritchie, J. M.: Non-medullated fibres in the saphenous nerve which signal touch. J. Physiol. (Lond.), *139*:385–399, 1957. Reprinted by permission.)

derived from axons that are physiologically active. Surprising amounts of activity of unmyelinated axons were evoked by gently stroking the skin with gauze (Fig. 17–16).

Since publication of this paper, numerous reports have appeared of somatic receptors that respond to nonnoxious stimuli and that pass their impulses through unmyelinated axons. The dynamic properties of cutaneous low-threshold mechanoreceptors with unmyelinated axons have recently been reviewed by Bessou and co-workers (1971). Using intracellular microelectrodes in the dorsal root ganglion, these workers confirmed the earlier reports of Iggo (1960), Ritchie, and others, and showed that the receptors had small receptive fields (approximately 4 × 2 mm.), exhibited after discharge following mechanical stimulation, and were excited by sudden cooling but not by heating. Bessou and associates (1971) showed that these receptors were much less capable than receptors associated with myelinated fibers of signaling rapid changes to a mechanical stimulus. They could not follow an oscillating stimulus above 1 Hz, and a long contact time was necessary to excite them.

Cutaneous receptors sensitive to nonnoxious thermal changes have been studied by Iggo (1969) and Stolwijk and Wexler (1971).

The properties of receptors with unmyelinated axons that respond to *maximum* stimuli have been analyzed by Bessou and Perl (1969). They found that low-threshold mechanoreceptors did not respond to noxious heat and irritant chemicals, but did respond briskly to cooling of the skin. A group of high-threshold receptors were not excited by low-threshold stimuli, but were polymodal in their response to noxious heat, irritant chemicals, or strong mechanical force. Of great interest is the observation of enhancement of response, so that some polymodal nocireceptors, after firing in response to damaging stimuli, would then fire again in response to a previously ineffective innocuous stimulus.

A further point against the concept that noxious stimuli are carried only in unmyelinated axons is the demonstration by Perl (1968) that such stimuli may be signaled through myelinated fibers conducting as fast as 30 to 49 m per second.

The whole field of visceral receptors with unmyelinated and myelinated afferents in the vagus nerve has been reviewed by Paintal (1973).

CENTRAL CONNECTIONS OF UNMYELINATED AFFERENT FIBERS

Stimulation of cutaneous unmyelinated axons can be shown to evoke prominent reflex discharges in the sympathetic trunk and in ventral roots, and excitatory actions in dorsolateral and anterolateral ascending tracts (for references see Gregor and Zimmermann, 1972). The interconnecting mechanisms from afferent unmyelinated axons to other systems within the nervous system originate in the dorsal horn.

Gregor and Zimmermann (1972) reported a detailed study of neurons in the cat dorsal horn responding to stimulation of cutaneous myelinated and unmyelinated axons. The effect of volleys in unmyelinated axons alone could be studied by blocking myelinated fibers in the nerve trunk by a steady direct current. These authors were able to show that about 50 per cent of dorsal horn cells that responded to myelinated fiber stimulation were also activated by volleys in unmyelinated axons. Only one cell of 36 studied

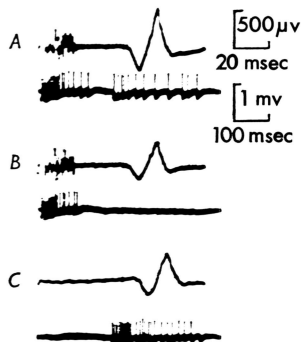

Figure 17–17 The effect of differential blocking of A fibers upon the activity of a cat dorsal horn neuron. *A, B,* and *C.* Paired records show the spike discharge of the cell (lower trace), and the simultaneously recorded compound action potential from the sural nerve in response to stimulation of the nerve (upper trace). Note different time scales for upper and lower traces. The A fiber volley was so large that it is off the screen in the upper traces in *A* and *B.* The stimulating shock was weaker in *B* than in *A.* Note that the C fiber component of the compound action potential has to reach a considerable size before the C fiber response of the neuron appears. When the sural nerve A fibers are blocked by transient polarization of the nerve proximal to the stimulus (*C*), the A fiber response of the neuron disappears, but the C discharge is increased. The stimulus was the same in *A* and *C.* (From Gregor, M., and Zimmerman, M.: Characteristics of spinal neurones responding to cutaneous myelinated and unmyelinated fibres. J. Physiol. (Lond.), *221*:555–576, 1972. Reprinted by permission.)

with supramaximal stimulation of unmyelinated axons could be shown to respond to stimulation of these axons alone. When sural myelinated fibers were blocked by polarizing current, the discharge of the neuron in response to the myelinated volley disappeared, but the discharge due to the unmyelinated volley at the same stimulation grew markedly larger (Fig. 17–17). The majority of the neurons responding to stimulation of unmyelinated axons were monosynaptically linked to the afferent fibers. Most of these cells discharged spontaneously, and most were excited by natural stimulation such as movement of hairs.

A similar study has been reported for the rhesus monkey (Wagman and Price, 1969). Again 48 of 70 units were excited by both myelinated and unmyelinated axons.

Apart from the synaptic mechanisms analyzed in the preceding paragraph, the effects of presynaptic termination of unmyelinated afferents on large myelinated afferents must also be considered. Both positive and negative dorsal root potentials have been recorded consequent on unmyelinated fiber input. A more direct analysis has been recently made by Hodge (1972), who made intracellular recordings within large myelinated afferent fibers just within the cord. Some fibers were neither depolarized nor hyperpolarized by a volley in any size afferents. Some fibers were depolarized in response to a volley in large-diameter afferents. Some of this second group showed no further change when the stimulus was increased to stimulate unmyelinated axons, but in other primary afferents hyperpolarization resulted, which would facilitate transmission of afferent input. This finding is compatible with the "gate" theory of the perception of pain in response to noxious stimulation.

Conduction in Unmyelinated Axons in Man

An estimate of the conduction velocity in human sympathetic nerve was given by Carmichael and co-workers (1941). They measured the differences in latency in the skin resistance response to remote electrical stimuli (the psychogalvanic response). The recording electrodes were placed on the front and back of the chest in the same dermatome, separated by about 40 cm. The difference in latency of about 200 msec gives a velocity of about 2 m per second. There was no distal slowing.

Compound action potentials from unmyelinated fibers can be recorded, with difficulty, through the skin of intact man. The strong stimulus currents necessary will make difficult the application of this procedure to clinical medicine, but proximal nerve block may be used to avoid pain. A direct recording of the compound unmyelinated fiber action potential in man, through a skin incision that exposed the sural nerve, was made by Collins, Nulsen, and Randt (1960). At stimuli sufficient to produce the unmyelinated component

the patients complained that the intensity was "unbearable." Multiple stimulation at this intensity was "always followed by the patient's refusal to continue." Fortunately recent advances in technique are likely to make such experiments unnecessary. Torebjörk and Hallin (1974) have recently described a technique in which percutaneous tungsten microelectrodes are used for recording C fiber unit responses from human nerves. Unitary C fiber responses can be distinguished from background noise by using signal processing and display techniques that show the response as a dot linked in time to the stimulus. The most interesting result so far from the early experiment using this technique is that repeated excitation of C fibers at 5 to 10 Hz results in considerable changes in latency and blocking of conduction. Such peripheral blocking may explain in part the decrease in pain *perception* during repetitive electrical intradermal stimulation. In further experiments, this technique can be used to study conduction velocity in normal and diseased nerves, and also to follow the effects of topical agents influencing neural activity under normal and pathologic conditions.

Dyck and Lambert (1966, 1969) have recorded action potentials in vitro from sural nerves of normal subjects and patients with neuropathy. This work is discussed later.

ABNORMAL PHYSIOLOGY

Degeneration in Unmyelinated Axons

FAILURE OF CONDUCTION

Tuckett, in 1896, showed that the postganglionic cervical sympathetic nerve of the rabbit lost its pupillodilator effect about 30 to 40 hours after section. Conduction in degenerating unmyelinated axons was studied by Heinbecker and colleagues, and by McLennan and Pascoe (both cited by Cragg, 1965), and in detail by Cragg (1965). He studied conduction and transmission in the degenerating rabbit cervical vagus nerve. Conduction was still present in some of the myelinated fibers at 67 hours after section, but not at 97 hours. The electrical responses of the unmyelinated axons, however, were still detectable over short distances at 144 hours, but not at 168 hours.

Hopkins and Lambert (1972a) carried out similar experiments on the rat cervical sympathetic trunk. They also found that degenerating axons still conducted up to six days after crush, but they did so for only short distances. Consequently, if conduction velocity is measured in a multifiber preparation between two electrodes, a false estimate of the velocity of the degenerating axons may be obtained, as the same axons do not necessarily contribute to both compound action potentials.

FAILURE OF TRANSMISSION

Cragg (1965) also studied the range of times after section at which transmission of an impulse to an effector organ failed. Transmission persists for longer in the less specialized endings (six days for the cat parotid or sweat gland and the rabbit stomach muscle) than for the cat or rabbit pupil or nictitating membrane, a multiunit muscle with specialized endings (two days). There was no relationship between time of failure and the type of transmitter released.

About two days after denervation of the feline nictitating membrane, the membrane becomes retracted. This contraction, and similar "degeneration contractions" in the rat vas deferens, supplied almost entirely by unmyelinated fibers, is probably due to sudden release of noradrenalin stores. Geffen and Hughes (1972) have recently investigated this problem in the isolated expansor secundariorum muscle of the chicken. The degeneration contraction is probably due to a sudden increase in permeability of the axon to calcium ion, causing discharge of transmitter. Withholding calcium ion from the medium abolishes the contraction, which can also be blocked by α-receptor antagonists. The contraction is contemporaneous with loss of specific histochemical fluorescence and with failure of transmission.

Regeneration in Unmyelinated Fibers

Observations on the reinnervation of the rabbit pupil, and the recordings of Hopkins (1970) suggest that unmyelinated axons regenerate at a rate of between 1 and 2 mm per day. The fastest regenerating sprouts at first conduct at about half normal velocity, and reach the lower limit of the normal range by 30 to 40 days after crush (Hopkins and

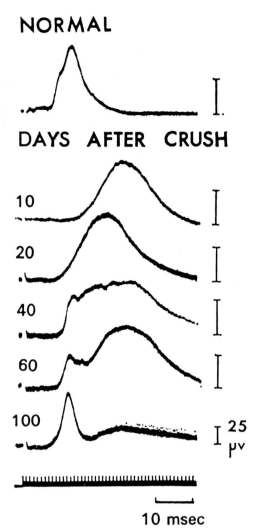

Figure 17–18 Monophasic compound action potentials recorded from the cervical sympathetic trunk of rats at various intervals after a crush, recorded about 11 mm distal to the site of the crush. The stimulating cathode was about 1 mm proximal to the site of the crush. Note the separation of the potential into two components from day 40. (From Hopkins, A. P., and Lambert, E. H.: Conduction in regenerating unmyelinated fibers. Brain, 95:213–222, 1972. Reprinted by permission.)

Lambert, 1972a). Velocity is certainly 100 per cent of normal by 100 days. This may be contrasted with myelinated fibers in which it has been shown that the velocity of regenerated fibers 12 months after the onset of regeneration does not exceed 75 per cent of the normal value (Cragg and Thomas, 1964).

Hopkins and Lambert (1972a) showed that if the compound action potential of regenerating rat cervical sympathetic fibers was recorded monophasically, the potential consistently had two peaks between 40 and 100 days (Fig. 17–18). The second peak is not an afterpotential, as the first component can be isolated on its own by using weaker stimuli. The second peak must be due to a group of axons of slower velocity and higher threshold than the first peak. These workers also showed that if they removed the superior cervical ganglion in addition to performing the crush, the first peak did not appear, suggesting that synaptic contact in the ganglion is necessary for conduction velocity to reach normal values. It may therefore also be assumed that synaptic connection is necessary for full increase in diameter of regenerating unmyelinated axons, as Aitken, Sharman, and Young (1947) showed to be true for myelinated fibers.

Conduction Changes in Unmyelinated Fibers in Neuropathy

As noted earlier, Dyck and Lambert in 1966 reported the compound action potentials recorded from sural nerve biopsies in humans. In seven normal controls, the amplitude of the unmyelinated fiber component ranged from 35 to 110 μv, the inflexion velocity ranging from 1.2 to 1.4 m per second. In one case of inherited sensory neuropathy the C potential was below the normal range (20 μv), but in this case no myelinated action potential could be recorded. As Hopkins and Lambert (1972b) point out, the absolute value of a potential recorded in this way from a biopsy depends upon whether the specimen is of whole nerve or of only a fascicle, and on the shunting conductance by moisture or connective tissue between the recording electrodes. There is no doubt, however, that Dyck and Lambert (1969) showed marked abnormalities of the unmyelinated fiber component in two cases of hereditary amyloidosis. In one patient no unmyelinated fiber component could be recorded, and in the other the potential was only 11 μv, though both had large myelinated fiber potentials (Fig. 17–19). This gross depression of the unmyelinated fiber component correlates with the already described marked reduction in numbers of unmyelinated axons in these nerves.

Figure 17–19 Compound action potentials of human sural nerve in vitro showing Aα, Aβ, and C fiber potentials from the sural nerve. *A.* Traces recorded from a healthy person. *B* and *C.* Traces from patients with amyloid neuropathy. Note the absence of a C component in *B* and the reduction in amplitude of the A components. (From Dyck, P. J., and Lambert, E. H.: Dissociated sensation in amyloidosis. Arch. Neurol., *20*:490–507, 1969. Copyright 1969, American Medical Association. Reprinted by permission.)

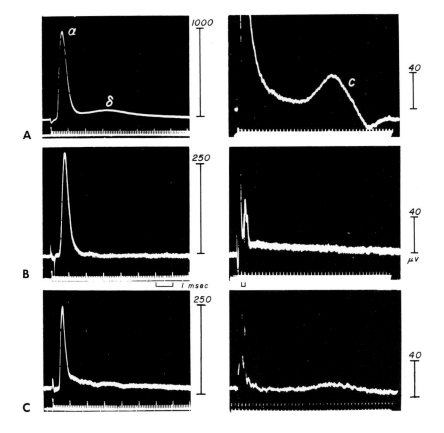

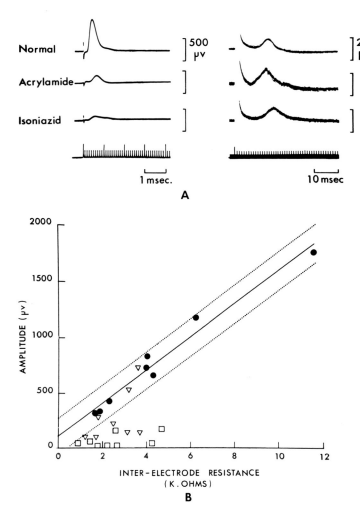

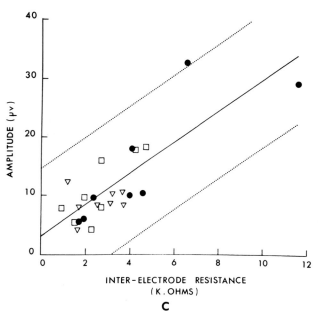

Figure 17–20 *A.* Monophasic compound action potentials of the sural nerves of normal rats and of rats intoxicated by acrylamide and isoniazid. Potentials were recorded at a point 8 mm above the calcaneus. The stimulating cathode was about 12 mm proximal to this point; the intensity of the stimulus was twice that necessary to evoke a maximal response of myelinated fibers (*left*) and unmyelinated fibers (*right*). *B.* Amplitude of the A fiber component of the sural nerve action potential of normal rats (●), and of rats intoxicated by acrylamide (□) or by isoniazid (△), plotted against the resistance between the recording electrodes. The calculated regression line for the normal rats has been drawn ± 2SE. *C.* The amplitudes of the C fiber component are plotted against the resistance between the recording electrodes. Note that the amplitudes of the A fiber component from the sural nerve of intoxicated rats is lower than normal (*B*), but the amplitude of the C fiber component is unchanged (*C*). (From Hopkins, A. P., and Lambert, E. H.: Conduction in unmyelinated fibres in experimental neuropathy. J. Neurol. Neurosurg. Psychiatry, *35*:163–169, 1972. Reprinted by permission.)

Hopkins and Lambert (1972b) have studied conduction in unmyelinated axons in experimental neuropathy in rats. Rats were intoxicated by isoniazid, which has been shown by Schröder (1970) to produce electron microscopic changes in unmyelinated fibers, and by acrylamide, which produces a profound clinical neuropathy in many animals (see Chapter 16). Figure 17–20 shows that although the myelinated fiber compound action potential was grossly reduced in intoxicated rats, there was no change in the amplitude of the C component.

Acknowledgments: Dr. Hopkins's experimental work described in this chapter was supported by a grant from the National Fund for Research into Crippling Diseases. While writing his portion of the chapter he was partly supported by a personal grant from the Epilepsy Research Fund of the British Epilepsy Association.

References

Abercrombie, M., and Johnson, M. L.: Quantitative histology of Wallerian degeneration. I. Nuclear population of rabbit sciatic nerve. J. Anat., *80*:37–50, 1946.

Abercrombie, M., Evans, D. H. L., and Murray, J. G.: Nuclear multiplication and cell migration in degenerating unmyelinated nerves. J. Anat., *93*:9–14, 1959.

Aguayo, A. J., Martin, J. B., and Bray, G. M.: Effects of nerve growth factor antiserum on peripheral unmyelinated nerve fibers. Acta Neuropathol. (Berl.), *20*:288–298, 1972a.

Aguayo, A. J., Terry, L. C., and Bray, G. M.: Spontaneous loss of axons in sympathetic unmyelinated nerves fibers of the rat during development. Brain Res., *54*:360–364, 1973a.

Aguayo, A. J., Peyronnard, J. M., and Bray, G. M.: A quantitative ultrastructural study of regeneration from isolated proximal stumps of transected unmyelinated nerves. J. Neuropathol. Exp. Neurol., *32*:256–270, 1973b.

Aguayo, A. J., Terry, L. C., and Bray, G. M.: Effects of nerve growth factor antiserum on axon–Schwann cell populations in developing unmyelinated nerve fibers. J. Neuropathol. Exp. Neurol., *33*:186, 1974.

Aguayo, A. J., Terry, L. C., and Bray, G. M.: Early ultrastructural effects of x-irradiation on autonomic nerves. In preparation, 1975.

Aguayo, A. J., Bray, G. M., Peyronnard, J. M., and Terry, L. C.: Analysis of single normal unmyelinated nerve fibers and their pathologic reactions. Trans. Am. Neurol. Assoc., *98*:70–72, 1973c.

Aguayo, A. J., Peyronnard, J. M., Martin, J. B., and Bray, G. M.: Responses of unmyelinated nerves to axonal transection and neuronal loss. *In* Desmedt, J. (ed.): New Developments in Electromyography and Clinical Neurophysiology. Vol. 2. Basel, S. Karger, 1973d, pp. 166–173.

Aguayo, A. J., Terry, L. C., Bray, G. M., and Martin, J. B.: Axonal loss in rat unmyelinated nerve fibers (UNF) during normal development and following administration of nerve growth factor antiserum (AS-NGF). Clin. Res., *20*:948, 1972b.

Aguayo, A. J., Terry, L. C., Peyronnard, J. M., Bray, G. M., and Martin J. B.: Peripheral control of axonal populations in developing rat cervical sympathetic trunks. Clin. Res., *21*:1064, 1973e.

Aitken, J. T.: The effects of peripheral connections on the maturation of regenerating nerve fibres. J. Anat., *83*:32–43, 1949.

Aitken, J. T., and Thomas, P. K.: Retrograde changes in fibre size following nerve section. J. Anat., *96*:121–129, 1962.

Aitken, J. T., Sharman, M., and Young, J. Z.: Maturation of regenerating nerve fibres with various peripheral connexions. J. Anat., *81*:1–22, 1947.

Angeletti, P. U.: Chemical sympathectomy in the newborn. *In* Steiner, G., and Schonbaum, E. (eds.): Immunosympathectomy. Amsterdam, Elsevier Publishing Co., 1972a, pp. 237–250.

Angeletti, P. U.: Antiserum to the nerve growth factor. *In* Steiner, G., and Schonbaum, E. (eds.): Immunosympathectomy. Amsterdam, Elsevier Publishing Co., 1972b, pp. 47–54.

Angeletti, P. U., and Levi-Montalcini, R.: Sympathetic nerve cell destruction in newborn mammals by 6-hydroxydopamine. Proc. Natl. Acad. Sci. U.S.A., *65*:114–121, 1970.

Angeletti, P. U., and Levi-Montalcini, R.: Growth inhibition of sympathetic cells by some adrenergic blocking agents. Proc. Natl. Acad. Sci. U.S.A., *69*:86–88, 1972.

Appenzeller, O., Arnason, B. G., and Adams, R. D.: Experimental autonomic neuropathy: an immunologically induced disorder of reflex vasomotor function. J. Neurol. Neurosurg. Psychiatry, *28*:510–515, 1965.

Bessou, P., and Perl, E. R.: Response of cutaneous sensory units with unmyelinated fibers to noxious stimuli. J. Neurophysiol., *32*:1025–1043, 1969.

Bessou, P., Burgess, P. R., Perl, E. R., and Taylor, C. B.: Dynamic properties of mechanoreceptors with unmyelinated (C) fibers. J. Neurophysiol., *34*:116–131, 1971.

Bielschowsky, M.: Die Silberimprägnation der Neurofibrillen. J. Psychol. Neurol. (Leipz.), *3*:169–189, 1904.

Birren, J. E., and Wall, P. D.: Age changes in conduction velocity, refractory period, number of fibers, connective tissue space and blood vessels. J. Comp. Neurol., *104*:1–16, 1956.

Bishop, G. H.: Neural mechanisms of cutaneous sense. Physiol. Rev., *26*:77–102, 1946.

Bishop, G. H.: My life among the axons. Ann. Rev. Physiol., *27*:1–18, 1965.

Black, I. B., Hendry, I. A., and Iversen, L. L.: Transsynaptic regulation of growth and development of adrenergic neurons in a mouse sympathetic ganglion. Brain Res., *34*:229–240, 1971.

Blümcke, S., Niedorf, H. R., and Rode, J.: Axoplasmic alterations in the proximal and distal stumps of transected nerves. Acta Neuropathol. (Berl.), *7*:44–61, 1966.

Blümcke, S., Niedorf, H. R., Rode, J., and Gehlen, E.: Die Degeneration peripherer aminergischer Nerven. Verh. Dtsch. Ges. Pathol., *52*:228–232, 1968.

Bray, G. M., and Aguayo, A. J.: Regeneration of peripheral unmyelinated nerves—fate of the axonal sprouts which develop after injury. J. Anat., *117*:517–529, 1974.

Bray, G. M., Aguayo, A. J., and Martin, J. B.: Immuno-sympathectomy: late effects on the composition of rat cervical sympathetic trunks and influence on axonal regeneration after crush. Acta Neuropathol. (Berl.), 26:345–352, 1973.

Bray, G. M., Peyronnard, J. M., and Aguayo, A. J.: Reactions of unmyelinated nerve fibers to injury—an ultrastructural study. Brain Res., 42:297–309, 1972.

Carmichael, E. A., Honeyman, W. M., Kolb, L. C., and Stewart, W. K.: Peripheral conduction rate in the sympathetic nervous system of man. J. Physiol. (Lond.), 99:338–343, 1941.

Clark, D., Hughes, J., and Gasser, H. S.: Afferent function in the group of nerve fibers of slowest conduction velocity. Am. J. Physiol., 114:69–76, 1935.

Collins, W. F., Nulsen, F. E., and Randt, C. T.: Relation of peripheral nerve fiber size and sensation in man. Arch. Neurol., 3:381–385, 1960.

Colquhoun, D., Henderson, R., and Ritchie, J. M.: The binding of labelled tetrodotoxin to non-myelinated nerve fibres. J. Physiol. (Lond.), 227:95–126, 1972.

Cottle, M. K., and Mitchell, R.: Degeneration time for optimal staining by Nauta technique. A study on transected vagal fibers of the cat. J. Comp. Neurol., 128:209–217, 1966.

Cragg, B. G.: Failure of conduction and of synaptic transmission in degenerating mammalian C fibres. J. Physiol. (Lond.), 179:95–112, 1965.

Cragg, B. G., and Thomas, P. K.: The conduction velocity of regenerated peripheral nerve fibres. J. Physiol. (Lond.), 171:164–175, 1964.

Cravioto, H.: The role of Schwann cells on the development of human peripheral nerves. An electron microscope study. J. Ultrastruct. Res., 12:634–651, 1965.

Dahlström, A.: Effects of vinblastine and colchicine on monoamine containing neurons of the rat with special regard to the axoplasmic transport of amine granules. Acta Neuropathol. (Berl.), Suppl. 5:226–237, 1971.

Dahlström, A., and Häggendal, J.: Studies on the transport of life span of amine storage granules in a peripheral adrenergic neuron system. Acta Physiol. Scand., 67:278–288, 1966.

Douglas, W. W., and Ritchie, J. M.: Non-medullated fibres in the saphenous nerve which signal touch. J. Physiol. (Lond.), 139:385–399, 1957.

Dyck, P. J., and Hopkins, A. P.: Electron microscopic observations on degeneration and regeneration of unmyelinated fibres. Brain, 95:223–234, 1972.

Dyck, P. J., and Lambert, E. H.: Numbers and diameters of nerve fibers and compound action potential of sural nerve; controls and hereditary neuromuscular disorders. Trans. Am. Neurol. Assoc., 91:214–217, 1966.

Dyck, P. J., and Lambert, E. H.: Dissociated sensation in amyloidosis. Arch. Neurol., 20:490–507, 1969.

Eames, R. A., and Gamble, H. J.: Schwann cell relationships in normal human cutaneous nerves. J. Anat., 106:417–435, 1970.

Eliasson, S. G.: Nerve conduction changes in experimental diabetes. J. Clin. Invest., 43:2353–2358, 1964.

Ellison, J. P., and Olander, K. W.: Simultaneous demonstration of catecholamines and acetyl cholinesterase in peripheral autonomic nerves. Am. J. Anat., 135:23–32, 1972.

Evans, D. H. L., and Murray, J. G.: Orientation of regenerating non-medullated nerves. J. Physiol. (Lond.), 120:52–53, 1953.

Evans, D. H. L., and Murray, J. G.: Regeneration of non-medullated nerve fibres. J. Anat., 88:465–480, 1954.

Falck, B., Hillarp, N. A., Thieme, G., and Torp, A.: Fluorescence of catecholamines and related compounds condensed with formaldehyde. J. Histochem. Cytochem., 10:348–354, 1962.

Franz, D. N., and Iggo, A.: Conduction failure in myelinated and non-myelinated axons. J. Physiol. (Lond.), 199:319–345, 1968.

Fullerton, P. M., Gilliatt, R. W., Lascelles, R. G., and Morgan-Hughes, J. A.: The relation between fibre diameter and internodal length in chronic neuropathy. J. Physiol. (Lond.), 178:26P–28P, 1965.

Gamble, H. J., and Eames, R. A.: An electron microscope study of the connective tissues of human peripheral nerve. J. Anat., 98:655–663, 1964.

Gasser, H. S.: Unmedullated fibers originating in dorsal root ganglia. J. Gen. Physiol., 33:651–690, 1950.

Gasser, H. S.: Discussion of a paper by B. Frankenhaeuser in Warren, K. B. (ed.): The Neuron. Cold Spring Harbor Symp. Quant. Biol., 17:32–36, 1952.

Gasser, H. S.: Properties of dorsal root unmedullated fibers on the two sides of the ganglion. J. Gen. Physiol., 38:709–28, 1955.

Gasser, H. S.: The post-spike positivity of unmedullated fibers of dorsal root origin. J. Gen. Physiol., 41:613–632, 1958.

Geffen, L. B., and Hughes, C. C.: Degeneration of sympathetic nerve in vitro and development of smooth muscle supersensitivity to nor-adrenalin. J. Physiol. (Lond.), 221:71–84, 1972.

Geffen, L. B., and Ostberg, A.: Distribution of granular vesicles in normal and constricted sympathetic neurons. J. Physiol. (Lond.), 204:583–592, 1969.

Greengard, P., and Straub, R. W.: After-potentials in mammalian non-myelinated nerve fibres. J. Physiol. (Lond.), 144:442–462, 1958.

Gregor, M., and Zimmermann, M.: Characteristics of spinal neurones responding to cutaneous myelinated and unmyelinated fibres. J. Physiol. (Lond.), 221:555–576, 1972.

Grundfest, H., and Gasser, H. S.: Properties of mammalian nerve fibers of slowest conduction. Am. J. Physiol., 123:307–318, 1938.

Haftek, J., and Thomas, P. K.: Electron microscope observations on the effects of localized crush injuries on the connective tissue of peripheral nerve. J. Anat., 103:233–243, 1968.

Hamori, J., Lang, E., and Simon, L.: Experimental degeneration of the preganglionic fibers in the superior cervical ganglion of the cat. Z. Zellforsch. Mikrosk. Anat., 90:37–52, 1968.

Hillarp, N. A.: The construction and functional organization of the autonomic innervation apparatus. Acta Physiol. Scand., 46: Suppl. 157, 1959.

Hodge, C. J.: Potential changes inside central afferent terminals secondary to stimulation of large- and small-diameter peripheral nerve fibers. J. Neurophysiol., 35:30–43, 1972.

Hoffman, H., and Springell, P. H.: An attempt at the chemical identification of "neurocletin" (the substance evoking axon-sprouting). Aust. J. Exp. Biol. Med. Sci., 29:417, 1951.

Hopkins, A. P.: Conduction in regenerating unmyelinated fibers. Physiologist, 13:225, 1970.

Hopkins, A. P., and Lambert, E. H.: Conduction in regenerating unmyelinated fibres. Brain, 95:213–222, 1972a.

Hopkins, A. P., and Lambert, E. H.: Conduction in unmyelinated fibres in experimental neuropathy. J. Neurol. Neurosurg. Psychiatry, 35:163–169, 1972b.

Hopkins, A. P., and Lambert, E. H.: Age changes in conduction velocity of unmyelinated fibers. J. Comp. Neurol., 147:547–552, 1973.

Iggo, A.: Cutaneous mechanoreceptors with afferent C fibres. J. Physiol. (Lond.), 152:337–353, 1960.

Iggo, A.: Cutaneous thermoreceptors in primates and sub-primates. J. Physiol. (Lond.), 200:403–430, 1969.

Iwayama, T.: Ultrastructural changes in the nerves innervating the cerebral artery after sympathectomy. Z. Zellforsch. Mikrosk. Anat., 109:465–480, 1970.

Janota, I.: Ultrastructural studies of an hereditary sensory neuropathy in mice. (dystonia musculorum). Brain, 95:529–536, 1972.

Joseph, J.: Absence of cell multiplication during degeneration of non-myelinated nerves. J. Anat., 81: 135–139, 1947.

Joseph, J.: Further studies in changes in nuclear population in degenerating non-myelinated and finely myelinated nerves. Acta Anat. (Basel), 9:279–288, 1950.

Kapeller, K., and Mayor, D.: An electron microscope study of the early changes proximal to a constriction in sympathetic nerves. Proc. R. Soc. Lond. [Biol.], 172:39–51, 1969a.

Kapeller, K., and Mayor, D.: An electron microscope study of the early changes distal to a constriction in sympathetic nerves. Proc. R. Soc. Lond. [Biol.], 172:53–63, 1969b.

King, R. H. M., and Thomas, P. K.: Electron microscope observations on aberrant regeneration of unmyelinated axons in the vagus nerve of the rabbit. Acta Neuropathol. (Berl.), 18:150–159, 1971.

Kirpekar, S. M., Prat, J. C., and Wakade, A. R.: Metabolic and ionic requirements for the intra-axonal transport of nor-adrenalin in the cat hypogastric nerve. J. Physiol. (Lond.), 228:173–179, 1972.

Lee, J. C-Y.: Electron microscopy of Wallerian degeneration. J. Comp. Neurol., 120:65–71, 1963.

Levi-Montalcini, R.: The morphological effects of immunosympathectomy. In Steiner, G., and Schonbaum, E. (eds.): Immunosympathectomy. Amsterdam, Elsevier Publishing Co., 1972b, pp. 55–78.

Levi-Montalcini, R.: The nerve growth factor. In Steiner, G., and Schonbaum, E. (eds.): Immunosympathectomy. Amsterdam, Elsevier Publishing Co., 1972a, pp. 25–46.

Levi-Montalcini, R., and Angeletti, P. U.: Nerve growth factor. Physiol. Rev., 48:534–569, 1968.

Levi-Montalcini, R., and Boeker, B.: Destruction of the sympathetic ganglia in mammals by an antiserum to the nerve-growth promoting factor. Proc. Natl. Acad. Sci. U.S.A., 46:384–391, 1960.

Masurovsky, E. B., Bunge, M. B., and Bunge, R. P.: Cytological studies of organotypic cultures of rat dorsal root ganglia following x-irradiation in vitro. J. Cell Biol., 32:497–518, 1967.

Mire, J. J., Hendelman, W. J., and Bunge, R. P.: Observations on a transient phase of focal swelling in degenerating unmyelinated nerve fibers. J. Cell Biol., 45:9–22, 1970.

Murray, J. G., and Thompson, J. W.: The occurrence and function of collateral sprouting in the sympathetic nervous system of the cat. J. Physiol. (Lond.), 135: 133–163, 1957.

Nageotte, J.: Sheaths of the peripheral nerves. Nerve degeneration and regeneration. In Penfield, W. (ed.): Cytology and Cellular Pathology of the Nervous System. Vol. 1. New York, Paul B. Hoeber, 1932, pp. 189–239.

Nathaniel, E. J. H., and Pease, D. C.: Degenerative changes in the rat dorsal roots during Wallerian degeneration. J. Ultrastruct. Res., 9:511–532, 1963.

Ochoa, J.: The sural nerve of the human foetus: Electron microscope observations and counts of axons. J. Anat., 108:231–245, 1971.

Ochoa, J., and Mair, W. G. P.: The normal sural nerve in man. I. Ultrastructure and numbers of fibres and cells. Acta Neuropathol. (Berl.), 13:197–216, 1969a.

Ochoa, J., and Mair, W. G. P.: The normal sural nerve in man. II. Changes in the axons and Schwann cells due to ageing. Acta Neuropathol. (Berl.), 13:217–239, 1969b.

Ohmi, S.: Electron microscopy of peripheral nerve regeneration. Z. Zellforsch. Mikrosk. Anat., 56: 625–631, 1962.

Olson, L.: Intact and regenerating sympathetic noradrenaline axons in the rat sciatic nerve. Histochemie, 17:349–367, 1969.

Orgel, M., Aguayo, A., and Williams, H. B.: Sensory nerve regeneration—an experimental study of skin grafts in the rabbit. J. Anat., 111:121–135, 1972.

Paintal, A. S.: Effects of temperature on conduction in single vagal and saphenous myelinated nerve fibres of the cat. J. Physiol. (Lond.), 180:20–49, 1965.

Paintal, A. S.: A comparison of the nerve impulses of mammalian non-medullated nerve fibres with those of the smallest diameter medullated fibres. J. Physiol. (Lond.), 193:523–533, 1967.

Paintal, A. S.: Vagal sensory receptors and their reflex effects. Physiol. Rev., 53:159–227, 1973.

Peebles, E. McC.: Functional recovery after section of the cervical sympathetic trunk in the cat. Anat. Rec., 118:340, 1954.

Peerless, S. J., and Yasargil, M. G.: Adrenergic innervation of the cerebral blood vessels in the rabbit. J. Neurosurg., 35:148–154, 1971.

Perl, E. R.: Myelinated afferent fibres innervating the primate skin, and their response to noxious stimuli. J. Physiol. (Lond.), 197:593–615, 1968.

Peters, A., and Muir, A. R.: The relationships between axons and Schwann cells during development of peripheral nerves of the rat. Q. J. Exp. Physiol., 44:117–130, 1959.

Peyronnard, J. M., and Aguayo, A. J.: Hereditary sensory neuropathy in mice. In Proceedings. Seventh Canadian Congress of Neurological Sciences, Banff, Canada, 1972.

Peyronnard, J. M., Aguayo, A. J., and Bray, G. M.: Internuclear distances of Schwann cells in normal and regenerating unmyelinated nerve fibers. Arch Neurol., 29:56–59, 1973.

Peyronnard, J. M., Terry, L. C., and Aguayo, A. J.: Schwann cell internuclear distances in developing rat unmyelinated nerve fibers. Arch. Neurol., 32:36, 1975.

Prestige, M. C.: Differentiation, degeneration and the role of the periphery: quantitative considerations. In Schmidt, F. O. (ed.): The Neurosciences. New York, Rockefeller University Press, 1970, pp. 73–82.

Prestige, M. C., and Wilson, M. A.: Loss of axons from ventral roots during development. Brain Res., 41: 467–470, 1972.

Ramón y Cajal, S.: Un sencillo método de coloración

selectiva del retículo protoplasmico. Trav. Lab. Recherch. Biol. Univ. Madrid, *2*:129–221, 1903.

Rang, H. P., and Ritchie, J. M.: On the electrogenic sodium pump in mammalian non-myelinated nerve fibres and its activation by various external cations. J. Physiol. (Lond.), *196*:183–221, 1968.

Ranson, S. W., and Billingsley, P. R.: The conduction of painful afferent impulses in the spinal nerves. Am. J. Physiol., *40*:573–584, 1916.

Recklies, A., Rathbone, M. P., and Hall, R. H.: Effect of prostaglandins on remote outgrowth from chick embryo sympathetic ganglia. Canada Physiol., *4*:47, 1973.

Reier, P. J., and Hughes, A.: Evidence for spontaneous axon degeneration during peripheral nerve maturation. Am. J. Anat., *135*:147–152, 1972.

Remak, R.: Observationes anatomicae et microscopicae de systematis nervosi structura. Berlin, Reimer, 1838.

Richardson, K. C.: The fine structure of autonomic nerve endings in smooth muscle of the rat vas deferens. J. Anat., *96*:427–442, 1962.

Roisen, F.: Environmental influences on development. *In* Regenerative Phenomena in the Central Nervous System. UCLA Brain Information Service. Report No. 25. 1972.

Romine, J. S., Bray, G. M., and Aguayo, A. J.: Schwann cell multiplication in crush injured unmyelinated nerves. J. Neuropathol. Exp. Neurol., in press, 1975.

Roth, C. D., and Richardson, K. C.: Electron microscopical studies on axonal degeneration in the rat iris following ganglionectomy. Am. J. Anat., *124*: 341–359, 1969.

Rushton, W. A. H.: A theory of the effects of fibre size in medullated nerve. J. Physiol. (Lond.), *115*:101–122, 1951.

Schröder, J. M.: Die Feinstruktur markloser (Remakscher) Nervenfasern bei der Isoniazid-Neuropathie. Acta Neuropathol. (Berl.), *15*:156–175, 1970.

Shelanski, M. L., and Wiśniewski, H.: Neurofibrillary degeneration induced by vincristine therapy. Arch. Neurol., *20*:199, 1969.

Shimozawa, A.: Quantitative studies of the deep petrosal nerve of the mouse with the electron microscope. Anat. Rec., *172*:483–488, 1972.

Stolwijk, J. A. J., and Wexler, J.: Peripheral nerve activity in response to heating the cat's skin. J. Physiol. (Lond.), *214*:377–392, 1971.

Taxi, J.: Etude au microscope électronique de la dégén-érescence Wallérienne des fibres nerveuses amyé-liniques. C. R. Acad. Sci. (Paris), *248*:2796–2798, 1959.

Terry, L. C., Bray, G. M., and Aguayo, A. J.: Schwann cell multiplication in developing rat unmyelinated nerves—a radioautographic study. Brain Res., *69*:144–148, 1974.

Thoenen, H., and Tranzer, J. P.: Chemical sympathectomy by selective destruction of adrenergic nerve endings with 6-hydroxydopamine. Naunyn Schmiedebergs Arch. Pharmakol., *261*:271–288, 1968.

Thomas, P. K.: The quantitation of nerve biopsy findings. J. Neurol. Sci., *11*:285–295, 1970.

Thomas, P. K.: The ultrastructural pathology of unmyelinated axons. *In* Desmedt, J. (ed.): New Developments in Electromyography and Clinical Neurophysiology. Vol. 2. Basel, S. Karger, 1973, pp. 227–239.

Thomas, P. K., King, R. H. M., and Phelps, A. C.: Electron microscope observations of unmyelinated axons following nerve section. J. Anat., *113*:279–280, 1972.

Tischner, K. H., and Schröder, J. M.: The effects of cadmium chloride on organotypic cultures of rat sensory ganglia. J. Neurol. Sci., *16*:383–399, 1972.

Torebjörk, H. E., and Hallin, R. G.: Responses in human A and C fibres to repeated electrical intradermal stimulation. J. Neurol. Neurosurg. Psychiatry, *37*:653–664, 1974.

Tuckett, I. L.: On the structure and degeneration of non-medullated nerve fibres. J. Physiol. (Lond.), *19*:267, 1896.

Wagman, J. H., and Price, D. D.: Responses of dorsal horn cells of M. mulatta to cutaneous and sural nerve A and C fiber stimuli. J. Neurophysiol., *32*:803–817, 1969.

Webster, H. deF.: Transient focal accumulation of axonal mitochondria during the early stages of Wallerian degeneration. J. Cell Biol., *12*:361–377, 1962.

Webster, H. deF., and Billings, S. M.: Myelinated nerve fibers in Xenopus tadpoles: in vivo observations and fine structure. J. Neuropathol. Exp Neurol., *31*: 102–111, 1972.

Yamada, K. M., Spooner, B. S., and Wessells, N. K.: Ultrastructure and function of growth cones and axons of cultured nerve cells. J. Cell Biol., *49*:614–635, 1971.

Zotterman, Y.: Touch, pain and tickling; an electrophysiological investigation on cutaneous sensory nerves. J. Physiol. (Lond.), *95*:1–28, 1939.

Chapter 18

TISSUE CULTURE IN THE STUDY OF PERIPHERAL NERVE PATHOLOGY

Richard P. Bunge *and* Mary Bartlett Bunge

The purposes of this brief chapter are to describe some of the types of cultures that have been prepared from the peripheral nervous system, to cite ways in which these preparations have been employed in studies of abnormalities of peripheral nervous tissues, and to suggest how these techniques may be useful in future neuropathologic research. The greater part concerns reaction to injury as observed in cultures prepared from normal peripheral nervous tissues. Studies of cultures prepared from abnormal tissues are also discussed, but with less emphasis. The chapter cannot be considered a complete catalog of all experimentation done with peripheral nerve in culture.

ADVANTAGES

Although some methods of long-term nerve tissue culture have become less complicated than previously (Bunge and Wood, 1973), the maintenance of nerve tissue in culture for long periods remains a substantial undertaking; its demanding rituals should be attempted only when it is possible to gain clear advantages over in vivo experimentation. Primary among these advantages is the opportunity to observe cellular components of ganglia and nerves directly and to record their interactions and responses. Modern nerve tissue culture differs from the in vitro dissection of fresh nerve, commonly used before the era of the microtome (and still very

useful), in that cultures provide tissues in a steady functional state rather than in a state of progressing degeneration. Experimental observations may thus be continued for days, weeks, or even months. Cultures also provide the opportunity to isolate a portion of the nervous system from the whole organism (and thus from the influence of vascular and systemic responses) as well as to treat tissues with exactly known amounts of reagents (and, if desirable, at levels that may be injurious or lethal if given to the whole animal). Finally, culture methods provide opportunities to dissociate and cultivate separately the individual cell types that constitute the peripheral nervous system. This has much appeal, for the hope is to elucidate the function of a particular cell by studying a pure population of that cell type. This approach has recently become feasible for certain normal cells, as is described later. The appeal dims somewhat, however, when experience reveals that much cellular activity in a mixed cell community depends upon interaction between cell types. Myelin cannot be studied, for example, without the presence of both the Schwann cell and the axon, which interact in the production of the myelin sheath; an earlier report that myelin was formed around artificial fibers in culture is not convincing (Ernyei and Young, 1966; see also Field et al., 1968). More recently there have been attempts to take advantage of the exposed membrane surfaces in tissue culture to learn more of the characteristics of the cell membrane (Pfenninger, 1972). Considering the compactness of central neural

391

tissues and the substantial ensheathment of elements of the peripheral nervous system in vivo, this advantage offered by tissue culture may prove invaluable in studies of the changes in membrane properties undoubtedly involved in nervous system development and disease.

METHODS

The many and divergent methods at present employed in peripheral nerve tissue culture are not discussed here. There are now available reviews of some of the principal methods used for both highly organized cultures (Murray, 1965) and dissociated cell techniques (Varon, 1970). In general highly organized long-term cultures (frequently termed organotypic) are prepared from embryonic or newborn avian or mammalian tissues and allowed a period of weeks or months to mature in culture. The aim is to obtain a facsimile of the parent tissue with the expression of as much normal cell interaction as possible.

As is discussed later, substantial degrees of differentiation do occur, but it should be noted that the facsimile obtained differs substantially from its parent tissue in at least two ways. First, there occurs along with the process of maturation and differentiation in culture a very substantial reduction in cell population (estimated to be between 75 and 95 per cent by Sobkowicz and co-workers, 1968), which exceeds the cell loss that is a normal event in nervous system development (Prestige, 1970). Thus the technique undoubtedly favors a portion of the starting cell population particularly adaptable to the condition of tissue culture, and these may not be entirely representative of the parent population. Second, tissue culture preparations are in many ways miniaturizations of their in vivo counterparts, for they cannot be exposed to the molding influences of body growth and reshaping. Data regarding this point are available from the cultured rat dorsal root ganglion and are discussed later.

Dissociated cell preparations also are generally started from embryonic or newborn tissues. The cells can be dissociated by enzymatic treatment or by mechanical means. They are generally a mixed population, but methods are becoming available to separate cell types either by differences in density or in adhesiveness (see Okun, 1972). The prepara-

tion of normal Schwann cells for culture is not difficult, for cultivation of segments of the nerve trunk will result in axon death with survival of Schwann cells although these are invariably mixed with connective tissue elements (see discussion by Cravioto and Lockwood, 1968). Neurons are generally taken after the period of mitosis has been completed. The yield is small because their number does not increase in culture, a disadvantage that is circumvented by using tumor cells, of which the neuroblastoma cell lines are most popular. Although malignant, these cells are known to express some of the physiologic and biochemical properties characteristic of neurons (Nelson et al., 1969; Harris and Dennis, 1970; Blume et al., 1970). This type of culture can be manipulated by cloning, i.e., selecting single cells and cultivating only their progeny, for considerable variation occurs in genotype in these rapidly growing populations. The advantages of this type of culture in biochemical studies of gene expression in neurons are obvious. A disadvantage is that tumor cells are known to have abnormal surfaces (Nicolson, 1971), which precludes their use in studying normal development and cell interactions.

PREPARATIONS AVAILABLE

It can now be said that representative portions of most major divisions of the peripheral nervous system and their basic connectivity have been established in long-term tissue culture. These now include the spinal cord (with the formation of ventral root fibers), the sensory ganglia, certain autonomic ganglia, and the expected synaptic connections between these structures. In addition, it has been demonstrated that neuromuscular junctions form between spinal cord neurites and skeletal muscle in culture and that autonomic ganglia are capable of innervating smooth muscle in vitro.

Historically, the autonomic and sensory ganglia were the tissues most intensively studied. As discussed by Murray (1965), autonomic ganglia may be taken from prenatal, postnatal, or adult animals and provide particularly hearty in vitro preparations. The dependence of these cultures upon the nerve growth factor and their use in its study are well known (Levi-Montalcini and Angeletti, 1963, 1968). As would be expected from their in vivo differentiation, the fibers of autonomic

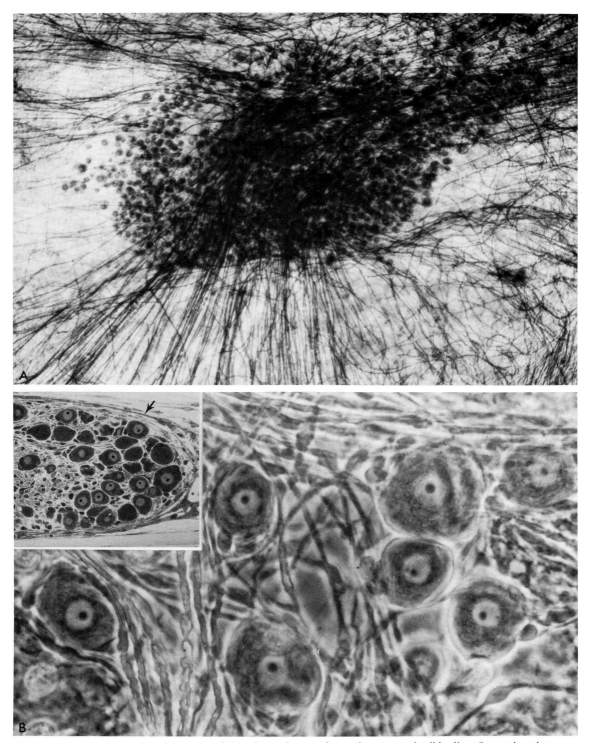

Figure 18–1 *A.* Clustered in the center of this photomicrograph are the neuronal cell bodies of a rat dorsal root ganglion that has matured in culture. Culture preparations of this type are prepared from fetal rats and require about six weeks to mature. They have been maintained for periods of up to one year. Radiating from the neuronal area are numerous myelinated nerve fibers. The particularly spread out neuronal grouping allows individual neurons to be visualized in this whole mount of an osmium tetroxide–fixed and Sudan black–stained culture. The neuronal domain is about 1 mm in diameter. *B.* Seven living neurons of a dorsal root ganglion that has matured in culture are shown in this phase contrast light micrograph. The light nucleus with a dense nucleolus, the variation in cell size, and the irregular somal outline formed by the nuclei of ensheathing satellite cells are all typical. Myelinated nerve fibers cross the field at various angles. The largest neuron is about 60 μm in diameter. *Inset*, The appearance of a similar, but much thicker, explant after fixation and sectioning. The capsule (arrow) surrounding the ganglion cell group is well shown, as are the nuclei of satellite cells closely applied to the neuronal somas.

ganglion neurons do not become myelinated in vitro; the fibers do, however, become related to Schwann cells as do unmyelinated nerve fibers in the body. Cultured sympathetic neurons are known to demonstrate their distinctive ultrastructural features (Masurovsky et al., 1970; Lever and Presley, 1971) and to retain their characteristic ability to concentrate catecholamine (England and Goldstein, 1969). It has recently been shown by Masurovsky and his associates (1972), among others, that cultured superior cervical ganglia contain not only the expected principal neurons but also the smaller, intensely fluorescent interneurons found in this ganglion in vivo (Eränkö and Eränkö, 1971). Silberstein and co-workers (1971) have shown that superior cervical ganglion neurons will provide a dense nerve plexus over iris muscle when these two tissues are grown together in organ culture.

The dorsal root ganglion taken from a prenatal or perinatal animal expresses its potential for differentiation in a remarkably organotypic manner under the proper long-term culture conditions (Fig. 18–1A and B) (Peterson and Murray, 1955; Bunge et al., 1967). The neuronal somas are of two types, either larger (and less dense) or smaller (and more dense), as in vivo. The somas are entirely surrounded by a mosaic of flattened satellite cells that in turn are embedded in a connective tissue framework containing a basal lamina as well as reticulin and collagen fibrils. With maturation the outgrowth contains both myelinated and unmyelinated nerve fibers with the expected Schwann cell relationships (see Fig. 18–6A). Winkler and Wolf (1966) have demonstrated that the trigeminal ganglion will also provide cultures of this type.

It should be noted that the organotypic nature of the sensory ganglion in culture is tempered by its miniaturization. Whereas large and small neurons are found, the largest are not as large as their counterparts in vivo. Also, the myelin segments formed are uniformly short, reflecting their residence in relation to small axons rarely more than 2 μm in diameter (Figs. 18–2 and 18–3). The failure of axons to attain larger diameters in

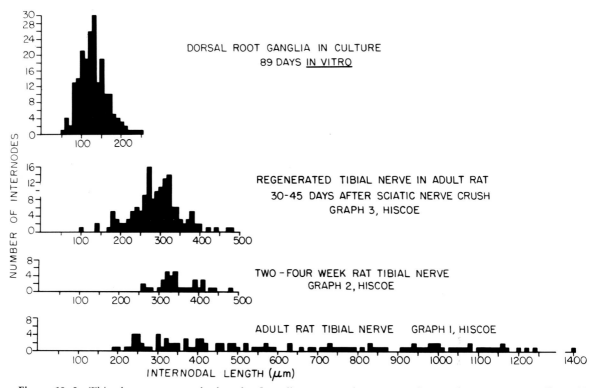

Figure 18–2 This chart compares the length of myelin segments in mature cultures of rat sensory ganglion with the lengths of myelin segments in vivo. The lower three graphs were prepared from data published by Hiscoe. (From Hiscoe, H. B.: Distribution of nodes and incisures in normal and regenerated nerve fibers. Anat. Rec., 99:447, 1947. Reprinted by permission.)

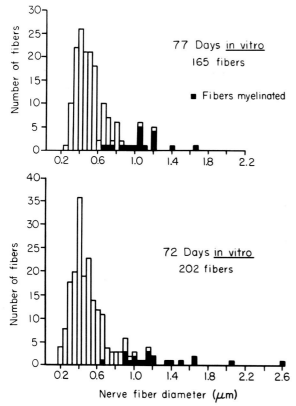

Figure 18–3 These two graphs chart the diameters of unmyelinated and myelinated nerve fibers in cultured rat dorsal root ganglia. Rat peripheral nerve in vivo contains axons up to 12 μm in diameter.

culture is thought to reflect the fact that cultured axons do not significantly increase in length after myelin formation has begun (Bunge and Bunge, 1966). The stability and the visibility of the components of the sensory ganglion, however, make it one of the most rewarding preparations for experimental study, as shown in the following section.

Spinal cord tissues have been cultured from many species and in many ways (see references given by Peterson et al., 1965, and Bunge and Wood, 1973). Of special interest here are those preparations in which circumscribed fascicles of neurites grow from segments of cultured fetal cord and form definitive ventral roots in culture (Fig. 18–4A and B). Sobkowitz, Guillery, and Bornstein (1968) have demonstrated the propensity of neurites to reform a ventral root in culture and have shown that the fibers in these roots arise from large neurons in the portion of the cord explant that was originally in the ventral position. It has now been demonstrated that these neurites that grow out from spinal cord explants in

culture have the ability to form typical neuromuscular junctions on skeletal muscle fibers grown in the same culture system (Fig. 18–5) (see discussions by Peterson and Crain, 1970, and Shimada and Fischman, 1973). The neuromuscular junction that forms in tissue culture has now been characterized in the electron microscope (James and Tresman, 1969; Pappas et al., 1971). Crain, Alfei, and Peterson (1970) have utilized the advantages of this culture system to demonstrate that rodent spinal cord neurites will form junctions on human skeletal muscle and that they exert a trophic influence on this muscle. It has also been demonstrated that single cells from dissociated spinal cord will also form junctions with striated muscle cells (Fischbach, 1972). It should be noted, however, that in these preparations only a small fraction of the isolated neurons form functional neuromuscular junctions (Fischbach, 1972); the problem of distinguishing the somatic motor neurons from the other dissociated cord neurons remains to be solved.

More recently it has been demonstrated that neurites from rat spinal cord explants will also innervate rat superior cervical ganglion neurons in culture (see Fig. 18–4B) (Olson and Bunge, 1973). These experiments provided anatomical evidence for spinal cord nerve fibers ending on the dendrites and somas of the principal cells of the superior cervical ganglion grown in proximity in organotypic culture. It was also demonstrated that entirely "foreign" neurons from cultured rat cerebral cortex did not provide synaptic input to the ganglion, indicating that a degree of synaptic specificity is retained by cultured nerve fibers.

Culture preparations of these various portions of the peripheral nervous system have also been studied for physiologic activity and connectivity. As summarized by Crain (1966), it has been shown that (1) cultured sensory ganglion cells possess physiologic properties similar to their in vivo counterparts, (2) spinal cord explants demonstrate physiologic properties indicative of intrinsic synaptic networks, (3) skeletal muscle contractions can be evoked by spinal cord stimulation, and (4) dorsal root ganglion neurons establish synaptic connections in spinal cord tissue.

Recently it has been demonstrated that two of the neuronal types just discussed may be maintained in culture in complete isolation from their normal supporting cell relation-

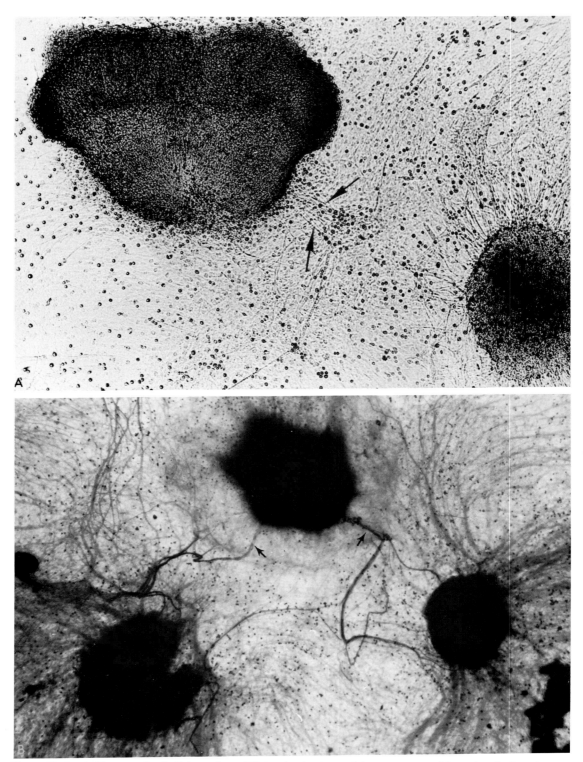

Figure 18–4 *A.* Photograph of a living culture (10 days in vitro) containing a segment of thoracic spinal cord at upper left and a portion of superior cervical ganglion at lower right. The bundle of neurites (between arrows) growing from the cord represents one ventral root. The neurites will invade the ganglion tissue in time. The distance between the two explants is about 1 mm. *B.* A preparation similar to that shown in *A*, after maturation in culture. Two ventral root regions (arrows) pass from the spinal cord segment above to approach the two superior cervical ganglion explants below. Many of the ventral root fibers are now myelinated. Some can be seen to enter the ganglia; others pass into the outgrowth to end among the various connective tissue elements there. These ganglia now contain synapses, which degenerate after cord removal. (From Olson, M. I., and Bunge, R. P.: Anatomical observations on the specificity of synapse formation in tissue culture. Brain Res., *59*:19, 1973. Reprinted by permission.)

396

ships. Isolated neurons of the superior cervical ganglia extend neurites and form complex networks when grown in isolation in culture (e.g., see Levi-Montalcini and Angeletti, 1963, and Bray, 1970). These preparations provide an opportunity for direct visualization of the growth cone in culture, and have provided information on the site of surface membrane addition in the growing nerve fiber (Bray, 1970) as well as material for electron microscopic analysis of the growth cone contents (Bunge, 1973). In rather similar preparations the effect of colchicine and cytochalasin on growth cone activity has been analyzed (Yamada et al., 1970, 1971).

Individual cells of sensory ganglia have been cultured in progressively greater degrees of isolation (Scott et al., 1969; Varon and Raiborn, 1971); a recent report illustrates isolated single mammalian dorsal root ganglion neurons completely free of associated supporting cells and demonstrates the excitability and conductile properties of neuronal processes under these circumstances (Okun, 1972). These single cell preparations from normal tissues have been developed too recently to have been employed in a significant number of experimental studies, and we must turn our attention again to organotypic cultures for a consideration of pathologic responses.

EXPERIMENTAL FINDINGS

It appears accurate to say that the seminal observation engendering the current enthusiasm for the use of nerve tissue culture in experimental studies was the demonstration in 1955 by Peterson and Murray that myelin sheath formation occurred in tissue culture. If nervous tissue could express its genetic potential to this degree in culture it was clear that this type of preparation would be highly useful. It was quite natural, then, that many early observations concerned the myelin sheath. Studies in culture have established that (1) Schmidt-Lanterman clefts were not artifacts of tissue preparation but could be directly visualized in living myelin (Peterson and Murray, 1961), (2) the Schwann cell nucleus appeared to circumnavigate the axon during the period of active myelin formation (Murray, 1965; Pomerat et al., 1967), and (3) choline incorporation occurred along the entire length of developing myelin segments

as well as into presumably mature myelin sheaths (Hendelman and Bunge, 1969). The clear visualization obtainable in cultured sensory neuronal somas allowed Deitch and Murray (1956) to demonstrate that Nissl bodies were not artifacts of preparation but did in fact exist in the living state, and Pomerat and co-workers (1967) to show that rapid particle movement occurred in lighter areas (between the Nissl bodies) of the neuronal cytoplasm. More recently these cultured neurons have been employed to study the sites of exogenous protein uptake (Holtzman and Peterson, 1969).

Response to Injury

Early studies on organotypic cultures also established that the response of myelinated fibers to axon amputation (wallerian degeneration) was similar to the pattern observed in vivo, except that it was considerably accelerated (Peterson and Murray, 1965). Taking advantage of the opportunity in tissue culture to control the cellular environment precisely, Schlaepfer and Bunge (1973) demonstrated that axon and myelin breakdown of amputated nerve fibers is substantially retarded in cultures maintained in media with decreased calcium levels.

Observations have also been made on the response of unmyelinated axons in culture to amputation or nutritional deprivation. Under direct continuous observation in culture it was found that these axons undergo a period of transient focal swelling as a part of their degenerative response (Fig. 18–6B) (Mire et al., 1970). When this swelling reaction occurs in response to glucose deprivation it can be rapidly reversed with the correction of the nutritional deficit. The authors suggested that this transient period of swelling occurs at a point at which the selective ion permeability of the axolemma is intact but the active extrusion of sodium ions is failing. Sensory ganglion cultures have also been employed in nutritional studies by Yonezawa and Iwanami (1966), who reported a complex response to thiamine deficiency.

Response to Toxic Agents

One of the early striking examples of the histiotypic fidelity of cultured peripheral

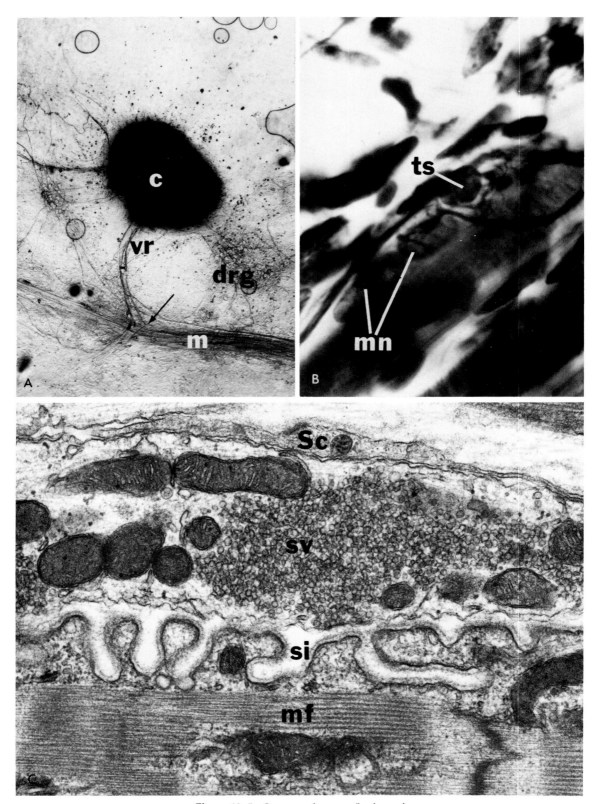

Figure 18–5 See opposite page for legend.

nerve was the demonstration that segmental demyelination occurred in response to diphtherial toxin in much the same pattern as it did in vivo (Peterson and Murray, 1965). Tissue culture allowed direct observation that the beginning of myelin damage occurred in the nodal regions and progressed toward the internode center. Direct participation by the involved Schwann cell in removing the myelin debris could also be observed.

Highly organized sensory ganglion cultures have also been utilized for a detailed study of the direct effects of x-rays in circumstances in which blood vessel response cannot contribute to the pathologic reaction (Masurovsky et al., 1967a, 1967b). These studies confirmed that the neuron is relatively resistant to damage by x-rays and illustrated some of the cytologic mechanisms engendered in damaged neurons. In addition, they demonstrated the sensitivity to ionizing irradiation of satellite cells and of the Schwann cells related to unmyelinated nerve fibers. The myelin-related Schwann cells were damaged in time by the irradiation, leading to a characteristic form of myelin breakdown. The same system was used to demonstrate the efficiency of radiation protective compounds (AET derivatives) in protecting against irradiation damage and the localization of these compounds within the tissue (Masurovsky and Bunge, 1969).

The results of direct interference with energy production in organotypic sensory ganglion cultures have been reported by Tischner and Murray (1972). Sodium azide application led to progressive and irreversible changes in neuronal cytoplasm beginning with mitochondrial damage and alterations in granular endoplasmic reticulum. With time the smooth endoplasmic reticulum of axons becomes diluted and nodes of Ranvier are lengthened. Major alterations in myelin oc-

curred later, concomitant with general tissue deterioration. Masurovsky and Bunge (1971) utilized the organized sensory ganglion cultures for a long-term study of tissue breakdown after acute cyanide poisoning. This approach permitted study of the breakdown of myelin sheaths after Schwann cell death without the intervention of phagocytic responses of any type. In the absence of viable Schwann cells myelin breakdown often occurred by a slowly progressive lamellar splitting with retention of the tubular form of the myelin segments.

Sensory ganglion cultures have also been advantageously used to study nervous tissue responses to the toxic effects of thallium. Peterson and Murray (1965) first demonstrated the distinctive swellings that occur in the paranodal regions of myelin in sensory ganglion cultures exposed to thallium. This response has now been shown to involve mitochondrial damage (Spencer et al., 1972). It should be noted that the production of large vacuoles within the perikaryal neuronal cytoplasm has also been observed in response to carefully selected doses of thallium (Hendelman, 1969). The similarity in size between the potassium and thallium ions may provide a clue to the particular sensitivity of nervous tissue to thallium.

Cultured sensory neurons have recently been noted to undergo a peculiarly selective (and reversible) response to the cardiac glycoside, ouabain. This potent inhibitor of the sodium and potassium–activated adenosinetriphosphatase, which is involved in sodium and potassium pumping, has little observable effect on the varied components of rodent peripheral nerve in culture even at high dosages, but it does cause a progressive swelling of the membranous compartments of the Golgi apparatus in the neuronal perikaryon (Fig.

Figure 18–5 These micrographs illustrate highly organized cultures containing a combination of spinal cord and striated muscle tissue. *A.* The remarkably histiotypic organization obtainable when cord and dorsal root ganglia are grown with a segment of striated muscle. The cord explant (c) was from a fetal mouse and was placed in culture with the dorsal root ganglion (drg) attached. Its outgrowing ventral root (vr) has coupled with regenerated muscle (m) derived from adult mouse skeletal muscle fibers. A portion of the ventral root nerve fibers arborize (arrow) as they contact the muscle; others pass over and loop back to the muscle. Living culture, 11 weeks in vitro. ×16. *B.* The complex arborization of a nerve terminal in a well-differentiated endplate structure. Note the terminal Schwann cell nucleus (ts) and the sole plate myonuclei (mn). Holmes' silver impregnation, nine weeks in vitro. ×900. *C.* An electron micrograph of a longitudinal section through a portion of motor endplate that has developed on regenerated adult mouse skeletal muscle. This muscle was grown with spinal cord tissue from a fetal mouse for a period of eight weeks. Schwann cell cytoplasm (Sc) typically caps the axon terminal, which contains an abundance of agranular synaptic vesicles (sv) approximately 40 to 50 nm in diameter. Secondary postsynaptic sarcolemmal infoldings (si) are conspicuous by this stage of development in culture. Fine structural features of well-developed striated muscle, including organized myofilament lattices (mf), are apparent. × 36,000. (This figure was generously provided by Edith Peterson (parts *A* and *B*) and Edmund Masurovsky (part *C*) of the Albert Einstein College of Medicine.)

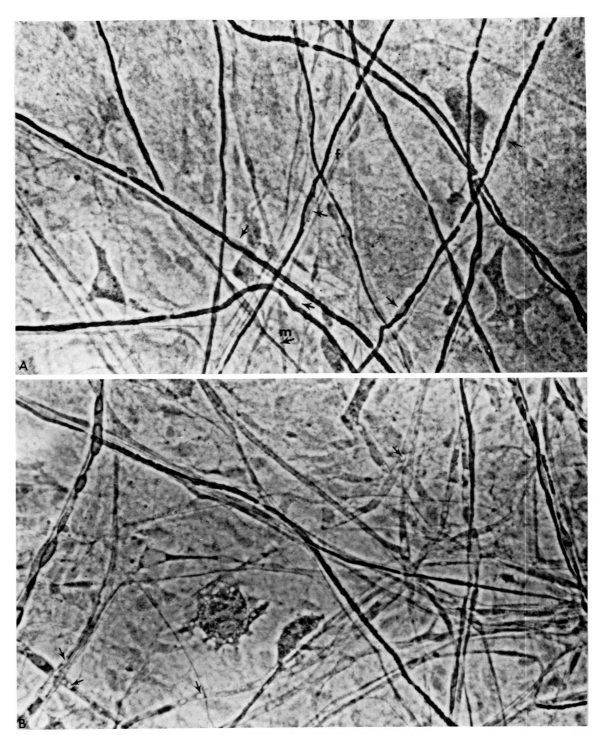

Figure 18–6 *A.* Control rat dorsal root ganglion that has matured in culture. The segments of myelin appear fairly regular in contour and are interrupted at the periodic nodes of Ranvier. Midway between the nodes are the Schwann cell nuclei (arrows), as is typical. Unmyelinated fibers are present in small fascicles (f). A myelin sheath in the process of formation is marked m. Whole mount fixed in osmium tetroxide and stained with Sudan black. × 400. *B.* Cultured rat dorsal root ganglion that has been damaged by transection (24 hours earlier) of some of the fibers that pass through this field. A myelinated fiber undergoing wallerian degeneration is seen on the left. The fascicles of unmyelinated nerve fibers contain characteristic small clear vacuole-like structures; the clearest examples are indicated by arrows. These clear regions are seen in the electron microscope to be focal swellings of the unmyelinated axons. Preparation as in *A.* × 400.

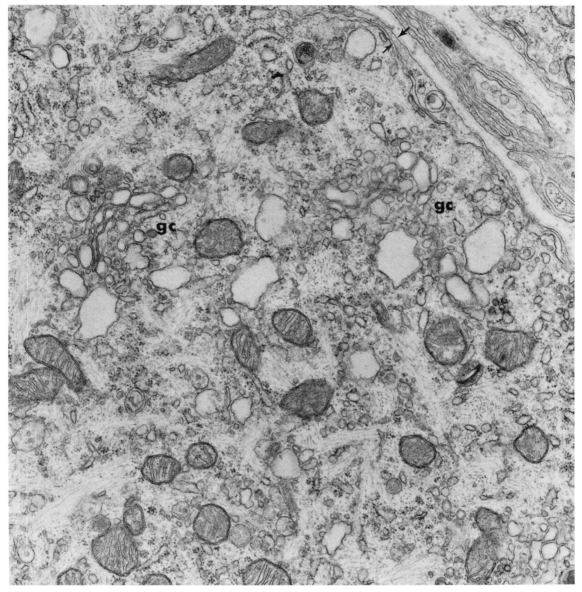

Figure 18–7   The effect of ouabain (5×10^{-5}M) administration to cultured mouse dorsal root ganglion neurons is illustrated in this electron micrograph. Some of the elements of the Golgi complex (gc) are swollen. Otherwise the cell appears normal. The typical covering of the neuronal soma by satellite cell cytoplasm (arrows) is shown at the upper right. Osmium tetroxide fixation. × 30,000.

18–7) (Whetsell and Bunge, 1969). It has been noted that this response may be related to the known activities of the Golgi region in concentrating material destined for cell export, but the real meaning of this particularly selective response in terms of neuronal function remains a mystery. The nature of this response may be related to (1) the observation that mice with the hereditary "wobbler" trait show changes in spinal cord motor neurons in the Golgi region that bear some resemblance to

the ouabain effect (Andrews and Maxwell, 1969) and (2) the fact that lithium ions also cause swelling of Golgi components (for discussion, see Whetsell and Mire, 1970).

Tissue cultures also permit observation of the direct effects of specific enzymes on living tissue components; a recent study indicates the potential usefulness (Yu and Bunge, in preparation). If fully developed myelinated peripheral nerve cultures were treated with a short (three hour) pulse of purified

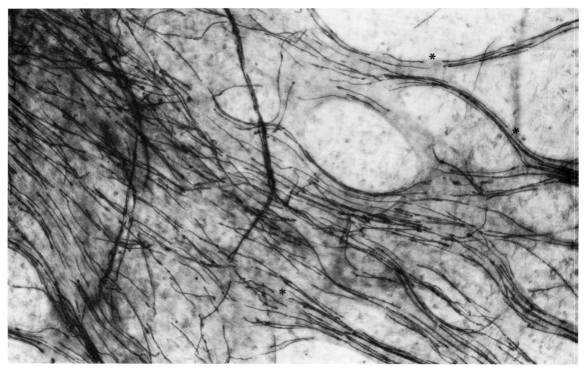

Figure 18–8   This whole mount illustrates the appearance of myelin sheaths 18 days after a three hour treatment with trypsin. Nodes (examples at *) are greatly lengthened everywhere, and the myelin bordering the node is thicker than usual as a result of the retraction that occurred during trypsin treatment. Osmium tetroxide fixation; Sudan black staining. × 100.

trypsin, the myelin segments retracted from the nodal regions, and as the node lengthened the myelin became "bunched up" in the paranodal areas; the neuronal cell body and axons were not visibly altered. Electron microscopy revealed that the myelin alterations involved loosening of the special Schwann cell–axolemmal contacts that occur near the node, but that over the next several weeks these contacts were repaired even though the induced deformation of the myelin segment was incompletely resolved (Fig. 18–8). In this instance long-term tissue culture allowed the direct observation that substantial myelin alteration or damage does not invariably lead to myelin breakdown and that after myelin damage some degree of repair of the retained myelin segment is possible.

Response to Drugs

The study of neuronal reaction to the widely used tranquilizer chlorpromazine pro-vides one of the clearest examples of the usefulness of tissue culture observations in understanding cellular responses. The fact that this drug is a fluorochrome was advantageously used by Murray, Peterson, and Loeser (1964) to demonstrate its uptake into the cytoplasm of cultured neurons. The fluorescence produced by the drug was at first diffuse, but within 24 hours it became particulate, suggesting localization within a cell organelle. Subsequent light and electron microscopic studies established that the increased cytoplasmic granularity induced by chlorpromazine as seen in the light microscope was due to the formation of large, multilaminated dense bodies in both neurons, as shown in Figure 18–9, and supporting cells (Brosnan et al., 1970). Histochemical studies indicated that lysosomal enzyme induction accompanied these changes. The authors concluded that chlorpromazine became concentrated in the multilaminated dense bodies that are a part of the lysosomal system of the cell. They also noted the similarity of this response to that observed after exposure to certain vital dyes. The appearance of large multilaminated bodies in neurons and supporting cells is also one of the effects of chloroquine administration to cultured dorsal root ganglia (Tischner, 1972).

Cultured neurons were also among the first nervous tissues to be used for morphologic studies of the effects of the plant alkaloids such as colchicine and its analogs (Peterson and Murray, 1966; Bunge and Bunge, 1968; Journey et al., 1968; Peterson and Bornstein, 1968; and Seil and Lampert, 1968). The response is dramatic and unique, as shown in Figure 18–10, and up to the stage illustrated it is slowly reversible. The speed at which the response is reversed depends upon the binding affinity of the particular alkaloid for the microtubule elements (Peterson, 1969). The

reaction involves a drastic rearrangement of neuronal cytoplasmic constituents concomitant with the disappearance of microtubules. It has also been demonstrated that this cytoplasmic response is accompanied by a substantial reduction in the centrifugal transport of proteins in cultured neurons (England et al., 1973). The response certainly involves the most fundamental properties involved in the organization of neuronal cytoplasm and the neuronal mechanisms for the intracellular transport of materials. This is an instance, however, in which similar studies can be carried out in vivo (see, for example, Gottschalk et al., 1968, and Schlaepfer, 1971), and tissue culture studies may be indicated only when precise control of the neuronal environment is desired.

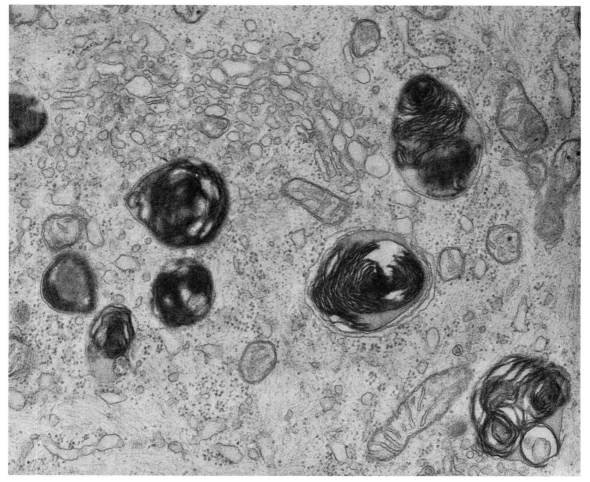

Figure 18–9 This electron micrograph shows a portion of cytoplasm of a cultured rat dorsal root ganglion neuron 24 hours after a six minute application of chlorpromazine (1.4×10^{-4}M). The outstanding change is the prominence of enlarged lysosomal bodies that contain myelin figures. Other organelles included here appear normal. Osmium tetroxide fixation. $\times$ 34,500. (From Brosnan, C. F., Bunge, M. B., and Murray, M. R.: The response of lysosomes in cultured neurons to chlorpromazine. J. Neuropathol. Exp. Neurol., 29:337, 1970. Reprinted by permission.)

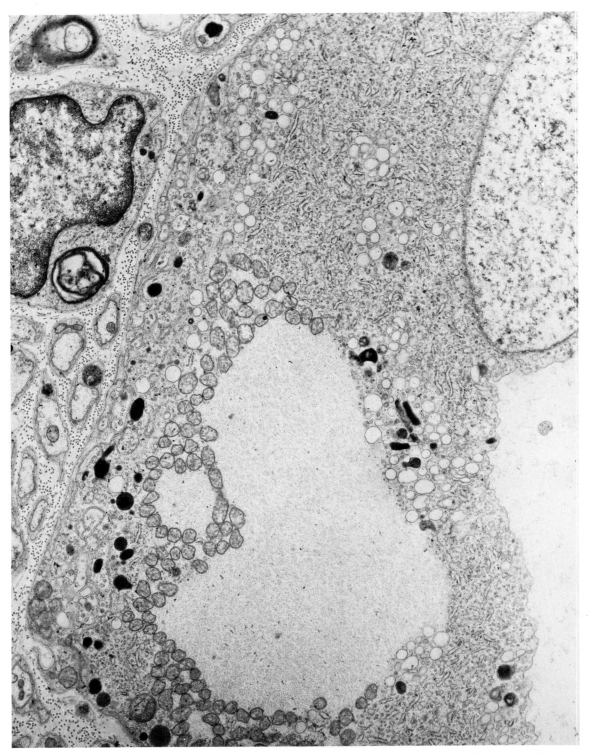

Figure 18–10 Cultured rat dorsal root ganglion neuron after three days in the presence of colchicine (0.5 μg per milliliter). The large light area in the lower center is filled with filaments. Mitochondria are clustered about them. Lysosomal and swollen Golgi elements are sequestered in certain areas, as is the Nissl substance. At higher magnification it can be seen that microtubules are no longer present. Part of a large cytoplasmic vacuole is at the right. Osmium tetroxide fixation. × 12,500.

An agent known to stabilize microtubules, deuterium oxide, has substantial effects on nervous tissue in culture (Murray and Benitez, 1968). These differ with various regions of the neuraxis, but generally involve an acceleration of growth, sometimes to the detriment of the cultured cells. Cultured sympathetic ganglia were the most greatly stimulated.

Immune Responses

The advantages of studying immune responses in isolated tissues in culture was early recognized. We shall consider here only studies on peripheral nervous tissue, though there are many parallel investigations on immune responses in the central nervous system.

From the time of its earliest description by Waksman and Adams (1955), the disease process in allergic neuritis has engendered considerable interest. The first electron microscopic study of affected peripheral nerve in rats indicated that an impressively active cellular process was involved in myelin breakdown in this disease. Mononuclear cells were observed to traverse the neurilemma, penetrate the outer mesaxon, push the Schwann cell aside, and surround and destroy the myelin sheath (Lampert, 1969). The question remained whether cell products alone in the absence of intact cells could attack the myelin sheath. Yonezawa and co-workers (1968) reported segmental demyelination, lysis, and phagocytosis of myelin sheaths after the application of sera from animals with experimental allergic neuritis to myelinated peripheral nerve cultures. Organotypic cultures of rat trigeminal ganglia were used to demonstrate that both lymph node and buffy coat cells and (less effectively) serum from sensitized animals caused the breakdown of myelin sheaths in culture (Arnason et al., 1969). Moreover, these authors were able to show that antiserum to an immunoglobulin inhibited the cell-mediated demyelination in these cultures (Winkler and Arnason, 1966).

This background proved to be most useful in clarifying the disease process in Guillain-Barré syndrome. Arnason, Winkler, and Hadler (1969) demonstrated that demyelination of cultured peripheral nervous tissue was caused by cells derived from the buffy coat layer of blood from patients with this syndrome. Cook and associates (1971) observed that serum from 26 of 31 patients with this syndrome caused demyelination of mouse sensory ganglia in culture. It was further established that the reaction was a primary demyelination rather than wallerian degeneration, was complement dependent, and was produced by both the 19S and 7S serum fractions. In these experiments, as in most others of this type performed in culture, sera from some patients with other neurologic disorders also caused demyelination. The fine structural aspects of the demyelination caused by sera from patients with Guillain-Barré syndrome have now been studied by Hirano and co-workers (1971), and their findings indicate that the pathologic process in this serum-induced demyelination is strikingly similar to that caused by invading cells in peripheral neuritis as mentioned earlier. These results demonstrated that both serum factors and buffy coat cells from patients with Guillain-Barré syndrome cause demyelination in culture and established this syndrome to be an immunologic phenomenon, with intriguing implications for central demyelinating conditions.

Virus Infections

The earliest work on virus effects on nervous tissue in culture was done with polio virus and brain cell cultures derived from human material (Hogue et al., 1955). This work proved to be of limited value in explaining the mechanism of this viral infection in nervous tissue, which may in part explain why the more highly developed organotypic cultures now available have been so little used in the study of neural virus infections. Also, because neurotypic viruses can now be grown on cells of nonneural origin, organized cultures are not necessary for studies of virus growth. These cultures should be useful, however, in studies of the cytopathologic changes accompanying virus infection. There is one report of a study of herpes simplex virus infection of organized peripheral nerve tissue cultures (Feldman et al., 1968). These workers demonstrated intracellular virus replication six to eight hours after inoculation of rat dorsal root ganglion cultures, with extracellular virus appearing 12 hours later. They also observed polykaryocyte formation involving Schwann cells but not neurons in these cultures. A progressive deterioration of neuronal somas beginning with nucleolar distortions and disintegration, margination of nuclear chromatin, and the appearance of intranuclear inclusions was observed. These changes have not been characterized at the electron microscopic level. A second report indicated that visna virus application to organotypic cultures of rat sensory ganglia produced little change, whereas the same virus preparation applied to mouse cerebellum cultures produced rapid and acute degenerative changes in the absence of virus multiplication (Bunge and Harter, 1969). It is clear that further work is needed to establish to what degree organotypic nerve tissue cultures will be useful in the study of virus infections of the peripheral nervous system.

Culture of Abnormal Tissues

If a segment of peripheral nerve is cultured without neuronal cell bodies, the axonal elements and myelin will degenerate, leaving a cellular outgrowth containing Schwann cells, fibroblasts, phagocytes and perhaps perineurial cells. This technique thus allows direct observation of Schwann cell form and activity in culture, and a comparison with these properties in cells derived from peripheral nerve tumors. It has been used to photograph normal Schwann cells serially and has led to the discovery that these cells (like the oligodendrocytes of the central nervous system) exhibit pulsatile activity in tissue culture (see recent discussion by Cravioto and Lockwood, 1968). This technique, when applied to tumors of peripheral nerve, has provided observations pertinent to the debate regarding the origin of the malignant cell (i.e., connective tissue vs. Schwann cell) in peripheral neuromas. The culture work favors the Schwann cell origin of these tumors (see Murray and Stout, 1940; Cravioto and Lockwood, 1969; among others). It would seem propitious in further studies of this type to search for unique enzymes or cellular components to use in clearly classifying the origin of the various cell types. The recent demonstration of the presence of a distinctive nervous tissue protein (S-100) in tumors derived from peripheral nerve tissue is a beginning step in this direction (Pfeiffer et al., 1972).

The foregoing parts of this chapter contain frequent references to studies on neuroblastoma cells in culture. The greater portion of these studies is at present mainly concerned with elucidating basic mechanisms of neuronal growth and metabolism. It is hoped that further work may lead to the design of effective therapeutic measures for this malignant tumor, as has recently been discussed by Goldstein (1972).

PROSPECTUS

The foregoing discussion indicates that nerve tissue culture has been useful in studying pathologic processes in peripheral nerve tissues. It is also clear, considering the complex culture systems available, that much more useful experimentation can now be done. Work on abnormalities of the neuromuscular junction or the spinal cord autonomic ganglion synapse is now possible. It should also be useful to employ the tissue combination cultures now available for the study of trophic interactions between tissues of the peripheral body regions, and a start in this direction has already been made (Harris et al., 1971; Peterson and Crain, 1972). The exploration of genetically abnormal peripheral nervous tissues in culture should prove rewarding, as has that of central nervous tissues (DeLong and Sidman, 1970). Finally, it should be noted that the recent dramatic increase in the availability of human fetal material should allow the types of experiments just discussed to be done with highly organized cultures from human sources (cf. Peterson et al., 1965).

SUMMARY

Some of the types of tissue cultures that are available from spinal cord, sensory ganglion, autonomic ganglion, and muscle tissues have been briefly described and illustrated, and their use in the study of a variety of pathologic responses discussed. These include the response of myelinated and unmyelinated axons to amputation from the neuronal soma and the response of the various cellular components of these cultures to diphtherial toxin, x-rays, cyanide, thallium, ouabain, and trypsin. Observations on the response to the drugs chlorpromazine and colchicine, immune responses in peripheral neuritis and the Guillain-Barré syndrome, and observations on herpes simplex and visna virus application have also been reviewed. From this discussion it seems clear that the culture systems that have been available for the study of peripheral nerve have been useful in clarifying pathologic processes and that the increasingly sophisticated culture systems now available should prove highly rewarding for future work.

Acknowledgments: Work in the authors' laboratory is supported by N.I.H. grant NS-09923 and grant 730 from the National Multiple Sclerosis Society. The authors are grateful to Dr. Mary I. Olson for providing Figure 18–4A and to Dr. Edmund Masurovsky for assembling Figure 18–5.

REFERENCES

Andrews, J. M., and Maxwell, D. S.: Motor neuron diseases in animals. *In* Norris, F. H., Jr., and Kurland, L. T. (eds.): Motor Neuron Diseases: Research in Amyotrophic Lateral Sclerosis and Related Disorders. Vol. 2. New York, Grune & Stratton, 1969, p. 369.

Arnason, B. G. W., Winkler, G. F., and Hadler, N. M.: Cell-mediated demyelination of peripheral nerve in tissue culture. Lab. Invest., *21*:1, 1969.

Blume, A., Gilbert, F., Wilson, S., Farber, J., Rosenberg, R., and Nirenberg, M.: Regulation of acetylcholinesterase in neuroblastoma cells. Proc. Natl. Acad. Sci. U.S.A., *67*:786, 1970.

Bray, D.: Surface movements during the growth of single explanted neurons. Proc. Natl. Acad. Sci. U.S.A., *65*:905, 1970.

Brosnan, C. F., Bunge, M. B., and Murray, M. R.: The response of lysosomes in cultured neurons to chlorpromazine. J. Neuropath. Exp. Neurol., *29*:337, 1970.

Bunge, M. B.: Fine structure of nerve fibers and growth cones of isolated sympathetic neurons in culture. J. Cell Biol., *56*:713, 1973.

Bunge, M. B., Bunge, R. P., Peterson, E. R., and Murray, M. R.: A light and electron microscope study of long term organized cultures of rat dorsal root ganglia. J. Cell Biol., *32*:439, 1967.

Bunge, R., and Bunge, M.: Electron microscopic observations on colchicine induced changes in neuronal cytoplasm. Anat. Rec., *160*:323, 1968.

Bunge, R. P., and Bunge, M. B.: An evaluation of some determinants of neuronal size and internode length in peripheral nerve. Anat. Rec., *154*:324, 1966.

Bunge, R. P., and Harter, D. H.: Cytopathic effects of Visna virus in cultured mammalian nervous tissue. J. Neuropathol. Exp. Neurol., *28*:185, 1969.

Bunge, R. P., and Wood, P.: Studies on the transplantation of spinal cord tissue in the rat. I. Methods for the culture of hemisections of fetal spinal cord. Brain Res., *57*:261, 1973.

Cook, S. D., Dowling, P. C., Murray, M. R., and Whitaker, J. N.: Circulating demyelinating factors in acute idiopathic polyneuropathy (Guillain-Barré). Arch. Neurol., *24*:136, 1971.

Crain, S. M.: Development of "organotypic" bioelectric activities in central nervous tissues during maturation in culture. Int. Rev. Neurobiol., *9*:1, 1966.

Crain, S. M., Alfei, L., and Peterson, E. P.: Neuromuscular transmission in cultures of adult human and rodent skeletal muscle after innervation in vitro by fetal rodent spinal cord. J. Neurobiol., *1*:471, 1970.

Cravioto, H., and Lockwood, R.: The behavior of normal peripheral nerve in tissue culture. Z. Zellforsch. Mikrosk. Anat., *90*:186, 1968.

Cravioto, H., and Lockwood, R.: The behavior of acoustic neuroma in tissue culture. Acta Neuropathol. (Berl.), *12*:141, 1969.

Deitch, A., and Murray, M.: The Nissl substance of living and fixed spinal ganglion cells. I. A phase contrast study. J. Biophys. Biochem. Cytol., *2*:433, 1956.

DeLong, G. R., and Sidman, R. L.: Alignment defect of reaggregating cells in cultures of developing brains of Reeler mutant mice. Dev. Biol., *22*:584, 1970.

England, J. M., and Goldstein, M. N.: The uptake and localization of catecholamines in chick embryo sympathetic neurons in tissue culture. J. Cell Sci., *4*:677, 1969.

England, J. M., Kadin, M., and Goldstein, M. N.: The effect of vincristine sulfate on axoplasmic flow of proteins in cultured chick sympathetic neurons. J. Cell Sci., *12*:549, 1973.

Eränkö, O., and Eränkö, L.: Small, intensely fluorescent granule containing cells in the sympathetic ganglion of the rat. Brain Res., *34*:39, 1971.

Ernyei, S., and Young, M. R.: Pulsatile and myelin-forming activities of Schwann cells in vitro. J. Physiol. (Lond.), *183*:469, 1966.

Feldman, L. A., Sheppard, R. D., and Bornstein, M. B.: Herpes simplex virus-host cell relationships in organized cultures of mammalian nerve tissues. J. Virol., *2*:621, 1968.

Field, E. J., Raine, C. S., and Hughes, D.: Failure to induce myelin sheath formation around artificial fibres with a note on toxicity of polyester fibres for nervous tissue in vitro. J. Neurol. Sci., *8*:129, 1968.

Fischbach, G. D.: Synapse formation between dissociated nerve and muscle cells in low density cell cultures. Dev. Biol., *28*:407, 1972.

Goldstein, M. N.: Growth and differentiation of normal and malignant sympathetic neurons in vitro. *In* Allin, P., and Viza, D. (eds.): Cell Differentiation. Copenhagen, Munksgaard, 1972, p. 131.

Gottschalk, P. G., Dyck, P. J., and Kiely, J. M.: Vinca alkaloid neuropathy: nerve biopsy studies in rats and in man. Neurology (Minneap.), *18*:875, 1968.

Harris, A. J., and Dennis, M. J.: Acetylcholine sensitivity and distribution on mouse neuroblastoma cells. Science, *167*:1253, 1970.

Harris, A. J., Heinemann, S., Schubert, D., and Tarakis, H.: Trophic interaction between cloned tissue culture lines of nerve and muscle. Nature, *231*:296, 1971.

Hendelman, W.: The effect of thallium on peripheral nervous tissue in culture. A light and electron microscopic study. Anat. Rec., *163*:198, 1969.

Hendelman, W., and Bunge, R.: Radioautographic studies of choline incorporation into peripheral nerve myelin. J. Cell Biol., *40*:190, 1969.

Hirano, A., Cook, S., Whitaker, J., Dowling, P. C., and Murray, M. R.: Fine structural aspects of demyelination "in vitro." The effects of Guillain-Barré serum. J. Neuropathol. Exp. Neurol., *30*:249, 1971.

Hiscoe, H. B.: Distribution of nodes and incisures in normal and regenerated nerve fibers. Anat. Rec., *99*:447, 1947.

Hogue, M. J., McAllister, R., Greene, A. E., and Coriell, L. L.: The effect of poliomyelitis virus on human brain cells in tissue culture. J. Exp. Med., *102*:29, 1955.

Holtzman, E., and Peterson, E. R.: Uptake of protein by mammalian neurons. J. Cell Biol., *40*:863, 1969.

James, D. W., and Tresman, R. L.: An electron-microscopic study of the de novo formation of neuromuscular junctions in tissue culture. Z. Zellforsch. Mikrosk. Anat., *100*:126, 1969.

Journey, L. J., Burdman, J., and George, P.: Ultrastructural studies on tissue culture cells treated with vincristine. Cancer Chemother. Rep., *52*:509, 1968.

Lampert, P. W.: Mechanism of demyelination in experimental allergic neuritis. Lab. Invest., *20*:127, 1969.

Lever, J. P., and Presley, R.: Studies on the sympathetic neuron in vivo. Progr. Brain Res., *34*:499, 1971.

Levi-Montalcini, R., and Angeletti, P. U.: Essential role of the nerve growth factor in the survival and maintenance of dissociated sensory and sympathetic embryonic nerve cells in vitro. Dev. Biol., *7*:653, 1963.

Levi-Montalcini, R., and Angeletti, P. U.: Biological aspects of the nerve growth factor. *In* Wolstenholme, G., and O'Connor, M. (eds.): Growth of the Nervous System. Boston, Little, Brown & Co., 1968, p. 126.

Masurovsky, E. B., and Bunge, R. P.: Radiation protection in mammalian spinal ganglion cultures treated with AET derivatives. Light and electron-microscopic autoradiographic studies. Acta Radiol. [Ther.] (Stockh.), *8*:38, 1969.

Masurovsky, E. B., and Bunge, R. P.: Patterns of myelin degeneration following the rapid death of cells in cultures of peripheral nervous tissue. J. Neuropathol. Exp. Neurol., *30*:311, 1971.

Masurovsky, E. B., Benitez, H. H., and Murray, M. R.: Development of interneurons in long-term organotypic cultures of rat superior cervical and stellate ganglia. J. Cell Biol., *55*:166a, 1972.

Masurovsky, E. B., Bunge, M. B., and Bunge, R. P.: Cytological studies of organotypic cultures of rat dorsal root ganglia following x-irradiation "in vitro." I. Changes in neurons and satellite cells. J. Cell Biol., *32*:467, 1967a.

Masurovsky, E. B., Bunge, M. B., and Bunge, R. P.: Cytological studies of organotypic cultures of rat dorsal root ganglia following x-irradiation "in vitro." II. Changes in Schwann cells, myelin sheaths and nerve fibers. J. Cell Biol., *32*:497, 1967b.

Masurovsky, E. B., Benitez, H. H., Kim, S. U., and Murray, M. R.: Origin, development and nature of intranuclear rodlets and associated bodies in chicken sympathetic neurons. J. Cell Biol., *44*:172, 1970.

Mire, J. J., Hendelman, W. J., and Bunge, R. P.: Observations on a transient phase of focal swelling in degenerating unmyelinated nerve fibers. J. Cell Biol., *45*:9, 1970.

Murray, M. R.: Nervous tissue in vitro. *In* Willmer, E. N. (ed.): Cells and Tissues in Culture. Vol. 2. New York, Academic Press, 1965, p. 373.

Murray, M. R., and Benitez, H. H.: Action of heavy water (D_2O) on growth and development of isolated nervous tissues. *In* Wolstenholme, G., and O'Connor, M. (eds.): Growth of the Nervous System. Boston, Little, Brown & Co., 1968, p. 148.

Murray, M. R., and Stout, A. P.: Schwann cell versus fibroblast as the origin of the specific nerve sheath tumor. Observations upon normal nerve sheaths and neurilemomas in vitro. Am. J. Pathol., *16*:41, 1940.

Murray, M. R., Peterson, E. R., and Loeser, C. N.: Localization of several fluorochromes in cultured neurons. *In* Cohen, M., and Snider, K. (eds.): Morphological

and Biochemical Correlates in Neural Activity. New York, Harper & Row, 1964, p. 225.

Nelson, P., Ruffner, W., and Nirenberg, M.: Neuronal tumor cells with excitable membranes grown in vitro. Proc. Natl. Acad. Sci. U.S.A., *64*:1004, 1969.

Nicolson, G.: Difference in topology of normal and tumour cell membranes shown by different surface distributions of ferritin-conjugated concanavalin A. Nature [New Biol.], *233*:244, 1971.

Okun, L. M.: Isolated dorsal root ganglion neurons in culture: cytological maturation and extension of electrically active processes. J. Neurobiol., *3*:111, 1972.

Olson, M. I., and Bunge, R. P.: Anatomical observations on the specificity of synapse formation in tissue culture. Brain Res., *59*:19, 1973.

Pappas, G. D., Peterson, E. R., Masurovsky, E. B., and Crain, S. M.: Electron microscopy of the *in vitro* development of mammalian motor end plates. Ann. N.Y. Acad. Sci., *183*:33, 1971.

Peterson, E. R.: Neurofibrillar alterations in cord-ganglion cultures exposed to spindle inhibitors. J. Neuropathol. Exp. Neurol., *28*:168, 1969.

Peterson, E. R., and Bornstein, M. B.: The neurotoxic effects of colchicine on tissue cultures of cord-ganglia. J. Neuropathol. Exp. Neurol., *27*:121, 1968.

Peterson, E. R., and Crain, S. M.: Innervation in cultures of fetal rodent skeletal muscle by organotypic explants of spinal cord from different animals. Z. Zellforsch. Mikrosk. Anat., *106*:1, 1970.

Peterson, E. R., and Crain, S. M.: Regeneration and innervation in culture of adult mammalian skeletal muscle coupled with fetal rodent spinal cord. Exp. Neurol., *36*:136, 1972.

Peterson, E. R., and Murray, M. R.: Myelin sheath formation in cultures of avian spinal ganglia. Am. J. Anat., *96*:319, 1955.

Peterson, E. R., and Murray, M. R.: The reality of Schmidt-Lanterman clefts. Observations in vitro. Abstracts of the First Annual Meeting of the American Society for Cell Biology, Chicago, 165, 1961.

Peterson, E. R., and Murray, M. R.: Patterns of peripheral demyelination in vitro. Ann. N.Y. Acad. Sci., *122*:39, 1965.

Peterson, E. R., and Murray, M. R.: Serial observations in tissue cultures on neurotoxic effects of colchicine. Anat. Rec., *154*:401, 1966.

Peterson, E. R., Crain, S. M., and Murray, M. R.: Differentiation and prolonged maintenance of bioelectrically active spinal cord cultures (rat, chick, human). Z. Zellforsch. Mikrosk. Anat., *66*:130, 1965.

Pfeiffer, S. E., Kornblith, P. L., Cares, H. L., Seals, J., and Levine, L.: S-100 protein in human acoustic neurinomas. Brain Res., *41*:187, 1972.

Pfenninger, K. H.: Freeze-cleaving of outgrowing nerve fibers in tissue culture. J. Cell Biol., *55*:203a, 1972.

Pomerat, C. M., Hendelman, W. J., Raiborn, C. W., Jr., and Massey, J. F.: Dynamic activities of nervous tissue in vitro. *In* Hyden, H. (ed.): The Neuron. New York, American Elsevier Publishing Co., 1967, p. 119.

Prestige, M. C.: Differentiation, degeneration, and the role of the periphery: quantitative considerations. *In* Schmitt, F. O. (ed.): The Neurosciences Second Study Program. New York, Rockefeller University Press, 1970, p. 73.

Schlaepfer, W.: Vincristine-induced axonal alterations in rat peripheral nerve. J. Neuropathol. Exp. Neurol., *30*:488, 1971.

Schlaepfer, W. W., and Bunge, R. P.: Effects of calcium

ion concentration on the degeneration of amputated axons in tissue culture. J. Cell Biol., 59:456, 1973.

Scott, B. S., Engelberg, V. E., and Fisher, K. C.: Morphological and electrophysiological characteristics of dissociated chick embryonic spinal ganglion cells in culture. Exp. Neurol., 23:230, 1969.

Seil, F. J., and Lampert, P. W.: Neurofibrillary tangles induced by vincristine and vinblastine sulfate in central and peripheral neurons in vitro. Exp. Neurol., 21:219, 1968.

Shimada, Y., and Fischman, D. A.: The morphological and physiological evidence for the development of functional neuromuscular junctions in vitro. Dev. Biol., 31:200, 1973.

Silberstein, S. D., Johnson, D. G., Jacobowitz, D. M., and Kopin, I. J.: Sympathetic reinnervation of the rat iris in organ culture. Proc. Natl. Acad. Sci. U.S.A., 18:1121, 1971.

Sobkowicz, H. M., Guillery, R. W., and Bornstein, M. B.: Neural organization in long term cultures of the spinal cord of the fetal mouse. J. Comp. Neurol., 132:365, 1968.

Spencer, P. S., Raine, C. S., and Peterson, E. R.: Effects of thallium on axonal mitochondria in cord-ganglion-muscle cultures. J. Cell Biol., 55:247a, 1972.

Tischner, K. H.: Chloroquine-induced alterations in rat sensory ganglia cultivated in vitro. A light and electron microscope study. Acta Neuropathol. (Berl.) 22:208, 1972.

Tischner, K. H., and Murray, M. R.: The effects of sodium azide on cultures of peripheral nervous system. J. Neuropathol. Exp. Neurol., 31:393, 1972.

Varon, S.: In vitro study of developing neural tissue and cells; past and prospective contributions. In Schmitt, F. O. (ed.): The Neurosciences Second Study Program. New York, Rockefeller University Press, 1970, p. 83.

Varon, S., and Raiborn, C.: Excitability and conduction in neurons of dissociated ganglionic cell cultures. Brain Res., 30:83, 1971.

Waksman, B. H., and Adams, R. D.: Allergic neuritis. An experimental disease of rabbits induced by the injection of peripheral nervous tissue and adjuvants. J. Exp. Med., 102:213, 1955.

Whetsell, W. O., and Bunge, R. P.: Reversible alterations in the Golgi complex of cultured neurons treated with an inhibitor of active Na and K transport. J. Cell Biol., 42:490, 1969.

Whetsell, W. O., and Mire, J. J.: Cytoplasmic vacuole formation in cultured neurons treated with lithium ions. Brain Res., 19:155, 1970.

Winkler, G. F., and Arnason, B. G.: Antiserum to immunoglobulin A: inhibition of cell mediated demyelination in tissue culture. Science, 153:75, 1966.

Winkler, G. F., and Wolf, M. K.: The development and maintenance of myelinated tissue cultures of rat trigeminal ganglion. Am. J. Anat., 119:179, 1966.

Yamada, K. M., Spooner, B. S., and Wessells, N. K.: Axon growth: Roles of microfilaments and microtubules. Proc. Natl. Acad. Sci. U.S.A., 66:1206, 1970.

Yamada, K. M., Spooner, B. S., and Wessells, N. K.: Ultrastructure and function of growth cones and axons of cultured nerve cells. J. Cell Biol., 49:614, 1971.

Yonezawa, T., and Iwanami, H.: An experimental study of thiamine deficiency in nervous tissue, using tissue culture techniques. J. Neuropathol. Exp. Neurol., 25:362, 1966.

Yonezawa, T., Ishihara, Y., and Matsuyama, H.: Studies on experimental allergic peripheral neuritis. I. Demyelination patterns studied in vitro. J. Neuropathol. Exp. Neurol., 27:453, 1968.

Yu, R., and Bunge, R. P.: Alterations in the peripheral myelin sheath and node of Ranvier produced by treatment with trypsin. In preparation.

Chapter 19

BIOPSY OF PERIPHERAL NERVES

J. Clarke Stevens, Eric P. Lofgren,
and Peter James Dyck

Although postmortem studies of peripheral nerve tissue have been made for many years, it is only recently that there has been widespread interest in the application of nerve biopsy to patients. The method of fascicular biopsy, the revival of the old technique of preparing single teased fibers, the development of methods for the quantitative analysis of nerve fiber populations, and the use of the electron microscope all have contributed to the upsurge in the use of nerve biopsy. New discoveries and methods for analysis of peripheral nerve myelin lipids, for measuring biochemical derangements, and for measuring axonal flow are being added to our armamentarium of investigational tools. In this chapter we discuss the choice of nerve for biopsy and the surgical technique, the postbiopsy symptoms, and the usefulness of nerve biopsy.

First, however, it is important to emphasize that nerve biopsy for diagnostic reasons is applicable to only a small number of patients who have peripheral nerve disorders. As in the case of liver or kidney biopsy, the decision to perform nerve biopsy should be made by a physician who has a special interest in the subject and who also has the training and equipment needed for full evaluation of the specimen. It is a great advantage also if one surgeon is able to perform all the biopsies done at an institution; in that way the specimen can be obtained without trauma or traction, and there will be fewer confusing artifacts.

Evaluation of the tissue requires fixation and staining for light and phase contrast microscopy, examination of suitably stained frozen sections, and preparation of single teased fibers. A knowledge of what constitutes the normal population of fibers and of the incidence of degenerative changes with age in the particular nerve studied is essential to avoid errors of interpretation. In certain situations, exact measurements of the internodes of many teased fibers are indicated for comparison with the normal indices. Quantitation of myelinated fiber density and of the spectrum of fiber diameter sizes also may be necessary to provide definitive answers. The results obtained depend on the kind and duration of fixation used, the age of the patient, the particular nerve sampled, and the portion (proximal or distal) of the nerve. Estimation of the changes in the number of and the pathologic alterations in unmyelinated fibers and ultrastructural alterations of nerve axons, Schwann cells, connective tissue, and other cellular elements can be made only with the electron microscope. The details of the preparation of the specimen for study and the application and execution of the various procedures just outlined are covered in another section. They are listed here only to make the point that the complete examination of a nerve biopsy specimen is a complex and time-consuming procedure best carried out at centers where there is a special interest in peripheral nerve histology and research. Conventional histopathologic techniques and sections of nerve frequently yield insufficient information to justify the procedure (Thomas, 1970).

CHOICE OF NERVE
FOR BIOPSY

Dyck and Lofgren (1966) listed six factors to be considered in the selection of the peripheral nerve for biopsy. The first and obvious point is that the nerve be affected by the neuropathy. The physical signs of peripheral neuropathy include diminished or altered sensation, trophic changes of the skin, muscle wasting and weakness, and diminution or absence of deep tendon reflexes. Methods are being developed for precise measurement of cutaneous, touch-pressure, pain, and temperature sensations to aid in diagnosis of and in detection of carriers of inherited neuropathies. At present, such sensory testing is time-consuming and is not suitable for routine use before nerve biopsy; however, automated procedures being explored may make such testing more practical in the future.

When possible, conduction velocity measurements of the nerve from which the specimen is to be taken are desirable, both to document the presence of a neuropathy and to correlate the conduction velocity and other changes found with the histologic appearance of the nerve. Needle electrode examination may reveal fasciculation, denervation, and neurogenic motor unit abnormalities when motor nerves are affected. If the neuropathy is predominantly sensory, biopsy of a sensory nerve is the logical choice. On the other hand, when motor fibers are predominantly or selectively affected, biopsy of a muscle nerve or a combined muscle and sensory nerve should be considered. In the case of arteritis with neuropathy or if neuropathy and myopathy coexist, it is convenient to choose a nerve located next to a muscle suitable for biopsy so that both may be obtained through a single incision.

Although a number of purely sensory nerves are available for biopsy, we do not have a method to obtain motor nerve fibers that are not intermingled with sensory fibers. Approximately a third to a half of the myelinated fibers in a muscle nerve (studied in cats) are composed of sensory afferents that can in no way be distinguished from motor fibers by histologic examination (Sherrington, 1894; Rexed and Therman, 1948). When only motor fibers seem to be affected, a solution may be to take specimens from a muscle nerve and an adjacent cutaneous nerve. If the sensory nerve appears normal on microscopic examination but fibers in the muscle nerve are degenerating, one can assume that the degenerating fibers are of motor origin. At autopsy, one can study motor fibers in isolation by obtaining sections of the ventral motor roots of the spinal cord (Corbin and Gardner, 1937; Rexed, 1944; Wohlfart and Swank, 1941).

Failure to obtain a specimen will be avoided if the nerve chosen is one that is constant in location and readily accessible. It also is important that the nerve be located where risk of damage to adjacent blood vessels, tendons, synovia, and joints is minimal.

The length of nerve fascicles removed will be determined by the extent of the studies planned. One to two centimeters of the same fascicle is sufficient for light and electron microscopy and for preparation of single teased fibers. In vitro nerve conduction studies and analysis of myelin lipids necessitate removal of longer portions of fascicles or of whole nerve. In most cases, fascicular biopsy is most desirable because the resulting sensory deficit is less than with full-thickness biopsy. When the primary pathologic problem is suspected to lie in the vasa nervorum, however, whole-nerve biopsy is required because the affected arterioles do not lie within the endoneurial area obtained with fascicular biopsy (Dyck et al., 1972).

To minimize the presence of unrelated degenerative changes the nerve chosen for biopsy should be located where peripheral entrapment and damage from recurrent trauma are not common. Nerve conduction velocity measurements may be helpful in this regard. For example, if branches of the common peroneal nerve are being considered for biopsy, it is prudent to make conduction velocity measurements above and below the head of the fibula.

The last factor to be considered is the availability of normative, statistically evaluated, histologic and teased-fiber measurements of the particular nerve to be examined. These values change, especially during growth and with advancing age. Accurate interpretation of the changes observed in the specimen is impossible without reference to data of this type.

Sural Nerve

The nerve of choice for biopsy in most instances is the sural nerve at the ankle level. It is the nerve most often used by other workers and, in regard to normal quantitative histometric values, it is the best-documented of the nerves discussed here (cf. Sunderland et al., 1949; Lavarack et al., 1951; Tomasch and Britton, 1956; Dyck and Lambert, 1966; Lascelles and Thomas, 1966; O'Sullivan and Swallow, 1968; Murai et al., 1969; Ochoa and Mair, 1969; Gutrecht and Dyck, 1970; Dyck et al., 1973). Except for unmyelinated autonomic fibers, the nerve is entirely sensory, supplying the skin of the lateral and posterior part of the lower one third of the leg, the lateral aspect of the heel and the lateral side of the foot and the fifth toe. It also contributes to the nerve supply of the ankle, the subtalar, and the calcaneocuboid joints. The sural nerve at this level is superficial and constant in location, lying between the Achilles tendon and lateral malleolus where it is relatively protected from injury. Because of this nerve's distal location in the lower extremity, it is particularly liable to be affected by a peripheral neuropathy. The long subcutaneous course of the nerve above the ankle permits removal of ample lengths of specimen if needed for special studies. At the ankle level, individual fascicles usually are easily distinguished, especially after the epineurium has been split longitudinally. This makes removal of fascicles, rather than whole nerve, practical and the procedure to be used routinely with the exceptions already mentioned.

When combined nerve and muscle biopsy is indicated, we often combine biopsy of the sural nerve at the midcalf level with biopsy of the underlying gastrocnemius muscle. Fascicular or whole-nerve biopsies of this nerve at both the ankle and midcalf levels have been used to study "dying back" neuropathies of the primary sensory neurons. In a few cases we have also removed the portion of the sural nerve between the ankle and midcalf biopsies to provide enough tissue for myelin lipid analysis.

There are few disadvantages to use of this nerve for biopsy. It is, perhaps, a larger nerve than might be desirable to sacrifice when whole-nerve biopsy is necessary. Although not subject to entrapment or pressure during most of its course, damage to its subcutaneous fibers in the foot by shoes and everyday trauma is possible. This can lead to retrograde changes in the nerve higher up (Aitken and Thomas, 1962). The possibility of accidental injury, however, applies to all superficial nerves supplying the distal extremities; the sural nerve probably is less affected than other lower limb nerves in this respect. Occasionally, fascicular biopsy is hampered by branching and interconnections between fascicles that make removal of long segments of a single fascicle difficult.

Superficial Peroneal Nerve

Fascicular biopsy of the superficial peroneal nerve above the ankle has been used as an alternative to sural nerve biopsy (Arnold and Harriman, 1970). The superficial peroneal nerve pierces the crural fascia at about the junction of the upper two thirds with the lower one third of the leg. Prior to or just after becoming subcutaneous, it divides into two branches—the medial and the intermediate dorsal cutaneous nerves—that are suitable for biopsy. The branches in this location overlie a handy source of muscle tissue, the peroneus brevis. Recently we have begun to take specimens from this nerve in conjunction with muscle nerve biopsy. The superficial peroneal nerve supplies a portion of the skin of the lower part of the leg, most of the dorsum of the foot, the dorsum of the toes except for the lateral side of the little toe, and the adjoining sides of the great and second toes. Several studies of this nerve, based on "normal" postmortem material and including the incidence of abnormality in teased-fiber preparations and quantitative histologic measurements, have been published (Arnold and Harriman, 1970; Stevens et al., 1973).

Deep Peroneal Nerve

The terminal sensory branches of the deep peroneal nerve on the foot have been used for biopsy and quantitative histologic studies (Greenfield and Carmichael, 1935; Aring et al., 1941; Garven et al., 1962; Swallow, 1966). It was concluded by Swallow (1966) that the wide variation in total fiber counts and in fiber density in healthy nerves from different persons limits the usefulness of this nerve for diagnosis. This is because a pathologic mild to moderate decrease in nerve fiber density might not be recognized.

Saphenous Nerve

The saphenous nerve has a long course in the lower extremity, making both proximal (upper thigh) and distal (ankle) biopsy attractive procedures for the study of simple atrophy or dying back neuropathies. Unfortunately, the nerve gives off many branches along its course, so that it is relatively small at the ankle level. This makes comparison of proximal and distal nerve fiber densities unreliable, but one can determine what percentage of fibers are degenerating at each level. In the neuropathies with axonal atrophy, fewer degenerating fibers are found in the proximal specimen. There are at present few data available about the normal composition of this nerve, although the fiber diameter spectrum appears to be fairly similar to that of the sural nerve (Dyck et al., 1974).

Superficial Radial Nerve

Biopsy of an upper limb cutaneous nerve is rarely indicated because the nerves of the lower limbs are more severely affected by most types of peripheral neuropathy. In addition, loss of sensation on the forearm, hand, or fingers is more noticeable than loss of sensation on the foot, and from a functional point of view one is hesitant to add to distal upper limb sensory loss. When only the upper limbs are affected or when venous stasis, edema, arterial vascular disease, or other factors are present and can be expected to interfere with the healing of an incision in the leg, biopsy of one of the nerves in the arm may be considered. The nerve most suitable is the superficial branch of the radial nerve (Ranson et al., 1935; Tsairis et al., 1972). The nerve is removed just after it emerges from under the brachioradialis tendon to become subcutaneous at about the junction of the middle and distal thirds of the forearm. Its terminal branches supply the skin on the lateral part of the dorsum of the wrist and hand, including a variable part of the dorsum of the thumb and of the lateral two and one half fingers. The

normal fiber density and spectrum of myelinated fiber diameters have been examined by several authors (Ranson et al., 1935; Sunderland et al., 1949; Lavarack et al., 1951; Tomasch and Schwarzacher, 1952; O'Sullivan and Swallow, 1968). Another advantage of this nerve is that conduction velocity studies can be carried out prior to biopsy.

Greater Auricular Nerve

Some hypertrophic neuropathies cause visible enlargement of the cutaneous branches of the cervical plexus, which suggests their use for biopsy. Biopsy of the enlarged greater auricular nerve has been done in the past (Thevenard and Berdet, 1958; Dyck et al., 1965); however, because of its proximal location and short course, this nerve is unlikely to be involved by most neuropathies. Aside from this, the nerve is too large, the fascicles are not separable for a sufficient length, and the scar may be considered unsightly, especially in women. Since the sural nerve is more affected by the hypertrophic neuropathies, use of the greater auricular nerve should be abandoned.

Combined Lateral Fascicles of Deep Peroneal and Superficial Peroneal Nerve

Muscle nerve biopsy for the investigation of disorders affecting the lower motor neuron has not been done in the past because of an understandable reluctance on the part of physicians to denervate any muscle permanently and so further impair the patient's motor function. The extensor digitorum brevis, a small muscle on the dorsum of the foot, is one that can be sacrificed with little functional impairment. Its tendons assist in extension of the medial four toes, along with the extensor hallucis longus and extensor digitorum longus. Innervation of the extensor brevis is provided by the lateral terminal branch of the deep peroneal nerve given off in front of the ankle. The lateral division also innervates the tarsal and metatarsophalangeal joints and sends a filament to the second dorsal interosseous muscle (Gardner and Gray, 1968). Exposure of the lateral terminal branch of the foot is difficult because of overlying tendons and the extensor retinacula, but the parent deep peroneal is easily approached through an incision above the ankle. At this location one can remove lateral fascicles of the nerve that form the lateral terminal branch several inches lower down. In theory, the fascicles left behind form the medial terminal branch of the deep peroneal nerve, which supplies cutaneous sensation to the adjacent sides of the great and second toes. Fascicular biopsy of the adjacent subcutaneous superficial peroneal nerve can be combined with lateral fascicle biopsy to determine if motor fibers only are affected. Peroneus brevis muscle biopsy also can be performed through the same incision.

Normative histologic and teased-fiber measurements on the lateral fascicles of the deep peroneal and on the superficial peroneal nerve at the same level are available (Stevens et al., 1973). Vizoso (1950) studied the changes, with age, in the relationship between internodal length and diameter of the anterior tibial nerve. Lateral fascicle biopsy has the advantage of providing fibers used for measurement of motor nerve conduction in the lower extremity. Prior to biopsy, nerve conduction studies should also be used to check for the presence of an accessory peroneal nerve, which supplies the lateral portion of the muscle in about 20 per cent of limbs (Lambert, 1969). If this accessory nerve is unilateral, the opposite side should be used for biopsy.

The disadvantages of lateral fascicle biopsy are that the deep peroneal nerve is more deeply situated than a cutaneous nerve and that it is difficult to obtain long lengths of nerve if needed for special studies. In addition, the motor fibers in the lateral fascicles are "diluted" since the nerve contains additional afferents to the joints, which are not present in a "pure" muscle nerve. Histochemical fiber typing of the extensor digitorum brevis and other lower limb muscles from normal adults showed grouping of fiber types only in the extensor brevis, indicating that the nerve supply to this muscle is more subject to injury than are other lower limb muscle nerves (Jennekens et al., 1971).

Combined Nerve to Peroneus Brevis and Superficial Peroneal Nerve

Another muscle nerve that has been studied in normal persons is the nerve to the peroneus brevis (Stevens et al. 1973). It is of the correct size and length for most nerve biopsy studies and also is conveniently located next to the superficial peroneal nerve, which is purely sensory in function after the nerve to the peroneus has been given off. It is an ideal nerve to study at autopsy, but its use in patients is severely limited by the fact that the peroneus brevis is a main evertor of the foot and is an important antagonist of the tibialis posterior (Duchenne, 1949; Steindler, 1955). This nerve can be considered for biopsy only when the patient has a permanent drop foot—for example, as occurs in the peroneal muscular atrophy of Charcot-Marie-Tooth. Occasionally, the nerve may be difficult to locate or it may lie deep in the leg, making the procedure painful under local anesthesia.

TECHNIQUE OF PERIPHERAL NERVE BIOPSY

For the peripheral nerve biopsy specimen to yield the greatest amount of information, it should be obtained with the least amount of surgical trauma. Also, the postoperative discomfort and the neurologic deficit should be minimal.

All nerve biopsies are performed under sterile conditions in the operating room, with the extremity shaved, scrubbed, disinfected, and draped as in any general surgical procedure. The surgical team wears gowns, masks, and gloves. Surgical instruments must be delicate and in good working order. Fine suture material, 4-0 or 5-0, and atraumatic needles are used to minimize foreign body reactions. Magnifying glasses are essential for visualizing the nerve fascicles and for accurate detection of bleeding vessels. We have found the Zeiss 2.2 power magnification glasses to be most suitable to our needs. An electrical nerve stimulator should be available to facilitate identification of sensory or motor components of a mixed nerve such as the deep peroneal nerve at the ankle and for accurate identification of the saphenous nerve at the femoral trigone (here, multiple muscle nerves to the thigh musculature are closely associated).

The research physician or technician is present in the operating room to receive the nerve specimen for immediate fixation. His advice is helpful to the surgeon in determining the extent of the biopsy specimen. Small weights are hung on the nerve ends to provide proper tension during fixation.

Because most patients are ambulatory outpatients, preanesthetic sedation is avoided. We prefer infiltration anesthesia with 0.5 per cent lidocaine (Xylocaine) without epinephrine. General anesthesia is rarely used, being reserved for the hyperactive adult or child.

Only the technique for sural nerve biopsy is described in detail here because the technique is similar for all peripheral nerve biopsies, once the nerve has been accurately identified and properly exposed.

Sural Nerve Biopsy

The sural nerve is most readily exposed at the ankle level. The patient lies prone on the operating table with the ankle, slightly everted, resting on a pillow so that the foot assumes a 90 degree relationship with the leg. This places the sural nerve at a normal tension. The skin is shaved from the knee to the ankle and scrubbed with germicidal soap (pHisoHex). Alcohol and thimerosal (Merthiolate) are applied. Sterile drapes are placed around the heel and on each side of the leg up to the knee. When the calf is compressed, the lesser saphenous vein becomes distended and may become visible or palpable in the trough between the external malleolus and the Achilles tendon. The saphenous vein is the most reliable anatomical landmark for locating the sural nerve, which lies immediately adjacent to the vein at this level.

Eight to ten milliliters of 0.5 per cent lidocaine is infiltrated in the skin and subcutaneous tissue, from just behind the external malleolus for a distance of 10 cm proximally. The incision is placed to overlie directly the course of the saphenous vein. As the tough semitransparent Scarpa's fascia is exposed, one sees the saphenous vein beneath it. When Scarpa's fascia directly over the vein is divided and the vein is retracted gently, the sural nerve comes into view, most commonly on the medial side of the vein. The bleeding points are now ligated; occasionally a tributary vein to the lesser saphenous at the malleolus requires division and ligation since it crosses over the sural nerve.

The epineurium is gently divided with fine sharp scissors for the full length of the exposed nerve. This allows the discrete fascicles to be teased apart. A long fascicle having minimal branching is selected for biopsy. Usually this fascicle is located on the posteromedial aspect of the nerve. A 5-0 silk suture is passed through the fascicle at the upper end and held as a loop retractor. The fascicle is transected just above this, and the patient experiences a brief twinge of pain, usually on the posterior aspect of the heel. By dissecting the fascicle free of the epineurium and occasionally dividing small nerve twigs, several segments 2 cm long are obtained. (These are suspended by the silk suture on one end, and a small weight is hooked onto the other end (Fig. 19-1). The specimen is placed in the appropriate fixative solution by the laboratory physician or technician.) Since the fascicle has been transected at the proximal end, further discomfort is not experienced by the patient if further lengths of the same fascicle are removed, as long as one carefully avoids trauma to the intact fascicles.

After meticulous hemostasis has been obtained by accurately ligating all bleeding points with fine absorbable sutures, Scarpa's fascia is reapproximated, with care taken not to pass the suture around the remaining nerve. The skin is approximated with vertical interrupted mattress sutures of 4-0 silk. A dry dressing is applied and held in place with a 4 inch elastic bandage. The patient may walk immediately after the procedure, but we prefer that he restrict his activity for one or two days. Analgesics generally are not necessary for postoperative discomfort, but the patient is forewarned that he may experience a twinge of pain if he stretches the sural nerve, as by stooping forward. The dressings are changed on the day after the procedure and then are left intact until the skin sutures are ready for removal on postoperative day 8, 9, or 10.

The entire diameter of the sural nerve may be removed in selected instances. If this is to be done, we first infiltrate the upper end of the exposed nerve with 0.5 per cent lidocaine to lessen the pain at the time of transection. Thereafter the entire nerve is removed as described for the fascicular biopsy.

The sural nerve is often exposed at the calf level in combination with the ankle-level nerve biopsy to obtain specimens for comparative study. The anatomical landmark at the mid-calf is the palpable groove between the heads of the gastrocnemius muscle. The skin is

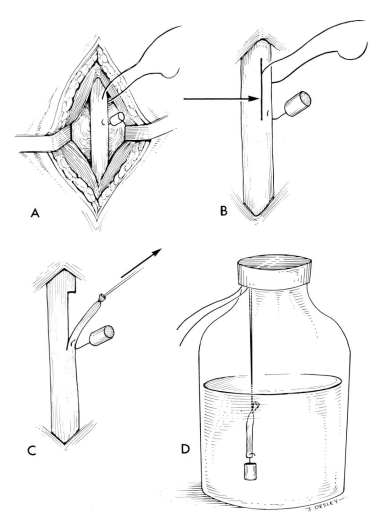

Figure 19–1 Surgical technique of sural nerve biopsy. (From Dyck, P. J., and Lofgren, E. P.: Method of fascicular biopsy of human peripheral nerve for electrophysiologic and histologic study. Mayo Clin. Proc., *41*:778, 1966.)

infiltrated with 0.5 per cent lidocaine and the longitudinal incision is carried down to the fascia. The lesser saphenous vein is visible beneath the deep fascia, but the sural nerve usually does not accompany the vein at this level. Some searching in the areolar tissue between the muscle heads beneath the vein, as much as 2 cm deep, is required. A useful maneuver in finding the nerve is to pull gently on the exposed sural nerve at the ankle wound while palpating its movement in the muscle interspace. Once the nerve is exposed, the biopsy technique is similar to that performed at the ankle. The intervening segment of sural nerve between the ankle and calf wounds may be required for biochemical analysis. This segment can be teased out in most instances by pushing a fine wire loop around the nerve in both directions, to free it. On occasion, the peroneal communicating branch of the common peroneal nerve joining the sural nerve deep in the calf may prevent this maneuver.

Deep Peroneal Nerve Biopsy

The anatomical landmarks for exposure of the peroneal nerve at the ankle level are the external malleolus, the lateral edge of the tibia, and the anterior edge of the fibula. In the adult, one infiltrates the skin with 0.5 per cent lidocaine, beginning about 6 cm proximal to the external malleolus, midway between the palpable bones, and extending for a distance of 10 cm proximally. The incision is placed longitudinally and carried down to the deep fascia. By gently elevating the posterior skin edge, the sensory branch of the peroneal nerve is found, usually in the areolar plane above the deep fascia. Suitable biopsy specimens can be obtained from this sensory branch. The deep fascia is then divided midway between the tibia and fibula, exposing the extensor hallucis longus. This muscle is gently retracted laterally away from the tibialis anterior muscle. Palpable in this groove is the anterior tibial artery, which lies adjacent to the deep peroneal nerve. The nerve is exposed by deepening the groove between the two muscles.

The epineurium is divided and the motor fascicles, most often found on the lateral edge of the nerve, are identified with the nerve stimulator. Fascicles may then be obtained by using the technique described for the sural nerve. The wound is closed with meticulous hemostasis and accurate approximation of the fascia, subcutaneous tissue, and skin.

The postoperative discomfort is somewhat greater than that from sural nerve biopsy, since the deep muscle compartment has been exposed, but analgesics generally are not required.

Saphenous Nerve Biopsy

Biopsy of the saphenous nerve is readily performed at the thigh and also at the ankle. The saphenous nerve accompanies the superficial femoral artery on its lateral side in the femoral trigone, where it crosses over the artery to lie on the medial side below the adductor canal. The skin incision is placed in the femoral trigone to overlie the superficial femoral artery, which is palpable in thin persons; this incision will expose the medial edge of the sartorius muscle. The muscle is retracted laterally, and the underlying femoral sheath is divided. The prominent saphenous nerve is found immediately lateral to the superficial femoral artery in the upper end of the incision, and it usually crosses over the artery before entering the adductor canal. Since there are motor branches of other nerves lateral to the femoral artery, positive identification of the saphenous nerve is obtained with the nerve stimulator (a sensory response at the inner aspect of the knee or leg, without muscle contraction). Biopsy of nerve fascicles and wound closure are by the techniques described for the sural nerve biopsy.

At the ankle level, the saphenous nerve accompanies the saphenous vein, usually being deep and medial to the vein. It is readily identified just above the medial malleolus. Since branching of the nerve has already occurred, the size of the nerve may vary at this level.

Biopsy of the gastrocnemius muscle may be done in the wound used for the upper sural nerve biopsy; similarly, specimens of the thigh muscles may be obtained in the femoral trigone incision for the saphenous nerve.

SYMPTOMS AFTER NERVE BIOPSY

Since 1966, a brief questionnaire has been sent to each patient 3 and 12 months after his biopsy to determine the morbidity following the procedure and to provide accurate information about symptoms following biopsy for the benefit of future patients (see Dyck and Lofgren, 1968). The patient is asked: Was there discomfort in the region of the biopsy greater than a similar region on the other side of the body? What was the nature of the discomfort and when did it come? Were there additional symptoms? Was the discomfort severe enough so that you think that biopsies should not be done?

The information that follows has been supplemented by follow-up questioning and examination of many patients.

Experience of Normal Subjects

In order to provide normative histometric and teased-fiber measurements, nine healthy paid volunteers between the ages of 20 and 46 years underwent sural nerve biopsy. Fascicles were removed from the ankle level in five and from the ankle and midcalf levels in four. Seven replied to questionnaires at three months and one year; two replied only to the three month questionnaire.

It might be expected that these subjects would be more likely to complain of after effects of biopsy than would patients who had peripheral sensory loss or impairment. In fact, the volunteers reported surprisingly few symptoms. Those with symptoms described them as minor or mild and as occurring "once in a while." None found the discomfort severe enough to make them think biopsies should not be done. Two of nine were without symptoms at three months, and four of seven were without symptoms at one year. The main symptoms reported were prickling, aching, and itching in the area of the incision or incisions. The midcalf incision did not appear to give rise to any more trouble than the ankle incision. A higher proportion of the volunteers (five of nine) noted loss of sensation in the sural nerve distribution on the foot and heel than did the patients.

One of the authors underwent fascicular biopsy of the sural nerve at the ankle, and the following is a detailed account based on that experience (Dyck and Lofgren, 1968). After injection of the local anesthetic, there was no discomfort until isolation of the fascicle. Immediately after the transection, a sharp, stinging, burning discomfort occurred in a region just below the lateral malleolus and across to the Achilles tendon. Although severe, the pain lasted only one or two seconds.

Through the first three or four days there was no spontaneous discomfort other than soreness at the site of the incision. Examination revealed a circular area of loss of sensation, about 3 cm in diameter, just below the lateral malleolus and including the skin overlying the insertion of the Achilles tendon. Additional symptoms began on the third postoperative day, reached their peak in about a week, and declined thereafter. When sitting, there was a mildly unpleasant, raw, burning discomfort in the anesthetized region. Upon arising, the first two or three steps were accompanied by a burning discomfort that radiated into the skin of the lateral heel. With continued walking, all discomfort disappeared completely. When the nerve was stretched, as occurs on bending forward with the knees held straight, a prickling, burning discomfort was felt in the region of the lateral heel and Achilles tendon. This ceased promptly after the stretch on the nerve was released. One month after nerve biopsy, all these symptoms had disappeared.

Later, a raw, unpleasant, poorly localized burning was experienced when the anesthetized area was touched. About a year after the biopsy, sitting for prolonged periods again caused a mild burning, raw, warm feeling in the anesthetized area. Activity put an end to it promptly, and after a week it ceased to recur. Approximately 15 months after biopsy, considerable return of light touch and superficial pain sensation had occurred in the formerly anesthetized area. Pinprick sensation in the area had a hyperpathic quality. Three years after biopsy, all symptoms had dis-

appeared, and about five years later, almost normal sensation had returned to the foot.

Experience of Patients

The experience of patients after sural nerve biopsy was derived from a review of 108 three month questionnaires and 97 one year questionnaires. These questionnaires represent the replies of 134 different patients, many of whom did not reply to both questionnaires. All those who underwent fascicular or whole-nerve biopsy at the ankle or ankle and midcalf levels were considered together. Questionnaires also were available from patients who had had biopsies of nerves other than the sural, but the number was small. It can, however, be stated that symptoms reported by patients after superficial peroneal and saphenous nerve biopsy have so far been similar to those reported by patients after sural nerve biopsy. Questionnaires were answered by eight patients who had had motor nerve biopsy or combined motor and sensory nerve biopsy. "Partial paralysis" of the great toe was noted by one patient who had had fascicular biopsy of the deep peroneal nerve in the middle third of the leg. This may have been due to weakness of the extensor hallucis brevis or, more likely, of the extensor hallucis longus. We now take the biopsy from the lateral fascicles of the deep peroneal that run to the extensor digitorum brevis just above the ankle, a level below the branch to the extensor hallucis longus.

Approximately 60 per cent of patients who had had diagnostic sural nerve biopsy claimed to be entirely free of symptoms at three months, 36 per cent reported some persisting discomfort and other symptoms, and 3 per cent had symptoms such as numbness or swelling but no discomfort (Table 19–1). The most frequent symptom in the region of incision was a feeling of prickling followed by a tight or drawing sensation, burning, aching, numbness, and swelling of the ankle. Loss of sensation was most often noted at the heel or side of the foot, but a few patients mentioned loss of sensitivity adjacent to the ankle incision. Miscellaneous symptoms listed by four patients were "electric shock–like feelings," "pains like the snap of a rubber band," and a "tingling and twitching in the region of the fifth toe." The parents of an eight year old child who had had sural biopsy at ankle and

TABLE 19–1 SUMMARY OF PATIENTS' ANSWERS TO QUESTIONNAIRES AFTER SURAL NERVE BIOPSY

	3 Months		12 Months	
	Number	*Per Cent**	*Number*	*Per Cent**
Discomfort or symptom				
Prickling	22	52	21	54
Tight or drawing sensation	20	48	12	31
Burning	12	29	9	23
Aching	8	19	5	13
Numbness	6	14	10	26
Swelling of ankle	3	7	1	3
Other	4	10	4	10
Number with discomfort and other symptoms	39		36	
Number with symptoms but no discomfort	3		3	
Number with no discomfort or other symptom	66		58	
Total number answering questionnaire	108		97	
Time of discomfort or symptom				
While moving	11	26	6	15
While sitting	8	19	12	31
During day	8	19	8	21
During night	6	14	5	13
Anytime	5	12	3	8
When incision is rubbed	4	10	1	3
When incision is bumped	4	10	1	3
Other	6	14	6	15

*Based on total with symptoms or discomfort.

midcalf levels wrote that the child had bad dreams about the biopsy. It was evident that those patients with a severe degree of sensory loss experienced little or no pain and paresthesia during or after the biopsy, but there were exceptions to this generalization. Ten of the 108 patients were motivated to add that they had annoying symptoms during the first few days or weeks after the biopsy, but these had subsided by the time the three month questionnaire arrived.

In analyzing the answers to the question, When does the discomfort come? it was apparent that no single activity was especially noteworthy in this regard. Discomfort came as often with movement as with sitting still. Some noted paresthesia or pain when the incision was rubbed or bumped; others said that the discomfort did not occur at any particular time. Three patients had symptoms when there was pressure over the incision, one when the leg was stretched while doing exercises to lengthen shortened muscles, and one each after a change of weather and after "heat and cold."

At one year after the procedure, approximately 40 per cent of the patients admitted to some discomfort or other symptoms that they attributed to the nerve biopsy. This percentage is almost the same as the percentage of patients answering affirmatively at three months. The complaints most common at three months were again most common at one year. The number of different symptoms reported by each patient was less than at three months. These data give the misleading impression that the majority of patients with symptoms at three months cannot look forward to further reduction of their symptoms. It is clear from talking to patients that their persisting symptoms appear much less frequently with the passage of time. In all but a few, the symptoms that remain are of a mild nature. Significantly, none of the patients had pain of the intensity called causalgia after biopsy, nor are we aware of any patient who had developed neuropathic joints consequent to the surgical loss of deep sensation.

Patients Who Think Nerve Biopsy Should Not Be Done

Perhaps the most important question asked of the patients was: Is the discomfort severe enough that you think that biopsies should not be done? At three months after biopsy, seven patients replied that biopsies should not be performed; three others were not sure about the answer to the question at three months, but nine months later, when their symptoms had diminished or disappeared, all replied that biopsies should be done. Ten of 97 patients (10 per cent) answering the one-year questionnaire also answered in the negative. The actual percentage of patients with significant discomfort is probably less than 10 per cent since those with persisting symptoms may have been more likely to return the questionnaire.

An interesting finding was that the type of biopsy done did not have much bearing on whether patients thought nerve biopsies should or should not be done. The breakdown according to type of biopsy among the group who said biopsies should not be done was as follows: fascicles at ankle level, 9 of 78 (11.5 per cent); fascicles at ankle and midcalf levels, none of 5 (0 per cent); whole nerve, at ankle level, 2 of 23 (8.7 per cent); whole nerve at ankle and midcalf levels, 2 of 28 (7.1 per cent). There is no doubt, however, that fascicular biopsy at one level results in a smaller area of sensory loss than does whole-nerve biopsy. It also must be remembered that fascicular biopsy at two levels can be the equivalent of whole-nerve biopsy since different fascicles might be taken at each level.

The reason for condemnation of the procedure most often was that the patients found the pain and paresthesia too bothersome. One patient lost three toenails, and another with a collagen vascular disease reported that the biopsy site required several months to heal. A 46 year old man with a profound peripheral neuropathy, whose teased fibers showed marked segmental demyelination, reported constant paresthesia and the belief that the leg on which biopsy was performed was not as good as the other since the operation. Two patients indicated by their comments that they were also unhappy that no specific etiologic diagnosis or effective treatment resulted from histologic examination of their sural nerves.

In summary, 60 per cent of patients will have no symptoms one year after sural nerve biopsy, 30 per cent will have intermittent mild persisting symptoms that can be expected to disappear, and 10 per cent will be troubled by significant pain or paresthesia. It is probable that some of the discomfort experienced by many of the patients is related to the neuropathic process and not to the biopsy. How much of the time this is a factor is a question that cannot be answered.

CONSENT FOR NERVE BIOPSY

The patient's informed consent is a prerequisite for nerve biopsy. He should be given an outline of the operative procedure itself and of the nature and duration of the symptoms that may follow. The procedure should be done under local anesthesia, since the added risk of general anesthesia is almost never justified. Histologic examination of the excised nerve does not ensure a specific diagnosis or curative treatment; awareness of this fact by the patient will avoid excessive disappointment when nonspecific changes are found. The physician, of course, is responsible for recommending nerve biopsy only when the history, physical findings, and laboratory studies suggest that the procedure may yield information of value in the diagnosis and management of the patient's illness.

Selected patients may be asked to consider volunteering for nerve biopsy for a clinical study, a trial of drug therapy, or a study of the pathogenesis of peripheral neuropathy as part of a basic research project involving several disciplines. In these situations, the patient must clearly understand that the biopsy is being done for research purposes and not for diagnosis.

The consent form for nerve biopsy for research purposes used at the Mayo Clinic follows. It is presented as a model and might need additions or modifications if used at other centers engaged in peripheral nerve research. Most of the content of the consent form would also be part of our discussion with a patient prior to diagnostic nerve biopsy.

MAYO FOUNDATION

Consent to Participate in Medical Research Study

The Neurology Department has a program in research into the cause and treatment of nerve diseases. Research involving human subjects with and without peripheral nerve diseases is necessary to answer questions which we hope will ultimately lead to an understanding and cure of these disorders. Study of nerve tissue is essential to this research.

This request by Dr. _____ of Mayo Clinic is for permission to perform a biopsy of your _____ nerve as part of a

research entitled _____
_____. In the following paragraphs we will explain what is being asked of you, how the procedure is done and what symptoms may come from it.

Procedure

Nerve biopsy will be performed as an outpatient procedure in the operating room of the _____ _____ Hospital by Dr. _____ _____, who is experienced in the performance of this procedure. In the operating room your _____ will be prepared by cleansing and disinfecting procedures conventionally used in operating rooms. A local anesthetic will be infiltrated into the skin. A _____ cm skin incision will be made. A small sliver (approximately one fourth of the thickness *or* the full thickness) of the nerve will be removed for study. The entire procedure will take approximately _____ hours. The sutures are to be left in for _____ days. You may walk about immediately after the procedure but are encouraged to elevate your leg intermittently.

Symptoms

Recognized symptoms from this procedure which you may have include a soreness at the region of the incision for the first few days, a small region of sensation loss approximately _____ inches square in size which may be permanent, and an intermittent unpleasant and sometimes painful numbness in the region of the incision and in the area of the sensory loss. The first symptom is of little concern since it almost invariably disappears in a few days. The loss of sensation also is probably not of great importance since we have performed many biopsies of _____ nerve and have not found that this sensory loss has resulted in a skin ulcer or other disability. One patient has lost three toenails following nerve biopsy. The unpleasant or even painful numbness which may occur is something you should know about. Some subjects or patients have experienced it while moving about, when rubbing their fingers on the upper part of the incision, on stretching the nerve as in bending with the knees held straight, on sitting for a prolonged period of time, and unrelated to a known event. Some degree of painful numbness occurs at some time in approximately 40 per cent of persons having nerve biopsy. It is greatest within the first week and gradually subsides thereafter. Even after a year about one third of such subjects or patients have had on occasion an unpleasant or painful numbness. Approximately 10 per cent of subjects and patients say that this discomfort is of sufficient severity that they wish they had not had the nerve biopsy. We have not had any subject or patient who required pain medication or surgery for pain relief as a result of nerve biopsy. A few patients have taken a mild analgesic such as aspirin in the immediate post-operative period. A few patients have reported mild ankle swelling following nerve biopsy, although serious complications such as infection or other medical events conceivably could occur at the time of nerve biopsy.

Consent

The procedure of nerve biopsy, the place on my body from which the biopsy will be taken, and the symptoms and potential results of nerve biopsy have been explained to me. In addition I have read this form, which outlines these matters. I have had an opportunity to ask questions concerning the study and my participation, and they have been answered to my satisfaction by _____ (name of physician). I am aware that this procedure is done as a research study and not for diagnosis or treatment. I understand that I may withdraw at any time from participation in this study. I agree to the procedure of nerve biopsy.

Date:_____

Signature of Subject or Patient:

_____

Signature of Investigator Obtaining Consent:

_____

USEFULNESS OF NERVE BIOPSY

The indications for nerve biopsy are not well defined (Thomas, 1970). Certainly the many patients in whom the etiologic diagnosis is relatively certain on clinical and laboratory grounds alone (e.g., diabetes, alcohol, heavy metal poisoning) do not require nerve biopsy. Conversely, there are many patients whose illness defies diagnosis even after the most thorough investigation. The yield of specific diagnoses from nerve biopsy in these cases remains disappointingly small, although other information of value to the patient may be obtained.

At present, the list of diseases producing specific histologic alteration is not large, but in most the diagnosis often can be strongly suspected, making nerve biopsy worthwhile in these patients. In metachromatic leukodystrophy, the presence of metachromatically staining sulfatides in the cytoplasm of Schwann cells will confirm the diagnosis. Ultrastructural changes in the peripheral nerves in other lipid storage diseases also have been described (Babel et al., 1970). The diagnosis of inherited or primary amyloidosis often can be made on the basis of deposits lying in the connective tissue of the fascicles or infiltrating vessels in the epineurium. Objective evidence of necrotizing angiopathy associated with collagen vascular diseases such as periarteritis nodosa or rheumatoid arthritis producing a peripheral neuropathy or mononeuritis multiplex may be found if biopsy of an affected nerve is performed. Combining whole-nerve biopsy with adjacent muscle biopsy will improve the chances of finding the vasculitis. In leprosy, appropriate stains will show that the Schwann cells contain Hansen's bacilli.

Nonspecific but distinctive patterns of histologic abnormality are important because they direct attention to certain diagnostic possibilities and because they may provide support for the clinical diagnosis. For example, in the absence of vasculitis, a central-fascicular pattern of fiber degeneration suggests that ischemia was the cause (Dyck et al., 1972). The onion bulb formations of hypertrophic neuropathy suggest the diagnosis of Dejerine-Sottas disease, hypertrophic neuropathy of Charcot-Marie-Tooth, Refsum's disease, or other neuropathies in which there has been repeated segmental demyelination and re-myelination.

Teased-fiber preparations will indicate whether the neuropathy is predominantly demyelinating or axonal in type and, by inference, whether it affects Schwann cells or the neuron itself. This simple division has been complicated by the knowledge that segmental demyelination along the length of certain fibers may be a manifestation of malfunction of the primary sensory neuron (Dyck et al., 1971). The severity of the degenerative process and the amount of regeneration present may have some prognostic value regarding the possibility and rapidity of recovery.

In most cases, nerve biopsy will easily settle the more fundamental question of whether neuropathy is or is not present. Histologically normal nerve can be obtained, however, when the primary sensory neuron is affected proximal to the dorsal root ganglion or if demyelination is confined to the proximal portions of peripheral nerves. Combined motor and sensory nerve biopsy will demonstrate whether the disorder is affecting the lower motor neuron exclusively or if sensory neurons are affected as well.

Quantitative assessment of the number of fibers present per unit of fascicular area provides information about the number of fibers that have been lost. The fiber diameter spectrum may show that the process preferentially affects a certain population of myelinated fibers as in Friedreich's ataxia, dominantly inherited amyloidosis, or hereditary sensory neuropathy (see Chapter 15). An absence of unmyelinated fibers has been discovered in patients with familial dysautonomia (Aquayo et al., 1971). Pathophysiologic correlations are possible when the patient's symptoms, sensory abnormalities, and motor deficits can be compared with the quantitative histologic and teased-fiber measurements and the in vitro recording of the compound nerve action potential. Lastly, nerve biopsy may be justified as a research procedure designed to provide the answers that will eventually lead to better methods of diagnosis and treatment.

REFERENCES

Aitken, J. T., and Thomas, P. K.: Retrograde changes in fibre size following nerve section. J. Anat., 96:121, 1962.

Aquayo, A. J., Nair, C. P. V., and Bray, G. M.: Peripheral nerve abnormalities in the Riley-Day syndrome. Arch. Neurol., 24:106, 1971.

Aring, C. D., Bean, W. B., Roseman, E., Rosenbaum, M., and Spies, T. D.: The peripheral nerves in cases of nutritional deficiency. Arch. Neurol., 45:772, 1941.

Arnold, N., and Harriman, D. G.: The incidence of abnormality in control human peripheral nerves studied by single axon dissection. J. Neurol. Neurosurg. Psychiatry, 33:55, 1970.

Babel, J., Bischoff, A., and Spoendlin, H.: Ultrastructure of the peripheral nervous system and sense organs. In Bischoff, A. (ed.): Atlas of Normal and Pathologic Anatomy. Stuttgart, Georg Thieme Verlag, 1970.

Corbin, K. B., and Gardner, E. D.: Decrease in number of myelinated fibers in human spinal roots with age. Anat. Rec., 68:63, 1937.

Duchenne, G. B.: Physiology of Motion: Demonstrated by Means of Electrical Stimulation and Clinical Observation and Applied to the Study of Paralysis and Deformities. (Translated and edited by E. B. Kaplan.) Philadelphia, J. B. Lippincott Co., 1949.

Dyck, P. J., Beahrs, O. H., and Miller, R. H.: Peripheral nerves in hereditary neural atrophies: number and diameters of myelinated fibers (abstract). (Sixth International Congress of Electroencephalography and Clinical Neurophysiology, Vienna, 1965.) In Clinical Neurophysiology: EEG-EMG. Communications. Vienna, Wiener Medizinische Akademie, 1965, pp. 673–677.

Dyck, P. J., Conn, D. L., and Okazaki, H.: Necrotizing angiopathic neuropathy. Mayo Clin. Proc., 47:461, 1972.

Dyck, P. J., Johnson, W. J., Lambert, E. H., and O'Brien,

P. C.: Segmental demyelination secondary to axonal degeneration in uremic neuropathy. Mayo Clin. Proc., *46*:400, 1971.

Dyck, P. J., Lais, A., and Offord, K. P.: The nature of myelinated nerve fiber degeneration in dominantly inherited hypertrophic neuropathy. Mayo Clin. Proc., *49*:34–39, 1974.

Dyck, P. J., and Lambert, E. H.: Numbers and diameters of nerve fibers and compound action potential of sural nerve: controls and hereditary neuromuscular disorders. Trans. Am. Neurol. Assoc., *91*:214, 1966.

Dyck, P. J., and Lofgren, E. P.: Method of fascicular biopsy of human peripheral nerve for electrophysiologic and histologic study. Mayo Clin. Proc., *41*:778, 1966.

Dyck, P. J., and Lofgren, E. P.: Nerve biopsy: choice of nerve, method, symptoms, and usefulness. Med. Clin. North Am., *52*:885, 1968.

Dyck, P. J., Schultz, P. W., and Lais, A. C.: Mensuration and histologic typing of teased myelinated fibers of healthy sural nerve in man. *In* Kakulas, B. K. (ed.): Clinical Studies in Myology. Int. Congr. Series. Amsterdam, Excerpta Medica, 1973.

Gardner, E., and Gray, D. J.: The innervation of the joints of the foot. Anat. Rec., *161*:141, 1968.

Garven, H. S. D., Gairns, F. W., and Smith, G.: The nerve fibre populations of the nerves of the leg in chronic occlusive arterial disease in man. Scott. Med. J., *7*:250, 1962.

Greenfield, J. G., and Carmichael, E. A.: The peripheral nerves in cases of subacute combined degeneration of the cord. Brain, *58*:483, 1935.

Gutrecht, J. A., and Dyck, P. J.: Quantitative teased-fiber and histologic studies of human sural nerve during postnatal development. J. Comp. Neurol., *138*:117, 1970.

Jennekens, F. G. I., Tomlinso, B. E., and Walton, J. N.: The sizes of 2 main histochemical fiber types in 5 limb muscles in man. J. Neurol. Sci., *13*:281, 1971.

Lambert, E. H. The accessory deep peroneal nerve: a common variation in innervation of extensor digitorum brevis. Neurology (Minneap.), *19*:1169, 1969.

Lascelles, R. G., and Thomas, P. K.: Changes due to age in internodal length in the sural nerve in man. J. Neurol. Neurosurg. Psychiatry, *29*:40, 1966.

Lavarack, J. O., Sunderland, S., and Ray, L. J.: The branching of nerve fibers in human cutaneous nerves. J. Comp. Neurol., *94*:293, 1951.

Murai, Y., Ota, M., Kuroiwa, Y., and Yamaqucki, K.: Sensory conduction velocity and biopsy findings of sural nerves in normal and neuropathic subjects. Brain Nerve (Tokyo), *21*:233, 1969.

Ochoa, J., and Mair, W. G.: The normal sural nerve in man. I. Ultrastructure and numbers of fibers and cells. Acta Neuropathol. (Berl.), *13*:197, 1969.

O'Sullivan, D. J., and Swallow, M.: The fibre size and content of the radial and sural nerves. J. Neurol. Neurosurg. Psychiatry, *31*:464, 1968.

Ranson, S. W., Droegemueller, W. H., Davenport, H. K., and Fisher, C.: Number, size and myelination of the sensory fibers in the cerebrospinal nerves. Assoc. Res. Nerv. Ment. Dis. Proc., *15*:3, ·1935.

Rexed, B.: Contributions to the knowledge of the postnatal development of the peripheral nervous system in man: a study of the bases and scope of systematic investigations into the fibre size in peripheral nerves. Acta Psychiatr. Scand. [Suppl.], *33*:1, 1944.

Rexed, B., and Therman, P.-O.: Calibre spectra of motor and sensory nerve fibres to flexor and extensor muscles. J. Neurophysiol., *11*:133, 1948.

Sherrington, C. S.: On the anatomical constitution of nerves of skeletal muscles with remarks on recurrent fibers in the ventral spinal nerve-root. J. Physiol. (Lond.), *17*:211, 1894.

Steindler, A.: Kinesiology of the Human Body: Under Normal and Pathological Conditions. Springfield, Ill., Charles C Thomas, 1955.

Stevens, J. C., Lofgren, E. P., and Dyck, P. J.: Histometric evaluation of branches of peroneal nerve: technique for combined biopsy of muscle nerve and cutaneous nerve. Brain Res., *52*:37, 1973.

Sunderland, S., Lavarack, J. O., and Ray, L. J.: The caliber of nerve fibers in human cutaneous nerves. J. Comp. Neurol., *91*:87, 1949.

Swallow, M.: Fibre size and content of the anterior tibial nerve of the foot. J. Neurol. Neurosurg. Psychiatry, *29*:205, 1966.

Thevenard, A., and Berdet, H.: Remarques sur l'hypertrophie des nerfs périphériques: intérêt de l'exploration clinique du plexus cervical superficiel en particulier de sa branche auriculaire et de son examen histologique après biopsie. Presse Méd., *66*:529, 1958.

Thomas, P. K.: The quantitation of nerve biopsy findings. J. Neurol. Sci., *11*:285, 1970.

Tomasch, J., and Britton, W. A.: On the individual variability of fibre composition in human peripheral nerves. J. Anat., *90*:337, 1956.

Tomasch, J., and Schwarzacher, H. G.: Die innere Struktur peripherer menschlicher Nerven im Lichte faseranalytischer Untersuchungen. Acta Anat. (Basel), Suppl. *16*:315, 1952.

Tsairis, P., Dyck, P. J., and Mulder, D. W.: Natural history of brachial plexus neuropathy. Arch. Neurol., *27*:109, 1972.

Vizoso, A. D.: The relationship between internodal length and growth in human nerves. J. Anat., *84*:342, 1950.

Wohlfart, G., and Swank, R. L.: Pathology of amyotrophic lateral sclerosis: fiber analysis of the ventral roots and pyramidal tracts of the spinal cord. Arch. Neurol. Psychiatry, *46*:783, 1941.

SECTION IV

*Nerve Conduction and
Measurement of
Cutaneous Sensation
in Diseases of
the Peripheral Nervous System*

Chapter 20

COMPOUND ACTION POTENTIALS OF SURAL NERVE IN VITRO IN PERIPHERAL NEUROPATHY

Edward H. Lambert *and* Peter James Dyck

Electrophysiologic evidence for the involvement of different fiber groups in neuropathies can be obtained by recording the compound action potential of the nerve. In this chapter compound action potentials of fascicles of sural nerve obtained by biopsy in a variety of neuropathies are presented together with clinical and histologic data.

When a maximal electrical stimulus is applied to a mixed nerve, the resulting compound action potential recorded several centimeters away is dispersed in time and has two or more peaks. The compound action potential is the classic demonstration that the nerve is composed of groups of fibers with different conduction velocities. The action potentials of the most rapidly conducting fibers appear first in the record and those of more slowly conducting fibers appear later. In their initial studies of frog sciatic nerve, Erlanger and Gasser used Greek letters (α, β, γ, and δ) to identify successive peaks of the action potential in order of decreasing conduction velocity (Erlanger, 1927; Erlanger and Gasser, 1937). Subsequently, two additional peaks produced by fibers of much lower conduction velocity were discovered and were called B (not found in mammalian peripheral nerves) and C. The early peaks designated by Greek letters and referred to collectively as the A potential are produced by myelinated fibers ranging from large to small diameters. In mammalian nerves the designation B is reserved for an elevation produced by preganglionic (small-diameter myelinated) fibers in autonomic nerves, although for a time it was

also applied to the elevation now called A delta (Bishop and Heinbecker, 1930; Bishop, 1965). The C potential is produced by unmyelinated fibers. In cutaneous nerves, these include both dorsal root and sympathetic C fibers.

Erlanger and Gasser demonstrated that conduction velocity, as well as excitability, amplitude of action potential, and certain other properties of a nerve fiber are proportional to the fiber diameter. Among fibers that produce the A potential, conduction velocity and external fiber diameter are related almost linearly. Hursh (1939) compared maximal conduction velocity and diameter of the largest fibers of various nerves of the cat and found that the slope of the relationship was 6 m per second per micron diameter. It has been customary to use this factor in estimating one variable from the other. Thus, a fiber of 10 μm diameter would have a conduction velocity of approximately 60 m per second. Similar conversion factors for alpha fibers have been reported by others, but Boyd and Davey (1968) found a smaller conversion factor for small than for large-diameter myelinated fibers in the same nerve (4.5 for gamma fibers and 5.7 for alpha fibers in motor nerve of cat).

In unmyelinated fibers also, the velocity of conduction varies directly with diameter of the fiber, but the conversion factor of 1.7 determined by Gasser (1950, 1955) for unmyelinated fibers is much smaller than that for myelinated fibers.

Compound action potentials of nerves with different functions have characteristic configu-

427

rations depending on the fiber composition of the nerve (Bishop and Heinbecker, 1930; Erlanger and Gasser, 1937; Boyd and Davey, 1968). The compound action potentials and fiber diameter spectra of cutaneous nerves such as the sural nerve are relatively simple and remarkably constant. The myelinated fibers produce an A potential with two peaks commonly designated alpha and delta, respectively. The unmyelinated fibers produce a later peak called C. There is still some confusion of terminology in the designation of peaks in the A potential of cutaneous nerves. The initial peak, called A alpha by Gasser (1960) because it was the first peak in the compound action potential, was called A beta by Erlanger (1927) because its conduction velocity was like that of the A beta peak in muscle nerves. An intermediate peak present in early records, called A gamma, was shown by Gasser (1960) to be an artifact that was absent when optimal monophasic recording was achieved. Gasser noted a bulge on the falling phase of the alpha peak in some nerves, but saw no reason to give it a special designation. In this chapter the terms alpha and delta are used for the two peaks of the A potential. The letter designations are used to refer not only to elevations of the compound action potential but also to the fibers themselves. In the fiber diameter spectrum, the A alpha fibers are myelinated fibers with an outside diameter generally over 6 μm, the A delta fibers are myelinated fibers with diameters less than 6 μm, and the C fibers are unmyelinated fibers that have diameters of 0.5 to 2 μm.

To avoid the confusion in letter designations of elevations in the compound action potential, Lloyd (1943) introduced a classification based on fiber diameter in which major afferent fiber groups are designated by Roman numerals: I (12 to 21 μm), II (6 to 12 μm), III (1 to 6 μm), and IV (C fibers). In this classification the A alpha fibers of cutaneous nerve are in group II, the A delta fibers in group III, and the C fibers in group IV.

RECONSTRUCTION OF THE COMPOUND ACTION POTENTIAL

To test the hypothesis that the conduction velocity of a nerve fiber is proportional to its diameter, Erlanger and Gasser attempted to predict the contour of the compound action potential of myelinated fibers from the spectrum of fiber diameters in the nerve (Erlanger, 1927). Their assumptions were that (1) conduction velocity of a fiber is directly proportional to its outside diameter, (2) the amplitude of the action potential of a nerve fiber is proportional to its cross sectional area, and (3) the action potential of all fibers has the same form and duration and can be approximated by a triangle in which the rising phase is one third of the total duration.

Reconstruction of a compound action potential was carried out by placing a triangle representing an action potential in its appropriate position along the abscissa for each myelinated fiber in the nerve. The position and amplitude of the triangle were determined by the fiber diameter. Summation of the triangles produced a contour that was a reasonable reproduction of the recorded compound action potential. More faithful reconstruction has been a challenge for many investigators; the classic one of the action potential of myelinated fibers of the cat saphenous nerve by Gasser and Grundfest (1939) was accomplished with a highly complicated technique. Recently Landau, Clare, and Bishop (1968) have described a simpler arithmetic method that employs corresponding fiber diameter histograms and is applicable to myelinated central nerve tracts as well as peripheral nerves.

Gasser (1950, 1955) was able to reconstruct the compound action potential of unmyelinated fibers from fiber diameter measurements by using a set of assumptions about the relation of conduction velocity and spike size to fiber diameter that was generally similar to that for myelinated fibers.

FIBER GROUPS AND SENSATION

In the early 1930's Heinbecker, Bishop, and O'Leary (1933, 1936) recorded the compound action potential of human nerves within 15 minutes to one hour after obtaining them from amputated limbs or from persons who died violently. In cutaneous nerves, they identified three potential elevations that they designated A or A beta-gamma (A alpha), B (A delta), and C. (The current designation of these elevations is given in parentheses.) The strengths of electrical stimuli required to excite the different fiber groups in excised nerve were compared with strengths of stimuli that produced sensations of different quality in vivo in unanesthetized man. In some instances observations were made on the same nerves before and after excision. Electrical stimulation of nerves in vivo caused only two sensations, touch and pain. Correlating thresholds for sensation and reflex effects with thresholds for the various components of the compound action potential and with histologic measurements of fiber diameter, these investigators concluded that stimuli that excited only the largest myelinated fibers (A alpha) produced tactile sensation, and stronger stimuli, which also excited A delta fibers, caused a pricking touch sensation. Repetitive stimulation of the latter fibers (3 to 7 shocks) caused pain. They failed to find a specific sensory effect from stimulation of the C fibers, but reactions to such strong stimuli were described as so violent that threshold determinations were not reliable.

Similar results were obtained by Collins, Nulsen, and Randt (1960), who stimulated the exposed sural nerve in nine conscious patients just prior to anterolateral thoracic cordotomy. The compound action potential recorded from the cut, crushed distal end of the nerve, in situ, had three major elevations designated Aβ-γ (A alpha), Aδ and C in order of increasing threshold and decreasing conduction velocity. Stimuli sufficient to excite only the A alpha fibers caused a tapping or thumping sensation. Neither single nor repetitive stimuli of this strength were painful. Increasing the strength of stimulus two to three times to excite the A delta fibers added a stinging or burning quality. Repetitive stimuli of this strength were always very painful. Further increase in the stimulus to 50 times the threshold for A alpha fibers excited C fibers. Even single stimuli that excited the C group caused unbearable pain. It was noted, however, that a stimulus of this intensity in addition to exciting C fibers caused repetitive firing of fibers of the A group.

A more definitive analysis of the sensory modalities mediated by fibers of different groups has been obtained by studies in animals. Single nerve fibers excited by adequate stimuli have been classified on the basis of their conduction velocity measured in situ. In such studies, fibers from mechanoreceptors are found in all fiber groups, A alpha and delta, and C. (Zotterman, 1939; Maruhashi et al., 1952; Douglas and Ritchie, 1957; Iggo, 1960; Iriuchijima and Zotterman, 1960). High-sensitivity mechanoreceptors that excite C fibers occur in hairy skin, but may be infrequent or absent in glabrous skin (Bessow et al., 1971).

Fibers activated by noxious stimuli, warmth, and cold are in both the A delta and C fiber groups, but not in the A alpha group.

Observations in man of the sensory abnormalities associated with disorders that cause a more or less selective loss of particular fiber groups support the view that touch-pressure, two-point recognition, joint position, and vibration sensations are mediated predominantly by fibers of the A alpha group, while sensations of pain, warmth, and cold are mediated by A delta and C groups (Dyck et al., 1971). There is as yet no evidence in man that small myelinated and unmyelinated fibers transmit impulses from high-sensitivity mechanoreceptors.

COMPOUND ACTION POTENTIALS OF SURAL NERVE IN PERIPHERAL NEUROPATHY

Recording the Compound Action Potential

A method for obtaining an ideal monophasic record of the compound action potential has not been found (Gasser, 1960). Several sources of distortion have been discussed in detail by Bishop, Erlanger, and Gasser (1926), Gasser and Grundfest (1939), Rushton (1949), Gasser (1960), and others. Some of these are as follows:

Shock strengths that are at threshold for delta fibers exceed by several times the threshold for alpha fibers. When the strength of stimulus is sufficient to excite the complete spectrum of A fibers, alpha fibers are excited further from the stimulating cathode than delta fibers, and the alpha elevation appears too early relative to the delta elevation in the compound action potential.

Strong shocks required to excite delta fibers may, particularly in fresh nerves, cause repetitive firing of alpha fibers, and the appearance of an extra elevation following the alpha potential. Similarly, strong stimuli required to excite C fibers may cause prolonged repetitive firing of A fibers whose action potentials may appear in the interval between the delta and C elevations.

Inadequate reduction of the diphasic artifact or lead separation effect (Gasser, 1960) may accentuate elevations or cause the appearance of artifactual elevations in the compound action potential.

Repetitive stimulation of C fibers at frequencies as low as 5 per second causes increase in the negative afterpotential of the C fibers and an increase in amplitude and duration of the C potential. Conduction velocity is decreased (Gasser, 1950; Ritchie and Straub, 1956; Brown and Holmes, 1956). The effect is reversible, but unless stimulation is infrequent, the C potential may be artificially enhanced.

A drop of fluid or fragment of tissue on the nerve between recording electrodes can cause distortion of the action potential (Bishop et al., 1926; Rushton, 1945). Changes in interelectrode resistance caused by drying of the nerve or by excess fluid on the nerve produce proportional changes in amplitude of the action potential. Drying does not change the conduction velocity until it is sufficient to damage the nerve fibers, causing a decrease in both amplitude and conduction velocity of the potential (Rud, 1961).

Method of Study

In most instances a fascicular biopsy of the sural nerve was obtained for study. The nerve was exposed from a point 1 to 2 cm above the lateral malleolus proximally for 10 to 15 cm. A bundle of 2 to 5 fascicles was dissected from the nerve; the distal 4 to 5 cm was used for histologic studies, and the proximal 4 to 6 cm was used for action potential recording. Immediately after excision the nerve was placed in cool Tyrode's solution, through which oxygen with 5 per cent carbon dioxide had been bubbled, and was taken from the operating room to the laboratory. Blood vessels, fat, and epineurium were cut away from the fascicles under a dissecting microscope. Cut or branching fascicles were removed. The nerve was placed on a series of silver electrodes in a chamber with an atmosphere of 5 per cent carbon dioxide in oxygen saturated with water vapor. The nerve was held under slight tension with an 0.5 to 0.9 gm weight hanging from each end. The chamber was sealed and immersed in a water bath at 37°C.

The nerve was stimulated at its distal end while the compound action potential was displayed on an oscilloscope and photographed. Monophasic records were made at several positions along the length of the nerve for determination of the conduction velocity of the various fiber groups, using maximal stimuli for each component of the action potential. Monophasic recordings were obtained by crushing the nerve between recording electrodes and applying 0.1 per cent procaine at the distal electrode. Optimal records for illustrating the contour of the compound action potential were obtained when the distance between recording electrodes was 5 to 10 mm (Gasser, 1960). For the illustrations that follow, the conduction distance (stimulating cathode to first recording electrode) was 20 to 22 mm, except for Figure 20–3 for which the distance was 30 mm.

Compound Action Potential and Fiber Diameter Spectrum

In normal nerves the contour of the compound action potential is determined by the relative numbers of excitable and conducting nerve fibers with various conduction velocities. Because conduction velocity and spike size are proportional to diameter of the fiber, one can in normal nerve, by using appropriate proportionality factors, make a reasonable prediction of the fiber diameter spectrum from the contour of the compound action potential. In this prediction, the amplitude of a component of the compound action potential (or the area of that component if its duration is not constant) is proportional to the density rather than to the total number of fibers that contribute to it. A much simplified model utilizing Ohm's law illustrates the basis of this relationship.

The current contributed by each fiber is $i = \frac{e}{R + r}$ in which e is the electromotive force generated by the fiber membrane, r is the internal resistance of the axis cylinder, and R is the external resistance, i.e., the resistance of the tissue and fluid surrounding the fiber. Since r is usually very large relative to R, because of the small diameter of the fiber, i is not greatly affected by small changes in external resistance (Gasser and Grundfest, 1939). The external resistance, however, is a particularly important factor affecting the amplitude of the action potential recorded by electrodes on the surface of the nerve. The amplitude (E) of the action potential recorded by surface electrodes is determined by the product of the action current flowing along the nerve between the two recording electrodes and the external (or interelectrode) resistance $(E = iR)$. Assuming that each nerve fiber of a particular diameter contributes an equal amount (i) to the action current, the total current contributed by that fiber group would be proportional to the total number of such fibers in the nerve ($I = ni$). A large nerve with a greater number of nerve fibers would have a greater action current than a small nerve. The larger nerve with the greater number of nerve fibers may not have a larger action potential, however, because as the diameter of the nerve increases, the external electrical resistance of the nerve decreases, and the product, $E = IR$, may remain the same. Thus, a whole nerve composed of many fascicles produces no larger an action potential than a single one of the fascicles dissected from the nerve, provided the composition of the fascicles is uniform. On the other hand, a nerve with many fibers per square millimeter of cross sectional area produces an action potential of higher amplitude than does a nerve with few fibers per square millimeter (ni or I is greater, but R is not proportionately lower). From these considerations it is apparent that the amplitude of a component of the compound action potential is roughly proportional to the density in the nerve of fibers that produce that component, rather than to the total number of those fibers in the nerve.

In neuropathy, changes in the contour of the compound action potential may result from changes in conduction velocity of the fibers either by demyelination or attenuation of fiber diameter, or by a disproportionate change in density of active nerve fibers in the different fiber groups by degeneration or inexcitability or block of conduction of fibers, or by both. A decrease in amplitude of all components of the compound action potential might occur from a proportional decrease in density of active fibers in all groups by degeneration, conduction block, or loss of excitability or by increase in relative amount of interstitial tissue.

Illustrative Compound Action Potentials and Fiber Diameter Histograms

NORMAL NERVE

The compound action potential has prominent A alpha, A delta and C components (Fig. 20–1*A*). The conduction velocity of the beginning of the alpha component was 61 m per second at 37°C. The peak of the delta component was conducted at 19 m per second and the

beginning and peak of the C potential were conducted at 1.6 and 1.1 m per second, respectively.

The histograms of fiber diameters in fascicles of the same nerve are plotted in two ways: the conventional way with increasing diameter from left to right on the abscissa as in Figure 20–1*B*, and the opposite way with decreasing diameter from left to right as in Figure 20–1*C*. In the conventional plot, the consecutive peaks of the histogram for myelinated fibers appear to correspond closely in relative amplitude and form with the alpha and delta peaks of the compound action potential. In fact, however, the large diameter fibers in the second peak on the right in the fiber diameter spectrum conduct impulses with the higher velocity and account for the alpha potential to the left in the compound action potential.

The histogram plotted in the opposite way presents the spectrum in order of decreasing diameter and conduction velocity, just as the components of the compound action potential occur in order of decreasing conduction velocity. The largest fibers present in significant numbers are 11 to 12 μm in diameter. If these fibers account for the beginning of the A alpha potential conducted at 61 m per second the ratio of conduction velocity to fiber diameter is about 5.3:1. Since varying amounts of shrinkage occur with the use of different histologic methods, this ratio may vary.

There is no discontinuity between the alpha and delta components of the A potential in cutaneous nerve. Similarly there is no discontinuity in the fiber diameter histogram between the distribution of large and small myelinated fibers. The alpha and delta peaks result from a high concentration of fibers in regions of a continuous spectrum of fiber diameters (Heinbecker et al., 1936; Bishop, 1965). From an evaluation of the amplitude and of the conduction velocity of various components of the compound action potential some inferences can be made about numbers, sizes, and abnormalities of fibers in the nerve evaluated.

It is usually assumed, in relating the compound action potential to the histogram of fiber diameters, that the diameter of fibers in a section is the same along the length of the nerve. Even in healthy nerve this is only approximately correct. In myelinated fibers of normal appearance considerable variability in diameter occurs along their length. The fiber usually has a greater diameter in paranodal regions and lesser diameters at nodes of Ran-

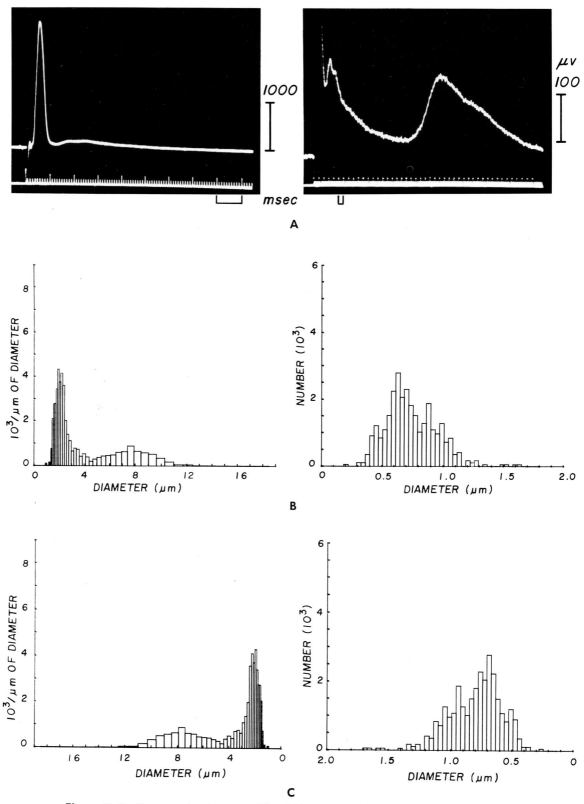

Figure 20–1 Compound action potential and histograms of fiber diameters of normal nerve.

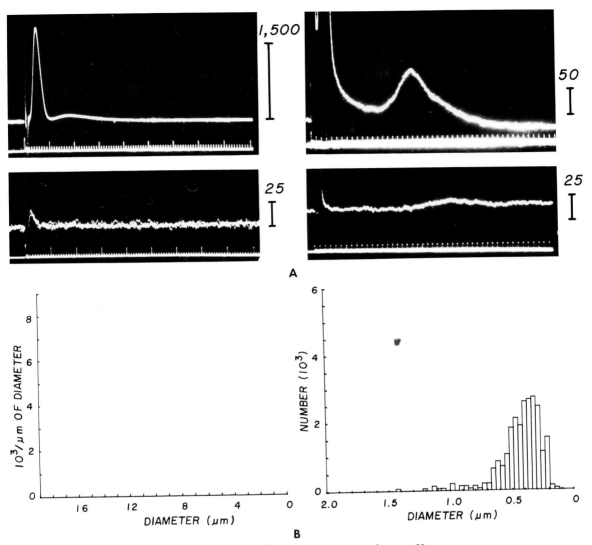

Figure 20–6   Hereditary sensory neuropathy type II.

D). The much higher density of myelinated fibers per square millimeter and the much lower frequency of teased fibers showing condition E in the sural nerve taken from the mid-calf as compared to the ankle level indicated that the pathologic alterations were much more severe in the distal parts of the nerve. This and other evidence favored the view that axonal atrophy and degeneration was primary (see Chapter 48).

RELAPSING INFLAMMATORY POLYRADICULONEUROPATHY

All components of the compound action potential probably are represented (Fig. 20–8A). The A component has a very small amplitude and is dispersed. Conduction velocity of the first wave is very slow (11 m per second). Presumably this is produced by A alpha fibers, but the rate of conduction in many of the A alpha fibers may be so low that their action potentials are mixed with those of the A delta fibers. The C fiber potential is normal in size. Some of the more slowly conducting, segmentally demyelinated A fibers may contribute to this potential, however, and may account for its unusual shape and irregularity.

The spectrum of fiber diameters does not correspond closely with the form of the compound action potential when there is segmental demyelination (Fig. 20–8B). The mean conduction velocity over the length of a myelinated fiber is determined by the mean of the velocity of conduction from one internode to the next over many internodes. When the internodes are uniform, as they usually are in

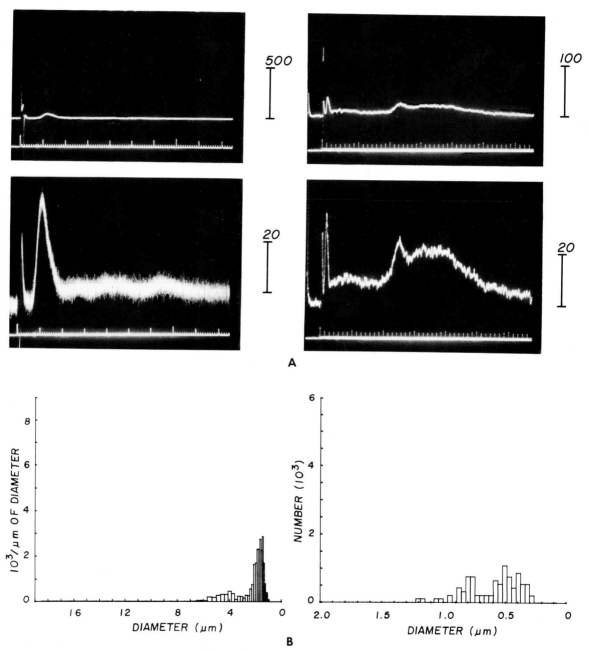

Figure 20–7 Uremic neuropathy.

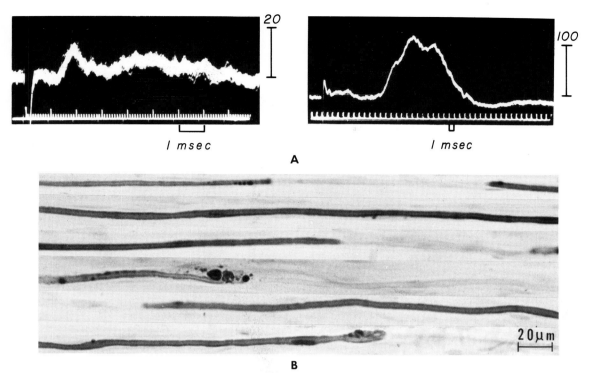

A

B

Figure 20–8 Relapsing inflammatory polyradiculoneuropathy.

healthy nerve, the diameter of the fiber at one internode may be representative of the fiber and be related to the mean conduction velocity (Fig. 20–9). When there is segmental demyelination and remyelination there may be a wide disparity between diameter of internodes. The diameter in a single section may not be representative of the fiber and therefore is not a reliable indicator of its conduction velocity.

HEREDITARY MOTOR AND SENSORY NEUROPATHY TYPE I (HYPERTROPHIC NEUROPATHY OF CHARCOT-MARIE-TOOTH TYPE)

The A alpha and delta potentials are reduced in size and increased in duration, but the C potential is essentially normal (Fig. 20–10). Conduction velocity of the A alpha and delta potentials is low. The velocity of the beginning of the A alpha potential is 17 m per second; that of the beginning of the C potential is normal, 1.1 m per second.

Although the transverse fascicular area of the sural nerves in this disorder is abnormally large, the total number and the density of myelinated fibers in the nerve is decreased. The largest myelinated fibers are smaller than normal, and evidence of segmental demyelination and remyelination is found with a variable

degree of "onion bulb" formation. The pathologic alterations in the myelinated fibers are sufficient to explain the abnormality of the A potential.

An example of the compound action potential in the hypertrophic neuropathy of the Dejerine-Sottas type is given in Chapter 41. In both these disorders, the apparent preservation of A alpha and delta elevations, in some cases despite marked slowing of conduction, suggests that there may be relatively uniform involvement of these two fiber groups.

COMMENTS

The conformation of the compound action potential of a nerve is determined by the relative density of functioning nerve fibers in different regions of the conduction velocity spectrum. In the evaluation of a patient with peripheral neuropathy, the compound action potential of a fascicular biopsy of sural nerve can give an indication of the populations of cutaneous nerve fibers that are affected and of the general nature of the pathologic alterations.

Acute degeneration of some myelinated nerve fibers may leave others whose conduction velocity remains essentially or nearly normal. Although the amplitude of the A poten-

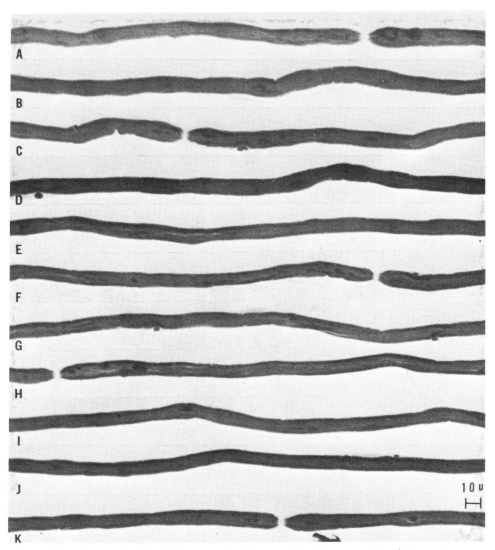

Figure 20-9 Uniform internodes in healthy nerve; the diameter of the fiber at one internode may be representative of that fiber and be related to the mean conduction velocity.

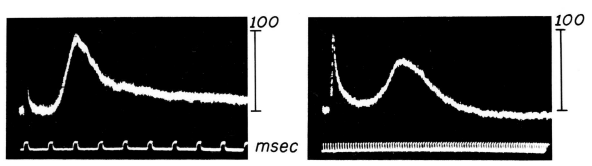

Figure 20-10 Hereditary motor and sensory neuropathy type I.

tial is smaller than normal, the alpha and delta elevations can be identified. If degenerating and nonconducting fibers can be excluded from the fiber diameter histogram, a reasonable correspondence between it and the compound action potential is found.

Widespread segmental demyelination and remyelination within nerve is associated with a low conduction velocity of myelinated fibers. The alpha and delta potentials may remain as discrete potentials if there is uniform involvement of all fiber groups. More often, however, there is disproportionate slowing of conduction in different fibers, and the alpha and delta potentials may be widely dispersed and merge so that alpha and delta elevations cannot be identified reliably. The potentials of alpha fibers are mixed with those of delta fibers. The fiber diameter histogram does not correlate well with the compound action potential because the wide variation in diameter of successive internodes of a nerve fiber prevents reliable prediction of its conduction velocity.

References

Bessow, P., Burgess, P. R., Perl, E. R., Taylor, C. B.: Dynamic properties of mechanoreceptors with unmyelinated C fibers. J. Neurophysiol., 34:116–131, 1971.

Bishop, G. H.: My life among the axons. In Hall, V. E. (ed.): Annual Review of Physiology. Palo Alto, Calif., Annual Reviews, Inc., 1965, p. 1.

Bishop, G. H., and Heinbecker, P.: Differentiation of axon types in visceral nerves by means of the potential record. Am. J. Physiol., 94:170, 1930.

Bishop, G. H., Erlanger, J., and Gasser, H. S.: Distortion of action potentials as recorded from the nerve surface. Am. J. Physiol., 78:592–609, 1926.

Boyd, I. A.: Differences in diameter and conduction velocity of motor and fusimotor fibres in nerves to different muscles in the hind limb of the cat. In Curtis, D. R., and McIntyre, A. C. (eds.): Studies in Physiology Presented to J. C. Eccles. Berlin, Springer Verlag, 1965, pp. 7–12.

Boyd, I. A., and Davey, M. R.: Composition of Peripheral Nerves. Edinburgh and London, Livingston Ltd., 1968, p. 57.

Brown, G. L., and Holmes, O.: The effects of activity on mammalian nerve fibres of low conduction velocity. Proc. R. Soc. Lond. [Biol.], 145:1–14, March, 1956.

Collins, W. F., Jr., Nulsen, F. E., and Randt, C. T.: Relation of peripheral nerve fiber size and sensation in man. A.M.A. Arch. Neurol., 3:381–385, 1960.

Douglas, W. W., and Ritchie, J. M.: Non-medullated fibres in the saphenous nerve which signal touch. J. Physiol., 139:385–399, 1957.

Dyck, P. J., and Lambert, E. H.: Compound nerve action potentials and morphometry. Electroencephalogr. Clin. Neurophysiol., 36:561–576, 1974.

Dyck, P. J., Lambert, E. H., and Nichols, P. C.: Quantitative measurement of sensation related to compound action potential and number and sizes of myelinated and unmyelinated fibers of sural nerve in health, Friedreich's ataxia, hereditary sensory neuropathy and tabes dorsalis. In Rémond, A. (ed.): Handbook of Electroencephalography and Clinical Neurophysiology, Vol. 9. Amsterdam, Elsevier Publishing Co., 1971, pp. 83–118.

Erlanger, J.: The interpretation of the action potentials in cutaneous and muscle nerves. Am. J. Physiol., 82:644–655, 1927.

Erlanger, J., and Gasser, H. S.: Electrical Signs of Nervous Activity. Philadelphia, University of Pennsylvania Press, 1937.

Gasser, H. S.: Unmedullated fibers originating in dorsal root ganglia. J. Gen. Physiol., 33:651–690, 1950.

Gasser, H. S.: Properties of dorsal root unmedullated fibers on the two sides of the ganglion. J. Gen. Physiol., 38:709–728, 1955.

Gasser, H. S.: Effect of the method of leading on the recording of the nerve fiber spectrum. J. Gen. Physiol., 43:927–940, 1960.

Gasser, H. S., and Erlanger, J.: The role played by the sizes of the constituent fibers of a nerve trunk in determining the form of its action potential wave. Am. J. Physiol., 80:522–547, 1927.

Gasser, H. S., and Grundfest, H.: Axon diameters in relation to the spike dimensions and the conduction velocity in mammalian A fibers. Am. J. Physiol., 127:393–414, 1939.

Heinbecker, P., Bishop, G. H., and O'Leary, J.: Pain and touch fibres in peripheral nerves. Arch. Neurol. Psychiatry, 29:771–789, 1933.

Heinbecker, P., Bishop, G. H., and O'Leary, J.: Functional and histologic studies of somatic and autonomic nerves of man. Arch. Neurol. Psychiatry, 35:1233–1255, 1936.

Hursh, J. B.: The conduction velocity and diameter of nerve fibers. Am. J. Physiol., 127:131–139, 1939.

Hursh, J. B.: The properties of growing nerve fibers. Am. J. Physiol., 127:140–153, 1939.

Iggo, A.: Cutaneous mechanoreceptors with afferent C fibres. J. Physiol. (Lond.), 152:337–353, 1960.

Iriuchijima, J., and Zotterman, Y.: The specificity of afferent cutaneous C fibres in mammals. Acta Physiol. Scand., 49:267–278, 1960.

Landau, W. M., Clare, M. H., and Bishop, G. H.: Reconstruction of myelinated nerve tract action potentials: an arithmetic method. Exp. Neurol., 22:480–490, 1968.

Lloyd, D. P. C.: Neuron patterns controlling transmission of ipsilateral hind limb reflexes in cat. J. Neurophysiol., 6:293–315, 1943.

Maruhashi, J., Mizuguchi, K., and Tasaki, I.: Action currents in single afferent nerve fibres elicited by stimulation of the skin of the toad and the cat. J. Physiol. (Lond.), 117:129–151, 1952.

Ritchie, J. M., and Straub, R. W.: The after-effect of repetitive stimulation on mammalian non-medullated fibres. J. Physiol. (Lond.), 134:698–711, 1956.

Rushton, W. A. H.: Resistance artefacts in action potential measurements. J. Physiol. (Lond.), 104:19 p, 1945.

Rushton, W. A. H.: The site of excitation in the nerve trunk of the frog. J. Physiol. (Lond.), 109:314–326, 1949.

Rud, J.: Local anesthetics. An electrophysiological investigation of local anesthesia of peripheral nerves with special reference to Xylocaine. Acta Physiol. Scand., 51, Suppl. 178, 1961.

Schaefer, H., and Schmitz, W.: Actionsstrom und Hullenleitfahigfeit. Arch. Gesamte Physiol., 234:737–747, 1934.

Zotterman, Y.: Touch, pain and tickling: an electrophysiological investigation on cutaneous sensory nerves. J. Physiol. (Lond.), 95:1–28, 1939.

Chapter 21

SENSORY POTENTIALS OF NORMAL AND DISEASED NERVES

Fritz Buchthal, Annelise Rosenfalck, *and* Friedrich Behse

Dawson (1956) was the first to record percutaneously from sensory nerve. He stimulated digital nerves and recorded sensory potentials at the wrist and at the elbow. Gilliatt and co-workers (1958, 1961, 1962) used sensory conduction time as a diagnostic aid in investigations of patients with peripheral nerve lesions. For the most part, they used differences in amplitude of the sensory potential as the indicator of involvement. Since it was not possible to record sensory potentials in half the patients, Buchthal and Rosenfalck (1966) improved the signal-to-noise ratio by adding a special input circuit and using electronic averaging. It thereby became possible to record sensory potentials at distal and proximal sites from nearly all diseased nerves. Fast as well as slow components of the potential were recorded, and their conduction velocities, amplitudes, and shapes were related to fiber caliber and to threshold of perception of touch. In systemic neuropathies the procedure was applied to obtain information about the histopathologic changes responsible for the abnormalities (Kaeser and Lambert, 1962; Gilliatt, 1966, 1969; Thomas, 1971; Buchthal and Rosenfalck, 1971a). In localized involvement, such as entrapment syndromes or traumatic lesions of peripheral nerves, the recording of sensory conduction allows the damage to be localized and local entrapment to be distinguished from root damage or systemic involvement (Payan, 1969).

METHODS

Stimulation

Sensory nerves were stimulated percutaneously or by needle electrodes placed near the nerve at sites where only sensory fibers were activated (Fig. 21–1) (Buchthal and Rosenfalck, 1966, 1971a; Behse and Buchthal, 1971). The stimulus was provided by a constant-current generator with a floating ground. To stimulate sensory fibers maximally with surface electrodes in normal nerve, 20 to 50 ma (0.2 msec) current was used. Activation of all fibers in diseased nerve may require up to 80 ma (cf. Fig. 21–10). Stimulation with needle electrodes requires current of 10 to 20 ma.

Recording

One of the recording electrodes (bared tip, 3 mm) was placed near the nerve, the remote electrode was placed at a transverse distance of 3 to 4 cm. The recording amplifier had a noise level lower than the noise produced by the electrodes (0.5 to 1 μv peak-to-peak, 20 to 4000 Hz) and a blocking time of less than 0.5 msec (Andersen and Buchthal, 1970). Averaging of 500 traces allowed components of 0.05 μv to be identified by their shape; with 1000 or more responses, 0.03 to 0.01 μv potentials could be distinguished from noise. The small components of the potential were

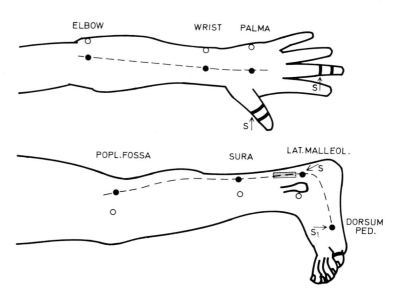

Figure 21–1 Placement of the "near-nerve" (•) and remote (○) needle electrodes to record from different segments of the median and sural nerve. S, stimulating cathode (surface or needle); S_1, cathode to stimulate the distal segment of the sural nerve. The shaded area shows the 3 cm segment taken in toto as biopsy.

identified by their shape when they increased in proportion to a calibration signal in subsequent averaging of, e.g., 250, 500, and 1000 responses (see also Figs. 21–3, 21–10, and 21–20).

Most recordings referred to in this chapter have been obtained by electronic averaging of many responses. Therefore a few remarks about the application of this technique seem appropriate. When averaging techniques are used it is assumed that interference from noise represents unpredictable stochastic variations superimposed on a deterministic response time locked to the stimulus. The response increases linearly with the number of stimuli (n); the root mean square of the amplitude of noise increases with the square of n, so the signal-to-noise ratio improves with the square root of n. When the noise is restricted to a narrow range of frequency (limitation of frequency band and amplitudes in the amplifier and interference by muscle action potentials), however, the square root function does not apply; the signal-to-noise ratio may be smaller or larger than the square root of n (Ten Hoopen and Reuver, 1972). Moreover, if the amplifier is overloaded by a muscle action potential the sweep is counted but not added. We introduced therefore a calibration signal, which is averaged together with the response, and compared its size with that of the response after averaging to estimate the amplitude (Buchthal and Rosenfalck, 1971a).

The maximum conduction velocity was determined from latency to the first positive peak of the potential and the minimum conduction velocity from latency to the first positive peak of the last component. Because of the change in conduction velocity with temperature (2 m per second per degree centigrade), the surface temperature of the extremity was kept constant at 35° to 37° C. This was obtained by a thermocouple placed on the extremity, which controlled an infrared heating element. When the velocity was calculated from latency to a single point of recording an increase in stimulus from submaximal to maximal may simulate an increase in distal velocity (Gilliatt et al., 1965; Buchthal and Rosenfalck, 1966, 1971b; Wiederholt, 1970). That the 2 to 5 per cent faster velocity was in fact due to proximal displacement of the point of stimulation was demonstrated by recording the conduction time as a function of stimulus strength at three different sites (wrist, elbow, axilla). The conduction time decreased equally at the three sites of recording.

THE SENSORY POTENTIAL OF NORMAL NERVE

Shape and Amplitude

The sensory potential evoked by stimulation of the digits and recorded at the wrist had a main triphasic component with an average range of 10 to 50 μv, followed by four or five small components of less than 0.5 μv (cf. Fig. 21–15). With longer distances of conduction the amplitude decreased and was from 3 to 20 μv at the elbow. At the same time temporal dispersion increased and there was less difference in the amplitude of both the main and the slower components (Buchthal and Rosen-falck, 1966, 1971a). The amplitude of the potential recorded at the ankle and in the popliteal fossa was about 5 to 10 per cent of that recorded at the wrist and at the elbow. The potential at the ankle, evoked by stimuli at the big toe and recorded from the super-ficial peroneal or posterior tibial nerve, nearly always consisted of 5 to 10 short spikes of 0.5 to 2 μv followed by several components of 0.5 to 0.1 μv. The potentials were less dispersed when the sural nerve was stimulated at the dorsum pedis and the potential was recorded at the lateral malleolus (cf. Fig. 21–7) (Behse and Buchthal, 1971).

Sensory Conduction and Caliber of Nerve Fibers

The conduction velocity increases with the external diameter of the nerve fiber (Gasser and Erlanger, 1927; Hursh, 1939; Rushton, 1951; Boyd and Davey, 1968). In the median nerve, in which sensory conduction was related to the distribution of fiber diameters in two nerves obtained at autopsy, the conver-sion factor was 5 and 5.7. The maximum sensory velocity corresponded to conduction along fibers 11 μm in diameter (Buchthal and Rosenfalck, 1966). In the sural nerve, in which conduction velocity and distribution of fiber diameters were determined in the same nerves, the first positive peak corresponded to fibers 12 to 13 μm in diameter (Fig. 21–2). Fibers of larger diameter conducted still faster; there were only a few and their responses were hidden in the rising phase of the initial posi-tive peak of the potential. The conversion factor was determined from the velocity of the fastest component and the largest fibers found in the same nerve (4.4 ± 0.1, n = 13). The fac-tor was the same for later components as long as the fibers were more than 7 μm in diameter (Behse et al., unpublished data).

The main phases of the potential in the sural nerve originated from about 1400 nerve fibers, 9 to 14 μm in diameter. They repre-sent 20 per cent of all myelinated fibers and 60 per cent of fibers 7 μm or more in diameter (group II). The slower components in the potential derived from the large group of myelinated fibers less than 7 μm in diameter (group III). The minimum velocity was de-termined from the latency to the last compo-

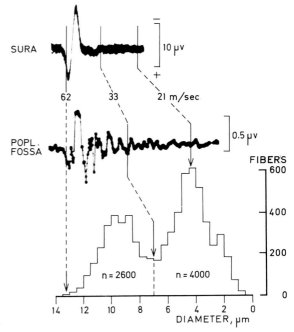

Figure 21–2 Components of the sensory potential and distribution of diameters of myelinated fibers in a normal sural nerve. *Top and middle.* The nerve was stimulated maximally at the lateral malleolus, and the potential was recorded 15 cm (sura, photographic superposition of 15 responses) and 50 cm (popliteal fossa, electronic averaging of 200 responses) proximally to it. The temperature near the nerve was 36° to 37° C. The dashed lines connect components conducted at the same velocity in the poten-tials recorded at the two sites, and point to the corre-sponding fiber diameter in the histogram below. The conversion factor (4.7) was determined from the com-ponents conducted at 62 m per second and the fibers of 13 to 13.5 μm in diameter. *Bottom.* Distribution of diame-ters of all myelinated fibers (n=6600) obtained from a biopsy of the same nerve taken 2 cm proximal to the lateral malleolus. The subject was a 14 year old boy (F.H.S.F.) without signs or symptoms of neuromuscular involvement in the legs. (From Behse, F., Buchthal, F., Carlsen, F., and Knappeis, G. G.: Light and electron microscopy as related to sensory conduction along normal and diseased sural nerve. Unpublished data.)

nent of the averaged response. Fifteen centi-meters proximal to the lateral malleolus the minimum velocity averaged 15 m per second, corresponding to fibers about 4 μm in diame-ter as shown in Figure 21–2 (Behse and Buchthal, 1971). In the median and ulnar nerves the minimum velocity recorded at the wrist averaged 16 m per second (0.05 μv; 95 per cent lower limit 12 m per second) (Buchthal et al., unpublished data).

In sural nerves with normal conduction velocity but a different number of myelinated fibers (including nerves from patients with axonal damage, as described later), the amplitude of the components of the sensory responses increased with the number of nerve fibers of corresponding caliber. From this relationship it can be deduced that a response of 0.1 μv originates from 5 to 10 fibers 10 μm or more in diameter.

Conduction in Unmyelinated Fibers

Conduction along unmyelinated fibers was slower (Fig. 21–3). Components conducted at less than 2 m per second originated probably from these fibers (C). To record them, stimuli of 40 to 80 ma had to be used, and the potentials were often obscured when microreflexes from muscle coincided with the potential (Bickford, 1966; Meier-Ewert et al., 1971). The amplitude of potentials from unmyelinated fibers was less than 0.1 μv.

Conduction in Different Segments of Nerves

The maximum conduction velocity was about 10 m per second slower in the distal than in the proximal segments of adult sensory nerves. Along the nerves of the leg conduction was 10 m per second slower than along the nerves of the upper extremity. This applied to both distal and proximal segments.

Sensory Conduction as a Function of Age

In adult nerve, maximum conduction velocity decreased with age. In the median nerve the decrease was uniform and was 2 m per second per decade. In the ulnar nerve the decrease was 1 m per second per decade from 20 to 55 years of age and 3 m per second per decade after 55 years of age. In the nerves of

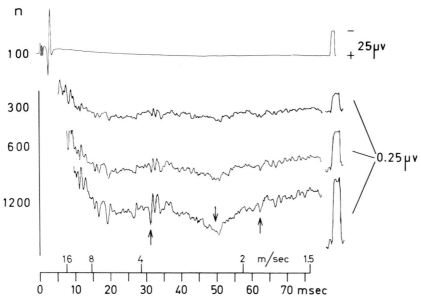

Figure 21–3 Sensory potentials from myelinated and unmyelinated fibers of the median nerve evoked by a maximal stimulus (40 ma.) to digit I. The maximum velocity to wrist was normal (48 m per second, *upper trace*). The slow components (*lower three traces*) were identified at high gain as they increased with the calibration signal (0.25 μv) in consecutive averages of 300, 600, and 1200 responses. The arrows below the trace indicate components conducted at 3.7 m per second, probably originating from myelinated fibers, and at 1.9 m per second, probably originating from unmyelinated fibers. The arrow above the trace indicates interference from a microreflex. The temperature near the nerve was 36° to 37° C. The patient was a 44 year old woman with a five year history of pain in the left thumb, probably due to arthrosis in the first metacarpal joint of digit I. There were no clear electrophysiologic abnormalities (normal maximum conduction along motor and sensory fibers of the median nerve, including the segment from palm to wrist; normal conduction along the ulnar nerve). This patient is included in the study because she tolerated painful stimuli without comment, allowing us to record potentials from unmyelinated fibers.

TABLE 21–1 MAXIMUM CONDUCTION VELOCITY AND AMPLITUDE OF SENSORY POTENTIALS IN NORMAL NERVE

Nerve	Number of Subjects	Stimulus	Velocity Segment	Regression Line* (m/sec) (15–80 yr)	S.D.† (m/sec)	Site of Recording	Amplitude Regression Line* (log μv) (15–80 yr)	S.D.† (log μv)
Median	185§	Dig. I	Dig. I–wrist	59.5–0.15 × age	4.6	Wrist	1.757–0.0060 × age	0.19
	84§	Dig. I	Wrist–elbow	74.7–0.22 × age	4.3	Elbow	1.222–0.0068 × age	0.20
	20	Dig. III	Dig. III–palm	71.2–0.25 × age	3.3	Palm	1.473–0.0024 × age	0.15
	20	Dig. III	Palm–wrist	68.9–0.18 × age	4.7			
	199§	Dig. III	Dig. III–wrist	67.4–0.18 × age	4.5	Wrist	1.311–0.0050 × age	0.21
	85§	Dig. III	Wrist–elbow	74.9–0.22 × age	4.4	Elbow	1.000–0.0056 × age	0.20
Ulnar‡ ≤ 54 yr	113	Dig. V	Dig. V–wrist	61.4–0.12 × age	5.5	Wrist	1.300–0.0037 × age	0.20
	44	Dig. V	Wrist–below sulcus	78.3–0.18 × age	5.5	Below sulcus	0.925–0.0015 × age	0.17
	46	Dig. V	Wrist–above sulcus	71.4–0.13 × age	4.3	Above sulcus	0.667+0.0018 × age	0.16
	44	Dig. V	Below–above sulcus	58.0	4.5			
≥ 55 yr	89	Dig. V	Dig. V–wrist	75.4–0.33 × age	4.5	Wrist	2.057–0.0172 × age	0.20
	27	Dig. V	Wrist–below sulcus	78.3–0.18 × age	5.5	Below sulcus	1.371–0.0123 × age	0.18
	38	Dig. V	Wrist–above sulcus	83.8–0.36 × age	4.4	Above sulcus	0.971–0.0072 × age	0.20
	27	Dig. V	Below–above sulcus	85.0–0.49 × age	5.6			
Radial	35	Dig. I	Dig. I–wrist	55.7	4.8	Wrist	1.102	0.18
	28	Dig. I	Wrist–elbow	68.8–0.12 × age	4.4	Elbow	0.725–0.0004 × age	0.17
	30	Wrist	Wrist–elbow	70.4–0.15 × age	3.0	Elbow	1.533–0.0016 × age	0.22
	14	Wrist	Elbow–axilla	67.5–0.02 × age	3.6	Axilla	1.018–0.0005 × age	0.19
Musculo-cutaneous	33	Elbow	Elbow–axilla	72.5–0.20 × age	3.1	Axilla	1.530–0.0010 × age	0.16
	32	Elbow	Axilla–Erb's point	69.4–0.15 × age	3.7	Erb's point	1.126–0.0069 × age	0.24
Sural	37	Dorsum pedis	Dorsum pedis–lateral malleolus	51.8–0.06 × age	4.6	Lateral malleolus	0.811–0.0057 × age	0.32
	58	Lateral malleolus	Lateral malleolus–Sura	57.4–0.05 × age	3.7	Sura	1.131–0.0046 × age	0.18
Superficial peroneal	47	Toe I	Toe I–superior retinaculum	47.8–0.10 × age	4.2	Superior retinaculum	0.187–0.0130 × age	0.30
	74	Superior retinaculum	Superior retinaculum–capitulum fibulae	58.0–0.08 × age	3.7	Capitulum fibulae	0.834–0.0078 × age	0.29
Tibial	38	Toe I	Toe I–medial malleolus	47.2–0.07 × age	3.4	Medial malleolus	0.808–0.0155 × age	0.33
	29	Toe I	Medial malleolus–popliteal fossa	57.6–0.06 × age	3.3	Popliteal fossa	0.162–0.0091 × age	0.32

*Regression line calculated by the method of least squares.
†Variation about the regression line.
‡Distances measured with the elbow extended and the forearm supinated.
§Forty subjects examined by Nielsen (1973).

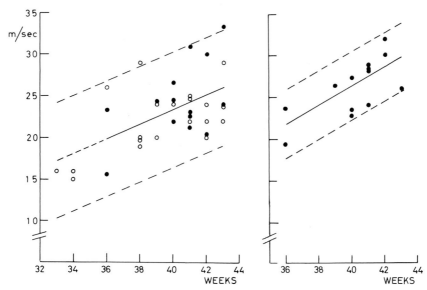

Figure 21-4 Maximum sensory conduction along the ulnar nerve of normal newborn infants as a function of conceptional age. *Left*. Digit V to wrist, 34 infants; *right*, wrist to elbow, 13 infants. ∘, data of Blom and Finnström, 1971; •, data of Wagner and Buchthal, 1972. The dashed lines give the scatter around the regression lines as two times the standard deviation. The temperature near the nerves was 36° C. (From Wagner, A. L., and Buchthal, F.: Motor and sensory conduction in infancy and childhood: reappraisal. Dev. Med. Child. Neurol., *14*:189, 1972. Reprinted by permission.)

the leg the variation with age was about 1 m per decade (Table 21–1).

Also the amplitude of the sensory potential decreased, the logarithm of amplitude decreasing linearly with increasing age. At 70 years of age the amplitude was about half that at 20 years. In the ulnar nerve the decrease in amplitude was greater after than before 55

years of age, probably because of a greater incidence of subclinical damage at the cubital sulcus in older subjects. The uniform change in conduction velocity and amplitude, which began at 20 years of age, cannot be attributed to loss of large fibers with increasing age. A decrease in fiber number and an increased incidence of fibers with segmental damage to

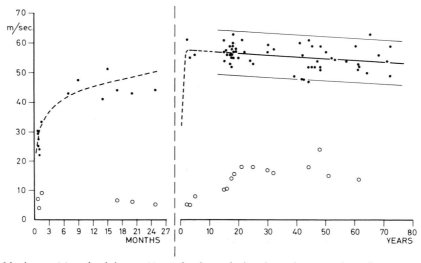

Figure 21-5 Maximum (•) and minimum (∘) conduction velocity along the normal sural nerve as a function of age. Dashed line, *left*, infants; *right*, infants and children. Solid line, adults. The thin lines denote the range delineated by plus or minus two times the standard deviation. The stimulus was applied to the nerve at the lateral malleolus, and the sensory potentials were recorded in infants 5 cm, in children 10 cm, and in adults 15 cm proximal to it. The temperature near the nerve was 36° C.

the myelin sheath were much more pronounced after than before 60 years of age (Lascelles and Thomas, 1966).

In the ulnar nerves of infants, maximum sensory conduction velocity increased with age from 20 m per second at a conceptional age of 33 weeks to 33 m per second at one month after term (Fig. 21–4) (Blom and Finnström, 1971; Wagner and Buchthal, 1972). From one month to four years the increase was 20 m per second. Along the sural nerve the maximum velocity increased from 30 m per second at one month after birth to 57 m per second at four years of age (Fig. 21–5). Average adult maximum conduction velocity was reached at eight years in the median nerve and at five years in the sural nerve. This increase reflects the increase in the number of large fibers from birth to eight years of age, when the number of large fibers is the same as in adult nerves (Wagner and Buchthal, 1972). Myelination is complete at five years of age

(Gutrecht and Dyck, 1970). Unlike adult nerve, the ulnar nerve in the infant has the same maximum conduction velocity in the proximal as in the distal segment (Wagner and Buchthal, 1972).

Within the first two months after birth, the main phase of the sensory potential of the ulnar and sural nerves had two separate peaks, indicating the presence of two groups of fibers with different degrees of maturation (Fig. 21–6). The fibers contributing to the second component conducted 20 to 30 per cent slower than the fibers of the first component. The amplitude of the second component was 20 to 30 per cent lower than that of the first component. The velocity of the slowest components, up to three years of age, was about 6 m per second, 10 m per second slower than the minimum velocity along adult nerve (cf. Fig. 21–5).

In view of the considerable changes in conduction velocity and amplitude of sensory potentials with age, in both adults and infants, all findings in diseased nerve were compared with those in normal nerve matched for age (see Table 21–1). Samples of normal sensory potentials in different nerves, along which conduction velocities were determined in a distal and a proximal segment, are shown in Figure 21–7.

Recruitment of Sensory Responses with Increasing Stimulus Strength

The maximum conduction velocity determined from responses recorded at wrist and at elbow evoked by a stimulus current at which each stimulus was just perceived (2 to 2.5 ma, one per second) was the same as the velocity of responses evoked by a maximal stimulus. Stimuli 30 to 50 per cent below threshold were either not perceived or gave false positive answers (Eijkman and Vendrik, 1964). They evoked potentials of between 0.04 and 0.1 μv conducted from wrist to elbow at the same rate as the responses to a maximal stimulus or from 3 to 9 m per second slower (Fig. 21–8). The greater slowing from digit to wrist was attributed to the longer rise time of the transmembrane potential at its threshold (Buchthal and Rosenfalck, 1966).

The responses recruited by subthreshold stimuli may well originate from proprioceptive fibers. They were among the largest fibers (10 μm in diameter) though not the

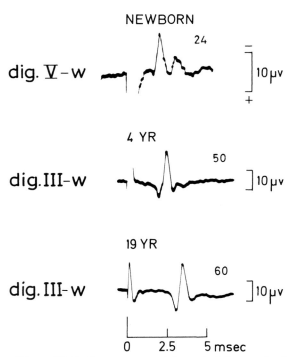

Figure 21–6 Sensory potentials evoked by maximal stimuli to digit V (*top*) and digit III (*middle and bottom*) and recorded with a needle electrode near the ulnar and median nerves at the wrist. The number above each trace denotes the maximum conduction velocity in meters per second. The subjects were a normal newborn at term and normal subjects 4 years and 19 years of age. The temperature near the nerves was 36° C. (From Wagner, A. L., and Buchthal, F.: Motor and sensory conduction in infancy and childhood: reappraisal. Dev. Med. Child. Neurol., *14*:189, 1972. Reprinted by permission.)

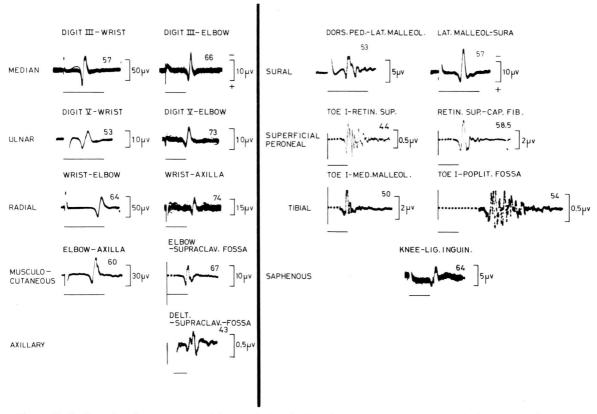

Figure 21–7 Samples of sensory potentials recorded at distal and proximal sites from normal adult nerves of the upper (left) and the lower (right) extremities. The figures above the traces give the maximum velocity in meters per second along the distal or proximal segments of the nerves. The dotted lines indicate a delay before sampling; the horizontal line below each trace denotes 5 msec. The temperature near the nerves was 36° to 37° C.

Figure 21–8 Recruitment of components in the sensory potential with increasing stimulus strength (ma). A stimulus current of 2.2 ma (1 per second) was just perceived. Note the sudden (all-or-none) appearance of fast and slow components (fibers) with a slight increase in stimulus current. Stimuli to digit III and simultaneous recording from wrist (*left*, 2 msec delay before sampling) and elbow (*right*, 5 msec delay before sampling) 1000 to 5000 responses per trace. The figures above each trace give the velocity of the fastest components distal to the site of recording in meters per second. The figures below the trace give the velocity of the slowest components. The subject (I.M.T.) was a normal woman 26 years old. The temperature near the nerve was 36° to 38° C.

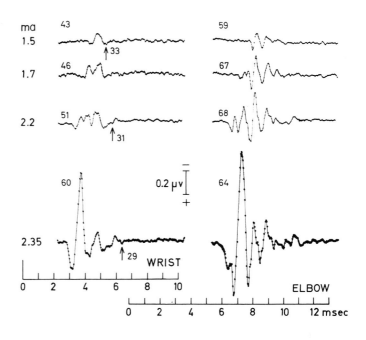

very largest. When the stimulus was just above threshold (2.5 to 3.0 ma) it also activated fibers as small as 6 μm in diameter (30 m per second). As the stimulus approached maximum (20 to 30 ma) the amplitude increased further and additional slow components were recruited (30 to 16 m per second) from fibers less than 6 μm in diameter in an all-or-none fashion (Rosenfalck and Buchthal, 1973).

In patients with neuropathy a greater electrical stimulus was required than in normal subjects. The fewer the fibers activated by maximal stimuli, the more pronounced was this effect. The response evoked by a threshold stimulus had the same amplitude as in normal subjects but contained many more components. Thus, more fibers had to be activated to transmit perception in neuropathy when loss of nerve fibers diminished the probability of summation of responses (Rosenfalck and Buchthal, 1973).

Mechanical and Electrical Stimuli

Sears (1959) recorded action potentials at the wrist, evoked by tapping the nail. Mechan-ical stimuli applied to the finger tips evoked nerve action potentials conducted with a maximal velocity of 50 m per second between two recording points (McLeod, 1966). A comparison of maximal mechanical and electrical stimuli in the same subject showed that the maximum velocity of sensory responses evoked by the touch probe was about 10 m per second slower (Rosenfalck and Buchthal, 1973).

A decrease in stimulus down to the strength at which each displacement of the skin was just perceived was not associated with a decrease in maximum velocity. The velocity of the slowest components evoked by mechanical stimuli was the same as with electrical stimulation, 30 m per second at threshold and 16 m per second at 10 times threshold. The subthreshold mechanical stimulus did not evoke a sensory potential. When the mechanical stimulus was increased to 10 times threshold, the amplitude of the sensory potential was still about 50 times lower than when the response was evoked by maximal electrical stimulus. The response evoked by the mechanical stimulus was split up in many components of about the same size (Fig. 21–9).

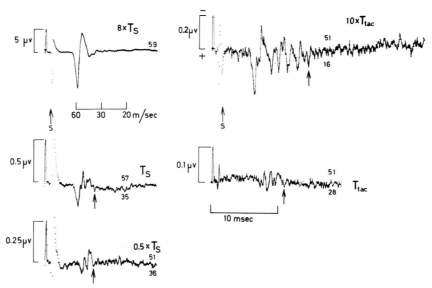

Figure 21–9 Sensory potentials evoked by electrical and by tactile stimuli to digit III recorded from the median nerve at wrist. *Left.* Responses to maximal (8 × T$_s$), threshold (T$_s$) and subthreshold (0.5 × T$_s$) electrical stimuli. *Right.* Responses to tactile stimuli above (10 × T$_{tac}$) and at threshold (T$_{tac}$). T$_s$ (2.5 ma) was the current and T$_{tac}$ (10 μm) the displacement of the probe when each stimulus was just perceived (one per second). S indicates the onset of electrical and the peak of the mechanical stimulus. The figures above each trace indicate the maximum velocity in meters per second, and the figures below each trace the minimum velocity (component at arrow). Electronic averaging of 500 to 3000 responses. The subject (I.M.P.) was 21 years old. The temperature on the skin was 35° C. (From Rosenfalck, A., and Buchthal, F.: Sensory potentials and threshold for electrical and tactile stimuli. *In* Desmedt, J. E. (ed.): New Developments in Electromyography and Clinical Neurophysiology. Vol. 2. Basel, Karger, 1973, pp. 45–51. Reprinted by permission.)

SENSORY POTENTIALS IN DISEASED MYELINATED NERVE

In polyneuropathy sensory potentials have an abnormal shape and diminished amplitude, either with or without slowing in conduction. Diminished amplitude may be due to loss of fibers, to block in conduction, or merely to an increase in the temporal dispersion of the compound potential associated with slowing in conduction in fibers of different caliber (Buchthal and Rosenfalck, 1971a).

Conduction in Wallerian Degeneration and in Regeneration

Data on sensory conduction during wallerian degeneration after transection of a nerve in man are not available. In the facial nerve the progressive decrease in amplitude of the evoked motor potential was concomitant with axonal degeneration. Excitable fibers conducted at normal velocity as long as there was any response at all (Gilliatt and Taylor, 1959).

In regeneration after complete transection of the nerve the sensory potential was severely diminished in amplitude, the maximum and minimum conduction velocities were diminished and the potential was extremely split up.

In the example shown in Figure 21–10, nine months after suture of a transected median nerve, the amplitude was 1 per cent of normal, and the maximum and minimum conduction velocities were less than one third of normal. Electrophysiologically there is no way of distinguishing between slowing in conduction in immature regenerating fibers and in demyelinated fibers. The speed of recovery may provide a clue, however, since regeneration proceeds much more slowly than remyelination (Trojaborg, 1970). From animal experiments it is known that regenerating nerve may reach 80 per cent of normal conduction that nerve fibers have a thinner axon and a thinner myelin sheath than normal, and that internodal distances are shorter (for references see Cragg and Thomas, 1964).

Polyneuropathy

The following data are derived from studies of sensory conduction along the median

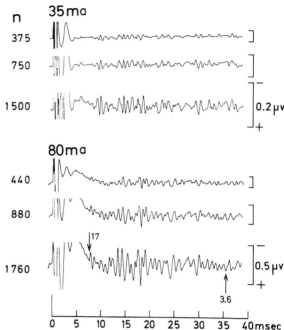

Figure 21–10 Sensory potentials in regenerating fibers after wallerian degeneration. The responses were evoked by stimulation of the proximal phalanx of digit III (upper three traces, 35 ma; lower three traces, 80 ma) and recorded at the wrist nine months after suture of the completely divided median nerve. The fastest (17 m per second) and slowest (3.6 m per second) components in the averaged responses were identified by their increase in amplitude in three consecutive averages of increasing number (n) of responses. The subject was a 20 year old woman (B.M.) with a complicated fracture at the wrist. Three centimeters of the median nerve was removed and the stumps reunited by suture. Four months later there was no motor or sensory response in the median nerve. Nine months after suture the distal motor latency was 9 msec (distance, 6 cm). Sensitivity to touch was present on the volar surface of the proximal phalanx of digit III and absent distal to it. The temperature near the nerve was 35° to 37° C.

nerves of 84 consecutive patients by Buchthal and Rosenfalck (1971a) and along the sural nerve of 63 other patients by Behse and co-workers (unpublished data).

PREDOMINANTLY AXONAL DEGENERATION

This lesion was characterized by a severe decrease in amplitude of the sensory potential, a less marked reduction in conduction velocity, and a normal or diminished temporal dispersion of the response (Fig. 21–11A). With these criteria we found a predominantly axonal lesion in the median nerve in 15 patients. The maximum conduction velocity (digit III to wrist) averaged 50 ± 2 m per second (88 per cent of normal), and the amplitude of the sensory potentials was 1.8 ± 0.5 μv (11 per cent of normal).

The *minimum conduction velocity* could even seem faster than normal when the amplitude of the slowest component was so low that it could not be distinguished from noise. Though the loss of many fibers resulted in an increased splitting up of the compound potential, there was no increase in temporal dispersion.

In patients in whom conduction was examined in the sural nerve, a biopsy was obtained of the same nerve, and amplitude and conduction velocity of the sensory potential were related to the number and caliber of large myelinated fibers. As in the median nerve the amplitude was markedly diminished. In 16 patients it averaged 0.4 ± 0.1 μv (5 per cent of normal). The maximum conduction velocity was normal or diminished to an extent corresponding to the loss of large fibers (> 9 μm); it averaged 49 ± 2 m per second (92 per cent of normal). The histogram of fiber diameters showed a decrease in the number of all fibers that contribute to the main phases of the sensory potential (Fig. 21–12). Thus the number of fibers more than

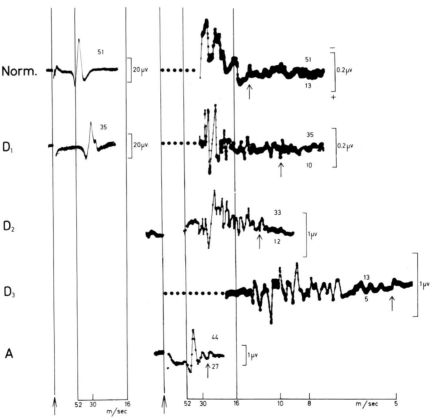

Figure 21–11 Sensory action potentials in polyneuropathies with predominantly segmental demyelination (D_1, D_2, D_3) or axonal damage (A). Maximal stimuli were applied to digit I, recording was from the median nerve at the wrist by electronic averaging of 500 responses (*right*) or photographic superposition of 15 traces (*left*). The responses from normal (Norm.) and from group D_1 were recorded both at low gain (*left*) and at a 150 times higher gain (*right*). The dotted lines indicate a delay before sampling. In groups D_1, D_2, and D_3 conduction was slowed. In group D_1 the 40 per cent decrease in amplitude can be accounted for by an increase in temporal dispersion. In groups D_2 and D_3 the severe decrease in amplitude required assumption of block in conduction, loss of fibers, or both, as well as temporal dispersion. In group A the maximum conduction velocity was nearly normal and the amplitude was severely reduced, corresponding to loss among fibers 7 μm or more in diameter. The figures above the traces give the maximum and those below the traces the minimum conduction velocity. Vertical lines indicate, at arrows, onset of stimulus; at 52 m per second, average maximum; and at 16 m per second, average minimum velocity along normal median nerve. The temperature near the nerves was 35° C. (Modified from Buchthal, F., and Rosenfalck, A.: Sensory potentials in polyneuropathy. Brain, *94*:241, 1971.)

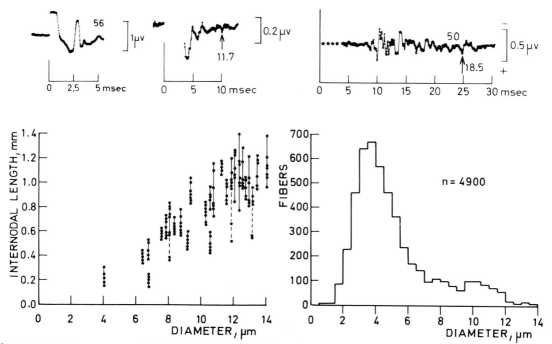

Figure 21–12   Sensory potentials in the sural nerve and biopsy findings in a patient with predominantly axonal neuropathy from lead poisoning. The maximum conduction velocity was normal, the minimum velocity borderline, and the amplitude of the sensory potential diminished by 90 per cent. *Top.* Sensory potentials evoked by stimulation at the lateral malleolus and recorded 12 cm proximally (sura, left trace, 270 averaged responses; middle trace, 500 responses) and 45 cm proximally (popliteal fossa, right trace, 500 responses). The figures above the traces give the maximum, and below the traces the minimum conduction velocities. The dotted line indicates a delay before sampling. The temperature near the nerve was 36° to 37° C. *Lower left.* Internodal length as a function of diameter in 48 teased fibers (26 fibers shown, plotted according to the method of Fullerton et al., 1965). Ten per cent of the fibers more than 7 μm in diameter had uniformly shortened segments indicating regeneration, and 13 per cent had both short and normal segments indicating remyelination. *Lower right.* Histogram of fiber diameters. The total number of myelinated fibers was at the lower limit of normal, the number of fibers of 7 μm or more in diameter was diminished by 70 per cent. Cf. case history 1. (From Behse, F., Buchthal, F., Carlsen, F., and Knappeis, G. G.: Light and electron microscopy as related to sensory conduction along normal and diseased sural nerve. Unpublished data.)

7 μm in diameter was 580 ± 140 (n = 9) as compared to 2300 ± 290 (n = 6) in normal nerve. The diminished maximum conduction velocity was seen in those nerves in which fiber loss was most severe.

CASE HISTORY 1

The patient (L.A.H.) was a 57 year old man (cf. Fig. 21–12).

Chief Complaint.   Crampy abdominal pain, weakness in arms and legs, paresthesia in hands.

History.   Since the age of 45 he had been exposed daily to lead in a metal factory. He was seen at 46 years of age for lassitude and abdominal pain, at which time he had no neurologic signs or symptoms. The blood count showed 12,900 red cells per million with punctate basophilia. The urine contained lead, 185 μg per liter. For the past year he had had increased abdominal pain, progressive weakness in arms and legs, and paresthesia in the hands.

Examination.   Muscle examination revealed weakness of the facial muscles; force of flexion of the neck and arms measured by dynamometer half of normal; and slight weakness of external rotation at the shoulder, extension of the fingers, and dorsiflexion of the feet (graded 4 on a 5 point scale, Medical Research Council, 1943). There were coarse fasciculations in the muscles of the shoulder.

Reflexes were absent in the arms, weak or absent in the legs. Mandibular reflex was normal.

Perception of touch and pinprick and vibratory and position sense were normal.

Laboratory Findings.   The blood contained 9200 red cells per million with punctate basophilia. The urine contained lead, 200 μg per liter; co-proporphyrin, 0.4 to 0.8 mg per liter; and delta-amino-levulinic acid, 0.09 g per liter.

Electromyography.   Left *abductor pollicis brevis* and *extensor digitorum communis muscles* showed moderate loss of motor unit potentials during full effort, normal amplitude, fibrillation potentials at three sites, increased incidence of polyphasic potentials (25 per cent, normal upper limit 12 per cent), and normal mean duration of motor unit potentials.

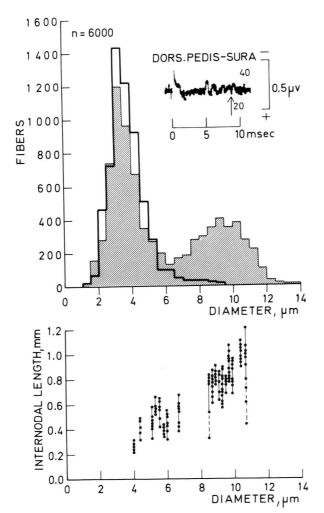

Figure 21–13 Number (n) and distribution of myelinated nerve fibers (thick line) and sensory potential in sural nerve in a patient with signs and symptoms of polyneuropathy (axonal type). *Top.* There were 130 fibers 7 μm or more in diameter compared to 2500 in normal nerve (hatched area in histogram). *Inset, upper right.* Maximum velocity of the sensory potential evoked by a stimulus to dorsum pedis and recorded at the lateral malleolus and 15 cm proximal to it (sura) was diminished to 40 m per second (figures above the trace) corresponding to the 20 largest fibers (9.5 μm in diameter) of the histogram (conversion factor 4.4). The minimum velocity (arrow and number below the trace) was normal. The amplitude of the sensory potential was diminished by 90 per cent. The temperature near the nerve was 36° C. *Bottom.* Internodal length as a function of diameter, determined in 27 fibers of the nerve (19 fibers shown). The internodal lengths were normal except for shortened segments (remyelination) in only two fibers, as can occur in normal nerve. Cf. case history 2. (From Behse, F., Buchthal, F., Carlsen, F., and Knappeis, G. G.: Light and electron microscopy as related to sensory conduction along normal and diseased sural nerve. Unpublished data.)

Nerve Conduction. The *radial nerve* showed normal motor latency and amplitude in extensor digitorum muscle; normal sensory conduction velocity in distal and proximal segments, amplitude of sensory potential 25 per cent of normal. In the *median nerve* distal motor latency was at the upper limit of normal; distal sensory conduction velocity at the lower limit of normal and amplitude of sensory potentials 15 to 30 per cent of normal.

Figure 21–13 illustrates how severe fiber loss can result in a decrease in conduction velocity by as much as 30 per cent. This patient had only 130 fibers more than 7 μm in diameter, and the largest fibers had a diameter of 9.5 μm. They can account for a maximum velocity of 40 m per second (conversion factor 4.4, as described earlier). In this nerve, as in the other nerve of this group, evidence of previous segmental demyelination was absent or the incidence resembled that of normal

nerve (up to 8 per cent, among fibers of 7 μm for more in diameter).

CASE HISTORY 2

The patient (B.N.J.) was a 38 year old woman (cf. Fig. 21–13).

Chief Complaint. Uncoordinated movements, hyperkinesia, and tingling sensation in the fingers.

History. Two years earlier the patient had had a brief febrile illness, cause unknown. When she recovered, she had weakness of all muscles and ataxia of arms and legs. Tendon jerks were absent, vibratory and position sense were absent in hands and feet, perception of touch and pinprick was normal. Spinal fluid protein level was elevated, 9.1 g per liter (normal 0.2 to 0.4 g per liter).

One year later muscle force was normal, tendon jerks were absent, vibratory and position sense were still absent. Spinal fluid protein was normal (0.4 g per liter).

Electromyography. *Abductor pollicis brevis muscle* showed normal pattern of discharge during full effort; duration of motor unit potentials was prolonged by 40 per cent; there were normal incidence of polyphasic potentials and positive sharp waves at two sites.

Nerve Conduction. The *median nerve* showed normal motor latency, sensory conduction slightly slowed, and amplitude of sensory potentials 1 per cent of normal.

The diminution of amplitude is a relatively insensitive indicator of early involvement. Owing to the interindividual scatter of amplitudes in normal nerves, the 95 per cent lower limit of normal is 30 to 40 per cent of the average. Therefore about one third of the fibers of 7 μm or more may be lost before a decrease in amplitude is significant. This is illustrated by the findings in the sural nerve shown in Figure 21–14. Though the number of fibers contributing to the potential was diminished to 1500 as compared to 2300 in normal nerve, the peak-to-peak amplitude recorded in the segment of the nerve examined later by biopsy was 3 μv, the 95 per cent lower limit of normal. The conduction velocity was just within the normal range. That the lesion was axonal was evidenced by findings in 83 teased fibers 7 μm or more in diameter: 27 per cent had uniformly diminished internodal lengths indicating regeneration after axonal degeneration (Hiscoe, 1947; Sanders, 1948; Vizoso and Young, 1948). Remyelination after segmental demyelination was as in normal nerve (7 per cent).

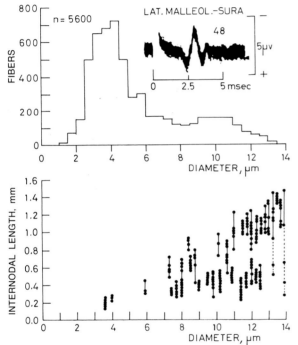

Figure 21–14 Sural nerve with histologic evidence of axonal degeneration that did not appear in the sensory potentials. *Top.* Histogram of diameters. The number of fibers larger than 7 μm was diminished by 30 per cent, the total number (n) of myelinated nerve fibers was normal. *Inset, upper right.* Sensory potential evoked by stimulus to sural nerve at lateral malleolus and recorded 15 cm proximally (sura) had an amplitude at the lower limit of normal and was conducted at normal maximum velocity (figure above the trace). The temperature near the nerve was 36° C. *Bottom.* Internodal length as a function of fiber diameter. One third of the fibers had uniformly shortened internodal lengths indicating regeneration after axonal degeneration. The incidence of segmental demyelination and remyelination (dashed lines) was as in normal nerve. Cf. case history 3. (From Behse, F., Buchthal, F., Carlsen, F., and Knappeis, G. G.: Light and electron microscopy as related to sensory conduction along normal and diseased sural nerve. Unpublished data.)

CASE HISTORY 3

S.A.E., a 64 year old man, was referred for ulnar palsy and polyneuropathy (cf. Fig. 21–14).

Chief Complaint. For the past 18 months the patient had had weakness in the left thumb, tingling in digits III, IV, and V.

History. He had a fracture of the medial epicondyle of the left humerus two years earlier.

Examination. There were weakness and wasting of the right and left adductor pollicis and abductor digiti quinti, uncertain sensory findings in the leg. The tendon jerks were normal in the arms and legs except the Achilles reflexes, which were weak. Sensation of touch and pinprick were diminished on the volar surface of both hands (mostly digits III, IV, and V). Glucose tolerance test results were normal.

Electromyography. Electromyography was performed in hand and foot with normal findings in the left abductor pollicis brevis muscle, a pattern of discrete activity of diminished amplitude in the left extensor digitorum brevis muscle, no fibrillation potentials.

Nerve Conduction. Distal sensory conduction along the median and radial nerves and distal motor latency in the median nerve were normal.

SEGMENTAL DAMAGE TO THE MYELIN SHEATH

Segmental demyelination is associated with slowing in conduction. In the single nerve fiber the conduction time of a demyelinated internodal segment was prolonged as much as 25 times before conduction was blocked (Rasminsky and Sears, 1972). In whole mixed nerve, segmental demyelination was associated with slowing in conduction, a normal number of nerve fibers, and a normal distribution of diameters (McDonald, 1963; Morgan-Hughes, 1968). Nevertheless, the amplitude of the sensory potential was diminished on account of (1) increase in temporal dispersion associated with slowing in conduction (Buchthal and Rosenfalck, 1971a) and (2) block of conduction in some fibers because the demyelinated segment had ceased to conduct. Comparison of the recorded and reconstructed potential indicated that a decrease in conduction velocity of all fibers more than 6 μm in diameter to about 80 per cent of normal could account for a reduction in amplitude of 40 per cent (Buchthal and Rosenfalck, 1971a).

Slowing in conduction to 80 per cent of normal with an amplitude about one third of normal was found in about one third of the patients with polyneuropathy in whom the median nerve was investigated (see Fig. 21–11, D_1). Since the slowed potentials were prolonged, it is unlikely that selective block of the largest fibers accounted for the diminished maximum conduction velocity. Nor could selective slight slowing of the fast fibers be responsible, since this would have resulted in an increased amplitude. Since histologic examination was not available, we cannot decide whether all components of the potential were conducted at diminished velocity or whether the fastest fibers (10 to 14 μm in diameter) conducted so slowly as to contribute to components throughout the range of velocities represented in the prolonged potential (Fig. 21–15).

Moderate slowing in maximum conduction (by 30 per cent; cf., Fig. 21–11, D_2) was associated with a reduction in amplitude to one fifth of normal, and severe slowing (by 70 per cent; cf. Fig. 21–11, D_3) with an amplitude of less than 1 μv (3 per cent of normal). The conduction of the slowest components was as slow as 4 m per second.

When distal slowing was slight, maximum sensory conduction in the proximal segment from wrist to elbow was normal. When distal slowing was moderate or severe, proximal slowing was less than distal, but there was a relatively greater increase in temporal dispersion from the distal to the proximal site of

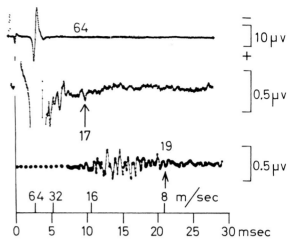

Figure 21–15 Fast and slow components of sensory potentials recorded at the wrist from normal and from probably demyelinated median nerve. *Top.* Electronic averaging of 20 responses in a normal subject (E.B.), male, 28 years old. *Middle.* Averaging of 500 responses at 50 times higher gain to distinguish slow components. *Bottom.* Averaging of 500 responses at high gain in a patient with polyneuropathy. Severe slowing of maximum and minimum conduction velocities (for clinical and other electrophysiologic data, see legend of Figure 21–16 and case history 4). Stimuli were administered to digit III. The figure above each trace give the maximum conduction velocity in meters per second, the figures below the traces give the minimum velocity (slowest component marked with arrow below the traces). The dotted line below indicates the delay before sampling. The upper scale below the potentials gives the conduction velocities, the lower scale the conduction times. The temperature near the nerve was 35° to 36° C.

recording in polyneuropathy than in normal nerve.

Abnormalities of the sensory potential in the median nerve were found in many patients with florid diabetic neuropathy in the legs but no clinical signs in the arms. An increase in temporal dispersion, manifest as prolonged duration and irregularities in shape, could then be the earliest sign of impairment when conduction along the fastest fibers and the amplitude of the sensory potential were still within the range of normal. Thus 5 of 30 patients with abnormalities in sensory conduction did not have electrophysiologic evidence of involvement of motor fibers (including fibrillation potentials), whereas all patients with distal slowing in motor fibers had abnormalities in sensory conduction. In six of the patients symptoms or signs of neuropathy appeared before or at about the time when the metabolic disturbance was diagnosed (Lamontagne and Buchthal, 1970).

We examined four pairs of monozygotic twins, the four probands with diabetic neuropathy and all four co-twins without diabetes or abnormal glucose tolerance; three of the four co-twins had slight abnormalities in sensory potentials of the median nerve with diminished conduction velocity of the slowest components (Behse and Buchthal, unpublished data). This is in keeping with the concept that diabetic neuropathy is an integral part of the metabolic defect rather than a secondary effect of a vascular disturbance (Ellenberg, 1964).

In polyneuropathy with prominent demyelination, maximum conduction along the sural nerve was slowed more than to be expected from the largest fibers found in the histogram of diameters (Fig. 21–16). The degree of slowing was roughly related to the incidence of fibers with demyelinated or remyelinated segments: When all the teased nerve fibers showed segmental damage the maximum conduction velocity along the segment of the nerve later examined by biopsy was 20 to 25 m per second as compared to 55 m per second in normal nerve (two patients with hypertrophic neuropathy, Dejerine-Sottas; two patients with a hypertrophic type of peroneal

muscular atrophy, Charcot-Marie-Tooth). When more than half of the teased fibers showed segmental damage the maximum velocity was decreased by 50 per cent. (See, however, the exceptional slowing along the nerve shown in Figure 21–16). When 15 to 30 per cent of the teased fibers showed segmental damage the decrease was 20 to 40 per cent. In addition to segmental damage to the myelin sheath, there was, in 16 of 18 nerves, loss by at least 50 per cent of fibers 7 μm or more in diameter. This contributes to the decrease in amplitudes of the sensory potential to 30 per cent of normal or less. The slowing in minimum conduction velocity was most pronounced when slowing in maximum velocity was severe, but was somewhat less than in the median nerve. Thus, not only may the same nerve show evidence of axonal degeneration and damage to the myelin sheath, but also electrophysiologic findings in the nerves of the arms and legs may indicate a different type of histopathologic change. In two thirds of our patients with electrophysiologic signs of axonal degeneration in the median and ulnar nerves, the same abnormality was found in the lateral popliteal or sural nerves, whereas in one third conduction along nerve

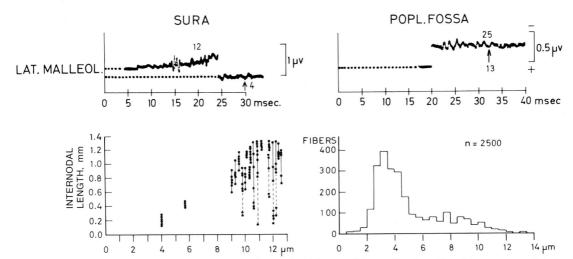

Figure 21–16 Severe slowing in sensory conduction and evidence of demyelination. *Top.* Sensory potentials in the sural nerve evoked by stimuli to the lateral malleolus and recorded 13 cm (sura) and 43 cm (popliteal fossa) proximally. The maximal conduction velocity was exceptionally low, 12 m per second to sura and 25 m per second from sura to the popliteal fossa (figures above the traces). The arrows and figures below the traces indicate the minimum conduction velocity calculated from the lateral malleolus. Electronic averaging of 500 responses. The dotted lines indicate a delay before sampling. *Lower left.* Internodal length as a function of fiber diameter, determined in 29 teased fibers and shown in 19. Half the teased fibers had segmental damage with long stretches of entirely denuded axons. *Lower right.* Histogram of diameters. The total number of myelinated nerve fibers (n) was reduced by 60 per cent. Note that there were 500 fibers larger than 7 μm and 15 fibers 12 μm or more in diameter, disproportionate with the severe slowing, a finding characteristic for demyelination. Cf. case history 4. (From Behse, F., Buchthal, F., Carlsen, F., and Knappeis, G. G.: Light and electron microscopy as related to sensory conduction along normal and diseased sural nerve. Unpublished data.)

fibers of the legs was slowed, indicating demyelination or remyelination in the legs and, thus, another kind of neuropathy than in the median nerve. In two patients impairment was acute and regeneration an unlikely cause of slowing (Buchthal and Rosenfalck, 1971a).

CASE HISTORY 4

The patient (G.P.) was a 62 year old man (cf. Fig. 21–16).

Chief Complaint. Paresthesia in hands and feet.

Present Illness. He had had a "prickling sensation" in hands and feet for nine months.

Examination. There was no weakness or wasting; tendon jerks were absent in the legs and weak in the arms. Perception of touch and pinprick and vibratory and position sense were diminished in hands and feet, most pronouncedly in the fingers and the toes.

Laboratory Examination. Spinal fluid protein was 0.96 g per liter; there were no cells. Serum vitamin B_{12} and glucose tolerance tests were normal.

Electromyography. Pattern of discharge was normal during full effort; duration of motor unit potentials was increased by 30 per cent, incidence of polyphasic potentials was markedly increased, and in the foot, there were fibrillation potentials at many sites.

Nerve Conduction. In the *peroneal nerve*, distal motor latency was much prolonged, as was the latency to the anterior tibial and long peroneal muscles, the velocity from capitulum fibulae to ankle was 30 m per second (normal average, 50 m per second). In the *superficial peroneal nerve*, the conduction velocity was diminished by 25 per cent and the potential was markedly desynchronized. In the *median nerve*, the distal motor latency was

prolonged; conduction from elbow to wrist was 30 m per second (normal, 61 m per second). The sensory conduction velocity from digits to wrist was diminished to 12 to 19 m per second (normal, 51 and 56 m per second) and between wrist and elbow was normal.

A group of neuropathies was studied in which neither axonal damage nor segmental demyelination accounted for the slowing in conduction (Behse et al., 1972). In hereditary neuropathy with liability to pressure palsy the maximum conduction of the clinically unaffected sural nerves was slowed by from 20 to 70 per cent, the potentials were split up more than normal, and the amplitude of the sensory potential was nearly normal or slightly reduced. In young patients, the incidence of segmental demyelination was as in normal nerve and could not account for the slowing in conduction; nor could a reduction in the number of nerve fibers 7 μm or more in diameter. The total number of myelinated fibers and the number per square millimeter were normal. The most conspicuous change was an abnormal growth of the myelin sheath, resulting in a lowered ratio of axonal diameter to external diameter. Although the number and the diameter of the fibers seemed normal when the external diameter was measured, 25 per cent of the largest fibers had axons of diminished diameter (Fig. 21–17). The thin axons of the largest fibers could account in part for the slowing in conduction. In addition there were multiple defects in the myelin sheath, often present along the entire length of the fiber.

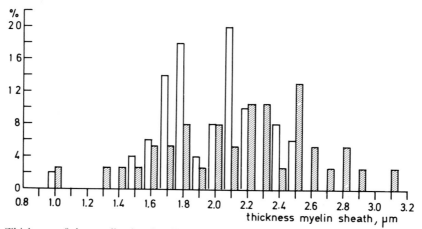

Figure 21–17 Thickness of the myelin sheath (Fibers 8 μm or more in external diameter) in sural nerves of patients with hereditary liability to pressure palsy (40 fibers, striped columns) and in normal sural nerves (50 fibers, white columns). The thickness of the myelin sheath was measured on electron micrographs. (From Behse, F., Buchthal, F., Carlsen, F., and Knappeis, G. G.: Hereditary neuropathy with liability to pressure palsies. Electrophysiological and histopathological aspects. Brain, *95*:777, 1972. Reprinted by permission.)

Similar myelin defects were rarely seen in nerves treated by the same method from normal persons or from those with other neuropathies and never as profusely as in the patients liable to pressure palsy. Since the defects resembled artifacts, we postulate that they may have been precipitated by fixation in nerves with preexisting damage that allowed leakage and caused slowing in conduction.

Sensory Conduction in Localized Lesions of Peripheral Nerve

In localized traumatic lesions and entrapment of peripheral nerves, sensory conduction helps to determine the site of the lesion and its type. To localize the lesion the potentials must be recorded both distally and proximally to the site of the lesion. Local slowing could be established more accurately by recording sensory potentials, since the difference in the rate of conduction along motor nerve fibers after stimulating above and below the site of the lesion could be distorted because of spread of the stimulating current.

A lesion of the *ulnar nerve* in *the cubital sulcus*, associated with slowing in sensory conduction across an area of compression was localized by comparison of conduction distally and proximally (Fig. 21–18) (Payan, 1969). The sensory potentials were diminished in amplitude at all sites of recording. When the potentials at the wrist were 1 μv or less the conduction velocity across the sulcus was severely diminished, to 40 m per second or less. A split up or prolonged potential proximal to the sulcus was an additional indicator of abnormality.

Sensory conduction may reveal abnormalities when motor conduction is normal. In fact, since the activity of one motor unit can be picked up by the recording electrode, one motor nerve fiber that conducts at a normal maximal rate is sufficient to make the maximum conduction velocity appear normal. On the other hand, a normal velocity in the sural nerve obtained without averaging of the initial positive peak of the sensory potential required normal conduction along about one quarter of the largest fibers 8 μm or more in diameter (Behse and Buchthal, 1971). Thus the maximum conduction velocity of the sensory potential is a more sensitive gauge of

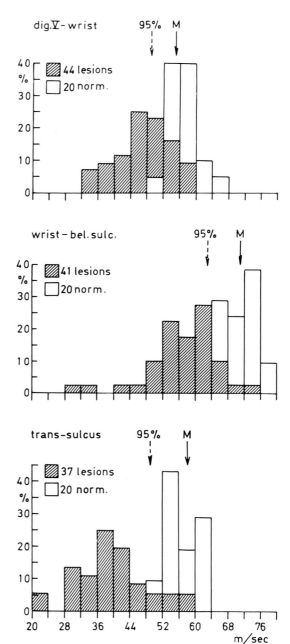

Figure 21–18 Sensory conduction velocity in three segments of ulnar nerve in patients with lesions of the ulnar nerve at the cubital sulcus (hatched columns) as compared to normal (white columns). The arrows denote the average (M) and the 95 per cent lower limit of normal conduction velocity. (From Payan, J.: Electrophysiological localization of ulnar nerve lesions. J. Neurol. Neurosurg. Psychiatry, 32:208, 1969. Reprinted by permission.)

impairment than conduction along motor fibers.

In 25 per cent of patients with *carpal tunnel syndrome* the distal latency from the wrist to the abductor pollicis brevis muscle was normal, and slowing in the sensory nerve established the site of the lesion (Kaeser, 1963; Thomas and Lambert, 1967; Buchthal et al., 1974). In mild involvement changes in the shape of the sensory potential were the earliest sign of abnormality. Borderline slowing from digit to wrist was nearly always associated with significant slowing from palm to wrist when the stretch of nerve where conduction was normal, from digit to palm, was excluded (Fig. 21–19) (Buchthal and Rosenfalck, 1971b). Across the region of compression the maximum velocity was as slow as 20 m per second and the minimum velocity as slow as 5 m per second. Slowing has been attributed to localized demyelination by Denny-Brown and Brenner (1944), to loss of the fastest fibers by Thomas and Fullerton (1963), or to both. In patients with the carpal tunnel syndrome the *same* fibers in which conduction was severely slowed across the flexor retinaculum conducted at a normal rate from wrist to elbow (Buchthal et al., 1974). This finding applied both to the

fastest and to the slow components of the sensory potential, and it indicates that the diminished conduction velocity was due to localized slowing (demyelination) rather than to loss of the largest fibers (Fig. 21–20). Diminished amplitude of the potential recorded at the wrist indicated that there was, in addition, loss or block of many fibers. In half the nerves of the 111 patients with carpal tunnel syndrome we have examined, the potential was less than 2 μv as compared to about 15 μv in normal nerve. Components conducting at 10 to 20 m per second were larger than normal because potentials were slowed from fibers that normally conduct fast, and the slowed potentials were superimposed on normally slow components. Conduction during remyelination or regeneration may also give rise to slow components that may occur in bursts. Distal to the site of compression the maximum conduction velocity was faster than across the region of compression, but often slower than normal (see Fig. 21–19). The slowing in the distal segment

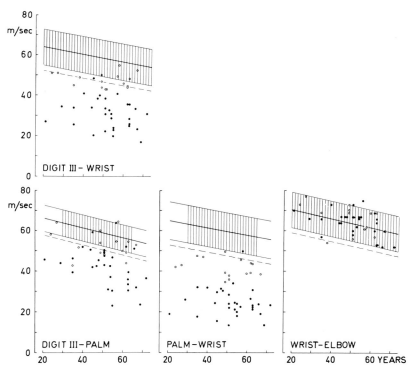

Figure 21–19   Carpal tunnel syndrome. *Upper left.* Maximum conduction velocity along sensory fibers of digit III to wrist (ordinate) and age (abscissa). The hatched area represents the range of velocities and age (two times standard deviation) in normal median nerves (cf. Table 21–1). The dashed line indicates the lower 99 per cent confidence limit of normal. *Below.* Same patients. Slow conduction from palm to wrist (*middle*), less slowing along the same fibers from digit III to palm (*left*) and normal conduction from wrist to elbow (*right*). Conduction velocity was slow from palm to wrist even when it was borderline from digit III to wrist (○, 16 patients); it was normal from wrist to elbow even when it was very slow from palm to wrist (•, 28 patients).

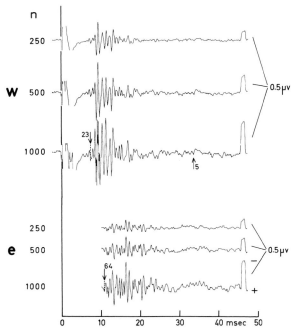

Figure 21–20 Slowed sensory conduction from digit III to wrist and normal conduction from wrist to elbow in a patient with a carpal tunnel syndrome. Stimulus 60 ma (0.2 msec) to digit III. Recording from median nerve at wrist (w) and at elbow (e). The three traces are consecutive averages of 250, 500, and 1000 responses (n) at each site to distinguish slow components from noise. The arrows and figures above and below the traces point to the components from which the maximum and minimum velocities were calculated. The temperature near the nerve was 36° C. Note that the increase in temporal dispersion from wrist to elbow was about the same as in normal nerve. Cf. case history 5.

could be explained by the constriction in diameter that occurs distal to the site of compression (Weiss and Hiscoe, 1948) or by inclusion of a short demyelinated stretch of the nerve in the distal segment.

We have observed the first signs of recovery in sensory conduction 15 days after surgical division of the flexor retinaculum at the wrist. The slow components of the sensory potential recorded from the median nerve at the wrist had longer latencies and higher amplitudes 30 days after than before decompression, compatible with remyelination and not with regeneration, as discussed in the section on conduction in wallerian degeneration and regeneration.

In *radial nerve palsy* caused by compression during sleep ("Saturday night palsy"), the velocity along the radial nerve was diminished from elbow to axilla by about 30 per cent in two thirds of the patients and recovered within 50 days. Conduction was normal distal to the site of compression, from wrist to elbow. With blunt injury either the sensory potential was abolished or conduction was normal; amplitudes were diminished, consistent with axonal damage (Trojaborg, 1970).

CASE HISTORY 5

The patient (K.D.F.) was a 44 year old woman (cf. Fig. 21–20).

Chief Complaint. Weakness in right thumb, pain and paresthesia in the thumb, digit II, and digit III of right hand radiating at times to the volar surface of the hand and forearm.

History. She had had diabetes since the age of 39 years, controlled by insulin. There were no clinical symptoms or signs of diabetic neuropathy or retinopathy.

Progressive symptoms in the right hand had persisted for the past year and a half.

Examination. Severe weakness and wasting of right abductor pollicis brevis muscle was force graded as 1 to 2. Perception of touch and pinprick were diminished on the volar surface of digit III. Otherwise perception of touch, pain, vibratory and position sense were normal in arms and legs. Tendon jerks were normal.

Electromyography. Right abductor pollicis brevis muscle showed discrete discharges of 2 mv during full effort, fibrillation potentials and positive sharp waves in eight sites, duration of motor unit potentials prolonged by 35 per cent, incidence of polyphasic potentials increased (19 per cent; normal upper limit, 12 per cent); flexor of the right forearm showed no abnormalities.

Nerve Conduction. In the right *median nerve*, distal motor latency was prolonged (6 msec, distance 6.5 cm), motor conduction velocity from elbow to wrist was 20 per cent below the average of normal. Sensory conduction from digits I and III to wrist was slowed (see Figure 21–20). The right *ulnar nerve* showed normal distal motor latency, sensory conduction velocity, and amplitudes of sensory potentials.

Entrapment of the *peroneal nerve* at the capitulum fibulae ("crossed legs palsy") was associated with slowing in conduction along the superficial peroneal nerve from below the capitulum fibulae to the popliteal fossa, diminished amplitude of the sensory potential, and normal or nearly normal conduction from the superior extensor retinaculum at the ankle to below the capitulum fibulae (Behse and Buchthal, 1971). In root compression (L4, L5) conduction and amplitude of the sensory potentials were normal in spite of

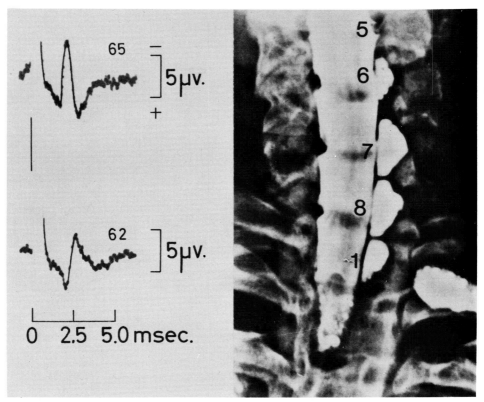

Figure 21–21   Sensory potentials along the radial and median nerves after root avulsion. *Left.* The potentials were evoked by stimuli to the proximal (radial nerve, above) and the distal (median nerve, below) phalanx of the thumb. Maximum sensory conduction was normal (figures above the traces are meters per second). The amplitudes of the sensory potentials were diminished to one fifth of normal. The temperature near the nerves was 37° C. *Right.* Myelography (Pantopaque) showed avulsion of roots C6, C7, C8, and T1. The patient, a 21 year old man (H.J.A.), was examined four months after a traffic accident. Perception of touch and pinprick and position sense were absent in the left arm and hand, and there was paralysis of the left arm and shoulder.

sensory loss as long as the dorsal root ganglion was spared. In *root avulsion* (C6 to T1) with total loss of sensory function in forearm and hand, the sensory potentials recorded from the median, ulnar, or radial nerves at the wrist were conducted at a normal rate and their amplitudes were normal or slightly reduced, indicating that all or most of the sensory axons were still connected with cells in the dorsal root ganglion (Fig. 21–21) (Bonney and Gilliatt, 1958). In traumatic lesions of the *brachial plexus*, the sensory potentials recorded from the nerves of the arm were conducted at a normal rate but were often diminished in amplitude. When compression of the brachial plexus was caused by an elongated transverse process from C7 or by a rudimentary cervical rib, sensory potentials recorded from the ulnar nerve at the wrist were absent, or when present, were conducted at a normal rate but were of diminished amplitude. Conduction velocity

and amplitude of the sensory potentials were normal when the median nerve was stimulated (Gilliatt et al., 1970).

Acknowledgments: We thank Dr. Blatt, Dr. Carlsen, Dr. Knappeis, and Dr. Trojaborg for allowing us to quote from unpublished work.

For permission to report findings from patients under their care, we are indebted to the Departments of Neuromedicine, Neurosurgery, Occupational Medicine and Orthopaedic Surgery, Rigshospitalet, Copenhagen; the Department of Neuromedicine, Bispebjerg Hospital, Copenhagen; the Department of Physical Medicine, Orthopaedic Hospital, Copenhagen; and Frederiksborg County Hospital, Esbønderup.

We thank the staff of the Department of Neurosurgery, Rigshospitalet, Copenhagen, for performing the biopsies of the sural nerves.

References

Andersen, V. O., and Buchthal, F.: Low noise a.c. amplifier and compensator to reduce stimulus artefact. Med. Biol. Eng., *8:*501, 1970.

Behse, F., and Buchthal, F.: Normal sensory conduction in the nerves of the leg in man. J. Neurol. Neurosurg. Psychiatry, *34*:404, 1971.

Behse, F., and Buchthal, F.: Electrophysiological findings in non-diabetic monozygotic co-twins of diabetic probands. Unpublished data.

Behse, F., Buchthal, F., Carlsen, F., and Knappeis, G. G.: Hereditary neuropathy with liability to pressure palsies. Electrophysiological and histopathological aspects. Brain, *95*:777, 1972.

Behse, F., Buchthal, F., Carlsen, F., and Knappeis, G. G.: Light and electron microscopy as related to sensory conduction along normal and diseased sural nerve. Unpublished data.

Bickford, R. G.: Human "microreflexes" revealed by computer analysis. Neurology, *16*:302, 1966.

Blom, S., and Finnström, O.: Sensible Nervenleitgeschwindigkeit bei neugeborenen Kindern. Z. Elektroencephalographie Elektromyographie, *2*:16, 1971.

Bonney, G., and Gilliatt, R. W.: Conduction after traction lesion of the brachial plexus. Proc. R. Soc. Med., *51*:365, 1958.

Boyd, J. A., and Davey, M. R.: Composition of peripheral nerves. Edinburgh and London, Livingstone Ltd., 1968.

Buchthal, F., and Rosenfalck, A.: Evoked action potentials and conduction velocity in human sensory nerves. Brain Res., *3*:1, 1966.

Buchthal, F., and Rosenfalck, A.: Sensory potentials in polyneuropathy. Brain, *94*:241, 1971a.

Buchthal, F., and Rosenfalck, A.: Sensory conduction from digit to palm and from palm to wrist in the carpal tunnel syndrome. J. Neurol. Neurosurg. Psychiatry, *34*:243, 1971b.

Buchthal, F., Rosenfalck, A., and Trojaborg, W.: Electrophysiological findings in entrapment of the median nerve at wrist and elbow. J. Neurol. Neurosurg. Psychiatry, *37*:340, 1974.

Cragg, B. G., and Thomas, P. K.: The conduction velocity of regenerated peripheral nerve fibres. J. Physiol. (Lond.), *171*:164, 1964.

Dawson, G. D.: The relative excitability and conduction velocity of sensory and motor nerve fibres in man. J. Physiol. (Lond.), *131*:436, 1956.

Denny-Brown, D., and Brenner, C.: Lesion in peripheral nerve resulting from compression by spring clip. Arch. Neurol. Psychiatry, *52*:1, 1944.

Eijkman, E., and Vendrik, A. J. H.: Detection theory applied to the absolute sensitivity of sensory systems. *In* Swets, J. A. (ed.): Signal Detection and Recognition by Human Observers. New York, Wiley, 1964, pp. 392–409.

Ellenberg, M.: Clinical concept of prediabetes. N.Y. State J. Med., *64*:2885, 1964.

Fullerton, P. M., Gilliatt, R. W., Lascelles, R. G., and Morgan-Hughes, J. A.: The relation between fibre diameter and internodal length in chronic neuropathy. J. Physiol. (Lond.), *178*:26P, 1965.

Gasser, H. S., and Erlanger, J.: The role played by the sizes of the constituent fibers of a nerve trunk in determining the form of its action potential wave. Am. J. Physiol., *80*:522, 1927.

Gilliatt, R. W.: Nerve conduction in human and experimental neuropathies. Proc. R. Soc. Med., *59*:989, 1966.

Gilliatt, R. W.: Experimental peripheral neuropathy. *In* The Scientific Basis of Medicine, Annual Reviews. London, The Athlone Press, 1969, pp. 202–219.

Gilliatt, R. W., and Sears, T. A.: Sensory nerve action potentials in patients with peripheral nerve lesions. J. Neurol. Neurosurg. Psychiatry, *21*:109, 1958.

Gilliatt, R. W., and Sears, T. A.: Peripheral nerve conduction in diabetic neuropathy. J. Neurol. Neurosurg. Psychiatry, *25*:11, 1962.

Gilliatt, R. W., and Taylor, J. C.: Electrical changes following section of the facial nerve. Proc. R. Soc. Med., *52*:1080, 1959.

Gilliatt, R. W., Goodman, H. V., and Willison, R. G.: The recording of lateral popliteal nerve action potentials in man. J. Neurol. Neurosurg. Psychiatry, *24*:305, 1961.

Gilliatt, R. W., Le Quesne, P. M., Logue, V., and Sumner, A. J.: Wasting of the hand associated with a cervical rib or band. J. Neurol. Neurosurg. Psychiatry, *33*:615, 1970.

Gilliatt, R. W., Melville, I. D., Velate, A. S., and Willison, R. G.: A study of normal nerve action potentials using an averaging technique (barrier grid storage tube). J. Neurol. Neurosurg. Psychiatry, *28*:191, 1965.

Gutrecht, J. A., and Dyck, P. J.: Quantitative teased-fiber and histologic studies of human sural nerve during postnatal development. J. Comp. Neurol., *138*:117, 1970.

Hiscoe, H. B.: Distribution of nodes and incisures in normal and regenerated nerve fibers. Anat. Rec., *99*:447, 1947.

Hursh, J. B.: Conduction velocity and diameter of nerve fibers. Am. J. Physiol., *127*:131, 1939.

Kaeser, H. E.: Diagnostische Probleme beim Karpaltunnelsyndrom. Dtsch. Z. Nervenheilkd., *185*:453, 1963.

Kaeser, H. E., and Lambert, E. H.: Nerve function studies in experimental polyneuritis. Electroencephalogr. Clin. Neurophysiol., Suppl. *22*:29, 1962.

Lamontagne, A., and Buchthal, F.: Electrophysiological studies in diabetic neuropathy. J. Neurol. Neurosurg. Psychiatry, *33*:442, 1970.

Lascelles, R. G., and Thomas, P. K.: Changes due to age in internodal length in the sural nerve in man. J. Neurol. Neurosurg. Psychiatry, *29*:40, 1966.

McDonald, W. I.: The effects of experimental demyelination on conduction in peripheral nerve: a histological and electrophysiological study. I. Clinical and histological observations. Brain, *86*:481, 1963.

McLeod, J. G.: Digital nerve conduction in the carpal tunnel syndrome after mechanical stimulation of the finger. J. Neurol. Neurosurg. Psychiatry, *29*:12, 1966.

Medical Research Council War Memorandum No. 7: Aids to the Investigation of Peripheral Nerve Injuries. London, H. M. Stationery Office, 1943.

Meier-Ewert, K., Dahm, J., and Niedermeier, E.: Optisch und elektrisch ausgelöste Mikroreflexe des Menschen. Z. Neurol., *199*:167, 1971.

Morgan-Hughes, J. A.: Experimental diphtheric neuropathy. A pathological and electrophysiological study. J. Neurol. Sci., *7*:157, 1968.

Nielsen, V. K.: Sensory and motor nerve conduction in the median nerve in normal subjects. Acta Med. Scand., *194*:435, 1973.

Payan, J.: Electrophysiological localization of ulnar nerve lesions. J. Neurol. Neurosurg. Psychiatry, *32*:208, 1969.

Rasminsky, M., and Sears, T. A.: Internodal conduction in undissected demyelinated nerve fibres. J. Physiol. (Lond.), *227*:323, 1972.

Rosenfalck, A., and Buchthal, F.: Sensory potentials and

threshold for electrical and tactile stimuli. *In* Desmedt, J. E. (ed.): New Developments in Electromyography and Clinical Neurophysiology. Vol. 2. Basel, Karger, 1973, pp. 45–51.

Rushton, W. A.: A theory of the effects of fibre size in medullated nerve. J. Physiol. (Lond.), *115*:101, 1951.

Sanders, F. K.: The thickness of the myelin sheaths of normal and regenerating peripheral nerve fibres. Proc. R. Soc. Lond. [Biol.] *135*:323, 1948.

Sears, T. A.: Action potentials evoked in digital nerves by stimulation of mechanoreceptors in the human fingers. J. Physiol. (Lond.), *148*:30P, 1959.

Ten Hoopen, M., and Reuver, H. A.: Aspects of average response computation by aperiodic stimulation. Med. Biol. Eng., *10*:621, 1972.

Thomas, J. E., and Lambert, E. H.: Electrodiagnostic aspects of the carpal tunnel syndrome. Arch. Neurol., *16*:635, 1967.

Thomas, P. K.: The morphological basis for alterations in nerve conduction in peripheral neuropathy. Proc. R. Soc. Med., *64*:295, 1971.

Thomas, P. K., and Fullerton, P. M.: Nerve fibre size in the carpal tunnel syndrome. J. Neurol. Neurosurg. Psychiatry, *26*:520, 1963.

Trojaborg, W.: Rate of recovery in motor and sensory fibres of the radial nerve: clinical and electrophysiological aspects. J. Neurol. Neurosurg. Psychiatry, *33*:625, 1970.

Trojaborg, W.: Motor and sensory conduction along the musculocutaneous nerve (unpublished data).

Vizoso, A. D., and Young, J. Z.: Internode length and fibre diameter in developing and regenerating nerves. J. Anat., *82*:110, 1948.

Wagner, A. L., and Buchthal, F.: Motor and sensory conduction in infancy and childhood: reappraisal. Dev. Med. Child Neurol., *14*:189, 1972.

Weiss, P., and Hiscoe, H. B.: Experiments on the mechanism of nerve growth. J. Exp. Zool., *107*:315, 1948.

Wiederholt, W. C.: Threshold and conduction velocity in isolated mixed mammalian nerves. Neurology, *20*:347, 1970.

Chapter 22

QUANTITATION OF CUTANEOUS SENSATION IN MAN

Peter James Dyck

The examination of cutaneous sensation at the bedside is imprecise and, if done poorly, may be misleading. This opinion is based on comparison of the reliability of determinations of the type and degree of sensory loss by conventional clinical methods to the reliability of these determinations by methods described in this chapter, correlated with the degree and kind of cutaneous nerve fiber loss (which can be reliably assessed by histometric evaluation of nerve biopsy specimens). There are many reasons for this lack of precision at the bedside: stimuli are variable, are not graded, and are not reproducible; the conditions of stimulation are variable and not controlled; the anatomical sites tested are not standardized; the number of trials at one site is too small to provide statistical validity; normative control values (specific for age, sex, and site) have not been determined; nonstimuli interspersed at random with stimuli are not systematically utilized to assess the reliability of the subject's responses; and the examination is subjective.

This surprising lack of clinical utilization of better methods for determining cutaneous sensation can be attributed to several causes. With the exception of the dolorimeter of Hardy, Wolff, and Goodell (1952), good instruments for measuring cutaneous sensation have not been commercially available. In addition, measurement of cutaneous sensation is extremely time-consuming and tedious. Finally and most important, neurologists may have thought that more precision in measurement of sensation would not provide a greater understanding, more accurate diagnosis, or

better treatment of their patients than was possible with traditional methods. They have also assumed, incorrectly I think, that because sensation is subjective it cannot be evaluated accurately.

In my view, quantitation of cutaneous sensation in persons with peripheral neuropathy is a necessary part of the clinical evaluation. It should be possible to establish, with a high degree of reliability, whether a modality of sensation is normal or not. An abnormality may provide information about which population of neurons is affected. As has been shown by Dyck and co-workers (1971), the type of sensory loss found in an affected region correlates reasonably well with the characteristics of the compound action potential and with the numbers and sizes of nerve fibers in the appropriate cutaneous nerve.

A further and important reason is that quantitation of sensation may be a sensitive method of following the severity of a neuropathy that affects the peripheral sensory neurons. It is now well known that, although of great value in the detection of abnormality within nerve fibers, the conduction velocity does not mirror very closely the clinical condition of the patient. To illustrate, in hypertrophic neuropathy the patient may be without symptoms and without clinical signs yet have markedly abnormal values of conduction velocity of motor and sensory fibers of limb nerves. Also, a patient may show marked clinical improvement from an episode of neuropathy without a comparable improvement in conduction velocity. Particularly in neuropathies characterized by low conduction velocities, there may be a long lag between clinical improvement and conduction velocity improvement.

Quantitative measurement of cutaneous sensation may be valuable in following the severity of many neuropathies in which distal axonal degeneration and atrophy of peripheral sensory neurons occurs. Comparative trials of medications and of treatment schedules may be possible, with the quantitated sensation used as one index of the severity of nerve fiber abnormality. As an example of this, in a study of patients with end-stage uremia, we are assessing two schedules of diet, fluid intake, and frequency of dialysis as they affect nerve function. Serial evaluations of touch-pressure, pain, and temperature sensations by the methods described in this chapter are providing serial data on the integrity of peripheral sensory neurons.

What constitutes a cutaneous sensation? This much discussed question is not considered in detail here. It should be realized, however, that it can be defined according to the nature of the stimulus, according to the nature of the physiologic or chemical event, or according to the subjective experience. The main purpose of this chapter is to acquaint the reader with the design of instruments that can be utilized for the quantitative measurement of cutaneous sensation, the methods for their use, the normative values obtained at various sites, the differences in threshold at various sites, and the possible reasons for these differences.

THRESHOLDS OF SENSATION FROM MECHANICAL DEFORMATION OF SKIN

Different subjective experiences or sensations may arise when the skin is deformed in different ways. When the skin is lightly stroked with cotton wool, the subject reports "touch," whereas when the skin is compressed with a blunt object he may report "pressure." The light application of two points of a caliper sufficiently spread apart may be reported as "two points," the light application of a tuning fork may be reported as "buzzing," "humming" or "vibration," and a numerical figure 5 drawn on the skin may be reported as "5." Common to all these different sensations

experienced by subjects is deformation of the skin and stimulation of mechanoreceptors. These mechanoreceptors, of various kinds, are situated at various depths and locations in the skin and deeper structures. From morphologic and physiologic characteristics, it is evident that there are different types of mechanoreceptors. These may vary in threshold, in response to phasic and tonic deformation, and in speed of adaptation.

From electrical recordings from small groups of fibers or from single fibers of cutaneous nerves, it is now known that fibers from mechanoreceptors are found in Aα, Aδ, and drC groups (Gasser and Erlanger, 1927; Adrian, 1930; Zotterman, 1939; Maruhashi et al., 1952; Douglas and Ritchie, 1957; Hunt and McIntyre, 1960; Iggo, 1960; Iriuchijima and Zotterman, 1960; Burgess and Perl, 1967; Bessou and Perl, 1969). These groups correspond to large myelinated, small myelinated, and unmyelinated fibers, respectively. When it is appreciated that cutaneous stimulation may involve these different groups of mechanoreceptors in different patterns of space and time and spinal cord mechanisms may influence the handling of this information, it is evident that there are sufficient mechanisms to explain the grading and differentiation that must underlie cutaneous sensation.

The simplest deformation of the skin might be a minute punctate indentation. Blix (1884) used a beam to which a horsehair stylus was attached so that the force of the stylus could be adjusted by a counterweight. Von Frey (1894) used calibrated horsehairs of various thicknesses and lengths, attached to a handle, to produce graded stimuli. The main, and serious, disadvantages of these methods are that (1) the instruments are hand held, which prevents precise placement and allows extraneous movement; (2) the rate of impact is variable; (3) the surface area of the stimulating stylus is greater when greater pressures are used; and (4) the wave form of deformation is variable and not defined.

A "baresthesiometer," using a spring-loaded hair, was devised by Eulenburg (1885), but it has the same defects as the von Frey hairs.

Instruments in which the stimulating stylus was dropped onto defined skin points were made by Benussi (1913), Dallenbach (1923), and Hulin (1929). The magnitude of the force and the rate and duration of the stimulus could be quantitated. The impact of falling seeds of various vegetables have been used to test touch sensation. In addition, drops of mercury and stainless steel balls of various sizes have been utilized. A recent instrument utilizing the principle of falling weights is that of Carmon and Dyson (1967). Because the deformation produced is critically dependent on the height of fall, these instruments are difficult to use. In addition, the pressure wave form was not accurately defined. A good mechanical instrument was devised by Nafe and Wagoner (1941). Its advantages are that the stimulus is superimposed on an initial load and that the variables of mechanical displacement of the skin can be quantitated.

More complex stimulation of mechanoreceptors occurs when deformation of the skin or of hairs traverses the surface of the skin. Fine jets of air moving across the skin were utilized by de Cillis (1944). The ability to recognize the roughness of sandpaper or to recognize a V-shaped groove has been used as an index of tactile sensation.

A novel approach, but one that does not depend on mechanical deformation of skin, is the use of electrical sparks.

The instruments that we use and that have been the most suitable for our studies are described in greater detail in the following paragraphs. These allow for exact placement of the stylus tip, standardization of stylus area, wide range of intensity of stimuli with defined and constant wave form, and relative ease of operation.

Touch-Pressure Instrument, Generation 1

The instrument consists of a square-wave generator that drives a motor and a stimulating stylus (Fig. 22–1) (Dyck et al., 1971). The voltage control is activated by a motor and reduction gear to increase or decrease the voltage. A square wave of 400 msec duration at a rate of 1 Hz is modified by a specially built power amplifier so that there is an exponential rise to full force and an exponential decay to the baseline, as shown in Figure 22–2; the pressure is exerted at the stylus tip of the pressure arm fastened to the shaft of a torque motor. The stylus tip is a 0.6 mm Teflon-coated steel ball. Controls on the power amplifier allow the touch-pressure arm to be raised or lowered with precision so that the stylus tip can be made to contact the skin surface at a force that cannot be felt by the subject. Coarse micrometer screws permit

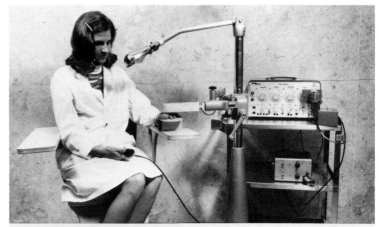
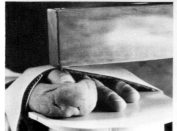
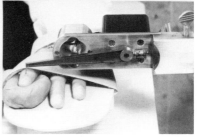

Figure 22–1 Touch-pressure instrument, generation 1, as described in text. (From Dyck, P. J., Lambert, E. H., and Nichols, P. C.: Quantitative measurement of sensation related to compound action potential and number and sizes of myelinated and unmyelinated fibers of sural nerve in health, Friedreich's ataxia, hereditary sensory neuropathy, and tabes dorsalis. *In* Rémond, A. (ed.): Handbook of Electroencephalography and Clinical Neurophysiology. Vol. 9. Amsterdam, Elsevier Publishing Co., 1971, p. 83. Reprinted by permission.)

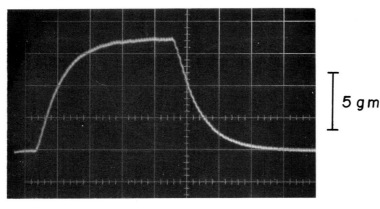

5 gm

400 msec

Figure 22–2 Oscilloscope tracing of 400 msec pressure wave form as recorded with strain gauge and amplifier. (From Dyck, P. J., Schultz, P. W., and O'Brien, P. C.: Quantitation of touch-pressure sensation. Arch. Neurol., 26:465, 1972. Copyright 1972, American Medical Association. Reprinted by permission.)

the stylus tip to be displaced forward, backward, and laterally.

The finger or toe to be tested is cradled in modeling clay. A grid with points separated by 1 mm is printed onto the skin. Sites tested have included the dorsal surface of the index finger just proximal to the base of the nail and a homologous site on the first great toe. Rows of points parallel to and beginning at the base of the nail are numbered with Roman numerals. Points within a row are numbered with Arabic numerals from left to right (as the subject sees the dorsum of his finger).

In the test situation, the force of the tapping of the stylus is increased by the motor-driven voltage control to the point at which the tapping is just felt. In a study of touch-pressure sensation of healthy subjects, 10 separate determinations of threshold were obtained at each of nine points (points 4, 5, and 6 of rows IV, V, and VI) (Dyck et al., 1972). The voltage values were converted to grams from a nomogram. The touch-pressure threshold was taken as the mean of the 90 determinations of threshold (Figs. 22–3 and 22–4). Table 22–1 shows the touch-pressure sensation thresholds of male and female subjects in three age groups.

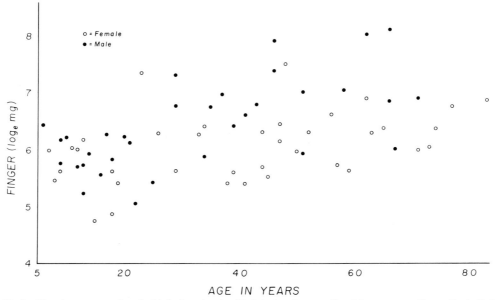

Figure 22–3 Touch-pressure threshold, in $\log_e$ (mg), of left index finger of healthy persons. (From Dyck, P. J., Schultz, P. W., and O'Brien, P. C.: Quantitation of touch-pressure sensation. Arch. Neurol., 26:465, 1972. Copyright 1972, American Medical Association. Reprinted by permission.)

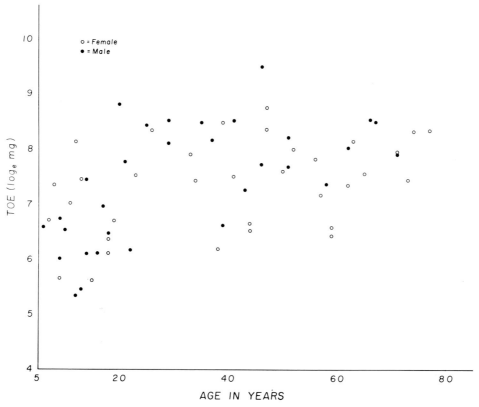

Figure 22–4   Touch-pressure threshold, in log$_e$ (mg), of left great toe of healthy persons. (From Dyck, P. J., Schultz, P. W., and O'Brien, P. C.: Quantitation of touch-pressure sensation. Arch. Neurol., 26:465, 1972. Copyright 1972, American Medical Association. Reprinted by permission.)

For both sexes and in all three age groups, thresholds were lower on the finger than on the toe (P values ranged from <0.0001 to <0.02). Male and female subjects did not differ significantly in touch-pressure sensation

TABLE 22–1   TOUCH-PRESSURE SENSATION THRESHOLDS OF HEALTHY SUBJECTS BY AGE*

Sex	Digit	Group 1 (6–20 yr) Mean	SD	Group 2 (21–40 yr) Mean	SD	Group 3 (>40 yr) Mean	SD
M	Fi	0.43	0.15	0.79	0.54	1.77	1.24
	T	1.29	1.85	3.59	2.14	5.93	4.95
F	Fi	0.34	0.14	0.67	0.59	0.64	0.32
	T	1.35	1.15	3.39	2.22	3.06	2.10

*Thresholds are given in grams, with Fi indicating finger, and T, toe. (From Dyck, P. J., Schultz, P. W., and O'Brien, P. C.: Quantitation of touch-pressure sensation. Arch. Neurol., 26:465, 1972. Copyright 1972, American Medical Association. Reprinted by permission.)

threshold except on fingers of subjects more than 40 years old. In this group, female subjects had a significantly lower threshold value than males ($P < 0.01$ for fingers; $P < 0.05$ for toes). For both fingers and toes of male and female subjects, the threshold values were higher in the oldest age group ($P < 0.01$); no statistically significant difference was observed between the thresholds in the middle and oldest age groups.

Touch-Pressure Instrument, Generation 2

This is a fully redesigned automated version of the generation 1 instrument with additional improvements (Ness et al., unpublished data). The pressure wave form is exactly the same, however, as that of the generation 1 instrument. One part of the instrument is shown in Figure 22–5. After mechanical alignment of the stimulator

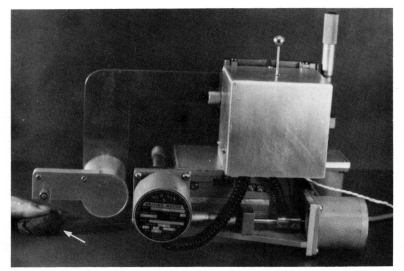

Figure 22–5 Touch-pressure instrument, generation 2, as described in text. Controller (not shown) has a hard-wired program for the conditions and sites of stimulation. These can be altered by controls on the panel. The stimulating unit on the right contains the three motors governing the traverse of the electromechanical stimulator, the stylus of which is shown by an arrow. This instrument was designed by A. Ness, P. Caskey, and P. J. Dyck.

portion of the instrument with the site to be tested, precise placement of the height and position of the stylus tip is controlled by a joy stick that activates three electric motors. After this initial alignment the program conditions are set and the program is begun. The stylus tip is lowered to rest on the skin at a static load of about 100 mg. After a short period of accommodation a stimulus routine is begun. Just prior to a test, an amber alerting light is turned on.

The instrument has been designed to produce 31 levels of stimulation between 8 and 0 g. The increments are based on a study of just-noticeable differences of touch-pressure with the generation 1 instrument (Stevens and Dyck, unpublished data). Stimulation at one skin point begins either with a nonstimulus or with a level-16 stimulus (whether a stimulus or a nonstimulus falls at a grid point has been determined by random selection). The next train of stimuli is always at level 16. If the subject feels the tapping at this level, he says so and the examiner presses a switch. The switch must be pressed during the train of stimuli. If the subject felt the tapping at level 16 and the switch was activated correctly, the next train of stimuli will be given at level 8. If the subject does not feel level-8 stimulation, the next train of stimuli will be given at level 12. If he feels level 12, a train of stimuli will be given at level 10. If he does not feel level-10 stimuli, the next train will be given at level 11. By using this binary logic, a threshold of touch-pressure can be determined at one point in just over one minute.

In addition, the subject's response is noted for a level-16 stimulus or a nonstimulus. The location of the grid point, the response to the level-16 stimulus or the nonstimulus, and the threshold are then printed on a tape. The instrument will automatically lift the stylus and move it to the next point, lower it to produce a static load of 100 mg, and after a period of accommodation, will stimulate the new point according to the routine just outlined. The stylus can be returned to the 0, 0 position at any time or be allowed to go to its maximum position of 7, 7 (49 grid points).

In scoring the results, an estimate is made of the percentage of responses to a nonstimulus, the percentage of responses to the level-16 stimulus, the percentage of the grid points at which a threshold could not be obtained, and the mean value and variability of the thresholds from the points at which it could be obtained.

Two-Point Discrimination

Tests of two-point discrimination are commonly utilized in the neurologic examination and in evaluation of patients with neuropathy. The necessary first condition for recognition of two points is that each of the points cause sufficient deformation of the skin to activate mechanoreceptors. In addition, however, the subject must be able to distinguish two points, so more complex neural events may be involved. It can be shown, for example, that "touch-sensitive spots" are closer together than the values obtained in the two-point discrimination test.

Clearly, the recognition of two points is affected, at least in part, by the magnitude of the punctate indentation made by each of the two points of the calipers. Furthermore, it is known that the wave of depression surrounding each of the points increases with the load. With increasing depression and with the points close together, the indentation might become contiguous and be experienced as one point. It is therefore apparent that the necessary conditions for determination of touch-pressure at one point should be met at each of two points. Ideally, the two points should rest on the skin with a static load, and a stimulus of graded magnitude and of known mechanical wave form should be superimposed. The points should be precisely placed and not hand held. An instrument that meets these criteria is not available, but one that fulfills them in part was devised by Ringel and Ewanowski (1965) for the determination of two-point discrimination in oral structures.

The results of two-point discrimination tests shown in Table 22–2 were taken from the work of Goldscheider (1885), Weber (1835), and Weinstein (1968); these measurements were made with hand-held calipers. From this table it is apparent that there are great differences in two-point discrimination at different cutaneous sites: tongue tip, lip, and finger tip have small values while other regions such as thigh and back have large values. These differences are usually considered to be due to differences in density of mechanoreceptors. Specific and reliable information on this point, however, is not available.

Vibration Sensation (Pallesthesia)

Weber, in 1846, wrote of a "vibration sense" (see Fox and Klemperer, 1941). Rumpf (1889) used no less than 14 tuning forks to assess this sensation (see Pearson, 1928). Pearson (1928) attempted to standardize the tuning fork test by use of a "constant blow" and timed the

TABLE 22–2 TWO-POINT DISCRIMINATION VALUES IN MILLIMETERS

Location	Value (mm)		
	By Goldscheider*	By Weber	By Weinstein†
Head			
Tongue, tip		1.1	
Lip, mucosa		4.5	
Lip, ectoderm		9.0	5.6
Gums		13.6	
Nose, tip	0.3	6.8	8.4
Forehead	0.5–1.0	22.6	16.8
Scalp, posterior	1.0–1.4	27.1	
Neck and trunk			
Cervical, anterior		33.9	
Sternum		40.7	
Belly			33.6
Chest, ventral	0.8		35.2
Spine, lumbar	4.0–6.0	64.2	40.4
Spine, sacral		40.7	
Upper limb			
Arm, middle		67.8	42.8
Hand, palm		11.3	10.5
Hand, back		31.6	
Finger, tip		2.3	2.8
Finger, dorsum, terminal phalanx	0.3–0.5	6.8	
Finger, pulp	0.1–0.2	6.8	
Lower limb			
Thigh, middle	3.0	67.8	43.6
Patella		36.2	
Leg, posterior calf			46.0
Great toe, tip		11.3	11.0
Foot, sole			21.0

*Probably based mainly on observations on the investigator himself.
†Based on evaluation of 24 men and 24 women.

duration during which the vibrations could be felt. For measurement of the sensitivity to mechanical vibration, Gilmer (1935) used an electronic oscillator and the coil of an electromagnetic speaker to produce vibration; the frequency and magnitude of the stimulus were assessed by using a piezoelectric pickup (Rochelle salt crystal). He tested the effects of size of skin contactor, of frequency, and of amplitude of skin displacement on threshold values. The frequency with the lowest threshold was 512 Hz; the highest frequency that was discernible was 2600 Hz (this also was the highest frequency tested). Some variability—in the range of 128 to 512 Hz—has been observed in the frequency with the lowest threshold (Gordon, 1936).

A series of observations has confirmed that the frequencies 64, 128, 256, and 512 Hz have approximately equal thresholds. In a good early review article on concepts of perception of mechanical vibration, Geldard (1940) pointed out that only a few instruments produced a vibration stimulus that was adequately controlled for frequency, amplitude, and wave form. In the instrument that he made with Fessard, these features were controlled and the degree of damping by the skin was recorded (see Geldard, 1940). Much of this article is a refutation of the arguments for vibration being a separate sense from touch-pressure.

It had been pointed out that a displacement of skin as small as 3 μm by mechanical vibration could be perceived, but such small displacements could not be recognized as pressure. Geldard pointed out that Fessard had shown that the mechanical displacement necessary for pressure to be felt was not much greater than that for vibration and that summation of repetitive impulses would explain the lower values for vibration in any case. It had also been reported by Treitel in 1897 that the tongue was insensitive to vibration yet possessed very good pressure discrimination (see Geldard, 1940). Geldard noted that the tongue does not have a rigid structure within it to act as a sounding board for vibration, as do conventional sites for vibration tests. It had been argued that vibration does not adapt readily while pressure does. Geldard summarized the work of several persons to demonstrate that adaptation did occur with vibration.

It had further been pointed out by clinical neurologists that vibration sensation in certain disorders was preserved while touch sensation was lost and vice versa. Geldard pointed out that in the first case this may be easily explained by the transmission of mechanical vibration along bones to

sensitive regions. The second situation he thought might be explained by the perceptual process.

A particularly strong argument had come from the work of Goldscheider and of Cummings (1938; see Geldard, 1940): intradermal injection of a local anesthetic virtually abolished pressure sensitivity without markedly affecting vibration thresholds. Geldard argued that these studies had been misconstrued. He pointed out that, if vibration were checked at punctate regions of skin with a needle and a similar load and amplitude of mechanical deformation, the skin would be as insensitive to vibration as to pressure. Geldard drew maps of spots at which he found the lowest thresholds for vibration (confirming von Frey's observation of punctate regions on skin where vibratory sensation of low intensity could be elicited) and for touch and found that the maps did not coincide, which he explained away as due to conduction of vibration away from the tested spot. Geldard therefore concluded that there was no justification for postulating a separate vibration sensation.

An important study on the physiology of vibration receptors was that by Hunt (1961). Using isolated pacinian receptors of the interosseous sheath of the leg of cats, stimulation by a glass stylus attached to a hearing aid mechanism driven by a sine-wave oscillator of variable frequency and amplitude, and recording from the appropriate nerve fiber, he showed that these receptors did not respond to frequencies less than 85 Hz and that they might respond to frequencies as high as 1000 Hz. Ineffectiveness of low frequencies of mechanical deformation could be attributed to rapid adaptation of these receptors. Hunt thought that the pacinian corpuscle was the only receptor in skin capable of following frequencies of vibration exceeding 150 Hz.

Clinical pathologic evidence had accumulated that posterior column lesions of the spinal cord abolish vibration sensation below the level of the lesion, while anterolateral cordotomy for pain relief does not (Fox and Klemperer, 1941).

From this brief review of sensation from mechanical vibration, it should be apparent that the testing of vibration as done at the bedside is inadequate. The stimulus of the tuning fork or of a commercially available instrument such as the bioesthesiometer (Bio Medical Instrument Co., Chagrin Falls, Ohio) is utilized in several ways. In clinical neurology, vibration sensation conventionally is assessed by holding the tuning fork firmly against the malleolus or some other bone. As pointed out by Geldard (1940), the bone underlying the site being tested acts as a sounding board, and it is difficult to know which receptors are activated. It is common experience to feel vibration in the fingers when the tuning fork is held against a bone protuberance at the elbow. There is no clinical instrument available for testing vibration sense at grid points of a skin surface that uses a stylus resting on the skin with defined and constant load and a sine wave whose amplitude and frequency can be varied and recorded precisely.

The bioesthesiometer is the only commercial instrument available. It is a simple device consisting of a voltage supply and an electromagnet that activates a spring-loaded stimulator; it is calibrated at the factory. The main drawbacks of the instrument are: (1) the amplitude of the vibrations decreases with an increase of the static load; (2) the movement of the stimulator is in more than one plane; (3) in the test situation, the rate of increase of the voltage is not controlled; and (4) it is a hand-held instrument. The first drawback is important because the amount of mechanical displacement of the skin appears to be a necessary factor for feeling vibration. The first and last objections can in part be remedied by modifying the instrument so that it is used at defined static loads. Even then, however, the amplitudes of displacement will not be what the manufacturer claims unless the instrument has been calibrated for such loads. The second and third objections cannot be resolved without redesigning the instrument. Because the voltage is increased by hand, the examiner must attempt to increase it at a uniform rate.

THRESHOLDS OF SENSATION FROM THERMAL STIMULI

The methods for testing thermal sensation at the bedside usually are so imprecise that only complete absence of thermal sensation can be determined with reliability. In contrast to this, there have been highly sophisticated studies of the physiology of cold and warm sensations with precisely graded thermal stimuli (Hensel, 1950).

There is now evidence from single-fiber studies that some receptors respond when they are cooled and others respond when they are warmed (Zotterman, 1939; Hunt and McIntyre, 1960; Iggo, 1960; Burgess and Perl, 1967; Bessou and Perl, 1969). Fibers from

such "warm receptors" and "cold receptors" are found in the drC and $A\delta$ groups of cutaneous nerves. From the mapping studies of the "warm" and "cold" spots of early investigators, it is known that there are differences in the distribution and density of "warm" and "cold" receptors (Blix, 1884; Goldscheider, 1885).

Instruments utilized at the bedside to measure warm and cold sensation usually consist of two small containers, each filled with water drawn from the hot or cold faucet. Sometimes a thermometer is used so that the temperature of each liquid can be determined. A variant of this approach is to heat or cool solid metal thermodes to known temperatures and to use these as stimuli. These methods do not, however, give the finely graded stimuli needed to measure the threshold of warm or cold sensation in healthy subjects or in patients with mild disorders of these neurons.

Very elaborate instruments have been devised consisting of a thermode that rests on the skin and through which a fluid at an accommodating temperature could be circulated (Kenshalo et al., 1960). A rapid change of temperature (Δ temperature) could then be introduced and a strip record kept of the change in temperature with time at the point of thermode contact with skin by using a small thermistor. In this way, small temperature differences with defined gradients could be given. These instruments are costly. In addition, a trial of a large number of stimuli of different temperature variations, at various sites and in an adequate sample of subjects, is prohibitively slow. With the two instruments described next, the thermal stimuli can be graded, the surface area of the thermode is constant, and the operation is rapid. They produce a reliable measurement of thermal sensation.

Measurement of Temperature Discrimination With Two Constant-Temperature Circulating Units

Two constant-temperature circulators (Model K-2/rd Lauda circulators, Brinkman Instruments, Inc., Westbury, N.Y.) are connected by silicone pressure hoses to a brass thermode whose area of contact with the skin is 7.1 cm² (Fig. 22–6). A slotted groove through the center of the base of the thermode contains a small thermistor, the resistance of which is measured in a bridge circuit. The

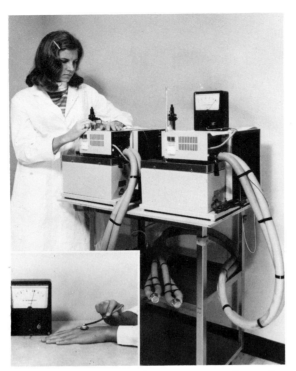

Figure 22–6 Instrument for measurement of cutaneous temperature discrimination as discussed in text. *Inset.* Skin thermometer with spring-loaded handle. (From Dyck, P. J., Lambert, E. H., and Nichols, P. C.: Quantitative measurement of sensation related to compound action potential and number and sizes of myelinated and unmyelinated fibers of sural nerve in health, Friedreich's ataxia, hereditary sensory neuropathy, and tabes dorsalis. *In* Rémond, A. (ed.): Handbook of Electroencephalography and Clinical Neurophysiology. Vol. 9. Amsterdam, Elsevier Publishing Co., 1971, p. 83. Reprinted by permission.)

thermistors in the thermodes are calibrated against the thermistor used for measuring skin temperature. The skin thermometer is a specially fabricated thermistor affixed to the end of the stalk mounted in a small cup-shaped device. The flanged edges of this device permit only a small indentation of the thermistor into the skin and, in addition, protect the skin from conduction currents. The skin thermometer is held against the skin by a spring-loaded handle (Fig. 22–6 *inset*).

In the test situation, the temperature of one thermode is adjusted to be a certain value higher than the recorded skin temperature (this will be the warm thermode). The temperature of the other thermode is adjusted to the same amount below the skin temperature (the cool thermode). Before a series of trials is begun at one temperature difference, the subject is blindfolded and each thermode

is held to the skin for 5 seconds while the subject is told which thermode is being presented. Then, a series of 50 warm or cool stimuli are presented in random fashion; an equal number of warm and cool stimuli are presented. Stimulus duration is approximately 5 seconds, and the time between consecutive stimuli is approximately 5 to 10 seconds. The subject is asked to report "warm," "cool," or "I don't know."

For healthy subjects, temperature differences of 2°, 1.6°, 1.2°, 0.8°, 0.4°, 0.2°, and 0.0° C were tried. In scoring, all the "I don't know" responses were marked as errors. Even when there was no difference of temperature, the subjects would say "warm" or "cool" more frequently than "I don't know," but the identification of the thermode called "warm" and the one called "cold" was on the average what it would have been by chance (guessing). Therefore, the threshold of recognition of the difference in temperature was set at the 75 per cent correct level. The probability of a subject guessing correctly at this level when 50 random stimuli are presented is less than 0.1 per cent.

In Figure 22–7 are shown the responses of a 23 year old woman to a series of cool and warm stimuli given in random sequence, at various differences of temperature, on blackened spots of the forehead, abdomen, and foot. The temperature discrimination threshold level is indicated by the broken line. On the forehead of this subject the threshold was less than 0.2° C, on the abdomen it was between 0.2° and 0.4° C, and on the dorsum of the foot it was between 0.4° and 0.6° C. Figure 22–8 shows the temperature discrimination thresholds on blackened skin of the dorsum of the foot of 10 healthy persons.

Minnesota Thermal Disks

This instrument, shown in Figure 22–9, has several commendable features. It is simple, inexpensive, and has no moving part; it does not require electricity or water; it can be carried in the physician's bag; and it delivers relatively constant graded thermal stimuli that can be quantitated. Four materials—copper, stainless steel, glass, and polyvinyl chloride—act as differential heat sinks when applied to the skin at ambient temperature. The copper would conduct away the most heat and would feel the coldest; the others would conduct

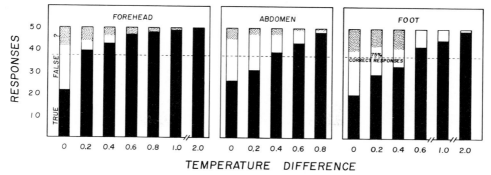

Figure 22–7 Responses of 23 year old healthy woman to series of cool and warm stimuli given in random sequence, at various differences of temperature, on blackened spots of forehead, abdomen, and foot. (From Dyck, P. J., Lambert, E. H., and Nichols, P. C.: Quantitative measurement of sensation related to compound action potential and number and sizes of myelinated and unmyelinated fibers of sural nerve in health, Friedreich's ataxia, hereditary sensory neuropathy, and tabes dorsalis. *In* Rémond, A. (ed.): Handbook of Electroencephalography and Clinical Neurophysiology. Vol. 9. Amsterdam, Elsevier Publishing Co., 1971, p. 83. Reprinted by permission.)

away less heat (and would feel less cold than the copper) in the order listed. Ballast is added to each of the stimulators so that they all rest on the skin with the same load. The surface area of the thermode is 10 cm².

In the test situation, the subject is blindfolded and the copper (C) thermode is placed on the skin. The subject is told that this is "cold." Next the polyvinyl (P) thermode is applied and the subject is told that this is not as cold and it will be called "warm." The "cold" and the "warm" thermodes are again presented and identified for the subject. The subject is told that after each presentation he must respond with "cold," warm," or "I don't know." First, 25 stimuli with the C thermode and 25 with the P thermode are presented in an order drawn by chance. Each stimulus is presented for two seconds; the interval between stimuli is eight seconds. The second series of stimuli uses 25 with the copper thermode and 25 with the glass (G) thermode. Then a third series of stimuli is given similarly with the copper and stainless steel (S) thermodes. In some studies a fourth series is used with 50 stimuli by copper (C_1 and C_2) thermodes; in this case the subject is told that C_1 is "cold" and C_2 is "warm" but not that both

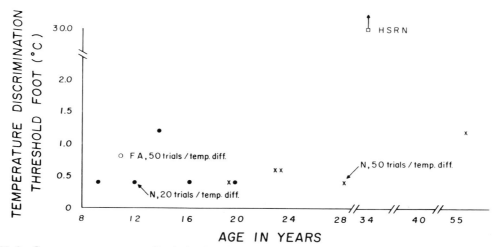

Figure 22–8 Cutaneous temperature discrimination thresholds on dorsum of the foot in 10 healthy subjects. N, normal; FA, Friedreich's ataxia; HSRN, hereditary sensory radicular neuropathy. (From Dyck, P. J., Lambert, E. H., and Nichols, P. C.: Quantitative measurement of sensation related to compound action potential and number and sizes of myelinated and unmyelinated fibers of sural nerve in health, Friedreich's ataxia, hereditary sensory neuropathy, and tabes dorsalis. *In* Rémond, A. (ed.): Handbook of Electroencephalography and Clinical Neurophysiology. Vol. 9. Amsterdam, Elsevier Publishing Co., 1971, p. 83. Reprinted by permission.)

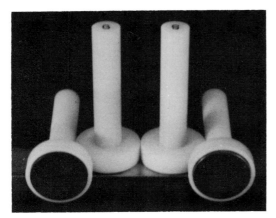

Figure 22–9 Minnesota thermal disks for testing cutaneous temperature discrimination as discussed in text. This instrument was designed by P. J. Dyck and D. Curtis.

thermodes are made of the same material. Again the options are "cold," "warm," and "I don't know."

The C_1 and C_2 thermodes are seldom acknowledged by the response "I don't know." On the average, about 50 per cent of stimuli will be correctly identified by chance. The value with 75 per cent correct responses was therefore chosen as the threshold.

It might be argued that, with the thermode at ambient temperature, approximately 10° C below skin temperature, the thermode temperature would quickly rise to the skin temperature and the subject would not be able to recognize differences between two thermodes. In fact, however, under the conditions in which the thermodes are utilized, the temperature of the thermode rises approximately 1° C and then remains at this temperature throughout the trial.

To determine the reproducibility of this method, we tested the responses of four

healthy subjects on 10 consecutive mornings. On each occasion, 50 stimuli were given for each of the combinations, in the order C and P, C and G, and C and S (Table 22–3).

In tests at multiple skin sites of four healthy subjects, series of 50 stimuli with the combinations C and P, C and G, and C and S were used in the order shown. All sites were on the left side of the body. The results of these studies are shown in Table 22–4.

In studies on the forehead, dorsum of the foot, and dorsum of the hand of 30 healthy subjects, 50 stimuli were presented at each of the three sites with the combinations C and P, C and G, and C and S in that order. Table 22–5 shows the results of these tests.

THRESHOLDS OF SENSATION FROM NOCICEPTIVE STIMULI

Pain sensation is commonly tested clinically with a sharpened thistle or pin. It is well known, however, that patients without pain sensation may on occasion be able to distinguish a sharp pointed object, such as the point of a pin, from a dull object, such as the head of the pin. Also, subjects or patients may be able to distinguish various sensations depending on the nature of the stimulation. The compression of a tendon produces a different quality of painful sensation than that of the deep prick of a pin. Although one can appreciate that the sensation produced is different, it is far from proved that the first is a measure of deep sensation of pain while the second is cutaneous sensation of pain.

An old, valid but time-consuming, approach was to identify pain spots by methodical exploration of the surface of the skin with a sharpened pin or thistle. Although there have

TABLE 22–3 REPRODUCIBILITY OF THRESHOLD OF THERMAL SENSATION DETERMINED WITH MINNESOTA THERMAL DISKS*

Stimulus Pair	Per Cent Correct Responses											
	F, 18			M, 22			M, 54			F, 58		
	C + P	C + G	C + S	C + P	C + G	C + S	C + P	C + G	C + S	C + P	C + G	C + S
Mean	100	93	62	99	95	60	99	92	63	99	88	63
Range	...	80–100	31–72	96–100	88–100	48–70	96–100	86–96	50–70	96–100	74–94	50–78
SD	0	5	9	1	4	6	1	3	6	1	6	9

*On 10 separate days; 50 trials per test per stimulus pair; all tests on forehead of four healthy subjects.

TABLE 22–4 THRESHOLD OF THERMAL SENSATION DETERMINED WITH MINNESOTA THERMAL DISKS AT MULTIPLE SITES

| | Per Cent Correct Responses[†] | | | | | | | | | | | |
| | F, 18 | | | M, 22 | | | M, 54 | | | F, 58 | | |
Site*	C + P	C + G	C + S	C + P	C + G	C + S	C + P	C + G	C + S	C + P	C + G	C + S
1	100	94	64	100	92	70	100	92	64	100	86	58
2	100	82	66	98	94	54	96	88	52	100	90	52
3	100	86	66	100	92	60	92	82	60	100	94	50
4	100	64	52	100	92	56	92	84	64	100	92	52
5	92	80	52	98	90	58	90	78	62	98	82	64
6	100	92	48	100	82	60	92	76	54	90	76	56
7	100	76	44	98	88	58	90	72	56	92	74	60
8	98	80	54	100	64	64	98	88	52	98	86	50
9	100	86	72	98	84	40	88	80	48	92	88	54
10	100	88	56	98	78	44	96	78	50	86	74	66
11	98	80	64	96	86	54	88	82	56	86	80	46
12	98	68	62	100	90	60	90	80	58	86	78	62
13	98	70	60	100	80	58	92	84	56	90	80	60
14	96	74	66	84	66	50	88	74	50	94	70	64
15	100	96	58	90	66	60	94	78	52	94	90	64
16	100	90	54	98	76	56	96	82	60	96	86	64
17	96	80	60	100	90	50	94	80	70	92	88	64
Mean	98	82	59	98	83	56	93	81	57	94	83	58
Range	88–100	64–96	44–72	84–100	64–94	40–70	88–100	72–92	48–70	86–100	70–94	46–66
SD	3	9	7	4	10	7	4	5	6	5	7	6

*Sites (all on left side of body): 1, forehead above the eyebrow; 2, cheek; 3, subclavicular region; 4, midabdomen; 5, anterior midthigh; 6, midmedial side of the leg (L4 dermatome): 7, midlateral side of leg (L5 dermatome); 8, dorsum of foot; 9, sole of foot; 10, back of calf; 11, midback of thigh; 12, posterior chest at eighth rib; 13, back of hand; 14, center of palm; 15, midvolar forearm; 16, midback of forearm; 17, skin over the deltoid muscle.

†With 50 trials of each pair at each site in each subject.

been a variety of ways devised to produce pain, few can be graded, used repetitively, and quantitated. Several workers have applied electrical currents to the skin to the point at which a sensation of pain was elicited. A good instrument for the measurement of pain sensation is the dolorimeter, which was produced by Hardy, Wolff, and Goodell (1952). This instrument can be calibrated precisely, a graded response can be given, and the test is reproducible. Extensive investigations have been performed with this instrument. A study of the pricking pain threshold, as defined by Hardy, Wolff, and Goodell, was done by us on a series of normal, healthy, untrained subjects (Fig. 22–10). For an extensive review of the instrument and its calibration, threshold values, and significance, the book by Hardy, Wolff and Goodell (1952) is recommended.

TABLE 22–5 THRESHOLD OF THERMAL SENSATION DETERMINED WITH MINNESOTA THERMAL DISKS AT THREE SITES*

| | Per Cent Correct Responses[†] | | | | | | | | |
| | Forehead | | | Hand | | | Foot | | |
	C + P	C + G	C + S	C + P	C + G	C + S	C + P	C + G	C + S
Mean	98	86	61	94	83	61	93	82	62
Range	88–100	44–98	48–80	82–100	66–98	34–91	78–100	62–98	40–96
SD	3	10	8	5	9	11	6	9	11

*In 30 healthy subjects (16 female; 14 male) of ages 8 to 78 years.
†In 50 trials for each stimulus pair.

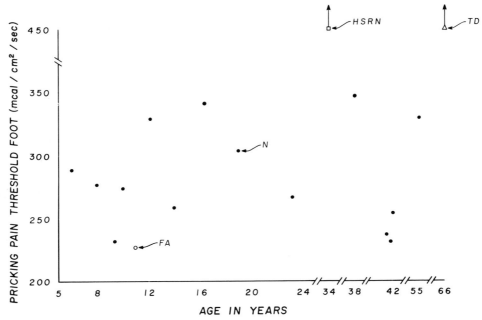

Figure 22–10   Pricking pain threshold on dorsum of foot of healthy subjects, determined by using dolorimeter devised of Hardy, Wolff, and Goodell. N, normal; FA, Friedreich's ataxia; HSRN, hereditary sensory radicular neuropathy; TD, tabes dorsalis. (From Dyck, P. J., Lambert, E. H., and Nichols, P. C.: Quantitative measurement of sensation related to compound action potential and number and sizes of myelinated and unmyelinated fibers of sural nerve in health, Friedreich's ataxia, hereditary sensory neuropathy, and tabes dorsalis. *In* Rémond, A. (ed.): Handbook of Electroencephalography and Clinical Neurophysiology. Vol. 9. Amsterdam, Elsevier Publishing Co., 1971, p. 83. Reprinted by permission.)

References

Adrian, E. D.: The effects of injury on mammalian nerve fibres. Proc. R. Soc. Lond., *106*:596, 1930.

Benussi, V.: Kinematohaptische Erscheinungen (Vorläufige Mitteilung über Scheinbewegungsauffassung auf Grund haptischer Eindrücke). Arch. Psychol. (Frankf.), *29*:385, 1913.

Bessou, P., and Perl, E. R.: Response of cutaneous sensory units with unmyelinated fibers to noxious stimuli. J. Neurophysiol., *32*:1025, 1969.

Blix, M.: Ueber Wirkung und Schicksal des Trichloräthyl- und Trichlorbutylalkohols im Thierorganismus. Z. Biol., *20*:141, 1884.

Burgess, P. R., and Perl, E. R.: Myelinated afferent fibres responding specifically to noxious stimulation of the skin. J. Physiol. (Lond.), *190*:541, 1967.

Carmon, A., and Dyson, J. A.: New instrumentation for research on tactile sensitivity and discrimination. Cortex, *3*:406, 1967.

Dallenbach, K. M.: Some new apparatus. Am. J. Psychol., *34*:90, 1923.

De Cillis, O. E.: Absolute thresholds for the perception of tactual movement. Arch. Psychol. *41*(Serial No. 294):1, 1944.

Douglas, W. W., and Ritchie, J. M.: Discharges in non-medullated afferent fibres in the cat's saphenous nerve in response to touch and to drugs (abstract). J. Physiol. (Lond.), *139*:9P, 1957.

Dyck, P. J., Lambert, E. H., and Nichols, P. C.: Quantitative measurement of sensation related to compound action potential and number and sizes of myelinated and unmyelinated fibers of sural nerve in health, Friedreich's ataxia, hereditary sensory neuropathy, and tabes dorsalis. *In* Rémond, A. (ed.): Handbook of Electroencephalography and Clinical Neurophysiology. Vol. 9. Amsterdam, Elsevier Press, Inc., 1971, p. 83

Dyck, P. J., Schultz, P. W., and O'Brien, P. C.: Quantitation of touch-pressure sensation. Arch. Neurol., *26*:465, 1972.

Eulenburg, A.: Zur Methodik der Sensibilitätsprüfungen, besonders der Temperatursinnsprüfung. Z. Klin. Med., *9*:174, 1885.

Fox, J. C., Jr., and Klemperer, W. W.: Vibratory sense: a quantitative study of its thresholds in nervous disorders. Trans. Am. Neurol. Assoc., *67*:171, 1941.

Gasser, H. S., and Erlanger, J.: The rôle played by the sizes of the constituent fibers of a nerve trunk in determining the form of its action potential wave. Am. J. Physiol., *80*:522, 1927.

Geldard, F. A.: The perception of mechanical vibration. I. History of a controversy. II. The response of pressure receptors. III. The frequency function. IV. Is there a separate "vibratory sense"? J. Gen. Psychol., *22*:243, 271, 281, 291, 1940.

Gilmer, B. v. H.: The measurement of the sensitivity of the skin to mechanical vibration. J. Gen. Psychol., *13*:42, 1935.

Goldscheider, A.: Nachtrag zu den Mitteilungen über die spezifischen Energien der Hautnerven. Mont. Prakt. Dermatol., *4*:5, 1885.

Gordon, I.: The sensation of vibration, with special reference to its clinical significance. J. Neurol. Psychopathol., *17*:107, 1936.

Hardy, J. D., Wolff, H. G., and Goodell, H.: Pain Sensations and Reactions. Baltimore, Williams & Wilkins Co., 1952.

Hensel, H.: Temperaturempfindung und intracutane Wärmebewegung. Pfluegers Arch., *252*:165, 1950.

Hulin, W. S.: A simplified electromagnetic aesthesiometer. Am. J. Psychol., *41*:476, 1929.

Hunt, C. C.: On the nature of vibration receptors in the hind limb of the cat. J. Physiol. (Lond.), *155*:175, 1961.

Hunt, C. C., and McIntyre, A. K.: Properties of cutaneous touch receptors in cat. J. Physiol. (Lond.), *153*:88, 1960.

Iggo, A.: Cutaneous mechanoreceptors with afferent C fibres. J. Physiol. (Lond.), *152*:337, 1960.

Iriuchijima, J., and Zotterman, Y.: The specificity of afferent cutaneous C fibres in mammals. Acta Physiol. Scand., *49*:267, 1960.

Kenshalo, D. R., Nafe, J. P., and Dawson, W. W.: A new method for the investigation of thermal sensitivity. J. Psychol., *49*:29, 1960.

Maruhashi, J., Mizuguchi, K., and Tasaki, I.: Action currents in single afferent nerve fibres elicited by stimulation of the skin of the toad and the cat. J. Physiol. (Lond.), *117*:129, 1952.

Nafe, J. P., and Wagoner, K. S.: The nature of pressure adaptation. J. Gen. Psychol., *25*:323, 1941.

Ness, A. B., Caskey, P. E., and Dyck, P. J.: Unpublished data.

Pearson, G. H. J.: Effect of age on vibratory sensibility. Arch. Neurol. Psychiatry, *20*:482, 1928.

Ringel, R. L., and Ewanowski, S. J.: Oral perception. 1. Two-point discrimination. J. Speech Hear. Res., *8*:389, 1965.

Stevens, J. C., and Dyck, P. J.: Unpublished data.

Von Frey, M.: Beitrage zur Physiologie des Schmerzsinns. Math. Phys. Ber., *46*:283, 1894.

Weber, E. H.: Ueber den Tastsinn. Arch. Anat. Physiol. Wissensch. Med., 1835, p. 152.

Weinstein, S.: Insensitive and extensive aspects of tactile sensitivity as a function of body part, sex and laterality. *In* Kenshalo, D. R. (ed.): International Symposium on the Skin Senses. Springfield, Ill., Charles C Thomas, 1968, p. 195.

Zotterman, Y.: Touch, pain and tickling: an electrophysiological investigation on cutaneous sensory nerves. J. Physiol. (Lond.), *95*:1, 1939.

Chapter 23

CEREBRAL EVOKED POTENTIALS

John E. Desmedt *and* P. Noël

Somatosensory cerebral potentials evoked by stimulation of the skin or of peripheral sensory nerves can be recorded from the intact human scalp. These small responses (0.2 to 10 μv) are embedded in the spontaneous electroencephalographic activity (10 to 100 μv) and other background noise, and they can only be displayed by averaging about 100 to 1000 sweeps to extract the stimulus-locked central response from the random noise; this can now be done with commercially available fixed program digital computers (Dawson, 1956). With appropriate precautions and careful design of the tests, consistent cerebral evoked potentials are obtained that offer exceptional opportunities for the study of somatic sensation and its disorders in neurologic diseases (cf. Halliday, 1967; Desmedt, 1971). The direct recording of sensory nerve action potentials with needle electrodes inserted through the skin in man also provides a wealth of data in the peripheral neuropathies (Dawson, 1956; Gilliatt and Sears, 1958; Kaeser, 1970; Gilliatt, 1973; Buchthal, 1973). It should be pointed out that recording of cerebral evoked potentials allows the studies of peripheral nerves to be extended to the proximal nerves, the spinal roots, and the central somatosensory pathway. This chapter reviews a number of diagnostic applications based on the features and latency of the early primary components of the cerebral potential reported by Desmedt and Noël (1973), but does not consider the changes in the later components observed in certain cerebral diseases.

METHODS

The methods for extracting satisfactory evoked potentials have been described in detail (Desmedt and Manil, 1970; Desmedt, 1971; Desmedt et al., 1973). The subject lies comfortably on a couch with a pillow under the neck and with the muscles relaxed. The room is electrically shielded and air-conditioned. The temperature of the skin overlying the limb studied is maintained above 34° C, as measured by a plate thermistor (Yellow Springs Instruments Co.); under such conditions the deep tissue temperature around the nerve can be assumed to be between 35° and 37° C (cf. Desmedt, 1973, p. 250). The stimulus is a square electric pulse of 100 μsec duration delivered either to the distal phalanx of one or more appropriate fingers or to a nerve trunk. The stimulus intensity is chosen between 2 and 60 ma and it is checked throughout the runs with a Hewlett-Packard model 1111A current probe. Sensory nerve potentials are recorded with two fine stainless steel needles, one inserted close to the nerve trunk and the other inserted 1 to 2 cm away, at a right angle to the nerve direction and at the same level on the limb. The insertion of such fine unvarnished needles is not painful and is quite safe, which makes it possible to study several nerves at different levels if necessary (cf. Desmedt, 1973, p. 246).

Cerebral responses are also recorded with fine subcutaneous needles, the active electrode being on the contralateral parietal focus for the hand or on the midline focus for the foot, while the reference electrode is generally on the mid upper forehead. Intervals between successive electrical stimuli can be reduced to 2 sec when the study deals with only the primary components of the cerebral response (Desmedt and Manil, 1970; Desmedt and Debecker, 1972). The frequency response of the whole system, amplifier and averager, should be flat from 2 to 1000 cps to avoid distortion of the rather fast early components (Desmedt, 1971). Our averaging computer is a FabriTek model 1062 with analog-to-digital conversion of 10 bits' accuracy and sweeps of 50 or 100 μsec per address, which satisfactorily resolves the fast peripheral nerve potentials or the early components of the cerebral response (Desmedt et al., 1974).

The tests generally last for one to three hours and they are not considered unpleasant. Mild sedation with diazepam (Valium) or secobarbital (Seconal) per os is used only in tense patients to help them achieve proper muscle and mental relaxation. Excess alpha rhythm in the background in the electroencephalogram is avoided by having the subjects remain alert with eyes open. Eye blinks are minimized by fixation of the gaze. In normal subjects 16 to 256 responses are averaged to obtain well-defined records on the X-Y plotter, but as many as 2048 responses may have to be averaged in some patients to resolve the reduced pathologic potentials from the background noise.

EVALUATION OF MAXIMUM CONDUCTION VELOCITY IN SENSORY FIBERS

The usual method for estimating the maximum sensory conduction velocity in peripheral nerves of intact human subjects is by recording the sensory nerve potentials evoked by an electrical stimulus to the fingers, which avoids activation of nerve fibers to and from the muscles (Dawson, 1956). This method sometimes fails in pathologic cases in which the nerve potentials are severely reduced or desynchronized proximally or both, even when an averaging method is used to enhance the signal-to-noise ratio (cf. Figs. 23–4 and 23–5). In some studies on pathologic nerves, the electrical stimuli were delivered, not to the fingers, but to the mixed

nerve trunk (at the wrist or the ankle) in order to obtain a large potential from the corresponding proximal nerve trunk. The latter procedure does not, however, provide unequivocal evidence, since the stimulus involves both motor axons and muscle afferents in addition to the skin and joint afferents (cf. Kaeser, 1970).

This difficulty can be avoided by recording average cerebral potentials from the scalp, where, even for stimuli delivered to mixed nerve trunks, the cerebral responses are evoked by the skin and joint afferents (cf. Desmedt and Noël, 1973). It is thus meaningful to compare the latencies of the cerebral responses to stimulation of the fingers and of the nerve trunk at various levels, since they are evoked by a similar class of afferent nerve fibers. The questions then arise whether the latency of the cerebral responses can be estimated with sufficient accuracy and whether the maximum sensory conduction velocity obtained by this method is consistent with that derived from direct recording of the sensory nerve potentials in normal subjects.

Upper Limb

When averaged with due precautions and on a fast computer, the latency of the early negative component N_1 of the cerebral response shows little, if any, variation in successive runs on the same subject and it can be estimated with an accuracy better than 0.5 msec (Desmedt et al., 1973). As shown in Figure 23–1, the cerebral responses of a normal young adult subject display fairly similar wave forms when the electrical stimulus is delivered either to fingers II and III or to the median nerve at the level of the axilla. In the latter run the intensity of the stimulus was just above threshold for eliciting a small muscle twitch. The latencies to the onset of the negative N_1 component of the cerebral responses were estimated as 19.5 and 10.8 msec respectively. The difference of 8.7 msec must correspond to the conduction time in afferent axons of the median nerve between the distal parts of fingers II and III and the axilla. In the same subject and with the same electrodes, a sensory nerve potential was recorded from the median nerve at the axilla and the latency of its negative-going phase was also 8.7 msec (cf. Buchthal and Rosenfalck, 1966).

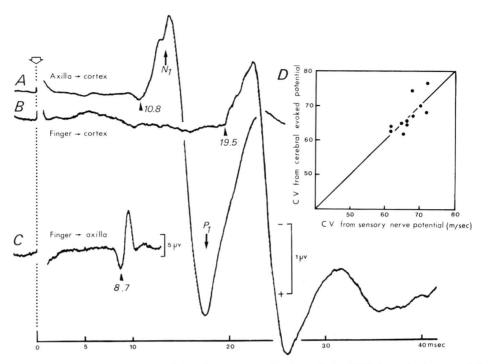

Figure 23–1 Evaluation of maximum peripheral sensory conduction velocity (CV) from the latency of the cerebral evoked potentials in normal adults. *A* and *B*. Average responses recorded from the contralateral parietal projection of the hand and evoked by electrical stimulation of either fingers II and III (*B*) or median nerve at the level of the axilla (*A*). The latency in milliseconds of the negative N_1 early component is indicated. *C*. Average sensory nerve potentials recorded from the median nerve at the axilla while stimulating fingers II and III in the same subject. Abscissa, time in milliseconds. Vertical calibration in microvolts. *D*. Pooled data of the maximum sensory conduction velocity of the median nerve from finger to axilla in 11 normal young adults. The diagram compares for each subject the maximum conduction velocity estimated by the two methods illustrated in *A*, *B*, and *C*, namely, by direct recording of sensory nerve potentials (abscissa) and by the latency difference of average cerebral potentials (ordinate). (From Desmedt, J. E., and Noël, P.: Average cerebral evoked potentials in the evaluation of lesions of the sensory nerves and of the central somatosensory pathway. *In* Desmedt, J. E. (ed.): New Developments in Electromyography and Clinical Neurophysiology. Vol. 2. Basel, S. Karger, 1973, pp. 352–371. Figure 1. Reprinted by permission.)

The same test performed in 11 normal adults 19 to 23 years of age gave consistent results as shown by the diagram in Figure 23–1*D* in which the maximum sensory conduction velocities estimated by the two methods are compared. The range extends from 62 to 77 m per second, and in any subject, for both methods, the conduction velocity tends to be either in the upper or in the lower part of the range. There seems to be no indication of a systematic deviation of the estimation by either of the methods. These studies are currently being developed in this laboratory. The results suggest that the maximum sensory conduction velocity in peripheral nerves can indeed be evaluated from the latency of cerebral evoked potentials, when the experimental conditions are adequate to provide clean and consistent responses. In this method the stimuli delivered at different levels along

the nerve should be adjusted roughly in order to evoke cerebral potentials of reasonably comparable size. The latter statement is kept somewhat vague because we realize that peripheral nerves with localized lesions may raise special problems in this respect.

It is of interest that the negative N_1 components compared in Figure 23–1*A* and *B* are quite similar in configuration, duration (4 msec), and voltage. The latency difference is indeed roughly the same for the onset and for the peak of N_1, and also for the peak of the subsequent positive P_1 component. This is not surprising because the two components are considered "primary" in nature, are fairly localized to the parietal projection for the contralateral hand, and presumably involve only few intracortical synapses (cf. Goff et al., 1962; Debecker and Desmedt, 1964; Halliday, 1967; Desmedt, 1971). The early negative N_1

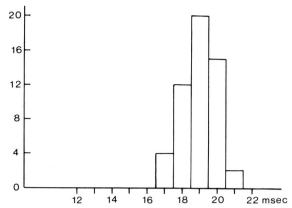

Figure 23-2 Latencies of onset of negative N_1 component of the cerebral potentials evoked by stimulation of finger II and III in 53 control subjects 16 to 50 years old who had no neurologic disease. Abscissa, time in milliseconds. Ordinate, number of subjects.

component has been found in recent years to represent a quite consistent feature of the cerebral response evoked from the contralateral upper limb in man, from birth to adulthood (Desmedt and Manil, 1970; Desmedt et al., 1973). Its latency varied within rather narrow limits, 16.5 to 21.0 msec, in 53 subjects aged 16 to 50 years with no neurologic disease (Fig. 23-2). We think that the remaining scatter of the latencies can be related at least in part to a size factor, namely the difference in length of the upper limb pathway from distal fingers to brachial plexus. Large subjects with long arms appear to contribute most of the longer N_1 latencies shown in Figure 23-1D.

Lower Limb

The method can also be used for the evaluation of maximum sensory conduction velocity in the lower limbs. This application is quite promising because the most common neuropathies involve predominantly the sensory fibers of the lower extremities and because sensory potentials are more difficult to record from these nerves (Gilliatt et al., 1961; Buchthal and Rosenfalck, 1966; Shiozawa and Mavor, 1969; Buchthal, 1973).

The electrical stimuli can be delivered along a sensory nerve like the sural nerve or along a mixed nerve. The cerebral potentials are recorded from the midline scalp, about 2 cm behind the vertex. Stimulation of the toes is possible but generally less convenient. Figure

23-3 shows the responses evoked in a normal 21 year old man by stimulating the sural nerve with bipolar needle electrodes on the upper aspect of the foot, behind the lateral malleolus, and at the lower third of the calf. The size and wave form of the three potentials are quite comparable. The early component is found to be surface-positive for lower limb stimulation (Desmedt, 1971; Noël, 1971; Tsumoto et al., 1972). The latencies of the cerebral responses are 36.5, 41.5, and 45.0 msec, respectively, and the calculated maximum sensory conduction velocities are 48 m per second from foot to ankle and 51 m per second from ankle to calf.

This method based on latency differences of cerebral potentials evoked from different levels along, say, the sural nerve gives results that are consistent with direct recordings of nerve potentials. It should be pointed out that the absolute value of the cerebral potential latency can vary a good deal between different normal subjects, even when the limb temperature is adequate, as explained in the section on methods. One of the parameters involved in these differences is the body size. Figure 23-3D compares the latencies of the cerebral potentials evoked by electrical stimulation of the sural nerve at the ankle in 12 normal subjects of 19 to 26 years. The scatter of latencies from 32 to 42 msec appears in first approximation to be linearly related to the body size plotted as the abscissa. We do not discuss here the respective contributions of the peripheral and central pathways to the cerebral latency (cf. Desmedt et al., 1973). In any case, the effect of body size, illustrated in Figure 23-3D, should be kept in mind when evaluating cerebral latencies in patients.

DIAGNOSTIC APPLICATIONS

Peripheral Neuropathies

Patients with peripheral nerve lesions, entrapment neuropathies, and metabolic or toxic neuropathies can be investigated by the method considered (Desmedt et al., 1966; Desmedt, 1971; Noël, 1973). Desmedt and Noël (1973) have recently reviewed the data. The latency differences of the cerebral response evoked by stimuli delivered at various levels along the limb may disclose a general or a localized slowing of the maximum sensory conduction velocity in one nerve. Studies of the cerebral responses evoked from different

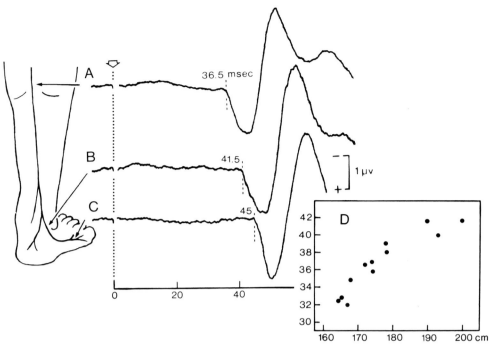

Figure 23–3 Evaluation of the maximum sensory conduction velocity in the sural nerve in normal adults. *A, B,* and *C.* Average cerebral responses were recorded from the midline focus in a normal subject 21 years old. The sural nerve was stimulated electrically at the base of the fifth toe (*C*), behind the lateral malleolus (*B*), and at the lower third of the calf (*A*). *D.* Pooled latencies of the cerebral responses evoked by stimulation of the sural nerve at the lateral malleolus in 12 normal adults. Abscissa, body size in centimeters. Ordinate, latency in milliseconds.

nerves of the same limb sometimes provide unique data for the detailed evaluation of nerve lesions, and positive findings have been obtained in patients who show no other evidence of damage to the motor axons. It is sometimes impossible to obtain a consistent sensory potential proximally in diseased peripheral nerves, even when using averaging techniques. In such cases of severe neuropathy, the position of the recording scalp electrodes is less critical than the position of a nerve recording electrode (cf. Gilliatt and Sears, 1958).

Figure 23–4 shows data obtained from a 50 year old male patient with poorly controlled diabetes of 10 years' duration and severe neuropathy. The lower limbs presented pseudotabetic signs. Touch and proprioceptive sensations were impaired, and deep reflexes were absent. In the upper limbs the deep reflexes were weak and position sense was impaired. During electrical stimulation of fingers II and III, no sensory potentials could be recorded from the median nerve at the wrist, even when many successive sweeps were averaged, as shown in Figure 23–4*A.* Yet the electrodes were ap-

parently close to the median nerve trunk, because stimulation through the same electrodes readily elicited motor responses in the abductor pollicis muscle. It is well known that desynchronization of the fiber action potentials in severely affected nerves makes it very difficult to record a sensory nerve potential, and such activity as remains is better displayed by recording the cerebral responses (Gilliatt and Sears, 1958). In this case, stimulation of fingers II and III elicited a definite cerebral potential of reduced voltage (0.55 μv for the first negative component) and increased latency (26.5 msec) (Fig. 23–4*B*). When the median nerve was stimulated at the wrist and at the axilla, the latencies of the cerebral potentials were respectively 18.8 and 11.8 msec. These figures allow the calculation of a maximum sensory conduction velocity of about 21 m per second from fingers to wrist and 47 m per second from wrist to axilla. Furthermore, the cervical latency for the axillary stimulation definitely exceeds the range of 9.5 to 11 msec found in adult normal control subjects (cf. Desmedt and Noël, 1973). This suggests that the fastest afferent fibers that can still be activated have some slowing

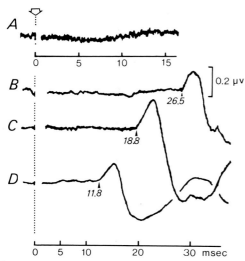

Figure 23–4   Evaluation of maximum sensory conduction velocity in severe diabetic neuropathy in a male patient 50 years old with insulin-dependent diabetes. *A.* Average record from the median nerve at the wrist during electrical stimulation of fingers II and III. No sensory nerve potential can be seen. *B, C,* and *D.* Average cerebral responses from the contralateral parietal hand focus evoked by electrical stimulation of fingers II and III (*B*), of the median nerve at the wrist (*C*), and at the axilla (*D*). (From Noël, P.: Sensory nerve conduction in the upper limbs at various stages of diabetic neuropathy. J. Neurol. Neurosurg. Psychiatry, *36*:786–796, 1973. Figure 7. Reprinted by permission.)

of conduction velocity proximally between the axilla and the spinal cord.

Lesions of Plexus and Spinal Roots

The usual nerve conduction studies cannot provide direct evidence in cases with proximal lesions involving the plexus or the spinal roots, whereas cerebral evoked potentials allow evaluation of the most proximal levels. Traction injuries of the brachial plexus usually result in avulsion of the anterior and posterior roots from the spinal cord, as these represent the mechanically weakest link in the plexus (Drake, 1964). This produces electromyographic signs of massive degeneration of motor axons. The sensory nerve potentials, however, may be recorded in spite of complete anesthesia of the extremity, because the sensory fibers generally remain in continuity with the dorsal root ganglion and do not degenerate (Bonney and Gilliatt, 1958; Warren et al., 1969). The stimulation of the nerves, of course, fails to evoke cerebral responses on the affected side.

In a patient with a lesion of the brachial plexus no sensory nerve potentials can be recorded in the limb, but electrical stimulation at a proximal level evokes genuine cerebral responses (Desmedt and Noël, 1973). Furthermore, evidence for regeneration of sensory axons from the proximal stump can be obtained by averaging cerebral responses evoked by stimuli delivered to the peripheral nerve stump, even at stages of axonal growth antedating the reinnervation of the denervated muscles. Regenerating human sensory axons were found, by this method, to conduct at 5 to 10 m per second (Desmedt et al., 1966; Desmedt and Noël, 1973).

Another example of diagnostic use of the evoked potential method in proximal nerve lesions is found in spinal root compression. A female patient, 26 years old, suffered from Hodgkin's disease, stage III, and had been undergoing chemotherapy for two years. She developed, progressively, pain and hypoesthesia with no motor deficit in the right femoral nerve distribution. Electrical stimulation in the affected skin area 5 cm below the patella elicited cerebral potentials whose early positive component was clearly delayed on the left side (latency 42 msec) and even more so on the right side (latency 52 msec) (Fig. 23–5). A cerebral potential recorded under similar conditions of femoral nerve stimulation in a normal adult subject of the same body size had a latency of 31.5 msec and is shown in the same figure. The data suggested a bilateral involvement presumably at spinal root level rather than a lesion restricted to the right femoral nerve. Subsequent progress of the disease necessitated surgical decompression, which confirmed epidural invasion by Hodgkin tissue at the level of the third lumbar vertebra.

Combined Involvement of Peripheral Nerve and Spinal Cord

The evoked potential method evaluates the entire somatosensory pathway, and it is possible to design the tests to distinguish between lesions located either in the peripheral nerve or in the dorsal column pathway or in both. Friedreich's ataxia provides a good example, since it involves both the degeneration of posterior columns in the spinal cord (Mott, 1907; Spiller, 1910; Lambrior, 1911) and a severe loss of the large fibers in dorsal

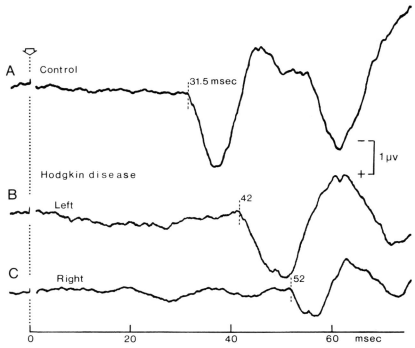

Figure 23–5 Comparison of cerebral potentials evoked by femoral nerve stimulation 5 cm below the patella. *A.* Responses in a normal 28 year old male subject. *B* and *C.* Responses in a 26 year old female patient with epidural invasion by Hodgkin tissue. The cerebral responses are recorded from the midline focus. Electrical stimulation was applied to the left leg in *A* and *B,* and to the right leg in *C.*

roots and sensory nerves (Dyck et al., 1968; Hughes et al., 1968). C fibers are preserved, and sural nerve biopsies studied in vitro indicate that they retain normal conduction (Dyck et al., 1971). Sensory nerve potentials in situ, however, are much reduced in size and generally fail to be recorded (Dyck et al., 1971; McLeod, 1971). Thus cerebral evoked potentials should provide useful data of sensory conduction in spite of the small size of the responses and of the difficulty in keeping the patients completely relaxed during long runs. Figure 23–6 shows data for a male patient 23 years old in whom signs of Friedreich's ataxia had been identified 11 years before the test. Averaging technique was used, but no sensory potential was recorded from the median nerve at the wrist, even with strong stimulation of the fingers. The same stimulus evoked cerebral potentials with a latency of 37.8 msec and fairly normal configuration that two separate runs show to be consistent. Electrical stimulation of the median nerve at the axilla elicited a response with abnormally prolonged latency of 23.2 msec and a larger

negative N_1 component. The latency difference indicates a maximal sensory conduction velocity of 31.5 m per second from fingers to axilla. If it is assumed that the same conduction velocity applies to the nerve segment from axilla to dorsal roots, the afferent volley would arrive at the spinal cord about 8 msec later, 15 msec before the onset of the cortical response seen in Figure 23–6D. According to the sort of calculation for lemniscal conduction discussed by Desmedt and his associates (1973), this would imply that the central pathway from spinal entry to cortex would be traveled by the earliest action potentials at a mean maximum velocity of about 20 m per second, which is much lower than the figures for normal adult subjects. This argues that there is abnormal central conduction, apart from and in addition to the peripheral slowing in maximum sensory conduction velocity, but it does not tell whether the central slowing is confined to the dorsal column or involves other structures in the somatosensory pathway. In any case these records show that direct physiologic study of the sensory pathway is

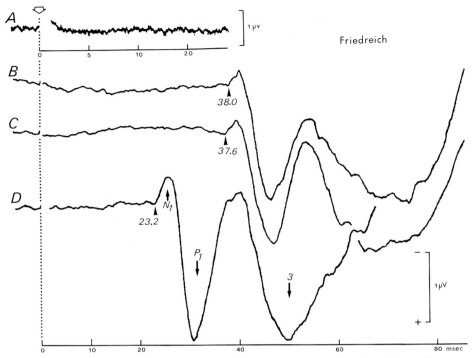

Figure 23–6 Male patient 23 years old with Friedreich's ataxia. *A.* Average record from the median nerve at the wrist shows no identifiable response to electrical stimulation of fingers II and III. *B* and *C.* Average cerebral potentials evoked by the same finger stimuli. Two successive runs are shown to indicate the consistency in latency and wave form. *D.* Average cerebral potential evoked by electrical stimulation of the median nerve at the axilla. The nomenclature of components is indicated as well as the latency of N_1. (From Desmedt, J. E., and Noël, P.: Average cerebral evoked potentials in the evaluation of lesions of the sensory nerves and of the central somatosensory pathway. *In* Desmedt, J. E. (ed.): New Developments in Electromyography and Clinical Neurophysiology. Vol. 2. Basel, S. Karger, 1973, pp. 352–371. Figure 5. Reprinted by permission.)

feasible in Friedreich's ataxia and that the afferent conduction is abnormal both peripherally and centrally.

Involvement of the Central Somatosensory Pathway

Symptoms and signs of multiple sclerosis are generally related to blocked or impaired conduction in central nerve fibers across areas of demyelination (Spiller, 1910; Lambrior, 1911). At least during the initial stages of the lesion, there are axons that are demyelinated but not destroyed and there is a loss of oligodendrocytes (Suzuki et al., 1969; Lumsden, 1970). In animal experiments, McDonald and Sears (1970) reported that a focal demyelinating lesion produced by local injection of diphtheria toxin reduced the conduction velocity in central axons in much the same way as it does in peripheral axons (McDonald, 1973).

Namerow (1968) showed that the cerebral potentials evoked by median nerve stimulation are abnormal and delayed in multiple sclerosis patients with impairment of either position or vibration sense or both. Conrad and Bechinger (1969) found that the maximum sensory and motor conduction velocities are within normal limits in the peripheral nerves of such patients, thus confirming that the disease involves only the central myelin sheaths, which are formed by oligodendroglia. These data have been confirmed and extended in our study of 17 patients with characteristic clinical signs of multiple sclerosis (Desmedt and Noël, 1973). Figure 23–7 shows that, in a female patient 41 years old who had had multiple sclerosis for 14 years, the sensory potentials evoked by finger stimulation and recorded from the median nerve at the level of the axilla and wrist have a normal configuration and a maximum conduction velocity of 63 m per second, within the normal adult

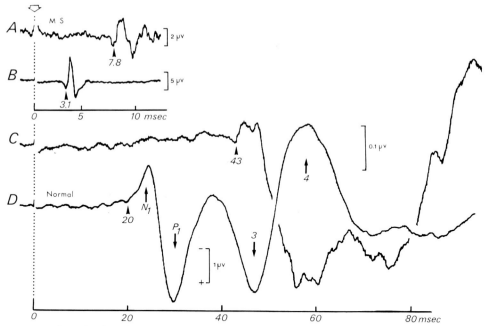

Figure 23–7   Female patient aged 41 years, with multiple sclerosis (MS) since 14 years (*A*, *B*, and *C*) compared with a normal adult subject (*D*). Electrical stimulation of distal fingers II and III on the right side. Sensory potentials recorded from the right median nerve at the axilla (*A*) and wrist (*B*) show maximum sensory conduction velocity in the normal range. *C* and *D*. Average cerebral potentials recorded from the parietal hand projection in the left hemisphere. The nomenclature of components is indicated for the normal response in *D*. The latency of N_1 is considerably increased in *C*. (From Desmedt, J. E., and Noël, P.: Average cerebral evoked potentials in the evaluation of lesions of the sensory nerves and of the central somatosensory pathway. *In* Desmedt, J. E. (ed.): New Developments in Electromyography and Clinical Neurophysiology. Vol. 2. Basel, S. Karger, 1973, pp. 352–371. Reprinted by permission.)

range. The background noise at the axilla is contributed mostly by the muscle activity related to spasticity in this patient. The same finger stimulation evokes a cerebral response with the considerable latency of 43 msec at the contralateral parietal projection, which can be compared to the 20 msec latency of the control response recorded in a normal adult subject. The nomenclature of evoked potential components is indicated on the latter record (see Desmedt et al., 1973). It is interesting that the cerebral response of this patient, although considerably reduced in voltage (see vertical calibrations shown in the figure) has a roughly preserved wave form. The initial negative component N_1 presents a duration of about 5 msec and the subsequent W-shaped positive deflection is similar except that it is, of course, shifted to the right along the time scale by about 25 msec. On this basis one could argue that the cerebral electrogeneses involved proceed with a fairly preserved intrinsic temporal organization and that the anomalous response associated with multiple sclerosis is largely restricted to a slowing and a reduction of the corticipetal volley in the central pathway.

The latency increases of the cerebral response can be compared to the clinically tested disturbance of the position sense of the same fingers. The latencies are generally much more increased when such a sensory defect is present, but it is interesting that significant latency increases can also be recorded when the position sense is normal (Desmedt and Noël, 1973). The evoked potential method thus provides useful evidence of a clinically silent lesion. Related observations have been made for the visual system with the evoked potential method (Halliday et al., 1972).

Vascular Lesions in the Brain Stem

Halliday and Wakefield, in 1963, and Halliday, in 1967, emphasized that the somatosensory cerebral evoked potentials cannot be recorded or are reduced in size in patients with severe loss of touch and position sense, while they are preserved in patients with loss of pain and thermal sensations as well as in those with congenital indifference to pain.

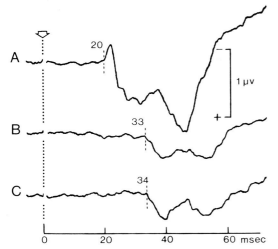

Figure 23-8 Cerebral potentials in a 43 year old male patient with a right thalamic syndrome of ischemic origin. *A*. Response recorded from the right parietal hand focus by stimulation of the fingers II and III on the left (normal) side. *B* and *C*. Responses of increased latency and reduced amplitude evoked by stimulation of the right fingers II and III and recorded from the left parietal hand focus. Two successive runs show the responses to be consistent.

This suggests that the afferent volley is conducted in the dorsal column pathway and in the medial lemniscus (cf. Desmedt, 1971). We recently found that the cerebral evoked potentials can provide useful data on the probable location of the lesions in patients with vascular disease of the brain stem (Noël and Desmedt, in press). Such data are particularly valuable when routine clinical sensory testing cannot be performed. Figure 23-8 illustrates unilateral changes of the cerebral evoked potentials in a male patient, 43 years old, with a vascular lesion in the left diencephalon. The tests were performed five days after the acute onset of a unilateral thalamic syndrome with hypoesthesia and hyperalgesia on the right side. Electrical stimuli of 18 ma delivered to fingers II and III of the left hand evoked a contralateral cerebral response of normal configuration with a latency of 20.0 msec. Identical stimuli of 18 ma on the right fingers were considered slightly painful by the patient and evoked cerebral responses of reduced voltage and with a latency augmented to 33 and 34 msec, respectively, in the two runs illustrated. Two separate runs are shown in order to document the consistency of the findings. It is also noticed that these responses have apparently no early negative component in this case. Such marked increases of the cortical latency are presumably related

to a localized slowing of axonal conduction in the lemniscal pathway at the diencephalic level due to compression by vascular hemorrhage and local edema.

COMMENTS

In this chapter, a number applications of the cerebral evoked potentials to the diagnosis of lesions of the somatosensory pathway have been considered. This method provides consistent data on the maximum sensory conduction velocity and thus assists current studies of the peripheral nerves. In applying the method to the evaluation of peripheral nerve lesions, a careful design of the test is necessary, and further studies will no doubt increase the range of such diagnostic applications. The examples quoted illustrate how the method can be used for identifying extensive or localized lesions in one or more peripheral nerves of the upper and lower limbs (for other examples, see Desmedt, 1971, and Desmedt and Noël, 1973). Studies of the sural nerve as shown in Figure 23-3 are of interest because of the prevalence of sensory neuropathies of the lower limb and because sural nerve biopsies are currently used for histologic and in vitro physiologic studies (Dyck et al., 1971). As a general statement it can be said that the direct recording of sensory nerve potentials is more useful in identifying the milder lesions (which produce desynchronization of the fiber action potentials and marked reductions of the sensory nerve response) while the cerebral evoked potentials are more valuable in assessing the cases with more severe neuropathy in which sensory nerve potentials cannot be recorded (cf. Figs. 23-4 and 23-5).

Cerebral evoked potentials also afford unique possibilities for the evaluation of lesions involving the proximal nerves, the plexus, the spinal roots, and the central pathway. In multiple sclerosis the peripheral nerve conduction is normal, but marked increases in the cerebral latency are recorded in patients with clinical disorders of somatic sensation, as shown in Figure 23-7; this is also true to a lesser extent in cases with subclinical involvement of the somatosensory pathway (Desmedt and Noël, 1973).

Vascular lesions of the brain stem can also be investigated this way in order to obtain data on the involvement of the lemniscal pathway; such data are of practical usefulness in unresponsive patients such as the man whose record is shown in Figure 23–8.

Acknowledgments: The research reported has been supported by grants from the National Institute of Neurological Disease and Stroke, National Institutes of Health, Bethesda, and from the Fonds de la Recherche Scientifique Médicale of Belgium.

REFERENCES

Bonney, G., and Gilliatt, R. W.: Sensory nerve conduction after traction lesion of the brachial plexus. Proc. R. Soc. Med., *51*:365–367, 1958.

Buchthal, F.: Sensory and motor conduction in polyneuropathies. *In* Desmedt, J. E. (ed.): New Developments in Electromyography and Clinical Neuropathology. Vol. 2. Basel, S. Karger, 1973, pp. 259–271.

Buchthal, F., and Rosenfalck, A.: Evoked action potentials and conduction velocity in human sensory nerves. Brain Res., *3*:1–122, 1966.

Conrad, B., and Bechinger, D.: Sensorisch und motorische Nervenleitgeswindigkeit und distale Latenz bei Multipler Sklerose. Arch. Psychiatr. Nervenkr., *212*:140–149, 1969.

Dawson, G. D.: The relative excitability and conduction velocity of sensory and motor nerve fibres in man. J. Physiol. (Lond.), *131*:436–451, 1956.

Debecker, J., and Desmedt, J. E.: Les potentiels évoqués cérébraux et les potentiels de nerf sensible chez l'homme. Utilisation de l'ordinateur numérique Mnémotron 400-B. Acta Neurol. Belg., *64*:1212–1248, 1964.

Desmedt, J. E.: Somatosensory cerebral evoked potentials in man. *In* Rémond, A. (ed.) Handbook of Electroencephalography and Clinical Neurophysiology. Vol. 9. Amsterdam, Elsevier Publishing Co., 1971, pp. 55–82.

Desmedt, J. E.: The neuromuscular disorder in myasthenia gravis. I. Electrical and mechanical responses to nerve stimulation in hand muscles. *In* Desmedt, J. E. (ed.): New Developments in Electromyography and Clinical Neurophysiology. Vol. 1. Basel, S. Karger, 1973, pp. 241–304.

Desmedt, J. E., Brunko, E., Debecker, J., and Carmeliet, J.: The system bandpass required to avoid distortion of early components when averaging somatosensory evoked potentials. Electroencephalogr. Clin. Neurophysiol., *37*:407–410, 1974.

Desmedt, J. E., and Debecker, J.: The somatosensory cerebral evoked potentials of the sleeping human newborn. *In* Clemente, C. D., Purpura, D. P., and Mayer, F. E. (eds.): Sleep and the Maturing Nervous System. New York, Academic Press, 1972, pp. 229–239.

Desmedt, J. E., and Manil, J.: Somatosensory evoked potentials of the normal human neonate in REM sleep, in slow wave sleep and in waking. Electroencephalogr. Clin. Neurophysiol., *29*:113–126, 1970.

Desmedt, J. E., and Noël, P.: Average cerebral evoked potentials in the evaluation of lesions of the sensory nerves and of the central somatosensory pathway. *In* Desmedt, J. E. (ed.): New Developments in Elec-

tromyography and Clinical Neurophysiology. Vol. 2. Basel, S. Karger, 1973, pp. 352–371.

Desmedt, J. E., Noël, P., Debecker, J., and Namèche, J.: Maturation of afferent conduction velocity as studied by sensory nerve potentials and by cerebral evoked potentials. In Desmedt, J. E. (ed.): New Developments in Electromyography and Clinical Neurophysiology. Vol. 2. Basel, S. Karger, 1973, pp. 52–63.

Desmedt, J. E., Franken, L., Borenstein, S., Debecker, J., Lambert, C., and Manil, J.: Le diagnostic des ralentissements de la conduction afférente dans les affections des nerfs périphériques: Intérêt de l'extraction du potentiel évoqué cérébral. Rev. Neurol. (Paris), *115*:255–262, 1966.

Drake, C. G.: Diagnosis and treatment of lesions of the brachial plexus and adjacent structures. Clin. Neurosurg., *11*:110–127, 1964.

Dyck, P. J., Lambert, E. H., and Nichols, P. C.: Quantitative measurement of sensation related to compound action potential and number and size of myelinated fibres of sural nerve. *In* Rémond, A. (ed.): Handbook of Electroencephalography and Clinical Neurophysiology. Vol. 9. Amsterdam, Elsevier Publishing Co., 1971, pp. 83–118.

Dyck, P. J., Gutrecht, J. A., Bastron, J. A., Karnes, W. E., and Dale, A. J. D.: Histologic and teased-fiber measurements of sural nerve in disorders of lower and primary sensory neurons. Mayo Clin. Proc., *43*:81–123, 1968.

Gilliatt, R. W.: Recent advances in the pathophysiology of nerve conduction. *In* Desmedt, J. E. (ed.): New Developments in Electromyography and Clinical Neurophysiology. Vol. 2. Basel, S. Karger, 1973, pp. 2–18.

Gilliatt, R. W., and Sears, T. A.: Sensory nerve action potentials in patients with peripheral nerve lesions. J. Neurol. Neurosurg. Psychiatry, *21*:109–118, 1958.

Gilliatt, R. W., Goodman, H. V., and Willison, R. G.: The recording of lateral popliteal nerve action potentials in man. J. Neurol. Neurosurg. Psychiatry, *24*:305–318, 1961.

Goff, W. R., Rosner, B. S., and Allison, T.: Distribution of cerebral somatosensory evoked responses in normal man. Electroencephalogr. Clin. Neurophysiol., *14*:697–713, 1962.

Halliday, A. M.: Changes in the form of cerebral evoked responses in man associated with various lesions of the nervous system. Electroencephalogr. Clin. Neurophysiol., Suppl. *25*:178–192, 1967.

Halliday, A. M., and Wakefield, G. S.: Cerebral evoked potentials with dissociated sensory loss. J. Neurol. Neurosurg. Psychiatry, *26*:211–219, 1963.

Halliday, A. M., McDonald, W. I., and Mushin, J.: Delayed visual evoked response in optic neuritis. Lancet, *1*:982–985, 1972.

Hughes, J. T., Brownell, B., and Hewer, R. L.: The peripheral sensory pathway in Friedreich's ataxia. Brain, *91*:803–818, 1968.

Kaeser, H. E.: Nerve conduction velocity measurements. *In* Vinken, P. J., and Bruyn, G. W. (eds.): Handbook of Clinical Neurology. Vol. 9. Amsterdam, North-Holland Publishing Co., 1970, pp. 217–309.

Lambrior, R. A.: Un cas de maladie de Friedreich avec autopsie. Rev. Neurol. (Paris), *21*:525–540, 1911.

Lumsden, C. E.: The neuropathology of multiple sclerosis. *In* Vinken, P. J., and Bruyn, G. W. (eds): Handbook of Clinical Neurology. Vol. 9. Amsterdam, North-Holland Publishing Co., 1970, pp. 217–309.

McDonald, W. I.: Experimental neuropathy. The use of diphtheria toxin. *In* Desmedt, J. E. (ed.): New Developments in Electromyography and Clinical Neurophysiology. Vol. 2. Basel, S. Karger, 1973, pp. 128–144.

McDonald, W. I., and Sears, T. A.: The effects of experimental demyelination on conduction in the central nervous system. Brain, *93*:583–598, 1970.

McLeod, J. G.: An electrophysiological and pathological study of peripheral nerves in Friedreich's ataxia. J. Neurol. Sci., *12*:333–349, 1971.

Mott, F. W.: Case of Friedreich's disease, with autopsy and systematic microscopical examination of the nervous system. Arch. Neurol., *3*:180–200, 1907.

Namerow, N. S.: Somatosensory evoked responses in multiple sclerosis patients with varying sensory loss. Neurology (Minneap.), *18*:1197–1204, 1968.

Noël, P.: Evaluation des troubles de la sensibilité dans le membre inférieur. Electromyography, *11*:137–141, 1971.

Noël, P.: Sensory nerve conduction in the upper limbs at various stages of diabetic neuropathy. J. Neurol. Neurosurg. Psychiatry, *36*:786–796, 1973.

Noël, P., and Desmedt, J. E.: Cerebral evoked potentials in brain stem infarction. In press.

Schiozawa, R., and Mavor, H.: In vivo human sural nerve action potentials. J. Appl. Physiol., *26*:623–629, 1969.

Spiller, W. G.: Friedreich's ataxia. J. Nerv. Ment. Dis., *37*:411–435, 1910.

Suzuki, K., Andrews, J. M., Walz, J. M., and Terry, R. D.: Ultrastructural studies of multiple sclerosis. Lab. Invest., *20*:444–454, 1969.

Tsumoto, T., Hirose, N., Nonaka, S., and Takahashi, M.: Analysis of somatosensory evoked potentials to lateral popliteal nerve stimulation in man. Electroencephalogr. Clin. Neurophysiol., *33*:379–388, 1972.

Warren, J., Gutmann, L., Figueroa, A. F., and Bloor, B. M.: Electromyographic changes of brachial plexus root avulsions. J. Neurosurg., *31*:137–140, 1969.

Weiss, P., and Hiscoe, H. B.: Experiments on the mechanism of nerve growth. J. Exp. Zool., *107*:315–396, 1948.

SECTION V

*Diseases of the
Peripheral Nervous System*

PART A

Symptomatology
and Differential Diagnosis
of Peripheral Neuropathy

Chapter 24

CLINICAL FEATURES
AND DIFFERENTIAL DIAGNOSIS

P. K. Thomas

The peripheral nervous system, in anatomical terms, consists of those parts of the nervous system in which neurons or their processes are related to the peripheral satellite cell, the cell of Schwann. It thus comprises the cranial nerves with the exception of the second, the spinal nerve roots, the dorsal root ganglia, the peripheral nerve trunks and their terminal ramifications, and the peripheral autonomic system. The junction with the central nervous system is marked by an abrupt transition where the Schwann cells are replaced by glial elements. This junction, the Obersteiner-Redlich zone (see Chapter 9), is not necessarily at the point of emergence of the cranial nerves or the spinal nerve roots from the neuraxis. For the eighth cranial nerve, in particular, the junction exists well external to the brain stem.

It is obvious from these considerations that the central processes of the dorsal root ganglion cells and the cell bodies of the motor axons lie within the central nervous system. The definition of a peripheral neuropathy must therefore be somewhat arbitrary in topographical terms. "Spinal muscular atrophies," in which the anterior horn cells undergo primary degeneration leading to loss of the motor axons in the peripheral nerves, are not customarily considered as peripheral neurop-

athies. Yet there is increasing evidence that in many disorders that produce degeneration of the peripheral portions of motor axons, the primary disturbance lies within their cell bodies (see Chapter 14), and thus the distinction may well be artificial.

A second reason for lack of certainty in the definition of peripheral neuropathy is operational. It is evident that many patients with diabetes or chronic renal failure, for example, who are neurologically asymptomatic, exhibit abnormalities when examined. Moreover, disturbances of nerve conduction may be demonstrable in the total absence of symptoms or abnormal signs on physical examination, both in diabetes and in uremia (Lawrence and Locke, 1961; Preswick and Jeremy, 1964; Thomas, 1973). These cases have been categorized as subclinical neuropathy. Yet alterations in nerve conduction do not necessarily indicate structural changes in the peripheral nerves. Patients receiving diphenylhydantoin therapy may develop reduced nerve conduction velocity at blood concentrations in excess of 30 mg per liter, rapid restoration to normal velocity taking place with reduction of the blood concentration of the drug (Birket-Smith and Krogh, 1971). This suggests that metabolic factors are responsible for the alterations in nerve conduction. A more dramatic demonstration of this is seen in relation to changes in plasma magnesium concentrations before and after hemodialysis in patients with chronic renal failure (Fleming, Lenman, and Stewart, 1972). The clinical use of the term "neuropathy" is therefore also to some extent an arbitrary decision, depending upon the level of functional disturbance at which it is decided to state that a patient has a peripheral neuropathy. In some situations, it has been held that the occurrence of symptoms is insufficient to merit a clinical label of neuropathy. In terms of clinical utility, Gilliatt (1965) suggested that, in cases of diabetic neuropathy, the term should be reserved for those patients who seek medical advice because of their symptoms. Yet such a decision clearly brings in considerations as to individual tolerance of discomfort or disability. These difficulties have undoubtedly contributed in large measure to the widely varying estimates for the incidence of diabetic neuropathy in different series (see Chapter 47). It is therefore important that in studies of this type, the criteria adopted for a diagnosis of neuropathy are adequately defined.

CLINICAL CATEGORIES OF NEUROPATHY

Polyneuropathy, Mononeuropathy, and Multiple Mononeuropathy

It is useful to distinguish two broad categories of peripheral neuropathy in terms of the pattern of involvement of the peripheral nervous system, as this often provides a guide to the causation. First, there are processes that result in a bilaterally symmetrical disturbance of function and that can be designated polyneuropathies. If it is wished to emphasize an involvement of the spinal roots, or involvement of both the roots and the peripheral nerve trunks, the terms "polyradiculopathy" or "polyradiculoneuropathy" are sometimes employed. A polyneuropathy tends to be associated with agents that act diffusely on the peripheral nervous system such as toxic substances, deficiency states, and certain examples of immune reaction.

The second category comprises isolated lesions of peripheral nerves (mononeuropathy) or multiple isolated lesions (multiple

mononeuropathy or "mononeuritis multiplex"). A qualifying statement must be made that with a widespread multiple mononeuropathy, the individual peripheral nerve lesions may summate to produce symmetrical involvement. Even in such cases, however, careful examination may reveal differential changes corresponding to the territory of individual nerves, or this may be indicated from the history of the onset of the symptoms. In some examples of multiple mononeuropathies that have a proximal distribution but do not follow a clear peripheral nerve pattern, it is likely that the lesions may also involve the limb girdle plexuses, as in the syndrome of "diabetic amyotrophy" (Garland, 1955), or "neuralgic amyotrophy" (see Chapter 32). Isolated or multiple isolated peripheral nerve lesions result from processes that produce localized damage, and include nerve entrapment, mechanical injuries (pressure, traction, direct blows, and penetrating wounds), thermal or electrical or radiation injury, vascular lesions, granulomatous or neoplastic or other infiltrative processes, and peripheral nerve tumors.

A number of diffuse polyneuropathies may be complicated by superimposed isolated nerve lesions as a consequence of an abnormal susceptibility to pressure palsies. This has been most clearly established for diabetic neuropathy (Gilliatt and Willison, 1962; Shahani and Spalding, 1969). In this condition, abnormalities of nerve conduction, in the absence of signs of nerve damage, tend to occur at the common sites of entrapment or pressure lesions (Mulder et al., 1961). An abnormal susceptibility to pressure has been demonstrated in experimental diphtheritic neuropathy (Hopkins and Morgan-Hughes, 1969). The reason for this increased vulnerability is not understood. The interesting hereditary neuropathy with liability to pressure palsies described by Earl and co-workers (1964) and others has been related to a defect of myelination in which localized areas display an increased number of myelin lamellae associated with axonal narrowing (Behse et al., 1972).

Distribution of Involvement

In severe symmetrical polyneuropathies, a generalized loss of peripheral nerve function may occur, and although this can be true of milder cases, the emphasis is then usually maximal distally in the limbs. A mixed motor and sensory polyneuropathy with a distal distribution results in weakness and wasting that is maximal peripherally in the arms and legs, loss of tendon reflexes affecting the ankle jerks before the knee jerks and those in the lower limbs before the upper, and distal sensory changes of "glove and stocking" distribution. It is probable that a variety of factors are involved in determining this selective distal distribution. In those neuropathies that involve "dying back" of the axons from the periphery (see Chapter 15), it is possible that the neurons that have the longest axons to maintain may be the first to suffer. In neuropathies in which there is selective damage to Schwann cells leading to demyelination, if this affects Schwann cells in a random manner, the fibers of greatest length have the greatest chance of being affected. Furthermore, there may be differences between the activity of proximal and distal Schwann cells. Majno and Karnovsky (1958) have demonstrated that the lipogenic activity of Schwann cells decreases progressively toward the periphery.

In symmetrical polyneuropathies, a proximal distribution of motor involvement may occasionally be observed. This is encountered in some examples of the Guillain-Barré syndrome and the polyneuritis related to infectious mononucleosis, occasionally in acute intermittent porphyria (see Chapter 46), and in rare cases of chronic progressive demyelinating neuropathy (Thomas and Lascelles, 1967). A proximal distribution of sensory loss is less frequent, but may be observed in acute intermittent porphyria (see Chapter 46) and in Tangier disease (Kocen et al., 1967, 1973). The explanation for selective proximal involvement is unknown. It has been stated that this can be related to an underlying polyradiculopathy, but a moment's reflection indicates that this explanation is unsatisfactory. A possible answer in some instances could lie in the fact that the proximal portions of the limbs are supplied by nerve fibers of larger diameter than those innervating the more distal regions and the trunk (Rexed, 1944); such fibers may have a differing susceptibility to metabolic change or immunologic insults. This explanation cannot be true for Tangier disease, in which the smaller myelinated fibers are affected to a greater degree than the larger (Kocen et al., 1973).

The first manifestations in symmetrical polyneuropathies are usually in the legs, but in occasional instances, the initial symptoms develop in upper limbs. Thus lead neuropathy may begin with a bilateral wrist drop before weakness in the lower limbs appears. The symptoms of the sensory polyneuropathy resulting from vitamin B_{12} deficiency may begin in the hands. In certain kinships with dominantly inherited amyloid neuropathy, the sensory loss characteristically begins in the hands as a result of compression of the median nerve in the carpal tunnels by amyloid deposits in the transverse carpal ligaments (Mahloudji et al., 1969).

Patchy involvement of the cranial nerves is seen most typically in sarcoidosis, but it may also be a feature in diabetes and in malignant infiltration of the nerves in cases of neoplastic invasion of the meninges or skull base. In these instances, the pattern is one of multiple mononeuropathy. Cranial nerve involvement may take place as part of a symmetrical polyneuropathy. Thus in the Guillain-Barré syndrome, bilateral facial palsy is a frequent accompaniment, and less commonly, a more widespread disturbance of cranial nerve function occurs, particularly affecting the bulbar musculature. In rare instances of what appears to be the Guillain-Barré syndrome, a symmetrical disturbance of cranial nerves may take place in the absence of involvement in the limbs ("polyneuritis cranialis"). In progressive polyneuropathies, the cranial nerves tend to be involved late in the evolution of the disease, symptoms distally in the legs and arms having preceded. Rarely, the reverse pattern is observed, with cranial nerve involvement being followed by proximal and later distal weakness in the limbs (Thomas and Lascelles, 1967).

In lepromatous leprosy, the pattern of neurologic deficit can be related to tissue temperature gradients (see Chapter 58). The proliferation of bacilli is greater in cooler tissues. In lead neuropathy, it has been suggested that the distribution and severity of muscle paralysis are directly related to the extent to which the affected muscles have been exercised.

Functional Selectivity

Most neuropathies give rise to a mixed sensorimotor disturbance, sometimes with associated autonomic features. Certain conditions produce a predominantly motor or predominantly sensory disturbance, and in others autonomic symptoms are obtrusive.

Predominantly motor involvement is observed in particular in the Guillain-Barré syndrome and in neuropathies associated with porphyria, lead intoxication, and diphtheria. It is also the usual pattern in peroneal muscular atrophy, both in the hypertrophic and neuronal forms (Dyck and Lambert, 1968a, 1968b), and in chronic relapsing and chronic progressive demyelinating polyneuritis of Guillain-Barré type (Thomas et al., 1969). It should be added that sensory changes are more easily overlooked than motor involvement, and their assessment is less easy. Predominantly sensory involvement may be a feature of neuropathy related to leprosy, diabetes mellitus, and amyloidosis; and virtually pure sensory changes typify the neuropathy of vitamin B_{12} deficiency and hereditary sensory neuropathy in both its dominantly and recessively inherited forms. A selective sensory neuropathy and sometimes a mainly motor neuropathy may occur as a nonmetastatic complication of carcinoma, although a mixed sensorimotor neuropathy is substantially more common (Croft and Wilkinson, 1965). Uremic neuropathy tends to be either purely sensory or sensorimotor in type, but pure motor forms may be observed (Thomas, 1973). Certain of the selective sensory neuropathies have been considered, on neuropathologic grounds, to represent degenerations of the dorsal root ganglion cells. This has been suggested in dominantly inherited sensory neuropathy, in diabetic sensory neuropathy, and in carcinomatous sensory neuropathy (Denny-Brown, 1948, 1951; Bosanquet and Henson, 1957), and it is known to underly the sensory loss in Friedreich's ataxia (Chapter 40). The question of selective loss of specific forms of sensation is considered later in this chapter.

Autonomic changes tend to be an early and troublesome feature in amyloid neuropathy (French et al., 1965), are often prominent in diabetic polyneuropathy (Keen, 1962), and may also occur in a variety of other neuropathies. They are the salient feature in the Riley-Day syndrome (familial dysautonomia), in which they may be associated with congenital insensitivity to pain (Dancis and Smith, 1966; Aguayo, Nair, and Bray, 1971).

Clinical Course

An abrupt onset, often with pain, is encountered in certain mononeuropathies and multiple mononeuropathies of ischemic origin, as in polyarteritis nodosa and rheumatoid arthritis, or in isolated neuropathies of presumed ischemic origin in diabetes mellitus, such as cranial nerve palsies or femoral neuropathy (Raff et al., 1968; Asbury et al., 1970). It is also observed in nerve compression resulting from hemorrhage into or around nerve trunks or from swelling within a restricted anatomical compartment, as in the anterior tibial syndrome. An abrupt onset of course characterizes nerve lesions resulting from direct external compression or penetrating wounds, thermal injury, and damage related to inadvertent injections into nerve trunks. It may also be encountered if a ganglion suddenly herniates against a nerve, e.g., the common peroneal nerve at the knee (Stack et al., 1965).

Neuropathy of somewhat less acute onset, but evolving over a matter of days, may be observed in some intoxications, such as that following the administration of thallium or tri-ortho-cresyl phosphate (TOCP); in conditions presumed to be related to disordered immune mechanisms, as in the Guillain-Barré syndrome; and in diphtheritic neuropathy. Certain neuropathies of metabolic origin may display a rapid onset, as in acute intermittent porphyria, and at times a relatively rapid onset is encountered in neuropathy related to diabetes, particularly when precipitated by treatment, and in uremia, when it can be precipitated by hemodialysis (Tenckhoff et al., 1965; Thomas et al., 1971). In some of these disorders there is a characteristic delay between the initiating process and the development of the neuropathy, which is particularly evident in the Guillain-Barré syndrome, in neuralgic amyotrophy, in diphtheritic neuropathy, and following tri-ortho-cresyl phosphate administration. In the Guillain-Barré syndrome, the delay between an antecedent viral infection or other initiating event is probably explicable in immunologic terms: a cell-mediated delayed hypersensitivity reaction is the likely basis of the disorder. The explanation for the delay in diphtheritic and tri-ortho-cresyl phosphate neuropathy has not yet been established.

A subacutely evolving course over weeks or months is seen in many neuropathies related to a maintained exposure to toxic agents, to a persisting nutritional deficiency, or to an abnormal metabolic state. Neuropathy occurring as a remote effect of malignant disease most often pursues this time course, as do occasional cases otherwise resembling the acute Guillain-Barré syndrome (Thomas et al., 1969).

A chronic course with an insidious onset and a slow progress occupying a time course of years typifies many genetic neuropathies, including peroneal muscular atrophy, hereditary hypertrophic neuropathy, dominantly inherited sensory neuropathy, and Refsum's syndrome. There is also a large group of chronic progressive neuropathies of uncertain etiology (Prineas, 1970). Certain inherited disorders with abnormalities present from birth, such as recessively inherited sensory neuropathy and the Riley-Day syndrome, may be substantially nonprogressive (Aguayo, Nair and Bray, 1971; Murray, 1973). It is possible that some of these represent a neuronal aplasia.

Of particular interest are those neuropathies with a recurrent or relapsing course. The Guillain-Barré syndrome may be recurrent, and other cases with similar clinical and pathologic features pursue a relapsing course over many years (Thomas et al., 1969). Refsum's disease (see Chapter 42) and occasional cases of dominantly inherited hypertrophic neuropathy may display a relapsing course (Thomas and Lascelles, 1967). The possible aggravation of Refsum's disease by dietary influences could provide a basis for the fluctuations in this disorder (Eldjarn et al., 1966).

The clinical course taken by a neuropathy is a reflection of the underlying pathologic changes. Acute generalized polyneuropathies with a rapid and full recovery, such as the Guillain-Barré syndrome or diphtheritic polyneuropathy, or cases of relapsing polyneuropathy of the type just discussed, are the manifestation of a widespread temporary conduction block related to demyelination. Recovery is associated with remyelination. A rapid and complete restoration of function in localized neuropathies is characteristically seen in the "Saturday night" paralysis of the radial nerve and in most cases of Bell's palsy; it is presumably related to a localized demyelination with conduction block, and subsequent remyelination and restoration of conduction. In contradistinction to such disorders, in neuropathies involving axonal destruction, provided that the causal process is reversible, recovery is associated with axonal regeneration or collateral sprouting from surviving axons. Restoration of function is therefore slow and often incomplete.

SYMPTOMS AND SIGNS OF NEUROPATHY

Motor Involvement

Paralysis of voluntary movement may result either from a conduction block in motor nerve fibers or from loss or interruption of the motor axons. Apart from temporary conduction blocks related to such events as the action of local anesthetics, cooling, or anoxia, a persisting conduction block is due to selective demyelination with preservation of axonal continuity. This has been demonstrated for demyelinating neuropathies by McDonald (1963) and Cragg and Thomas (1964), and in experimental tourniquet paralysis by Denny-Brown and Brenner (1944) and Mayer and Denny-Brown (1964) and by Ochoa, Fowler, and Gilliatt (1972).

Characteristic examples of a localized conduction block are "Saturday night" paralysis of the radial nerve, "crossed legs" paralysis of the peroneal nerve, and a large proportion of cases of Bell's palsy. Axonal continuity and preservation of conduction distal to the lesion is indicated by muscular contraction on stimulation of the nerve distal to the lesion. Some disuse wasting of the affected muscles may ensue, but denervation atrophy does not take place since the "trophic action" of the motor axons on the muscle fibers is maintained. Recovery, which accompanies remyelination, occurs over a matter of weeks and takes place more or less simultaneously throughout the distribution of the nerve.

Examples of neuropathies in which the paralysis is largely attributable to demyelination are diphtheritic neuropathy and the less severe examples of the Guillain-Barré syndrome. As is true for localized demyelinating lesions, muscle bulk is maintained, electromyographic signs of denervation do not appear unless there is coexistent axonal interruption, and recovery is characteristically rapid and complete.

Interruption of motor axons, either from a localized nerve lesion or as part of a widespread neuropathy, in addition to causing motor paralysis, leads to denervation atrophy of the muscle. Clinically evident atrophy appears within a few weeks and is then progressive. Loss of muscle fibers in denervated human muscle fibers begins after six to nine months, and few remain after about three years (Bowden and Gutmann, 1944). Complete restoration of function is usually possible, however, if reinnervation is established within 12 months (Sunderland, 1950). Thereafter it becomes increasingly less satisfactory.

Fasciculation, Muscle Cramps, and Generalized Muscular Stiffness

Fasciculation is not uncommonly observed in peripheral neuropathies and occasionally may be extensive enough to lead to cases of motor neuropathy being diagnosed as motor neuron disease of progressive muscular atrophy type. Muscle cramps are again a more obtrusive symptom in spinal muscular atrophy, but may feature in cases of peripheral neuropathy. They are particularly common in uremic neuropathy, in which their relationship to dialysis suggests that they may at times be provoked by alterations in fluid and electrolyte balance (Thomas, 1973).

Occasional cases have been recorded with generalized muscular stiffness and fasciculation that have been shown to be associated with continuous motor unit activity in the electromyogram (Isaacs, 1961, 1967). The activity has been considered to arise in the peripheral motor axons and nerve terminals. In one case, motor nerve conduction velocity was slightly reduced and degenerative changes in myelinated nerve fibers were found in a sural nerve biopsy (Wallis et al., 1970). These findings were taken as supportive evidence for a peripheral nerve disorder.

Tendon Areflexia

Loss of tendon reflexes is common in peripheral neuropathy, but may not develop until the late stage of some neuropathies, as is often true in that due to amyloidosis. This has sometimes led to the diagnosis of such cases as hysterical when the distal sensory loss in the limbs was unaccompanied by other demonstrable evidence of peripheral nerve disorder (Andrade, 1952).

Loss of the afferent fibers from the muscle spindles may be responsible for areflexia and is likely to be the explanation in Friedreich's ataxia. In motor neuropathies in which the smaller fibers are affected, denervation of the intrafusal muscle fibers could provide an explanation. A further mechanism, which may well be operative in neuropathies in which

nerve conduction velocity is reduced, is temporal dispersion of conduction (Gilliatt and Willison, 1962). The tendon reflexes are likely to depend upon the ability of the peripheral nerves to transmit a synchronous volley of impulses, and this is not possible when there is unequal slowing of conduction in the component fibers of the nerve.

Sensory Loss

Loss of sensation in peripheral neuropathy may involve all sensory modalities, or the impairment may be restricted to particular forms of sensation. The latter situation provides the interesting possibility of making correlations between the sensory loss and the pattern of fiber size depletion. Two patterns of preferential sensory loss have been recognized (Dyck et al., 1972). In one, a selective loss of pain and temperature sensibility develops, and in the other, of touch-pressure, two-point discrimination, and joint position sense. A third pattern of loss is the simultaneous involvement of all modalities.

Cases of dissociated pain and temperature loss in the legs, often on a familial basis, have been recognized since the latter part of the last century (see Spillane and Wells, 1969). They were initially attributed to "lumbosacral syringomyelia" and other unconfirmed pathologic conditions, but this interpretation was called into question by Thévenard (1942). It is now clear that such cases are likely to have been examples of hereditary sensory neuropathy (Denny-Brown, 1951). Denny-Brown in 1937 performed an autopsy on a member of a family originally reported by Hicks (1922) and demonstrated dorsal root ganglion cell degeneration. This was considered to be the primary pathologic lesion, and amyloid deposits that were also noted in the dorsal root ganglia were believed to be a secondary phenomenon. Dyck, Lambert, and Nichols (1972) showed in a case of hereditary sensory neuropathy in which all modalities of sensation were affected that there was a diffuse loss of myelinated axons, but particularly those of smaller diameter, and there was also a substantial loss of unmyelinated axons. More recently Sluga (1975), in an early case in which the sensory loss was limited to pain and temperature appreciation, found that the myelinated fiber depletion was limited to those of smaller caliber.

The further recognition of a neuropathy that produces dissociated pain and temperature sensory loss beginning in the legs was provided when Andrade (1952) recognized the existence of hereditary amyloid neuropathy. The pattern of fiber loss in this disorder has also been shown to involve a selective reduction in the population of small myelinated and unmyelinated axons (Dyck and Lambert, 1969; Thomas, 1973). Another similar instance has recently been established by Kocen and co-workers (1973). Two cases of Tangier disease were described, in both of which selective pain and temperature loss was a feature of the earlier stages of the neuropathy. A predominant loss of the smaller myelinated fibers and a gross loss of unmyelinated axons was demonstrated. Both cases had initially been diagnosed as syringomyelia.

In Friedreich's ataxia, which involves a degeneration of the primary afferent neuron (see Chapter 40), joint position sense and vibration sense are lost and touch-pressure sensibility is impaired, whereas pain and temperature sensation is preserved. Dyck, Lambert, and Nichols (1972) found that this could be related to a selective disappearance of the larger myelinated fibers.

It is possible that loss of vibration sense may occur because of temporal dispersion of conduction rather than from loss of the afferent fibers concerned. As seems likely for the tendon reflexes, the perception of vibration would be expected to depend upon the ability of the peripheral nerves to conduct a synchronous volley of impulses, which may not be possible in demyelinating neuropathies (Gilliatt and Willison, 1962).

Paresthesias, Hyperesthesia, and Hyperpathia

Paresthesias, most often of a tingling or thermal nature, are a frequent accompaniment of a sensory or a mixed sensorimotor neuropathy. They may be felt in the territory of an individual peripheral nerve; in a symmetrical polyneuropathy, they usually exhibit a distal "glove and stocking" distribution in the limbs. The mechanism of their origin is largely obscure. The factors involved in the attacks of nocturnal paresthesias that occur in the carpal tunnel syndrome are considered later.

A sensory symptom of some interest is the phenomenon of "restless legs" (Ekbom, 1970). Affected individuals experience an uncomfortable sensation in the feet and lower legs when they are at rest, particularly at night. Patients usually experience difficulty in describing the nature of the sensation, but it is generally characterized by a creeping or dull tingling quality, felt deep within the limb, which induces an irresistible desire to move the limb. Movement produces temporary relief. Although there are clearly multiple causes for this symptom, in which the particular personality of the individual may play a part, "restless legs" may be a feature of certain neuropathies. They have been recognized most consistently in uremic neuropathy (Callaghan, 1966; Thomas, 1973). It is also noteworthy that they may be a prominent symptom in hypercapnic states (Spillane, 1970).

The terms "hyperesthesia" and "hyperpathia" have been employed in a variety of ways, but both, in general, refer to an unpleasant quality that is added to cutaneous sensation. In peripheral neuropathies, this is constantly associated with a raised sensory threshold, and it has therefore been suggested that the term "hyperpathia" is preferable to "hyperesthesia" (Walters, 1969). Tactile stimuli that are normally neutral or even pleasant in affective tone may be uncomfortable or sometimes excruciatingly unpleasant. Such sensations are more often evoked by light moving stimuli than by firm sustained pressure. With a painful stimulus such as a pinprick, the threshold will be found to be elevated, but repeated application of the stimulus at the same site leads to a steadily increasing unpleasant stinging or burning pain that radiates diffusely from the site of stimulation. These phenomena are encountered, for example, following partial peripheral nerve injuries or during recovery from nerve injuries, in the hyperesthetic soles of the feet in alcoholic neuropathy, and in the affected areas of skin in postherpetic neuralgia. Attempts have been made to relate cutaneous hyperesthesia to a selective loss of large nerve fibers with a preservation of small diameter fibers, both myelinated and unmyelinated (Wortis et al., 1942; Weddell et al., 1948; Noordenbos, 1959; Lourie and King, 1966; Ochoa, 1970). A simple relationship of this type is unlikely. In some of these reports, the small fibers may have been derived by regeneration from fibers of larger diameter, although this possibility was excluded in the study by Ochoa (1970). It is noteworthy that the selective larger fiber loss in Friedreich's ataxia, to which reference has already been made, is unassociated with hyperesthesia (Dyck et al., 1972).

Pain and Causalgia

Pain may constitute a troublesome symptom in a variety of neuropathies. Certain localized peripheral nerve lesions may be accompanied by pain. Although this can be within the territory of distribution of the nerve, as instanced by the burning pain of meralgia paresthetica, in some situations it may arise locally in the nerve (see Chapter 9). The local pain and tenderness in the nerve in ulnar neuropathy at the elbow is probably of this nature, arising in endings in the neural connective tissues. At other times, localized nerve lesions result in widely radiating pain. The pain accompanying the nocturnal attacks of acroparesthesia in the carpal tunnel syndrome may spread up the arm as far as the shoulder or even to the root of the neck. Historically, this fact was partly responsible for the insistence by some authorities that this condition was due to "costoclavicular compression" or other anatomical derangements affecting the brachial plexus (Walshe, 1945).

Some generalized neuropathies are uniformly painless; others are attended by pain of various types. This may be felt as a generalized deep-seated aching sensation, typified by the nocturnal pains in the lower legs in diabetic sensory neuropathy or in ischemic neuropathy, or by the aching in the thighs, again particularly at night, in diabetic amyotrophy. Lancinating pains similar to tabetic lightning pains also occur. These may be experienced in diabetic sensory neuropathy and sometimes in dominantly inherited sensory neuropathy. Myeloma neuropathy is frequently painful (Davis and Drachman, 1972). Of particular interest is the pain that forms such an important aspect of Fabry's disease. Affected hemizygous males experience attacks of intense pain in the extremities, this often being aggravated by emotional factors.

The events that lead to the occurrence of pain in certain neuropathies are as yet unknown. Melzack and Wall (1966) advanced the view that pain may result from an imbalance between the large and small fiber input to the dorsal horn of the spinal cord. It was postulated that the substantia gelatinosa functions as a gate control system that modulates the afferent input before it influences transmission cells that project centrally. Both large and small fibers were believed to activate the transmission cells, but the large fibers were thought also to have an inhibitory effect on the transmission cells through a negative feedback system involving the substantia gelatinosa. From this it would be predicted that stimulation of the larger fibers in the peripheral nerves might relieve painful neuropathies, and there is some evidence that electrical stimulation of nerve trunks may have this effect (Wall and Sweet, 1967; Meyer and Fields, 1972). It might also be predicted that the selective loss of larger fibers would result in pain. Yet the differential loss of large afferents in Friedreich's ataxia and uremic neuropathy is not associated with pain (Thomas et al., 1971; Dyck et al., 1972), and pain may be a feature in neuropathies in which there is selective loss of small myelinated fibers as in Fabry's disease (Kocen and Thomas, 1970).

The definition of causalgia has given rise to difficulty. As advocated by Seddon (1972), this term is best restricted to pain resulting from injury to a nerve trunk that is severe and persistent, that usually but not always possesses a burning quality, and that frequently radiates beyond the territory of the injured nerve. The pain is characteristically aggravated by emotional stimuli. It is encountered most often following proximal lesions of the median nerve, the tibial division of the sciatic nerve, or the lowest trunk of the brachial plexus, and usually occurs after partial lesions. The onset may be within 24 hours of the injury or be delayed for periods of up to 45 days. Sympathectomy has been found to give relief in up to 70 to 80 per cent of cases (Seddon, 1972). Its pathogenesis is obscure. Doupe, Cullen, and Chance (1944) suggested that it was the result of ephaptic transmission between efferent autonomic fibers and afferent sensory fibers mediating pain, which would account for its relief by sympathectomy. Although interaction between nerve fibers has been demonstrated experimentally following acute nerve injury by Granit, Leksell, and Skoglund (1944), this has not been shown as a persistent phenomenon.

Ataxia

Sensory ataxia in the limbs may result from proprioceptive deafferentation and is typified by cases of "diabetic pseudotabes." When the deafferentation affects the upper limbs, this may be reflected in the occurrence of pseudo-athetoid movements of the fingers when the hands are held outstretched with the eyes closed. Ataxia in the limbs and tremor of the outstretched hands is sometimes observed in neuropathies in the absence of detectable loss of postural or movement sensibility. This may be a feature in recovering cases of the Guillain-Barré syndrome, in patients with hereditary hypertrophic neuropathy and in cases of chronic relapsing demyelinating neuropathy (Thomas et al., 1969). The regularity of the action tremor in these cases often mimics that of cerebellar disease. Its explanation is uncertain. There is no evidence to implicate a central lesion. It is possible that it results from a loss of muscle spindle afferent impulses, but with the preservation of those that reach consciousness. It is perhaps significant that these cases all have in common a greatly reduced nerve conduction velocity. The possibility that there is an increased conduction time in the peripheral servoloops must be entertained, but this cannot be the sole explanation since tremor is not found consistently in this situation.

Autonomic Involvement

The symptoms arising from disturbances of the parasympathetic components of the cranial nerves (III, VII, IX, X, XI) are discussed in the relevant chapters. This section is therefore limited to the effects of disturbances of the sympathetic system and of the sacral parasympathetic outflow that may occur in peripheral nerve disorders.

Horner's syndrome may develop from localized lesions affecting the first thoracic nerve root or of the cervical sympathetic chain, but the ocular sympathetic innervation is not often involved in generalized neuropathies. The commonest type of pupillary disturbance in diabetic autonomic neuropathy is a sluggish response to illumination (Friedman et al., 1967). Occasionally, the pupillary responses are of Argyll Robertson type.

Orthostatic hypotension may be the pre-senting symptom of an autonomic neuropathy in amyloidosis (Kyle et al., 1966). Estimates as to its frequency in diabetic subjects have varied considerably and its explanation has given rise to dispute (see Aagenaes, 1962). Sharpey-Schafer and Taylor (1960) considered that it was likely to be due to damage to baroreceptor pathways, whereas Aagenaes (1962) concluded that it was probably the result of a defect in the vasomotor innervation of blood vessels. Defects of vasomotor function have also been demonstrated in porphyria, in alcoholic neuropathy and the Guillain-Barré syndrome, and in neuropathy related to carcinoma and myelomatosis (Appenzeller and Marshall, 1963; Barraclough and Sharpey-Schafer, 1963).

Anhidrosis related to deficient sudomotor innervation may occur in the cutaneous territory of a peripheral nerve in mononeuropathies. In polyneuropathies that affect the autonomic system, it displays a symmetrical distribution and initially affects the lower legs. It is encountered particularly in diabetic subjects (Martin, 1953; Berge et al., 1956; Goodman, 1966) and when extensive may lead to heat intolerance and excessive sweating over the upper parts of the body (Rundles, 1945; Goodman, 1966). The anhidrosis is the result of a postganglionic lesion of the sympathetic sudomotor nerve fibers and is often accompanied by defective piloerection (Bárány and Cooper, 1956).

Disturbances of genitourinary function are also most often encountered in diabetic and amyloid neuropathy. With respect to vesical function, a dilated atonic bladder develops. Initially the patients may notice that the intervals between voiding increase, that voiding is difficult and the stream intermittent, and that postmicturition dribbling occurs. Later, retention with overflow incontinence follows, usually first noticed at night. Cystometry demonstrates a large atonic bladder with a flat pressure curve on filling until the bladder capacity is achieved. There is a lack of awareness of bladder filling, and these changes primarily result from sensory denervation of the bladder wall. When impotence develops, failure of erection from interference with the parasympathetic innervation usually precedes failure of ejaculation. An interesting symptom sometimes encountered in diabetic subjects is retrograde ejaculation (Greene et al., 1963; Ellenberg and Weber, 1966).

Despite normal erection and orgasm, seminal emission does not occur, and semen is subsequently found in the urine. This is assumed to be due to a failure of the normal closure of the internal sphincter of the bladder neck during ejaculation, although both this sphincter and the seminal vesicles are innervated by sympathetic fibers.

Symptoms related to disturbances of the innervation of the upper alimentary tract are considered in Chapter 29. Disturbances of large bowel function have been described in cases of autonomic neuropathy, e.g., the occurrence of colonic dilatation in diabetic neuropathy (Paley et al., 1961; Berenyi and Schwarz, 1967). Although this was attributed to autonomic denervation, this has not been verified histologically. Hirschsprung's disease (congenital megacolon) is known to be related to abnormalities of the myenteric plexus. The contracted segment contains a network of abnormal unmyelinated nerve fibers, but is devoid of ganglion cells, and those of the dilated segment are morphologically abnormal (Smith, 1972). Megacolon is also a feature in infection with *Trypanosoma cruzi* (Chagas's disease) and results from destruction of the ganglion cells in the colonic myenteric plexus (Smith, 1972).

Deformity

Chronic neuropathies developing before the cessation of the growth period frequently give rise to foot, hand, and spinal deformity, sometimes of grotesque proportions. Austin (1956) stated that foot deformity had been recorded in 30 per cent of all cases of hypertrophic neuropathy that had been reported up to that date and spinal deformity in 20 per cent. A "claw hand" and clawing of the toes may develop in a chronic neuropathy that commences at any age, but the presence of pes cavus or of spinal deformity indicates an onset in childhood, a point that is sometimes of diagnostic importance.

In the feet, a cavus deformity with clawing of the toes is the most frequent abnormality and in more severe instances is associated with a fixed equinovarus position. More rarely, pes planus results. Kyphoscoliosis is the usual spinal deformity. The causation of foot deformity in neuropathy can in most cases be reasonably attributed to muscle weakness. In peroneal muscular atrophy and hereditary hypertrophic neuropathy, the muscle weakness in the legs is commonly greatest in the anterolateral group in the lower leg and in the intrinsic foot muscles. The equinovarus position of the foot, the cavus deformity, and the clawing of the toes can thus be attributed to the preservation of the activity of the long flexors of toes, the plantar flexors of the foot, and the ankle invertors. Tyrer and Sutherland (1961) suggested that in cases of spinocerebellar degeneration the foot deformity might be the result of cerebellar disease. Spillane and Wells (1969) extended this concept by suggesting that the foot deformity in hereditary neuropathy might ensue upon "postural hypotonia" related to deafferentation of muscles and joints. Yet foot deformity is not an obtrusive feature in hereditary sensory neuropathy in the absence of muscle weakness.

"Trophic" Changes

The term "trophic change" is in many ways unsatisfactory, but it has been hallowed by long usage. It refers to alterations that follow denervation, but it is evident that the causes are often complex and multiple. The concept of specific trophic nerve fibers involved in the maintenance of the structural integrity of tissues and organs can no longer be upheld. Yet it is becoming increasingly evident that in certain instances, the normal innervation has a crucial part to play in tissue differentiation and in the subsequent maintenance of normal structure and activity. The nerve fibers innervating skeletal muscle have been shown to be involved in determining many of the structural and functional properties of muscle fibers (Buller et al., 1960). Moreover, loss of muscle innervation leads to denervation atrophy of the fibers, although the effects of trauma may be important in causing the degeneration and ultimate disappearance of denervated muscle fibers (Adams et al., 1962). Taste buds are known to undergo atrophic changes following loss of their sensory innervation (see Zelená, 1964). Lewis and Pickering (1936) held that the alterations in the skin, nails, and subcutaneous tissues that follow denervation, instead of being the result of the loss of a specific "trophic" function by nerve fibers, were due to the effects of disuse, alterations in blood supply, and sensory loss; no convincing evidence has since been adduced to alter the view.

The effects of denervation following peripheral nerve injury have been documented and critically appraised by Sunderland (1968). Apart from their occurrence in diabetic neuropathy, trophic changes consequent upon peripheral neuropathy are most often encountered in leprosy, hereditary sensory neuropathy (Denny-Brown, 1951), peroneal muscular atrophy with prominent sensory loss (England and Denny-Brown, 1952; Thomas et al., 1974), and hereditary amyloid neuropathy (Andrade, 1952). The changes are usually most evident at the periphery, which led Spillane and Wells (1969) to employ the term "acrodystrophic neuropathy" to describe cases of sensory and sensorimotor neuropathy of mixed etiology in which there was distal trophic ulceration; bony changes also tend to begin distally. The radiographic appearances include generalized or focal loss of density of bone, thinning of the phalanges, pathologic fractures, and the development of neuropathic arthropathy. Osteomyelitic changes may be superimposed.

It is generally accepted that the salient factor responsible for the appearance of trophic ulcers and neuropathic joint degeneration is loss of pain sensation, which exposes the tissues to the risk of repeated injury. It has been suggested by Spillane and Wells (1969) that loss of other joint and muscle afferent impulses may be important, but this is as yet unsubstantiated. In diabetic neuropathy, ischemia and the liability of diabetic tissues to infection may also be significant.

Nerve Thickening

Palpable or visible enlargement of nerve trunks is encountered in a variety of peripheral neuropathies and its detection may be helpful in diagnosis. Yet assessment of nerve thickening is often difficult. Nerves of normal size may be readily visible in thin subjects, particularly when the overlying skin is stretched, and they may then mistakenly be considered enlarged. This is particularly likely to happen in the case of the great auricular nerve in the neck and the superficial peroneal nerve in front of the ankle or on the dorsum of the foot.

In leprous neuropathy, in the lepromatous, tuberculoid, and borderline forms, enlargement of nerves is often a conspicuous feature. In lepromatous leprosy, in which

peripheral nerve symptoms occur late in relation to the appearance of cutaneous lesions, there tends to be a firm smooth enlargement limited to the most superficial nerve trunks. This is most easily detectable in the great auricular nerve in the neck, the supraclavicular nerves as they cross the clavicles, the ulnar nerve just above the elbow, the common peroneal nerve at the neck of the fibula, and the superficial peroneal nerve over the anterior aspects of the ankles or the dorsa of the feet. The infrapatellar branch of the saphenous nerve on the medial aspect of the knee is sometimes noticeably enlarged before there is detectable thickening elsewhere. In tuberculoid leprosy, the enlargement may be uniform or nodular. Rarely, a localized cystic swelling develops along a nerve, at times reaching substantial dimensions, related to caseous abscess formation. Nerves may be locally enlarged in the vicinity of cutaneous lesions. In patients who present with localized peripheral nerve lesions, such as ulnar palsy, enlargement of the affected nerve may be evident or thickening of other nerves may be demonstrable. A diagnostic point that may be helpful in the differentiation from a simple entrapment neuropathy of the ulnar nerve at the elbow is that in leprosy the enlargement usually extends for a greater distance up the arm or may be maximal some distance proximal to the elbow. In a simple entrapment neuropathy, the enlargement is usually restricted to a few centimeters in and above the ulnar groove. In borderline leprosy, widespread enlargement of nerves is also present before any neurologic symptoms or cutaneous lesions appear.

In hypertrophic neuropathy, both in the inherited and the acquired forms, nerve thickening constitutes an important physical finding. In the inherited forms, it tends to be a uniform and symmetrical enlargement, and is of greater degree in the recessively inherited Dejerine-Sottas disorder than in the dominantly inherited hypertrophic form of peroneal muscular atrophy. In sporadic cases, such as those of late onset described by Roussy and Cornil (1919a, 1919b), the enlargement may be nodular. Sometimes it is extraordinarily localized: in a case recorded by Webster and co-workers (1967), the enlargement was confined to the brachial plexus.

Other examples of conditions in which nerve enlargement may be found are the acute Guillain-Barré syndrome and chronic relapsing polyneuritis, amyloid neuropathy, and acromegaly (Reisner and Spiel, 1952; Austin, 1958; Chambers et al., 1958; Stewart, 1966). Although the enlargement in acromegaly has been referred to as hypertrophic neuropathy, it is important to realize that it is the result of connective tissue overgrowth and that concentric Schwann cell proliferation, which is the hallmark of both the inherited and acquired cases of hypertrophic neuropathy, does not occur to any significant degree.

In neurofibromatosis, apart from the more usual localized swellings subcutaneously or in relation to nerve trunks, diffuse peripheral nerve enlargement may occur (Thomas and Eames, 1969). Localized nerve enlargement may also indicate the presence of a schwannoma or other solitary peripheral nerve tumor (see Chapter 67).

Intermittent Symptoms

In general, symptoms in polyneuropathies are persistent in character, but transient symptoms may occur and are of considerable practical and theoretical interest. Their occurrence may be of assistance diagnostically and they may provide a convenient opportunity for the investigation of pathophysiologic mechanisms. Examples are the nocturnal attacks of intermittent paresthesias in the carpal tunnel syndrome, those that develop on elbow flexion in the cubital tunnel syndrome, and the burning paresthesias of meralgia paresthetica that occur on standing and that may be relieved by walking. Pain may also occur intermittently, most strikingly in trigeminal neuralgia (Chapter 26) and in the lightning pains of some polyneuropathies. Other examples of intermittent pain are the nocturnal aching in the lower limbs in diabetic and ischemic neuropathy, cold-induced pain following peripheral nerve injury, and the aggravation of causalgic pain by emotional factors. Intermittency of motor symptoms, apart from muscle cramps and fasciculation, is less common. Isaacs (1960) described attacks of cold-induced weakness in the legs in a patient with hypertrophic neuropathy, and an interesting example of cold-induced facial paralysis is on record (Kinsbourne and Rushworth, 1966).

Moderate elevations in temperature are known to cause conduction block in demyelinated axons (Rasminsky, 1973); it has been

suggested that this may be implicated in the worsening of symptoms in multiple sclerosis that follows hot baths or exercise. If this is true, it is perhaps surprising that weakness or sensory loss produced by warming has not been described in demyelinating neuropathies.

Lewis, Pickering, and Rothschild (1931) demonstrated that the application of a tourniquet at greater than arterial pressure around the upper arm in normal subjects, after first giving rise to ischemic paresthesias, leads to sensory loss and paralysis after an interval of about 20 minutes. This is rapidly reversible when the cuff is released. Recovery is associated with postischemic paresthesias. That these effects are due to ischemia of the nerve distal to the cuff and not to a direct pressure effect by the tourniquet was neatly shown by inflating a second cuff below the first after sensory loss had developed. On release of the upper cuff, the sensory loss persisted. The transient symptoms experienced by most people as a result of localized nerve compression are likely to be of this nature. Persisting symptoms may well be related to mechanical effects of the type shown to occur in experimental tourniquet paralysis (Ochoa et al., 1972).

The attacks of paresthesia that constitute an important aspect of the symptomatology of the carpal tunnel syndrome, which characteristically occur at night, have been subjected to a number of investigations (Gilliatt and Wilson, 1953, 1954; Fullerton, 1963). This work convincingly established that in such cases the median nerve is abnormally susceptible to ischemia produced by inflation of a pneumatic cuff around the arm. Gilliatt and Wilson found that median nerve sensory loss appeared with abnormal rapidity, and Fullerton showed that conduction in motor fibers failed with abnormal rapidity because of a conduction block in fibers distal to the wrist. Gilliatt and Wilson also noted that the patients reported that the symptoms produced by ischemia were similar to their spontaneous attacks. All these observations suggest that the attacks of paresthesia are related to episodes of ischemia. Personal observations on a patient with frequent nocturnal attacks of paresthesias revealed that these occurred when she slept on her side with arms flexed, but failed to develop when she slept with her elbows extended. Obstruction of the vascular supply by kinking of the brachial artery at the elbow that produced partial ischemia of the median nerve at the wrist may therefore have been involved. This patient's symptoms could readily be reproduced by obliteration of the circulation in the upper arm with a pneumatic cuff.

DIFFERENTIAL DIAGNOSIS

Disorders Simulating Peripheral Neuropathy

Primary diseases of muscle do not commonly give rise to difficulty, and in cases of doubt, electromyography is usually helpful in their differentiation. Where the onset is gradual, the proximal distribution of muscle involvement is unlike most neuropathies. Acute polymyositis, if there is no muscle tenderness or involvement of other systems, could be mistaken for an acute Guillain-Barré syndrome with proximal weakness. Rare cases of chronic polymyositis display a distal distribution of weakness and wasting in the limbs and clinically may resemble a chronic motor polyneuropathy or chronic distal spinal muscular atrophy (Hollinrake, 1969). Of the muscular dystrophies, the rare distal myopathy gives rise to a somewhat similar clinical picture but, in contradistinction to most neuropathies, usually commences in the upper limbs. (Welander, 1951). Dystrophia myotonica also affects the distal musculature in the limbs, and clinically detectable myotonia may be absent; however, selective atrophy of the sternomastoid muscles is likely to coexist, and other features of the disorder may be evident.

Myasthenia gravis is not usually confused with peripheral neuropathy, except for occasional cases of acute onset in childhood with proximal weakness in the limbs and little bulbar involvement. These may superficially resemble the Guillain-Barré syndrome. The Eaton-Lambert syndrome (Lambert and Rooke, 1965) is more likely to give rise to difficulty. The weakness is usually most marked in the limbs, and ocular, facial, and bulbar weakness may not be evident. There may be generalized depression of the tendon reflexes. It is of importance that these can often be obtained following vigorous contraction of the muscle under examination, this being a reflection of the pronounced posttetanic facilitation exhibited in this disorder. Confirmation of the diagnosis may be obtained

by electrophysiologic demonstration of this phenomenon.

Spinal muscular atrophies are often difficult to differentiate from predominantly motor neuropathies. The tendon reflexes may be depressed and although muscle fasciculation may occur, this does not necessarily imply anterior horn cell disease. This diagnostic problem arises in occasional cases of motor neuron disease of progressive muscular atrophy type, particularly in those that begin with bilateral foot drop and in which the ankle jerks are lost. It also arises in cases of hereditary distal spinal muscular atrophy (McLeod and Prineas, 1971). Careful sensory testing and the examination of sensory nerve action potentials is required. Acute anterior poliomyelitis formerly gave rise to occasional diagnostic confusion at the time of epidemics and still may do so in unimmunized individuals who have returned after visiting areas where the disease remains endemic. The acute onset, the total absence of sensory loss, the constitutional upset with fever, and the cerebrospinal fluid pleocytosis should indicate the correct diagnosis, and confirmation may be sought by virologic studies.

Tabes dorsalis may present clinical resemblances to a sensory neuropathy, and in particular to that related to diabetes. In both, the tendon reflexes are depressed or abolished, and there may be sensory ataxia of gait. Loss of pain sensibility may result in perforating ulcers in the feet and neuropathic arthropathy, although the distribution of joint involvement differs between the two disorders (see Chapter 47). Aching or lancinating pains in the legs occur in both, as may autonomic disturbances, including bladder atony, impotence, and pupillary disturbances. Differentiation between tabes dorsalis and a sensory neuropathy is not difficult. Impairment of tactile sensation is not a feature in tabes, and the pattern of sensory loss is often characteristic. Only minor abnormalities of the sensory nerve action potentials are detectable, whereas in a sensory neuropathy of equivalent clinical severity marked changes would be expected. Confirmation may be obtained by serologic tests for syphilis.

Spinal cord disorders sometimes mimic a sensory neuropathy by giving rise to distal paresthesias in the legs or in all four extremities. This situation may arise in multiple sclerosis or in cervical myelopathy from spondylosis, or occasionally from extramedullary tumors in the cervical region. If such symptoms develop before signs of long tract damage make their appearance, diagnostic difficulty may arise. Studies of sensory nerve conduction usually resolve matters. Inquiry should be made for Lhermitte's sign, which, if present, indicates cervical cord disease.

Cerebral lesions rarely give rise to difficulty. As originally pointed out by Foerster, it is of interest that cerebral tumors occasionally present with sensory or motor symptoms of a radicular or peripheral nerve disturbance (Thomas and Fullerton, 1963). The explanation is possibly to be found in the summation of a preexisting subclinical peripheral nerve or radicular lesion with the developing cerebral lesion.

Hysterical symptoms are generally readily identified as such. The inconstant and fluctuating character of hysterical weakness, its improvement by encouragement, and the lack of reflex change typify the situation. A "glove and stocking" distribution is a favored pattern of hysterical sensory loss and this may simulate a peripheral neuropathy, but inconsistencies or physical absurdities revealed by testing and the preservation of sensory nerve action potentials will indicate the nature of the disturbance. The occurrence of tingling paresthesias in the extremities is a not infrequent reason for patients with anxiety and a suspected diagnosis of a sensory neuropathy to be referred to a neurologist. Although hyperventilation is not always noticed or admitted by the patient, the evanescent nature of the symptoms and again the preservation of sensory nerve action potentials will exclude structural changes in the nerves.

Neuropathies Simulating Other Conditions

In the preceding section, the conditions most commonly mistaken for peripheral neuropathies have been considered. Conversely, certain neuropathies are likely to masquerade as other disorders. The instance of "diabetic pseudotabes" has already been cited, as has that of acute neuropathies with proximal muscle weakness that can be mistaken for acute polymyositis. This distribution of involvement may occur in the Guillain-Barré syndrome and porphyric neuropathy, in both of which sensory changes may be un-

obtrusive or absent. In neuropathies that present with cranial nerve involvement, particularly if the onset is insidious, a diagnosis of myasthenia gravis may be entertained (Thomas and Lascelles, 1967). Interesting but rare examples of a neuropathy that may mimic spinal cord disease are those cases of Tangier disease that present with muscle wasting in the upper limbs, loss of tendon reflexes, and dissociated pain and temperature sensory loss with a central distribution (Kocen et al., 1973). The ascription of cases of hereditary sensory neuropathy to "lumbosacral syringomyelia," to which allusion was made earlier in this chapter, has now been abandoned. Finally, the monotonous regularity with which the weakness of porphyric neuropathy is attributed to hysteria is emphasized in Chapter 46.

DIAGNOSIS OF PERIPHERAL NEUROPATHY

Confirmation of the diagnosis of peripheral neuropathy when this has been suspected on clinical grounds is usually best achieved by nerve conduction studies, useful both in detecting localized peripheral nerve lesions and in establishing the presence of generalized polyneuropathies. In broad terms, generalized polyneuropathies can be subdivided into those in which the primary disturbance is axonal degeneration and those in which it involves widespread segmental demyelination, although this distinction is now known not to be as clearly defined as was at first believed (Gilliatt, 1966; Thomas, 1971). The group in which demyelination is prominent is characterized by a substantial reduction in nerve conduction velocity, whereas in those in which the changes primarily affect axons, conduction velocity tends to be within normal limits or only slightly reduced. In the latter, the examination of motor nerve conduction velocity may not be helpful in distinguishing them from anterior horn cell disease, in which nerve conduction is similarly affected. In most peripheral neuropathies of this type, however, sensory nerve conduction, even if sensation is clinically normal, is likely to be abnormal. This statement requires the qualification that in lesions affecting the sensory roots central to the dorsal root ganglion cells, conduction in sensory fibers in the limbs is preserved even if there is total sensory loss. In brachial plexus injuries (see Chapter 32), this may be useful in distinguishing between avulsion of roots from the cord and lesions in the plexus distal to the dorsal root ganglia (Bonney and Gilliatt, 1958). In such cases, axon responses, demonstrated for example by the intradermal injection of histamine, will be preserved (Bonney, 1954). In cases of Guillain-Barré polyradiculopathy in which the demyelinating process is confined to the roots and in which axonal destruction has not occurred, sensory (and motor) conduction will be normal in the limbs.

The quantitative assessment of the structural integrity of peripheral nerves is possible by nerve biopsy, but the use of biopsy to substantiate a diagnosis of neuropathy is rarely necessary (Thomas, 1970). The procedure may be helpful in some instances in defining the nature of the disorder.

In patients in whom there may be difficulty in distinguishing between a myopathic process and a motor neuropathy, electromyography is usually decisive. An elevated serum creatine kinase level is more likely to indicate a myopathy, although a slight or moderate elevation may occur at times in cases of denervation atrophy. Increase of the cerebrospinal fluid protein content may also point to a neuropathic condition, and the degree of increase can sometimes be of assistance in defining the nature of the disorder.

The clinical features of the different categories of peripheral neuropathy are detailed in the succeeding chapters of this section and need not be enumerated here. It may be appropriate, however, to outline a few general aspects related to establishing the cause of a peripheral neuropathy. The analysis of the clinical history and of the abnormalities revealed by physical examination either may suggest the likely diagnosis or may narrow down the diagnostic possibilities, thus facilitating subsequent investigation. As discussed earlier in this chapter, the range of diagnostic possibilities differs in a case of multiple mononeuropathy as compared with a symmetrical polyneuropathy. In the latter, the distribution of involvement (that is, whether it is motor or sensory or mixed, or whether it is proximal or distal) can provide useful information, as may the rapidity of its onset and the previous clinical course in established cases. The age of the patient is important: a neuropathy of insidious onset in childhood is highly likely to be of genetic origin, whereas in later life a carcinomatous basis would figure high in the list of diagnostic possibilities. The country of origin may provide useful information. The presentation of an isolated ulnar neuropathy in an individual who was born in an area where leprosy is endemic should alert the clinician to this possibility and lead to a careful search for thickening of other nerves and for cutaneous changes. It needs no emphasis that the presence of abnormalities in other systems is often of crucial diagnostic value.

Estimates of the frequency with which an etiologic diagnosis was achieved in cases of peripheral neuropathy that were made 20 years ago yielded the gloomy conclusion that in a high proportion the explanation remained uncertain (Elkington, 1952; Matthews, 1952). Since then, a substantial amount of activity has been directed toward the investigation of peripheral nerve disorders. Yet it remains embarrassingly true that in many neuropathies, particularly those with a chronic progressive course, no satisfactory explanation for their occurrence can be given (Prineas, 1970).

REFERENCES

Aagenaes, Ö.: Neurovascular examinations on the lower extremities, with special reference to the autonomic neuropathy. Copenhagen, C. Hamburgers Bogtrykkeri, 1962.

Adams, R. D., Denny-Brown, D., and Pearson, C. M.: Diseases of Muscle: A Study in Pathology. 2nd edition. New York, Hoeber Div., Harper & Row, 1962.

Aguayo, A. J., Nair, C. P. V., and Bray, G. M.: Peripheral nerve abnormalities in the Riley-Day syndrome. Arch. Neurol., 24:106, 1971.

Andrade, C.: Peculiar form of peripheral neuropathy; familial atypical generalized amyloidosis with special involvement of peripheral nerves. Brain, 75:408, 1952.

Appenzeller, O., and Marshall, J.: Vasomotor disturbances in Landry-Guillain-Barré syndrome. Arch. Neurol., 9:368, 1963.

Asbury, A. K., Aldredge, H., Hershberg, R., and Fisher, C. M.: Oculomotor palsy in diabetes mellitus: a clinico-pathological study. Brain, 93:555, 1970.

Austin, J. H.: Observations on the syndrome of hypertrophic neuritis (the hypertrophic interstitial radiculoneuropathies). Medicine, Baltimore, 35:187, 1956.

Austin, J. H.: Recurrent polyneuropathies and their corticosteroid treatment. Brain, 81:157, 1958.

Bárány, F. R., and Cooper, E. H.: Pilomotor and sudomotor innervation in diabetes. Clin. Sci., 15:533, 1956.

Barraclough, M. A., and Sharpey-Schafer, E. P.: Hypotension from absent circulatory reflexes. Effects of alcohol, barbiturates and other mechanisms. Lancet, *1*:1121, 1963.

Behse, F., Buchthal, F., Carlsen, F., and Knappeis, G. G.: Hereditary neuropathy with liability to pressure palsies: electrophysiological and histopathological aspects. Brain, *95*:777, 1972.

Berenyi, M. R., and Schwarz, G. S.: Megasigmoid syndrome in diabetes and neurologic disease. Am. J. Gastroenterol., *47*:311, 1967.

Berge, K. G., Wollaeger, E. E., Scholz, D. A., Rooke, E. D., and Sprague, R. G.: Steatorrhoea complicating diabetes mellitus with neuropathy. Report of two cases without apparent external pancreatic insufficiency. Diabetes, *5*:25, 1956.

Birket-Smith, E., and Krogh, E.: Motor nerve conduction velocity during diphenylhydantoin intoxication. Acta Neurol. Scand., *47*:265, 1971.

Bonney, G.: Value of axon responses in determining site of lesion in traction injuries of brachial plexus. Brain, *77*:588, 1954.

Bonney, G., and Gilliatt, R. W.: Sensory nerve conduction after traction lesions of the brachial plexus. Proc. R. Soc. Med., *51*:365, 1958.

Bosanquet, F. D., and Henson, R. A.: Sensory neuropathy in diabetes mellitus. Folia Psychiatr. Neerl., *60*:107, 1957.

Bowden, R. E. M., and Gutmann, E.: Denervation and reinnervation of human voluntary muscle. Brain, *67*:273, 1944.

Buller, A. J., Eccles, J. C., and Eccles, R. M.: Interactions between motoneurones and muscles in respect of the characteristic speeds of their responses. J. Physiol. (Lond.), *150*:417, 1960.

Callaghan, N.: Restless legs syndrome in uremic neuropathy. Neurology (Minneap.), *16*:359, 1966.

Cavanagh, J. B.: The significance of the "dying-back" process in experimental and human neurological disease. Int. Rev. Exp. Pathol., *3*:219, 1964.

Chambers, R. A., Medd, W. E., and Spencer, H.: Primary amyloidosis, with special reference to involvement of the nervous system. Q.J. Med., *27*:207, 1958.

Cragg, B. G., and Thomas, P. K.: Changes in nerve conduction in experimental allergic neuritis. J. Neurol. Neurosurg. Psychiatry, *27*:106, 1964.

Croft, P. B., and Wilkinson, M.: The incidence of carcinomatous neuromyopathy in patients with various types of carcinoma. Brain, *88*:427, 1965.

Dancis, J., and Smith, A. A.: Familial dysautonomia. N. Engl. J. Med., *274*:207, 1966.

Davis, L. E., and Drachman, D. B.: Myeloma neuropathy. Arch. Neurol., *27*:507, 1972.

Denny-Brown, D.: Primary sensory neuropathy with muscular changes associated with carcinoma. J. Neurol. Neurosurg. Psychiatry, *11*:73, 1948.

Denny-Brown, D.: Hereditary sensory radicular neuropathy. J. Neurol. Neurosurg. Psychiatry, *14*:237, 1951.

Denny-Brown, D., and Brenner, C.: Paralysis of nerve induced by direct pressure and by tourniquet. Arch. Neurol. Psychiatry, *51*:1, 1944.

Doupe, J., Cullen, C. H., and Chance, G. Q.: Post-traumatic pain and causalgic syndrome. J. Neurol. Neurosurg. Psychiatry, *7*:33, 1944.

Dyck, P. J., and Lambert, E. H.: Lower motor and primary sensory neuron diseases with peroneal muscular atrophy. I. Neurologic, genetic, and electrophysiologic findings in hereditary polyneuropathies. Arch. Neurol., *18*:603, 1968a.

Dyck, P. J., and Lambert, E. H.: Lower motor and primary sensory neuron diseases with peroneal muscular atrophy. II. Neurologic, genetic, and electrophysiological findings in various neuronal degenerations. Arch. Neurol., *18*:619, 1968b.

Dyck, P. J., and Lambert, E. H.: Dissociated sensation in amyloidosis. Arch. Neurol., *20*:490, 1969.

Dyck, P. J., Lambert, E. H., and Nichols, P. C.: Quantitative measurement of sensation related to compound action potential and number and sizes of myelinated and unmyelinated fibers of sural nerve in health, Friedreich's ataxia, hereditary sensory neuropathy, and tabes dorsalis. *In* Cobb, W. A. (ed.): Handbook of Electroencephalography and Clinical Neurophysiology. Vol. 9. Amsterdam, Elsevier Publishing Co., 1972, p. 83.

Earl, C. J., Fullerton, P. M., Wakefield, G. S., and Schutta, H. S.: Hereditary neuropathy, with liability to pressure palsies. Q.J. Med., *33*:481, 1964.

Ekbom, K. A.: Restless legs. *In* Vinken, P. J., and Bruyn, G. W. (eds.): Handbook of Clinical Neurology. Vol. 8. Amsterdam, North Holland Publishing Co., 1970, p. 311.

Eldjarn, L., Try, K., Stokke, O., Munthe-Kaas, A. W., Refsum, S., Steinberg, D., Avigan, J., and Mize, C.: Dietary effects on serum-phytanic-acid levels and on clinical manifestations in heredopathia atactica polyneuritiformis. Lancet, *1*:691, 1966.

Elkington, J. St. C.: Recent work on the peripheral neuropathies. Proc. R. Soc. Med., *45*:661, 1952.

Ellenberg, M., and Weber, H.: Retrograde ejaculation in diabetic neuropathy. Ann. Intern. Med., *65*:1237, 1966.

England, A. C., and Denny-Brown, D.: Severe sensory changes and trophic disorder in peroneal muscular atrophy (Charcot-Marie-Tooth type). A.M.A. Arch. Neurol. Psychiatry, *67*:1, 1952.

Fleming, L. W., Lenman, J. A. R., and Stewart, W. K.: Effect of magnesium on nerve conduction velocity during regular dialysis treatment. J. Neurol. Neurosurg. Psychiatry, *35*:342, 1972.

French, J. M., Hall, G., Parish, D. J., and Smith, W. T.: Peripheral and autonomic nerve involvement in primary amyloidosis associated with uncontrollable diarrhoea and steatorrhoea. Am. J. Med., *39*:277, 1965.

Friedman, S. A., Feinberg, R., Podolak, E., and Bedell, R. H. S.: Pupillary abnormalities in diabetic neuropathy. Ann. Intern. Med., *67*:977, 1967.

Fullerton, P. M.: The effect of ischaemia on nerve conduction in the carpal tunnel syndrome. J. Neurol., Neurosurg. Psychiatry, *26*:385, 1963.

Garland, H.: Diabetic amyotrophy. Br. Med. J., *2*:1287, 1955.

Gilliatt, R. W.: Clinical aspects of diabetic neuropathy. *In* Cumings, J. N., and Kremer, M. (eds.): Biochemical Aspects of Neurological Disorders. 2nd series. Oxford, Blackwell Scientific Publications, 1965, p. 117.

Gilliatt, R. W.: Nerve conduction in human and experimental neuropathies. Proc. R. Soc. Med., *59*:989, 1966.

Gilliatt, R. W., and Willison, R. G.: Peripheral nerve conduction in diabetic neuropathy. J. Neurol. Neurosurg. Psychiatry, *25*:11, 1962.

Gilliatt, R. W., and Wilson, T. G.: A pneumatic-tourniquet test in the carpal-tunnel syndrome. Lancet, *2*:595, 1953.

Gilliatt, R. W., and Wilson, T. G.: Ischaemic sensory loss in patients with peripheral nerve lesions. J. Neurol. Neurosurg. Psychiatry, *17*:104, 1954.

Goodman, J. I.: Diabetic anhidrosis. Am. J. Med., *41*:831, 1966.

Granit, R., Leksell, L., and Skoglund, C. R.: Fibre interaction in injured or compressed region of nerve. Brain, 67:125, 1944.

Greene, L. F., Kelalis, P. P., and Weeks, R. E.: Retrograde ejaculation of semen due to diabetic neuropathy. Report of 4 cases. Fertil. Steril., 14:617, 1963.

Hicks, E. P.: Hereditary perforating ulcer of the foot. Lancet, 1:319, 1922.

Hollinrake, K.: Polymyositis presenting as distal muscle weakness: a case report. J. Neurol. Sci., 8:479, 1969.

Hopkins, A. P., and Morgan-Hughes, J. A.: The effect of local pressure in diphtheritic neuropathy. J. Neurol. Neurosurg. Psychiatry, 32:614, 1969.

Isaacs, H.: Familial chronic hypertrophic polyneuropathy with paralysis of the extremities in cold weather. S. Afr. Med. J., 34:758, 1960.

Isaacs, H.: Syndrome of continuous muscle fibre activity. J. Neurol. Neurosurg. Psychiatry, 24:319, 1961.

Isaacs, H.: Continuous muscle fibre activity in an Indian male with additional evidence of terminal motor fibre activity. J. Neurol. Neurosurg. Psychiatry, 30:126, 1967.

Keen, H.: Autonomic nerve involvement in diabetes. In Pyke, D. A. (ed.): Disorders of Carbohydrate Metabolism. London, Pitman & Sons, 1962, p. 177.

Kinsbourne, M., and Rushworth, G.: Fluctuating and intermittent facial weakness following a local anesthetic. J. Neurol. Neurosurg. Psychiatry, 29:367, 1966.

Kocen, R. S., and Thomas, P. K.: Peripheral nerve involvement in Fabry's disease. Arch. Neurol., 22:81, 1970.

Kocen, R. S., Thomas, P. K., Kind, R. H. M., and Haas, L. F.: Nerve biopsy findings in two cases of Tangier disease: Acta Neuropathol., 26:317, 1973.

Kocen, R. S., Lloyd, J. K., Lascelles, P. T., Fosbrooke, A. S., and Williams, D.: Familial α-lipoprotein deficiency (Tangier disease) with neurological abnormalities. Lancet, 1:1341, 1967.

Kyle, R. A., Kottke, B. A., and Schirger, A.: Orthostatic hypotension as a clue to primary systemic amyloidosis. Circulation, 34:833, 1966.

Lambert, E. H., and Rooke, E. D.: Myasthenic state and lung cancer. In Brain, R. L., and Norris, F. H., Jr. (eds.): The Remote Effects of Cancer on the Nervous System. New York, Grune & Stratton, 1965, p. 67.

Lawrence, D. G., and Locke, S.: Motor nerve conduction velocity in diabetes. Arch. Neurol., 5:483, 1961.

Lewis, T., and Pickering, G. W.: Circulatory changes in the fingers in some diseases of the nervous system with special reference to the digital atrophy of peripheral nerve lesions. Clin. Sci., 2:149, 1936.

Lewis, T., Pickering, G. W., and Rothschild, P.: Centripetal paralysis arising out of arrested blood flow to the limb, including notes on a form of tingling. Heart, 16:1, 1931.

Lourie, H., and King, R. B.: Sensory and neurohistological correlates of cutaneous hyperpathia. Arch. Neurol., 14:313, 1966.

Mahloudji, M., Teasdall, R. D., Adamkiewicz, J. J., Hartman, W. H., Lambird, P. A., and McKusick, V. A.: The genetic amyloidoses, with particular reference to hereditary neuropathic amyloidosis, type II (Indiana or Rukavina type). Medicine, Baltimore, 48:1, 1969.

Majno, G., and Karnovsky, M. L.: A biochemical and morphologic study of myelination and demyelination. II. Lipogenesis in vitro by rat nerves following transection. J. Exp. Med., 107:475, 1958.

Martin, M. M.: Involvement of autonomic fibres in diabetic neuropathy. Lancet, 1:560, 1953.

Matthews, W. B.: Cryptogenic polyneuritis. Proc. R. Soc. Med., 45:667, 1952.

Mayer, R. F., and Denny-Brown, D.: Conduction velocity in peripheral nerve during experimental demyelination in the cat. Neurology (Minneap.), 14:714, 1964.

McDonald, W. I.: The effects of experimental demyelination on conduction in peripheral nerve: a histological and electrophysiological study. II. Electrophysiological observations. Brain, 86:501, 1963.

McLeod, J. G., and Prineas, J. W.: Distal type of chronic spinal muscular atrophy: clinical, electrophysiological and pathological studies. Brain, 94:703, 1971.

Melzack, R., and Wall, P. D.: Pain mechanisms: a new theory. Science, 150:971, 1966.

Meyer, G. A., and Fields, H. L.: Causalgia treated by selective large fibre stimulation of peripheral nerve. Brain, 95:163, 1972.

Mulder, D. W., Lambert, E. H., Bastron, J. A., and Sprague, R. G.: The neuropathies associated with diabetes mellitus: a clinical and electromyographic study of 103 unselected diabetic patients. Neurology (Minneap.), 11:275, 1961.

Murray, T. J.: Congenital sensory neuropathy. Brain, 96:387, 1973.

Noordenbos, W.: Pain. Amsterdam, Elsevier Publishing Co., 1959.

Ochoa, J.: Isoniazid neuropathy in man. Brain, 93:831, 1970.

Ochoa, J., Fowler, T. J., and Gilliatt, R. W.: Anatomical changes in peripheral nerves compressed by a pneumatic tourniquet. J. Anat., 113:433, 1972.

Paley, R. G., Mitchell, W., and Watkinson, G.: Terminal colonic dilatation following intractable diarrhea in a diabetic. Gastroenterology, 4:401, 1961.

Preswick, G., and Jeremy, D.: Subclinical polyneuropathy in renal insufficiency. Lancet, 2:731, 1964.

Prineas, J.: Polyneuropathies of undetermined cause. Acta Neurol. Scand., 46:Suppl. 46, 1970.

Raff, M. C., Sangalang, V., and Asbury, A. K.: Ischemic mononeuropathy multiplex associated with diabetes mellitus. Arch. Neurol., 18:487, 1968.

Rasminsky, M.: The effects of temperature on conduction in demyelinated single nerve fibers. Arch. Neurol., 28:287, 1973.

Reisner, H., and Spiel, W.: Zur Frage der Polyneuritis hypertrophicans. Wien. Z. Nervenheilkd., 5:388, 1952.

Rexed, B.: Contributions to the knowledge of the postnatal development of the peripheral nervous system in man. Acta Psychiat., Suppl. 33, 1944.

Roussy, G., and Cornil, L.: Un cas de névrite hypertrophique progressive non familiale de l'adulte. Rev. Neurol. (Paris), 35:590, 1919a.

Roussy, G., and Cornil, L.: Névrite hypertrophique progressive non familiale de l'adulte. Ann. Méd., 6:296, 1919b.

Rundles, R. W.: Diabetic neuropathy: general review with report of 125 cases. Medicine, Baltimore, 24:111, 1945.

Seddon, H. J.: Surgical Disorders of the Peripheral Nerves. Edinburgh, Churchill Livingstone, 1972.

Shahani, B., and Spalding, J. M. K.: Diabetes mellitus presenting with bilateral foot drop. Lancet, 2:930, 1969.

Sharpey-Schafer, E. P., and Taylor, P. J.: Absent circulatory reflexes in diabetic neuritis. Lancet, *1*:559, 1960.

Sluga, E.: Correlations of electrophysiological and morphological methods in neuropathies. *In* Kunze, K., and Desmedt, J. E. (eds.): Studies on Neuromuscular Diseases. Proceedings of the International Symposium on Neuromuscular Diseases, April 1973, in Giessen. Basel, S. Karger, 1975.

Smith, B.: The Neuropathology of the Alimentary Tract. London, Edward Arnold, 1972.

Spillane, J. D.: Restless legs syndrome in chronic pulmonary disease. Br. Med. J., *4*:796, 1970.

Spillane, J. D., and Wells, C. E. C.: Acrodystrophic Neuropathy. London, Oxford Medical Publications, 1969.

Stack, R. E., Bianco, A. J., Jr., and MacCarty, C. S.: Compression of the common peroneal nerve by ganglion cysts: report of nine cases. J. Bone Joint Surg., *47A*:773, 1965.

Stewart, B. M.: The hypertrophic neuropathy of acromegaly: a rare neuropathy associated with acromegaly. Arch. Neurol., *14*:107, 1966.

Sunderland, S.: Capacity of reinnervated muscles to function efficiently after prolonged denervation. Arch. Neurol. Psychiatry, *64*:755, 1950.

Sunderland, S.: Nerves and Nerve Injury. Edinburgh, E. & S. Livingstone, 1968.

Tenckhoff, H. A., Boen, S. T., Jebsen, R. H., and Spiegler, J. H.: Polyneuropathy of chronic renal insufficiency. J.A.M.A., *192*:1121, 1965.

Thévenard, A.: L'acropathie ulcéro-mutilante familiale. Rev. Neurol. (Paris), *74*:193, 1942.

Thomas, P. K.: The quantitation of nerve biopsy findings. J. Neurol. Sci., *11*:285, 1970.

Thomas, P. K.: The morphological basis for alterations in nerve conduction in peripheral neuropathy. Proc. R. Soc. Med., *64*:295, 1971.

Thomas, P. K.: Metabolic neuropathy. J. R. Coll. Phys. Lond., *7*:154, 1973.

Thomas, P. K., and Eames, R. A.: Neurofibromatous neuropathy. *In* Serratrice, G., and Roux, H. (eds.): Actualités de Pathologie Neuro-musculaire: Advances in Neuromuscular Diseases. Paris, Riker, 1969, p. 612.

Thomas, P. K., and Fullerton, P. M.: Nerve fibre size in the carpal tunnel syndrome. J. Neurol. Neurosurg. Psychiatry, *26*:520, 1963.

Thomas, P. K., and Lascelles, R. G.: Hypertrophic neuropathy. Q. J. Med., *36*:223, 1967.

Thomas, P. K., Calne, D. B., and Stewart, G.: Hereditary motor and sensory polyneuropathy (peroneal muscular atrophy). Ann. Hum. Genet., *38*:111, 1974.

Thomas, P. K., Lascelles, R. G., Hallpike, J. F., and Hewer, R. L.: Recurrent and chronic relapsing Guillain-Barré polyneuritis. Brain, *92*:589, 1969.

Thomas, P. K., Hollinrake, K., Lascelles, R. G., O'Sullivan, D. J., Baillod, R. A., Moorhead, J. F., and Mackenzie, J. C.: The polyneuropathy of chronic renal failure. Brain, *94*:761, 1971.

Tyrer, J. H., and Sutherland, J. M.: The primary spinocerebellar atrophies and their associated defects, with a study of the foot deformity. Brain, *84*:289, 1961.

Wall, P. D., and Sweet, W. H.: Temporary abolition of pain in man. Science, *155*:108, 1967.

Wallis, W. E., van Poznak, A., and Plum, F.: Generalized muscular stiffness, fasciculations, and myokymia of peripheral nerve origin. Arch. Neurol., *22*:430, 1970.

Walshe, F. M. R.: On "acroparaesthesia" and so-called "neuritis" of hands and arms in women; their relation to brachial plexus pressure by probable normal first ribs. Br. Med. J., *2*:596, 1945.

Walters, A.: The differentiation of causalgia and hyperpathia. Can. Med. Assoc. J., *80*:105, 1969.

Webster, H de F., Schröder, J. M., Asbury, A. K., and Adams, R. D. The role of Schwann cells in the formation of "onion bulbs" found in chronic neuropathies. J. Neuropathol. Exp. Neurol., *26*:276, 1967.

Weddell, G., Sinclair, D. C., and Feindel, W. H.: An anatomical basis for alterations in the quality of pain sensibility. J. Neurophysiol., *11*:99, 1948.

Welander, L.: Myopathia distalis tarda hereditaria. Acta Med. Scand., *141*:Suppl. 265, 1951.

Wortis, H., Stein, M. H., and Jolliffe, M.: Fiber dissociation in peripheral neuropathy. Arch. Intern. Med., *69*:222, 1942.

Zelená, J.: Development, degeneration and regeneration of receptor organs. Prog. Brain Res., *13*:175, 1964.

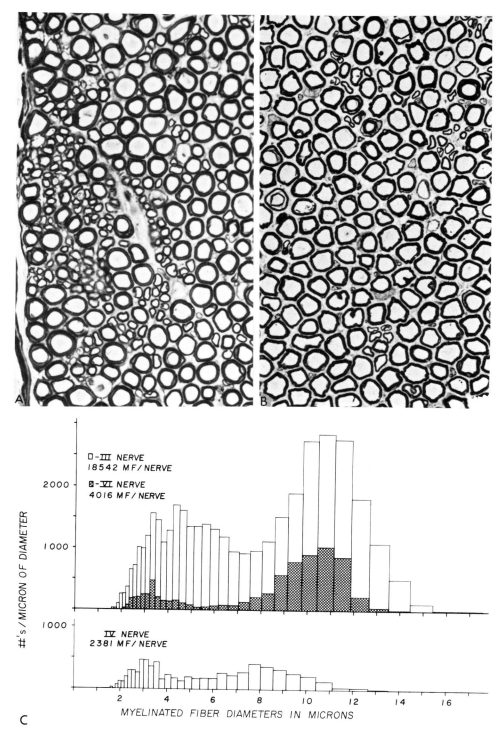

Figure 25–2 *A.* Normal nerve VI, × 500. *B.* Normal nerve III, × 500. *C.* Myelinated fiber spectra of nerves III and VI (*top*) and myelinated fiber spectrum of nerve IV (*bottom*). Counts were made on phase contrast enlargements of intracranial portion of normal nerves at site of contact with dura.

medial and medial aspects of nerve III with a gradually descending position within the nerve as it passes anteriorly. The accommodative fibers appear to be intimately associated with the pupillomotor fibers.

Figure 25–2 illustrates the numbers of myelinated fibers as well as the spectrum of fiber diameter within normal cranial nerves III, IV, and VI. The measurements were made on photographic enlargements of 1.5 μm transverse sections of each nerve at its intracranial-dural junction. This method for evaluating peripheral nerves has been described by Dyck and co-workers (1968). The oculomotor nerve that was examined was 2.33 mm² in transverse area and contained 18,542 fibers; the trochlear nerve measured was 0.19 mm² and contained 2381 fibers; and the abducens nerve measured was 0.56 mm² and contained 4016 fibers. Among the myelinated fibers, large fibers were predominant. In nerves III and VI the mean diameter of these large fibers was approximately 14 μm; in nerve IV the mean diameter for the large fibers was slightly less. There is also a strong suggestion that nerve III contains a third population of intermediate-size fibers; this is not evident in nerves IV and VI. Whether these fibers represent the parasympathetic fibers of nerve III remains to be proved. In the sections examined there were essentially no unmyelinated fibers detected.

CONGENITAL DEFECTS

Congenital abnormality of ocular movements may be due to defects of the nuclei of nerves III, IV, or VI and of the peripheral nerve. The literature of the nineteenth century contains several reports of such defects (Hoyt and Nachtigäller, 1965). These include unilateral or bilateral absence of cranial nerve VI, either alone or associated with abnormalities of other cranial nerves, as well as total or partial aplasia of the brain stem nuclei. Of interest also are a few reports of aberrant innervation of extraocular muscles, such as the lateral rectus muscle being innervated by a branch of nerve III in the absence of nerve VI.

In 1905, Duane described patients with congenital deficiency of abduction. These patients appeared to have complete paralysis of the lateral rectus muscle except for the associated features. On adduction, the globe

usually retracted, the lid fissure narrowed, and occasionally the globe moved up. There are several variations of Duane's syndrome. It occurs more frequently in females. It may be either unilateral or bilateral, with the left eye reportedly affected more often than the right. Subjectively, the patients usually have no disturbing symptoms; although they may be aware of their inability to move the eye or eyes laterally, they usually are not aware of diplopia.

In 1957, Breinin demonstrated abnormal electromyographic patterns of the extraocular muscles of patients with Duane's syndrome. It is now well established that in most cases the extraocular muscles are present and that the apparently paretic lateral rectus muscle usually has a functioning, although anomalous, nerve supply. Electromyographic tracings have shown a cocontraction pattern of the medial and lateral rectus muscles on attempted adduction and absence of electrical response of the lateral rectus muscle on attempted abduction (Blodi et al., 1964). This results in abnormal adduction with retraction of the globe and an absence of abduction. Further electromyographic studies have shown several anomalous innervational patterns in patients with Duane's syndrome or related congenital oculomotor retraction syndromes. Hoyt and Nachtigäller (1965) correlated several of the anatomical anomalies of peripheral nerves with various electromyographic data and concluded that at least some of these cases may be due to anatomical anomalies of the peripheral cranial nerves supplying the extraocular muscles.

Moebius (1888, 1892) reviewed the literature on cranial nerve palsies in children and classified 43 cases into six groups. Although he was wrong in his conclusion that the congenital and acquired palsies were fundamentally the same, his name has continued to be used to classify patients who present with facial diplegia and ocular palsy usually consisting of bilateral abducens paralysis. In 1939, Henderson reviewed 61 cases of congenital facial diplegia and noted external ocular palsies, including ptosis, to be present in 50 cases. Abducens palsy was present in 45 patients; it was bilateral in all but 2 of these patients and was the only ocular palsy in 31. Half these patients manifested convergence strabismus. Ptosis and paralysis of nerve III were less frequent, and internal ophthalmoplegia was not observed. All these congenital cranial nerve palsies are stationary from birth.

In addition to the facial diplegia and ocular palsy, patients with Moebius' syndrome may also show paralysis and atrophy of the anterior part of the tongue as well as other congenital defects such as hearing loss, clubfoot, or other skeletal deformities. Henderson noted only three reports of pathologic studies. These cases strongly support the view that the basis for the cranial nerve palsies is nuclear hypoplasia. The nerve roots of the affected cranial nerve were either absent or sparsely developed, depending on the degree of ganglion cell loss. The cause for this nuclear loss is obscure; only occasionally can a hereditary factor be traced in Moebius' syndrome or in other types of congenital ocular palsies except congenital ptosis.

Congenital horizontal gaze palsy may be seen as an isolated cranial nerve defect. It differs from the ocular palsy of Moebius' syndrome in that there usually is no convergent strabismus and no facial paralysis. Zweifach, Walton, and Brown (1969) described five children with complete absence of abduction on attempted conjugate gaze to either side; four of these five children substituted convergence and cross fixation for lateral eye movements. This substitution phenomenon has been reported in both congenital and acquired conjugate gaze paralysis (Burian et al., 1965). The sparing of vertical gaze with severe impairment of horizontal gaze is similar to that seen with acquired midline pontine lesions, which would suggest a congenital defect in this region.

EFFECTS OF TRAUMA

Trauma to the head frequently results in injury to cranial nerves III, IV, and VI. In 2000 cases of acquired ocular paralysis reviewed by Rucker (1958, 1966), 307 were due to head trauma: nerve III, 85; nerve IV, 47; nerve VI, 112; nerves III and IV, 16; nerves III and VI, 25; nerves IV and VI, 1; and nerves III, IV, and VI, 21. Bielschowsky (1939) earlier reported that 15 per cent of all cases of ocular paralysis had a traumatic etiology.

Cranial nerve VI is frequently affected because of its long course along the basiocciput, its firm attachment as it enters the dura over the clivus, its right angle as it arches over the ridge of the petrous bone, and its close association with the rigid petrosphenoidal ligament and the lateral branches of the basilar artery. Contusion, tearing, or traction may occur at any of these points owing to sudden displacement of the brain stem. Fractures through the temporal bone or through the posterior clinoids may injure the nerve directly or may be associated with sufficient hemorrhage to cause either unilateral or bilateral pressure paralysis. Schneider and Johnson (1971) have reported cases of bilateral abducens palsy after severe hyperextension injury to the head and associated cervical spinal column fractures. The mechanism postulated by them was an upward and posterior displacement of the brain, causing avulsion of nerve VI under the rigid petrosphenoid ligaments.

Most compression and contusion injuries of nerve VI heal spontaneously within two to five weeks, although a severe injury may require as long as four to six months to reach the full extent of recovery. If paresis of nerve VI with diplopia persists after four to six months, surgical treatment may be indicated.

Although protected by the tentorium, cranial nerve IV is vulnerable to trauma because of its long course and its delicate structure. Trauma has been reported to be the most frequent cause of acquired nerve IV paralysis (Burger et al., 1970; Jefferson, 1962; Rucker, 1958, 1966). This is often associated with an oblique frontal impact and loss of consciousness (Burger et al., 1970). On impact, the brain stem may be thrust against the lateral edge of the tentorium, resulting in contusion and hemorrhage of the dorsolateral midbrain and pons. The injury may then involve either the peripheral or the fascicular portion of one or both nerves. Bilateral symmetrical nerve IV paralysis has been reported after severe head injury and coma. Burger, Kalvin, and Smith (1970) postulated that the damage to the nerves is in the region of the anterior medullary velum where the nerves emerge from the midbrain. The prognosis for recovery of function after bilateral nerve IV paralysis is poor, and surgical treatment may be needed to correct the persistent diplopia on downward gaze. Bilateral tenotomy or recession of the inferior oblique muscles may be effective.

Cranial nerve III is vulnerable to injury at several sites: between the rigid posterior cerebral and superior cerebellar arteries, at the free edge of the reflected leaf of the tentorium, at its dural attachments on entering the cavernous sinus, and within the cavernous sinus. Weiner and Porro (1965) reviewed the mechanisms of nerve III palsy in trauma and described one case in which traumatic subdural hemorrhage resulted in total nerve III paralysis.

Meyer (1920) first described various herniations of brain substance. He found that the uncus of the temporal lobe was most likely to herniate through the incisura of the tentorium. Jefferson (1938) emphasized the tentlike form of the tentorium with its anteroposterior convex upper surface and a lateral decline that normally causes the temporal lobes to slide away from the incisura. With a unilateral mass or increased pressure on the temporal lobe, however, as occurs with a subdural or intracerebral hemorrhage or tumor, there may be sufficient force to push the medial hippocampal gyrus up and over the free edge of the tentorium. This may result in direct pressure on the ipsilateral nerve III and may also push the brain stem against the opposite edge of the tentorium. Kernohan and Woltman (1929) called attention to the ipsilateral paresis of the extremities from pressure on the contralateral cerebral peduncles, and Jefferson (1938) called attention to the ipsilateral paresis of nerve III in such cases. Transtentorial herniation causes a unilateral dilated pupil, either by direct pressure on the more superficially placed small parasympathetic fibers within nerve III or by indirect kinking of the nerve by the posterior cerebral and superior cerebellar arteries. Magoun and co-workers (1936) were unable to produce unilateral pupillary constriction with midbrain stimulation.

Plum and Posner (1966) described two clinical pictures of brain stem decompensation due to supratentorial lesions. The first is due to herniation of the uncus and is accompanied by signs of compression of the ipsilateral nerve III and contralateral cerebral peduncle. The second is due to central compression of the midbrain, which causes progressive bilateral parenchymal damage to the midbrain. The latter results in disorders of consciousness, respiration, and pupillary and ocular function as well as of motor function. The pupils initially may be small or unequal, and progressively change to become semidilated and fixed in the late stage of

brain stem decompensation. Bilateral ptosis or lid retraction and loss of upward gaze may be present along with other signs of involvement of the oculomotor nuclei.

Gosch, Gooding, and Schneider (1970) recorded the movement of the brain in the lexan calvarium on sudden impact. With displacement of the brain there was a concomitant compression of the intracranial contents followed by engorgement of cortical veins and diapedesis with petechial hemorrhages. The greater damage occurred at sites of fixation, and larger hemorrhages occurred in the upper spinal cord and in the brain stem. Hemorrhage within the brain stem may result in damage either to the nuclei or to the intramedullary fascicular portion of the cranial nerves. Lesions of the abducens nucleus produce paralysis of conjugate gaze to the same side rather than isolated paralysis of the lateral rectus as seen with lesions of the fascicular or peripheral portion of cranial nerve VI.

Cranial nerve involvement is frequent and expected in severe trauma, particularly when the midbrain has been injured. Jefferson (1962) has, however, described cases of head injury without loss of consciousness but with profound abnormalities of eye movements. He presented evidence that sufficient motion of the brain stem can occur in relation to the free edge of the tentorium so that at times trivial trauma may injure small vessels to the midbrain and result in disorders of eye movements.

Intracranial bleeding, as a result of trauma, occurs not infrequently in the postnatal period of life. Hollenhorst and associates (1957) noted an incidence of about 1 case per 4000 children per year and reported on 47 cases of intracranial bleeding. Of the 47 patients, 31 had subdural hematoma, 10 had subarachnoid hemorrhage, and 6 had subdural hygroma. The majority of these children were less than one year of age, and there was a probable history of trauma in 49 per cent of the cases. Seven presented with cranial nerve palsies, five affecting nerve VI (two bilaterally) and two affecting nerve III. Four of these seven patients with ocular palsies were left with permanent impairment of binocular vision. Intracranial bleeding in infants is usually attributed to tears in the veins of the poorly developed middle structures, due to shifting of the brain within the relatively rigid skull.

Prognosis

The prognosis for acquired traumatic palsies of cranial nerves III, IV, and VI depends on the degree of injury. Most of the patients who recover from an injury to the brain stem that has produced ocular disorders tend to recover ocular function, some rather rapidly and others over a period of several months. After injuries to the peripheral nerves, the nerve fibers regenerate at a rate of about 2.5 cm per month (Jefferson, 1962). When there has been total paralysis due to avulsion of the nerve, the prognosis for recovery of function is poor.

Aberrant Regeneration of Nerve III

When the axons of nerve III have been damaged, regeneration may occur with new axons developing from the severed ends or from collateral uninjured axons. This results in more axons within the regenerating nerve than were originally present. The new axons grow into the distal Schwann sheaths in a spurious manner and may terminate in ocular muscles other than those that they originally innervated. Walsh (1957) described the classic misdirection syndrome after total nerve III paralysis as totally random regeneration so that, on stimulation of nerve III, there is "mass movement" of all the muscles supplied by the nerve. This results in elevation of the upper lid, voluntarily or involuntarily, absence of vertical movement of the eye (because of cocontraction of the superior and inferior recti), adduction of the eye, and constriction of the pupil. There may be a small degree of retraction of the globe or enophthalmus in the fully developed syndrome. On abduction, the upper lid droops while the eye fully abducts.

More frequent than the classic mass movement are partial forms of aberrant regeneration in which fewer axons become misdirected, resulting in different patterns of eye movements in response to stimulation of nerve III. For example, should axons of the inferior rectus be misdirected into the iris sphincter or to the levator of the upper lid, on attempts to look down, the pupil would constrict or the upper lid would elevate.

Aberrant regeneration occurs most frequently after injury of nerve III by an aneurysm or by trauma. It is infrequent after nerve III paralysis due to neoplasm, inflammatory disease, or ischemic vascular disease. Cogan (1956) stated that it is unlikely to occur if recovery takes place within six weeks. Aberrant regeneration of nerve III is permanent and often results in loss of binocular vision because of the resultant diplopia.

NEOPLASMS

Whereas trauma accounts for about 15 per cent of acquired paralyses of cranial nerves III, IV, and VI, neoplasms account for about 20 to 25 per cent of such paralyses. In Rucker's (1958, 1966) series of 2000 cases of acquired ocular palsies, 428 were due to neoplasms: 241 involved nerve VI, 85 involved nerve III, and 10 involved nerve IV. This is comparable to a series of 3000 cases reported by Zielinski (1959) in which he found nerve VI affected in 66.3 per cent of his cases, nerve III affected in 20.3 per cent, and nerve IV affected in 1.3 per cent. Zielinski found a combined paralysis of nerves III, IV, and VI in 12.1 per cent of the cases.

Neoplasms involving the midbrain affect the nuclei and the intramedullary portion of the cranial nerves directly. Examples of such tumors are pontine gliomas, medulloblastomas, hemangiomas, and metastatic tumors. A lesion of the rostral midbrain producing progressive nerve III paralysis is well illustrated by the unique case of a patient with a solitary metastasis to the midbrain from a primary adenocarcinoma of the breast, reported by Stevenson and Hoyt (1963). The sequence began with abrupt bilateral ptosis, minimal oculomotor involvement, and normal pupils and progressed to complete extraocular paralysis and terminal pupillary paralysis. Coma and death resulted from extensive destruction of the mesencephalic reticular formation. Autopsy revealed a large solitary metastatic lesion extending through the entire anteroposterior extent of the quadrigeminal plate and adjoining tegmentum.

Parinaud in 1883 described lesions of the midbrain that produced paralysis of conjugate upward gaze and convergence. In 1903, Koerber described retractory nystagmus, although it remained for Salus and Elschnig, a few years later, to describe the complete clinical picture of nystagmus retractorius, paralysis of upward gaze, pupillary abnormalities, and papilledema associated with "malignant tumor" in the region of the pineal gland and the posterior third ventricle. Although this symptom complex allows for good localization to the rostral midbrain and pineal region, the exact physiology and pathways of the paraaqueductal gray matter are too poorly understood to explain the precise pathogenesis of this syndrome. From his study of gliomas limited to the quadrigeminal plate, Balthasar (1968) concluded that such tumors do not produce ocular disorders; it is only when such tumors extend beyond the quadrigeminal plate to the tegmentum or to the paraaqueductal gray matter that ocular disorders occur.

Pontine gliomas are a relatively frequent cause of acquired nerve VI paralysis as well as of horizontal gaze paralysis. This is especially true in children. Robertson, Hines, and Rucker (1970) reported on 133 cases of acquired esotropia in children; 52 cases were due to neoplasms, and 40 of these were identified as pontine gliomas. Excluding the cases of obvious severe trauma (evidenced by skull fractures or unconsciousness), intracranial tumors accounted for about half the cases reviewed. Other primary posterior fossa tumors encountered were meningioma, pinealoma, hemangioendothelioma, hemangioma, and craniopharyngioma. Nerve VI paralysis was the presenting sign in one fourth of these cases, with other neurologic signs appearing within a few weeks to a few months in the majority of the cases.

This is in contrast to a group of 12 cases of benign nerve VI palsy reported by Knox, Clark, and Schuster (1967). These children exhibited nerve VI palsy 1 to 3 weeks after a febrile illness, and in all but one it cleared within 10 weeks. From this experience, when nerve VI paralysis develops in a child after a febrile or an exanthematous disease, it would seem reasonable to observe the child for several weeks before beginning a more intensive diagnostic search for a brain tumor. As Bailey and associates (1939) have stressed, however, the development of multiple cranial nerve palsies in a child without an antecedent history of exanthematous disease strongly suggests an intracranial neoplasm.

Cushing (1910) proposed that lesions of the brain stem or subtentorial structures tend to stretch the arteries encircling the brain stem, particularly the anteroinferior cerebellar and anterior auditory arteries, to produce vascular strangulation of nerve VI. Supratentorial tumors may similarly displace the brain stem downward sufficiently to stretch nerve VI at its points of fixation or against the more rigid arterial branches of the basilar artery. Supratentorial tumors may cause the uncinate gyrus to herniate through the incisura and indirectly produce nerve III palsy. Not infrequently, with increased intracranial pressure, nerve III or VI or, more rarely, nerve IV is paralyzed; therefore, in the presence of papilledema, nerve III or nerve VI paralysis has to be evaluated with caution because it may be a false localizing sign. Gassel (1961) reported 40 cases of nerve III paralysis and 14 cases of nerve VI paralysis due to either a contralateral or a far-distant tumor in a series of 250 meningiomas. Meningiomas are often associated with false localizing signs because they are discrete tumors that tend to compress and displace structures of the central nervous system rather than to infiltrate cerebral and cranial nerve tissue. False localizing signs tend to be late manifestations of intracranial tumor and are usually associated with papilledema.

Contrary to the foregoing axiom—that, in the presence of an intracranial tumor, nerve VI paralysis has no localizing value—was the observation by Rucker (1966) that in 90 cases of nerve VI palsy due to primary intracranial neoplasm, 80 of them were due to an infratentorial tumor. In this series, 89 per cent of the intracranial tumors were near enough to affect nerve VI directly.

Tumors in the region of the cerebellopontine angle affect the nerves to the ocular muscles. Pool and Pava (1957) reported 18 cases of transient diplopia in 135 cases of acoustic neuroma. Palsies of the ocular muscles occur late in the course of an acoustic neuroma and are usually on the side of the tumor, although rarely they may be bilateral or on the opposite side. Nerve VI is affected most frequently. The ocular palsy is usually incomplete and often results secondarily from increased intracranial pressure rather than from direct growth of the tumor. The most frequent tumor of the cerebellopontine angle is the acoustic neurofibroma; it accounts for about 70 per cent of these tumors (Nager, 1967). Classically, it is composed of spindle-shaped fibroblasts arranged in a palisade formation. When there is a familial history of the disease, the acoustic neurofibroma may be considered as a manifestation of von

Recklinghausen's disease; rarely bilateral tumors may be present (Gardner and Frazier, 1930). Other cerebellopontine angle tumors may show characteristics of both a neurofibroma and a glioma; less frequently, meningiomas, gliomas, ependymomas, cholesteatomas, cysts, and aneurysms may occur in this location.

Neoplasms that occur in the region of the clivus affect the ocular nerves early in their course. An example of such a neoplasm is the chordoma, a tumor derived from remnants of the notochord and more frequently found in the sacrococcygeal region but occasionally presenting as an intracranial neoplasm. Intracranial chordomas account for about 1 per cent of intracranial tumors and occur predominantly in young men (Sassin and Chutorian, 1967). Although the tumor is a midline tumor of the clivus, there is a curious tendency for it to produce unilateral cranial nerve palsies, with nerves III and IV affected more frequently on the left side than bilaterally. The reason for this is not apparent. Nerve VI is most often affected, and this often is the initial sign of the tumor. Givner (1945) stated that an unexplained paralysis of nerve VI in a patient in his thirties, with progression to chiasmal signs and headaches but without evidence of pituitary disorder, should suggest a chordoma. The differential diagnosis must also include a nasopharyngeal tumor; rarely the chordoma may invade the nasopharynx.

Minor head injury without loss of consciousness or fracture rarely causes ocular palsy. Eyster, Hoyt, and Wilson (1972) reported three cases of parasellar or clival tumors in which the initial sign, paralysis of nerve III in two patients and of nerve VI in the third patient, was precipitated by a mild blow to the head (no skull fracture or loss of consciousness). In two cases the underlying tumor was a chordoma of the clivus; the third case proved to be a meningioma of the middle fossa. In contrast to the transient ocular palsies following minor trauma reported by Jefferson (1962), the ocular palsies in these tumor patients persisted for years after the initial injury before other signs and symptoms prompted more complete study and discovery of the underlying tumor. The late signs and symptoms mimicked subarachnoid hemorrhage from an intracranial aneurysm in all three patients, pain and nerve III paralysis in two, and increased intracranial pressure and bloody cerebrospinal fluid in one. Because of this experience, investigation for a basal tumor is advisable in cases of ocular palsy that occur after minor trauma, particularly when the palsy persists beyond a month or two.

In 1872, Bartholow first called attention to ocular palsies and trigeminal disturbances occurring with lesions within the cavernous sinus. Tumors of the pituitary gland may extend laterally into the cavernous sinus or, by their generally expanding size, may compress the cavernous sinus sufficiently to cause paresis of the cranial nerves within it. Nerve III, lying within the superior lateral wall of the cavernous sinus, is particularly liable to compression against the rigid interclinoid ligament. It is the most frequently affected, although nerves IV and VI as well as the ophthalmic branch of nerve V also may be affected.

Reported incidences of ophthalmoplegias caused by pituitary tumors vary considerably. Chamlin, Davidoff, and Feiring (1955) reported 8 cases of ophthalmoplegia in a series of 109 cases of pituitary tumors and also reported an incidence rate of about 10 per cent in other series that they reviewed. Pituitary adenomas accounted for 51 of the 428 cases of acquired ocular palsies due to neoplasms reported by Rucker (1958, 1966). German and Flanigan (1962) reported that Cushing had noted 24 instances of extraocular muscle palsies in 50 consecutive cases of pituitary tumor. Kearns and co-workers (1959) reported on 122 cases of Cushing's syndrome due to adrenal hyperplasia and found 12 cases of chromophobe pituitary adenoma that occurred after adrenalectomy. Of these 12 patients, 6 developed ocular symptoms, and 4 of these 6 developed oculomotor paresis due to parasellar extension of the tumor into the cavernous sinus. One of these patients died from metastatic spread of the chromophobe adenoma to the posterior fossa, lumbosacral plexus, and liver. Malignant tumors of the pituitary gland are unusual (Kearns et al., 1959; Walsh and Hoyt, 1969).

A sudden hemorrhage within a pituitary tumor may result in a rapid onset of loss of vision and ophthalmoplegia of one or both eyes. This is usually accompanied by severe headache in the classic "pituitary apoplexy." In such cases the prognosis for recovery of ocular muscle function is good after immediate surgical evacuation of the hemorrhagic tumor. Walsh and Hoyt (1969) reported on a patient, described by David, who developed almost complete bilateral ophthalmoplegia with normal visual acuity and only questionable temporal field defects after an acute hemorrhage into a pituitary adenoma. After surgical treatment there was rapid recovery from the left ophthalmoplegia; however, recovery from the right oculomotor paralysis was in an aberrant manner.

François and Neetens (1968) have stated that oculomotor paralysis usually occurs at a late stage in cases of pituitary tumor; however, they described 40 cases in the literature and 2 cases of their own in which the oculomotor paralysis occurred at an early stage and was the initial symptom of a pituitary tumor. Usually, this was a partial paralysis of nerve III and probably was due to backward and upward extension of a portion of the tumor into the cavernous sinus, compressing the nerve against the dura at its entrance into the sinus. Again, the prognosis is good after surgical treatment, and the ocular palsy usually disappears promptly. Of interest is the report of an isolated nerve III paralysis, with normal visual fields, due to a pituitary tumor in a patient who presented with acute ptosis and pain in the eye resulting from acute angle closure glaucoma secondary to the dilated pupil and internal ophthalmoplegia (Miller and Colton, 1968).

The nasopharynx is a not infrequent site for neoplasms that extend intracranially, often into the cavernous sinus, where they affect the cranial nerves to the extraocular muscles. Godtfredsen and Lederman (1965) reported on 672 cases of malignant tumors of the nasopharynx, of which 240 presented with symptoms of intracranial involvement. Of the 672, 3 per cent presented with ophthalmoplegia; this is similar to the 45 cases of acquired ocular palsies in a series of 2000 reported by Rucker (1958, 1966) as due to nasopharyngeal tumors. Among the ocular palsies, that of nerve VI is the most frequent; in the series of 381 patients evaluated by Thomas and Waltz (1965), this nerve was involved in 68 per cent of the patients. Other cranial nerves traversing the middle fossa are also susceptible to injury because Rosenmüller's fossa, the classic site of origin for nasopharyngeal tumors, lies directly beneath the foramen lacerum. Malignant tumors in this region spread easily into the middle fossa or cavernous sinus through the foramen lacerum or the foramen ovale. In Godtfredsen

and Lederman's experience, nerve V was more frequently involved than nerve VI; Thomas and Waltz found the reverse. A combination of trigeminal face pain and ophthalmoplegia, the classic cavernous sinus syndrome, occurred in 20 per cent of the total 672 cases of nasopharyngeal tumors. Jefferson (1953) noted the corollary to this also to be true — that is, 20 per cent of the cases of cavernous sinus syndrome were due to malignat nasopharyngeal tumors. Thus a malignant nasopharyngeal tumor becomes a significant and frequent cause for painful ophthalmoplegia.

All unexplained nerve VI palsies require a thorough examination of the nasopharynx, especially when there is simultaneous occurrence of ophthalmoplegia and facial pain. Repeated examination of the nasopharynx may be necessary to detect the tumor, as well as roentgenograms of the base of the skull and biopsies of suspected cervical lymph nodes. Occasionally, a blind biopsy of the nasopharynx may be worth consideration.

The prognosis for patients with nasopharyngeal tumors that have extended into the cranial cavity is extremely poor. Thomas and Waltz (1965) reported a 24 per cent five year survival rate, and Godtfredsen and Lederman (1965) reported a 17 per cent 10 year survival rate in all patients followed who had nasopharyngeal tumors. Of those with neurologic deficits and cranial nerve involvement, each series included only one patient who survived longer than 10 years. Thomas and Waltz noted that more than one third of patients died within the first year after the onset of nervous system complications. Tumors encountered most frequently within the nasopharynx are squamous cell carcinomas, lymphoepitheliomas, and lymphosarcomas, all of varying degrees of radiosensitivity (Scanlon et al., 1958).

Intracranial metastatic tumors account for about 40 per cent of the neoplasms that affect nerves III, IV, and VI. The most frequent primary source is the nasopharynx. The other sources for metastatic tumors are widely scattered throughout the body and include the breast, thyroid, lung, and lymphoid tissue. Frequently, metastatic disease affects the cranial nerve by direct infiltration. Rubinstein (1969) evaluated 13 patients in whom nerves V and XII were affected as the first evidence of intracranial metastases and found direct meningeal or cranial nerve infiltration by the tumor. In 8 of these 13 patients, the involvement progressed to other cranial nerves (nerves VI and III most frequently), and all the patients had an active primary neoplasm at the time the cranial nerves became involved. The cranial nerve symptoms responded to chemotherapy or radiotherapy of the underlying disease as well as of the cranial nerve involvement, although the median length of survival after the onset of cranial nerve involvement was only three months. Robertson, Hines, and Rucker (1970) reported an average survival of five months in six children with disease metastatic to the posterior fossa (three neuroblastomas, one small-cell carcinoma of the nasopharynx, one lymphosarcoma of the nasopharynx, and one rhabdomyosarcoma invading nerve VI after extension from the inner ear).

Whisnant, Siekert, and Sayre (1956) noted involvement of the central nervous system in 10 to 25 per cent of patients with lymphomas; reticulum cell sarcomas invaded the central nervous system most frequently. Occasionally, a reticulum cell sarcoma or a lymphosarcoma will first manifest itself by neurologic signs and symptoms. Direct extension from the nasopharynx or cervical lymph nodes may invade basal structures and frequently affect the cranial nerves by diffuse infiltration of the meninges as well as by cranial nerve infiltration. Schwab and Weiss (1935) found that 30 per cent of patients with leukemia involving the central nervous system had cranial nerve involvement.

Neurologic syndromes associated with carcinoma but not due to metastatic lesions or to direct involvement of the central nervous system take several forms and involve any level of the nervous system. Carcinomatous neuromyopathies occur and result in proximal muscle weakness and wasting of muscle associated with loss of tendon reflexes; clinically, it is difficult to distinguish this from a lower motor neuron lesion or a minor degree of myopathy. Paralysis of the extraocular muscles may be seen as a part of the neuromyopathy or with other cerebellar or brain stem signs. Rarely, if ever, however, does isolated paralysis of cranial nerve III, IV, or VI occur as a result of a distant extracranial malignant neoplasm.

The cause of the neurologic manifestations of distant malignant tumors is unknown. Carcinoma of the lung, and in particular the oat cell carcinoma, accounted for more than 50 per cent of the cases reported by Croft and Wilkinson (1965). A review of the incidence of neuropathy associated with bronchogenic carcinoma cited two reported series with incidence rates of 1.7 per cent and 1.3 per cent, and stated that Brain and Henson (1958) had estimated that 5 per cent of all bronchogenic carcinomas are associated with neuromuscular disorders (Greenberg et al., 1964). An excellent brief review of this topic was published by Diamond (1961).

VASCULAR DISEASE AND ANEURYSMS

Acquired ocular palsies are frequently the result of vascular disease. Within the brain stem the nuclei are supplied by end arteries arising from the posterior cerebral or basilar artery without significant collateral circulation; therefore, thrombosis of or hemorrhage from these vessels results in varying degrees of ocular palsy. Arteriosclerosis is an important factor in the cause of such ophthalmoplegias. Weber (1971) stated that 50 per cent of cases of nerve III palsy occur in patients with hypertension and arteriosclerosis. The acute ocular palsies seen in infections and toxic diseases also may be the result of vascular lesions.

Ocular palsies due to vertebral-basilar arterial disease usually are associated with other signs and symptoms of brain stem and cerebellar involvement; rarely, partial or complete ophthalmoplegia may be the only evidence (Harel et al., 1967). Minor and associates (1959) reviewed 183 cases of vertebral-basilar artery disease and noted varying degrees of paralysis of cranial nerves III, IV, and VI in 27 per cent. Masucci (1965) described 5 cases of bilateral ocular palsy in 200 cases of stroke due to vertebral-basilar artery disease.

The association of ocular palsies and diabetes mellitus in well recognized. Rucker (1958, 1966) found nerves III and VI to be about equally affected and nerve IV less frequently affected. The acute oculomotor palsy associated with diabetes is characterized by sudden onset of ptosis and paralysis of the extraocular muscles supplied by nerve III. Initially there may be severe pain within or behind the orbit in the distribution of the ophthalmic division of nerve V. The pupillomotor fibers within nerve III are frequently spared, and the response to light and accommodation are normal. A normal pupil was found in 75 per cent of the 110 cases of oculomotor palsy attributed to vascular disease by Rucker (1958, 1966); this has been the experience of others as well. Recovery usually begins in a few weeks and is usually complete within six to eight weeks. Only rarely does an oculomotor palsy associated with diabetes recover in an aberrant manner. Walsh (1957) reported only four cases of aberrant regeneration of nerve III in patients with diabetes.

Demyelination with some loss of axons within the central portion of the peripheral part of nerve III has been the essential finding in three reports describing the clinicopathologic features of oculomotor palsy in diabetes mellitus. Dreyfus, Hakim, and Adams (1957) noted a focal zone of myelin sheath and axon destruction within the intracavernous portion of the nerve. Although they were unable to find any occluded vessels in the many sections they studied, they concluded that the lesion was ischemic in origin and postulated an occluded nutrient vessel remote from the site of fiber degeneration. Asbury and co-workers (1970) also found a circumscribed patch of demyelination within the intracavernous portion of nerve III. Its borders were sharply demarcated on the proximal edge and less distinct on the distal edge. There was a paucity of axonal degeneration distally and an absence of central chromatolysis in the cell bodies of the nerve III nucleus, both features consistent with a demyelinating process and with the rapid and complete recovery seen in most cases of oculomotor palsy associated with diabetes mellitus. Weber, Daroff, and Mackey (1970) reported similar demyelination with some loss of central axons within the subarachnoid portion of nerve III. Hyalinization of the intraneural arterioles was evident, but no occluded vessels were found.

Relevant to the ischemic theory for diabetic neuropathy is the study by Dyck, Conn, and Okazaki (1972) of the peripheral nerves of patients with necrotizing angiopathy and neuropathy. Similar central fascicular fiber degeneration was noted, with only an occasional occluded vessel in the vicinity of the fiber degeneration. They postulated that there were areas within the peripheral nerves examined (the mid–upper arm and midthigh levels) that represented watershed zones of poor perfusion. Under these conditions the ischemic effects would be greatest within the most remote portion of a region supplied by a specific epineurial vessel or vessels, and the typical picture of an infarct with softening and necrosis would not be seen even though the underlying mechanism might be occlusive vascular disease.

All three studies of the pathology of nerve III noted a relative sparing of the peripheral fibers (Asbury et al., 1970; Dreyfus et al., 1957; Weber et al., 1970). Dreyfus, Hakim, and Adams (1957) hypothesized that the superficial position of the fine "parasympathetic" fibers protected them from the effects of ischemia. The same argument is used for their greater susceptibility to injury from external pressure.

Oculomotor palsy secondary to an aneurysm may have a clinical picture similar to that of the oculomotor palsy associated with diabetes, except that the pupil is only rarely normal in nerve III paralysis due to an aneurysm. Rucker (1966) observed only 4 cases in which the pupil was normal in 114 cases of nerve III palsy resulting from aneurysms. The retroorbital pain associated with an aneurysm is similar to although more constant than that in diabetic nerve III palsy. The duration of the paralysis caused by an aneurysm is more prolonged, and recovery is frequently associated with aberrant regeneration (Walsh, 1957).

The most common cause of sudden onset of nerve III paralysis in an adult, with headache and a dilated fixed pupil, is an aneurysm at the junction of the posterior communicating artery and the internal carotid artery (Smith, personal communication). This is especially true in women more than 40 years old. In a cooperative study of subarachnoid hemorrhages, it was noted that 56 per cent of the subarachnoid hemorrhages due to a bleeding aneurysm occurred in women and that the aneurysm was located at the posterior communicating–internal carotid junction more than twice as frequently in women as in men (Sahs et al., 1969).

Of the 2672 bleeding aneurysms reported in the cooperative study, 94.5 per cent arose from the internal carotid artery. The region of the anterior communicating artery was the most common site of the aneurysm, as noted previously by Henderson (1956). Aneurysms in this location do not affect the cranial nerves to the ocular muscles directly, but may result in ocular palsies secondary to the hemorrhage and increased intracranial pressure. Aneurysms at the junction of the posterior communicating and internal carotid arteries accounted for 25 per cent of the bleeding aneurysms and made up the majority of the unruptured symptomatic aneurysms reported in the cooperative study. These aneurysms are in close proximity to nerve III and frequently affect this nerve. Nerve VI is affected less frequently, and only rarely is nerve IV affected by an aneurysm.

Only a small percentage of patients with aneurysms have symptoms prior to their first subarachnoid hemorrhage. In the cooperative study, unruptured aneurysms constituted 5 per cent of the group. The majority of these patients presented with headache, orbital pain, and varying degrees of oculomotor palsy.

Reports on the prognosis for recovery of ocular function after treatment of an intracranial aneurysm have varied. Jefferson (1947) and Troupp, Koskinen, and af Björkesten (1958) reported a poor prognosis with frequent incomplete or aberrant regeneration of an incapacitating degree. Others (Hepler and Cantu, 1967; Johnston and Pratt-Johnston, 1963) have reported much more favorable results. Hepler and Cantu (1967) described the follow-up of a typical patient in this way:

. . . a 59 year old woman who developed her acute third nerve paralysis associated with an aneurysm at or near the origin of the posterior communicating artery seven years prior to [their] evaluation. She now enjoys good general health, but is reminded of the previous illness by occasional diplopia. In addition, she or those about her note minor peculiarities in the movement of her upper eyelid. Upon examination she displays pupillary abnormalities, as well as involvement of the levator palpebrae superioris and extraocular muscles in aberrant regeneration of the third nerve. Adduction, depression and particularly elevation of the involved globe are limited.

Aneurysms within the cavernous sinus are infrequent, accounting for only 1.9 per cent of the aneurysms reported in the cooperative study. Intracavernous aneurysms produce symptoms of an expanding mass, with headache, sensory impairment over the distribution of the ophthalmic division of cranial nerve V, and slowly progressive ipsilateral ophthalmoplegia often followed by loss of vision on the same side. A significant case report is that by Keane and Talalla (1972) describing a patient with a posttraumatic intracavernous aneurysm who responded well to surgical occlusion of the internal carotid artery above and below the aneurysm. The importance of recognizing such a lesion is attested to by the fact that in 50 per cent of the reported cases the patient died from profuse nasal hemorrhage before the diagnosis was established. The diagnosis should be suspected in any patient who has sustained a major head injury, who had loss of vision at the time of the injury or shortly thereafter with involvement of ipsilateral cranial nerve III, IV, V, or VI, and who then begins to have repeated nosebleeds of increasing severity and frequency. Angiography should reveal the aneurysm within the cavernous sinus and extending into the sphenoid sinus. Prompt surgical treatment can be lifesaving.

INFECTIONS AND TOXINS

Acquired ocular palsies are infrequent manifestations of infectious disease. In several of the neurotropic viral encephalitides, such as St. Louis encephalitis or Eastern and Western equine encephalitis, ocular palsies are extremely rare; in von Economo's encephalitis and bulbar poliomyelitis, ophthalmoplegia may occur. Paralyses of cranial nerves III, IV, and VI are less frequent in bulbar poliomyelitis than are paralyses of cranial nerves VII, X, XI, and XII. In other viral diseases, ocular palsies are much less frequent than other signs of meningitis and encephalitis and, when present, are often a late manifestation occurring two to three weeks after the febrile illness.

Postinfectious encephalitis most frequently occurs after rabies vaccination; it may be seen infrequently after other immunizations as well as after infections such as smallpox, vaccinia, varicella, measles, infectious mononucleosis, herpes zoster, influenza, and pertussis. The incidence of neurologic manifestations after measles, for example, is reported to range from 1 to 50 per 10,000 cases (Aita, 1964). The majority of these patients present with signs of encephalitis. Only a small percentage present with signs of a polyradiculitis with extraocular paralysis. Schnell and co-workers (1966) reviewed 1285 cases of infectious mononucleosis and found only 12 with neurologic manifestations; of these 12 cases, only 1 had involvement of cranial nerves III and IV. The pathogenesis of the postinfectious ophthalmoplegia remains obscure. A few clinicopathologic studies have shown evidence of neuronal degeneration within the nuclei of nerves III, IV, and

VI, as well as swelling and demyelination of the peripheral nerves (Bergin, 1960; Dolgopol and Husson, 1949; Peters et al., 1947).

Ocular palsies are more frequent with bacterial infections, particularly when the meninges are involved. Impaired ocular movement was the most frequent sign of cranial nerve dysfunction in 147 cases of acute bacterial meningitis reported by Swartz and Dodge (1965). In this group there were 26 cases of ocular palsy, equally divided between cranial nerves III and VI. The ocular palsies tended to be transient and to disappear shortly after recovery from the meningitis. Walsh and Hoyt (1969) reported a case of bilateral nerve III paralysis in a patient with acute pneumococcal meningitis who recovered completely without any evidence of aberrant regeneration. This is in contrast to the damage often sustained by nerve VIII; permanent hearing loss is an important sequela of acute bacterial meningitis. Usually there is perineural inflammation that extends into the substance of the peripheral nerve; this is most often seen in the purulent meningitis due to Meningococcus, Pneumococcus, or *Haemophilus influenzae.*

Although the antibiotic era has brought about a remarkable change in the spectrum of diseases, unfortunately it has not eliminated the infectious diseases. One of the more ubiquitous organisms, *Treponema pallidum,* continues to account for a significant number of cases of acquired ocular palsy. Duke-Elder (1971) stated that syphilis in one form or another used to account for 40 per cent of the ocular palsies, and even as recently as 1964, Green, Hackett, and Schlezinger reported that 12 of 130 cases of oculomotor paresis were due to syphilis. Shrader and Schlezinger (1960) presented 104 cases of abducens palsy of which 10 were due to syphilis, although Rucker (1966) was only able to attribute 1 case of oculomotor palsy to syphilis in his second series of 1000 cases of acquired ocular palsy collected between the years 1958 and 1964. Patient selection may well be a factor in the low incidence observed by Rucker.

In basilar meningitis due to syphilis, the branches of the cranial nerves are often affected as they emerge from the brain stem. Nerve III is most commonly affected, although nerves IV and VI as well as other cranial nerves may be affected within the meningeal spaces. The paralysis is often incomplete,

with the pupillomotor fibers and the fibers to the medial recti seeming to be particularly vulnerable to basilar inflammation. The inflammatory process may extend forward to the superior orbital fissure and there result in paresis of nerves III, IV, and VI as well as the ophthalmic division of nerve V. The ocular palsies of meningovascular syphilis usually respond favorably to antibiotic therapy.

Tuberculosis involving the meninges may affect the cranial nerves in a similar manner. The pupillomotor fibers of nerve III are more often affected than are the fibers to the extraocular muscles.

The finding of a low glucose concentration in cerebrospinal fluid usually leads to an initial consideration of pyogenic, tuberculous, or mycotic meningitis. When only a few cells are present, the diagnosis usually is between tuberculosis or mycotic meningitis. Swartz and Dodge (1965) pointed out that neoplasms such as carcinomas, gliomas, melanomas, sarcomas, or lymphomas may also be associated with hypoglycorrhachia and that a decreased cerebrospinal fluid glucose value in association with increased intracranial pressure, mental deterioration, meningeal irritation, and multiple cranial nerve signs in the absence of infection strongly suggests the diagnosis of a diffuse meningeal tumor.

There are a number of entities that affect the cranial nerves to the ocular muscles for which the cause is not clearly evident; infections may play a role but are not directly the cause of these ocular palsies.

In 1904, Gradenigo described a "special syndrome" of external rectus paralysis in children and adolescents with signs of inflammation within the mastoid or inner ear. These patients may experience pain in or about the ipsilateral eye and have facial weakness on the same side together with photophobia, lacrimation, and decreased corneal sensation. Symonds (1944) proposed that some patients with "Gradenigo's syndrome" may develop increased intracranial pressure and papilledema due to aseptic thrombophlebitis of the lateral sinus with extension into the inferior petrosal sinus and involvement of nerve VI lying adjacent to the inferior petrosal sinus within Dorello's canal. This he called "otitic hydrocephalus," a term that is infrequently used at the present time. The pathologic features are more often those of inflammatory petrositis with involvement of nerve VI in its extradural course in this region. Bilateral abducens paresis may occur, particularly in those patients with papilledema. The clinical picture is much too benign for meningitis or a brain abscess, which the signs may suggest, and recovery is usually spontaneous although antibiotics are indicated for the mastoiditis or inner ear infection.

In 1954, Tolosa described a patient who presented with retroorbital pain, vomiting, paralysis of cranial nerves III, IV, and VI, and a diminished corneal reflex. Similar symptoms had occurred three years before with complete recovery. Angiography had shown a narrowing of the carotid siphon just distal to the cavernous sinus. The patient died three days after a negative surgical exploration; autopsy revealed the intracavernous portion of the carotid artery to be wrapped in granulomatous tissue that was not obstructing the lumen of the sinus but was affecting the adjacent cranial nerves. In 1961, Hunt and co-workers described six cases of recurrent painful ophthalmoplegia that, they thought, represented a clinical entity similar to that described by Tolosa. Since then there have been a number of reports attesting to the reality of such a clinical entity but demonstrating no cause (Mathew and Chandy, 1970; Smith and Taxdal, 1966). A recent paper by Hallpike (1973) indicates that the Tolosa-Hunt syndrome is probably part of a spectrum that includes orbital "pseudotumor" and also that angiographic changes may be found. Hunt and associates (1961) described the following criteria for the syndrome: (1) pain may precede the ophthalmoplegia by several days or may not appear until sometime later; (2) there is paresis of nerves III, IV, and VI, the first division of nerve V, and the periarterial sympathetic and the optic nerves; (3) symptoms last for days or weeks; (4) spontaneous remissions occur, sometimes with residual neurologic defects; (5) attacks recur at intervals of months or years; and (6) exhaustive studies, including angiography and surgical exploration, show no evidence of involvement of structures outside the cavernous sinus. There usually is no systemic reaction. Although systemic administration of steroids may produce dramatic relief of symptoms, it is not wise to use this as a diagnostic criterion. Thomas and Yoss (1970) pointed out the hazard of doing so, noting that neoplasms may also respond favorably to steroids temporarily. The diagnosis is wisely made only after carefully excluding other more serious causes of painful ophthalmoplegia.

Guillain-Barré syndrome, an acute symmetrical polyneuritis of unknown etiology first described by Landry in 1859, is characterized by a rapidly ascending involvement of the peripheral nerves, with motor involvement more pronounced than sensory involvement. As the flaccid paralysis ascends to the bulbar region, the cranial nerves may be affected, although frequently this stops short of the cranial nuclei within the pons and midbrain. Papilledema may accompany a markedly increased spinal fluid protein concentration. There are variants in which involvement of the cranial nerves is the predominant feature. In 1956, Fisher described three patients who developed progressive total ophthalmoplegia as well as ataxia and areflexia after an upper respiratory tract infection. All three had a benign course with full recovery in three to six weeks. Thomas and associates (1969) reported five cases of recurrent and chronic relapsing polyneuritis of the Guillain-Barré type and reviewed the clinicopathologic features of the disease. Segmental demyelination, with little destruction of axons, and foci of perivascular lymphocytes were seen in the peripheral nerves as well as within the ventral and dorsal roots. The similarity to recent studies of chronic relapsing experimental allergic neuritis in animals was discussed. In none of these cases was cranial nerve III, IV, or VI affected.

Acquired ocular palsies may be the result of cranial nerve involvement by cranial arteritis, although more commonly the extraocular muscles are primarily affected.

In multiple sclerosis, Ivers and Goldstein (1963) noted that 11 per cent of patients presented with diplopia, and Rucker reported that 50 of his 1000 cases of acquired ocular palsies were due to multiple sclerosis, nerve VI being affected most often.

Sarcoidosis involving the central nervous system often causes symptoms of recurrent cranial nerve palsy. The facial nerve (cranial nerve VII) is affected much more frequently than are cranial nerves III, IV, and VI. In 118 cases reviewed by Colover (1948), the facial nerve was involved in 58 cases; there were only 6 cases of ptosis, 3 of nerve III paralysis, and 1 of nerve IV paralysis. Peripheral neuropathies, both spinal and cranial, may be the earliest manifestation of sarcoidosis, and usually recovery is complete.

Toxic effects on the cranial nerves to the ocular muscles are best illustrated by the acute loss of accommodation and mydriasis seen with botulism. The ocular symptoms occur from 12 hours to several days after ingestion of contaminated food. Internal ophthalmoplegia is common also in diphtheria and may progress to a more complete nerve III paralysis, although total ophthalmoplegia is rare. The site of action of the neurotoxic substance may be the oculomotor nuclei, within the peripheral nerve, or the motor endplate of the muscle.

References

Aita, J. A.: Neurologic Manifestations of General Diseases. Springfield, Ill., Charles C Thomas, 1964.

Asbury, A. K., Aldredge, H., Hershberg, R., and Fisher, C. M.: Oculomotor palsy in diabetes mellitus: a clinicopathological study. Brain, 93:555, 1970.

Bailey, P., Buchanan, D. N., and Bucy, P. C.: Intracranial Tumors in Infancy and Childhood. Chicago, University of Chicago Press, 1939, pp. 188, 238–239.

Balthasar, K.: Gliomas of the quadrigeminal plate and eye movements. Ophthalmologica, 155:249, 1968.

Bartholow, R.: 1872. Cited by Chamlin, M., Davidoff, L. M., and Feiring, E. H.

Bielschowsky, A.: Lectures on motor anomalies. XI. Etiology, prognosis, and treatment of ocular paralyses. Am. J. Ophthalmol., 22:723, 1939.

Bergin, J. D.: Fatal encephalopathy in glandular fever. J. Neurol. Neurosurg. Psychiatry, 23:69, 1960.

Blodi, F. C., Van Allen, M. W., and Yarbrough, J. C.: Duane's syndrome: a brain stem lesion; an electromyographic study. Arch. Ophthalmol., 72:171, 1964.

Brain, R., and Henson, R. A.: 1958. Cited by Greenberg, E., Divertie, M. B., and Woolner, L. B.

Breinin, G. M.: Electromyography: a tool in ocular and neurologic diagnosis. II. Muscle palsies. Arch. Ophthalmol., 57:165, 1957.

Burger, L. J., Kalvin, N. H., and Smith, J. L.: Acquired lesions of the fourth cranial nerve. Brain, 93:567, 1970.

Burian, H. M., Van Allen, M. W., Sexton, R. R., and Baller, R. S.: Substitution phenomena in congenital and acquired supranuclear disorders of eye movement. Trans. Am. Acad. Ophthalmol. Otolaryngol., 69:1105, 1965.

Chamlin, M., Davidoff, L. M., and Feiring, E. H.: Ophthalmologic changes produced by pituitary tumors. Am. J. Ophthalmol., 40:353, 1955.

Cogan, D. G.: Neurology of the Ocular Muscles. 2nd Edition. Springfield, Ill., Charles C Thomas, 1956.

Colover, J.: Sarcoidosis with involvement of the nervous system. Brain, 71:451, 1948.

Croft, P. B., and Wilkinson, M.: The incidence of carcinomatous neuromyopathy in patients with various types of carcinoma. Brain, 88:427, 1965.

Cushing, H.: Strangulation of the nervi abducentes by lateral branches of the basilar artery in cases of brain tumour: with an explanation of some obscure palsies on the basis of arterial constriction. Brain, 33:204, 1910.

Diamond, M. T.: Carcinomatous neuropathy. Ann. Intern. Med., 54:1259, 1961.

Dolgopol, V. B., and Husson, G. S.: Infectious mono-

nucleosis with neurologic complications. Arch. Intern. Med., 83:179, 1949.

Dreyfus, P. M., Hakim, S., and Adams, R. D.: Diabetic ophthalmoplegia: report of case, with postmortem study and comments on vascular supply of human oculomotor nerve. Arch. Neurol., 77:337, 1957.

Duane, A.: Congenital deficiency of abduction, associated with impairment of adduction, retraction movements, contraction of the palpebral fissure and oblique movements of the eyes. Arch. Ophthalmol., 34:133, 1905.

Duke-Elder, S.: System of Ophthalmology. Vol. 12. St. Louis, C. V. Mosby Co., 1971, p. 759.

Dyck, P. J., Conn, D. L., and Okazaki, H.: Necrotizing angiopathic neuropathy: three-dimensional morphology of fiber degeneration related to sites of occluded vessels. Mayo Clin. Proc., 47:461, 1972.

Dyck, P. J., Gutrecht, J. A., Bastron, J. A., Karnes, W. E., and Dale, A. J. D.: Histologic and teased-fiber measurements of sural nerve in disorders of lower motor and primary sensory neurons. Mayo Clin. Proc., 43:81, 1968.

Elschnig, A.: Cited by Wolf, J. K.: The Classical Brain Syndromes. Springfield, Ill., Charles C Thomas, 1971, p. 155.

Eyster, E. F., Hoyt, W. F., and Wilson, C. B.: Oculomotor palsy from minor head trauma: an initial sign of basal intracranial tumor. J.A.M.A., 220:1083, 1972.

Fisher, M.: An unusual variant of acute idiopathic polyneuritis (syndrome of ophthalmoplegia, ataxia, and areflexia). N. Engl. J. Med., 255:57, 1956.

François, J., and Neetens, A.: Oculomotor paralyses and tumors of the pituitary gland. Confin. Neurol., 30:239, 1968.

Gardner, W. J., and Frazier, C. H.: Bilateral acoustic neurofibromas: a clinical study and field survey of a family of five generations with bilateral deafness in thirty-eight members. Arch. Neurol. Psychiatry, 23:266, 1930.

Gassel, M. M.: False localizing signs: a review of the concept and analysis of the occurrence in 250 cases of intracranial meningioma. Arch. Neurol., 4:526, 1961.

German, W. J., and Flanigan, S.: Pituitary adenomas: a follow-up study of the Cushing series. Clin. Neurosurg., 10:72, 1962.

Givner, I.: Ophthalmologic features of intracranial chordoma and allied tumors of the clivus. Arch. Ophthalmol., 33:397, 1945.

Godtfredsen, E., and Lederman, M.: Diagnostic and prognostic roles of ophthalmoneurologic signs and symptoms in malignant nasopharyngeal tumors. Am. J. Ophthalmol., 59:1063, 1965.

Gosch, H. H., Gooding, E., and Schneider, R. C.: The lexan calvarium for the study of cerebral responses to acute trauma. J. Trauma, 10:370, 1970.

Gradenigo, G.: A special syndrome of endocranial otitic complications (paralysis of the motor oculi externus of otitic origin). Ann. Otol. Rhinol. Laryngol., 13:637, 1904.

Green, W. R., Hackett, E. R., and Schlezinger, N. S.: Neuroophthalmologic evaluation of oculomotor nerve paralysis. Arch. Ophthalmol., 72:154, 1964.

Greenberg, E., Divertie, M. B., and Woolner, L. B.: A review of unusual systemic manifestations associated with carcinoma. Am. J. Med., 36:106, 1964.

Hallpike, J. F.: Superior orbital fissure syndrome: some clinical and radiological observations. J. Neurol. Neurosurg. Psychiatry, 36:486–490, 1973.

Harel, D., Lavy, S., and Schwartz, A.: Ophthalmoplegia

as a manifestation of basilar artery disease. Am. J. Ophthalmol., 63:519, 1967.

Henderson, J. L.: The congenital facial diplegia syndrome: clinical features, pathology and aetiology; a review of sixty-one cases. Brain, 62:381, 1939.

Henderson, J. W.: Intracranial artery aneurysms: a study of 119 cases, with special reference to the ocular findings. Trans. Am. Ophthalmol. Soc., 53:349, 1956.

Hepler, R. S., and Cantu, R. C.: Aneurysms and third nerve palsies. Arch. Ophthalmol., 77:604, 1967.

Hollenhorst, R. W., Stein, H. A., Keith, H. M., and MacCarty, C. S.: Subdural hematoma, subdural hygroma and subarachnoid hemorrhage among infants and children. Neurology (Minneap.), 7:813, 1957.

Hoyt, W. F., and Nachtigäller, H.: Anomalies of ocular motor nerves: neuroanatomic correlates of paradoxical innervation in Duane's syndrome and related congenital ocular motor disorders. Am. J. Ophthalmol., 60:443, 1965.

Hunt, W. E., Meagher, J. N., LeFever, H. E., and Zeman, W.: Painful ophthalmoplegia: its relation to indolent inflammation of the cavernous sinus. Neurology (Minneap.), 11:56, 1961.

Ivers, R. R., and Goldstein, N. P.: Multiple sclerosis: a current appraisal of symptoms and signs. Proc. Staff Meet. Mayo Clin., 38:457, 1963.

Jefferson, A.: Ocular complications of head injuries. Trans. Ophthalmol. Soc. U.K., 81:595, 1962.

Jefferson, G.: The tentorial pressure cone. Arch. Neurol. Psychiatry, 40:857, 1938.

Jefferson, G.: Isolated oculomotor palsy caused by intracranial aneurysm. Proc. R. Soc. Med., 40:419, 1947.

Jefferson, G.: The Bowman lecture: concerning injuries, aneurysms and tumours involving the cavernous sinus. Trans. Ophthalmol. Soc. U.K., 73:117, 1953.

Johnston, A. C., and Pratt-Johnston, J. A.: The ocular sequelae of third cranial nerve palsy. Can. Med. Assoc. J., 89:871, 1963.

Keane, J. R., and Talalla, A.: Posttraumatic intracavernous aneurysm. Arch. Ophthalmol., 87:701, 1972.

Kearns, T. P., Salassa, R. M., Kernohan, J. W., and MacCarty, C. S.: Ocular manifestations of pituitary tumor in Cushing's syndrome. Arch. Ophthalmol., 62:242, 1959.

Kernohan, J. W., and Woltman, H. W.: Incisura of the crus due to contralateral brain tumor. Arch. Neurol. Psychiatry, 21:274, 1929.

Kerr, F. W. L., and Hollowell, O. W.: Location of pupillomotor and accommodation fibres in the oculomotor nerve: experimental observations of paralytic mydriasis. J. Neurol. Neurosurg. Psychiatry, n.s. 27:473, 1964.

Knies, M.: Ueber die centralen Störungen der willkürlichen Augenmuskeln. Arch. Augenheilkd., 23:19, 1891.

Knox, D. L., Clark, D. B., and Schuster, F. F.: Benign VI nerve palsies in children. Pediatrics, 40:560, 1967.

Koerber, H.: 1903. Cited by Wolf, J. K.: The Classical Brain Syndromes. Springfield, Ill., Charles C Thomas, 1971, p. 155.

Landry, O.: Note sur la paralysie ascendante aiguë. Gaz. Hebd. Méd. Chir., 6:472, 1859.

Magoun, H. W., Atlas, D., Hare, W. K., and Ranson, S. W.: The afferent path of the pupillary light reflex in the monkey. Brain, 59:234, 1936.

Masucci, E. F.: Bilateral ophthalmoplegia in basilar-vertebral artery disease. Brain, 88:97, 1965.

Mathew, N. T., and Chandy, J.: Painful ophthalmoplegia. J. Neurol. Sci., 11:243, 1970.

Meyer, A.: Herniation of the brain. Arch. Neurol. Psychiatry, 4:387, 1920.

Miller, W. W., and Colton, R. P.: Oculomotor paralysis without visual field loss in pituitary tumor: case report. Trans. Pac. Coast Otoophthalmol. Soc., 49:243, 1968.

Minor, R. H., Kearns, T. P., Millikan, C. H., Siekert, R. G., and Sayre, G. P.: Ocular manifestations of occlusive disease of the vertebral-basilar arterial system. Arch. Ophthalmol., 62:84, 1959.

Moebius, P. J.: 1888, 1892. Cited by Henderson, J. L.

Nager, G. T.: Gliomas involving the temporal bone: clinical and pathologic aspects. Laryngoscope, 77:454, 1967.

Parinaud, M. H.: Paralysie des mouvements associés des yeux. Arch. Neurol. (Paris), 5:145, 1883.

Perlia: Die Anatomie des Oculomotoriuscentrums beim Menschen. Graefe's Arch. Ophthalmol., 35:287, 1889.

Peters, C. H., Widerman, A., Blumberg, A., and Ricker, W. A., Jr.: Neurologic manifestations of infectious mononucleosis: with special reference to the Guillain-Barré syndrome. Arch. Intern. Med., 80:366, 1947.

Plum, F., and Posner, J. B.: The Diagnosis of Stupor and Coma. Philadelphia, F. A. Davis Co., 1966.

Pool, J. L., and Pava, A. A.: The Early Diagnosis and Treatment of Acoustic Nerve Tumors. Springfield, Ill., Charles C Thomas, 1957.

Robertson, D. M., Hines, J. D., and Rucker, C. W.: Acquired sixth-nerve paresis in children. Arch. Ophthalmol., 83:574, 1970.

Rubinstein, M. K.: Cranial mononeuropathy as the first sign of intracranial metastases. Ann. Intern. Med., 70:49, 1969.

Rucker, C. W.: Paralysis of the third, fourth, and sixth cranial nerves. Am. J. Ophthalmol., 46:787, 1958.

Rucker, C. W.: The causes of paralysis of the third, fourth and sixth cranial nerves. Am. J. Ophthalmol., 61:1293, 1966.

Sahs, A. L., Perret, G. E., Lochsey, H. B., and Nicioka, H.: Intracranial Aneurysms and Subarachnoid Hemorrhage: A Cooperative Study. Philadelphia, J. B. Lippincott Co., 1969.

Salus, R.: Cited by Wolf, J. K.: The Classical Brain Syndromes. Springfield, Ill., Charles C Thomas, 1971, p. 155.

Sassin, J. F., and Chutorian, A. M.: Intracranial chordoma in children. Arch. Neurol., 17:89, 1967.

Scanlon, P. W., Devine, K. D., and Woolner, L. B.: Malignant lesions of the nasopharynx. Ann. Otol. Rhinol. Laryngol., 67:1005, 1958.

Schneider, R. C., and Johnson, F. D.: Bilateral traumatic abducens palsy: a mechanism of injury suggested by the study of associated cervical spine fractures. J. Neurosurg., 34:33, 1971.

Schnell, R. G., Dyck, P. J., Bowie, E. J. W., Klass, D. W., and Taswell, H. F.: Infectious mononucleosis: neurologic and EEG findings. Medicine (Baltimore), 45:51, 1966.

Schwab, R. S., and Weiss, S.: The neurologic aspect of leukemia. Am. J. Med. Sci., 189:766, 1935.

Shrader, E. C., and Schlezinger, N. S.: Neuro-ophthalmologic evaluation of abducens nerve paralysis. Arch. Ophthalmol., 63:84, 1960.

Smith, J. L.: Personal communication.

Smith, J. L., and Taxdal, D. S. R.: Painful ophthalmoplegia: the Tolosa-Hunt syndrome. Am. J. Ophthalmol., *61*:1466, 1966.

Stevenson, G. C., and Hoyt, W. F.: Metastasis to midbrain from mammary carcinoma: cause of bilateral ptosis and ophthalmoplegia. J.A.M.A., *186*:514, 1963.

Sunderland, S., and Hughes, S. R.: The pupillo-constrictor pathway and the nerves to the ocular muscles in man. Brain, *69*:301, 1946.

Swartz, M. N., and Dodge, P. R.: Bacterial meningitis: a review of selected aspects. I. General clinical features, special problems and unusual meningeal reactions mimicking bacterial meningitis. II. Special neurologic problems, postmeningitic complications and clinicopathological correlations. N. Engl. J. Med., *272*:898, 1003, 1965.

Symonds, C. P.: Discussion. Proc. R. Soc. Med., *37*:386, 1944.

Thomas, J. E., and Waltz, A. G.: Neurological manifestations of nasopharyngeal malignant tumors. J.A.M.A., *192*:95, 1965.

Thomas, J. E., and Yoss, R. E.: The parasellar syndrome: problems in determining etiology. Mayo Clin. Proc., *45*:617, 1970.

Thomas, P. K., Lascelles, R. G., Hallpike, J. F., and Hewer, R. L.: Recurrent and chronic relapsing Guillain-Barré polyneuritis. Brain, *92*:589, 1969.

Tolosa, E.: Periarteritic lesions of the carotid siphon with the clinical features of a carotid infraclinoidal aneurysm. J. Neurol. Neurosurg. Psychiatry, n.s. *17*:300, 1954.

Troupp, H., Koskinen, K., and af Björkesten, G.: Ophthalmoplegia caused by intracranial aneurysm: prognosis after intracranial surgery. Acta Ophthalmol. (Kbh.), *36*:79, 1958.

Walsh, F. B.: Third nerve regeneration: a clinical evaluation. Br. J. Ophthalmol., *41*:577, 1957.

Walsh, F. B., and Hoyt, W. F.: Clinical Neuro-ophthalmology. Vols. 2 and 3. 3rd Edition. Baltimore, Williams & Wilkins Co., 1969, pp. 1411, 2132, 2228, 2390.

Warwick, R.: A study of retrograde degeneration in the oculomotor nucleus of the rhesus monkey, with a note on method of recording its distribution. Brain, *73*:532, 1950.

Warwick, R.: Representation of the extra-ocular muscles in the oculomotor nuclei of the monkey. J. Comp. Neurol., *98*:449, 1953.

Warwick, R.: The ocular parasympathetic nerve supply and its mesencephalic sources. J. Anat., *88*:71, 1954.

Warwick, R.: The so-called nucleus of convergence. Brain, *78*:92, 1955.

Warwick, R.: Oculomotor organisation. Ann. R. Coll. Surg. Engl., *19*:36, 1956.

Weber, R. B.: Cranial neuropathies and diabetes. Lancet, *1*:645, 1971.

Weber, R. B., Daroff, R. B., and Mackey, E. A.: Pathology of oculomotor nerve palsy in diabetics. Neurology (Minneap.), *20*:835, 1970.

Weiner, L. P., and Porro, R. S.: Total third nerve paralysis: a case with hemorrhage in the oculomotor nerve in subdural hematoma. Neurology (Minneap.), *15*:87, 1965.

Whisnant, J. P., Siekert, R. G., and Sayre, G. P.: Neurologic manifestations of the lymphomas. Med. Clin. North Am., *40*:1151, 1956.

Wolff, E.: Anatomy of the Eye and Orbit: Including the Central Connections, Development and Comparative Anatomy of the Visual Apparatus. 6th Edition. (Revised by R. J. Last.) London, H. K. Lewis & Co., Ltd., 1968, pp. 286, 293.

Zielinski: 1959. Cited by Duke-Elder, S., p. 778.

Zweifach, P. H., Walton, D. S., and Brown, R. H.: Isolated congenital horizontal gaze paralysis: occurrence of the near reflex and ocular retraction on attempted lateral gaze. Arch. Ophthalmol., *81*:345, 1969.

Chapter 26

DISEASES OF THE FIFTH CRANIAL NERVE

George Selby

The fifth cranial nerve, the trigeminal, contains both motor and sensory fibers. The sensory part of the nerve is much larger than the motor portion and has the important function of protecting the head, the seat of the brain and of the special sense organs, from local injury. The dense network of cutaneous sensory receptors of the face, the size of the semilunar (gasserian) ganglion—the largest sensory ganglion in man—and the complexity of the central connections of the sensory trigeminal pathways reflect the functional significance of this nerve.

ANATOMY

As the anatomy of the trigeminal nerve and its connections is described in all standard texts on anatomy and is reviewed in a more clinical context by Brodal (1969), this discussion is confined to specific aspects relevant to diseases of the trigeminal nerve and to some recent anatomical, histologic, and physiologic studies.

The cutaneous areas supplied by the three peripheral divisions of the trigeminal nerve—the ophthalmic, the maxillary, and the mandibular—show only very little overlap, and the borders between the trigeminal and upper cervical sensory fields are exceptionally sharp. This is in contrast to the overlapping of sensory dermatomal areas in other parts of the body. The trigeminal nerve also innervates the mucous membranes of the nasal and oral cavities and of the maxillary and frontal sinuses. It sends meningeal branches to the

dura, with the exception of the infratentorial dura in the posterior cranial fossa (Brodal, 1969). Further details of the trigeminal contribution to dural innervation can be found in the studies of Penfield and McNaughton (1940), Feindel, Penfield, and McNaughton (1960), and Wirth and Van Buren (1971).

Semilunar Ganglion

The semilunar (gasserian) ganglion is sickle-shaped. The three peripheral divisions of the nerve enter on the convexity, while the root bundles leave from the concavity. On its concave side the ganglion is folded over and has an upper and lower lip that bound the ganglion sinus. The sinus is within an arachnoidal sac protruding from the middle cranial fossa and containing cerebrospinal fluid (Fig. 26–1). The arachnoid is attached to the lips of the ganglion and is firmly fused to its convexity. The root bundles of the triangular part of the sensory root are covered by pia mater and bathed in cerebrospinal fluid, just as the compact part of the sensory root, which runs through the lateral pontine cistern, is surrounded by cerebrospinal fluid.

At the trigeminal pore, where the sensory root enters the middle cranial fossa, the dura mater of the posterior cranial fossa loosely invaginates under the dura of the middle fossa and forms a pouch surrounding the triangular part of the sensory root and fused with the gasserian ganglion (Ferner, 1970).

Examination of the semilunar ganglion by light microscopy shows a characteristic ar-

533

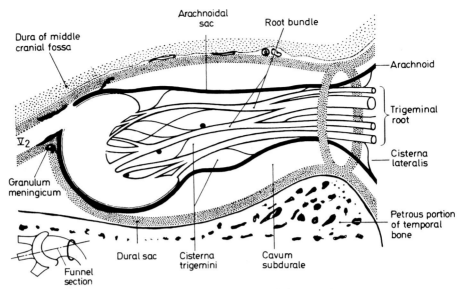

Figure 26-1 Schematic diagram of the trigeminal cistern. V₂, second division of nerve. (From Ferner, H.: Zur Anatomie der intrakranialen Abschnitte des Nervus trigeminus. Z. Anat., *114*:108-122, 1948. Berlin, Springer Verlag. Reprinted by permission.)

rangement of pseudounipolar ganglion cells in clusters, separated by bundles of axons (Kerr, 1970). These axons arise from the cell body as a single fiber, which initially is greatly convoluted (the glomerulus of Cajal), then acquires a myelin sheath and follows a straight or slightly curved course to the nearest bundle of axons, where it bifurcates into a central process directed toward the pons and a usually thicker peripheral branch (Fig. 26-2).

Electron microscopic studies of the semi-lunar ganglion of various animal species and from human autopsies showed neurons of varying size, surrounded by satellite cells and often grouped in clusters (Moses, 1967; Moses et al., 1965; Beaver et al., 1965a; Kerr, 1970). They have a large vesicular nucleus with a prominent nucleolus. Cytoplasmic organelles include mitochondria, lysosome-like structures, Golgi complexes, and a variety of inclusions such as dense bodies, pigment granules, lipofuscin, and other granular and lipid components. Each neuron is completely invested by the cytoplasmic processes of surrounding satellite cells, and some of these form interdigitations with the neuronal

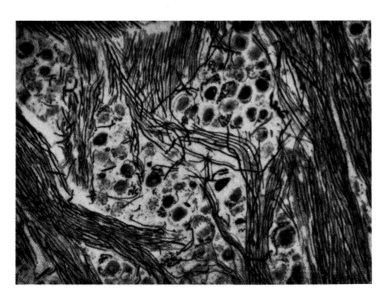

Figure 26-2 Trigeminal ganglion showing clusters of ganglion cells separated by bundles of nerve fibers. Numerous glomeruli of the initial portion of the axon are seen. Satellite cells appear as small spherical bodies surrounding the neurons. Winkelmann silver stain × 80. (From Kerr, F. W. L.: Fine structure and functional characteristics of the primary trigeminal neuron. *In* Hassler, R., and Walker, A. E. (eds.): Trigeminal Neuralgia, Pathogenesis and Pathophysiology. Stuttgart, Georg Thieme Verlag, 1970. Reprinted by permission.)

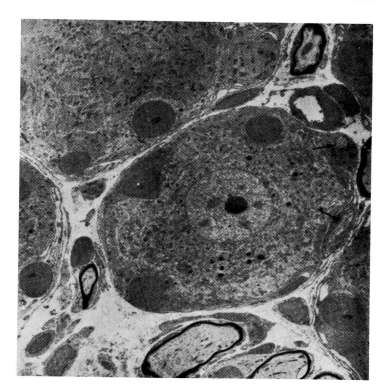

Figure 26–3 Low-magnification electron micrograph of trigeminal ganglion. The small neuron in the center shows all the characteristic features. The satellite cells, which can be distinguished by the greater electron density of the cytoplasm and nuclei, are so intimately associated with the neuron that their respective cytoplasms appear to blend at this low power. The initial unmyelinated portion of the axon is seen at the arrows. In the lower part of the figure the myelinated portion of another axonal glomerulus is seen. × 2500. (From Kerr, F. W. L.: Fine structure and functional characteristics of the primary trigeminal neuron. *In* Hassler, R., and Walker, A. E. (eds.): Trigeminal Neuralgia, Pathogenesis and Pathophysiology. Stuttgart, Georg Thieme Verlag, 1970. Reprinted by permission.)

limiting membrane (Fig. 26–3). Myelinated and unmyelinated axons, capillaries, fibroblasts, and collagen fibrils occupy the area between neurons. The unmyelinated axons are usually small and completely or partly surrounded by Schwann cells; myelinated axons are generally larger, though of varying size, and have different degrees of myelination.

In human autopsy material the changes of advancing age include more numerous and larger lipid globules within the ganglion cells, but degeneration of ganglion cells is unusual.

Trigeminal Sensory Root

The fibers of the trigeminal sensory root leave the concavity of the sinus of the semilunar ganglion as a triangular plexus, but then converge to form the compact part of the sensory root at the trigeminal porus, where the root enters the posterior cranial fossa (see Fig. 26–1). There are wide differences in the arrangement of fibers; in some cases they are arranged in parallel bundles with few anastomoses, in others they mingle extensively and form anastomoses between fiber bundles from different divisions (Fig. 26–4) (Ferner, 1970; Gudmundsson et al., 1971). Fibers from the

mandibular division occupy a posterolateral position throughout the course of the sensory root from ganglion to pons, the ophthalmic fibers are dorsomedial, and the maxillary fibers lie in an intermediate position. This somatotopic localization is maintained in spite of the prominent anastomosis behind the ganglion. Aberrant sensory rootlets frequently arise from the pons, separately from the main sensory root, and most of these join the root fibers from the first (ophthalmic) division (Jannetta and Rand, 1967a). There is no anatomical evidence that these accessory rootlets are concerned with only a single sensory modality. In the majority of nerves there are also anastomoses between the motor and sensory roots, but the functional significance of these is uncertain (Gudmundsson et al., 1971).

Nerve cells, similar to ganglion cells, were recently observed in the compact (pontine) part of the sensory root and in the motor root of the human trigeminal nerve. They suggest the possibility of an accessory relay station for trigeminal sensory fibers, and their presence in the motor root may imply that it carries afferent fibers (Mira et al., 1971).

On microscopic examination the sensory root is seen to consist of medium-sized and

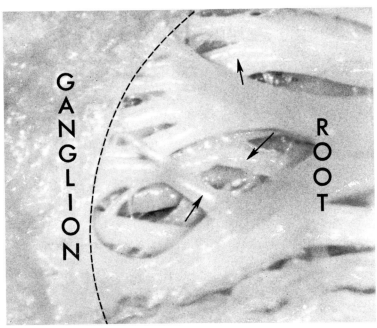

Figure 26–4   Magnified view of the trigeminal ganglion (*left*) and the posterior trigeminal root (*right*). The broken line marks the junction between the root and ganglion. Significant anastomosis (arrows) between the filaments is present immediately posterior to the ganglion. (From Gudmundsson, K., Rhoton, A. L., Jr., and Rushton, J. G.: Detailed anatomy of the intracranial portion of the trigeminal nerve. J. Neurosurg., 35:592–600, 1971. Reprinted by permission.)

small myelinated fibers, and of a moderate number of unmyelinated fibers in a proportion similar to that found in other sensory roots (Kerr, 1970). At a distance of less than 10 mm from the pons, there is an abrupt transition from the peripheral Schwann cell investment to the central sheath system formed by oligodendroglia (Maxwell, 1967).

Trigeminal Nuclei

On entering the pons, almost half the fibers of the sensory trigeminal root divide into an ascending branch ending in the main sensory nucleus, and a descending branch that terminates in the nucleus of the spinal tract (Brodal, 1969). Olszewski (1950) has shown that the nucleus of the spinal tract can be subdivided into three regions, which differ in cytoarchitectonics and are called the nucleus caudalis, the nucleus interpolaris, and the nucleus oralis. Within each of these nuclei different subgroups can further be distinguished, suggesting a functional differentiation of various parts of the nucleus of the spinal tract.

The long-held concept that the ophthalmic fibers extend most caudally, while the maxillary and mandibular fibers are disposed successively more rostrally in the spinal tract and nucleus, has been challenged by recent studies. Kerr (1963a), in cats and monkeys, found that the spinal tract terminates at the midpoint of the second cervical level, and that in both the spinal tract and nucleus the ophthalmic fibers lie ventrolaterally, the mandibular fibers lie dorsomedially, and the maxillary fibers occupy an intermediate position. The fibers from each division remain segregated with little or no overlap. Some third division fibers leave the spinal tract and enter the nucleus of the tractus solitarius, suggesting that the trigeminal nerve may contain some visceral afferent fibers from glands and vascular structures of the nose, mouth, and teeth, and some that could be concerned with taste.

The termination of fibers in the main sensory nucleus shows the same dorsoventral somatotopic organization as in the spinal tract and nucleus (Kerr, 1963a). Emmons and Rhoton (1971) corroborated these findings in the monkey, but observed degenerative changes in the spinal tract and nucleus down to the level of the C3 dorsal horn after section of the whole sensory root or of individual divisions. They found that the medial cuneate nucleus receives fibers from each of the three trigeminal divisions and may, therefore, be a site for convergence of proprioceptive impulses from the head and upper part of the body. They could not discover a component of the posterior root that projected specifically to the main sensory or spinal trigeminal nucleus, and dispute the concept that the main sensory nucleus is concerned with touch and the spinal nucleus with pain and temperature sensation. Neurophysiologic studies have confirmed that units responding to tactile stimuli are present in the main nucleus, as well as in all subdivisions of the spinal nucleus (see Darian-Smith, 1966, for references). Although there is abundant clinical evidence for the relief of facial pain after medullary trigeminal tractotomy (Sjöqvist, 1938; Kunč, 1970), physiologic experiments in animals have so far failed to demonstrate any cells or fibers within the sensory trigeminal nuclei that are specifically concerned with pain perception. Wall and Taub (1962) found, in the cat, that small peripheral nerve fibers failed to reach the caudal part of the spinal nucleus, and that this caudal nucleus has large receptive fields that respond to light pressure. The main sensory nucleus, on the other hand, contained cells with large receptive fields that respond to a wide range of pressure stimuli with little adaptation. They suggest the hypothesis that pain reactions are elicited by a massive spatial and temporal summation of many impulses from the primary nuclei on deeper, presumably second-order, neurons. Surgical section of the descending spinal tract would reduce this integrated maximum discharge.

The structural and functional similarity of the nucleus caudalis to the spinal relay of the anterolateral system and the functional homology of the main sensory nucleus and nucleus oralis with the medial lemniscal relay in the dorsal columns were recently confirmed by Darian-Smith (1970a). While fibers from various mechanoreceptor endings project to all nuclei of the ipsilateral trigeminal complex, responses to cutaneous vibratory stimuli applied to the face were recorded only from second-order relay neurons in the nucleus oralis. Cells in this nucleus have the capacity to relay to the thalamus information about the intensity of a tactile stimulus with only negligible loss of accuracy, whereas no gradation of stimulus intensity is possible from the limited information relayed by cells in the nucleus caudalis.

The descending tract of the fifth nerve and its caudal nucleus are a direct continuation of the dorsolateral tract of Lissauer and of the substantia gelatinosa of the cervical segments. Denny-Brown and Yanagisawa (1970) found that trigeminal anesthesia resulting from section of the descending tract at the first cervical segment, in the monkey, could be abolished by the administration of subconvulsive doses of strychnine. Differential section of the dorsal part of the lower descending tract produced a sensory loss similar to that following total section. In contrast, section of the ventral part of the tract failed to produce anesthesia, but resulted in an expansion of the area of both trigeminal and vagal skin sensation, corresponding to the increase in area caused by strychnine. These observations suggest that the dorsal part of the descending tract is concerned mainly with facilitation, while the ventral part is concerned with inhibition, which can be abolished by strychnine. A similar situation applies to the medial (facilitatory) and lateral (inhibitory) segments of Lissauer's tract in the spinal cord. Further observations after additional section of the upper three cervical dorsal roots permit the assumption that the descending tract of the fifth nerve provides a mechanism for intersegmental sensory facilitation between the trigeminal and upper cervical segments. Interstitial cells at all levels, sending axons up and down the tract, are the anatomical substrate for this mechanism.

In the course of this study, Denny-Brown and Yanagisawa found that an oval area including the side of the nose, the lower eyelid and cheek, the medial two thirds of the upper lip, and the most medial parts of the alveolar margin escaped the sensory loss following on section of the whole descending tract. This helps to explain the concentric, onion skin pattern of sensory loss that may occur in some cases of syringomyelia.

Further evidence suggesting the existence of inhibitory fibers in the substantia gelatinosa trigemini was provided by the electron microscopic observations of Hassler and Bak (1970). They described presynaptic axoaxonal contacts, which may subserve presynaptic inhibition. On the basis of pharmacologic studies involving changes in dense-core vesicles, they postulated that serotonin acts as one of the synaptic transmitter substances in the descending trigeminal nucleus.

Physiologic studies have shown that stimulation of peripheral branches of the trigeminal nerve evokes both an immediate and a delayed response; the latter arises from cells in the nucleus caudalis and is conducted centrifugally into peripheral components of the trigeminal nerve. This trigeminal dorsal root reflex can be activated at the same threshold as touch fibers. It is abolished by caudal tractotomy and is greatly enhanced by injection of alumina gel or strychnine into the caudal nucleus (King et al., 1956). From a series of recent experiments it was deduced that, in the normal state, cells in the nucleus caudalis have a hyperpolarizing (inhibitory) effect on primary afferent preterminals in the rostral (oralis) nucleus. Trigeminal tractotomy or the application of conditioning stimuli to cells in the nucleus caudalis decreases this inhibition, whereas the application of strychnine or alumina gel at the caudal nucleus augments it. An ascending system of fibers between the caudal nucleus and the rostral relay nuclei of the trigeminal system, and axoaxonal junctions at presynaptic positions are the anatomical substrate for this functional relationship between the caudal and rostral parts of the trigeminal nuclei (King, 1970). Further studies of excitability changes in primary afferent preterminals established that nonnoxious stimuli to the face produce primary afferent depolarization, while noxious stimuli result in an initial period of depolarization of low amplitude followed by a more prolonged period of primary afferent hyperpolarization (inhibition) maximal in the nucleus oralis. This preterminal inhibition of noxious stimuli in the nucleus oralis is again augmented by the application of strychnine to the caudal nucleus and abolished by medullary tractotomy. On the basis of these findings, Young and King (1972) suggested the hypothesis that the direct relay of sensory information from the face, including painful stimuli, may occur mainly in the rostral parts of the spinal trigeminal nuclei, and that one of the functions of the nucleus caudalis is to modulate the transfer of information through these rostral nuclei.

Apart from primary trigeminal sensory fibers, the spinal tract contains some afferent fibers from the intermediate, glossopharyngeal, and vagus nerves as well as dorsal root fibers from the upper cervical roots. There are also in this tract fibers that pass from the nucleus caudalis to the more rostral nuclei, including the main sensory nucleus.

All the subdivisions of the spinal nucleus, as well as the main nucleus, receive descending fibers from the primary sensory cortex and from the reticular formation; these appear to be concerned with presynaptic inhibition of trigeminal impulses relayed by the nuclei (see Brodal, 1969, for references).

The mesencephalic nucleus differs in many respects from the spinal and main nuclei. It consists chiefly of pseudounipolar cells, similar to those of the semilunar and other ganglia; their peripheral fibers form the mesencephalic root of the trigeminal nerve. Most of them are large myelinated fibers and travel peripherally in the motor root and then in the mandibular division, though a few fibers have been traced also into the ophthalmic and maxillary divisions. They supply mainly the muscles of mastication via pterygoidal, temporal, and masseteric branches of the mandibular nerve, but innervate also the palate and periodontal membrane through palatine and superior and inferior alveolar branches, which run in the maxillary and mandibular divisions (Corbin, 1940).

The termination of fibers from the mesencephalic nucleus on muscle spindles in the masticatory muscles is evidence for their proprioceptive function; they also provide the afferent arc for the jaw reflex. Mesencephalic root fibers passing in the second and third sensory divisions of the trigeminal nerve are assumed to be concerned with control of the force of the bite and with reflex control of mastication (Corbin, 1940).

The significance of the mesencephalic nucleus for the proprioceptive innervation of extrinsic ocular muscles is still a subject of controversy. Brodal (1969) summarized some of the anatomical and physiologic evidence for this function. Recent experimental observations in three mammalian species by Manni, Palmieri, and Marini (1971) have shown, however, that proprioceptive fibers from extraocular muscles arise from cells in the semilunar ganglion, with peripheral processes in the ophthalmic division, and central processes projecting, via the sensory root, to the ipsilateral descending tract and nucleus oralis. Cerebellar projections from this nucleus oralis appear to contribute to this proprioceptive function.

Ascending Connections to Thalamus

The ascending connections from the trigeminal nuclei to the thalamus and somatosensory cortex have not yet been fully elucidated. Current anatomical and physiologic concepts were reviewed by Brodal (1969), and Hassler (1970). Although physiologic studies have failed to demonstrate neurons responding specifically to pain (Grubel, 1970), it is assumed from the clinical results of medullary tractotomy that cells in the nucleus caudalis are the second-order neuron concerned primarily with transmission of pain from the face. Hassler (1970) postulated two distinct trigeminal pain pathways, one cortical, the other subcortical, which interact with each other. If the cortical pathway is interrupted, the subcortical pathway may be released from inhibition.

More precise information is available about the transmission of tactile information from the face than about the anatomical pathways and physiologic mechanisms concerned with pain. A somatotopic representation of tactile stimuli from different parts of the face, including the tongue and teeth, is maintained from the primary cutaneous afferent fiber, through the relay nuclei in the brain stem and thalamus, to the three cortical (SI, SII, SIII) somatosensory areas (Darian-Smith et al., 1963). The degree of convergence at successive synaptic levels is limited by both presynaptic and postsynaptic inhibitory mechanisms, which help to maintain a sharp spatial and temporal "image" of the location and duration of the peripheral tactile stimulus. These include presynaptic "surround" inhibition as well as a cortical inhibitory feedback, both acting on the relay cells within the brain stem trigeminal nuclei (Darian-Smith, 1965). There is evidence also of a positive feedback mechanism of postsynaptic facilitation from the somatosensory cortex on neurons in the trigeminothalamic (lemniscal) projection (Wiesendanger et al., 1970).

Motor Division

The motor division of the trigeminal nerve is not nearly as complex as its sensory components and, therefore, has not been so extensively studied. The motor nucleus is situated medial to the main sensory nucleus in the middle of the pons. Its fibers leave the pons as the motor root (portio minor), which is composed of up to 14 separately originating rootlets, which usually join about 1 cm from the pons (Gudmundsson et al., 1971). Anas-

tomoses between the motor and sensory roots are commonly present. The motor fibers run toward the periphery beneath the ganglion and then join the mandibular division to supply the masticatory muscles as well as the tensor tympani, the tensor palati, the mylohyoid, and the anterior belly of the digastric muscle. Cells in the motor nucleus have reflex connections with central fibers of the mesencephalic trigeminal nucleus and, via intercalated cells, with other cranial nerves. The motor nucleus also receives corticobulbar afferent fibers (Brodal, 1969).

The vast literature concerned with the anatomy and physiology of the trigeminal somatic afferent system reflects its complexity and importance. It is hoped that the small fraction of the many valuable publications just reviewed will contribute to a better understanding of the pathophysiology of trigeminal pain.

PERIPHERAL LESIONS OF TRIGEMINAL NERVE

The peripheral divisions of the fifth nerve mediate sensation from an extensive area including the skin of the face and scalp as far back as the lambdoid suture; the cornea, conjunctiva, and iris; the mucous membrane of the nose, lips, mouth, and frontal and maxillary sinuses; the anterior wall of the external auditory meatus and anterior part of the tympanic membrane; the mucosa of the anterior two thirds of the tongue; and the teeth of both upper and lower jaws and most of the hard and soft palate. It is, therefore, concerned in transmission of pain caused by a large variety of traumatic, inflammatory, and neoplastic lesions of the face, eye, ear, nose, paranasal sinuses, oral cavity, tongue, and teeth.

Trauma and Infection

The supratrochlear, supraorbital, and infraorbital nerves are frequently involved in craniofacial trauma, but the result is more often anesthesia than pain. Partial regeneration of the injured nerve may cause a constant pain, usually confined strictly to the distribution of the nerve. Such pain can be relieved by surgical section of the nerve, which, however, has a remarkable capacity for regeneration and consequent return of pain. Traumatic lesions of the mandibular division occur in fractures of the skull base and cause both anesthesia and paralysis of the muscles innervated by the trigeminal motor root.

Pain of dental origin, though often not precisely localized to the offending tooth, only very rarely extends to involve the dermatome of the mandibular or maxillary division. Trauma to alveolar branches, incurred during complicated extractions of impacted wisdom teeth or during excision of dentigerous cysts, may cause protracted facial neuralgia. This pain is generally constant, of burning quality, and associated with unpleasant dysesthesias, but on occasions it may be paroxysmal and excited by triggers identical to those that operate in "genuine" trigeminal neuralgia. Harris (1950) strongly favored trauma to dental nerves as an important pathogenetic mechanism for major trigeminal neuralgia; he cited the case of a young woman who developed typical tic douloureux after a difficult extraction of four teeth from the lower jaw, complicated by a fracture of the mandible. This patient subsequently enjoyed remissions from pain varying from 18 months to six years.

Infective neuritis of the infraorbital nerve, secondary to maxillary sinusitis, can cause pain that continues long beyond the cure of the sinus infection but is never paroxysmal.

Tumors and Vascular Disorders

Involvement of the peripheral branches of the trigeminal nerve may result from primary or metastatic malignant tumors of the face, mouth, tongue, paranasal sinuses, and base of the skull. In rare instances such tumors can produce symptomatic trigeminal neuralgia, confined to a single division and precipitated by the usual triggers. This was observed in a patient with a metastasis at the foramen ovale (Selby, unpublished data). Primary carcinoma of the nasopharynx not infrequently presents with pain, numbness, and objective sensory changes along the mandibular dermatome, often months or even years before the malignant nasopharyngeal tumor is, in spite of diligent search, discovered. Trigeminal motor paralysis is often only a late development. Some of these patients experience symptomatic trigeminal neuralgia in addition to a constant dull ache, presumably owing to com-

pression or distortion of trigeminal fibers from the surrounding neoplasm. The discovery of objective sensory defects and the absence of prolonged remissions from pain distinguish such cases from "genuine" tic douloureux.

The ophthalmic division is particularly vulnerable in the cavernous sinus and may be the first, or the only, part of the trigeminal nerve affected in thrombosis of this sinus or in aneurysms of the distal part of the internal carotid artery at its junction with the posterior communicating artery. In most patients with with such aneurysms, complete third nerve palsy occurs in association with pain in a first division distribution.

Toxins

The trigeminus appears to be relatively immune to the many toxins and drugs that can affect peripheral nerves. It is, however, specifically vulnerable to stilbamidine and to trichlorethylene or, more probably, one of its breakdown products (see Chapter 60).

Progressive and persistent numbness and paresthesias, mainly in the form of pruritus and formication, confined to the face, may appear from two to five months after the administration of stilbamidine (Smith and Miller, 1955). The mechanism of this neuropathy is unknown, but Collard and Nevin (1946) postulated lesions of the trigeminal nuclei and central gray matter of the spinal cord.

After trichlorethylene had been implicated as a cause of trigeminal palsy in German industrial workers, Humphrey and McClelland (1944) and Carden (1944) attributed the multiple cranial nerve palsies that occurred after general anesthesia to a breakdown product, dichloracetylene. This substance is the product of a chemical reaction between trichlorethylene and soda-lime in closed-circuit anesthetic apparatus. In all the reported cases the trigeminal nerves were predominantly and bilaterally involved, in some including the motor fibers; in several cases other cranial nerves, but excluding those that mediate the special senses, were also affected. The initial symptoms, appearing 12 to 24 hours after administration of the general anesthetic, were numbness and paresthesias around the mouth, which spread to involve the entire distribution of the fifth nerve on both sides over the next few days. In the more severely affected cases recovery was incomplete, even after many months. It is of some interest that in 10 of the 15 cases reported by the authors just cited, the cranial nerve lesions were associated with labial herpes. Buxton and Hayward (1967) reported on four men who were exposed to trichlorethylene in an industrial accident. Two developed severe multiple cranial nerve palsies, and in both the sensory parts of the trigeminal nerves were the most severely affected, though the trigeminal motor root did not escape. An autopsy of one of these patients showed most striking changes of demyelination and axonal damage in the trigeminal sensory roots and descending tracts. Severe nerve cell loss was seen in both the main and spinal trigeminal nuclei, and the changes were bilateral and symmetrical. Several other cranial nerve nuclei were involved to a lesser extent.

Systemic Disease

Trigeminal neuropathy has been reported in progressive systemic sclerosis (generalized scleroderma) and dermatomyositis by Ashworth and Tait (1971), in systemic lupus erythematosus by Bailey, Sayre, and Clark (1956) and Lewis (1965), and in Sjögren's syndrome by Kaltreider and Talal (1969). In progressive systemic sclerosis the neuropathy is always preceded by Raynaud's phenomenon and appears with an acute or subacute onset within three years from the first manifestations of the systemic disease. It is confined to the sensory portion of the nerve, may be bilateral, is completed within a few days or weeks, and then neither progresses nor remits. All sensory modalities are affected. Pain is prominent and sometimes persistent; numbness is invariably present and may involve only two or all three divisions of the nerve. Objective sensory defects can always be demonstrated, but the corneal reflex need not be lost. Pathologic evidence of the site and nature of the lesion is lacking, but Ashworth and Tait (1971) assumed that it may be in the ganglion or root and secondary to pathologic changes in small vessels. As the sensory manifestations follow the distribution of divisions of the trigeminal nerve, the lesion cannot be situated in the peripheral sensory receptors of the subcutaneous connective tissue.

Two instances of trigeminal involvement in the course of neuritis associated with systemic lupus erythematosus were described by Bailey, Sayre, and Clark (1956). Both patients were found to have hypalgesia over a unilateral fifth nerve distribution, but neither complained of pain. Autopsy examination of the gasserian ganglion in one case showed inflammatory changes, diffuse degeneration of ganglion cells, and proliferation of capsular cells. From a review of the literature presented by Lewis (1965), it appears that trigeminal involvement is very rare in the mixed polyneuropathy associated with systemic lupus. The only evidence for a trigeminal lesion in his patient was a subjective numbness of the tongue.

Kaltreider and Talal (1969) found four cases of trigeminal neuropathy among 10 patients suffering from Sjögren's syndrome associated with peripheral nerve involvement. In three of these, there were also signs of a sensory or mixed peripheral neuropathy that affected mainly the lower limbs. An impairment of taste sensation in three of these patients may be attributed, at least partly, to xerostomia. Trigeminal nerve involvement was bilateral in one case, and affected either two or all three sensory divisions of the nerve. Acute or chronic vasculitis or perivasculitis was found in biopsies from sural nerves or muscle, and the authors concluded that the lesion was probably situated in the peripheral divisions of the nerve.

Sarcoidosis, which may affect the nervous system without any of its more common systemic manifestations, can involve any of the cranial nerves, most often the seventh. Jefferson (1957) described one instance of trigeminal sensory impairment among seven cases of sarcoidosis with lesions in the central or peripheral nervous system. Colover (1948) was able to find 7 cases with sarcoid trigeminal lesions in a review of 115 cases from the literature. In five of these, only the sensory components of the nerve were affected, and in two there was paresis of the muscles of mastication. In a further three cases diminution or loss of corneal reflexes was noted, but this might well have resulted from facial paralysis. It would appear then that trigeminal involvement is uncommon, compared to the many other neurologic lesions associated with sarcoidosis.

Spillane and Wells (1959) presented a careful study of 16 cases of isolated trigeminal neuropathy of undetermined etiology, collected over a period of eight years. The age at onset varied from 30 to 64 years. Sensory impairment in the territory of one or more divisions of the fifth nerve was the predominant dysfunction in 15 cases, and in 4 of these it was bilateral. Trigeminal motor paresis was found, in association with sensory defect, in only one case that differed from all others in that complete recovery occurred after 12 months. In seven patients the initial symptom, often of abrupt onset, was pain; in the others the illness began with numbness or paresthesias. In all, numbness or altered sensations of the face dominated the clinical picture in the later stages of the disease. Some described the face as "swollen" or the skin as "unduly thick," while others complained of burning or abnormal feelings of warmth of the face. Similar dysesthesias are a frequent sequel to sensory root section for tic douloureux. The ophthalmic division was involved in six cases, and an additional five patients had diminution or loss of the corneal reflex. In 19 instances (including those with bilateral lesions) the maxillary division was affected, and lesions of the mandibular division occurred in 16. Initially the abnormal sensations were felt mainly around the mouth, on the cheek, and on the chin, and six patients complained of burning dysesthesias in the tongue. In nine patients, sensory loss within the oral cavity interfered with eating. Impairment or loss of taste on the affected side was found in seven cases and could be attributed to involvement of fibers of the chorda tympani in their course in the mandibular nerve. As an alternative explanation, Spillane and Wells quoted the views expressed by Rowbotham (1939) that ageusia after various surgical procedures for the relief of tic douloureux can be interpreted as a central disorder of perception, due to a loss of a "background of common sensations" of the fifth nerve, rather than a peripheral loss of specific sensation. A similar view was later expressed by Harris (1952), who proposed "that there is a correlation or welding of the sensibility of the tongue and palate supplied by the fifth nerve with the true gustatory sensations from the chorda and petrosal nerves."

Three of the patients with isolated trigeminal neuropathy had partial or complete Horner's syndrome, and one suffered a gross, bilateral disturbance of autonomic function that eventually resulted in a trophic destruction of her nose. This patient, however, also suffered from Sjögren's syndrome, which may

have been the cause of the trigeminal neuropathy and could have contributed to the "trophic" necrosis of the nose (cf. Kaltreider and Talal, 1969). With the exception of the single case in which both motor and sensory divisions were affected, no recovery was found at follow-up examinations from 15 months to nine years after onset of the disease. Examination revealed that pain sensation was more often impaired than other modalities, and analgesia was always more dense than thermanesthesia; deep pressure and vibration sense were spared in all cases. The cerebrospinal fluid was examined in 10 cases and showed no abnormality, and the Wassermann reaction in the blood was negative in all 16 patients.

Spillane and Wells had no autopsy or biopsy confirmation for the site, nature, and extent of the pathologic lesion underlying their cases of trigeminal neuropathy. They inferred from clinical evidence — particularly from the fact that deep pressure and vibration sense are not involved — that the lesion is not in the brain stem and that it may be situated in either the root, ganglion, or proximal (intracranial) part of the three primary divisions.

Hill (1954) referred to 12 cases that may be of a similar nature, though his paper provided clinical details of only two of these. As several had Horner's syndrome on the side of the trigeminal neuropathy, he postulated a peripheral extension of the lesion to include fibers arising from the ciliary ganglion. Most of his cases showed some degree of motor paresis, and some enjoyed partial recovery. Hughes (1958) reported a further five cases of chronic benign trigeminal paresis, followed up for periods ranging from 11 months to 12 years. The clinical features of his cases appear to be identical to those described by Spillane and Wells (1959) and were confined to the sensory portion of the nerve. Trigeminal sensory root section, in an effort to relieve pain and paresthesias, afforded an opportunity for macroscopic and microscopic examination of the root and ganglion in three cases. The sensory root appeared to be reduced to a few wisps of nerve fibers, embedded in a considerably thickened arachnoid that extended to the side of the pons. On histologic examination, degenerative changes were seen in the remaining fibers of the root, associated with collections of lymphocytes. Ganglion cells also showed degenerative changes with satellitosis.

There was a marked increase of fibrous tissue showing hyaline changes.

Blau, Harris, and Kennett (1969) have described 10 cases of trigeminal sensory neuropathy without pain. The age of onset varied from 27 to 54 years, and six patients were less than 40 years old. All complained of painless numbness; this was confined to the second division in one case, the third division in three cases, and the second and third simultaneously in five cases, while all three divisions were affected in only one case. Absence or alteration of taste on the homolateral side featured in three patients in whom the third division was affected. Trigeminal motor function was never involved. In five subjects examination revealed partial or complete blunting of sensation confined to the distribution of the affected branch of the trigeminal nerve; in the remainder there was only a subjective sensory difference. In no case was the corneal reflex lost. No other abnormal neurologic signs were found. Five subjects made a complete recovery after three weeks to four and a half months; three enjoyed only partial recovery, and one of these developed trigeminal neuralgia some three years later; in the remaining two cases no change was recorded after two years. Appropriate investigations excluded compressive lesions, luetic infection, and malignant nasopharyngeal tumors. No biopsy or autopsy confirmation is available, but the authors considered that the lesion is most probably distal to the gasserian ganglion. They drew a comparison to the isolated and transient neuropathies of the sixth and seventh cranial nerves.

This chronic benign sensory neuropathy of the trigeminal nerve is probably more common than would appear from the few cases reported in the literature. The diagnosis can be established only after compressive lesions have been excluded by thorough investigations, repeated over months or years, and the records of such patients may then be filed away as "undiagnosed." The etiology need not be the same for all cases. Spillane and Wells (1959) had considered the possibility of infection with herpes simplex or a related virus. One of their patients has now died, and postmortem examination has revealed localized amyloid trigeminal neuropathy (Urich, 1974).

Five cases of trigeminal neuritis reported by Harris (1950) differ from those just considered in that all of them developed a paroxysmal trigeminal tic 3 to 12 years after the onset of complete anesthesia of the ipsilateral side of the face, which had persisted for six weeks to four years and had then recovered for varying intervals of time before the tic appeared. One of these patients developed unequivocal signs of multiple sclerosis 18 years after the episode of trigeminal anesthesia and 11 years after the onset of her tic.

The selective vulnerability of different parts of the central and peripheral nervous systems in various metabolic disorders is again exemplified by the absence of trigeminal lesions in uremic and diabetic neuropathies. It is possible, however, that the occasional, painful, isolated oculomotor paralysis in diabetes may include involvement of some first division trigeminal fibers (see Chapter 47). In contrast to the common involvement of the facial nerve, the trigeminus is usually spared in the Guillain-Barré syndrome. Spillane and Wells (1959), however, quoted Guillain's description of residual trigeminal hypesthesia following the rare cranial form of the Guillain-Barré syndrome (Guillain and Kreis, 1937).

LESIONS OF THE TRIGEMINAL GANGLION

The most important pathologic afflictions of the trigeminal ganglion are infection with the virus of herpes zoster, primary neurinoma, and involvement from neighboring expanding or metastatic processes.

Infections

In herpes zoster the semilunar ganglion appears to be more frequently infected than any other sensory ganglion. Hope-Simpson (1965) found 25 cases of trigeminal herpes in a series of 192 cases of shingles seen in a general practice. In accord with general experience, the frequency of involvement of the ophthalmic division exceeded that of either the second or third division by a ratio of almost 4:1. This selective vulnerability of the ganglion cells and fibers of the first division is of considerable interest but has so far defied explanation. Simultaneous involvement of all three trigeminal dermatomes is rare, but has been reported in patients in whom the herpetic infection spread into the neighboring intermedius, glossopharyngeal, and vagus nerves and into the upper cervical dermatomes (Steffen and Selby, 1972).

Histologic examination by light microscopy usually reveals degenerative changes in both axons and myelin, and perivascular inflammatory infiltrates between fiber bundles in the peripheral divisions of the nerve. Similar inflammatory changes and varying degrees of ganglion cell degeneration or necrosis are seen in the affected part of the semilunar ganglion. The trigeminal tract and nuclei in the brain stem are not involved.

In a recent study of a patient who died four days after the onset of ophthalmic herpes zoster, both histologic changes typical of zoster infection and virus particles were found in epidermal cells. Degenerate axons and myelin were seen in some fiber bundles of peripheral twigs of the nerve, and virus particles were present in both cytoplasm and nuclei of some Schwann cells. In parts of the trigeminal ganglion, there was severe gangglion cell degeneration and disarray of satellite cells, and both of these cell types contained virus particles in their nuclei and cytoplasm. Viral antigen was detected by immunofluorescent techniques in only a small proportion of fibers of the ophthalmic nerve and of one of its branches (Esiri and Tomlinson, 1972).

Ophthalmic zoster not infrequently attacks the cornea, and in rare instances may be associated with optic neuritis or with paralysis of the third, fourth, and sixth cranial nerves.

The incidence of postherpetic dysesthesias appears to be similar to that occurring after herpes in other areas. The pathogenetic mechanisms that cause postherpetic pain remain a mystery. This pain, though subject to exacerbations, is never truly paroxysmal, nor can it be relieved by alcohol injection, by surgical section of the trigeminal root, or by medullary tractotomy.

In Gradenigo's syndrome, in which infection spreads from the middle ear or mastoid to the petrous apex and thence to the inferior petrosal sinus, the semilunar ganglion as well as the abducens nerve may become involved in the infective process. Pain, often confined to the distribution of the ophthalmic division, will then occur together with the characteristic lateral rectus palsy.

Tumors

Neurinoma (schwannoma) of the trigeminal ganglion is a rare tumor and accounts for no more than 1.5 per cent of intracranial neurinomas. This contrasts with the vastly more frequent occurrence of acoustic neurinomas, which represent about 98 per cent of these tumors (Morniroli, 1970). The pathologic and clinical features characteristic of trigeminal neurinoma and neurofibroma were fully reviewed by Jefferson (1955), Olive and Svien (1957), and Morniroli (1970) and are discussed in Chapter 68. In the majority of cases symptoms begin in middle life, though five of the seven patients reported by Jefferson (1955) were under 30 years of age. The initial complaint is more often a change in the sensibility of the face—numbness, paresthesias, or a feeling of stiffness—than pain. In the subsequent course of the illness, however, most patients experience pain or painful dysesthesias, often confined to one division at first, but later extending to involve most or all of the trigeminal dermatome. Sensory loss can usually be demonstrated over two or all three divisions, but in a few instances is restricted to diminution or loss of the corneal reflex. Signs of involvement of trigeminal motor fibers were noted in less than half the cases reported by the authors just quoted. In 2 of the 13 cases described by Olive and Svien (1957), in 1 of Jefferson's (1955) 7 cases, and in 1 of Morniroli's (1970) 7 patients, no objective signs of a trigeminal lesion were found. In none of the reported cases was the pain paroxysmal or provoked from cutaneous trigger zones. Love and Woltman (1942) had also stressed that, in tumors of the ganglion, pain is constant, sometimes intense, but never affected by eating, talking, or shaving.

The majority of gasserian neurinomas arise from the medial (radicular) part of the ganglion, but Cuneo and Rand (1952) and Morniroli (1970) each published a case in which the tumor appeared to arise from the mandibular nerve. These neoplasms, though slow growing, can reach a large size; most present in the middle cranial fossa, some are situated in the posterior fossa, and a few are dumbbell-shaped and extend both above and below the tentorium. Compression of neighboring structures is common, particularly involving the abducens nerve, whereas the oculomotor nerve tends to escape. Some patients may present with signs of a posterior fossa lesion, and five of Morniroli's seven cases had developed such signs before they came to operation.

In contrast to the usually high protein level in the cerebrospinal fluid of patients with acoustic neurinoma, less than half the cases of trigeminal neurinoma reported by the authors cited had an increased cerebrospinal fluid protein content. Radiologic demonstration of erosion of the petrous apex and, in some cases, enlargement of the foramen ovale, assist in the diagnosis of trigeminal neurinoma. Surgical excision of the tumor is not unduly hazardous, though portions of its capsule, which adhere to the cavernous sinus or internal carotid artery, may have to be left behind.

The gasserian ganglion can also be the site of origin of primary neurocytoma, glioma, and ganglioneuroma. Daly, Love, and Dockerty (1957) have recorded a case of primary amyloid tumor of the gasserian ganglion with an 11 year history of trigeminal numbness, paresthesias, and pain. The ganglion may be compressed or infiltrated by gumma, by malignant metastases, or by tumors arising from the skull base, such as chondroma, sarcoma, and chordoma (Jefferson, 1955; Morniroli, 1970). These malignant tumors tend to cause a more dense sensory loss and run a more rapidly progressive course than ganglion neurinomas. Meningiomas arising from the dura in or near Meckel's cave were reported to cause classic paroxysmal trigeminal tic (Ver Brugghen, 1952; Ruge et al., 1958), but in such cases the tumor may have affected the sensory root more than the ganglion. On rare occasions, meningiomas originating from the sphenoid wing or from the tentorium may extend to involve the ganglion.

It is of considerable interest that pathologic lesions confined to the ganglion or to its immediate vicinity tend to cause numbness, various dysesthesias, and constant pain, but not the triggered brief paroxysms of pain so characteristic of tic douloureux.

LESIONS OF THE TRIGEMINAL ROOT

In most older textbooks, and in some reports published up to 50 years ago and cited for their historical interest by Penman (1968),

syphilis is mentioned as a cause of trigeminal neuritis and neuralgia. Nonparoxysmal facial pain, hyperesthesia of skin and mucosae, and conversely, trigeminal and corneal anesthesia were described in tabes (Wilson, 1947).

Inflammatory changes in the sensory root of obscure etiology were found in the three cases of chronic benign trigeminal paresis reported by Hughes (1958); details of these cases were described earlier in the section on lesions of the trigeminal nerve in systemic disease.

The sensory root can be invaded, stretched, distorted, or compressed by a variety of vascular malformations and tumors in its neighborhood. In the course of 215 operations for the relief of trigeminal neuralgia via a posterior fossa approach, Dandy (1934) found "aberrant" branches of the superior cerebellar artery or free arterial loops compressing the sensory root or lifting it away from the brain stem in 66 cases; in the same series of patients he also discovered six aneurysms and five angiomas in contact with the root. Gardner (1968) explored the cerebellopontine angle of 18 patients who had suffered recurrence of typical trigeminal neuralgia after previous root section via the middle fossa; he came across arterial loops "compressing, encircling or transfixing the nerve root" in six cases and a cirsoid aneurysm of the basilar artery in one case. Two patients with extensive angiomatous malformations in the posterior cranial fossa are described by Hierons (1953), and by Abbott and Killeffer (1970). Paroxysmal remitting pain involving either the second or the second and third divisions, with precipitating factors characteristic of trigeminal neuralgia, preceded the onset of other symptoms by four years. The pain then became constant, and Hierons' patient developed signs of brain stem and cerebellar dysfunction. Eisenbrey and Hegarty (1956) reported a similar case of arteriovenous malformation in which the patient began to complain of trigeminal neuralgia at the age of 12 years, but signs of involvement of the medulla and cerebellum did not appear until 16 years later. In five consecutive operations for trigeminal neuralgia by a transtentorial approach, Jannetta and Rand (1967b) found, with the aid of the dissecting microscope, that the trigeminal root was compressed and distorted by one or more small tortuous arteries, which appeard to be branches of the superior cerebellar artery. They were so small as to be barely visible to the naked eye. Similar anomalous vessels, compressing the trigeminal root, were not seen in patients undergoing posterior fossa craniotomy for other reasons, nor in any of 56 fresh cadavers from subjects without a history of facial pain. The literature contains several more reports referring to vascular compression of the sensory root from ectatic or redundant loops of the basilar artery as a cause of tic douloureux.

Acoustic neurinomas, meningiomas in the posterior cranial fossa, cholesteatomas, invasive adenomas of the pituitary gland, and metastatic tumors may irritate or invade the trigeminal sensory root.

Diminution or loss of the corneal reflex is a common finding in patients with acoustic neurinoma. Constant pain, sometimes confined to the ophthalmic division, occurs less often; paroxysmal pain typical of tic douloureux was a feature of 16 of Dandy's 154 cases of this tumor (Gonzalez Revilla, 1947).

Meningiomas may also present with classic paroxysmal trigeminal neuralgia, which can persist for several years before the pain becomes constant and objective neurologic signs appear (Ver Brugghen, 1952; Abbott and Killeffer, 1970; Morniroli, 1970). Tic douloureux occurred in 5 of 13 cases of posterior fossa meningioma reviewed by Gonzalez Revilla (1948). As was mentioned earlier, some of these tumors arise near Meckel's cave, but it appears from the available data that it is involvement of the root rather than the ganglion that is apt to produce trigeminal tic.

Cholesteatomas (epidermoids) are more likely to cause tic douloureux than any other tumors in the posterior fossa. Four of Olivecrona's (1949) seven cases of cholesteatoma in the cerebellopontine angle had suffered from typical tic for periods varying from one to seven years before the tumor was discovered and removed. The patients' ages ranged from 22 to 32 years; pain was confined to the mandibular division in three cases and involved both the second and third divisions in one. Apart from a diminished corneal reflex in one case, no abnormal neurologic signs were found. Although the tumor had reached the size of a walnut in two cases and was usually situated between the fifth and eighth cranial nerves, symptoms were confined to the trigeminus in all patients. Tic douloureux also occurred in 10 of the 13 cases of posterior fossa cholesteatomas reviewed by Gonzalez Revilla (1948). These

tumors may also arise in Meckel's cave, where they displace or distort the sensory root, again causing a typical paroxysmal tic (Mehta et al., 1971). In three cases reported by Baumann and Bucy (1956), however, very large extradural epidermoid tumors had produced complete sensory and motor trigeminal paralysis, as well as involving neighboring cranial nerves in two of these patients.

Three examples of invasion of the trigeminal root by invasive adenomas of the pituitary gland, confirmed by autopsy, were given by Jefferson (1940). Only brief clinical descriptions, referring to spasmodic pain and trigeminal anesthesia, are provided.

There are records of cases of trigeminal neuralgia in which the trigeminal root was compressed between the petrous bone and the pons as a result of displacement of the pons by a tumor in the contralateral posterior fossa (Hamby, 1947; Gardner, 1968).

Analysis of the case reports just cited justifies the conclusion that "typical" trigeminal neuralgia is more prone to occur with compressive lesions of the root than with those affecting the ganglion or peripheral divisions. A slow rate of growth of the tumor, such as that of cholesteatomas and meningiomas, which displaces and stretches the root rather than invading it, may, however, be a more important factor than the exact anatomical situation of the lesion.

CENTRAL LESIONS OF THE TRIGEMINAL PATHWAYS

The central connections of the trigeminal nerve may be involved in vascular and neoplastic lesions of the pons, medulla, and upper three cervical segments of the spinal cord, in syringobulbia and related developmental malformations at the craniocervical junction, and in multiple sclerosis. No reference could be found to trigeminal involvement in brain stem encephalitis.

Lesions of Pons, Medulla, and Upper Cord Segments

The descending trigeminal tract and nucleus are affected in lateral medullary infarction due to thrombosis of the posterior inferior cerebellar artery or of one vertebral artery. In these cases the initial sensory loss may be confined to the first two trigeminal divisions, and pain and temperature sensation are usually, but not always, more severely affected than touch. Severe, persistent, and spontaneous pain and painful dysesthesias may subsequently develop in a proportion of these patients and are most intractable. Harris (1950) states that this pain cannot be relieved by alcohol injection into the gasserian ganglion, an observation that may be significant in the consideration of the pathogenesis of trigeminal neuralgia.

Intrinsic tumors of the pons and medulla almost never cause pain and only rarely include trigeminal sensory loss among the many and variable signs that result from involvement of brain stem nuclei and tracts. In a review of 48 brain stem tumors in childhood, Bray, Carter, and Taveras (1958) found trigeminal sensory loss in 31 cases, but none of these patients had pain.

Syringobulbia, or syringomyelia involving the uppermost cervical segments and thus the descending trigeminal tract and nucleus, causes a dissociated anesthesia for pain and thermal sensation; touch is usually spared, though the corneal reflex may be lost. In some cases analgesia is initially confined to the posterior parts of the face and then gradually advances forward in a concentric, onion skin pattern that may spare the tip of the nose and the medial portions of the upper lip and upper alveolar margin. A rare association between syringomyelia and tic douloureux was mentioned by Penman (1968), who quoted two French studies, both published in 1933 (Alajouanine and Thurel, 1933; Schaeffer and Pelland, 1933). The lack of reference to this association in the literature of the past 40 years implies that it must be very rare indeed.

Multiple Sclerosis

In multiple sclerosis, tic douloureux occurs with a frequency sufficient to make a chance association extremely unlikely. In a review of 1735 cases of trigeminal neuralgia and 3880 cases of multiple sclerosis seen at the Mayo Clinic over a 15 year period, 35 patients were found in whom the two diseases occurred in conjunction. Thus, about 2 per cent of patients with trigeminal neuralgia had multiple sclerosis, and 1 per cent of patients with multiple sclerosis suffered from trigeminal

neuralgia (Rushton and Olafson, 1965). In an earlier series of 2083 cases of tic douloureux, Harris (1952) had discovered 66 with signs of multiple sclerosis, an incidence of about 3.1 per cent. A much higher incidence rate, about 8 per cent (10 of 124 patients with tic douloureux), was reported by Chakravorty (1966).

In 80 to 90 per cent of cases documented, symptoms of multiple sclerosis preceded the onset of trigeminal neuralgia by intervals varying from 1 to 29 years; in the remainder the paroxysmal tic was the first symptom, and the signs of multiple sclerosis appeared from one month to six and a half years later (Rushton and Olafson, 1965; Penman, 1968). There are even some cases on record in which clinical signs of multiple sclerosis were "accidentally" discovered during the examination of a patient suffering from tic douloureux. Harris (1950) referred to rare cases of multiple sclerosis with prolonged episodes of numbness or paresthesias of one side of the face, including loss of taste, but free from pain. He cited one case in which tic appeared seven years after such an episode of numbness; signs of multiple sclerosis became apparent 11 years later. Harris (1936) also first pointed out that bilateral trigeminal neuralgia is much more common in patients with multiple sclerosis than in the "genuine" form of the disease. In his later series of 1443 cases of tic douloureux, bilateral involvement was reported in 5.3 per cent of those without multiple sclerosis, but in 14 per cent of those with it (Harris, 1940). Rushton and Olafson confirmed this view, as in 4 of their 35 patients (11 per cent) the neuralgia was bilateral. The intervals between involvement of the two sides of the face varied from four months to six years. In contrast, only 70 of their 1700 patients with uncomplicated trigeminal neuralgia (4 per cent) had bilateral pain. The same authors drew attention to the fact that 505 of their series of 3845 patients with multiple sclerosis (13.1 per cent) experienced paresthesias in the face in the course of the disease, yet did not suffer from trigeminal neuralgia while under their observation. The mean age of onset of tic douloureux is generally lower in patients with multiple sclerosis than in those with "genuine" tic. The frequency of involvement of individual divisions of the trigeminal nerve in Chakravorty's (1966) 10 cases did not differ significantly from that found in "genuine" trigeminal neuralgia. In only one of his cases, however, was mention made of trigger factors. Harris (1950) had stressed that "triggers" were not invariably present in patients with trigeminal neuralgia and multiple sclerosis; Rushton and Olafson (1965) made no specific comment on this point except that a "common occurrence of trigger zones and trigger mechanisms" was one of four criteria used for the diagnosis of trigeminal neuralgia. In all other respects the clinical characteristics of trigeminal neuralgia in multiple sclerosis, including prolonged remissions and relapses, are identical to those of "genuine" tic. There is a conspicuous lack of objective sensory defects in the face, though a mild hypalgesia was found in one of the 10 cases described in detail by Chakravorty (1966). The presence of disseminated sclerosis has no influence on the result of treatment of tic douloureux by carbamazepine or by alcohol injection or section of the sensory root; the incidence of postoperative recurrence of pain is also similar for the two conditions.

There are few autopsy studies of cases of trigeminal neuralgia with multiple sclerosis. A critical review of six previously recorded cases and precise clinical and pathologic observations of a seventh case were presented by Olafson, Rushton, and Sayre (1966). Their patient suffered from typical paroxysmal trigeminal neuralgia confined to the second division of the right trigeminal nerve. Autopsy revealed a plaque on the right sensory root where it penetrated the arachnoid and entered the pons; it involved the greater part of the entering fibers. While no abnormality was found along the intrapontine distribution of the *left* fifth nerve, a sclerotic plaque involved the region of the mesencephalic root and the beginning of the descending tract of the *left* trigeminus. There was no record of facial pain on the left side during the patient's life. In each of the six previous autopsy studies recorded in the literature since 1911, a plaque was found on the sensory root of one trigeminal nerve near the site of its entrance into the pons. In two of these cases, however, a plaque was found on only one nerve root, though the patients had suffered from bilateral neuralgia. In all seven recorded cases, plaques were shown to involve the trigeminal descending root bilaterally, a finding that could not be correlated with the patients' pain during life. It would appear then, in accord with the views expressed by Harris in 1950, that the sclerotic plaque at the pontine root

entry zone is the likely factor in the production of pain.

Vascular Anomalies

In the course of 42 medullary tractotomy operations for the relief of trigeminal neuralgia, Sunder-Plassmann, Grunert, and Böck (1971) observed an elongated posterior inferior cerebellar artery, which formed loops extending caudally over the lateral surface of the medulla, in 10 cases. In most of these the arterial wall was sclerotic, and in eight it was attached to the lateral surface of the medulla, over the region of the trigeminal descending tract, by fine fibrous strands; these arteries produced visible indentations on the medulla. The authors considered that such extramedullary arterial anomalies could be a contributing factor in the pathogenesis of trigeminal neuralgia.

The literature concerned with lesions of the trigeminal nerve and its connections has expanded considerably in recent years. A specific, though cryptogenic, form of trigeminal neuropathy has been defined, and the involvement of the trigeminus in various connective tissue disorders has received attention. Of even greater importance is the increasing recognition that vascular anomalies and various slowly growing tumors that compress, deform, or stretch the sensory root can cause a paroxysmal trigeminal neuralgia indistinguishable in every respect from "genuine" tic douloureux. The dictum of Stookey and Ransohoff (1959) that "in trigeminal neuralgia organic signs are not present" is no longer tenable. The demonstration of sclerotic plaques at the root entry zone in cases of disseminated sclerosis associated with trigeminal neuralgia supports the impression that pathologic changes in the sensory root, of various types and degrees, may contribute to the pathogenesis of paroxysmal neuralgia. The length of the sensory root compared to spinal posterior roots and the abruptness of transition from the peripheral Schwann cell investment of axons to the central sheath system formed by oligodendroglia before the root enters the pons may be factors that make the root susceptible to minor trauma. It must not be forgotten, however, that well-documented cases are on record in which injury or compression of peripheral branches or of the

doubtful whether much reliance can be placed on this finding. In a few cases trigeminal neuralgia, sometimes bilateral, may be associated with Paget's disease of the skull, and minor degrees of basilar impression were found more often in Gardner's (1968) patients with trigeminal neuralgia than in control subjects.

The results of masticator electromyography in tic douloureux were reported recently by Saunders, Krout, and Sachs (1971). Fibrillation potentials and signs of denervation in the masseter and temporalis muscles were observed in 7 of 18 patients; only one of the patients with an abnormal electromyogram had been treated by alcohol injection, and one had associated multiple sclerosis. Similar studies on a large series of patients are needed to assess the value of electromyography in the investigation of difficult cases of trigeminal neuralgia. Involvement of the motor root, disclosed by an abnormal electromyogram, could be a sign of a compressive lesion and thus an indication for exploratory surgery.

Examination of the cerebrospinal fluid has little value. The fluid is normal in "idiopathic" trigeminal neuralgia and may be equally normal in "symptomatic" cases in which the root is compressed by benign tumors, as noted earlier in the section on tumors of the trigeminal ganglion and sensory root.

Differential Diagnosis

The experienced neurologist should have little difficulty in distinguishing trigeminal neuralgia from "atypical facial pain," which usually occurs in depressed or neurotic individuals who present with a vague and variable, though greatly elaborated, history of incessant, intolerable, and usually bilateral pain. Emotion is the only factor that aggravates this pain, and there are none of the triggers so characteristic of tic douloureux.

Pain of dental origin is also constant and has neither the quality nor the radiation or precipitating factors of trigeminal neuralgia. Temporomandibular joint dysfunction causes a constant pain, often of only moderate intensity. It may radiate from the region of the joint along the mandibular division, but frequently also spreads into the side of the neck. It is aggravated by chewing, rarely by talking, and cannot be provoked by tactile stimuli. The joint is usually tender to firm pressure from without or from the oral cavity.

Migrainous facial neuralgia and cluster headache are distinguished from tic douloureux by the longer duration of pain, seldom less than 15 to 30 minutes; by the absence of precipitants, and by the frequent tendency to involve the other side of the face in some attacks. Cluster headaches often follow a remarkably specific time pattern, and profuse watering of the eye and nostril on the side of the pain is a common feature.

Glossopharyngeal neuralgia may at times be difficult to differentiate from tic douloureux. Coughing and swallowing, which are the main triggers of ninth nerve neuralgia, will only very rarely precipitate trigeminal tic. Radiation of pain to the tongue, palate, and eardrum may occur in both conditions, but the tonsillar area, which is a common site of pain in glossopharyngeal neuralgia, is hardly ever involved in tic douloureux. If paroxysms are frequent, painting the affected side of the throat with a 5 per cent solution of cocaine will relieve glossopharyngeal neuralgia temporarily and thus aid in the distinction.

The clinical features of some trigeminal neuropathies were described earlier in this chapter; as the pain is constant and objective signs are almost always found, they should not present diagnostic problems.

Pathology

Opinions are still divided about the significance of various pathologic changes observed in the semilunar ganglion and trigeminal sensory root. In many of the studies published during the past 75 years no abnormalities were found. Smith (1954) stated:

> In 3 of the cases I examined there was major trigeminal neuralgia or tic douloureux. In none of these cases have I found changes in the peripheral nerves, the semilunar ganglion, the sensory root, the sensory nuclei or any other part of the sensory pathway including the thalamus, which could be attributed to any other cause but the treatment given.

Pathologic findings reported by others were not universally accepted because some of the changes could be attributed to postmortem artifact and many were present also in the ganglia and roots from elderly people who had never suffered from trigeminal neuralgia. For example, distention of ganglion cells, mixed lymphocytic and plasmocytic infiltrations, and an increase in fibrous tissue were observed in some, but not all, gasserian ganglia from 52 subjects who had no complaints referable to the trigeminal nerves (Opalski, 1930). Thickening and irregularity of many of the myelin sheaths and segmental demyelination have been described in trigeminal sensory roots from aged people without any history of trigeminal disease (Kerr, 1967a). Such alterations may well be the result of mechanical trauma prior to fixation. It therefore becomes obvious that histopathologic changes in trigeminal neuralgia have to be interpreted with caution.

Biopsy material of the trigeminal ganglion, obtained during sensory root section for tic douloureux, showed thickening and disorganization of myelin sheaths, segmental demyelination of some fibers, and thinning or even complete disappearance of some axons when examined by light microscopy (Kerr, 1967b). Electron microscopic observations revealed "degenerative hypermyelination," demyelination and enlargement of axis cylinders, sometimes with "microneuroma" formation (Beaver et al., 1965b; Kerr and Miller, 1966; Kerr, 1967b). Ganglion cells were intact, apart from peculiar vacuoles in the Nissl substance, to which Beaver, Moses, and Ganote (1965b) attributed little significance as they may be an artifact produced by intracellular fluid shifts. The changes in the axons and myelin must also be treated with suspicion, as entirely similar changes may be produced by trauma (Thomas, 1970).

Treatment

While the cause of idiopathic trigeminal neuralgia remains obscure its treatment cannot be specific; at present only symptomatic relief from pain can be achieved by either pharmaceutical or surgical methods.

MEDICAL TREATMENT

During the past four centuries attempts to relieve the pain of tic douloureux have ranged from dental extraction to partial resection of the colon, from local galvanic stimulation to electroconvulsive therapy. Poisons such as hemlock, arsenic, strychnine, and venoms of the bee and of various snakes were in vogue until the beginning of the present century. They were then replaced by trichlorethylene and stilbamidine, toxins with a selective action on the trigeminal nerve. Stilbamidine abolishes

pain by producing a sensory trigeminal neuropathy, but usually causes bilateral facial dysesthesias as intolerable as the original tic (Smith and Miller, 1955). The literature abounds with uncritical reports of therapeutic triumphs in small series of patients who were temporarily relieved of pain by thiamine (vitamin B_1) or cyanocobalamin (vitamin B_{12}), by vasodilators or vasoconstrictors. None of these therapeutic endeavors was based on rational thought, and temporary successes can be attributed only to natural remissions of the disease.

For a more detailed and entertaining review of our ancestors' efforts to treat tic douloureux, the reader is referred to Penman (1968).

Simple analgesics such as aspirin or paracetamol (acetaminophen), alone or in combination with codeine, are inadequate for the severe pain of trigeminal neuralgia; the risk of addiction in a chronic recurrent disorder precludes the use of morphine, pethidine (meperidine), and similar drugs.

Diphenylhydantoin and carbamazepine are the only drugs at present available for the control of pain paroxysms in trigeminal neuralgia. Diphenylhydantoin has been used sporadically since 1942, though at first on the erroneous assumption that tic douloureux represented an "epileptic" discharge of trigeminal sensory neurons.

There is experimental evidence that diphenylhydantoin increases the threshold to electrical stimulation of nerve endings of A fibers of peripheral nerves and that it may exert its effect on the membrane properties of peripheral nerves (Morrell et al., 1958; Iannone et al., 1958). A central action of the drug, however, may be more significant: Kugelberg and Lindblom (1959) have shown that this drug raises the threshold for tactile stimuli from the trigger zones and shortens the duration of the attack by diminishing its tendency to self-maintenance. Both Blom (1963a) and Fromm and Landgren (1962) were able to demonstrate in the experimental animal that diphenylhydantoin inhibits synaptic transmission in the trigeminal pathway.

From the literature and from personal experience, it is known that diphenylhydantoin in doses ranging from 300 to 600 mg per day is effective in less than 50 per cent of patients with trigeminal neuralgia (Braham and Saia, 1960; Taverner, 1968). In a considerable proportion of cases in which the drug is initially successful, the pain paroxysms tend to become refractory to it within 12 months.

Carbamazepine is the drug of choice for the treatment of tic douloureux. It is an iminostilbene derivative, chemically related to imipramine hydrochloride. Like diphenylhydantoin it is an anticonvulsant, and Blom (1963b) has shown that it also inhibits the polysynaptic nociceptive linguomandibular reflex in decerebrate cats. Many clinical trials conducted in various parts of the world testify that carbamazepine controls the pain of trigeminal neuralgia in about 70 per cent of cases. In our series of 70 patients the attacks were completely abolished in 41 per cent, controlled to the patients' satisfaction in 29 per cent, and partially relieved in a further 4 per cent. Analysis of a further 198 cases reported in the literature prior to 1965 supported our findings (Burke et al., 1965), and more recent publications provide further confirmation (Bonduelle and Lormeau, 1966; Krayenbühl, 1969; Heyck, 1970).

Carbamazepine usually controls pain within 12 to 48 hours, and cessation of treatment produces an equally rapid recurrence. After the justly enthusiastic early reports, long-term follow-up studies have shown that this drug may lose its effect, even in large and potentially toxic doses, after two years of successful treatment in 10 to 30 per cent of patients (Heyck, 1970). The reasons why some patients do not respond to carbamazepine at all, and others become refractory to it after months or years, are unknown. The cause may not lie in the pathologic mechanisms producing the pain, but may be found in the pharmacodynamics of the drug, such as an accelerated induction of enzymes that metabolize it.

The age of the patient, the duration of his trigeminal neuralgia, the division of the nerve involved, and previous treatment by alcohol injection or surgery do not appear to influence the initial effect of carbamazepine or the later emergence of drug resistance (Burke and Selby, 1965).

Side effects include temporary drowsiness in about 40 per cent of patients, giddiness and ataxia in 10 to 15 per cent, and skin rashes in less than 10 per cent. A few patients experience gastrointestinal upsets, but only 2 of 70 in our series abandoned the drug because of side effects (Burke and Selby, 1965). Leukopenia and aplastic anemia were reported in isolated cases, but can be prevented by appropriate clinical and hematologic supervision. Virolainen (1971) described a single case in which blast cells increased significantly in the peripheral blood.

It is of particular interest that carbamazepine relieves only the pain of trigeminal and glossopharyngeal neuralgia, and that the proportion of successful results is lower in symptomatic than in idiopathic trigeminal neuralgia. The drug is ineffective against postherpetic dysesthesias and atypical facial neuralgias (Selby, unpublished observations; Krayenbühl, 1969), although Carnaille and associates (1966) and Westerholm (1970) have reported partial therapeutic successes in a few of these patients.

Once the diagnosis of idiopathic trigeminal neuralgia is established the initial treatment should be with carbamazepine. Careful clinical supervision reduces to insignificant levels the risk of toxic reactions. If the drug is effective, the patient is spared the facial numbness and dysesthesias that can be so distressing after alcohol injection or rhizotomy.

Minor side effects can be minimized by gradual increases in dosage, beginning with 100 mg twice daily. The average effective dose ranges from 600 to 800 mg per day, and only a few people will tolerate a daily dose of 1200 mg. If carbamazepine in the maximum tolerated dose does not control pain within 72 hours, therapeutic failure must be conceded. A few patients, however, respond better to a combination of carbamazepine and diphenylhydantoin than to either drug alone.

SURGICAL TREATMENT

The history of surgery of the trigeminal nerve, since the first attempts were made to cure tic douloureux by denervation of the face more than 200 years ago, is comprehensively and critically reviewed by Penman (1968). It is beyond the scope and purpose of this chapter to describe details of the different surgical methods or to discuss the vast literature that has accumulated on this subject. The astute and authoritative reviews of Stookey and Ransohoff (1959), Falconer and Harris (1968), and Krayenbühl (1969) are recommended to the interested reader. The discussion here is confined to a summary of current surgical techniques and a critical appraisal of their success, limitations, and complications.

ALCOHOL INJECTION

Alcohol injection into the supraorbital or infraorbital nerve rarely produces analgesia and relief from neuralgia for more than 6 to 12 months. Only 5 of 287 patients were free of pain five years after infraorbital alcohol injection (Henderson, 1967). This procedure should, therefore, be reserved for very debilitated patients and for those who initially refuse any other approach.

Injection of the mandibular division at the foramen ovale is relatively devoid of risk, but recurrence of pain within two years is the rule. Only 10 per cent of Henderson's (1967) 165 patients, who received a total of 227 injections, were still pain-free after five years; in one third of his cases an undesired sensory loss extended into the second and sometimes into the first division.

Injection of the second division in the sphenopalatine fossa is technically difficult and entails the risk of damage to the third, fourth, and sixth cranial nerves; even blindness due to destruction of the optic nerve has been reported.

The arachnoid pouch, called the trigeminal cistern, which surrounds the gasserian ganglion and triangular part of the trigeminal root (see Fig. 28–1), would cause any alcohol injected into the ganglion to spread via the cerebrospinal fluid into sensory root bundles (Ferner, 1970). Petř (1970) and Henderson (1967) state that these postganglionic fibers have to be reached for a successful injection. In a patient who died six days after alcohol injection into the ganglion, Smith (1954) found marked degeneration in the sensory root that could be traced into the main sensory nucleus. In another case in which death occurred three months after alcoholic destruction of the ganglion, autopsy revealed degenerative changes extending into the descending trigeminal tract and, transsynaptically, into the secondary ascending axons (Penman and Smith, 1950).

As it is generally held that functional regeneration of destroyed fibers does not occur in the central nervous system, the effect of "complete" alcohol destruction of the sensory root should be permanent. Failures may be attributed largely to technical difficulties allowing the survival of a sufficient number of root fibers.

In a follow-up study of 457 patients who had been successfully treated by alcohol injection, mostly into the gasserian ganglion, 316 (69 per cent) remained free of neuralgic tic for three years or longer (Harris, 1940). In 31 per cent of these 316 cases pain did not recur for 10 years or more, and 10 patients enjoyed relief for 20 to 31 years. Immediate total sensory loss was achieved in 81 per cent of 196 alcohol injections into the sensory root of 165 patients (Henderson, 1967). Eighty-six of these were reexamined after intervals varying from 1 to 17 years; almost two thirds remained free of pain, though only one third were found to have total anesthesia. Pain and touch sensibility tended to return most often in the mandibular division. In other follow-up studies, only 15.2 per cent of 248 patients, who had 427 alcohol injections, were free from pain for more than one year (Peet and Schneider, 1952), and the average duration of freedom from pain was only 7.23 months in another series of 298 cases subjected to 821 alcohol injections (Ruge et al., 1958). The exact site of alcohol injection is not stated in either of the aforementioned series, though the short duration of relief permits the assumption that peripheral divisions rather than the ganglion or root were the target in the majority of cases.

Apart from the inevitable ipsilateral numbness of the face, and the consequent dribbling of food and saliva from the anesthetic side of the mouth, undesirable sequelae of alcohol injection include crawling or burning dysesthesias in from 33 to 48 per cent of cases, exposure keratitis in from 10 to 20 per cent, and more rarely chronic ulceration and atrophy of the ala nasi (Peet and Schneider, 1952). Masticatory paralysis usually recovers after six to nine months. Anesthesia dolorosa may develop in about 4 per cent of cases (Falconer and Harris, 1968). Herpetic lesions around the mouth and ala nasi appear during the first few days after alcohol injection in about one third of patients.

In an effort to diminish the loss of cutaneous sensibility and to avoid some of these complications, Jefferson (1963) has used phenol in glycerin or iophendylate in place of alcohol; a high recurrence rate has prevented wide adoption of this method.

THERMAL DESTRUCTION OF TRIGEMINAL GANGLION AND SENSORY ROOT

Electrocoagulation of the gasserian ganglion was introduced by Kirschner in 1933. In 45 per cent of patients so treated pain recurred within two years, and in 61 per cent within 10 years (Bues, 1967). The incidence of postoperative complications is similar to that after alcohol injection, and this method has not found wide favor among neurosurgeons.

On the assumption that the finely myelinated A-delta and unmyelinated C fibers might be selectively destroyed by heat, Sweet and Wepsic (1970) have applied radiofrequency heat lesions with a hollow electrode introduced into the ganglion and sensory root through the foramen ovale. Electrical stimulation permits some localization of root fibers and their selective destruction. They have treated 68 patients with trigeminal neuralgia and succeeded in preserving some touch sensibility throughout the trigeminal field in about 85 per cent of these. The procedure had to be repeated in 15 per cent of their cases, and the long-term recurrence rate has yet to be assessed.

PERIPHERAL NEURECTOMY

Avulsion of the supraorbital and supratrochlear nerves is now only rarely performed because the area of denervation is usually insufficient to relieve first division pain and because regeneration of the nerve is the rule. Avulsion of the infraorbital nerve has a place in the treatment of elderly, debilitated patients with neuralgia confined to the maxillary division, particularly if a previous alcohol injection into the nerve has given some months of relief. In a follow-up study of 55 patients treated by section of the supraorbital or infraorbital nerve, freedom from pain ranged from five months to eight years, with an average of 33.2 months (Grantham and Segerberg, 1952). This compared favorably with the average duration of only 15.5 months of relief after alcohol injection into these nerves.

FRACTIONAL SECTION OF SENSORY ROOT

In recent years most surgeons have employed Frazier's operation and exposed the floor of the middle cranial fossa by a temporal craniectomy. An extradural approach is generally favored, though some surgeons prefer to open the dura (Henderson, 1967; Krayenbühl, 1969). Lasting relief from pain is achieved only if three quarters to four fifths of the fibers of the sensory root are divided. Selective section of posterolateral fibers usually suffices for neuralgia confined to the mandibular division, while dorsomedial fibers must be cut if pain involves the ophthalmic division; the maxillary fibers occupy an intermediate position. The motor root can usually be spared in this operation.

From an analysis of eight large series of cases reported over the past 50 years and comprising a total of 4259 patients, the operative mortality rate ranges from 0.26 to 2.5 per cent (Cushing, 1920; Frazier and Russell, 1924; Grant, 1938; Peet and Schneider, 1952; Ruge et al., 1958; Henderson, 1967; Krayenbühl, 1969; Kalyanaraman and Ramamurthi, 1970). Considering that the majority of patients are of advanced years, and that many have concomitant cardiovascular and other diseases, this mortality rate is remarkably low.

The incidence of relapse of pain in the area involved before operation varies from 1.1 per cent of the total rhizotomies performed by Ruge, Brochner, and Davis (1958) to 12.6 to 15 per cent of fractional root sections (Peet and Schneider, 1952; Henderson, 1967; Krayenbühl, 1969). These recurrences may be attributed to anatomical variations in the length and thickness of the trigeminal root, and to the fact that not all the fibers of the affected division were cut.

Corneal sensation can be preserved in about four fifths of cases of fractional root section (Henderson, 1967), yet some of the authors just cited quote an incidence of exposure keratitis varying from 4 to 15 per cent. Postoperative facial paralysis occurs in 6 to 16 per cent, usually appears only after one to six days following operation, and almost invariably recovers within a few months (Falconer and Harris, 1968).

Paresthesias in the analgesic part of the face are probably experienced by all patients, though most learn to accept them as a small price for the relief from their pain. A sensation of numbness and swelling of the lips, tongue, and cheek, and loss of feeling on one side of the mouth are usual complaints, and a proportion of people are troubled by intermittent unpleasant crawling or burning dysesthesias, or by a feeling of tightness of the face. These sequelae must be frankly discussed with the patient before operation so that he will not come to interpret them as a result of surgical failure. Personality traits and stressful environmental circumstances contribute to the degree of suffering caused by these paresthesias. Anesthesia of one side of the mouth and tongue inevitably allows food to collect on the numb side or to drop from the corner of the mouth. Most people soon learn precautionary maneuvers to prevent this.

Anesthesia dolorosa, which may develop in up to 5 per cent of cases after posterior rhizotomy, is probably the most distressing complication (Stookey and Ransohoff, 1959; Krayenbühl, 1969). It usually begins only weeks or months after operation and consists of constant unpleasant dysesthesias described as feelings of tightness, burning, cold, or itching, which may become intolerable. The pathogenesis is as obscure as that of post-herpetic dysesthesias, and no successful treatment has been discovered; trigeminal tractotomy and stereotactic coagulation of the thalamic sensory nuclei have proved to be equally ineffective (Falconer and Harris, 1968).

Herpetic eruptions around the angle of the mouth and lips occur as often after rhizotomy as after alcohol injections, and trophic erosion of the ala nasi is a relatively rare complication.

Partial or complete section of the trigeminal sensory root near its entry into the pons by a posterior fossa approach was recommended by Dandy (1932). His claims for preservation of cutaneous sensibility and of the corneal reflex were not substantiated by others. This operation, however, affords a better view of the compact portion of the trigeminal root, and Dandy's (1934) description of 12 tumors and 77 vascular anomalies encircling or compressing the root in a series of 215 cases is of considerable importance. Gardner (1968) found a tumor, vascular anomaly, or adherence of the root to the pons in 12 of 18 patients in whom a Dandy operation was performed for recurrence of trigeminal neuralgia after a rhizotomy in the middle fossa.

Dandy's suboccipital approach is technically more difficult and carries a higher mortality risk than Frazier's operation. For these reasons most neurosurgeons employ it only in selected cases, either if a compressive lesion is suspected clinically or if a previous middle fossa procedure has failed.

Recently Jannetta and Rand (1967a) have devised a subtemporal transtentorial operative approach to the trigeminal root at the pons. With the aid of the binocular dissecting microscope they were able to identify and spare the intermediate fibers of the trigeminal root. Although partial to complete section of the major portion of the sensory root was accomplished with resultant analgesia or hypalgesia, perception of light touch and corneal sensation were preserved in all five patients subjected to this operation. In these five cases the trigeminal root was found to be mildly to severely compressed and distorted by small tortuous arteries that were barely visible to the naked eye.

DECOMPRESSION OR COMPRESSION OF THE TRIGEMINAL GANGLION AND ROOT

As at least one fifth of patients remain distraught by numbness and unpleasant dysesthesias after trigeminal rhizotomy, several attempts have been made to discover a surgical procedure for the relief of neuralgia with preservation of normal cutaneous sensibility. On the reasonable assumption that compression of the ganglion or root was a factor in the pathogenesis of tic douloureux, Taarnhøj (1952) recommended decompression of the posterior part of the ganglion and adjoining root by dividing the overlying dura and the superior petrosal sinus at the point where the trigeminal root passes over the edge of the petrous bone into the posterior fossa. Other neurosurgeons have adopted various modifications of Taarnhøj's operation, but long-term follow-up of over 400 cases has revealed a recurrence rate of from 33 to 75 per cent within three to eight years after operation (for references see Stender and Grumme, 1969).

Surgical efforts were then directed at producing some degree of trauma to the ganglion while also decompressing it, in the hope that such injury to ganglion cells and their axons might reduce the high recurrence rate after simple decompression procedures. Shelden and co-workers (1955) rubbed the ganglion at operation, a procedure they described as "compression" of the ganglion. Five years later they reported their results in a series of 115 patients: postoperative herpes occurred in 52 per cent of them, and the neuralgia recurred within five years in 20 per cent. Postoperative dysesthesias were reported in only seven instances (Shelden et al., 1960). Decompression of the ganglion, which some surgeons called "gangliolysis," may be combined with the direct application of 70 per cent alcohol to the sensory root. Although this produced a more pronounced sensory loss, and the rate of relapse of neuralgia was proportional to the degree of postoperative hypoesthesia, Stender and Grumme (1969) found that the long-term results after the application of alcohol were no better than those of simple gangliolysis. They report a recurrence rate of 33 per cent after five years and 50 per cent after nine years in a series of 115 patients, but there were no instances of exposure keratitis or anesthesia dolorosa. Fargueta (1968) applied a 7.5 per cent solution of phenol in a radiopaque medium to the exposed sensory root and obtained initial satisfactory results in 81 per cent of his cases. Evaluation of this method must await long-term review. On present evidence it would appear that lasting relief from tic douloureux can be achieved only at the expense of analgesia, though not necessarily loss of touch sensibility, in the affected part of the face.

MEDULLARY TRIGEMINAL TRACTOTOMY

This operation was introduced by Sjöqvist (1938) and aims to interrupt pain and temperature conducting fibers in the descending trigeminal tract while preserving touch and proprioceptive sensation. Sjöqvist divided the tract in the lateral part of the medulla about 8 to 10 mm above the level of the obex. Difficulties with the operative technique and a high rate of complications, including cerebellar ataxia of the ipsilateral limbs and laryngeal palsy, prevented general acceptance of this method. While Penman (1968) strongly condemned medullary tractotomy on the grounds of high morbidity, mortality, and relapse rates, Kunč (1970) reports a mortality rate of only 0.85 per cent, and a recurrence rate of 17.5 per cent after 275 tractotomies, 240 of which were for trigeminal neuralgia. Kunč (1970) modified Sjöqvist's approach and cut the descending trigeminal tract some 5 to 8 mm below the obex (or about 12 to 15 mm above the first filament of the second cervical sensory root) just rostral to the upper edge of the nucleus caudalis. With the patient under local anesthesia, he was able to define the borders of the trigeminal tract and the limits of each division within it, by stimulation with a thin needle, before cutting the affected divisions. Recurrences were attributed to imperfect section of the tract. Postoperative herpes was observed frequently, and patients were troubled by dysesthesias, but their exact frequency was not stated.

A valuable by-product of Kunč's (1970) studies is confirmation of a lamellar "onion peel" representation of the face in the descending trigeminal tract. The ala nasi, lips,

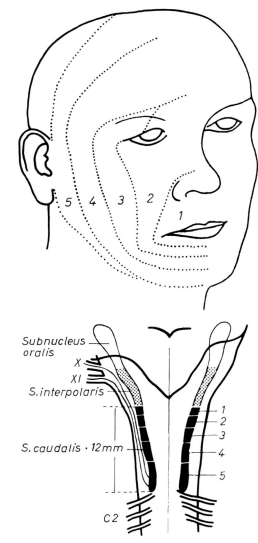

Figure 26–6 The lamellar "onion peel" representation of the face in the subnucleus caudalis of the spinal trigeminal nucleus. Numbers 1 to 5 in the lower diagram of the nucleus correspond with the numbers for the sensory segments of the face. (From Kunč, Z.: Significant factors pertaining to the results of trigeminal tractotomy. *In* Hassler, R., and Walker, A. E. (eds.): Trigeminal Neuralgia, Pathogenesis and Pathophysiology. Stuttgart, Georg Thieme Verlag, 1970. Reprinted by permission.)

and angle of the mouth are represented uppermost in the nucleus caudalis, the majority of second division fibers terminate next in the upper segments, while most of the first and third division fibers end in the lower parts of this nucleus (Fig. 26–6). In patients in whom tractotomy was performed a few millimeters below the rostral end of the nucleus caudalis, pain sensation was preserved in an oval area including the nose, inner canthus, and medial part of the cheek and lips, similar to the area where pain sensation is retained in some cases of syringobulbia.

The success of Kunč's modification of medullary tractotomy shows that the operation still has a useful place in the treatment of tic douloureux, particularly in the rare cases in which both sides of the face are involved and only tractotomy, at least on one side, can prevent the disabling bilateral loss of touch and proprioceptive sensibility of the mouth and jaw. In the very rare instances in which trigeminal and glossopharyngeal neuralgia are combined, medullary tractotomy is the operation of choice.

The merits, risks, and complications of each of the commonly used surgical procedures for the treatment of trigeminal neuralgia have been summarized to help the reader formulate a plan of treatment for the individual patient. The first essential step is the correct diagnosis of idiopathic tic douloureux. If carbamazepine fails to give lasting relief, retrogasserian fractional rhizotomy is the best operation; the recent transtentorial approach to the pontine part of the root with sparing of intermediate fibers may prove to offer the best prospects of cure with relatively few complications. In view of the almost certain recurrence of pain, peripheral alcohol injection and peripheral neurolysis should be offered only to the very young or very old, or to those people who, after patient and intelligent explanation of all facts, prefer the strong probability of recurrence to the relatively small risks of complications from root section. Alcohol injection into the ganglion or root can provide more lasting freedom from pain, but carries a higher risk of exposure keratitis and of recurrence of neuralgia than fractional rhizotomy. Compression and decompression operations offer no clear advantages, and the long-term success of selective and partial destruction of the ganglion and root by heat has not yet been established.

The mere fact that so many different procedures are commonly used—and some that enjoyed only a short vogue or were employed in a small number of cases are not included in this review—is evidence that the ideal treatment for trigeminal neuralgia has yet to be discovered. We still have no universally accepted explanation of why sensory denervation of the face can abolish this pain; a better understanding of its pathogenesis is needed for further therapeutic progress.

Etiology and Pathophysiology

The cause of trigeminal neuralgia is still unknown and a subject of controversy. Discussion of the many theories of etiology has been left to the end of this chapter so that the reader may consider the merits of such theories with reference to the characteristic clinical features—including the success of different therapeutic procedures—in this syndrome.

STRUCTURAL CAUSES

Trigeminal neuralgia is not a specific disease, but a symptom that can be produced by various pathologic processes. A review of the extensive literature has shown that a variety of small, benign, slow-growing tumors, as well as vascular malformations and even tiny "aberrant" arteries encircling or compressing the trigeminal sensory root, can cause tic douloureux, which is in every respect—including long remissions—indistinguishable from the "idiopathic" form of the syndrome. All the responsible pathologic lesions were only distorting, compressing, or stretching the root, whereas larger tumors or those invading it tended to produce more constant pain, numbness, and paresthesias. The trigeminal root, and particularly its compact part near the pons, was much more often the site of compression than the ganglion.

Cases of tic douloureux consequent on trauma to dental nerves are so exceedingly rare that they can be dismissed from pathogenetic consideration (Harris, 1950).

Dandy's (1934) finding of 11 large vascular malformations and 66 "aberrant" vessels in contact with the root in a series of 215 posterior fossa operations for trigeminal neuralgia was not confirmed by other surgeons. This may simply be because the vast majority of patients were treated by either alcohol injection or by Frazier's middle fossa operation, and the trigeminal root in the posterior fossa could not be inspected. More recently Jannetta and Rand (1967b) have again drawn attention to these anomalous vessels, so small that they are seen only with the operating microscope.

The somatotopic localization of peripheral divisions within the sensory root permits a selective involvement of different branches from mild external compressive forces. Aberrant sensory rootlets, which leave the pons separately from the main sensory root and join the fibers from the ophthalmic division, could explain why this branch is so rarely affected alone (Jannetta and Rand, 1967a). The even rarer simultaneous involvement of the first and third divisions agrees also with the anatomy of the root, where their fibers are separated by those of the maxillary branch.

As the evidence derived from the often incomplete observations at operation or autopsy failed to reveal structural lesions in most cases, various anomalies of the bone and dura in the region of the petrous apex and Meckel's cave were considered responsible for compressing or stretching the ganglion and root. Olivecrona (1941) suggested that the contents of the posterior fossa tend to sag toward the foramen magnum with advancing years, and that this causes stretching and angulation of the sensory root over the petrous crest. Gardner (1968) postulated that such kinking of the root over the petrous tip may be due to mild degrees of basilar impression, which can be caused by postmenopausal osteoporosis, These theories fail to take account of the fact that bilateral tic occurs in only 4 to 5 per cent of cases (Harris, 1940; Rushton and Olafson, 1965), nor can they explain the even greater rarity of isolated involvement of the first division. Gardner's (1968) observation of an elevated petrous ridge on the side of the tic is more consistent with the predominantly unilateral pain, though in 20 per cent of his cases the neuralgia occurred on the side of the lower petrous ridge.

The concept of compression of the ganglion and adjoining root by its dural sheath and by the superior petrosal sinus motivated Taarnhøj's decompression operation. This concept was recently extended by Malis (1967), who described a fibrous band stretching from the anterior clinoid process over the trigeminal root to the apex of the petrosal bone. He postulated that increasing elevation of the petrous pyramid with age alters the angle of this dural band and narrows the opening into Meckel's cave. Kerr (1963b) relates the occurrence of tic in old age to a decreased density of the fascial reinforcement covering the lacuna in the roof of the carotid canal. This exposes the inferior surface of the ganglion and of the adjoining divisions and root to the minor repeated trauma of carotid pulsation. He supports his argument by the more frequent involvement of the maxillary and man-

dibular divisions, whereas the ophthalmic division, situated in the cavernous sinus, is cushioned by venous blood. Another possible source of irritation of the ganglion or root was raised by O. Hassler (1967), who found very small round calcifications, composed mainly of calcium hydroxyapatite with a little tricalcium phosphate, scattered through the arachnoid membrane, but most pronounced in the floor of the arachnoid pouch surrounding the trigeminal ganglion and root. As none of the 80 patients from whom this autopsy material was derived had suffered from trigeminal neuralgia during life, the etiologic significance of such calcifications is highly speculative.

All the foregoing theories are based on the idea that mild external irritation of the ganglion or root is capable of causing the pain of tic douloureux. Other hypotheses, attributing it to intrinsic lesions of these structures, have received less support.

The frequent occurrence of herpes simplex eruptions on the lips or face after alcohol injection or operations on the trigeminal pathway (including decompression procedures and medullary tractotomy) has stimulated the proposal that chronic latent infection of the gasserian ganglion with the herpes virus could be the cause of trigeminal neuralgia (Knight, 1954; Behrman and Knight, 1956). Cogent arguments against this thesis include the vast number of people who suffer from recurrent herpes simplex of the lips and never develop tic douloureux, the not infrequent occurrence of similar herpetic eruptions after craniotomy for various other indications, and the fact that herpes virus could not be isolated from the trigeminal ganglion or root (Carton and Kilbourne, 1952).

The age incidence of tic douloureux is the only justification for considering ischemia due to atherosclerotic narrowing of arteries supplying the gasserian ganglion as a possible causal factor. As tic has not been reported after thrombosis or ligation of the internal carotid artery, and as its incidence cannot be correlated with cerebral or coronary or peripheral arterial disease, this theory has little to recommend it. Furthermore, histologic examination of biopsy and autopsy material has failed to show ischemic changes restricted either to the involved portion of the ganglion or even to the ganglion on the affected side (Kerr, 1963b).

The only intrinsic pathologic process capable of causing paroxysms of trigeminal neuralgia, identical to those of the "idiopathic" form, is multiple sclerosis in which the plaques of demyelination were always shown to involve the fibers of the trigeminal root at their zone of entry into the pons (Olafson et al., 1966).

There is no convincing evidence that a pathologic lesion central to the pontine root entry zone can be the *primary* cause of tic douloureux. Paroxysmal tic-like pain has never been reported in lateral medullary infarction, syringobulbia, or tumors of the brain stem that invaded the descending trigeminal tract and nucleus. A thalamic lesion was postulated by Lewy and Grant (1938), even though such a lesion was ipsilateral to the neuralgia in each of their five cases in which autopsy was performed; their finding of cerebral atrophy and vascular lesions in the corona radiata was similarly unrelated to the site of the patients' pain. Apart from the tenuous arguments used by these authors, there are no reports of thalamic infarcts or of stereotactic lesions in thalamic sensory nuclei, including the arcuate nucleus, that have produced the paroxysmal pain characteristic of tic douloureux.

From the evidence just summarized, we may conclude that mild external injury to the sensory root, and less often to the ganglion, as well as a plaque of demyelination in the root near its entry into the pons, can cause the clinical syndrome of trigeminal neuralgia. It might, therefore, be speculated that at a microscopic level partial demyelination and loss of some axons may be implicated in the pathogenetic mechanism.

If we accept the validity of such structural causation, we still have to account for the spontaneous, and often prolonged, remissions so characteristic of the natural history of trigeminal neuralgia. Similar remissions of varying duration are equally typical of multiple sclerosis, so that remyelination could be considered as an event contributing to the termination of a bout that has persisted for days, weeks, or months. The intracranial contents, including the trigeminal root, are not rigidly fixed; their position may be influenced by movements of the head and neck, by arterial pulsations, and by changes in the cerebrospinal fluid pressure. Such dynamic forces could cause sufficient minor trauma to a trigeminal root, already compromised by intrinsic degenerative changes and by extrinsic stretching or compression, to precipitate a new series of pain paroxysms.

The peripheral structural lesions we have so far considered do not provide a sufficient explanation for many of the highly specific features of the pain of trigeminal neuralgia.

PATHOPHYSIOLOGIC MECHANISMS

A valid theory of the pathogenesis of tic douloureux must account for each of the following characteristics of this syndrome: (1) the brief, paroxysmal nature and intensity of the pain; (2) triggering of some, though not necessarily all, attacks by minute tactile or proprioceptive stimuli; (3) occurrence of trigger spots in the majority of cases and their predominant location in the central (most anterior) parts of the face; (4) radiation of pain along linear tracks that are usually confined to one or two divisions, but hardly ever diffuse over an entire dermatome; (5) absence of demonstrable neurologic deficit; (6) natural history of remissions and relapses, and tendency to progression of the frequency, duration, and severity of relapses; (7) relief from sensory denervation of the face by destruction of fibers of the primary sensory neuron; (8) immediate, though often temporary, relief from decompression or compression operations on the ganglion and root; (9) frequent occurrence of dysesthesias, and rarely of anesthesia dolorosa, after sensory denervation of the face; and (10) the similarity of trigeminal and glossopharyngeal neuralgia and the occasional concurrence of these two syndromes.

The paroxysmal character of trigeminal and glossopharyngeal tic is unlike any other painful affliction of man, with the possible exceptions of intermedius neuralgia and vagal neuralgia, which are so rare that some doubt has been cast on their very existence (Wegner, 1968; Crue and Todd, 1968). The only common denominator for these neuralgias is the anatomical convergence of their exteroceptive afferent fibers in the nucleus caudalis of the spinal tract and nucleus of the trigeminal nerve.

Gardner (1968) considered the paroxysm of tic douloureux to be a reflex phenomenon on the following grounds: it is evoked by a stimulus, and the response is self-limited but outlasts the stimulus; it is followed by a refractory period and is abolished when the afferent arm of the reflex arc is interrupted. He attributed this reflex to "cross stimulation" or "ephaptic" transmission across intact trigeminal axons that have become approximated and partly denuded of their myelin sheaths as a result of compression. Kerr

(1967c) offered a similar hypothesis of short-circuiting between demyelinated surfaces of two adjacent axons, or from a large demyelinated fiber to an intact unmyelinated axon that has lost its Schwann cell envelope. Such short-circuiting would continue as long as the denuded fibers remain viable, and cease as soon as one of the axons degenerates. Further slight trauma to the vulnerable, partly degenerated sensory root fibers again causes demyelination in some of them, and so starts the next cycle of pain paroxysms. This is an attractive theory in that it provides a tentative explanation for spontaneous remissions from pain; it presupposes that both compression and decompression operations inflict sufficient trauma on the exposed surviving axons to arrest their short-circuiting. It is interesting in this context that Falconer and Harris (1968) have cited a case in which a compression operation aggravated the neuralgia.

Kerr's hypothesis was criticized by Darian-Smith (1970b) on the grounds that the concept of ephaptic transmission between adjacent fibers rests on a fragile foundation; he proposed that a differential loss of large myelinated fibers may be of greater importance than the loss of myelin insulation of surviving axons. This large-fiber input may have a sustained inhibitory influence on transmission in the earliest relays of the nociceptive anterolateral pathways—a "gating" of the input as suggested by Melzack and Wall (1965). The nociceptive pathway, therefore, becomes "sensitized" by the differential loss of these inhibitory fibers so that pain can be evoked by a stimulus that would normally elicit only a tactile sensation.

If cross stimulation between fibers of the sensory root were an adequate cause of the paroxysmal pain of tic douloureux, why does a similar pain never result from compression of the spinal posterior roots? It is reasonable to assume that during the early stage of spinal posterior root irritation, from whatever cause, the degree of damage to afferent sensory fibers must be similar to that in the trigeminal root. Even when no objective sensory deficit can be demonstrated by clinical examination, patients complain of paresthesias and a constant aching pain, but never of a paroxysmal neuralgia of the intensity and nature of tic douloureux. As was implied by Darian-Smith (1970b), a heightened state of excitability of the central relays, which may occur exclusively in the trigeminal nociceptive pathways, must be responsible.

List and Williams (1957) suggested that an attack of tic douloureux represents a pathologic multineuronal reflex in the trigeminal nuclei of the brain stem. This may be initiated by the trigeminal dorsal root reflex in which antidromic impulses from the spinal nucleus are conducted back to the periphery, and then reexcite, orthodromically, the central trigeminal connections, with recruitment of additional neurons. Such a process of self-exciting after-discharge can be repetitive until the firing neurons become refractory. Much of this theory has received support from later physiologic experiments.

Kugelberg and Lindblom's (1959) study of 50 patients with trigeminal neuralgia defined the relationship between a paroxysm of pain and stimuli applied to cutaneous trigger zones. They found that touch and tickle, rather than pain or temperature, are the adequate stimulus for eliciting an attack. While rapid displacement of a single hair was sometimes sufficient, a larger spatial and temporal summation of impulses was necessary to trigger a paroxysm in the majority of cases. With a weak stimulus, summation times of 15 to 30 seconds were often observed. Cessation of the stimulus was followed by a rapid decrease in excitability, although it remained above the resting value for up to 20 seconds in three patients. A refractory period of up to two to three minutes, depending on the duration and intensity of the pain, follows the attack. Stimulation at higher intensities could elicit pain during the refractory interval, but this pain tended to be shorter and of less severity. The anticonvulsant drugs lidocaine and hydantoin raised the threshold for the effective stimuli, and shortened the duration of the attack by diminishing its tendency to self-maintenance. From these findings Kugelberg and Lindblom (1959) deduced that the pathophysiologic mechanism responsible for the paroxysmal pain of tic douloureux is centrally situated, probably in the spinal trigeminal nucleus.

At the beginning of this chapter current physiologic concepts of the transmission of touch and pain in trigeminal pathways were reviewed. It was shown that units responding the tactile stimuli are present in all subdivisions of the spinal nucleus as well as in the main nucleus, and that animal experiments had failed to demonstrate any cells or fibers within the sensory trigeminal nuclei and tract specifically concerned with pain perception.

Physiologic experiments have indicated that the delayed antidromic wave of the trigeminal dorsal root reflex may be due to activity of short-chain neurons in a multisynaptic central internuncial pool (Crue et al., 1968). There is further experimental evidence that this delayed antidromic wave may itself evoke orthodromic activity from cutaneous endings in the affected peripheral trigeminal dermatome. This complex concept agrees with List and Williams's (1957) earlier hypothesis of a repetitive, self-exciting after-discharge.

While caudal tractotomy abolishes this dorsal root reflex, a tractotomy rostral to the nucleus caudalis augments it, a response that can be interrupted by hydantoin. Mild graded pressure on the trigeminal sensory root will also interrupt conduction of the dorsal root reflex at the site of pressure so that the impulse no longer reaches the cutaneous terminals. As yet only little information is available concerning the existence of the dorsal root reflex in man. King (1967) referred to two patients with paroxysms of trigeminal neuralgia felt near the frontal vertex in the dermatome of the first division but elicited from trigger zones in the second division; in each instance an injection of procaine above the eyebrow interrupted the radiation of pain distally to the vertex, whereas pain in the upper eyelid and eyebrow persisted.

The concept of the dorsal root reflex, evoked by tactile stimuli and capable of generating a repetitive, self-exciting after-discharge, provides a tentative explanation for the tactile triggers and for the brief repetitive bursts of pain so characteristic of tic douloureux. The theory of a *central mechanism* (though not primary cause) of this pain receives further support from the findings of Young and King (1972) that nonnoxious stimuli to the face produce primary afferent depolarization (excitation), while noxious stimuli result in an initial period of depolarization of low amplitude followed by a more prolonged period of primary afferent hyperpolarization (inhibition), maximal in the nucleus oralis. These authors further propose the theory that one of the functions of the nucleus caudalis is to modulate the transfer of information through the rostral subnuclei of the spinal trigeminal nuclear complex. As the nucleus caudalis is functionally homologous to the substantia gelatinosa of the spinal cord, this view agrees with Melzack and Wall's (1965) theory of a gate control system mediated by the substantia gelatinosa.

The evidence for a purely peripheral pathogenesis of trigeminal neuralgia is further weakened by the fact that a trigger zone in one division can elicit pain in another, and that the vast majority of trigger spots are situated in the central part of the face. The anatomical substrate for these clinical characteristics may be the concentric onion skin pattern of sensory representation in the nucleus caudàlis, and the projection of fibers from the central regions of the face to the most rostral part of this nucleus (see Fig. 26–6).

From the anatomical and physiologic data just reviewed, a working hypothesis of the pathophysiology of tic douloureux can be constructed. Mild mechanical trauma to the trigeminal root, or a plaque of demyelination in multiple sclerosis, results in a partial and differential loss of some large myelinated axons. This reduces the normal inhibitory influence of these fibers on the earliest relays in the nucleus caudalis. The "gate" has been opened, and the secondary and internuncial neuron pools in the rostral parts of the spinal trigeminal nucleus are now in a deranged excitatory state. This augments the self-exciting, repetitive discharge of the trigeminal dorsal root reflex, so that a barrage (summation) of afferent impulses is consciously appreciated as a pain paroxysm. The long latent period between the trigger stimulus and the onset of pain, and the subsequent refractory period are consistent with such a hypothesis. It does not explain, however, why a bout of pain terminates, or why, during such a temporary remission, stimulation of the trigger zone fails to evoke another paroxysm. This is analogous to the enigma of the cessation of an epileptic seizure while the irritative epileptogenic focus persists. The balance between excitation and inhibition is obviously very unstable; either exhaustion of the excitatory synaptic transmitter or accumulation of an inhibitory transmitter would provide an explanation. Remyelination and regeneration of a sufficient number of damaged fibers restores the normal inhibitory state and allows for a prolonged remission. A "subliminal" degree of disinhibition of the central neuron pool in the spinal nucleus, however, persists. Further mechanical trauma to the root can thus evoke the next attack more readily, and relapses become progressively more frequent, prolonged, and severe. Surgical destruction of fibers of the primary sensory neuron (including the descending trigeminal tract) prevents the summation of afferent impulses required to elicit a pain paroxysm. Trauma to sensory root fibers from compression or decompression operations would act in a similar manner, or interrupt the antidromic wave of the trigeminal dorsal root reflex at the point of compression.

The conscious appreciation of pain, and its precise localization must involve the connections between the trigeminal nuclei and the thalamus and somatosensory cortex. The role of the various presynaptic and postsynaptic inhibitory and facilitatory feedback mechanisms on the complex physiology of pain is still obscure (see the earlier discussion of the ascending connections to the thalamus). They may be implicated in the rare instances in which trigeminal tic is triggered by remote sensory impulses from a limb, by eye movement, or by visual, auditory, or emotional stimuli. Further evidence for the significance of these central connections is the experimental observation that conditioning stimuli applied to many different parts of the central nervous system can materially inhibit the excitability of the central terminals of primary afferent trigeminal neurons (King, 1967).

Animal experiments have demonstrated that spontaneous neuronal hyperactivity appears in the medullary trigeminal nucleus some 2 to 10 days after posterior rhizotomy and then increases progressively for at least a month (Anderson et al., 1971). This could account for the common occurrence of facial dysesthesias after sensory denervation by alcohol injection or root section, while some of the thalamic or cortical inhibitory feedback relays may be concerned in the causation of anesthesia dolorosa.

The tentative hypotheses presented here are a gross oversimplification of highly complex and constantly fluctuating physiologic events. They are handicapped by our inadequate knowledge of the physiology of pain in general. The unique qualities of trigeminal tic provide some clues for further study of peripheral and central mechanisms in chronic pain syndromes. On present evidence it would seem that more effective treatment of trigeminal neuralgia will have to await the discovery of pharmacologic agents that can either suppress synaptic excitation or enhance inhibition.

In spite of the spectacular advances in the medical sciences during the past 200 years, we can conclude this chapter with the words of Fothergill (1771-6):

What, therefore, I had to offer upon the nature of this disease is rather submitted for your consideration as matter of further inquiry than as opinions sufficiently established.

References

Abbott, M., and Killeffer, F. A.: Symptomatic trigeminal neuralgia. Bull. Los Angeles Neurol. Soc., *35*:1–10, 1970.

Alajouanine, T., and Thurel, R.: Sur la pathogénie de la névralgie faciale. Rev. Neurol. (Paris), *2*:658–661, 1933 (quoted by Penman, 1968).

Ameli, N. O.: Avicenna and trigeminal neuralgia. J. Neurol. Sci., *2*:105–107, 1965.

Anderson, L. S., Black, R. G., Abraham, J., and Ward, A. A., Jr.: Neuronal hyperactivity in experimental trigeminal deafferentation. J. Neurosurg., *35*:444–452, 1971.

Ashworth, B., and Tait, G. B. W.: Trigeminal neuropathy in connective tissue disease. Neurology (Minneap.), *21*:609–614, 1971.

Bailey, A. A., Sayre, G. P., and Clark, E. C.: Neuritis associated with systemic lupus erythematosus. A.M.A. Arch. Neurol. Psychiatry, *75*:251–259, 1956.

Baumann, C. H. H., and Bucy, P. C.: Paratrigeminal epidermoid tumors. J. Neurosurg., *13*:455–467, 1956.

Beaver, D. L., Moses, H. L., and Ganote, C. E.: Electron microscopy of the trigeminal ganglion. II. Autopsy study of human ganglia. Arch. Pathol., *79*:557–570, 1965a.

Beaver, D. L., Moses, H. L., and Ganote, C. E.: Electron microscopy of the trigeminal ganglion. III. Trigeminal neuralgia. Arch. Pathol. *79*:571–582, 1965b.

Behrman, S., and Knight, G.: Decompression and compression operations for trigeminal neuralgia. Neurology (Minneap.), *6*:363–367, 1956.

Blau, J. N., Harris, M., and Kennett, S.: Trigeminal sensory neuropathy. N. Engl. J. Med., *281*:873–876, 1969.

Blom, S.: The effects of diphenylhydantoin and lidocaine on the linguomandibular reflex in decerebrate cats. Arch. Neurol., *8*:506–509, 1963a.

Blom, S.: Tic douloureux treated with new anticonvulsant. Experiences with G 32883. Arch. Neurol., *9*:285–290, 1963b.

Bonduelle, M., and Lormeau, G.: Les algies faciales et leurs thérapeutiques. Thérapie, *21*:1123–1144, 1966.

Braham, J., and Saia, A.: Phenytoin in the treatment of trigeminal and other neuralgias. Lancet, *2*:892–893, 1960.

Bray, P. F., Carter, S., and Taveras, J. M.: Brainstem tumors in children. Neurology (Minneap.), *8*:1–7, 1958.

Brihaye, J., Périer, O., Smulders, J., and Franken, L.: Glossopharyngeal neuralgia caused by compression of the nerve by an atheromatous vertebral artery. J. Neurosurg., *13*:299–302, 1956.

Brodal, A.: Neurological Anatomy. New York, Oxford University Press, 1969, pp. 411–429.

Bruzstowicz, R. J.: Combined trigeminal and glossopharyngeal neuralgia. Neurology (Minneap.), *5*:1–10, 1955.

Bues, E.: A simplified method of coagulating the Gasserian ganglion and follow-up review of 200 cases of trigeminal neuralgia. Excerpta med. (Amst.), International Congress Series, *139*:104, 1967.

Burke, W. J. G., and Selby, G.: Trigeminal neuralgia. A therapeutic trial of Tegretol. Proc. Aust. Assoc. Neurol., *3*:89–96, 1965.

Burke, W. J. G., Grant, J. M. F., and Selby, G.: The treatment of trigeminal neuralgia: A clinical trial of carbamazepine ("Tegretol"). Med. J. Aust., *1*:494–497, 1965.

Buxton, P. H., and Hayward, M.: Polyneuritis cranialis associated with industrial trichloroethylene poisoning. J. Neurol. Neurosurg. Psychiatry, *30*:511–518, 1967.

Carden, S.: Hazards in the use of the closed-circuit technique for trilene anaesthesia. Br. Med. J., *1*:319–320, 1944.

Carnaille, H., De Coster, J., Tyberghein, J., and Dereymaeker, A.: Étude statistique de près de 700 cas de facialgies traitées par le Tégrétal. Acta Neurol. Belg., *66*:175–196, 1966.

Carton, C. A., and Kilbourne, E. D.: Activation of latent herpes simplex by trigeminal sensory root section. N. Engl. J. Med., *246*:172–176, 1952.

Chakravorty, B. G.: Association of trigeminal neuralgia with multiple sclerosis. Arch. Neurol., *14*:95–99, 1966.

Collard, P., and Nevin, S.: Affection of the trigeminal nerve nucleus and central gray matter of the spinal cord following the administration of stilbamidine. Proc. R. Soc. Med., *40*:87–88, 1946.

Colover, J.: Sarcoidosis with involvement of the nervous system. Brain, *71*:451–475, 1948.

Corbin, K. B.: Observations on the peripheral distribution of fibers arising in the mesencephalic nucleus of the fifth cranial nerve. J. Comp. Neurol., *73*:153–177, 1940.

Crue, B. L., and Todd, E. M.: Vagal neuralgia. *In* Vinken, P. J., and Bruyn, G. W. (eds.): Handbook of Clinical Neurology. Vol. 5. Amsterdam, North-Holland Publishing Co., 1968, pp. 362–367.

Crue, B. L., Todd, E. M., and Carregal, E. J. A.: Cranial neuralgia. Neurophysiological considerations. *In* Vinken, P. J., and Bruyn, G. W. (eds.): Handbook of Clinical Neurology. Vol. 5. Amsterdam, North-Holland Publishing Co., 1968, pp. 281–295.

Cuneo, H. M., and Rand, C. W.: Tumors of the Gasserian ganglion. Tumor of the left Gasserian ganglion associated with enlargement of the mandibular nerve. A review of the literature and case report. J. Neurosurg., *9*:423–431, 1952.

Cushing, H. W.: The major trigeminal neuralgias and their surgical treatment based on experiences with 332 Gasserian operations; varieties of facial neuralgia. Am. J. Med. Sci., *160*:157–184, 1920.

Daly, D. D., Love, J. G., and Dockerty, M. B.: Amyloid tumor of the Gasserian ganglion. J. Neurosurg., *14*:347–352, 1957.

Dandy, W. E.: The treatment of trigeminal neuralgia by the cerebellar route. Ann. Surg., *96*:787–795, 1932.

Dandy, W. E.: Concerning the cause of trigeminal neuralgia. Am. J. Surg., *24*:447–455, 1934.

Darian-Smith, I.: Tactile sensory pathways from the face. Proc. Aust. Assoc. Neurol., *3*:27–39, 1965.

Darian-Smith, I.: Neural mechanisms of facial sensation. Int. Rev. Neurobiol., *9*:301–395, 1966.

Darian-Smith, I.: The neural coding of "tactile" stimulus parameters in different trigeminal nuclei. *In* Hassler, R., and Walker, A. E. (eds.): Trigeminal Neuralgia. Pathogenesis and Pathophysiology. Philadelphia, W. B. Saunders Co., 1970a, pp. 59–72.

Darian-Smith, I.: Discussion for chapter 23 (Peripheral versus central factors in trigeminal neuralgia, by F. W. L. Kerr). *In* Hassler, R., and Walker, A. E. (eds.): Trigeminal Neuralgia. Pathogenesis and Pathophysiology. Philadelphia, W. B. Saunders Co., 1970b, pp. 187–188.

Darian-Smith, I., Proctor, R., and Ryan, R. D.: A single-neurone investigation of somatotopic organization within the cat's trigeminal brain-stem nuclei. J. Physiol. (Lond.), *168*:147–157, 1963.

Denny-Brown, D., and Yanagisawa, N.: The descending trigeminal tract as a mechanism for intersegmental sensory facilitation. Trans. Am. Neurol. Ass., *95*: 129–133, 1970.

Eisenbrey, A. B., and Hegarty, W. M.: Trigeminal neuralgia and arteriovenous aneurysm of the cerebello-pontine angle. J. Neurosurg., *13*:647–649, 1956.

Emmons, W. F., and Rhoton, A. L., Jr.: Subdivision of the trigeminal sensory root. Experimental study in the monkey. J. Neurosurg., *35*:585–591, 1971.

Esiri, M. M., and Tomlinson, A. H.: Herpes zoster. Demonstration of virus in trigeminal nerve and ganglion by immunofluorescence and electron microscopy. J. Neurol. Sci., *15*:35–48, 1972.

Falconer, M. A., and Harris, L.: Surgical treatment of the cranial neuralgias. *In* Vinken, P. J., and Bruyn, G. W. (eds.): Handbook of Clinical Neurology. Vol. 5. Amsterdam, North-Holland Publishing Co., 1968, pp. 386–404.

Fargueta, J. S.: A new conservative surgical treatment for trigeminal neuralgia: "phenol root-painting." Acta Neurochir. (Wien), *18*:1–14, 1968.

Feindel, W., Penfield, W., and McNaughton, F.: The tentorial nerves and localization of intracranial pain in man. Neurology (Minneap.), *10*:555–563, 1970.

Ferner, H.: The anatomy of the trigeminal root and the gasserian ganglion and their relations to the cerebral meninges. *In* Hassler, R., and Walker, A. E. (eds.): Trigeminal Neuralgia, Pathogenesis and Pathophysiology. Philadelphia, W. B. Saunders Co., 1970, pp. 1–6.

Fothergill, J.: Of a painful affection of the face. *In* Medical Observations and Inquiries by a Society of Physicians in London. London, T. Cadell, 1771–6, Vol. 5:129–142 (quoted by King, 1967).

Frazier, C. H., and Russell, E. C.: Neuralgia of the face; an analysis of seven hundred and fifty-four cases with relation to pain and other sensory phenomena before and after operation. Arch. Neurol. Psychiatry, *11*:557–563, 1924.

Fromm, G. H., and Landgren, S.: Effect of diphenyl-hydantoin on single cells in the spinal trigeminal nucleus. Neurology (Minneap.), *12*:302, 1962.

Gardner, W. J.: Trigeminal neuralgia. Clin. Neurosurg., *15*:1–56, 1968.

Gonzalez Revilla, A.: Neurinomas of cerebellopontile recess. A clinical study of one hundred and sixty cases including operative mortality and end results. Bull. Johns Hopkins Hosp., *80*:254–296, 1947.

Gonzalez Revilla, A.: Differential diagnosis of tumors at the cerebellopontile recess. Bull. Johns Hopkins Hosp., *83*:187–212, 1948.

Grant, F. C.: Results in the operative treatment of major trigeminal neuralgia. Ann. Surg., *107*:14–19, 1938.

Grantham, E. G., and Segerberg, L. H.: An evaluation of palliative surgical procedures in trigeminal neuralgia. J. Neurosurg., *9*:390–394, 1952.

Grubel, G.: The physiology of single neurons of the trigeminal nuclei. *In* Hassler, R., and Walker, A. E. (eds.): Trigeminal Neuralgia, Pathogenesis and Pathophysiology. Philadelphia, W. B. Saunders Co., 1970, pp. 73–77.

Gudmundsson, K., Rhoton, A. L., Jr., and Rushton, J. G.: Detailed anatomy of the intracranial portion of the trigeminal nerve. J. Neurosurg., *35*:592–600, 1971.

Guillain, G., and Kreis, B.: Sur deux cas de polyradiculo-névrite avec hyperalbuminose du liquide céphalo-rachidien sans réaction cellulaire. Paris Méd., *2*: 244–247, 1937 (quoted by Spillane and Wells, 1959).

Hamby, W. B.: Trigeminal neuralgia due to contralateral tumors of the posterior cranial fossa. Report of 2 cases. J. Neurosurg., *4*:179–182, 1947.

Harris, W.: Bilateral trigeminal tic. Its association with heredity and disseminated sclerosis. Ann. Surg., *103*:161–172, 1936.

Harris, W.: An analysis of 1433 cases of paroxysmal trigeminal neuralgia (trigeminal-tic) and the end-results of Gasserian alcohol injection. Brain, *63*: 209–224, 1940.

Harris, W.: Rare forms of paroxysmal trigeminal neuralgia, and their relation to disseminated sclerosis. Br. Med. J., *2*:1015–1019, 1950.

Harris, W.: The fifth and seventh cranial nerves in relation to the nervous mechanism of taste sensation. A new approach. Br. Med. J., *1*:831–836, 1952.

Hassler, O.: Calcifications in the intracranial arachnoid. A microradiological and histological study of the occurrence and appearance of calcifications, with special reference to the trigeminal nerve. J. Neurosurg., *27*:336–345, 1967.

Hassler, R.: Dichotomy of facial pain conduction in the diencephalon. *In* Hassler, R., and Walker, A. E. (eds.): Trigeminal Neuralgia, Pathogenesis and Pathophysiology. Philadelphia, W. B. Saunders Co., 1970, pp. 123–138.

Hassler, R., and Bak, I. J.: The fine structure of different types of synapses and their circuit arrangement in the substantia gelatinosa trigemini. *In* Hassler, R., and Walker, A. E. (eds.): Trigeminal Neuralgia, Pathogenesis and Pathophysiology. Philadelphia, W. B. Saunders Co., 1970, pp. 50–58.

Henderson, W. R.: Trigeminal neuralgia: the pain and its treatment. Br. Med. J., *1*:7–15, 1967.

Heyck, H.: Drug therapy of trigeminal pain. *In* Hassler, R., and Walker, A. E. (eds.): Trigeminal Neuralgia, Pathogenesis and Pathophysiology. Philadelphia, W. B. Saunders Co., 1970, pp. 115–122.

Hierons, R.: Brain-stem angioma confirmed by arteriography. Relapsing symptoms and signs strongly suggestive of disseminated sclerosis. Proc. R. Soc. Med., *46*:195–196, 1953.

Hill, T. R.: Two cases of trigeminal neuropathy. Proc. R. Soc. Med., *47*:914–915, 1954.

Hope-Simpson, R. E.: The nature of herpes zoster: a long-term study and a new hypothesis. Proc. R. Soc. Med., *58*:9–20, 1965.

Hughes, B.: Chronic benign trigeminal paresis. Proc. R. Soc. Med., *51*:529–531, 1958.

Humphrey, J. H., and McClelland, M.: Cranial-nerve palsies with herpes following general anaesthesia. Br. Med. J., *1*:315–318, 1944.

Iannone, A., Baker, A. B., and Morrell, F.: Dilantin in the treatment of trigeminal neuralgia. Neurology (Minneap.), *8*:126–128, 1958.

Jannetta, P. J., and Rand, R. W.: Gross (mesoscopic) description of the human trigeminal nerve and ganglion. J. Neurosurg., *26*(Suppl.):109–111, 1967a.

Jannetta, P. J., and Rand, R. W.: Arterial compression of the trigeminal nerve at the pons in patients with trigeminal neuralgia. J. Neurosurg., *26*(Suppl.):159–162, 1967b.

Jefferson, A.: Trigeminal root and ganglion injections using phenol in glycerine for the relief of trigeminal neuralgia. J. Neurol. Neurosurg. Psychiatry, *26*: 345–352, 1963.

Jefferson, G.: Extrasellar extensions of pituitary adenomas. Proc. R. Soc. Med., *33*:433–458, 1940.

Jefferson, G.: Trigeminal neurinomas with some remarks on the malignant invasion of the Gasserian ganglion. Clin. Neurosurg., *1*:11–54, 1955.

Jefferson, M.: Sarcoidosis of the nervous system. Brain, *80*:540–556, 1957.

Kaltreider, H. B., and Talal, N.: The neuropathy of Sjögren's syndrome: trigeminal nerve involvement. Ann. Intern. Med., *70*:751–762, 1969.

Kalyanaraman, S., and Ramamurthi, B.: Trigeminal neuralgia—a review of 331 cases. Neurol. India, *18*(Suppl. 1):100–108, 1970.

Kerr, F. W. L.: The divisional organization of afferent fibers of the trigeminal nerve. Brain, *86*:721–732, 1963a.

Kerr, F. W. L.: The etiology of trigeminal neuralgia. Arch. Neurol., *8*:15–25, 1963b.

Kerr, F. W. L.: Correlated light and electron microscopic observations on the normal trigeminal ganglion and sensory root in man. J. Neurosurg., *26*(Suppl.): 132–137, 1967a.

Kerr, F. W. L.: Pathology of trigeminal neuralgia: light and electron microscopic observations. J. Neurosurg., *26*(Suppl.):151–156, 1967b.

Kerr, F. W. L.: Evidence for a peripheral etiology of trigeminal neuralgia. J. Neurosurg., *26*(Suppl):168–174, 1967c.

Kerr, F. W. L.: Fine structure and functional characteristics of the primary trigeminal neuron. *In* Hassler, R., and Walker, A. E. (eds.): Trigeminal Neuralgia, Pathogenesis and Pathophysiology. Philadelphia, W. B. Saunders Co., 1970, pp. 11–21.

Kerr, F. W. L., and Miller, R. H.: The pathology of trigeminal neuralgia. Electron microscopic studies. Arch. Neurol., *15*:308–319, 1966.

King, R. B.: Evidence for a central etiology of tic douloureux. J. Neurosurg., *26*(Suppl.):175–180, 1967.

King, R. B.: Electrophysiology of trigeminal neurons under normal and epileptogenic conditions. *In* Hassler, R., and Walker, A. E. (eds.): Trigeminal Neuralgia, Pathogenesis and Pathophysiology. Philadelphia, W. B. Saunders Co., 1970, pp. 78–85.

King, R. B., Meagher, J. N., and Barnett, J. C.: Studies of trigeminal nerve potentials in normal compared to abnormal experimental preparations. J. Neurosurg., *13*:176–183, 1956.

Kirschner, M.: Die Punktionstechnik und die Elektro-koagulation des Ganglion Gasseri. Arch. Klin. Chir., *176*:581–620, 1933.

Knight, G.: Herpes simplex and trigeminal neuralgia. Proc. R. Soc. Med., *47*:788–790, 1954.

Krayenbühl, H.: Idiopathic trigeminal neuralgia. Acta clinica No. 9, Documenta Geigy. Basle, Switzerland, J. R. Geigy S. A., 1969.

Kugelberg, E., and Lindblom, U.: The mechanism of the pain in trigeminal neuralgia. J. Neurol. Neurosurg. Psychiatry, *22*:36–43, 1959.

Kunč, Z.: Significant factors pertaining to the results of trigeminal tractotomy. *In* Hassler, R., and Walker, A. E. (eds.): Trigeminal Neuralgia, Pathogenesis and Pathophysiology. Philadelphia, W. B. Saunders Co., 1970, pp. 90–100.

Lewis, D. C.: Systemic lupus and polyneuropathy. Arch. Intern. Med., *116*:518–522, 1965.

Lewy, F. H., and Grant, F. C.: Physiopathologic and pathoanatomic aspects of major trigeminal neuralgia. Arch. Neurol. Psychiatry, *40*:1126–1134, 1938.

List, C. F., and Williams, J. R.: Pathogenesis of trigeminal neuralgia. A review. A.M.A. Arch. Neurol. Psychiatry, 77:36–43, 1957.

Love, J. G., and Woltman, H. W.: Trigeminal neuralgia and tumors of the Gasserian ganglion. Proc. Mayo Clin., 17:490–496, 1942.

Malis, L. I.: Petrous ridge compression and its surgical correction. J. Neurosurg., 26(Suppl.):163–167, 1967.

Manni, E., Palmieri, G., and Marini, R.: Extraocular muscle proprioception and the descending trigeminal nucleus. Exp. Neurol., 33:195–204, 1971.

Maxwell, D. S.: Fine structure of the normal trigeminal ganglion in the cat and monkey. J. Neurosurg., 26(Suppl.):127–131, 1967.

Mehta, D. S., Malik, G. P., and Dar, J.: Trigeminal neuralgia due to cholesteatoma of Meckel's cave. J. Neurosurg., 34:572–574, 1971.

Melzack, R., and Wall, P. D.: Pain mechanisms: a new theory. Science, 150:971–979, 1965.

Mira, K. M., Elnaga, I. A., and El-Sherif, H.: Nerve cells in the intracranial part of the trigeminal nerve of man and dog. Anatomical study of the fifth cranial nerve. J. Neurosurg., 34:643–646, 1971.

Morniroli, G.: Das Trigeminus neurinom. Schweiz. Arch. Neurol. Neurochir. Psychiatr., 107:47–86, 1970.

Morrell, F., Bradley, W., and Ptashne, M.: Effect of diphenylhydantoin on peripheral nerve. Neurology (Minneap.), 8:140–144, 1958.

Moses, H. L.: Comparative fine structure of the trigeminal ganglia, including human autopsy studies. J. Neurosurg., 26(Suppl.):112–126, 1967.

Moses, H. L., Beaver, D. L., and Ganote, C. E.: Electron microscopy of the trigeminal ganglion. I. Comparative ultrastructure. Arch. Pathol., 79:541–557, 1965.

Olafson, R. A., Rushton, J. G., and Sayre, G. P.: Trigeminal neuralgia in a patient with multiple sclerosis. An autopsy report. J. Neurosurg., 24:755–759, 1966.

Olive, I., and Svien, H. J.: Neurofibromas of the fifth cranial nerve. J. Neurosurg., 14:484–505, 1957.

Olivecrona, H.: Die Trigeminusneuralgie und ihre Behandlung. Nervenarzt, 14:49–57, 1941.

Olivecrona, H.: Cholesteatomas of the cerebello-pontine angle. Acta Psychiatr. Neurol. Scand., 24:639–643, 1949.

Olszewski, J.: On the anatomical and functional organization of the spinal trigeminal nucleus. J. Comp. Neurol., 92:401–413, 1950.

Opalski, A.: Zur normalen und pathologischen Anatomie des Ganglion Gasseri. Z. Gesamte Neurol. Psychiatr., 124:383–419, 1930.

Peet, M. M., and Schneider, R. C.: Trigeminal neuralgia. A review of six hundred and eighty-nine cases with a follow-up study on sixty five per cent of the group. J. Neurosurg., 9:367–377, 1952.

Penfield, W., and McNaughton, F.: Dural headache and innervation of the dura mater. Arch. Neurol. Psychiatry, 44:43–75, 1940.

Penman, J.: Trigeminal neuralgia. In Vinken, P. J., and Bruyn, G. W. (eds.): Handbook of Clinical Neurology. Vol. 5. Amsterdam, North-Holland Publishing Co., 1968, pp. 296–322.

Penman, J., and Smith, M. C.: Degeneration of the primary and secondary sensory neurones after trigeminal injection. J. Neurol. Neurosurg. Psychiatry, 13:36–46, 1950.

Petr̃, R.: Discussion of paper by H. Ferner. In Hassler, R., and Walker, A. E. (eds.): Trigeminal Neuralgia, Pathogenesis and Pathophysiology. Philadelphia, W. B. Saunders Co., 1970, p. 5.

Rowbotham, G. F.: Observations on the effect of trigeminal denervation. Brain, 62:364–380, 1939.

Ruge, D., Brochner, R., and Davis, L.: A study of the treatment of 637 patients with trigeminal neuralgia. J. Neurosurg., 15:528–536, 1958.

Rushton, J. G., and Olafson, R. A.: Trigeminal neuralgia associated with multiple sclerosis. Report of 35 cases. Arch. Neurol., 13:383–386, 1965.

Saunders, R. L., Krout, R., and Sachs, E., Jr.: Masticator electromyography in trigeminal neuralgia. Neurology (Minneap.), 21:1221–1225, 1971.

Schaeffer, H., and Pelland, M.: Deux cas de névralgie trigéminale dans la syringobulbie. Le caractère de la douleur dans les algies faciales d'origine centrale et leur traitement. Rev. Neurol. (Paris), 40:699–703, 1933 (quoted by Penman, 1968).

Shelden, C. H., Crue, B. L., and Coulter, J. A.: Surgical treatment of trigeminal neuralgia and discussion of compression operation. Postgrad. Med., 27:595–601, 1960.

Shelden, C. H., Pudenz, R. H., Freshwater, D. B., and Crue, B. L.: Compression rather than decompression for trigeminal neuralgia. J. Neurosurg., 12:123–126, 1955.

Sjöqvist, O.: Studies on pain conduction in trigeminal nerve; contribution to surgical treatment of facial pain. Acta Psychiatr. Neurol., Suppl. 17:1–139, 1938.

Smith, G. W., and Miller, J. M.: The treatment of tic douloureux with stilbamidine. Bull. Johns Hopkins Hosp., 96:146–149, 1955.

Smith, M. C.: Discussion on facial pain. Proc. R. Soc. Med., 47:783–790, 1954.

Spillane, J. D., and Wells, C. E. C.: Isolated trigeminal neuropathy. A report of 16 cases. Brain, 82:391–416, 1959.

Steffen, R., and Selby, G.: "Atypical" Ramsay Hunt syndrome. Med. J. Aust., 1:227–230, 1972.

Stender, A., and Grumme, T.: Late results of gangliolysis as a treatment for trigeminal neuralgia. J. Neurosurg., 31:21–24, 1969.

Stookey, B., and Ransohoff, J.: Trigeminal Neuralgia, Its History and Treatment. Springfield, Ill., Charles C Thomas, 1959, p. 86.

Sunder-Plassmann, M., Grunert, V., and Böck, F.: Zur Frage der vaskulären Kompression des Tractus spinalis Nervi trigemini als mögliche Ursache der Trigeminusneuralgie. Nervenarzt, 42:323–325, 1971.

Sweet, W. H., and Wepsic, J. G.: Relation of fiber size in trigeminal posterior root to conduction of impulses for pain and touch: production of analgesia without anesthesia in the effective treatment of trigeminal neuralgia. Trans. Am. Neurol. Assoc., 95:134–139, 1970.

Taarnhøj, P.: Decompression of the trigeminal root and the posterior part of the ganglion as treatment in trigeminal neuralgia: preliminary communication. J. Neurosurg., 9:288–290, 1952.

Taverner, D.: Drug treatment of the cranial neuralgias. In Vinken, P. J., and Bruyn, G. W. (eds.): Handbook of Clinical Neurology. Vol. 5. Amsterdam, North-Holland Publishing Co., 1968, pp. 378–385.

Thomas, P. K.: The quantitation of nerve biopsy findings. J. Neurol. Sci., 11:285–295, 1970.

Urich, H.: Personal communication, 1974.

Ver Brugghen, A.: Paragasserian tumors. J. Neurosurg., 9:451–460, 1952.

Virolainen, M.: Blast transformation of vivo and in vitro in carbamazepin hypersensitivity. Clin. Exp. Immunol., 9:429–435, 1971.

Wall, P. D., and Taub, A.: Four aspects of trigeminal nucleus and a paradox. J. Neurophysiol., 25:110–126, 1962.

Wegner, W.: Nervus intermedius (Hunt's) neuralgia. In Vinken, P. J., and Bruyn, G. W. (eds.): Handbook of Clinical Neurology. Vol. 5. Amsterdam, North-Holland Publishing Co., 1968, pp. 337–343.

Westerholm, N.: Treatment of facial pain with G 32883 (Tegretol Geigy). Scand. J. Dent. Res., 78:144–148, 1970.

Wiesendanger, M., Hammer, B., and Hepp-Reymond, M. C.: Corticofugal control mechanisms of somatosensory transmission in the spinal trigeminal nucleus of the cat. In Hassler, R., and Walker, A. E. (eds.): Trigeminal Neuralgia, Pathogenesis and Pathophysiology. Philadelphia, W. B. Saunders Co., 1970, pp. 86–89.

Wilson, S. A. K.: Neurology. London, Edward Arnold & Co., 1947.

Wirth, F. P., Jr., and Van Buren, J. M.: Referral of pain from dural stimulation in man. J. Neurosurg., 34: 630–642, 1971.

Young, R. F., and King, R. B.: Excitability changes in trigeminal primary afferent fibers in response to noxious and nonnoxious stimuli. J. Neurophysiol., 35:87–95, 1972.

Chapter 27

DISEASES OF THE SEVENTH CRANIAL NERVE

William E. Karnes

ANATOMY

Nerve

Sir Charles Bell (1821, 1829) established the functional and anatomical distinctions between the fifth and seventh cranial nerves, countering the notion held by Willis and surgeons of the day and serving to end the practice of cutting nerve VII in treating trigeminal neuralgia. Bell considered nerve VII to be a nerve of respiration ("respiratory nerve of the face"), as he did the long thoracic nerve ("great external respiratory nerve") and the phrenic nerve ("great internal respiratory nerve"). His name is still associated with the former two.

For this discussion, nerve VII is defined as the central and peripheral extensions of the fibers contained in its two roots at the level of their entry into the brain stem. It is important to establish such a definition because in the course of these fibers, both centrally and peripherally, there are numerous close relationships and interconnections with the fibers of other cranial nerves. Thus, at points along its course, the nerve may not only have lost some fibers through terminal branching but also have gained others through communicating branching. These interrelationships, the large number of functions subserved by its fibers, and its long and tortuous interosseous course make nerve VII unique and one of the more complex cranial nerves.

EMBRYOLOGY

Nerve VII is associated with the development of the second (hyoid) branchial arch and supplies its motor and sensory components. It is analogous to cranial nerves V, IX, and X, which supply the remaining arches. Its motor root arises from neuroblasts beneath the third neuromere of the rhombencephalon. In early development its fibers pass laterally, rostral to the nucleus of nerve VI. Later, as the nucleus of nerve VI moves rostrally and that of nerve VII moves caudally and laterally, the internal genu of nerve VII is formed (Arey, 1946).

The geniculate ganglion is formed from cells that separate from the acousticofacial primordium, which also gives rise to the vestibular and spiral ganglia.

Components of the second branchial arch evaginate to overlap the lower arches during the sixth week of development. Later, the primordial muscle tissue of the second arch enters the skin of the face, thereby overlying the masticatory muscles of the first branchial arch and underlying its cutaneous sensory distribution (Braus-Eltze, 1940). These migrations of the second arch with respect to adjacent arches probably explain the complex interconnections between the respective cranial nerves in the adult.

ANATOMY OF CENTRAL CONNECTIONS

Nerve VII generally is described as consisting of two roots, although they are often not easily distinguished (Sunderland and Cossar, 1953). The larger is the medially placed motor division, and the smaller lateral division, the nervus intermedius of Wrisberg, lies between the motor division and nerve VIII (Fig. 27–1). The two roots enter the caudolateral aspect of the pons in the cerebellopontine angle (Gray, 1973).

Motor Division. Fibers of the motor division arise from the facial (and probably the accessory facial) nucleus, which lies in the lateral tegmentum of the caudal portion of the pons, ventromedial to the spinal tract of nerve V. They pass rostrally and dorsally (the ascending root) to the level of the nucleus of nerve VI, sweep around it dorsally and rostrally (internal genu), and then pass ventrally, laterally, and caudally to the point of emergence from the brain stem (the

descending root). The facial nucleus averages 3.5 mm in length (Olszewski and Baxter, 1954). Caudally it lies in the same line as the nucleus ambiguus, with which it is analogous; rostrally it reaches the level of the caudal end of the nucleus of nerve VI dorsomedially and the motor nucleus of nerve V laterally. The smaller accessory facial nucleus is found at this level. The facial and accessory facial nuclei consist of large multipolar cells having an appearance typical of motor neurons. They are congregated into consistent, distinct groups. Although there is almost certainly some somatotopic localization within the nucleus, there is disagreement about its description (see Papez, 1927; Pearson, 1946; Szentágothai, 1948; Jacobs, 1970).

Nervus Intermedius of Wrisberg. This portion of nerve VII contains preganglionic parasympathetic fibers destined for the submandibular ganglion, with postganglionic connections to the submandibular and sublingual glands, and for the pterygopalatine ganglion, with postganglionic connections to the glands of the palatal and nasal mucosa and lacrimal glands. The nervus intermedius also contains several kinds of sensory fibers, the

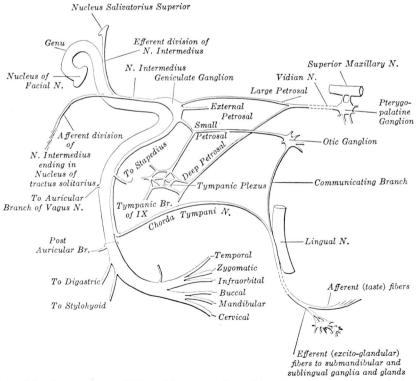

Figure 27–1 Plan of facial nerve (nerve VII) and its connections with other nerves. (From Gray, H.: Anatomy of the Human Body. 29th Edition. Edited by C. M. Goss. Philadelphia, Lea & Febiger, 1973, pp. 904, 924–931. Reprinted by permission.)

cell bodies of which are in the geniculate ganglion. Some afferent fibers supply the taste buds of the anterior two thirds of the tongue; other afferent fibers supply the mucous membranes of the pharynx, nose, and palate; and still others supply a portion of the skin of the external auditory meatus, ear, and mastoid area.

The efferent fibers of the nervus intermedius arise from cell clusters along the descending facial root, collectively termed "the superior salivatory nucleus." A group of these has been identified as giving rise to preganglionic fibers destined for the lacrimal gland (Crosby and DeJonge, 1963).

Some afferent fibers (probably gustatory) enter the area of the nucleus tractus solitarii. A number of these ascend and end in the rostral portion of this nucleus (Rhoton, 1968). Others descend in the tractus solitarius with fibers from nerves IX and X and synapse mostly in the ventromedial portion of the nucleus as far caudally as the obex (Kerr, 1962). Other afferent fibers descend in the spinal tract of nerve V in company with similar fibers from nerves IX and X. Nerve VII fibers are situated in the dorsomedial angle of the tract and end in its nucleus as far caudally as the lower part of C1. Small numbers of afferent fibers (touch from ear?) ascend to end in the medial part of the main sensory nucleus of nerve V (Rhoton, 1968), while other fibers (proprioceptive?) may have their cell bodies in the caudal end of the mesencephalic tract of nerve V (Allen, 1919).

ANATOMY OF PERIPHERAL COURSE

Posterior Fossa and Internal Acoustic Meatus. On emerging from the brain stem, nerve VII passes laterally in company with nerve VIII for a distance of 23 to 24 mm before entering the internal meatus, and continues for a distance of 7 to 8 mm within the internal auditory canal (Jepsen, 1965). At the fundus of the meatus it is anterior to the superior vestibular nerve and is separated from the cochlear and inferior vestibular nerves below by a horizontal bony process, the crista falciformis. In this region, interconnections and vestibular ganglion neurons are occasionally found between the nervus intermedius and the vestibular nerve (Van Buskirk, 1945).

Labyrinthine Segment. Nerve VII enters the facial canal and turns anterolaterally to pass above the labyrinth for 3 to 4 mm to reach the geniculate ganglion. An evagination of the arachnoid accompanies the nerve for a variable distance, sometimes as far as the ganglion (Perlman and Lindsay, 1939).

External Genu. At the geniculate ganglion, nerve VII turns abruptly posteriorly to form the external genu. This segment has three branches: the large petrosal nerve, the external petrosal nerve, and a communication with the small petrosal nerve. The *large petrosal nerve* passes anteriorly through the hiatus of the facial canal to the floor of the middle fossa. En route to the pterygopalatine ganglion, it unites with the deep petrosal nerve (from the superior sympathetic ganglion and tympanic plexus of nerve IX) to become the vidian nerve. At the pterygopalatine ganglion there are communications with the second division of nerve V via two pterygopalatine branches. Sensory fibers of nerve V pass downward via these branches through the ganglia, are joined by sensory fibers of nerve VII in the palatine nerves, and supply mucous membranes of the palate and nasal cavity. Postganglionic fibers descend with these branches to supply glands in the nasal and palatal mucosa, and ascend in the pterygopalatine branches to join the superior maxillary nerve, eventually reaching the lacrimal gland. Two smaller branches of nerve VII also arise at or near the geniculate ganglion. The *external petrosal nerve* communicates with the sympathetic plexus on the middle meningeal artery. The small petrosal nerve passes from the tympanic plexus of nerve IX to the otic ganglion.

Horizontal or Tympanic Segment. From the geniculate ganglion, nerve VII travels posteriorly and somewhat laterally for 12 to 13 mm. The impression of this segment is sometimes visible on the medial wall of the middle ear below the prominence of the horizontal semicircular canal and above the oval window.

Vertical or Mastoid Segment. At the posterior aspect of the middle ear, nerve VII again changes course and passes inferiorly for 10 to 14 mm. This segment has three branches. The nerve to the stapedius muscle arises near the upper end of the segment. The site of origin of the *chorda tympani* is quite variable, being anywhere from 10.9 mm proximal to 1.2 mm distal to the stylomastoid foramen; the average point is 5.3 mm proximal (Cawthorne, 1941; Kullman et al., 1971). The chorda tympani travels within the facial canal to the point of its exit through an aperture on the posterior wall of the middle ear. It passes forward on the medial surface of the tympanic membrane to emerge from the middle ear anteriorly. It has a small communication with the otic ganglion and joins the lingual branch of the third division of nerve V. Some chorda tympani fibers synapse in the submandibular ganglion, and postganglionic fibers reach the submandibular and sublingual glands. Other fibers end in taste buds on the anterior two thirds of the tongue.

Parotid Segment. Nerve VII leaves the facial canal at the stylomastoid foramen. Near its exit it gives rise to the posterior auricular, digastric, and stylohyoid branches, which supply the posterior auricular, occipital, posterior belly of the digastric, and stylohyoid muscles. Near this point, nerve VII or these branches communicate with nerves IX and X, with the auriculotemporal branch of nerve V, and with the great auricular and lesser occipital branches of the cervical plexus. Nerve VII then passes forward through the parotid gland for about 15 to 20 mm, where it terminates in the zygomatic, buccal, mandibular, and cervical branches. These supply the muscles of expression and have a number of further communications with branches of nerve V and the cervical plexus.

MICROSCOPIC ANATOMY

Results of various cell and fiber counts are summarized in Table 27–1. In some cases the values are inconsistent because they are data obtained by different authors in different species. In other cases values have been rounded off for clarity.

Neurons of the geniculate ganglion are of the unipolar type. They extend a variable distance proximally along the nervus intermedius and distally along the large petrosal nerve.

Large Petrosal Nerve. Foley and DuBois (1943) called attention to the difference in afferent fiber size in the large petrosal nerve compared with the chorda tympani, noting that fibers larger than 6.5 μm were the rule in the former. Van Buskirk (1945) found that most of the fibers in the large petrosal nerve of man were smaller than 2 μm but some were in the range of 6 to 8 μm. In a study of human fetuses, Larsell and Fenton (1928) noted that the small myelinated fibers reached the ptery-

gopalatine ganglion, where they synapsed, whereas the larger "sensory type" fibers passed through the ganglion without synapsing, to reach the palatine nerves and probably other branches to the nose and pharynx.

Communication With Small Petrosal Nerve. Fiber counts of nerve VII just proximal and just distal to the geniculate ganglion (where the distal count includes the large petrosal nerve) have shown about 334 "extra" fibers in the distal segment (Foley et al., 1946). The apparent discrepancy was not explained until Vidić and Woźniak (1969), in a study of human fetuses, noted that fibers from nerve X reached nerve VII via a twig near the stapedius muscle and ascended almost to the geniculate ganglion before departing via the communication with the small petrosal nerve.

Vertical Segment of Nerve VII. Sunderland and Cossar (1953) found that this portion of nerve VII consists of a single more or less homogeneous bundle of fascicles down to the lower end, where there is a rather complex interchanging fascicular pattern in which the individual grouping of fibers has little relationship to distal branchings. This seems to contradict the observations by Miehlke (1960), who described a "typical fascicular arrangement." Sunderland and Cossar admitted the possibility of distinct localization of function within nerve VII at this level, despite their inability to define it by fascicular arrangement. A group of sensory fibers was shown by Saito, Ruby, and Schuknecht (1970) to be consistently localized, and these probably represent the afferent contribution to the chorda tympani. Foley (1945) estimated that 60 to 65 per cent of chorda tympani fibers in cats and dogs were afferent in origin.

"Muscular" Branches. In tracing fibers of geniculate ganglion origin to the "muscular" branches over the face, Bruesch (1944) found them to be small and to terminate in free endings in the adventitia of blood vessels.

Sheath

The sheath of nerve VII as described by otologic surgeons probably consists of three layers, although the terminology offered by different authors is confused (Sunderland and Cossar, 1953; Anson et al., 1970). The outermost layer is the endosteum of the canal wall and is so thin that it may not appear as a

TABLE 27–1   CELL AND FIBER COUNTS

Site	Fibers/Cell		Size	
	Count	*Source**	*Range (μm)*	*Source**
Nucleus	6811	6	15–50	6
Accessory nucleus	131	6		
Proximal to geniculate ganglion	11,624	6		
Motor division	6999	6	3–14	6
Nervus intermedius				
Motor	2509	6		
Sensory	2116	6	1.5–10	3
Geniculate ganglion	2129	6	5–50	3, 6
Large petrosal nerve	1173	6		
Motor	(853)†			
Sensory	320	1		
Communication with small petrosal nerve‡	334	4		
Vertical	19,000	5	1.2–14	5
Chorda tympani	3250	5		
Motor	(1220)		1.5–2.5	3
Sensory	(2030)			
Communication with auricular branch, nerve X	2000	1		
Postauricular				
"Muscular" branches, sensory fibers	139	1	1.5–6	1

*Sources: 1, cat, Bruesch (1944); 2, cat, Foley (1945); 3, cat, Foley and DuBois (1943); 4, cat, Foley et al. (1946); 5, man, Kullman et al. (1971); 6, man, Van Buskirk (1945).

†Parentheses indicate value deduced from other data.

‡See text for explanation.

separate entity. The next layer, termed "epineurium" by Sunderland and Cossar, is the vessel-bearing connective tissue layer and, although voluminous, is so diffuse as not to be easily dissectable. The third layer, termed "perineurium" by Sunderland and Cossar, is more dense and better defined, and best qualifies as the "sheath proper." There is general agreement that the sheath of nerve VII is thin and delicate at the internal auditory meatus and becomes progressively thicker, more dense, and better defined distally, particularly in the vertical segment. According to James (1961), the sheath is formed by concentric layers of collagen fibers in the vertical segment and by elastic fibers in the horizontal and proximal segments. Chapter 9, by Thomas and Olsson, should be reviewed for a more recent discussion of the structure and function of the perineurium. Sunderland and Cossar noted that the perineurium invests the entire nerve throughout most of its interosseous course but splits to invest separate interwoven fascicles near the distal end of the vertical course. When incising the perineurium of normal nerves, Sunderland (1946) noted bulging

or herniation of the underlying nerve fibers. This did not occur when the incision was limited to the epineurium. Although some have described a strong fibrous collar constricting nerve VII at the stylomastoid foramen, this was not noted by Sunderland and Cossar (cf. McGovern and Hansel, 1961).

Vasculature

GROSS ANATOMY

That portion of nerve VII between the brain stem and the stylomastoid foramen is supplied primarily from three sources (Fig. 27–2) (Nager and Nager, 1953). Proximally, a loop, usually of the *anterior inferior cerebellar artery*, approaches or enters the internal auditory meatus in close association with nerves VII and VIII, gives rise to the internal auditory and subarcuate arteries, and runs back to the cerebellum (Mazzoni, 1969). Fine branches of these arteries supply nerve VII as far distally as the geniculate ganglion (Blunt, 1954).

OF NERVE VII IN MAN AND ANIMALS

| Size | | Myelinated | | Per Cent of Fibers | | | |
| | | | | All Nerve VII (6) | From Geniculate Ganglion (1, 3) | From Nervus Intermedius (Motor) (3) | From Auricular Branch, Nerve X (1) |
Mode (μm)	Source*	Per Cent	Source*				
17/25/40	6						
		76	6				
7–10	6	Most	6	58			
1.5–2.5	3			24			
2–4	3	93	4	18			
25–40	6						
		68	6				
<2		(56)				70	
>6.5	3	100			25		
		60	4				
2–4 / 6–8	5						
2–3	5						2
		80	2			30	
<6.5	3	82	2		50		
					15		88
					10		10

The *petrosal branch* of the middle meningeal artery approaches nerve VII with the large petrosal nerve via the hiatus of the facial canal. It supplies the region of the geniculate ganglion and divides into an ascending branch that supplies the proximal segment of nerve VII and a descending branch that accompanies the nerve as far as the stylomastoid foramen.

The *stylomastoid branch* of the posterior auricular artery enters the facial canal at the stylomastoid foramen and ascends a short distance before dividing into ascending and descending branches. The descending branch returns to the stylomastoid foramen and accompanies the posterior auricular nerve. The ascending branch accompanies nerve VII to the level of the geniculate ganglion.

Sunderland and Cossar (1953) noted that the territories of the three arteries supplying nerve VII overlapped, at least two supplying any given level, and they doubted that occlusion of any one would compromise the blood supply of nerve VII. They did not at first report anastomoses between these arteries, although Blunt (1956) quoted them as having demonstrated them subsequently. This brought their observations into line with his own, in contrast to those of Hilger (1949) that

"there was little or no collateral supply to relieve the ischemia" in nerve VII.

Most macroscopically visible arteries and veins in the facial canal lie in the epineurium. Anson and co-workers (1970) noted "capacious veins of a circumneural plexus and . . . numerous, though smaller, arteries" in this layer, particularly in the vertical segment. They also noted numerous anastomoses with the marrow spaces of surrounding bone and with a rich vascular plexus of the middle ear, which has components from the internal maxillary, posterior auricular, and ascending pharyngeal arteries.

MICROSCOPIC ANATOMY

By contrast with the large and prominent vessels of the epineurium, the vasculature of the perineurium consists of smaller arterioles and capillaries arranged in a longitudinal network interconnected at intervals with transverse vessels (Blunt, 1954). Although anastomoses between the epineurial and perineurial vessels were not demonstrated by the macroscopic techniques of Anson and his associates (1970), Bosatra (1956) reported

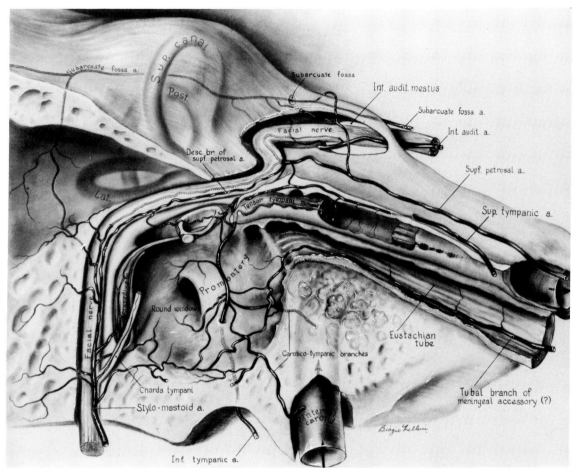

Figure 27–2   Blood supply of nerve VII. (From Nager, G. T., and Nager, M.: The arteries of the human middle ear, with particular regard to the blood supply of the auditory ossicles. Ann. Otol. Rhinol. Laryngol., 62:923, 1953. Reprinted by permission.)

them in all segments of nerve VII. He also described intima cushions containing smooth muscle at bifurcations of the larger arteries and suggested that they might have a vascular autoregulatory function.

Canal and Adjacent Structures

In the human fetus, Anson and his co-workers (1970) observed that the structures of the vertical portion of the facial canal are grouped into a triad consisting of nerve, muscle (stapedius), and arteriovenous complex. At four to five months of gestation, these structures occupy a sulcus in the posterior wall of the middle ear. By seven months, surrounding mesenchymal tissue has differentiated into connective tissue, and the sulcus has been partly closed by growth of bone. By nine

months, the canal is completed and petrous in texture.

Although described as "neatly rounded" by Cawthorne and Haynes (1956), variability in size and shape of the canal has been stressed by others (Lindeman, 1960). Variability of the course of the canal and the thickness of its walls was pointed out by Yates (1936), and dehiscence (failure of development) of portions of the facial canal has been shown to occur in as many as 55 per cent of specimens examined by Baxter (1971), most commonly in the horizontal segment near the oval window. Hall, Pulec, and Rhoton (1969) observed absence of a bony roof over the geniculate ganglion in 15 per cent of specimens and over the proximal segment of the large petrosal nerve in an additional 15 per cent (as noted later in the discussion of surgical trauma). Lindeman (1960) found no narrowing of the canal at the stylomastoid foramen.

The recent development of tomographic techniques for visualizing minute changes in the wall of the bony canal makes preoperative assessment of these variations possible, as well as allowing accurate localization of sites of nerve VII involvement by fractures, foreign bodies, surgical trauma, tumors, or infections (Wright and Taylor, 1972).

Although the canal is obviously filled by tissue of some sort at every level, the proportion occupied by nerve VII itself varies from nearly 100 per cent in the proximal portion of the horizontal segment to 25 to 50 per cent in the vertical segment. The remainder of the space is occupied by epineurial connective tissue, blood vessels, and, for a portion of the vertical segment, stapedius muscle. According to Anson and co-workers (1970), variations in size, shape, and structure of the canal are related to the pattern of vascular communications through the canal wall, the chorda tympani, and the stapedius muscle. The latter two structures may be partially compartmentalized by semicanals.

FUNCTIONS AND THEIR MEASUREMENT

Special Visceral Efferent (Branchiomeric, Skeletal Motor) Fibers

CLINICAL EXAMINATION

Strength of the facial muscles is assessed by having the patient mimic various facial movements while the examiner observes the symmetry and degree of movement. With paralysis of the posterior belly of the digastric muscle, the jaw deviates to the healthy side when opened widely (Tschiassny, 1955); with paralysis of the pterygoids, the opposite is true. The characteristic upward deviation of the eyes with attempted eye closure (Bell's phenomenon) is readily apparent with paralysis of the orbicularis oculi.

A loss of symmetry of the face at rest may be the result of flaccidity in acute paralysis, with flattening of the nasolabial folds and widening of the palpebral fissure, or to contracture, in older cases with incomplete re-

covery. One should look closely for adventitious movements such as synkinesis and myokymia (discussed later under Aberrant Function).

ELECTRODIAGNOSIS*

Several fundamental observations are the basis for applying these tests to the study of nerve VII function and dysfunction. As with nerves elsewhere in the body, nerve VII injury may be of three degrees, alone or in combination (Seddon, 1943). In *neurapraxia*, the nerve's function is paralyzed, but there is no distal wallerian degeneration and, as a rule, recovery is prompt and complete. In *axonotmesis*, there is interruption of the axis cylinders, but the supporting architecture is intact; recovery must await regeneration but is generally of good quality. In *neurotmesis*, there is disruption of both the axis cylinders and the supporting architecture; recovery not only must await regeneration but rarely is of good quality.

With neurapraxia, distal trophic effects persist despite absence of nerve impulses, the endplate and muscle do not atrophy (Denny-Brown and Brenner, 1944a), and peripheral conductivity is preserved. Even with complete section of a nerve, there is normal distal excitability and conductivity for 48 hours, with some excitability persisting for four to six days. Gilliatt and Taylor (1959) noted that conduction velocity did not slow significantly prior to the loss of excitability in complete lesions. These physiologic observations correlate well with the anatomical changes of wallerian degeneration. Endplate degeneration is not apparent for 5 to 10 days after nerve section, and reaction of degeneration may be delayed for 10 days (Adams et al., 1962). Although fibrillation potentials may occur (rarely) as early as four days, they usually are not seen for 7 to 21 days (Taverner, 1955).

All the examinations described in this section test the function of the distal segment of nerve VII, and abnormalities usually reflect degenerative changes distal to a site of axonotmesis.

Each of the electrodiagnostic tests mentioned may have special advantages and disadvantages in the study of particular disorders of nerve VII, and none is without its short-

---

*See also Section IV.

comings. Specific applications of some are mentioned subsequently in the discussions of individual diseases of nerve VII.

Reaction of Degeneration. For many years it has been observed that, with denervation of a muscle, a galvanic (direct current) stimulus applied at the motor point produces a sluggish contraction. This reaction of degeneration is not elicitable until 10 to 14 days after nerve section.

Intensity-Duration Curve. This determination can be thought of as a refinement of the galvanic and faradic tests—the longer duration stimulus is comparable to the galvanic test, and the shorter duration stimulus is comparable to the faradic test (Richardson, 1963). This refinement helps to quantitate the state of denervation but is still a late indicator (Yanagihara and Kishimoto, 1971).

Electromyogram. The conventional electromyogram may serve as an early semiquantitative measure, to supplement the clinical examination, by showing a decreased number or absence of motor unit action potentials at maximal effort; again, abnormal insertion activity and fibrillation potentials are late indicators of denervation. In addition, patterns of motor unit discharge may help in the diagnosis of such disorders as synkinesis, hemifacial spasm, facial myokymia, or blepharospasm (see the section on aberrant function).

Nerve Conduction. The short length of the facial nerve accessible for electrophysiologic study limits the assessment of nerve conduction time to a latency measurement. A stimulus is applied to the facial nerve near the stylomastoid foramen, and the onset of the muscle action potential is recorded at a standard site or at a measured distance away by means of surface or concentric needle electrodes (Langworth and Taverner, 1963; Yanagihara and Kishimoto, 1972). The conduction latency is expressed in milliseconds, and the normal range depends on the test conditions used. Langworth and Taverner found an average latency of 2.7 msec in healthy subjects with an interelectrode distance of 3.5 cm, and they considered a latency of 4 msec or greater to be abnormal. If the findings of Gilliatt and Taylor, cited earlier, are valid, one might anticipate that measurement of conduction latency would have little value in sudden complete lesions of nerve VII, but still could be of possible use in evolving or incomplete lesions (see discussion of prognostic indicators under Idiopathic Facial Paralysis).

Nerve Excitability Threshold. Duchenne (1872) claimed that, when facial muscle contractility to nerve stimulation was absent, facial palsy would persist despite treatment. At present the test has been refined to allow determination of excitability threshold. Short-duration (0.1 to 1.0 msec) rectangular pulses are applied to nerve VII near the stylomastoid foramen at increasing strengths of stimulus until a twitch or evoked action potential can just be detected (Richardson, 1963; Yanagihara and Kishimoto, 1972). The threshold may be elevated as early as 48 hours after complete section of nerve VII. Nelson (1971) found the test to be reliable, objective, and descriptively valid. Unfortunately, the threshold may be normal in some cases of incomplete denervation while, on the other hand, the regenerated nerve may remain inexcitable to conventional testing and yet be functional (McGovern, 1970b).

Maximal Action Potential. This is an extension of the test for determining the nerve excitability threshold in which the stimulus strength is increased progressively until the amplitude of the evoked response is maximal. In cats, May, Harvey, and Marovitz (1971) observed a decrease in the maximal action potential as early as the first day after section or ligation of nerve VII.

STETHOSCOPE LOUDNESS IMBALANCE TEST

This test is for assessment of stapedius muscle dysfunction. It had long been known that some patients with nerve VII paralysis complained of hypersensitivity to loud noise in the ipsilateral ear. In 1929, Lüscher observed contraction of the human stapedius tendon in response to acoustic stimuli that were usually considerably above threshold.

Applying earlier observations by Perlman (1938), Tschiassny (1953) developed the stethoscope loudness imbalance test to simplify assessment of stapedius muscle function. With a stethoscope in place in the patient's ears, a tuning fork is activated and placed near the bell. The sound of a strongly activated tuning fork lateralizes to the side of stapedius paralysis, while the sound of a lightly activated tuning fork fails to lateralize. He found that lateralization occurred with intensities as low as 45 db. These findings differ from those of the recruitment response, which also can be tested by this technique (stethoscope loudness *balance* test). Objective measurement of stapedius dysfunction by acoustic impedance testing is beyond the scope of this chapter (cf. Djupesland, 1969).

General Visceral Efferent Fibers

LACRIMAL FUNCTION

Jepsen (1965) gave reasons to conclude that the excess tearing so often observed in facial paralysis might often be more apparent than real. First, Horner's muscle, which dilates the lacrimal sac, usually is paralyzed. Second, there may be outward displacement of the opening of the nasolacrimal duct due to orbicularis oculi weakness (paralytic ectropion). Third, absence of blinking may lead to corneal irritation and normal reflex tearing. Jepsen thought a history of "dry eye" was equally unreliable, and he stressed the importance of quantitative testing of lacrimal function.

Zilstorff-Pedersen (1959) described a technique for quantifying the nasolacrimal reflex. He used Schirmer's (1903) blotting paper test in which a fold is made near one end of a piece of filter paper (0.5 by 10 cm) and the short segment is placed over the lower lid. Benzene vapor is then injected into the ipsilateral nostril for 30 seconds by using an olfactometer. The filter paper is left in place for an additional 30 seconds and then removed, and the length of the moistened portion is measured. The procedure is done separately on each side. A difference of 74 per cent or more occurred in only 1 per cent of normal subjects. The test is apparently a sensitive measure of nerve VII dysfunction in cerebellopontine angle tumors. Zilstorff-Pedersen (1965) found decreased reflex lacrimation in 41 per cent of his cases. Other authors have used simpler modifications of this test (Cawthorne and Haynes, 1956).

SUBMANDIBULAR SALIVARY FLOW

A quantitative test of submandibular secretory function has been described by Magielski and Blatt (1958). After each Wharton's duct is probed and dilated, no. 60 polyethylene catheters are inserted for a distance of 3 to 4 cm. The patient then sucks a slice of lemon for 60 seconds, and the secretion rate, in drops per minute, is determined for each gland. The uninvolved side serves as the normal control, and the rate on the involved side is expressed as a percentage of normal. With section of the chorda tympani, the rate is generally at or near 0 per cent.

In addition to supplying lacrimal, submandibular, and sublingual glands, postganglionic parasympathetic fibers of nerve VII origin have also been shown, in monkeys, to be involved in the maintenance of intraocular pressure and vasodilatation (Ruskell, 1970, 1971).

Special Visceral Afferent (Taste) Fibers

For many years, taste function was assessed only by means of solutions of substances representing the four taste qualities. The results were often inconsistent because coarse testing techniques either allowed the solutions to extend beyond the intended area or else caused the general sensibility of the tongue to be stimulated (Krarup, 1958a). Even the more consistent semiquantitative methods lacked sensitivity (Börnstein, 1940). This led to the development and adaptation of electrogustometry for clinical use by Krarup (1958b). The method is based on the observation that anodal galvanic stimulation of the tongue is perceived as an acidic or metallic taste. The test apparatus is designed to deliver a direct-current stimulus of variable intensity. Although there are wide variations in taste threshold from individual to individual, the threshold is normally equal on the two sides in a given individual.

General Visceral and Somatic Afferent Fibers

Although there may be pain or vesicle formation of the skin and mucous membranes in a characteristic distribution in geniculate herpes zoster, as reported by Hunt (1907), a consistent general sensory loss is not usually apparent with nerve VII lesions, probably owing in part to overlapping supply by adjacent cranial nerves.

PRESSURE PAIN (DEEP PAIN)

The finding by Bruesch (1944) that about 8 per cent of geniculate ganglion fibers accompany the peripheral branches to the facial muscles is not entirely surprising, since Sherrington (1894–1895) had long before demonstrated that from one third to one half of the myelinated fibers of all "motor" nerves he studied were of afferent origin. Sherrington found large fibers terminating in muscle spindles and smaller ones terminating in free fibrils. Bruesch demonstrated only smaller afferent fibers in the "motor" branches of nerve VII, however, and concluded that they subserved pressure pain function. It is known that stimulation of nerve VII at the parotid gland is painful (Hollinshead, 1968). Most reports of human or animal lesions support the thesis that pressure pain, as measured by such devices as the Cattel algometer, is subserved at least in part by afferent fibers of nerve VII (Maloney and Kennedy, 1911; Davis, 1923), although Carmichael (1933) suspected that faulty testing technique might account for "preservation" of pressure pain appreciation in patients with sensory lesions of nerve V. Although cats still "react" to painful pressure stimuli after section of the spinal tract of nerve V, as reported by Gerard (1923), man does not (Smyth, 1939). The anatomical evidence that afferent fibers of nerves V and VII descend in the spinal tract of nerve V has already been cited. Hunt (1937) suggested that some cases of head pain, such as "atypical facial pain" and Sluder's (1927) or vidian neuralgia (Vail, 1932), may be the result of dysfunction of these neurons. There is no disagreement that pressure *touch* on the face, as measured by the aesthesiometer of Holmes, is mediated entirely by nerve V (Maloney and Kennedy, 1911).

PROPRIOCEPTION

Kadanoff (1956) demonstrated classic spindles and spiral endings in the facial muscles of man, but several years later Taverner failed to find them after an extensive search, so they must be few in number (cf. Jongkees et al., 1965). The question of their innervation is unanswered. As noted earlier, those few geniculate ganglion fibers that have been demonstrated in the muscular branches of nerve VII are small and are unlikely to be proprioceptive afferents. Could a few larger geniculate ganglion fibers have been overlooked by these investigators? Or do the large fibers of nerve V that accompany the branches of nerve VII innervate the spindles seen by

Kadanoff? The occasional afferent fibers of nerve VII that reach the vicinity of the mesencephalic root of nerve V (Pearson, 1947) resemble the proprioceptive afferents of nerve V whose cell bodies are there (Allen, 1919).

LOCALIZATION OF SITE OF LESION (TOPOGNOSIS)

Tschiassny (1953) proposed a scheme that, he claimed, allowed the localization of eight levels of involvement on the basis of distinctive syndromes associated with facial paralysis. The first or supranuclear syndrome is distinguished mainly by sparing of the forehead musculature and absence of Bell's phenomenon. The seven remaining syndromes and their distinctive findings are summarized in Table 27–2.

Tschiassny's scheme is valid if we make several assumptions: first, that the anatomy of the components of nerve VII in the case in question fits the standard description; second, that the pathologic lesion responsible for the facial paralysis is sharply localized to a particular level; third, that the lesion affects all the components of nerve VII at that level to an equal extent; and fourth, that the techniques used in measuring the various functions of nerve VII are reliable. Unfortunately, exceptions to each of these assumptions have already been or are pointed out later in this chapter. Despite the exceptions, there certainly are cases in which sharply defined severe lesions can be accurately localized by Tschiassny's scheme, thereby assisting in diagnosis and therapy. Careful and complete assessment of patterns of dysfunction in cases of nerve VII paralysis would seem desirable in any event, to add to the understanding of its various diseases.

TABLE 27–2 THE SEVEN SYNDROMES OF LOWER MOTOR FACIAL PARALYSIS*

Level	Chin in Midline†	Taste	Stapedius Reflex	Lacrimation
Nuclear	No	Yes	No	Yes
Suprageniculate	No	Yes	No	No
Transgeniculate	No	No	No	No
Suprastapedial	No	No	No	Yes
Infrastapedial	No	No	Yes	Yes
Infrachordal	No	Yes	Yes	Yes
Infraforaminal	Yes	Yes	Yes	Yes

*Modified from Tschiassny (1955).
†Refers to effect of posterior belly of the digastric muscle on jaw opening.

ABERRANT FUNCTION

Thus far the functions of the components of nerve VII have been discussed in quantitative terms; that is, is the function normal or reduced? There are malfunctions of nerve VII, however, that are not easily explained in these terms. For this discussion, these malfunctions are defined as "aberrant."

Pathophysiologic Mechanisms of Aberrant Function

The two mechanisms most frequently cited to explain the various signs of aberrant function of nerve VII are faulty regeneration and ephaptic transmission at sites of injury.

FAULTY REGENERATION

Lipschitz (1906) presented a theory to explain the phenomenon of the synkinesis that frequently complicates recovery from facial paralysis. He hypothesized a haphazard intermingling of regenerating axons at the site of injury so that isolated movement of a given part of the face is no longer possible. In a study of experimental nerve VII injury in monkeys, Howe, Tower, and Duel (1937) demonstrated branching of axons at the site of injury, and they also observed a phenomenon in the regenerated facial field that they likened to the axon reflex. After sectioning of the regenerated facial nerve trunk proximal to the site of original injury and of one of the three main branches of the nerve, they stimulated the proximal stump of the branch and noted contraction of muscles in the distribution of the other two branches. They interpreted this as a result of antidromic propagation of the impulse to the site of original injury followed by orthodromic propagation to the remainder of the facial field by way of the abnormal branching observed. Fowler (1939) also found that branching of axons invariably occurs at the site of severe nerve VII injury, whether mechanical or toxic in origin, and he thought that this explained the development of synkinesis with recovery. He found that improper rerouting of nerve bundles could not account for this because, in monkeys, when two bundles were sectioned and then sutured together in reverse manner,

reeducation took place and no synkinesis occurred.

EPHAPTIC TRANSMISSION AND SPONTANEOUS ACTIVITY

Adrian (1930) made a series of in vitro observations on the electrical potentials arising at the site of acute injury in mammalian nerves. He observed spontaneous discharges that followed one of several patterns in individual axons. Small sensory axons usually were involved. Sometimes, repetitive discharges became synchronized in different axons. He concluded that depolarization at the site of injury acted as a stimulus to the intact portion of the fiber, and that the action potential in one fiber was capable of exciting adjacent fibers in the area of injury. In short-term experiments in cats, Granit, Leksell, and Skoglund (1944) demonstrated ephaptic transmission ("artificial synapse") at the site of compression in a nerve that was still capable of transmitting impulses across the site.

Kugelberg (1946, 1948) demonstrated an acute, reversible phenomenon in the peripheral nerve of man. After producing ischemia by means of pneumatic cuffs, he demonstrated the development of foci of spontaneous, repetitive, and synchronized discharges, both during the ischemia and after release of the cuff. When the spontaneous activity ceased in the postanoxic period, it could be retriggered by the passage of an action potential or a constant current through the involved segment of the nerve. One pattern of activity he observed consisted of bursts of grouped impulses, the groups repeating at 1 per second, and the impulses repeating at 100 to 180 per second. A proximal shock stimulus led to a burst of synchronized discharges after a latent period of 7 msec, and an antidromic stimulus led to bursts that reflected back down the nerve—a phenomenon Kugelberg referred to as a "pseudoreflex." By a series of ingenious experiments, Kugelberg and Cobb (1951) showed that the abnormal discharges arose in the trunk of the nerve itself and not at its central or peripheral endings. Although the bulk of the observations were made on motor fibers as reflected in the electromyogram, Kugelberg thought that sensory fibers were more sensitive to postanoxic excitation, and he used his observations to explain paresthesias of peripheral origin in neuropathy as well as in hyperventilation and hypocalcemia.

Oppenheim (1911) wrote, "A physician whom I treated for facial paralysis with ageusia, with the commencement of improvement there occurred on every effort at movement of the paralyzed muscles the sensation of a metallic taste on the corresponding side of the tongue." This observation is difficult to interpret physiologically except by ephaptic transmission at the site of injury.

Signs and Syndromes of Aberrant Function

SYNKINESIS

In general, synkinesis (associated movements, mass action, blinking tic) is an abnormal synchronization of movement, occurring with voluntary or reflex activity, of different muscles that normally do not contract together. Although it is sometimes noted symmetrically about the nose or chin with blinking in otherwise normal individuals, it occurs most frequently in cases of recovered facial paralysis. In its subtlest form, it may consist of no more than a tiny twitch of the chin that accompanies blinking on the side of prior paresis, and its detection may require close, purposeful observation. In more severe cases there may be eye closure with smiling or gross contraction about the mouth with blinking, and it may be so prominent as to be cosmetically disabling.

The electromyogram of lower facial muscles in such cases shows the so-called blink burst, which is nothing more than an electrographic reflection of the clinical phenomenon. Magun and Esslen (1959) made the point that the *form* of nerve impulse conduction is not so much impaired in such cases as are its *pathways*.

Although most authors attribute synkinesis to faulty regeneration or aberrant innervation, Wartenberg (1946) presented lengthy arguments to the contrary, thinking that it probably was a release phenomenon, although he suggested ephaptic transmission could also play a role. Woltman and co-workers (1951) and Williams and co-workers (1952) noted synkinesis in some cases of hemifacial spasm in which there was no history of paralysis. They also observed its disappearance with decompressive surgery that resulted in little or no weakness of facial muscles. They thought these two observations suggested that, in these

cases at least, the synkinesis was more likely due to ephaptic transmission than to misdirection of regenerating nerve fibers.

It seems certain that aberrant regeneration occurs after severe injury to nerve VII, and it seems likely that the explanation of synkinesis after facial paralysis rests at least in part on this basis. It cannot be concluded, however, that ephaptic transmission is not also a factor in its production, particularly in cases of hemifacial spasm without prior paralysis.

CROCODILE TEARS

This term refers to inappropriate unilateral lacrimation while eating, a phenomenon noted on recovery from facial paralysis in some cases. According to Chorobski (1951), the term was first used by Bogorad in 1928 and is based on the theme of one of many "scientific" anecdotes of Pliny the Elder that "the crocodile . . . will weep over a man's head after he has devoured the body, and then will eat the head, too." The phenomenon is to be distinguished from paralytic ectropion, which occurs in the acute stage of facial paralysis. Thought of as analogous to synkinesis by Oppenheim (1911), it has been attributed by most authors to faulty regeneration, with nerve fibers that originally supplied the submandibular and sublingual glands being rerouted to the lacrimal gland via the large petrosal nerve (Taverner, 1955). Chorobski presented the alternative possibility of ephaptic transmission as the responsible mechanism. In either case, it seems probable that the responsible lesion must involve the nervus intermedius proximal to the origin of the large petrosal nerve.

CONTRACTURE

With recovery from peripheral facial paralysis, as well as in the intervals between paroxysms of hemifacial spasm, the affected side "may present a drawn appearance, as though it were in a state of constant spasm" (Woltman et al., 1951). The nasolabial fold may be deeper, the palpebral fissure narrower, and the angle of the mouth higher than on the normal side. Whether it is the result of permanent shortening of tissue, as its name implies, or is the result of active contraction of muscle fibers is still argued. Spiller (1919) suggested that a gradual shortening of muscle fibers is brought on by overstimulation of the affected facial muscles that results from aberrant regeneration. Bratzlavsky and Vander Eecken (1971) also concluded that it is not an active phenomenon because electrical silence was observed with voluntary effort at relaxation in their cases, yet observable contracture persisted. These authors explained contracture on the basis of "fautive [sic] neurotrophic influences" of misdirected nerve fibers. The view that contracture is the result of active muscle contraction is supported by observations by Marinesco, Kreindler, and Jordanesco (1931) that a procaine block of nerve VII abolishes it. Taverner (1955) observed that it was associated with electromyographic findings of "continuous low frequency firing of single motor units with no recognizable pattern." A different form of contracture is discussed later in the paragraph on facial myokymia.

HEMIFACIAL SPASM

Gowers (1888) presented a detailed description of the syndrome (clonic facial spasm, tic convulsif). Ehni and Woltman (1945) found 106 examples of cryptogenic hemifacial spasm among 663 patients with abnormal facial movements of all sorts. In their analysis they excluded cases of known cause (symptomatic). The condition was marked by paroxysms of rapid, irregular, clonic twitching, although a tonic phase was sometimes a feature. The paroxysms almost always started about the eyes and spread to a variable extent to involve other facial muscles on the same side, but never beyond the muscles innervated by nerve VII. They lasted for up to five minutes. The syndrome was bilateral in only six cases, and in these the twitching was asynchronous and unequal in severity and extent on the two sides. Paroxysms occurred spontaneously or in response to voluntary or reflex movement of the facial muscles.

The twitching was more severe in periods of tension and fatigue, was sometimes observed during sleep, and occurred only in adults (more commonly in women). The patients had no compulsion to produce the movements, they were unable to mimic the movements within a paroxysm, and once the movements started, they were unable to stop them. Only 9 of the 106 patients had remissions. Although facial weakness was noted in 16 cases and contracture was observed frequently, Ehni and Woltman did not describe synkinesis in the cryptogenic form. They even suggested the sign be used to differentiate it from the symptomatic form. Later, however, Williams, Lambert, and Woltman (1952) noted synkinesis in some cases even in the absence of prior paralysis.

Postparalytic Hemifacial Spasm. Hemifacial spasm has been reported as a sequel to facial paralysis, but Ehni and Woltman found only two such cases in their series. In the 100 cases of Taverner (1955), the 85 cases of Hauser and co-workers (1971), and the 140 cases of Wigand and associates (1972), no case of hemifacial spasm was observed. One must conclude that hemifacial spasm as described by Ehni and Woltman is a rare sequel to facial paralysis, and the continuing mention of this association in the literature may be partly attributable to confusion about the definitions of the terms "hemifacial spasm," "contracture," and "synkinesis."

Associated Pathologic Changes.   Since the time of Gowers, it has been recognized that hemifacial spasm as here defined has often been found associated with lesions of nerve VII. Most frequently described have been cases of tumors or aneurysms in the cerebellopontine angle, which compressed or angulated nerve VII in its subarachnoid course. Gardner and associates (1962, 1966) demonstrated what they considered to be "responsible lesions" in the cerebellopontine angle in 36 of 42 cases. In 19 surgical cases, a "definite pathologic process" was found in 7, and a redundant arterial loop compressed nerve VII in 7 others. In only five cases was no apparent compression of the nerve found.

Using microsurgical techniques, Jannetta, Hackett, and Ruby (1970) explored the cerebellopontine angle in nine patients and found "apparently significant neurovascular compression-distortion of the facial nerve" in all nine. Fascicular biopsies of the nerve were taken in three cases and examined by electron microscopy. The authors described "excess myelin" around many fibers, "disruption" of myelin in most areas with "naked axons . . . (abutting) against each other," and a "break down" of myelin sheath on one side, exposing axons in some areas. Unfortunately, there were no supporting photomicrographs, and no confirmation of these amazing findings is in the literature. Eckman, Kramer, and Altrocchi (1971) described arteriographic evidence of a vascular abnormality in the cerebellopontine angle near nerve VII in each of four cases they studied. It is interesting to note that in 14 of Ehni and Woltman's 106 "cryptogenic" cases of hemifacial spasm there was ipsilateral hearing loss. Pathologic lesions in this syndrome have been observed less frequently in the intratemporal course of nerve VII.

Electromyography. Williams, Lambert, and Woltman (1952), Magun and Esslen (1959), and Fisch and Esslen (1972b) presented the electromyographic findings in hemifacial spasm; these are characteristic if not pathognomonic of the condition. The electromyogram is characterized by (1) bursts of high-frequency impulses, 150 to 400 impulses per second; (2) rhythmic or irregular repetition of the bursts at a rate of 5 to 20 per second, each burst consisting of 2 to 12 impulses; (3) synchronization of impulses in widely separated facial muscles; and (4) the induction of typical bursts by means of antidromic stimulation of nerve VII.

Pathophysiologic Mechanism. Woltman, Williams, and Lambert (1951), Denny-Brown (1953), Magun and Esslen (1959), and most subsequent authors have noted the striking resemblance of this syndrome, particularly in its electrophysiologic features, to the phenomena described as ephaptic transmission. In addition to ephaptic transmission and spontaneous and induced activity, Gardner and Dohn (1966) hypothesized a peripheral reverberating short circuit between afferent (proprioceptive) and efferent fibers at a point of compression. Such a "circuit" was not a part of the basic observations of either Adrian or Kugelberg, and the idea is unsupported by the available evidence. Wigand and associates (1972) studied 18 patients with "facial spasm" and used computer techniques to process the electromyograms. Their recordings showed rhythmic electrical patterns that they interpreted as more consistent with a central than a peripheral origin for the phenomenon. Although this conclusion would be in keeping with the older theories, the weight of evidence favors the theory of a peripheral ephaptic mechanism.

Treatment. Prompted by the idea that hemifacial spasm might be the result of fibrous constriction of nerve VII in its vertical segment, Williams, Lambert, and Woltman (1952) attempted surgical neurolysis in seven patients. They interpreted the resolution of symptoms, despite only minimal postoperative weakness, as evidence that ephaptic transmission in the treated segment of nerve VII had been corrected. Their results were disappointing, however, because of recurrence of symptoms in most cases. Since then, various surgical approaches have been described. Gardner and Sava (1962) and Jannetta, Hackett, and Ruby (1970) reported a lower recurrence rate with decompressive surgery in the posterior fossa, but Fisch and Esslen (1972b) also reported good results with peripheral sectioning of branches of nerve VII, the particular branches being selected on the basis of the severity of involvement.

FACIAL MYOKYMIA

Described by Bernhardt (1902), the condition consists of fine, continuous, fibrillary or undulating movements of facial muscles, giving an appearance suggesting a "bag of worms." It is a subtle disorder and sometimes is detected only on close inspection. It often is associated with apparent sustained contraction of facial muscles and sometimes also with facial weakness on the side of the involvement. Many cases have been reported in association with multiple sclerosis, in which the disorder is usually self-limited and lasts for six weeks on average (Andermann et al., 1961). It has also been seen with intrinsic tumors of the brain stem; in these cases, the sign is more persistent, and associated contraction of the side of the face is more prominent. Espinosa, Lambert, and Klass (1967) noted that the contraction of facial muscles was so prominent in some cases that myokymia was obscured clinically, but the characteristic electromyographic findings were still present. They suspected that the cases described by Sogg, Hoyt, and Boldrey (1963) under the name "spastic paretic facial contracture" were of the same type.

The electromyogram shows independent, intermittent firing of neighboring motor units (Lambert et al., 1961). Each unit fires rhythmically at a rate of 30 to 70 times per second; bursts last for 0.2 to 2 seconds and occur at intervals of from 0.8 to 7 seconds. The rate, duration, and interval of bursts for a given unit tend to be consistent, and it is the independent action of neighboring units with differing firing characteristics that results in the unique clinical appearance. With few exceptions, the cases reported have had intrinsic brain stem lesions.

ABNORMAL FACIAL MOVEMENTS NOT OF FACIAL NERVE ORIGIN

A few movements of this type are mentioned briefly to distinguish them from the disorders just described.

Blepharospasm (Facial Paraspasm, Bilateral Facial Spasm). In this condition there is involuntary spasmodic eye closure, spreading variably to other facial and cranial musculature, often worse with exposure to bright light, and often suppressed by whistling, singing, or chewing (Ehni and Woltman, 1945). The condition is sometimes a feature of extrapyramidal disorders such as Parkinson's disease and its variants. It is distinguished by its symmetry of involvement. The electromyogram shows that the individual contractions are synchronous on the two sides but the motor units making up the contractions are not (Fisch and Esslen, 1972b).

Tic (Habit Spasm). This usually has its onset in childhood. The movements may be simple or consist of a complex series of individual components that are repetitive and stereotyped. There usually is also an involvement of muscles outside the distribution of nerve VII. The patient has the compulsion to perform the movements, can reproduce them voluntarily, and can inhibit them for a length of time.

Focal Cortical Seizures. When the face is involved by a focal seizure, the movements are usually gross clonic ones that often spread beyond the distribution of nerve VII. After such a seizure, there may be transient postictal facial paralysis of the supranuclear type (sparing the forehead muscles).

PERIPHERAL FACIAL PARALYSIS

The published incidence rates of the various causes of "unselected" cases of facial paralysis vary with the source of the patients studied, the experience and specialty of the investigator, the system of classification, and the tenacity and skill invested in the search for a cause. Despite the advances in techniques that allow the definition and localization of dysfunction of nerve VII, the majority of cases in most series are still designated "idiopathic." The recent study by Adour and Swanson (1971) can serve as an example. They studied 403 patients and found "idiopathic" facial

paralysis in 77 per cent, an infectious origin (including herpes zoster and otitis media) in 14 per cent, and a traumatic cause (including skull fractures and surgical trauma) in 6 per cent; genetic and newborn cases accounted for about 2 per cent. The reader is also referred to the papers by Park and Watkins (1949), Cawthorne and Haynes (1956), Blatt and Freeman (1966), Hauser and associates (1971), and May and Lucente (1972). The last report is of particular interest because the cases were drawn from a series of 160 diagnosed as "Bell's palsy" and referred to the authors; in this group, about 17 per cent were reclassified as to etiology. Half of these patients had neoplasms involving nerve VII.

Similar series representing pediatric age groups show a higher proportion of patients whose disease is not in the "idiopathic" category and a much higher proportion of congenital and newborn cases (Lloyd et al., 1966; Manning and Adour, 1972).

Idiopathic Facial Paralysis (Bell's Palsy, Rheumatic Facial Paresis)

HISTORICAL BACKGROUND

Kindler (1970) collected a number of examples of ancient sculpture depicting obvious peripheral facial paralysis. Sir Charles Bell (1821, 1829) drew on cases of known structural lesions of nerve VII or nerve V to support his arguments as to their anatomical and functional distinctions. He indicated that with this knowledge the physician could be:

. . . better able to distinguish between that paralysis which proceeds from the brain, and that partial affection of the muscles of the face, when, from a less alarming cause, they have lost the controuling influence of the respiratory nerve.

Cases of this partial paralysis must be familiar to every medical observer. It is very frequent for young people to have what is vulgarly called a blight; by which is meant, a slight palsy of the muscles on one side of the face, and which the physician knows is not formidable (Bell, 1821).

Although in the latter part of the nineteenth century it was customary to refer to all cases of peripheral facial paralysis as "Bell's palsy," regardless of cause, the term has been recently applied only to cases of unknown cause.

EPIDEMIOLOGY

In a population study in Rochester, Minnesota, Hauser and co-workers (1971) found an annual incidence rate of 22.8 per 100,000. The rate was lower in children, increased with age until the fourth decade, and remained steady thereafter. There was no clustering of cases or seasonal variation. Melotte's (1961) incidence rates were similar, but most other authors have reported lower rates, perhaps because of incomplete case retrieval. Leibowitz (1969) and Vassallo and Galea-Debono (1972) reported an apparent clustering of cases revealed by statistical analysis, suggesting "epidemics" of Bell's palsy, and El-Ebiary (1971a) suggested a seasonal clustering in August and December. Since these and most other studies are based on referral practices, the possibility of unrecognized selection bias cannot be excluded.

Diabetes Mellitus. Ten per cent of the patients in the Rochester series were known diabetics, but the incidence rate of known diabetes mellitus in the population, particularly when matched for age and sex, was not known. Adour and Bell (1971) reported a similar incidence. Korczyn (1971a) reported known diabetes in 14 per cent of 130 patients with Bell's palsy but a total incidence increased to 66 per cent as defined by abnormality in glucose tolerance tests. A greater incidence of diabetes (29 per cent) was diagnosed in patients more than 40 years old as compared with age-matched control subjects in the series of Vassallo and Galea-Debono. Aminoff and Miller (1972), also using glucose intolerance as the criterion for diagnosis, found diabetes in only 6 per cent of their cases, which led them to conclude that, at least in England, diabetes mellitus was not a common etiologic factor in the development of Bell's palsy.

Hypertension. Hauser and associates found the incidence rate of known hypertension to be 8 per cent in their cases of Bell's palsy. This is less than the incidence of hypertension in the Framingham population (Kannel et al., 1969). Vassallo and Galea-Debono (1972) found that 36 per cent of their patients who had Bell's palsy and were more than 40 years old had hypertension, significantly more than in the age-matched controls. This was not true of their patients less than 40 years old. Lloyd, Jewitt, and Still (1966) reviewed all the cases of severe hypertension and all the cases of facial palsy seen at a London pediatric hospital in a 10 year period and found that 20 per cent of those with hypertension had facial palsy, and that 7 per cent of those with facial palsy had severe hypertension.

Pregnancy and Post Partum. In the study by Hauser and associates, Bell's palsy developed in three patients during pregnancy and in two others on the first postpartum day. This was not significantly different from the expected incidence, three cases, during any 10 month period in women of childbearing age. Adour (1970) also found no correlation with pregnancy, but Korczyn (1971b) reported evidence to suggest a correlation, particularly in the time near parturition.

From the conflicting reports cited, well-controlled population studies are still needed in order to establish possible concordance of Bell's palsy with diabetes mellitus, hypertension, or pregnancy.

CLINICAL FEATURES

Acute Symptoms. Taverner (1955) suggested that the following criteria must be met for the diagnosis of Bell's palsy: (1) sudden onset of unilateral complete or partial paralysis of the facial muscles on one side; (2) absence of symptoms or signs of disease of the central nervous system; and (3) absence of symptoms or signs of ear or posterior fossa disease. The paralysis may appear suddenly and be complete from the time it is first noted, or it may progress over a period of several days to complete or incomplete paralysis. About half the patients complain of pain in or about the mastoid in the first few days. Many complain of excess tearing (as described under Lacrimal Function), and a few of inadequate tearing. About one third will admit to a disturbance of taste perception, but usually only direct questioning will bring this out. Some have hyperacusis, and in rare cases there is vertigo. Although many patients complain of "numbness" of the side of the face, it seems that they use the term in most instances to indicate a lack of mobility rather than a lack of sensation.

Physical Signs and Laboratory Findings. The most obvious finding, of course, is the facial weakness, which is partial in 30 per cent of cases and complete in 75 per cent of cases (Cawthorne, 1952b). About one third to half the patients have stapedius dysfunction (Djupesland, 1969). Only 6 per cent had decreased lacrimation in the series of Zil-storff-Pedersen (1965), but Fisch and Esslen (1972a) described lacrimal disturbance in all 12 of their cases. Although Blatt (1965) implied that submandibular salivary flow was decreased, to some extent at least, in all cases of Bell's palsy, May and Harvey (1971) found it to be 80 to 100 per cent of normal in 5 of 16 cases. Peiris and Miles (1965) found that 48 per cent of their patients with Bell's palsy had a decreased threshold to anodal galvanic stimulation of the tongue, if tested within 14 days of onset.

Less commonly recognized findings include the following. Hilger (1949) described injection of vessels of the posterior aspect of the external auditory meatus and adjacent tympanic membrane in some of his cases in the first few days. Kime (1958) observed that nicotinic acid produced the usual cutaneous flush everywhere except on the paretic side of the face and that a gradual return of normal flushing in succeeding days heralded early recovery. Philipszoon (1962) observed positional nystagmus in 10 of 12 cases, and in 6 of the 9 cases he tested the caloric response was decreased or absent on the paretic side. Spinal fluid examinations in 24 patients showed increased protein in 7 and pleocytosis in 3 (Park and Watkins, 1949). Pantopaque cisternography in two cases reported by Fisch and Esslen (1972a) revealed findings similar to those in an intrameatal acoustic neuroma, presumably based on edema of nerve VII.

Course and Residual Abnormalities. Recovery usually follows one of two patterns. It can be rapid and complete, or it can be delayed and partial with signs of aberrant function. A positive correlation between the speed and extent of recovery was noted by Hauser and co-workers (1971). Taverner (1959) found that about half the patients recovered completely, and these patients began to show improvement in an average of 10 days and returned to normal in an average of one and a half months. Those patients whose recovery was never complete began to improve in about two months on the average, and recovery stabilized within nine months in almost all cases. This, of course, is an oversimplification. The course and extent of recovery in individual patients actually falls along a continuum from one extreme to the other.

Depending to some extent on how closely they are looked for, residual abnormalities consist of synkinesis in 50 to 75 per cent of cases, weakness in 25 to 50 per cent, contracture in 10 to 35 per cent, and crocodile tears in about 6 per cent. At least minimal signs of residua could be detected in 76 per cent of the cases of Hauser and associates, but in only 14 per cent were abnormalities obvious on casual observation; 79 per cent of these patients graded their own recovery as 95 per cent or better. Taverner (1959, 1968) indicated that only 10 to 15 per cent of his patients were dissatisfied with their recovery, usually because of crocodile tears or contracture.

Prognostic Indicators. The difference in patterns of recovery suggests a difference in degree of injury to nerve VII, with neurapraxia occurring at the one extreme and axonotmesis or even neurotmesis at the other. If Seddon's (1943) observations are applicable to Bell's palsy, one might conclude that effective therapy should antedate and prevent the more severe degrees of nerve injury. Assuming for the moment the availability of such therapy, it may be that it is too risky or too inconvenient to use indiscriminately in all cases. For this reason, the earliest possible identification of patients with poor prognosis is of more than academic interest.

Age. Older age at onset of Bell's palsy correlated with greater residual abnormalities in the series of Hauser and associates (1971). Taverner (1959) found the average age of patients who recovered "completely" to be 34.4 years as contrasted with 44.8 years for those who had permanent residua. Also, of 14 patients under age 10 in his series, 13 recovered completely, whereas of 18 patients over age 70, only 5 recovered completely.

Degree of Weakness. Taverner and co-workers (1959, 1971) reported that incomplete paralysis suggested a favorable prognosis, and Jongkees (1970) found that 85 to 95 per cent of patients with incomplete paralysis could be expected to recover completely. The correlation of tearing in the acute stages with poorer prognosis may be simply a reflection of degree of paralysis and paralytic ectropion (Hauser et al., 1971).

Pain. Hauser and co-workers found no correlation between pain at the onset of Bell's palsy and ultimate prognosis, nor did Jongkees (1970). Taverner's finding (1959) that 43 per cent of his patients who recovered completely had pain at the onset as compared with 58 per cent of those whose recovery was incomplete may be statistically significant but seems of little practical use.

TASTE. Peiris and Miles (1965) noted that, when patients with Bell's palsy were tested in the first 14 days, 95 per cent of those who had equal thresholds to anodal galvanic stimulation on the two sides of the tongue had "complete" recoveries, and that 100 per cent of those whose thresholds were decreased on the side of paralysis had incomplete recoveries. The favorable category represented 52 per cent of the total group.

SUBMANDIBULAR SALIVARY FLOW. Blatt (1965), May (1970), and Diamant, Ekstrand, and Wiberg (1972) examined the relationship between submandibular salivary flow and ultimate recovery from Bell's palsy, and the results were comparable in the three studies. In general, if the flow rate was greater than 50 per cent of normal, complete recovery could be expected; a flow rate of less than 10 to 25 per cent of normal presaged incomplete recovery.

It is interesting to speculate on the mechanism for dissociation of taste and salivary function from branchiomeric motor function in those cases in which it is observed. The proponents of the topognosis scheme argue that the site of the lesion in such cases must be distal to the chorda tympani. May (1970) wondered if the pathologic process had a differential effect based on fiber size, the smaller fibers being more resistant to presumed compressive ischemia. Denny-Brown and Brenner (1944b), however, noted that the relative resistance of function of sensory fibers to spring clip pressure on peripheral nerves was not related to fiber size but seemed to be a functional property of the axoplasm itself. Sensory impulses were conducted past the site of compression despite localized demyelinization, while motor impulses were not.

ELECTRODIAGNOSTIC TESTS. It has been appreciated for many years that the tests mentioned earlier under Functions and Their Measurement, such as galvanic and faradic stimulation for reaction of degeneration, the intensity-duration curve, and detection of fibrillation in the conventional electromyogram, were helpful prognostic indicators (Park and Watkins, 1949; Taverner, 1955). Their results parallel the recovery patterns already described and confirm the suggestion that Seddon's observations do indeed apply to Bell's palsy. The test results become abnormal only after one to two weeks, however.

Measurement of *conduction latency* accurately divided Bell's palsy cases into three prognostic groups (Langworth and Taverner, 1963). Patients with complete denervation had the worst prognosis, and in keeping with the observations by Gilliatt and Taylor (1959), there was a loss of nerve excitability by the fifth day without antecedent slowing of conduction. The second group had partial denervation, with slowing of conduction appearing by the seventh day; recovery was generally satisfactory in this group. The third group had normal conduction latencies throughout the period of observation; their paralyses were presumably based on neurapraxia, and their recoveries were complete.

The *nerve excitability threshold* has also been a reliable indicator of prognosis, particularly at the two extremes of excitability (Campbell et al., 1962). In general, those patients with equal thresholds on the normal and paretic sides recovered completely, while those with absence of excitability had permanent residua. The critical threshold difference between sides appeared to be 3.5 ma (Laumans, 1965). According to Mechelse and co-workers (1971), nerve excitability thresholds never increased after the second week, while Richardson (1963) and El-Ebiary (1971b) reported occasional delays in threshold increases to as late as 21 and 32 days, respectively.

May and associates (1971) found that the test for *maximal action potential* not only was an earlier indicator of denervation but also was more reliable in predicting prognosis when compared to nerve excitability threshold.

SUMMARY. Younger patients with incomplete paralysis, preservation of taste perception and submandibular salivary flow, and electrodiagnostic evidence of an intact distal segment of nerve VII have a better prognosis. Measures of taste perception and salivary flow have the advantage of indicating whether these particular functions of nerve VII may still be intact despite a loss of branchiomeric motor function. The available evidence appears to indicate a relative resistance of fibers subserving these functions to the pathologic process, and the better that taste and salivation are preserved, the less the chances of axonal degeneration of fibers to facial muscles. In other words, the two tests of function anticipate axonal degeneration. Results of the electrodiagnostic tests become abnormal only after there is at least some degree of axonal degeneration. Only to the extent that the pathologic process is a dynamic one, acting over a given period, can even the earliest indicator of degeneration hope to anticipate further degeneration in time for preventive therapy. Some cases do show evidence of progression clinically and by physiologic measures for as long as two weeks or more. Unfortunately, those cases with poorest prognosis have the most rapidly developing degeneration, and even the test for maximum action potential may show abnormalities only after complete degeneration has occurred.

PATHOLOGY

Autopsy Findings. The pertinent details of autopsy reports of 10 cases of idiopathic facial paralysis are summarized in Table 27-3. Only in Alexander's (1902) case were clear-cut parenchymatous inflammatory changes noted; one wonders whether this could have been an unrecognized case of herpes zoster. At that time, Hunt (1907) had not yet described "geniculate zoster."

The case of Reddy and co-workers (1966) showed some inflammatory changes in adjacent mastoid cells and around the walls of arteriosclerotic arteries. Those of Dejerine and Theohari (1897) and André-Thomas (1907) were temporally related to herpes zoster, but inflammatory neuropathy was not described in the former case and was specifically denied in the latter. In the two case reports in which Dejerine participated, "parenchymatous neuritis" was the term used to describe the pathologic features, but no inflammation was described (Dejerine and Theohari, 1897; Mirallie and Dejerine, 1906).

The site of major involvement in most cases seemed to extend from either side of the geniculate ganglion to the vertical segment of nerve VII, with gradually increasing degrees of involvement more distally. Flatau's (1897) case is a notable exception—but the intratemporal course was not examined, and the degenerative changes he described within the brain stem are difficult to interpret in terms of present concepts of neuropathology. Also, the locus of major involvement in the two cases of Dejerine was thought to be peripheral, but the petrous segments were not examined in one case.

Fowler's (1963) case, in which extensive examination by modern neuropathologic techniques was carried out, was the only one in which intraneural hemorrhage and venous dilatation were described. The patient of Monier-Vinard and Puech (1930) had an intracanalicular hemorrhage. Hypertension was present in both these cases.

Surgical Findings. Many otologic surgeons have described abnormalities in the appearance of nerve VII or the surrounding tissue at the time of surgical decompression. Cawthorne (1946) described constriction of the nerve at the stylomastoid foramen in most cases, with swelling of the nerve and longitudinal hemorrhagic streaks (never extending more than 1 cm above the foramen) in acute cases. When operation was delayed more than six months, he noted a shrunken appearance of the nerve. Jongkees (1972) found that the vessels on the nerve were swollen to two to three times normal caliber. Kettel (1959) described bulging of the vertical segment of the nerve upon incision of its sheath, which Jongkees found did not extend into the horizontal segment. Pulec (1972) found no evidence of hemorrhage but noted that the nerve sometimes swelled to two or three times its normal size when the sheath was incised, while the normal nerve did not. Sadé, Levy, and Chaco (1965) noted bulging of the nerve upon incision of the perineurium in its horizontal as well as its vertical segments and suggested, along with Sunderland (1946), that this was a normal phenomenon. Kettel found aseptic necrosis in adjacent bone near the stylomastoid foramen in a few cases, but Cawthorne did not (Jongkees et al., 1965). Miller (1967) wrote,

Recalling similarly graphic descriptions of the operative appearances of the sciatic nerve in syndromes which we now know to have had their origin at a much higher level from disc prolapse, the physician may be pardoned an unworthy suspicion that the surgeon who describes the swollen and congested facial nerve observed at operation for decompression is less likely to be familiar with the appearance of the entirely normal nerve under similar circumstances.

Blatt and Freeman (1966) excised segments of the chorda tympani in 15 cases and described white plaques on the surface of the nerve and edema in all cases. Microscopic examination revealed "infiltration of mononuclear and inflammatory cells with phagocytosis by histiocytes," which they interpreted as "clear evidence of an inflammatory process." They concluded that Bell's palsy was the result of retrograde extension of this process. The written description and supporting illustrations of the histopathologic features, however, seem to be compatible with simple wallerian degeneration. McGovern (1970a) found swell-

TABLE 27-3 AUTOPSY FINDINGS

Author (see references)	Age (yr)	Duration (wk)*	Cause of Death	Site and Extent of Degeneration†			
				Brain Stem	Roots and Internal Auditory Canal	Labyrinthine Segment	Genu
Minkowski (1891)	27	8	Ingestion of HCl	−	−	−	−
Flatau (1897)	34	9	TB	+	3+	NE	NE
Dejerine and Theohari (1897)	81	13	Ca, uterus	+	0	+	+
Alexander (1902)	56	4	Ca, esophagus	−	+	−	3+
Mirallie and Dejerine (1906)	76	6	Pulmonary congestion	+	−	NE	NE
André-Thomas (1907)	75	2½	Pulmonary congestion	+	0	0 to +	−
Mills (1910)	80	1½	Ca, stomach	−	+	+	2+
Monier-Vinard and Puech (1930)	21	4	Chronic nephritis	0	−	−	−
Fowler (1963)	60	2	Dissecting aortic aneurysm	0	0/3	3+	3+
Reddy et al. (1966)	71	2½	Renal cell carcinoma; pulmonary embolism	−	−	−	−

*Interval from onset to death.
†NE, not examined.
‡Upper < lower.

ing of the chorda tympani but no inflammatory response in his two cases. Biopsies of the sheath of nerve VII itself showed no inflammatory response (Sadé et al., 1965).

After exploration of the vertical segment of nerve VII showed it to be normal in four cases, Cawthorne (1965) found subsequently that the patients had decreased lacrimation. He reoperated and exposed the nerve in the region of the geniculate ganglion where he found the nerve "swollen and discolored." Fisch and Esslen (1972a) found morphologic changes proximal to the geniculate ganglion in 11 of 12 cases, which they described as "pronounced, edematous, red swelling with marked vascular injection," observed after splitting of the sheath. In 8 of 11 cases the nerve was two to three times normal size, and it compressed the superior division of the vestibular nerve at the level of the fundus of the internal auditory meatus.

Animal Models. Working with white rats,

Sullivan and Smith (1950) found that application of ice to the shaven face of the animal for 20 minutes resulted in a slight accumulation of systemically administered trypan blue in nerve VII 24 hours later. When a suture, tied just tightly enough to block venous drainage, was placed around nerve VII distal to the stylomastoid foramen, edema spread proximally to block the foramen completely.

Coassolo (1952, 1953a, 1953b) placed ice on the mastoid region of rabbits sensitized to horse serum, with unsensitized rabbits serving as controls. Facial paralysis developed only in the sensitized rabbits, and the nerves were described grossly as enlarged and red. Microscopically, there was evidence of blood extravasation, infiltration with leukocytes, and myelin fragmentation and absorption. The changes did not occur in sensitized animals that were given procaine intravenously prior to the application of ice. Coassolo interpreted this as evidence of inhibition of an allergic

Large Petrosal Nerve	Horizontal Segment	Vertical Segment	Chorda Tympani	Distal Segment	Inflammation	Additional Comment
+	+	3+	−	−	No	...
NE	NE	NE	NE	0 to +	None described	Pathologic description detailed but seemingly inconsistent
−	+	+	−	2+‡	None described	Ipsilateral cervical plexus "vaste zona" 3 months before onset; nerve VII not squeezed in its petrous course; "parenchymatous neuritis"
3+	3+	3+	3+	3+	Yes	Small cell infiltration of endoneurium following course of nerve fibers and vasculature, mainly at and beyond geniculate ganglion; spared perineurium and epineurium
NE	NE	NE	NE	2+‡	None described	Paresis improving by 4 weeks after onset; "parenchymatous neuritis"
−	2+	2+	−	2+	No	"Zona intercostal" 3 weeks before onset
0	2+	3+	0	3+	No	...
−	−	−	−	−	No	Hemorrhage in facial canal
3+	3+	3+	2+	−	No	Hypertension; family history of nerve VII palsy; intraneural hemorrhages, dilated veins, normal arteries and arterioles
−	+	2+	−	−	Mastoid and perivascular	Hypertension; diabetes; dense connective tissue in vertical segment; inflammatory changes in some mastoid cells; arteries sclerotic with perivascular inflammatory cells

mechanism through interference with the release of histamine. McGovern and Hansel (1961) were unable to produce more than transient paralysis of nerve VII in dogs by using Coassolo's techniques.

Jain and Sharma (1964) infused saline into nerve VII within the facial canal of rabbits and found that, at a constant infusion pressure, the resulting paralysis lasted for a period proportional to the duration of compression. Infusion of nerve VII outside of its canal had no effect. McGovern, Edgemon and Konigsmark (1972) compared the effects of injecting epinephrine or saline into the facial canals of normal dogs and of dogs sensitized to horse serum. Although all dogs receiving injections had neuropathic changes in the nerve, the changes were more severe in sensitized dogs receiving epinephrine injections. McGovern thought that pressure ischemia from the injection was the common denominator but that both prior serum sensitization and vasoconstriction induced by epinephrine potentiated the effects. The pathologic changes in the nerve were noninflammatory, more in line with those reported in Bell's palsy than in experimental allergic neuritis.

Hazama and co-workers (1972) were not able to induce facial paralysis in rabbits sensitized to horse serum when they injected horse serum and Freund's adjuvant into the stylomastoid foramen. When they applied a spring clip to nerve VII just distal to the foramen in normal rabbits for various periods, they observed changes in the appearance and function of the nerve. Paralysis began within 90 seconds and was complete within five minutes in all animals. When the clip was removed, dilatation of small vessels and redness and swelling of the sheath were always observed. The hyperemia subsided in 7 minutes, but swelling persisted for 60 minutes. When the spring clip was removed within 20 minutes, recovery began within the subsequent 30 minutes and was complete within three hours. If the clip was left in place for more than 30 minutes, recovery was delayed for more than a month.

Pathophysiology and Etiology. Most authors accept the general thesis that in Bell's palsy a vicious circle of edema and compressive ischemia involves nerve VII within its bony canal (Hilger, 1949; Blunt, 1956). Most of the differences in opinion expressed in the literature concern the relative importance of several factors in this pathophysiologic process.

POSSIBLE UNIQUENESS OF VASCULAR SUPPLY. As already noted, and contrary to the ideas reported in the earlier literature, the arterial supply of nerve VII is rich with anastomoses and collateral channels, and it seems unlikely to be any more susceptible to arterial occlusive ischemia acting alone than is any other peripheral nerve. Anson and his associates (1970) noted prominence of the venous plexus surrounding nerve VII.

SHEATH VERSUS BONY CANAL AS FACTOR IN COMPRESSION. As noted previously, many surgeons have pointed out the relative disproportion of cross sectional areas of the vertical segment of nerve VII as compared with its canal, while stressing the swelling of the nerve that occurs in Bell's palsy when the sheath is incised. It should be recognized, however, that the extra "space" in the canal is occupied by tissue that, for practical purposes, is incompressible, and any increase in volume in one compartment of the canal must be balanced by a proportional decrease in volume of another. For example, if tissue fluid increases (edema), then intravascular blood volume must decrease, in arteries, in capillaries, or in veins. In this context, the canal of nerve VII is comparable to the cranial vault. The "sheath" of nerve VII, on the other hand, is not unique as compared with that of other peripheral nerves (Sunderland and Cossar, 1953).

SITE OF INVOLVEMENT. Although there may be a site of initial and maximal involvement, the weight of pathologic evidence suggests that in most cases the process extends a considerable distance on either side of this, once it is under way.

DURATION OF ACTIVE PROCESS. It would seem from the evidence cited that the process is almost never an "instantaneous" one, but is dynamic, with the degree of resultant nerve injury depending on the combined factors of duration and severity.

TRIGGERING MECHANISMS. Facial paralysis can be induced by a variety of methods in animals; it seems possible also that a variety of different factors may serve as triggers in man, setting off the vicious circle of edema and

ischemia in "idiopathic" facial paralysis (Sadé, 1972).

Zülch (1970) discussed exposure to cold as a factor and noted that in about one third of 149 cases "it was clear that the lesion was the direct result of chill." Such chilling was attributed to such things as winter wind, air conditioning, ocean breezes, driving in open automobiles, sleeping in front of a fan, and having the hair shampooed. If a comparable group of individuals without Bell's palsy were questioned about such exposure, would the proportion of affirmative replies differ significantly? I know of no such study.

Hilger (1949) hypothesized that an autonomic nervous impulse to the vasa nervorum resulted in vasoconstriction, ischemia, capillary dilatation, tissue edema, compression, and so forth. He noted that his patients with Bell's palsy also frequently had other evidence of vasomotor instability such as vasomotor rhinitis, migraine, and labyrinthitis. Philipszoon (1962) thought that Ménière's disease, vestibular neuritis, Bell's palsy, and some cases of supposed "herpes zoster" without skin lesions were all expressions of the same disease, citing as support the electronystagmographic findings in his Bell's palsy cases. The case of Fowler (1963) and the surgical findings of Fisch and Esslen (1972a) support the idea of a proximal process that may involve nerves VII and VIII together.

The possibility that some cases may be of viral origin is discussed in a subsequent section of this chapter.

Evidence is still incomplete regarding the possible correlation of Bell's palsy with diabetes, hypertension, and pregnancy, but it does suggest an increased incidence of the disease in children with severe hypertension and in women near the time of parturition.

A possible triggering mechanism not discussed in the literature is suggested by the autopsy findings in the case of Fowler (1963). The prominence of venous distention, hemorrhage, and nerve degeneration suggests venous hemorrhagic infarction. Acute, noninflammatory venous thrombosis is not easy to recognize histologically and might have been overlooked in this case and perhaps in others.

TREATMENT

Nonsurgical Methods.   In their analysis of 500 cases of Bell's palsy, Park and Watkins

(1949) found no evidence that decongestant treatment, heat, massage, or electrical stimulation altered the course of recovery. They did think those patients who cooperated with facial exercises had a more rapid recovery after the initial return of function. Zülch (1970), however, found that exercise before a mirror had no effect on the prevention of mass movements. Despite the evidence of Gutmann and Guttmann (1944) that galvanic exercise decreased the degree of atrophy in denervated rabbit muscle and resulted in greater recovery with reinnervation, Mosforth and Taverner (1958) found it ineffective in Bell's palsy in a controlled trial. Fearnley and co-workers (1964) found cervical sympathetic blockade ineffective in another controlled study. Kime (1958) claimed that intramuscular injection of nicotinic acid resulted in full recovery within three weeks in 72 of 74 cases, when given within 14 days of onset of Bell's palsy; earlier treatment resulted in still more rapid recovery. I could find no other study in the literature confirming these amazing results.

Although Taverner (1954) reported failure of cortisone acetate to alter the outcome in a controlled study, there were only 26 patients in the series and they were accepted as late as the ninth day after the onset of paralysis. Taverner and his co-workers subsequently found that corticotropin therapy resulted in better recovery than "expected" on the basis of previous experience with untreated cases (Taverner, 1959, 1968; Taverner et al., 1966). Treatment was started within six days of onset and consisted of 80 units of corticotropin daily for the first five days, the dosage then being tapered over the next five days. In a subsequent study, they compared the effects of corticotropin (60 units per day for five days with tapering over four days) with prednisolone therapy (80 mg per day for five days with tapering over four days) in a randomized series (Taverner et al., 1971). They reported significantly better recovery in the group receiving the steroid.

Adour and co-workers (1972) started a double-blind study of the effects of prednisone therapy (40 mg per day for four days with tapering over four days) in Bell's palsy, but interrupted the study when it became apparent that pain was relieved dramatically in the treated group within 24 hours. The 194 patients who ultimately received treatment had better recovery than the 110 untreated patients. These authors suggested that, when steroid treatment was not contraindicated, all patients with Bell's palsy should receive 60 mg of prednisone daily for four days with the dosage tapered over the subsequent six days.

Surgical Methods. Ballance and Duel (1932), noting that others had recommended the removal of the damaged portion of nerve VII and suture of the cut ends in patients who did not recover spontaneously, observed, "but surely, in Bell's palsy only decompression would be necessary." They suggested that most patients would respond to a facial sling, massage, and galvanism. Cawthorne (1946), Kettel (1959), McGovern (1969), and Jongkees (1970) have been strong advocates of surgical decompression of the vertical segment of nerve VII in selected cases, although their criteria for selection of patients and timing of decompression differ in detail. Jongkees observed, "I am afraid I cannot prove statistically that an operation improves the prognosis of well-chosen cases of Bell's paralysis, but I have good reason to believe it does." Giancarlo and Mattucci (1970) and Yanagihara and Kishimoto (1972) compared surgical and nonsurgical results and reported the former to be better.

Groves (1965), on the other hand, reported no benefit from surgical treatment in his series, and Harrison (1970) gave up surgical decompression because he found it to be ineffective. Mechelse and associates (1971) and Adour and Swanson (1971) reported controlled series, comparing surgical and nonsurgical treatment, that showed no benefit from the operation.

Fisch and Esslen (1972a) suggested a wider decompression, presenting evidence of a more proximal lesion in Bell's palsy. Blatt and Freeman (1968) suggested chorda tympani neurectomy as a cure for Bell's palsy, giving as their reasons (1) prevention of spread of inflammatory neuropathy back to nerve VII, and (2) a "physiological decompression" of the vertical segment of nerve VII as a result of retrograde degeneration of fibers of the chorda tympani after its section in the middle ear. McGovern (1970a) found chorda tympani resection ineffective in his cases.

In summary, clinical studies have suggested that corticotropin has a beneficial effect on the outcome in Bell's palsy when given early, and other studies have shown steroids to be equally or even more effective. Thus far, the evidence that surgical decompression is ever of use in Bell's palsy is less convincing, and a number of otologic surgeons have given up the procedure for treating this condition.

Infectious and Granulomatous Facial Paralysis

CEPHALIC HERPES ZOSTER

Hunt (1907) noted that herpes zoster with eruptions in and behind the ear was sometimes associated with acute facial paralysis and concluded that the geniculate ganglion was affected in these cases in a manner analogous to the involvement of the posterior root ganglia in spinal zoster. He also used the association as one of his arguments in support of the "sensory field" of nerve VII. It is interesting to note that the geniculate ganglion was lost in his first case, and he failed to demonstrate its involvement by the pathologic process in any of his subsequent cases. Hunt classified cephalic herpes zoster according to its clinical manifestations. In the first type the only manifestation was the appearance of vesicles in the "sensory field" of nerve VII. In the second type there were vesicles anywhere on the head, combined with facial paralysis. In the third type there were these two features plus auditory or vestibular involvement.

The reported incidence of cephalic zoster among patients with acute facial paralysis (Ramsay Hunt syndrome) varies from 5 per cent (Taverner, 1959) to nearly 30 per cent (Aitken and Brain, 1933; Tomita et al., 1972a). From 80 to 100 per cent of such patients have increased titers of antibodies to herpes zoster (Aitken and Brain, 1933; Peitersen and Caunt, 1970; Tomita et al., 1972a), but up to 25 per cent of patients with facial paralysis without vesicles also have increased titers. The incidence of associated pain and acousticovestibular symptoms was greater in those with increased titers, whether or not they had zoster vesicles. Tomita and co-workers (1972b) found taste function impaired in all their cases of the Ramsay Hunt syndrome, although it tended to recover more quickly than in idiopathic facial paralysis. The prognosis for recovery of motor function in the syndrome is generally good (Jongkees, 1969), although Taverner (1959) found that the syndrome was more often associated with nerve degeneration than with conduction block.

The pathologic features of "geniculate" herpes zoster parallel those of the spinal form. Denny-Brown, Adams, and Fitzgerald (1944) reviewed the literature on herpes zoster and added several cases of their own, including one with facial paralysis. In their view, the essential features were inflammatory ganglionitis with pannecrosis, posterior poliomyelitis, leptomeningitis, and mononeuritis, all of which tended to show segmental localization. Especially when it affects the cranial nerves, however, herpes zoster often involves two or more segments of the neuroaxis; even Hunt's classification does not include all the many combinations of involvement that have been described. Because of this, Blackley, Friedman, and Wright (1967) thought that the term "cephalic zoster" was more appropriate than "geniculate ganglionitis," especially since there was, and still is, no report in the literature describing ganglionitis and pannecrosis affecting the geniculate ganglion. Their case, in which autopsy was performed 214 days after the onset of symptoms, still showed an inflammatory response with lymphocytic infiltration of nerves VII and VIII and perivascular cuffing.

Although Crabtree (1968) suggested that cephalic zoster with facial paralysis should be treated by surgical decompression of nerve VII from the geniculate ganglion to the stylomastoid foramen, most authors think that surgical decompression is contraindicated (Jongkees et al., 1965). Harner, Heiny, and Newell (1970) reviewed the literature with respect to steroid treatment of herpes zoster, which they used in their two cases of cephalic zoster. They suggested giving 80 mg of prednisone daily for seven days and tapering the dosage over the subsequent three weeks.

OTHER VIRAL DISEASES

Tomita, Hayakawa, and Hondo (1972a) found a significant increase in titer of antibodies to herpes simplex in 6 per cent of their cases of facial paralysis. McCormick (1972) presented an interesting argument for the thesis that the herpes simplex virus could be the cause of a large proportion of Bell's palsy cases. Allison (1950) found only seven instances of facial paralysis associated with 1805 cases of infectious mononucleosis in the literature. It was the only neurologic sign in two cases and was a part of the Guillain-Barré syndrome in two others. The comprehensive reviews by Wolf (1956) and Schnell and co-workers (1966) refer to a few additional cases associated with infectious mononucleosis.

Engler and Missal (1955) reviewed 500 cases of anterior poliomyelitis, 112 of which were of the bulbar form. They found that nerve VII was involved alone in 55 cases, second in frequency only to nerves IX and X. It was involved in combination with other cranial nerves in 45 other cases.

OTITIS MEDIA

From 0.5 to 1.0 per cent of all cases of acute otitis media are complicated by facial paralysis (Riskaer, 1946; McGovern and Fitz-Hugh, 1956), and about 8 per cent of cases of facial paralysis occur in association with acute otitis media. According to Cawthorne and Riskaer, all these patients recover, and surgical intervention is not indicated (1946). The incidence of facial paralysis is about the same in chronic otitis media, but the prognosis is less uniformly favorable although most patients still recover (Riskaer, 1946). Cawthorne, and later Jongkees (1970), suggested immediate surgical intervention in facial paralysis associated with chronic otitis media. When cholesteatoma is present the prognosis is less favorable, with or without surgical intervention.

OTHER INFECTIONS

Leprosy often involves nerve VII and may present with facial paralysis (Bosher, 1962; Van Droogenbroeck, 1970; McGovern, 1972). It is a common cause of facial paralysis in endemic areas. Syphilis sometimes involves nerve VII, and is perhaps secondary to involvement of adjacent structures of the temporal bone (Goodhill, 1939; Jongkees, 1969). In a similar way, nerve VII may be involved by osteomyelitis, petrositis, or acute bacterial or tuberculous meningitis.

GRANULOMATOUS DISEASE

Sarcoidosis of Besnier, Boeck, and Schaumann was first related to the syndrome of uveoparotid fever of Heerfordt (1909) by Pautrier (1937). Colover (1948) found 115 cases of sarcoidosis with nervous system involvement in the literature; in 50 per cent of them there was facial paralysis. The paralysis was bilateral in one third of the cases although both sides were not always affected at the same time. In 17 per cent, taste impairment was reported. Wilson (1957) observed marked edema of the nerve when he decompressed its vertical segment in one case.

Garland and Thompson (1933) thought that the facial paralysis that often occurred in Heerfordt's syndrome was due to direct involvement of nerve VII by the parotid lesion. Lambert and Richards (1964) argued that the facial canal was the more likely site of involvement because of the loss of taste function and hyperacusis in some cases, the absence of associated parotitis in some, and the absence of facial paralysis in association with the parotitis of mumps. They noted that in most cases (87 per cent of those reviewed by Wilson) there was complete or nearly complete recovery in five months. They suggested steroid therapy followed, if not effective, by surgical decompression.

Traumatic Facial Paralysis

CLOSED HEAD INJURY

Davis (1928) noted that 46 per cent of patients with middle fossa fractures had associated facial paralysis, apparent at first examination in some cases (immediate) and developing hours or days after the trauma in others (delayed). Those in whom it was delayed recovered more rapidly. Grove (1939) presented a detailed study of 211 cases of skull fractures involving the ear. His classification included longitudinal fractures of the temporal bone (parallel to the long axis of the pyramid) and transverse fractures. Longitudinal fractures were more difficult to detect in routine roentgenograms of the skull. They occurred in 146 of his cases, while transverse fractures occurred in only 16. Complicating facial paralysis occurred with 19 per cent of the longitudinal fractures and with 31 per cent of the transverse fractures. On follow-up, one fifth of the cases of facial paralysis showed no recovery of function. Cases of delayed onset (up to two weeks after injury) had the better prognosis.

Turner (1944) followed 70 consecutive cases of facial paralysis associated with closed head injuries (36 of immediate onset and 34 delayed). In the former group, 75 per cent of the patients recovered completely, but three had no recovery at all. In the group with delayed onset, only two patients failed to recover completely; one remained totally paralyzed. At exploration in two cases of delayed traumatic paralysis, Jongkees (1965) found that nerve VII had been severed. He stressed the importance of reliable observations of facial function in these cases.

Jongkees (1965), Kettel (1950, 1959), and Cawthorne (1952a) reported extensive experience with surgical treatment of traumatic facial paralysis and suggested that in patients with the immediate type in particular, surgical exploration is advisable. Their results, however, are not obviously different from the expected course (70 to 80 per cent of Jongkees's patients had "good improvements" with operation). There are no controlled studies testing the efficacy of surgical treatment in such cases. If no recovery has occurred in six months, traumatic severance of nerve VII can be assumed; if the site of severance can be localized and is accessible, an attempt to anastomose or graft the nerve would seem reasonable (see Krekorian, 1971).

Briggs and Potter (1971) found previously that, in 38.5 per cent of head injury cases with bleeding from the ear and roentgenologic evidence of fractures of the petrous temporal bone, delayed facial paralysis would develop. When they treated 50 consecutive patients with corticotropin (80 units daily for three days with tapering over the subsequent five days) they found delayed facial paralysis in only four cases (8 per cent). They pointed out that the treatment may not have altered the ultimate outcome in their cases because the natural course is so favorable.

SURGICAL TRAUMA

Riskaer (1946) followed 47 cases of facial paralysis complicating surgery of the ear. In 18, the paralysis was immediate, and it persisted in 16 of these. In 29, the paralysis was delayed, and most of these patients recovered. Miehlke (1969) and Jongkees (1970) stressed the importance of early recognition of immediate operative facial paralysis despite the tendency for surgeons not to "see" their complications. Many cases of immediate paralysis are due to unrecognized severance of the nerve, and immediate reoperation and anastomosis are simpler and the results better than if operation is delayed. Both Riskaer and Miehlke noted occurrence rates of just over 1 per cent for this complication in otologic surgery, with higher rates for more complex procedures or reoperation.

Love and Svien (1954) noted the complication of facial paralysis in 16 of 100 consecutive operations for subtemporal decompres-

sion of the gasserian ganglion for trigeminal neuralgia via an extradural approach. The finding by Hall, Pulec, and Rhoton (1969) that there was incomplete bony covering of the geniculate ganglion in 15 per cent of the temporal bones they dissected may be a lead toward understanding this surgical complication.

Newborn and Congenital Facial Paralysis

Neuropathic facial paralysis that is apparent at birth was divided, by Hepner (1951), into four groups: that due to trauma of intrapartum compression, that due to intrauterine posture, that due to forceps trauma, and that due to nuclear aplasia. The nuclear aplasia group includes Möbius' syndrome and a restricted form of lower facial paralysis often associated with congenital heart disease, the cardiofacial syndrome.

INTRAPARTUM COMPRESSION

In a study of 1000 consecutive deliveries, from which 125 were excluded from further analysis (stillborn, breech, and premature), Hepner found 56 cases (6.4 per cent) of unilateral facial weakness. The side of paralysis correlated with the position of presentation and direction of external version at delivery in all but two. He concluded that pressure of the prominence of the maternal sacrum on nerve VII in the parotid region was responsible. The majority of these patients recover with few or no residua. This strikingly large incidence and association with presentation at delivery has not been confirmed by others.

INTRAUTERINE POSTURE

Parmelee (1931) described a case of facial paralysis in a newborn infant in which the face and jaws were asymmetrical, with upward and inward compression of the mandible on the side of the paralysis. He thought the condition was due to extreme intrauterine flexion of the head that caused pressure of the shoulder against the jaw. There was one such case in Hepner's series.

in the cat: afferent connections. Arch. Neurol., 6:264, 1962.

Kettel, K.: Peripheral facial paralysis in fractures of the temporal bone: indications for surgical repair of the nerve; report of cases in which the Ballance and Duel operation was used. Arch. Otolaryngol., 51:25, 1950.

Kettel, K.: Peripheral Facial Palsy: Pathology and Surgery. Springfield, Ill., Charles C Thomas, 1959.

Kime, C. E.: Bell's palsy: a new syndrome associated with treatment by nicotinic acid; a guide to adequate medical therapy. Arch. Otolaryngol., 68:28, 1958.

Kindler, W.: Die Fazialislähmung in der darstellenden Kunst seit mehr als 4 jahrtausenden. Z. Laryngol. Rhinol. Otol., 49:1, 1970.

Klaus, S. N., and Brunsting, L. A.: Melkersson's syndrome (persistent swelling of the face, recurrent facial paralysis, and lingua plicata): report of a case. Proc. Staff Meet. Mayo Clin., 34:365, 1959.

Korczyn, A. D.: Bell's palsy and diabetes mellitus. Lancet, 1:108, 1971a.

Korczyn, A. D.: Bell's palsy and pregnancy. Acta Neurol. Scand., 47:603, 1971b.

Krarup, B.: Electro-gustometry: a method for clinical taste examinations. Acta Otolaryngol. (Stockh.), 49:294, 1958a.

Krarup, B.: On the technique of gustatory examinations. Acta Otolaryngol. [Suppl.] (Stockh.), 140:195, 1958b.

Krekorian, E. A.: The repair of combat-injured facial nerves. Laryngoscope, 81:1926, 1971.

Kugelberg, E.: "Injury activity" and "trigger zones" in human nerves. Brain, 69:310, 1946.

Kugelberg, E.: Activation of human nerves by ischemia: Trousseau's phenomenon in tetany. Arch. Neurol. Psychiatry, 60:140, 1948.

Kugelberg, E., and Cobb, W.: Repetitive discharges in human motor nerve fibres during the post-ischaemic state. J. Neurol. Neurosurg. Psychiatry, 14:88, 1951.

Kullman, G. L., Dyck, P. J., and Cody, D. T. R.: Anatomy of the mastoid portion of the facial nerve. Arch. Otolaryngol., 93:29, 1971.

Lambert, E. H., Love, J. G., and Mulder, D. W.: Facial myokymia and brain tumor: electromyographic studies (abstract). Am. Assoc. Electromyogr. Electrodiagn. News Letter, 8:8, 1961.

Lambert, V., and Richards, S. H.: Facial palsy in Heerfordt's syndrome. J. Laryngol. Otol., 78:684, 1964.

Langworth, E. P., and Taverner, D.: The prognosis in facial palsy. Brain, 86:465, 1963.

Larsell, O., and Fenton, R. A.: The embryology and neurohistology of sphenopalatine ganglion connections: a contribution to the study of otalgia. Laryngoscope, 38:371, 1928.

Laumans, E. P. J.: Nerve excitability tests in facial paralysis. Arch. Otolaryngol., 81:478, 1965.

Leibowitz, U.: Epidemic incidence of Bell's palsy. Brain, 92:109, 1969.

Lindeman, H.: The fallopian canal: an anatomical study of its distal part. Acta Otolaryngol. [Suppl.] (Stockh.), 158:204, 1960.

Lipschitz, R.: Beiträge zur Lehre von der Facialislähmung nebst Bemerkungen zur Frage der Nervenregeneration. Monatsschr. Psychiatr. Neurol., 20 Suppl.:84, 1906.

Lloyd, A. V. C., Jewitt, D. E., and Still, J. D. L.: Facial paralysis in children with hypertension. Arch. Dis. Child., 41:292, 1966.

Love, J. G., and Svien, H. J.: Results of decompression operation for trigeminal neuralgia. J. Neurosurg., 11:499, 1954.

Lüscher, E.: Die Funktion des Musculus stapedius beim Menschen. Z. Hals- Nasen- Ohrenheilkd., 23:105, 1929.

Magielski, J. E., and Blatt, I. M.: Submaxillary salivary flow: a test of chorda tympani nerve function as an aid in diagnosis and prognosis of facial nerve paralysis. Laryngoscope, 68:1770, 1958.

Magun, R., and Esslen, E.: Electromyographic study of reinnervated muscle and of hemifacial spasm. Am. J. Phys. Med., 38:79, 1959.

Maloney, W. J., and Kennedy, R. F.: The sense of pressure in the face, eye, and tongue. Brain, 34:1, 1911.

Manning, J. J., and Adour, K. K.: Facial paralysis in children. Pediatrics, 49:102, 1972.

Marinesco, G., Kreindler, A., and Jordanesco, L.: Chronaximetrische Untersuchungen über die Kontraktur nach peripherer Facialislähmung (ein Beitrag zum physiopathologischen Mechanismus dieser Kontraktur). Dtsch. Z. Nervenheilkd., 120:87, 1931.

Masaki, S.: Congenital bilateral facial paralysis. Arch. Otolaryngol., 94:260, 1971.

May, M.: Facial paralysis, peripheral type: a proposed method of reporting. (Emphasis on diagnosis and prognosis, as well as electrical and chorda tympani nerve testing.) Laryngoscope, 80:331, 1970.

May, M., and Harvey, J. E.: Salivary flow: a prognostic test for facial paralysis. Laryngoscope, 81:179, 1971.

May, M., and Lucente, F. E.: "Bell's palsy" caused by basal cell carcinoma. J.A.M.A., 220:1596, 1972.

May, M., Harvey, J. E., Marovitz, W. F., and Stroud, M.: The prognostic accuracy of the maximal stimulation test compared with that of the nerve excitability test in Bell's palsy. Laryngoscope, 81:931, 1971.

Mazzoni, A.: Internal auditory canal arterial relations at the porus acusticus. Ann. Otol. Rhinol. Laryngol., 78:797, 1969.

McCormick, D. P.: Herpes-simplex virus as cause of Bell's palsy. Lancet, 1:937, 1972.

McGovern, F. H.: Management of Bell's palsy: experimental aspects. Arch. Otolaryngol., 89:144, 1969.

McGovern, F. H.: Chorda tympani neurectomy for Bell's palsy. Arch. Otolaryngol., 92:189, 1970a.

McGovern, F. H.: The return of function after damage to the facial nerve. Eye Ear Nose Throat Mon., 49:451, 1970b.

McGovern, F. H.: Facial paralysis (letter to the editor). Arch. Otolaryngol., 96:92, 1972.

McGovern, F. H., and Fitz-Hugh, G. S.: Diseases of the facial nerve. Laryngoscope, 66:187, 1956.

McGovern, F. H., and Hansel, J. S.: Decompression of the facial nerve in experimental Bell's palsy. Laryngoscope, 71:1090, 1961.

McGovern, F. H., Edgemon, L. J., and Konigsmark, B. W.: Experimental ischemic facial paralysis: further studies. Arch. Otolaryngol., 95:331, 1971.

Mechelse, K., Goor, G., Huizing, E. H., Hammelburg, E., van Bolhuis, A. H., Staal, A., and Verjaal, A.: Bell's palsy: prognostic criteria and evaluation of surgical decompression. Lancet, 2:57, 1971.

Melkersson, E.: Ett fall av recidiverande facialispares i samband med angioneurotiskt ödem. Hygiea, 90:737, 1928.

Melotte, G.: Idiopathic paralysis of the facial nerve. Practitioner, 187:349, 1961.

Miehlke, A.: Die Chirurgie des Nervus facialis. München, Urban & Schwarzenberg, 1960.

Miehlke, A.: Typical sites of facial-nerve lesions. Arch. Otolaryngol., 89:122, 1969.

Miehlke, A., and Partsch, C. J.: Ohrmissbildung, Facialis-

und Abducenslähmung als Syndrom der Thalidomidschädigung. Arch. Ohren- Nasen- Kehlkopfheilkd., *181*:154, 1963.

Miescher, G.: Über essentielle granulomatöse Makrocheilie (Cheilitis granulomatosa). Dermatologica, *91*:57, 1945.

Miescher, G.: Cheilitis et pareitis granulomatosa ohne Facialisparese bei Vorhandensein einer Lingua scrotalis. Dermatologica, *112*:536, 1956.

Miller, H.: Facial paralysis. Br. Med. J., *3*:815, 1967.

Mills, C. K.: The sensory functions attributed to the seventh nerve. J. Nerv. Ment. Dis., *37*:273, 1910.

Minkowski: Zur pathologischen Anatomie der rheumatischen Facialislähmung. Berl. Klin. Wochenschr., *28*:665, 1891.

Mirallie, C., and Dejerine, M.: Paralysie faciale périphérique: autopsie. Rev. Neurol. (Paris), *14*:702, 1906.

Möbius, P. J.: Ueber angeborene doppelseitige Abducens-Facialis-Lähmung. Munchen Med. Wochenschr., *35*:91, 1888.

Monier-Vinard, and Puech, P.: Néphrite chronique et paralysie faciale. Bull. Mem. Soc. Med. Hop. Paris, *1*:977, 1930.

Mosforth, J., and Taverner, D.: Physiotherapy for Bell's palsy. Br. Med. J., *2*:675, 1958.

Nager, G. T., and Nager, M.: The arteries of the human middle ear, with particular regard to the blood supply of the auditory ossicles. Ann. Otol. Rhinol. Laryngol., *62*:923, 1953.

Nelson, R. M.: Facial nerve excitability: its reliability, objectivity, and descriptive validity. Phys. Ther., *51*:387, 1971.

New, G. B., and Kirch, W. A.: Permanent enlargement of the lips and face secondary to recurring swellings and associated with facial paralysis: a clinical entity. J.A.M.A., *100*:1230, 1933.

Olson, W. H., Bardin, C. W., Walsh, G. O., and Engel, W. K.: Moebius syndrome: lower motor neuron involvement and hypogonadotrophic hypogonadism. Neurology (Minneap.), *20*:1002, 1970.

Olszewski, J., and Baxter, D.: Cytoarchitecture of the Human Brain Stem. Philadelphia, J. B. Lippincott Co., 1954.

Oppenheim, H.: Text-Book of Nervous Diseases for Physicians and Students. (Translated by A. Bruce.) Vol. 1. 5th Edition. London, T. N. Foulis, 1911.

Pape, K. E., and Pickering, D.: Asymmetric crying facies: an index of other congenital anomalies. J. Pediatr., *81*:21, 1972.

Papez, J. W.: Subdivisions of the facial nucleus. J. Comp. Neurol., *43*:159, 1927.

Park, H. W., and Watkins, A. L.: Facial paralysis: analysis of 500 cases. Arch. Phys. Med., *30*:749, 1949.

Parker, N.: Dystrophia myotonica presenting as congenital facial diplegia. Med. J. Aust., *2*:939, 1963.

Parmelee, A. H.: Molding due to intra-uterine posture: facial paralysis probably due to such molding. Am. J. Dis. Child., *42*:1155, 1931.

Pautrier, L.-M.: Syndrome de Heerfordt et maladie de Besnier-Boeck-Schaumann: Parotidite, irido-cyclite, paralysie faciale d'origine périphérique, paralysie due récurrent, éruption confluente de grosses sarcoïdes des bras et des cuisses, érythrodermie sarcoïdique des jambes et des plantes des pieds. Bull. Mém. Soc. Méd. Hôp. Paris, *2*:1608, 1937.

Pearson, A. A.: The development of the motor nuclei of the facial nerve in man. J. Comp. Neurol., *85*:461, 1946.

Pearson, A. A.: The roots of the facial nerve in human

embryos and fetuses. J. Comp. Neurol., *87*:139, 1947.

Peiris, O. A., and Miles, D. W.: Galvanic stimulation of the tongue as a prognostic index in Bell's palsy. Br. Med. J., *2*:1162, 1965.

Peitersen, E., and Caunt, A. E.: The incidence of herpes zoster antibodies in patients with peripheral facial palsy. J. Laryngol. Otol., *84*:65, 1970.

Perlman, H. B.: Hyperacusis. Ann. Otol. Rhinol. Laryngol., *47*:947, 1938.

Perlman, H. B., and Lindsay, J. R.: Relation of the internal ear spaces to the meninges. Arch. Otolaryngol., *29*:12, 1939.

Philipszoon, A. J.: Nystagmus and Bell's palsy. Pract. Otorhinolaryngol. (Basel), *24*:233, 1962.

Pitner, S. E., Edwards, J. E., and McCormick, W. F.: Observations on the pathology of the Moebius syndrome. J. Neurol. Neurosurg. Psychiatry, *28*:362, 1965.

Pulec, J.: Discussion. Arch. Otolaryngol., *95*:414, 1972.

Rainy, H., and Fowler, J. S.: Congenital facial diplegia due to nuclear lesion. Rev. Neurol. Psychiatry, *1*:149, 1903.

Reddy, J. B., Liu, J., Balshi, S., and Fisher, J.: Histopathology of Bell's palsy. Eye Ear Nose Throat Mon., *45*:62, 1966.

Rhoton, A. L., Jr.: Afferent connections of the facial nerve. J. Comp. Neurol., *133*:89, 1968.

Richardson, A. T.: Electrodiagnosis of facial palsies. Ann. Otol. Rhinol. Laryngol., *72*:569, 1963.

Richter, R. B.: Unilateral congenital hypoplasia of the facial nucleus. J. Neuropathol. Exp. Neurol., *19*:33, 1960.

Riggs, E. H.: Discussion. J. Neuropathol. Exp. Neurol., *17*:520, 1958.

Riskaer, N.: The course of otitic facial palsy under adequate treatment of the disease of the ear. Acta Otolaryngol. (Stockh.), *34*:280, 1946.

Rosenthal, C.: Klinisch-erbbiologischer Beitrag zur Konstitutionspathologie: Gemeinsames Auftreten von (rezidivierender familiärer) Facialislähmung, angioneurotischem Gesichtsödem und Lingua plicata in Arthritismus-Familien. Z. Neurol. Psychiatr., *131*: 475, 1930–1931.

Rossolimo, G. J.: Recidivirende Facialislähmung dei Migräne. Neurol. Zentralbl., *20*:744, 1901.

Ruskell, G. L.: An ocular parasympathetic nerve pathway of facial nerve origin and its influence on intraocular pressure. Exp. Eye Res., *10*:319, 1970.

Ruskell, G. L.: Facial parasympathetic innervation of the choroidal blood-vessels in monkeys. Exp. Eye Res., *12*:166, 1971.

Sadé, J.: Pathology of Bell's palsy. Arch. Otolaryngol., *95*:406, 1972.

Sadé, J., Levy, E., and Chaco, J.: Surgery and pathology of Bell's palsy. Arch. Otolaryngol., *82*:594, 1965.

Saito, H. S., Ruby, R. R. F., and Schuknecht, H. F.: Course of the sensory component of the nervus intermedius in the temporal bone. Ann. Otol. Rhinol. Laryngol., *79*:960, 1970.

Schirmer, O.: Studien zur Physiologie und Pathologie der Tränenabsonderung und Tränenabfuhr. Albrecht von Graefes Arch. Ophthalmol., *56*:197, 1903.

Schnell, R. G., Dyck, P. J., Bowie, E. J. W., Klass, D. W., and Taswell, H. F.: Infectious mononucleosis: neurologic and EEG findings. Medicine (Baltimore), *45*:51, 1966.

Seddon, H. J.: Three types of nerve injury. Brain, *66*: 237, 1943.

Sherrington, C. S.: On the anatomical constitution of

nerves of skeletal muscles: with remarks on recurrent fibres in the ventral spinal nerve-root. J. Physiol. (Lond.), *17*:211, 1894–1895.

Sluder, G.: Nasal Neurology: Headaches and Eye Disorders. St. Louis, C. V. Mosby Co., 1927, p. 93.

Smyth, G. E.: The systemization and central connections of the spinal tract and nucleus of the trigeminal nerve: a clinical and pathological study. Brain, *62*:41, 1939.

Sogg, R. L., Hoyt, W. F., and Boldrey, E.: Spastic paretic facial contracture: a rare sign of brain stem tumor. Neurology (Minneap.), *13*:607, 1963.

Spiller, W. G.: Contracture occurring in partial recovery from paralysis of the facial nerve and other nerves. Arch. Neurol. Psychiatry, *1*:564, 1919.

Sprofkin, B. E., and Hillman, J. W.: Moebius's syndrome — congenital oculofacial paralysis. Neurology (Minneap.), *6*:50, 1956.

Sullivan, J. A., and Smith, J. B.: The otological concept of Bell's palsy and its treatment. Ann. Otol. Rhinol. Laryngol., *59*:1148, 1950.

Sunderland, S.: The effect of rupture of the perineurium on the contained nerve-fibres. Brain, *69*:149, 1946.

Sunderland, S., and Cossar, D. F.: The structure of the facial nerve. Anat. Rec., *116*:147, 1953.

Szentágothai, J.: The representation of facial and scalp muscles in the facial nucleus. J. Comp. Neurol., *88*:207, 1948.

Taverner, D.: Cortisone treatment of Bell's palsy. Lancet, *2*:1052, 1954.

Taverner, D.: Bell's palsy: a clinical and electromyographic study. Brain, *78*:209, 1955.

Taverner, D.: The prognosis and treatment of spontaneous facial palsy. Proc. R. Soc. Med., *52*:1077, 1959.

Taverner, D.: The management of facial palsy. J. Laryngol., *82*:585, 1968.

Taverner, D., Cohen, S. B., and Hutchinson, B. C.: Comparison of corticotrophin and prednisolone in treatment of idiopathic facial paralysis (Bell's palsy). Br. Med. J., *4*:20, 1971.

Taverner, D., Fearnley, M. E., Kemble, F., Miles, D. W., and Peiris, O. A.: Prevention of denervation in Bell's palsy. Br. Med. J., *1*:391, 1966.

Tomita, H., Hayakawa, W., and Hondo, R.: Varicella-zoster virus in idiopathic facial palsy. Arch. Otolaryngol., *95*:364, 1972a.

Tomita, H., Okuda, Y., Tomiyama, H., and Kida, A.: Electrogustometry in facial palsy. Arch. Otolaryngol., *95*:383, 1972b.

Tschiassny, K.: Eight syndromes of facial paralysis and their significance in locating the lesion. Ann. Otol. Rhinol. Laryngol., *62*:677, 1953.

Tschiassny, K.: Topognosis of lesions of the facial nerve. J. Int. Coll. Surg., *23*:381, 1955.

Turner, J. W.: Facial palsy in closed head injuries: the prognosis. Lancet, *1*:756, 1944.

Vail, H. H.: Vidian neuralgia. Ann. Otol. Rhinol. Laryngol., *41*:837, 1932.

Van Buskirk, C.: The seventh nerve complex. J. Comp. Neurol., *82*:303, 1945.

Van Droogenbroeck, J. B. A.: The surgical treatment of lower facial palsy in leprosy. Ann. Soc. Belg. Med. Trop., *50*:653, 1970.

Vassallo, L., and Galea-Debono, A.: Aetiology of Bell's palsy (letter to the editor). Lancet, *2*:383, 1972.

Vidić, B., and Woźniak, W.: The communicating branch of the facial nerve to the lesser petrosal nerve in human fetuses and newborns. Arch. Anat. Histol. Embryol. (Strasb.), *52*:369, 1969.

Wallis, P. G.: Creatinuria in Möbius syndrome. Arch. Dis. Child., *35*:393, 1960.

Wartenberg, R.: Associated movements in the oculomotor and facial muscles. Arch. Neurol., *55*:439, 1946.

Wigand, M. E., Spreng, M., Bumm, P., and Mederer, R.: Electronic evaluation of electromyograms in facial nerve paralysis. Arch. Otolaryngol., *95*:324, 1972.

Williams, H. L., Lambert, E. H., and Woltman, H. W.: The problem of synkinesis and contracture in cases of hemifacial spasm and Bell's palsy. Ann. Otol. Rhinol. Laryngol., *61*:850, 1952.

Wilson, H. L.: Facial paralysis in the uveoparotid fever of Boeck's sarcoid. Ann. Otol. Rhinol. Laryngol., *66*:164, 1957.

Wolf, G.: Die infektiöse Mononukleose und das Nervensystem. Fortschr. Neurol. Psychiatr., *24*:167, 1956.

Woltman, H. W., Williams, H. L., and Lambert, E. H.: An attempt to relieve hemifacial spasm by neurolysis of the facial nerves: a report of two cases of hemifacial spasm with reflections on the nature of the spasm, the contracture and mass movement. Proc. Staff Meet. Mayo Clin., *26*:236, 1951.

Wright, J. W., Jr., and Taylor, C. E.: Facial nerve abnormalities revealed by polytomography. Arch. Otolaryngol., *95*:426, 1972.

Yanagihara, N., and Kishimoto, M.: Nerve conduction study in facial palsy. Arch. Klin. Exp. Ohren Nasen Kehlkopfheilkd., *198*:339, 1971.

Yanagihara, N., and Kishimoto, M.: Electrodiagnosis in facial palsy. Arch. Otolaryngol., *95*:376, 1972.

Yates, A. L.: The anatomy of the middle ear. J. Laryngol. Otol., *51*:476, 1936.

Zilstorff-Pedersen, K.: Quantitative measurements of the naso-lacrimal reflex. Acta Otolaryngol. (Stockh.), *50*:501, 1959.

Zilstorff-Pedersen, K.: Quantitative measurements of the nasolacrimal reflex: in the normal and in peripheral facial paralysis. Arch. Otolaryngol., *81*:457, 1965.

Zülch, K. J.: "Idiopathic" facial paresis. *In* Vinken, P. J., and Bruyn, G. W. (eds.): Handbook of Clinical Neurology. Vol. 8. New York, American Elsevier Publishing Co., Inc., 1970, pp. 241–302.

Chapter 28

DISEASES OF THE EIGHTH CRANIAL NERVE

Ellis Douek

This cranial nerve is distinguished by its dual nature. It consists of two separate divisions that carry the impulses set up by the two entirely different sensory stimuli of hearing and balance. This functional distinctness does not apply to its pathology or to the symptomatology of the diseases that disturb it. It is, indeed, common for the senses of balance and hearing to be affected together because of the proximity to each other not only of the nerve fibers but also of the sense organs and of the nuclei in the brain stem. The complex nature of this nerve, the possibilities for study that its sensory qualities offer, and the evidence for the diagnosis of intracranial lesions that they provide have made it the sole object of interest of an active specialty.

COURSE AND NUCLEI OF THE NERVE

The fibers of the vestibular division arise from the large bipolar cells of the vestibular or Scarpa's ganglion, which lies at the distal end of the internal auditory canal. Two types of fiber are recognized. Type I fibers are ultimately associated with a chalice-shaped plexus around the receptor hair cells of the organ of equilibrium. These lie in the ampullary cristae of the semicircular canals as well as in the maculae of the saccule and utricle. Type II fibers are less well understood, do not end in the same manner, and probably serve an efferent function. In the internal auditory canal, the vestibular division lies above the cochlear division and gradually becomes more medial. The facial nerve is anterosuperior to the eighth nerve in this canal.

The vestibular fibers enter the brain posterior to the facial nerve in the groove between pons and medulla and mostly end in the vestibular nuclei. These number four on each side and are clustered in the pons and medulla just beneath the floor of the fourth ventricle. The lateral nucleus receives fibers principally from the macula of the utricle, and for the most part its efferents form the vestibulospinal tract. Fibers from the canal cristae end mainly in the medial and inferior nuclei, while the saccular fibers reach the inferior nucleus. Other efferent fibers form the medial longitudinal bundle and establish connections with the nuclei of the third, fourth, and sixth cranial nerves, while others reach the cerebellum, the reticular substance, and higher levels. Descending fibers from reticular centers also influence the vestibular nuclei.

The cochlear division of the eighth nerve also consists of two types of fiber. The vast majority are associated with the hair cells of the auditory receptor organ and originate in the bipolar cells of the spiral ganglion. They tend to be smaller than the vestibular ganglion cells and are placed along a bony canal that winds its way down the length of the cochlea. Fibers of the second types are very few in number and represent efferents arising from the superior olivary nucleus. They reach the cochlear nerve by an unexpected anastomotic connection from the vestibular nerve. The cochlear division accompanies the vestibular, entering the brain stem just posterior to the lower border of the pons and close to the inferior cerebellar peduncle, lying lateral and inferior to the vestibular division.

The cochlear nerve divides into two groups of fibers as soon as it enters the brain stem, and these end in two nuclei, the ventral and dorsal cochlear nuclei, which lie in close relationship to the inferior cerebellar peduncle. The second neuron fibers take a complex pathway to the higher auditory centers.

DIAGNOSTIC TECHNIQUES

Before discussing in more detail the diseases that affect the eighth nerve, certain points concerning the assessment of eighth nerve function are to be considered.

In the first place, these diseases produce two separate sets of symptoms. Damage to the cochlear portion produces a disturbance of hearing. This may be deafness, distortion, or tinnitus. Damage to the vestibular portion causes loss of equilibrium of varying degree, described either as attacks of giddiness or as a sense of unsteadiness.

Second, these same symptoms can be caused by lesions at any level along the auditory or vestibular pathways. If the lesion is in the receptor organ, it is likely to be benign in nature. A lesion of the eighth nerve itself may well be due to a tumor in the cerebellopontine angle and require surgical treatment, whereas a lesion of the nuclei in the brain stem is often associated with a disorder carrying a worse prognosis. Clearly it is essential to be able to distinguish one from the other, and techniques that allow us to do so form the basis of neurootology.

Assessment of the Auditory Pathway

In the recent past there was little pathologic verification of clinical assessment by otologists, and clinical impression remained generally unconfirmed. The few cases in which the diagnosis was fairly certain that reached the otologist became the models for descriptions of symptomatology. In this way, Ménière's disease became the prototype of end organ lesions and contributed to the belief that sudden loss of hearing was caused by disease at that level, whereas cerebellopontine angle tumors suggested that nerve lesions were slow and progressive. Over the past few years a series of subjective and objective tests have been devised to establish the site of a lesion of the auditory pathway. Their importance is now such that, taken together, they are probably more valuable than clinical history, and the main area of controversy regards the contribution that each test can make relative to the others.

PURE TONE AUDIOMETRY

The pure tone audiogram is the simplest and most commonly used quantitative test of hearing. It is essential as the first step in the investigation of any hearing problem and will give the degree of deafness and demonstrate which frequencies of the auditory spectrum are most affected. Patients who suffer from a disease of the auditory nerve have a neurosensory or perceptive type of hearing loss, so the first step must be to exclude those who have a conductive hearing loss. Further help in distinguishing nerve deafness from that caused by a cochlear or brain stem lesion is difficult to obtain from the pure tone audiogram. Hereditary cochlear deafness may be demonstrated by testing the relatives; the hearing in Ménière's disease often fluctuates and the noise-induced type of cochlear deafness shows a particular drop in hearing for those frequencies at around 4 kHz. A bilaterally symmetrical perceptive hearing loss may suggest a brain stem rather than a nerve or cochlear lesion, particularly if other symptoms such as giddiness are present.

SPEECH AUDIOMETRY

The aim of speech audiometry is to test the patient's ability to discriminate words. The most common method is to use monosyllabic words produced at increasing intensity and to plot the percentage of those recognized against the loudness. Language reception is such a complex problem, however, that new tests, aimed at studying different aspects of the problem, are constantly being added.

Although speech audiometry is often tedious, important information can be obtained. Thus in lesions of the eighth nerve, the word discrimination scores may be very poor compared with the pure tone audiogram, and a combination of these two tests is then of considerable significance. In cochlear lesions, on the contrary, there is a better correlation between the degree of deafness and word discrimination, but often the distortion is increased with increasing loudness.

LOUDNESS BALANCE TESTS

An increasingly intense sound signal is perceived by the ear as increasing in loudness. Some ears, generally those affected by a sensorineural hearing loss, perceive a more rapid increase in loudness than would normally be expected. They are said, therefore, to exhibit recruitment. This phenomenon can be demonstrated and measured in a number of ways, the most popular being the alternate binaural loudness balance test (Fig. 28–1) (Fowler, 1936). Tests for recruitment are probably the most reliable for the diagnosis of eighth nerve lesions, as these disorders are not associated with recruitment. Cochlear lesions have long been known to show recruitment, and recently Dix and Hood (1973) have demonstrated that it also occurs in brain stem lesions. As loudness balance requires one good ear for comparison it is difficult to use the test when damage is bilateral. The loudness discomfort level can be used instead, although it is a sensitivity index and may not exactly represent the same phenomenon.

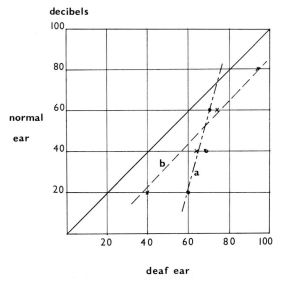

Figure 28–1 Loudness balance test. The loudness perceived in the deaf ear is compared with that in the normal and shows recruitment in (a) and an absence of recruitment in (b).

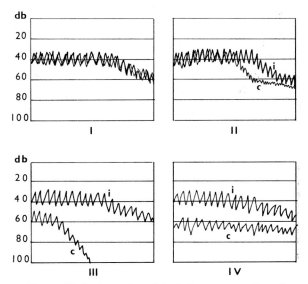

Figure 28–2 Jerger's original four types of audiometric tracing. Type I, presbyacusis; type II, end organ lesion; types III and IV, neuronal lesions. A fifth type in which the continuous tone gives a lower threshold occurs in functional deafness. i, Interrupted tone (pulsed); c, continuous tone.

TONE DECAY

This is the decrease in threshold sensitivity that results from stimulation with a barely audible sound. It has also been termed "fatigue" and "per-stimulatory adaptation," although these terms are not synonymous (Hood, 1956). Abnormal threshold tone decay occurs commonly in lesions of the auditory nerve, even when there is only slight hearing loss, and it is therefore an important test of retrocochlear disease.

SISI TESTS AND BÉKÉSY AUDIOMETRY

Other tests are also in use. The short increment sensitivity index (SISI) is widely used to exclude cochlear lesions, and a whole system of automatic measurement of continuous and interrupted signals known as Békésy audiometry after its originator is now of recognized value. The patient is asked to try to maintain a tone at threshold level by pressing a loudness control button himself. The tone is continuous and varies in frequency; the loudness level produced by the patient is then given as a tracing. This has the appearance of a series of peaks representing the patient's subjective recognition of what he can hear. Jerger (1960) divided these tracings into five types.

Types III and IV strongly suggest a lesion of the eighth nerve (Fig. 28–2).

EVOKED AUDITORY RESPONSES

For the past decade, averaging computers have been employed to record the electroencephalographic potentials evoked by auditory stimuli. These techniques have been used mainly as means of objective audiometry, but Shimizu (1968) demonstrated that in eighth nerve lesions there was a longer latency than normal or than in cochlear lesions. Auditory stimuli produce electrical changes in muscles throughout the body (Bickford et al., 1963). Kiang and co-workers (1963) described the muscle response from the postaural region, which is generally believed to be of purely cochlear origin. No clinical use for this response was found until recently when some important features were observed (Douek et al., 1973). The fact that this postaural myogenic electrical response to auditory stimuli was bilateral and consensual suggested that it may be altered by lesions within the brain stem (Figs. 28–3 and 28–4). This was found to be true in a number of proved cases, and the name of "crossed acoustic response" was given to emphasize its clinically important features. The crossed acoustic response, then, can separate cases in which auditory symptoms are due to interruption of the pathways within the brain stem from those in which they are due to lesions outside. The full evaluation of the different types of abnormalities still remains to come.

ELECTROCOCHLEOGRAPHY

This technique, recently applied clinically by Portmann and Aran (1971), measures the electrical potentials induced by sound stimuli in the auditory nerve. A transtympanic electrode is necessary in order to do this, but lesions of the eighth nerve can be demonstrated by the response pattern obtained.

The approach that these complex tests provide has been described as a "battery" system of diagnosis. There are few situations in which investigations are more important in diagnosis than those aimed at demonstrating auditory nerve lesions.

Assessment of the Vestibular Pathway

The preceding section has demonstrated the high degree of precision now possible in assessing the different aspects of auditory nerve function. The same cannot be said of the vestibular nerve. Nevertheless, tests of vestibular function are of considerable help in localization and exclusion.

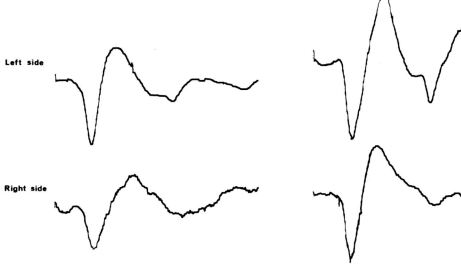
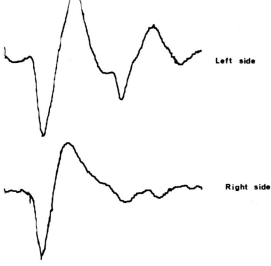

Figure 28–3 Normal crossed acoustic response (70 db, 4 kHz, 100 msec scan).

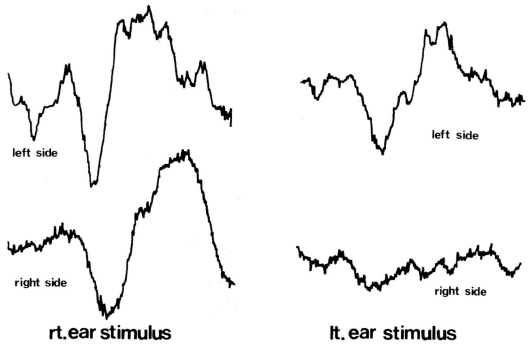

left side

right side

rt. ear stimulus

left side

right side

lt. ear stimulus

Figure 28–4   Abnormal crossover in a case of multiple sclerosis.

Observation of spontaneous nystagmus in different situations is of prime importance; it should be understood, however, that when the balance between the right and left vestibular potentials is disrupted, eye movements that produce nystagmus are initiated, but the neuromuscular processes leading to the ocular deviation are the same whatever the initial cause.

ELECTRONYSTAGMOGRAPHY

This has been in use for some years but its value remains controversial. Its main contribution is probably that it allows us to observe nystagmus with the eyes shut or in the dark and to compare it with that present with the eyes open. In this way, a lesion of the peripheral neuron can be distinguished from a nuclear or a more central lesion because the nystagmus tends to be enhanced when optic fixation is abolished by darkness.

Spontaneous nystagmus, even that induced by gaze or positioning, may not be present, and yet a hidden imbalance remains. It is to demonstrate this that tests involving induced nystagmus have been devised.

CALORIC TESTING

The caloric test is the most commonly used procedure. The head is raised to an angle of 30 degrees from the horizontal so that the lateral semicircular canal lies in a vertical plane. The stimulus consists of temperature alterations, which are obtained by irrigating the external auditory canal with water. In the bithermal test of Fitzgerald and Hallpike (1942), the temperatures used are 30° C and 44° C. Irrigation is maintained for 40 seconds, and the length of time the nystagmus persists is recorded. The most common abnormality in lesions of the vestibular nerve is a reduction or an absence of response (Fig. 28–5). Indeed, it would be difficult to make a diagnosis of a lesion of this type if there were no alteration of the caloric response.

OPTOKINETIC STIMULATION

This also induces nystagmus that is very similar to that produced by a vestibular stimulus. Although it is, of course, not identical in development, it will summate with the imbalance produced by a vestibular nerve lesion and show a directional preponderance.

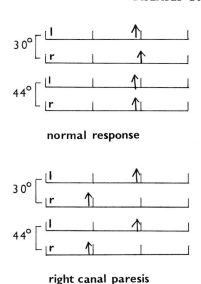

normal response

right canal paresis

Figure 28–5 Caloric test.

ROTATIONAL TESTS

Rotation can also induce nystagmus, but this is a cumbersome procedure and provides little help in the diagnosis of eighth nerve lesions.

If these tests of vestibular function are compared with those of auditory function, it is clear that although they can demonstrate a lesion of the peripheral neuron of the vestibular nerve, there is no way of separating a lesion of the nerve from that of the end organ. If all the tests of auditory and vestibular function are taken together, however, it is usually possible to reach a relatively accurate localization of the site of an eighth nerve lesion.

DISEASES OF THE EIGHTH NERVE

Because of the only relatively recent development of localizing techniques and because of lack of histologic material, it has rarely been possible to separate neural deafness from that due to damage of the sensory epithelium. Although this is now gradually being remedied, the term "neurosensory deafness" has to remain in general use. The following lesions have been described as affecting the eighth nerve, but a critical viewpoint should be taken unless undoubted evidence is offered.

Congenital and Hereditary Lesions

There are many types of inherited deafness, some of which form part of complex syndromes, and theoretically, abnormalities of the eighth nerve may occur in some. It should be emphasized, however, that in the expanding number of cases in which histologic examination is available, gross abnormalities of the end organ are usually found.

A totally different situation exists in hemolytic disease of the newborn, in which degeneration of the cochlear nuclei has been shown (Gerrard, 1952) as well as of the proximal auditory pathways (Dublin, 1951), but without damage to the cochlea. A similar state exists in the anoxia produced by birth trauma in which neuronal damage occurs around specific foci.

It is likely that with the new techniques of electrocochleography and the crossed acoustic response, it will quite soon be possible to distinguish beyond doubt those patients whose lesions are neuronal and who have an adequate cochlea. The importance of this possibility is already apparent, because the only techniques available at present for teaching such children to speak require amplification. This in its turn may well damage the cochlea and so increase the deafness.

The manifestations of the hereditary condition that Refsum described as "heredopathia atactica polyneuritiformis" include deafness (see Chapter 42). Since one of the principal features of the disorder is a hypertrophic neuropathy, it might be anticipated that the same changes would be present in the eighth nerve and be responsible for the deafness. Hallpike (1967) described one instance of a man whose case appears to be typical, although not confirmed biochemically. The clinical findings were severe and widespread peripheral neuropathy with visual impairment and the onset of sudden deafness some years before his death. Histologic examination showed gross diffuse thickening of the spinal nerves involving both the anterior and the posterior roots. Inspection of the auditory system, however, showed that the damage was virtually confined to the cochlea and saccule and included degeneration of their sense organ. Hallpike suggested that these changes could be explained by gene action alone, but as deafness occurred suddenly and late in the course of the disease, this is difficult to accept.

Hallpike (1967) also reported on the otologic findings in a case of hereditary sensory neuropathy with associated deafness and absence of caloric responses. Surprisingly, the cochlear nerve and spiral ganglion were found to be normal except for some cell loss in the basal part of the ganglion. The organ of Corti showed degenerative changes with severe involvement of the limbus cells. There were, however, considerable cell loss in the vestibular ganglion and fiber depletion in the vestibular nerve.

Trauma

Trauma to the eighth cranial nerve can occur during head injury. Deafness and vestibular dysfunction are not uncommon following an injury that involves loss of consciousness, and occasionally they result from even minor blows. In most cases, however, it is an injury to the cochlea and labyrinth that is responsible for loss of function, and it is only in extensive fractures of the petrosal bone that the nerve is directly injured.

The weakest part of the temporal bone is at the junction of the petrous and squamous portions, and only rarely is the fracture line directed longitudinally along the petrosal bone toward the internal auditory meatus. Usually in such a case, the fracture involves the anteromedial part of the cochlea and also disrupts the middle ear. Often it extends outward so that bleeding from the ear is present, and occasionally cerebrospinal fluid otorrhea occurs. In fractures of this type, tearing of the eighth nerve will cause deafness, vertigo, and usually an accompanying facial palsy. The deafness and vertigo are severe, and the chances of recovery of function are almost nonexistent.

Management is not surgical unless an attempt has to be made to restore continuity of the facial nerve or of the ossicular chain. If there is bleeding from the ear, no attempt should be made to clean the external auditory canal; antibiotics must be given. Cerebrospinal fluid otorrhea usually ceases within one to two weeks, but should it not do so, neurosurgical intervention is necessary. Recently attempts have been made to approach a damaged nerve through the middle cranial fossa in order to decompress it and even to provide a blood supply by inserting a muscle flap. There is no evidence that any of these attempts have been successful, and although the theoretical possibility remains that a crushed nerve could be freed in this way, there is still no known indication for such an operation.

Infections

Virus infections are often held responsible for perceptive deafness and vertigo that are of sudden onset. The vertigo invariably subsides, although this is often simply due to compensation, as caloric tests frequently continue to show canal paresis. The deafness classically covers all the frequencies with some predilection for the higher tones. As the deafness is often total, audiology cannot distinguish between a cochlear and a neural origin. In the cases in which some hearing has been retained, either type is possible. The vast majority are unilateral. It should be stressed here that no valid figures are available because few cases are properly investigated or reported; those patients seen in sophisticated centers are a very select group, and the label "viral" is usually the result of circumstantial evidence based on varying criteria. Enough cases of usually unilateral perceptive deafness have occurred during the course of a mumps illness to justify making the association, but in many children with unilateral deafness of unknown etiology, it has been wrongly labeled on the grounds that they have had mumps in the past. The same applies to deafness and vertigo that follow febrile illness due to other respiratory viruses or enteroviruses. Post-infective encephalitis occurs, in rare instances, after varicella, measles, pertussis, influenza, and infectious mononucleosis. Deafness and vertigo also occur, in rare instances, among other neurologic manifestations. It was during the Second World War that the association between deafness and typhus became well known. Daggett (1946) pointed out that it was one of the earliest signs but that complete recovery was to be expected. The eighth nerve is affected together with the seventh in otitic herpes, producing both deafness and vertigo.

Two types of association with bacterial infections were described in the past. In the first instance, the concept of "focal sepsis" was widespread. No evidence that bears scrutiny was ever produced, and with the advent of the antibiotic era, cases in which eighth nerve function was believed to have been damaged by toxins produced in distant bacterial foci have gradually ceased to be reported. On the other hand, eighth nerve dysfunction frequently occurs with bacterial meningitis. Before the development of antibiotics, 20 per cent of cases of acquired deafness in small children were due to meningitis (Shambaugh, 1930). Although less common today, hearing loss still occurs from meningococcal, pneumococcal, streptococcal, and *Hemophilus influenzae* meningitis, mainly in small children and neonates (Buch, 1967). One etiologic problem is that these children have often been treated with large doses of ototoxic antibiotics that may damage the cochlea. It is therefore difficult to know whether the major part of the deafness is of cochlear origin or due to the perineural inflammation resulting from the meningitis, which may extend into the nerve substance or give rise to vascular changes. The prognosis regarding recovery of hearing is poor, and in this type of case, the loss is often bilateral. Although there may also be vestibular dysfunction, the compensatory mechanisms are such that no symptoms or signs are apparent as soon as the initial vertigo has subsided. Tuberculous meningeal infections infiltrate the eighth nerve sheath, but following treatment with streptomycin, it is not possible exactly to apportion the blame for the severe sensorineural hearing loss that results.

Deafness due to syphilis is now uncommon. It is rare to find children with its congenital form in schools for the deaf in England, whereas before World War II their numbers could reach the level of 23 per cent (Rodger, 1940). The disease can affect the hearing and vestibular mechanism anywhere from the middle ear to the brain stem. Basilar meningitis is often present in the early congenital form and in the secondary and tertiary stages of the acquired type. This is associated with damage to the nerve trunk and labyrinthitis leading to atrophy of the neuroepithelial elements.

There is usually a sudden onset of sensorineural deafness that is fluctuating and quickly becomes bilateral. Vestibular symptoms, though present initially, quickly disappear, but in the later stages when both labyrinths and vestibular nerves have lost their function, these patients may have considerable difficulty keeping their balance in the dark. Treatment may arrest the progression of the deafness if it is still fluctuating. Large doses of ampicillin or penicillin, together with corticosteroids, have been found useful in a number of cases (Kerr et al., 1973).

Toxic Agents and Metabolic Disorders

It has been known for many years that drugs may cause sensorineural hearing loss as well as disturbance of vestibular function. Gradually the list has lengthened from quinine, the salicylates, and certain antibiotics such as streptomycin and kanamycin to include the diuretic agents ethacrynic acid and furosemide, and the antiheparin agent hexadimethrine bromide. As interest has grown in this important subject as well as in the effects of chemical agents in general, experimental work has shown that the histopathologic changes are mainly to be found in the end organ. Although some changes also occur in the ganglion cells and nerve fibers as well as in the central nuclei, it is probably more justifiable to consider toxic effects such as deafness and vertigo as resulting from an attack directed mainly against the end organ unless other neuropathies are also present.

Tobacco has often been incriminated as a cause of neural deafness, but little supporting evidence is available. A high rate of alcohol intake is frequently associated, but its effects may be due to vitamin deficiency. Although most vitamins have been prescribed at one time or another for deafness, it is only in deficiencies of the B group of vitamins such as in beri-beri and pellagra that this type of treatment has been successful. Recognition of these effects came during the Second World War when Denny-Brown (1947) found that among those prisoners of war who had neurologic disturbances, 10 per cent were deaf. Demyelination of the cochlear nerve was present as well as end organ changes.

Hypothyroidism can affect the hearing in three different ways. In children with endemic cretinism or with Pendred's syndrome (nonendemic goiter) the cochlea is affected, but when hypothyroidism occurs in adults, neuronal changes are present and audiometric tests tend to show retrocochlear deafness. This type of hearing loss responds well if treatment is not delayed too long. Deafness may also occur in diabetes. Eighth nerve involvement in this disorder is discussed in Chapter 47.

Vascular Changes

Ischemia is often blamed for vertigo and occasionally for deafness. This is usually related to brain stem vascular disease, but some cases of isolated unilateral deafness and vertigo of sudden onset have been ascribed to a vascular lesion affecting the eighth nerve.

Diseases of Unknown Etiology

Recurrent cranial nerve palsies may occur in sarcoidosis, often before other manifestations of the disease. The most commonly affected nerve is the facial, but the eighth is not infrequently involved. The deafness that results is bilateral and not very severe, with a likelihood of complete recovery.

As temporary deafness is associated with bilateral uveitis in both, sarcoidosis must be differentiated from the rare Vogt-Koyanagi syndrome. In this syndrome patchy alopecia, as well as whitening of the eyelashes and vitiligo, appears later.

Vestibular Neuronitis

This condition has to be given a special place, as it is probably the commonest diagnosis made in patients who suffer from vertigo. There is considerable doubt, however, regarding both its etiology and its existence as an entity.

The first cases were probably those reported by Nylen in 1924, but it was Hallpike who described the syndrome in 1949 and then, with Dix, studied 100 cases (Dix and Hallpike, 1952). The clinical picture is one of acute vertigo usually following a mild pyrexial illness. This invariably recovers, but the patient may be left with a residual canal paresis revealed by caloric testing. There is no sign of other neurologic disturbance or of cochlear abnormalities. It is obvious that these symptoms could be indicative of a number of different conditions, but basing their views on testing with galvanic stimuli, Dix and Hallpike believed that the lesion was central to the labyrinth. Histologic material has been very scant, and although there appear to be neuronal changes (Lindsay and Hemenway, 1956), neuroepithelial changes have also been observed (Morgenstein and Hong, 1971). A further difficulty in the interpretation of the latter findings is that there had been long-standing deafness before the vestibular illness occurred.

Compression of the Eighth Nerve

Tumors in the cerebellopontine angle usually produce slowly progressive symptoms and signs. Deafness may be so slow in its development that it may be very severe before it is noticed. Occasionally it is more sudden and accompanied by tinnitus. Audiometric tests suggest retrocochlear deafness and relatively poor speech discrimination. The electrocochleogram shows a characteristic response. True vertigo is rare, but in the vast majority of cases, the patient complains of a vague imbalance. Response to caloric tests is often absent, but this is not necessarily the case in lesions other than acoustic neurinoma. Although there may not be any other manifestations initially, nystagmus may be present, especially when there is compression of the cerebellum or brain stem, and positional nystagmus is common. Eventually other neurologic features appear; usually there is trigeminal sensory involvement and later facial weakness. Signs of cerebellar involvement appear and intracranial pressure may be raised.

Acoustic neurinoma is described in Chapter 66. Neurinomas of the eighth nerve are less common. Progressive facial palsy is the first sign, but deafness may occur. Occasionally a tumor of the ninth nerve may produce confusing symptoms (see Chapter 29). Posterior fossa meningiomas may produce similar symptoms, as may arachnoid cysts. Congenital or primary cholesteatomas may also present in this way, although with them facial weakness is usually an early sign.

Compression of the eighth nerve fibers within the temporal bone occurs in Paget's disease, and this is worsened by the conductive deafness that results from ossicular fixation.

REFERENCES

Bickford, R. G., Jacobson, J. L., and Galbraith, R. F.: A new audiomotor system in man. Electroencephalogr. Clin. Neurophysiol., *15*:922, 1963.

Buch, N.: Hearing loss in meningitis. Antibiotic News, *3*:2, 1967.

Daggett, W. I.: Discussion on war deafness and the care

of deafened ex-servicemen. J. Laryngol. Otol., *61*: 508, 1946.

Denny-Brown, D.: Neurological conditions resulting from prolonged and severe dietary restrictions. Medicine (Baltimore), *26*:41, 1947.

Dix, M. R., and Hallpike, C. S.: The pathology, symptomatology and diagnosis of certain common disorders of the vestibular system. Ann. Otol. Rhinol. Laryngol., *61*:987, 1952.

Dix, M. R., and Hood, J. D.: Personal communication, 1973.

Douek, E., Gibson, W., and Humphries, K.: The crossed acoustic response. J. Laryngol. Otol., *87*:711, 1973.

Dublin, W. B.: Neurologic lesions of erythroblastosis fetalis in relation to nuclear deafness. Am. J. Clin. Pathol., *21*:935, 1951.

Fitzgerald, G., and Hallpike, C. S.: Studies in human vestibular function. Brain, *65*:115, 1942.

Fowler, E. P.: A method for the early detection of otosclerosis. Arch. Otolaryngol., *24*:731, 1936.

Gerrard, J.: Kernicterus. Brain, 75:526, 1952.

Hallpike, C. S.: The pathology and differential diagnosis of aural vertigo. *In* Proceedings: Fourth International Congress of Otolaryngology, London, 1949. Vol. 2. London, British Medical Association, 1951, p. 514.

Hallpike, C. S.: Observations on the structural basis of two rare varieties of hereditary deafness. *In* de Reuck, A. V. S., and Knight, J. (eds.): Ciba Foundation Symposium on Myotatic, Kinesthetic and Vestibular Mechanisms. London, J. & A. Churchill Ltd., 1967, p. 285.

Hood, J. D.: Fatigue and adaptation of hearing. Br. Med. Bull., *12*:125, 1956.

Jerger, J.: Responses to continuous and interrupted stimuli in automatic audiometry. J. Speech Hear. Res., *3*:275, 1960.

Kerr, A. G., Smyth, G. D. L., and Cinnamond, M. J.: Congenital syphilitic deafness. J. Laryngol. Otol., *87*:1, 1973.

Kiang, N. Y-S., Crist, A. M., French, M. A., and Edwards, A. G.: Postauricular electrical response to acoustic stimuli in humans. Research Laboratory of Electronics, Massachusetts Institute of Technology, Quarterly Progress Report, *68*:218, 1963.

Lindsay, J. R., and Hemenway, W. G.: Postural vertigo due to unilateral sudden loss of vestibular function. Ann. Otol. Rhinol. Laryngol., *65*:692, 1956.

Morgenstein, K. M., and Hong, I. S.: Vestibular neuronitis. Laryngoscope, *81*:131, 1971.

Nylen, C. O.: Some cases of ocular nystagmus due to certain positions of the head. Acta Otolaryngol., *6*:106, 1924.

Portmann, M., and Aran, J. M.: Electrocochleography. Laryngoscope, *8*:899, 1971.

Rodger, T. R.: Syphilis as seen by the aural surgeon. J. Laryngol. Otol., *55*:168, 1940.

Schimizu, H.: Evoked responses in VIII nerve lesions. Trans. Am. Acad. Ophthalmol. Otolaryngol., *72*:596, 1968.

Shambaugh, G. E.: Statistical studies of the children in public schools for the deaf. Arch. Otolaryngol., *12*:190, 1930.

Chapter 29

DISEASES OF THE NINTH, TENTH, ELEVENTH, AND TWELFTH CRANIAL NERVES

J. Newsom Davis, P. K. Thomas, J. M. K. Spalding,
and M. Spencer Harrison

THE GLOSSOPHARYNGEAL NERVE

Anatomy

The nerve has five or six slender fila or rootlets as it emerges from the medulla oblongata in a sulcus at the dorsal border of the inferior olive. After the fila have united, the nerve is separated from the tenth nerve by a dural isthmus as it passes through the jugular foramen. Its ganglia are the superior and petrous. In the upper neck, the nerve lies in front of the tenth nerve and passes between the internal carotid artery and internal jugular vein before passing superficially to the internal carotid artery behind the styloid process. Thereafter it follows the posteroinferior part of the stylopharyngeus muscle, traveling across the lateral surface of this muscle and between the constrictors of the pharynx. Finally, before it divides, its course lies deep to the hyoglossus muscle. The nerve contains motor, parasympathetic, and sensory fibers.

Motor Fibers. Motor fibers innervate the stylopharyngeus muscle, which has some part in the elevation of the pharynx. Their cells of origin form part of the nucleus ambiguus; studies in the cat show that these neurons form a compact mass of cells lying level with, but ventrolateral to, the rostral tip of the main column of the nucleus (Lawn, 1966). Occasionally, the superior constrictor of the

pharynx is supplied by this nerve rather than by the vagus.

Parasympathetic Fibers. The parasympathetic fibers mediate secretion of the parotid gland and have their cells of origin in the inferior salivary nucleus. They leave the main body of the nerve as the tympanic nerve, passing through the tympanic plexus and reaching the otic ganglion as the lesser superficial petrosal nerve. Here the fibers synapse with the postganglionic fibers to the parotid gland. Occasionally, however, the gland may be innervated by a nerve other than the glossopharyngeal (Davie and Bourke, 1967).

Sensory Fibers. Visceral afferent fibers convey general sensation from the posterior third of the tongue, fauces, tonsils, nasopharynx, inferior surface of the soft palate, uvula, eustachian tube, and tympanic cavity. In addition, the nerve innervates a small cutaneous area in front of the tragus together with a little of the adjacent anterior wall of the outer auditory meatus (Bues, 1963). Taste afferents in the glossopharyngeal nerve supply the posterior third of the tongue and taste buds in the pharynx. The cell bodies of these afferent fibers lie in the petrous ganglion. Studies in cat and monkey have shown that these fibers terminate in the nucleus of the tractus solitarius, mainly in its rostral part but with a considerable caudal extension and with a connection to the contralateral commissural nucleus (Kerr, 1962; Rhoton et al., 1966). The fibers terminating rostrally probably serve gustatory function, while those serving visceral function terminate more caudally.

Carotid Sinus Nerve. The carotid sinus nerve, another branch of the glossopharyngeal nerve, contains the primary afferent fibers of chemoreceptors in the carotid body and of baroreceptors lying in the carotid sinus wall. These fibers project to the middle third of the nucleus of the tractus solitarius (Cottle, 1964), but some also terminate on large neurons of the paramedial reticular formation of the medulla (Miura and Reis, 1969). Recent evidence suggests the presence of an efferent supply to the carotid body carried in the carotid sinus nerve (see Biscoe, 1971). The baroreceptors are concerned in the regulation of blood pressure; the chemoreceptors are responsible predominantly for the ventilatory response to hypoxia, but also to a lesser extent for the response to hypercapnia.

Clinical Features of Glossopharyngeal Nerve Lesions

It is extremely rare for this nerve to be affected in isolation, the vagus almost always being involved as well. The symptoms relating to the latter nerve usually dominate the clinical picture. The patient may be aware of difficulty in swallowing and of disturbance in taste. On examination, sensation is found to be impaired on the affected side over the soft palate, pharynx, fauces, and posterior third of the tongue, and the gag reflex to be reduced or absent. Taste is lost over the ipsilateral posterior third of the tongue. Salivary secretion from the parotid gland is usually reduced or absent, although in some cases it can be increased. Interference with the chemoreceptor fibers does not seem to cause symptoms. Acute section of the glossopharyngeal nerves bilaterally causes transient hypertension (Whisler and Voris, 1965). In glossopharyngeal neuralgia, pain is experienced behind the angle of the jaw, deep within the ear, and in the side of the throat, as is described later.

Tests of Function

The integrity of taste perception on the posterior third of the tongue is most readily tested by galvanic stimulation. The parasym-pathetic secretomotor function can be assessed by measuring the secretion from Stenson's duct over a five minute period after intravenous injection of pilocarpine. In healthy subjects, the secretion is equal on the two sides but the quantity varies from 3 to 15 ml. Asymmetrical amounts may indicate impairment of the secretory fibers. Chemoreceptor function can be examined by assessing the ventilatory response to mild hypoxia or to a few breaths of pure oxygen (Dejours, 1962). Baroreceptor function can be tested by observing the blood pressure changes in response to tilting.

Lesions Affecting the Glossopharyngeal Nerve

INTRAMEDULLARY LESIONS

Lesions affecting the nuclei of the glossopharyngeal nerve commonly also involve the tenth and eighth nerves and may cause vertigo, dysphagia, dysarthria, and contralateral hemiplegia as well as the features of ninth nerve dysfunction (Bonnier's syndrome). Causes include vascular, neoplastic, and inflammatory lesions, and rarely, syringobulbia.

EXTRAMEDULLARY LESIONS

The ninth nerve can be involved by lesions in the cerebellopontine angle in which the eighth nerve deficit usually dominates the clinical picture. A neurinoma here may mimic an acoustic tumor (Naunton et al., 1968). More peripherally, the nerve can be affected by lesions in the jugular foramen where the tenth and eleventh nerves will also be involved, giving rise to the features of the jugular foramen syndrome (Vernet's syndrome). Glomus tumors are probably the commonest cause, but a ninth nerve neurinoma may arise at this site (Gejrot, 1964). Other tumors involving the nerve here include metastases and chordomas. The nerve may be damaged with basal fractures of the skull. Paralysis may occur in diphtheria. Neoplastic or inflammatory involvement of the meninges may affect the ninth nerve as part of a polyneuritis cranialis, and the nerve is occasionally affected in acute polyneuritis (Guillain-Barré syndrome).

In tabes dorsalis and diabetes, the baro-receptor reflex may be reduced or absent because of involvement of carotid and aortic baroreceptor afferents (Sharpey-Schafer, 1956; Sharpey-Schafer and Taylor, 1960). Recently, an impaired ventilatory response to hypoxia has been demonstrated in patients with these diseases, implying involvement of the chemoreceptor afferent fibers (Evans et al., 1971).

GLOSSOPHARYNGEAL NEURALGIA

This condition may be idiopathic or second-ary to a local structural lesion. Weisenburg first described the tic in 1910 in a patient with a cerebellopontine angle tumor. The idio-pathic form was termed glossopharyngeal neuralgia by Harris in 1921.

The clinical features of the disorder are described in detail in series of 18 and 10 patients respectively reported by Bohm and Strang (1962) and Chawla and Falconer (1967). The pain is stabbing in quality and almost always unilateral. It is usually situated at the base of the tongue and faucial region on one side, but may radiate into the vagal territory. Thus the pain may be felt in or behind the external auditory meatus and beneath the angle of the jaw. For this reason, some authorities have preferred the term vagoglossopharyngeal neuralgia (White and Sweet, 1969).

A hawking cough may accompany the paroxysms, perhaps as an attempt to relieve the pain, and pain may be precipitated by swallowing, talking, pressure on the tragus of the auricle, sneezing, coughing, and moving the head. Salivation, flushing, sweating, tinnitus, lacrimation, tachycardia, hyperten-sion, and even vertigo may be associated (Bohm and Strang, 1962). Cardiac asystole and seizures have also been reported (Garretson and Elvidge, 1963).

Bouts of pain occur on average two or three times a year and last from a few minutes to up to several days. With the passage of time, the bouts tend to increase in frequency.

The etiology of the idiopathic form of glossopharyngeal neuralgia is obscure. The possible significance of "cross talk" resulting from ephaptic excitation is discussed in a theoretical paper by Gardner (1966). The symptomatic or secondary type is commonly due to tumor. Dandy (1927) estimated that tumors in the peripheral distribution of the nerve or in the posterior fossa accounted for a quarter of the cases. Other reported causes include local infection, trauma to the neck, and elongation of the styloid process.

The disorder is usually cured by nerve section. Medullary tractotomy has also been employed (Kunč, 1965). Carbamazepine has been effective in a few cases in which it has been tried (Ekbom and Westerberg, 1966).

CAROTID SINUS SYNCOPE

The carotid sinus reflex, elicited by mechan-ical stimulation of the carotid body, is charac-terized by bradycardia or asystole, a fall in blood pressure and, according to Weiss and Baker (1933), independent changes in cerebral circulation. If asystole exceeds about seven seconds, electroencephalographic changes may be observed (Thomas, 1969). The carotid sinus reflex is usually regarded as hyperactive if asystole exceeds three seconds in duration or if the fall in blood pressure exceeds 50 mm of mercury. Hyperactive reflexes are com-mon in patients with cardiovascular disease, and sensitivity is further enhanced by digitalis (Thomas, 1969). Other predisposing disorders are local tumor infiltration, Takayashu's dis-ease, and vagal lesions. Eliciting the carotid sinus reflex is hazardous, and fatal ventricular fibrillation may occur (Alexander and Ping, 1966). The risks cannot be wholly avoided, and it has recently been suggested that this maneuver should be abandoned as a routine assessment procedure in patients with vascular disease (Brodie and Dow, 1968). Only a minority of those with hyperactive reflexes experience syncope (Thomas, 1969). Carotid sinus syncope may be precipitated by turning the head, wearing a tight collar, or stretching the skin of the neck during shaving, but the diagnosis is often difficult to substantiate clinically.

Several forms of treatment have been tried in carotid sinus syncope. Atropine and more recently propantheline have been found effective (Palmer, 1971). Surgical denervation of the carotid sinus has been performed in some patients, but this procedure may lead to uncontrollable hypertension, as mentioned earlier. Intracranial section of the nerve and irradiation have also been advocated. In the last two years, reports have appeared of the use of demand cardiac pacemakers in this disorder (von Maur et al., 1972).

Swallow syncope is a related disorder that is

largely dependent on vagal reflex pathways but is sometimes associated with pathologic changes in the glossopharyngeal nerve. The literature has been reviewed by Levin and Posner (1972), who describe a case of interest in the context of this discussion. Postmortem examination of their patient showed neoplastic infiltration of the glossopharyngeal nerve as well as degenerative changes in the vagus nerve.

THE VAGUS AND CRANIAL ACCESSORY NERVES

Anatomy

The cranial accessory nerve can be considered to constitute an aberrant bundle of the vagus nerve and the two are therefore discussed together. The rootlets of the vagus nerve emerge from the medulla at a sulcus immediately dorsal to the prominence of the inferior olive and unite to form the nerve trunk. The rootlets of the cranial accessory nerve emerge slightly more caudally and fuse with the spinal accessory nerve, which has ascended through the foramen magnum, although they remain as a discrete fascicle.

The vagus nerve emerges from the skull through the jugular foramen within the same dural sleeve as the accessory nerve, at which site is situated the jugular ganglion. The auricular branch of the nerve leaves distal to the ganglion; it traverses the mastoid process and finally supplies cutaneous sensory fibers to the concha of the external ear. The larger nodose ganglion lies on the nerve just below the jugular foramen, and at this site the vagus is joined by the internal ramus of the accessory nerve, which constitutes its cranial component. At this point also, the vagus nerve gives rise to its pharyngeal branch, which joins the pharyngeal plexus and is distributed to the levator veli palatini muscle and the three paired constrictors of the pharynx.

In the neck, the nerve lies within a sheath that also encloses the internal carotid artery and the internal jugular vein. The cardiac fibers are given off at about the level of the thoracic inlet. They join the sympathetic postganglionic fibers from the three cervical sympathetic ganglia, and these autonomic nerves with the corresponding nerves from the other side form the cardiac plexus on the anterior aspect of the bifurcation of the trachea from which the heart receives its nerve supply.

On the right side the rest of the vagus nerve passes behind the innominate vein and then behind the superior vena cava to lie on the right side of the trachea. On the posterior aspect of the root of the right lung it splits into a posterior and a smaller anterior part that together form an important part of the pulmonary plexus that provides the lung with its vagal innervation. At the lower edge of the lung root the nerve re-forms, passes down close to the esophagus, and at the level of the diaphragm is almost on the posterior aspect. On the left side the nerve, after entering the chest, crosses the lateral aspect of the aortic arch and continues beside the trachea to take part in the pulmonary plexus as on the right side. After re-forming at the lower edge of the lung root, it passes down close to the esophagus and at the level of the diaphragm is largely on the anterior aspect. There is, however, substantial interchange between the vagi as they accompany the lower esophagus.

The upper part of the esophagus has striated muscle in its wall. The lower part has smooth muscle that is innervated from the vagus as it passes down beside it, the preganglionic fibers synapsing with the ganglion cells of the esophageal plexus. In the abdomen the vagus supplies the stomach, liver, gallbladder, bile ducts, small intestine, pancreas, and colon almost to the splenic flexure. In the intestines the preganglionic fibers synapse in the enteric plexuses.

The superior laryngeal nerve arises from the vagus in the region of the nodose ganglion and subdivides into the external laryngeal branch, which supplies the cricothyroid muscle, and the internal laryngeal branch, which pierces the thyrohyoid membrane and delivers sensory fibers to the larynx. The recurrent laryngeal nerve follows a different course on the two sides. On the right, it arises in the root of the neck and passes deep to the subclavian artery; on the left, it arises in the upper thorax and passes deep to the aortic arch. On both sides it gains the groove between the trachea and the esophagus and ascends the neck to reach the larynx, where it supplies all the laryngeal muscles with the exception of the cricothyroid. It divides outside the larynx into two to six motor (anterolateral) and sensory (posteromedial) branches (Williams, 1954). There appears to be no constant intraneural topography within the recurrent laryngeal nerve (Sunderland and Swaney, 1952); separate nerve bundles to different muscles have not been traced (Bowden, 1955). Humphreys (1972), in a study of the recurrent laryngeal nerve during thyroidectomy in 1615 patients, found that this nerve arose from the vagus at the level of the larynx and pursued a nonrecurrent course in 11 cases.

The vagus nerve is structurally complex, with somatic sensory and visceral afferent and efferent components.

Somatic Sensory Fibers. Somatic sensory fibers are distributed to the skin of the concha of the external ear and travel in the auricular branch. This nerve in the cat contains a high proportion of myelinated fibers of large diameter whose cells of origin appear to be in the jugular ganglion (DuBois and Foley, 1937). On entering the brain stem they reach the trigeminal sensory nucleus.

Visceral Afferent Fibers. Visceral afferent fibers carry impulses from the pharynx, larynx, trachea, esophagus, and the thoracic and abdominal viscera, including a small gustatory contribution from the epiglottis and vallecula. Those carrying pain from the larynx probably terminate in the spinal nucleus of the trigeminal nerve (Brodal, 1947), the remainder mainly being distributed to the nucleus of the tractus solitarius. Their cell bodies lie in the nodose ganglion. The sensory innervation of the larynx has given rise to discussion, but it is now evident that spindles are present in all the laryngeal muscles of man (Lucas Keene, 1961) and that tendon organs and joint endings are also present (Bowden, in press). Their presence had been doubted because of the unimodal distribution of fiber diameter in the recurrent laryngeal nerve. However, Scheuer (1964) found fibers greater than 12 μm in diameter in both the internal and recurrent nerves in man and obtained a bimodal distribution if the values for the two nerves were combined. She considered that muscle afferents might travel centrally in both these nerves in man. Their central connections are uncertain. Their cell bodies are situated mainly in the nodose ganglion in the cat and rabbit (Bowden, in press).

Visceral Efferent Fibers. Motor fibers take origin in the nucleus ambiguus that are often referred to as "special visceral efferents," since they supply striated musculature derived from the branchial arches. Some of the fibers leave the medulla in the cranial portion of the eleventh nerve and reach the tenth nerve through the internal ramus of the eleventh nerve. They innervate striated muscle in the palate, pharynx, larynx, and upper esophagus. The laryngeal muscles are supplied by cells from the caudal part of the nucleus ambiguus, and there is evidence to indicate cell groupings related to individual laryngeal muscles (Szenthágothai, 1943; Lawn, 1966). Some fibers cross the midline to emerge with the nerves of the opposite side (Mitchell and Warwick, 1955).

The preganglionic parasympathetic fibers of this nerve that are distributed to the heart arise in cells close to the nucleus ambiguus. The remaining preganglionic autonomic fibers arise in the dorsal nucleus of the vagus in the floor of the fourth ventricle (Mitchell, 1953; Mitchell and Warwick, 1955). This nucleus is especially concerned with the alimentary tract and is immediately inferior to the inferior salivary nucleus from which the parotid gland is innervated through the ninth cranial nerve. Superior to the inferior salivary nucleus is the superior salivary nucleus concerned in innervation of the submandibular and sublingual salivary glands through the seventh cranial nerve.

The cardiac fibers pass backward at first from the vicinity of the nucleus ambiguus toward the floor of the fourth ventricle. They then pass laterally with the noncardiac fibers, and all emerge from the medulla in the rootlets of the vagus nerve.

Clinical Features of Vagus Nerve Lesions

PALATAL AND PHARYNGEAL PARALYSIS

During swallowing, the nasopharynx is occluded by elevation of the palate, and at the same time, the epiglottis is raised and the inlet to the larynx is closed. Food projected from the mouth into the oropharynx is then transferred to the esophagus by the peristaltic action of the pharyngeal constrictors.

Damage to the vagus nerve central to its ganglia, or lesions of the pharyngeal branches, result in paralysis of the levator veli palatini muscles and of the pharyngeal constrictors.

Unilateral palatal paralysis gives rise to defective elevation of the palate on phonation and movement of the uvula toward the affected side. It is usually asymptomatic, but may lead to snoring at night and slight alterations in phonation if it occurs in singers. With bilateral palatal palsy, the nasopharynx is not closed during swallowing or phonation, leading to nasality of speech, nasal regurgitation during swallowing, and snoring when asleep.

Unilateral pharyngeal paralysis produces drooping of the pharyngeal wall on the affected side and a "curtain" movement of the pharynx to the opposite side on phonation. There may be slight difficulty in clearing secretions from the throat and some interference with swallowing. Bilateral lesions give rise to severe dysphagia.

LARYNGEAL PARALYSIS

The larynx opens to allow breathing and closes during swallowing. Abduction of the vocal cords takes place during inspiration; the cords are adducted during phonation and coughing. The normal separation of the cords during respiration is about 13.5 mm, but in the fully adducted paramedian position there is a narrow separation only. The position assumed by the completely paralyzed cords (cadaveric position) is almost halfway between abduction and adduction, leaving a gap of approximately 7 mm.

Unilateral Paralysis. Unilateral lesions of the recurrent laryngeal nerve result in paralysis of all the laryngeal muscles with the exception of the cricothyroid. It may be entirely asymptomatic or give rise to transient or sometimes persistent hoarseness of the voice. The occurrence of hoarseness depends upon the ability of the opposite cord to compensate if the paralyzed cord is not in a median position. The affected cord usually adopts a median or paramedian position and, since the superior laryngeal nerve is intact, the cricothyroid muscle is able to exert action as a tensor of the cord and also, to some extent, as an adductor.

With partial lesions of the recurrent laryngeal nerve, movements of abduction may be abolished before those of adduction (Semon's law). Suggestions that the fibers innervating the abductor muscles occupy a particular position in the nerve that may be more vulnerable have not been confirmed by anatomical studies (Sunderland and Swaney, 1952). Ellis (1954) has argued that whether the cord adopts a paramedian position or not depends upon the activity of the cricothyroid muscle and upon individual variations in the anatomy of the larynx. The relative bulk of the abductors and the adductors may be important, the weight of the abductors being only a quarter of that of the adductors (Bowden and Scheuer, 1960). When there is persisting paralysis of the cord, because of fibrotic contracture, the cord almost invariably comes ultimately to lie near the midline and at a lower level than the unparalyzed cord.

If the superior laryngeal nerve is involved in addition, total paralysis of the cord on the affected side results, the cord lying in the cadaveric position. Under these circumstances, there is usually associated palatal and pharyngeal paralysis, as the lesion is likely to be central to the nodose ganglion. The voice is weak and husky, and tires easily. An isolated lesion of the superior laryngeal nerve must be a very rare eventuality, but has been described as a consequence of surgical or accidental trauma.

Bilateral Paralysis. The consequences of bilateral lesions of the recurrent laryngeal nerves depend upon the degree of approximation of the cords. Close approximation of the cords tends to result from acute lesions, such as follow thyroidectomy, whereas lesions of insidious onset tend to give rise to a less close apposition. The nearer the cords are to the midline, the better is the voice but the greater is the limitation of the airway. Acute lesions may necessitate tracheostomy, whereas insidious lesions may merely result in dyspnea and stridor on exertion, although the voice will be more severely affected.

Bilateral lesions affecting the superior laryngeal nerves usually imply damage above the nodose ganglia, and there is associated palatal and pharyngeal paralysis. The cords lie in the cadaveric position. Phonation is almost absent and is associated with much air wastage, and vocal pitch cannot be altered. There is an adequate airway for normal activities. Coughing is inefficient.

AUTONOMIC (PARASYMPATHETIC) DYSFUNCTION

Tests of Vagal Function. Although the vagus nerve supplies so many organs in the chest and abdomen, there are rather few tests of its function.

HEART RATE. Normally at rest vagal inhibition slows the heart rate, and atropine by paralyzing the vagus causes an increase in heart rate. If this increase occurs, it is evidence that the vagus was active, but it is necessary to give an adequate dose of atropine (3.0 mg). It is convenient to give 1.2 mg in the first instance, if there is no change in heart rate in five minutes to repeat it, and if there is still no change to give the remaining 0.6 mg. Pressure on the carotid sinus or on the eyeballs causes bradycardia by increasing vagal activity. These tests should, however, be used with caution, for the response may be severe, causing fainting or even death (Nelson and Mahru, 1963). If vagal activity is being examined in connection with a circulatory problem, it is valuable to observe whether bradycardia occurs in response to a rise in arterial blood pressure. It normally occurs as a reflex from baroreceptors, the efferent pathway being in the vagus. The hypertensive part (phase IV) of the normal response of the arterial blood pressure to Valsalva's maneuver may give this information. Alternatively a pressor agent such as noradrenaline or angiotensin may be infused to produce varying degrees of hypertension, which may then be related to heart rate to give a quantitative assessment of the baroreceptor reflex (Pickering et al., 1968).

GASTRIC ACID SECRETION. Hypoglycemia (50 mg per 100 ml or less) causes acid secretion in the stomach, but only if the vagal supply to the stomach is intact. If an insulin test meal (0.1 unit of insulin per kilogram of body weight) produces no increase in gastric acidity although the blood sugar level falls below 50 mg per 100 ml, it is evidence to suggest severe vagal failure (Hollander, 1946).

ESOPHAGEAL MOVEMENT. Denervation of the esophagus makes its muscle unduly sensitive to cholinergic drugs, a usual response to denervation (Cannon, 1939; Cannon and Rosenblueth, 1949). Methacholine (1.5 to 10 mg) is given by subcutaneous injection and the motility of the esophagus is observed radiologically or by manometry (Kramer and Ingelfinger, 1951; Palmer, 1957). In a patient with achalasia of the cardia there will be a strong but uncoordinated contraction of the esophagus, but in a normal subject or a patient with esophageal dysfunction from another cause there is no change in motility.

Disorders of Vagal Autonomic Function

ABNORMAL REGENERATION. If the vagus nerve is damaged, it may regenerate wrongly and in particular it may come to innervate sweat glands, to the distress of the patient. The vagus is cholinergic and this prevents functional regeneration along many sympathetic pathways for they are largely adrenergic. It can, however, functionally innervate sympathetic structures by innervating either preganglionic sympathetic nerves or postganglionic nerves to sweat glands, for both ganglia and sweat glands are cholinergic. The result can be *gustatory sweating,* that is, sweating in circumstances that normally produce salivary and gastric secretions. This may be best known from lesions in the neighborhood of the parotid gland where parasympathetic fibers from the glossopharyngeal nerve may innervate sweat glands through the auriculotemporal nerve, as mentioned earlier, and may be seen in diabetic neuropathy (Aagenaes, 1962; Watkins, 1973). Gustatory sweating mediated through the vagus is liable to occur after operations on the root of the neck or thoracotomy, as both vagus and sympathetic nerves may be damaged (Herxheimer, 1958). It may involve the ipsilateral side of the face, neck and shoulder, and as this is a substantial area, it may mean that even to pick up an appetizing menu causes enough sweating to require a change of clothes. Atropine by mouth an hour before meals may solve the problem. Local application of a cholinergic blocking agent (Laage-Hellman, 1957) and irradiation of the skin have also been recommended (Glaister et al., 1958). Surgical section of the sympathetic pathway gives good immediate results, but relapse may occur.

OVERACTIVITY OF THE VAGUS. Overactivity of the vagus and the consequent bradycardia are important in some forms of fainting, including emotional faints and carotid sinus syncope. Reflex overactivity can be induced by pressure on the eyeballs, and occasionally the bradycardia can be so severe as to cause loss of consciousness or even death (Nelson and Mahru, 1963).

UNDERACTIVITY OF THE VAGUS. Evidence has recently been presented for the occurrence of vagal denervation of the heart in diabetic neuropathy (see Chapter 47). Interference with the nerve supply of the alimentary tract supplied by the vagus may affect its function. Most patients who have had vagotomy at the cardia have satisfactory alimentary function. Some, however, are liable to intermittent diarrhea lasting one or two days and occurring every one or two weeks. This is severe enough to be a troublesome symptom in about 5 per cent of patients. If the lesion affects the intramural plexus rather than the (preganglionic) vagus nerve itself, the effect is to interfere with peristalsis and produce dilatation. The best-known example of dilatation from a lesion of the enteric plexus is Hirschsprung's disease, congenital megacolon. This is outside the territory of the vagus, but similar disorders can occur in the vagal territory. It is probably the basis of achalasia of the cardia (Smith, 1972), although some have regarded the abnormalities of the enteric plexus as being secondary to the esophageal distention. It can also occur in Chagas' disease (*Trypanosoma cruzi* infection) and cause dilatation of the esophagus as well as any part of the gastrointestinal tract including the bile passages (Koberle, 1956, 1958; Ferreira-Santos, 1961). Patients with diabetes, usually of long standing, may develop alimentary symptoms that have been attributed to autonomic neuropathy. These include esophageal dysfunction, gastric dilatation and nocturnal diarrhea and are considered in greater detail in Chapter 47.

VAGAL AFFERENTS

Laryngeal Receptors. The vagus supplies sensation to the mucous membrane of the larynx. This, with the corresponding sensory innervation of the tracheobronchial tree, provides the afferent pathway for the cough reflex. Unilateral anesthesia is usually symptomless. Bilateral anesthesia is generally part of a more widespread neurologic deficit. With bilateral lesions, the laryngeal and tracheobronchial reflexes are absent, and inhalation of secretions and food materials is likely to occur.

Pulmonary Receptors. Pulmonary stretch activity in the vagus is present at the resting expiratory position and it increases with inspiration. In man, however, during normal resting breathing vagal blockade does not affect the breathing (though it does so in some animals) (Widdicombe, 1963; Guz et al., 1970). The major role in monitoring tidal volume in man at rest appears to lie with receptors in the chest wall concerned with stretch and the load on inspiratory muscles, rather than with the vagal pulmonary stretch receptors. In non-resting breathing, however, vagal blockade reduces the ventilatory response to carbon

dioxide and makes respiration slower and deeper. This suggests that vagal stretch receptors may be concerned in the control of the pattern of breathing when the breathing is vigorous (Guz and Widdicombe, 1970). Deflation of the lung may cause an increase in respiratory rate and force, but in man the deflation has to be of the severity that occurs in pneumothorax. The effect is abolished in animals by vagotomy, and it is likely that it is also mediated by the vagus in man.

Animal experiments indicate that in addition to pulmonary stretch receptors there are vagal lung irritant receptors (Mills et al., 1970). They respond to many noxious stimuli such as toxic substances (ammonia, cigarette smoke) in the airways, overinflation or marked deflation of the lungs, or pulmonary congestion or microembolism. Unlike the pulmonary stretch activity, activity in these nerves does not adapt quickly if stimulation is continued, and they are probably concerned in unpleasant respiratory sensations in man.

Vascular Receptors. Baroreceptors in the aorta and the venae cavae, the right atrium, and other vessels are supplied by the vagus nerve. They play a part in controlling the circulation, both reflexly and by affecting blood volume.

Lesions Affecting the Vagus Nerves

INTRAMEDULLARY LESIONS

As already stated, lesions within the brain stem commonly affect other lower cranial nerves and long tracts simultaneously, and may be due to vascular (as in the lateral medullary syndrome), neoplastic and inflammatory causes, and sometimes syringobulbia (Melerovich and Liande, 1957). Lesions at this site usually produce palatal, pharyngeal, and laryngeal paralysis, but if the upper part of the nucleus ambiguus is selectively involved, there may be sparing of laryngeal function (palatopharyngeal syndrome of Avellis). The cells of the nucleus may be involved in progressive bulbar palsy (motor neuron disease) or poliomyelitis.

EXTRAMEDULLARY LESIONS

Damage to the tenth nerve intracranially after its emergence from the medulla may occur within the posterior fossa from tumors or in meningovascular syphilis, in which case other lower cranial nerves are often also involved, or it may occur after the nerve leaves the skull from the same types of disease as enumerated for the ninth nerve. The three nerves that emerge through the jugular foramen (IX, X, and XI) may simultaneously be involved, usually by a neoplasm, in Vernet's syndrome, or with more extensive lesions the twelfth nerve may also be affected (Collet-Sicard syndrome). Other combinations have been defined, including the syndromes of Schmidt (involving nerves X and XI) and of Hughlings Jackson (involving nerves X, XI, and XII).

The vagus nerves may be affected as part of a polyneuritis cranialis, particularly in sarcoidosis (see Chapter 59) and in occasional examples of the Guillain-Barré syndrome (see Chapter 56). Palatal palsy may complicate pharyngeal diphtheria (see Chapter 63). A recurrent laryngeal nerve palsy may occur as a rare involvement in cases of shoulder girdle neuritis (neuralgic amyotrophy).

The recurrent laryngeal nerves are liable to damage by a variety of intrathoracic lesions, particularly on the left because of the longer course of the nerve on that side. Neoplastic involvement of mediastinal lymph glands from carcinoma of the bronchus or esophagus is the commonest explanation, although in the past aortic aneurysm or enlargement of the left atrium in mitral stenosis figured as possible causes. The recurrent laryngeal nerves may also be involved in the neck from carcinoma of the esophagus or thyroid gland, or neoplastic invasion of the cervical lymph glands. Operative damage to the nerves is now considerably less frequent than formerly; a delayed postoperative laryngeal palsy may also occur. Williams (1958) analyzed his findings for 100 benign goiters. Preoperative inspection of the vocal cords revealed no paralysis, nor was any instance of immediate postoperative paralysis detected. Unilateral cord paralysis developed after four to five days in seven cases, however, and in two it was permanent. Since it was known that the nerves had not been transected or crushed during the operation, postoperative edema was considered to be the probable cause. Hawe and Lothian (1960) exposed the recurrent laryngeal nerves in 1011 operations. No paralysis was present preoperatively, but occurred following operation in 28, in only three of which was it permanent. If laryngoscopy at the termination of the operation revealed paraly-

sis, the nerve on the affected side was immediately explored. In two cases the nerve had been included in a ligature, but subsequent recovery occurred in both. Blackburn and Salmon (1961) reported their findings in 250 thyroidectomies in which preoperative and postoperative inspection of the larynx had been made. There were four instances of temporary and five of permanent unilateral recurrent laryngeal nerve paralysis.

Bilateral recurrent laryngeal damage usually follows thyroidectomy. In a series of 22 cases reported by Williams (1959), this was so in 18. In two, it was part of a polyneuropathy, and in two others it was the result of carcinoma, of the thyroid gland and esophagus respectively.

About one quarter to one third of all cases of isolated recurrent laryngeal palsy have no discoverable cause according to Huppler and associates (1956) and Ballantyne (1971), although other writers have given a lower incidence rate for "idiopathic" cases (Kecht, 1965). Males are affected twice as often as females, the left side is involved more frequently than the right, and a peak incidence occurs in the third decade (Huppler et al., 1956). A series of 21 such cases has recently been reported by Blau and Kapadia (1972). Five recovered completely and another five improved within a few months of the onset. The remainder developed no major disease over a follow-up period of one to eight years.

THE SPINAL ACCESSORY NERVE

Anatomy

This nerve is largely efferent. It emerges as a linear series of rootlets extending from the last of the rootlets of the cranial accessory nerve as far as the fifth or sixth segments of the spinal cord. It is derived from a column of cells in the posterolateral part of the anterior horn, which in their most cranial portion are relatively isolated and approach the caudal termination of the nucleus ambiguus (Pearson, 1938). The rootlets emerge from the lateral column of the cord posterior to the ligamenta denticulata and unite to form a bundle that passes through the foramen magnum. It is then joined by the cranial portion of the accessory nerve and leaves the skull through the jugular foramen. The cranial portion of the accessory nerve separates as the internal ramus and joins the vagus nerve.

Having left the skull, it descends between the internal carotid artery and the internal jugular vein and penetrates the sternomastoid muscle, which it supplies. It emerges just above the middle of the posterior border of this muscle and crosses the posterior triangle of the neck in its fascial roof to reach the trapezius muscle, which it also supplies. During its course, it receives communications from the third and fourth cervical nerves through the cervical plexus.

The spinal accessory nerve also contains some afferent fibers whose cell bodies lie within the nerve trunk in its intracranial portion (Windle, 1931; Pearson, 1938). These fibers are probably muscle afferents (Yee et al., 1939).

Clinical Features of Spinal Accessory Nerve Lesions

Damage to the spinal accessory nerve deep to the sternocleidomastoid muscle or intracranially leads to weakness of this muscle and also of the upper part of the trapezius muscle. Lesions in the posterior triangle result only in weakness of this portion of the trapezius. The lower fibers of the trapezius are supplied from the third and fourth cervical roots through the cervical plexus, although there is some variability; occasionally the whole trapezius is supplied by these roots (Coleman and Walker, 1950).

Following an accessory nerve lesion, there is weakness of rotation of the head to the opposite side because of paresis of the sternocleidomastoid muscle. Involvement of the trapezius gives rise to weakness of elevation of the shoulder and inability to lift the arm above the horizontal. It also leads to drooping of the shoulder, together with moderate winging of the scapula when the arms are hanging at the side. The winging is accentuated when the patient attempts to elevate the arm laterally. This is in contradistinction to the winging seen with serratus anterior weakness, which is minimal at rest, but becomes pronounced on forward elevation of the arm.

Lesions of the Spinal Accessory Nerve

The cells of origin in the spinal cord may be involved in motor neuron disease, polio-myelitis, syringomyelia, and spinal tumors. In the intraspinal and intracranial portion and in the region of the skull base, the nerve may be affected by the same disorders that have been described for the ninth and tenth nerves, including posterior fossa meningiomas (Cherington, 1968) and neurinomas (see Chapter 66). Its superficial position in the neck renders it liable to damage during surgical procedures and from external compression and injury (Schneck, 1960; Bell, 1964; Bateman, 1967).

Isolated unexplained lesions of the accessory nerve occasionally occur from which spontaneous recovery may take place (Eisen and Bertrand, 1972). They may be heralded by pain felt along the posterior border of the sternocleidomastoid muscle and in the sub-occipital region. This pain possibly arises in the nerve itself (see Chapter 9). After a few days, the severe pain subsides, to be replaced by a dull ache in the region of the shoulder, at which time the weakness is noticed. Such lesions are possibly instances of benign mononeuropathies of the type that may affect various other cranial nerves, of which Bell's palsy is the most frequent example (Foley, 1969).

Electromyography and measurement of the latency of the muscle response on nerve stimulation may be useful for confirmation of the diagnosis (Cherington, 1968; Eisen and Bertrand, 1972).

THE HYPOGLOSSAL NERVE

Anatomy

The hypoglossal nerve carries motor fibers to the intrinsic tongue muscles, and to the hyoglossus, styloglossus, genioglossus, and geniohyoid muscles. These fibers originate from the hypoglossal nucleus, which consists of a longitudinal arrangement of neurons lying beneath the floor of the fourth ventricle and extending caudally to the lower limit of the medulla. In their intramedullary course, the fibers traverse the reticular formation and the medial part of the inferior olive before leaving the medulla in the lateral ventral sulcus. The nerve emerges as several filaments, uniting into two bundles that pass separately through the dura and the anterior condyloid foramen (hypoglossal canal). Outside the skull, the nerve passes vertically downward to the level of the angle of the jaw where it turns forward to innervate the ipsilateral half of the tongue. Sympathetic fibers travel in association with the nerve.

There is now no doubt that the hypoglossal nerve contains afferent fibers, a view supported by both anatomical and physiologic evidence. The earlier literature is reviewed by Blom (1960). Muscle spindles have been identified in the human tongue by Cooper (1953) and by Walker and Rajagopal (1959) and in that of other primates. The fiber caliber spectrum of the hypoglossal nerve in man shows a peak at 7 to 9 μm, the largest fiber size being 11 to 13 μm (Rexed, 1944). In the rhesus monkey, the caliber spectrum of the distal portion of the nerve is consistent with a significant component from spindle afferents although this is not the case more proximally in the nerve, suggesting that spindle afferents reach the central nervous system by a different route (Egel et al., 1968). Physiologic studies in the same species indicate that this route involves the second and third cervical nerve roots (Bowman and Combs, 1969). This finding accords with the earlier work of Corbin and Harrison (1939), who demonstrated that the cells of origin for proprioceptive fibers from the tongue in the rhesus monkey lie in the dorsal root ganglion of C2.

A small ganglion is found along the course of the hypoglossal nerve in some species, and nerve cells have been identified in the extracranial portion of the hypoglossal nerve in the human fetus by Wózniak and Young (1968), who suggested that these cells, because of their morphologic similarities, may have migrated from those of the inferior ganglion of the vagus nerve.

Electrical stimulation of the hypoglossal nerve in the cat was shown by Downman (1939) to cause pupillary dilatation and a rise in blood pressure, and in the dog such stimulation evokes efferent activity in thoracic and renal sympathetic nerves (Whitwam et al., 1969). Stimulation at an adequate intensity to excite group III afferent fibers evokes in the cat responses in muscles innervated by the facial nerve (Lindquist and Mårtensson, 1969). Hanson and Widén (1970) have demonstrated a reflex response in the styloglossus muscle to stimulation of the central cut end of a peripheral branch of the nerve. Afferent impulses have also been recorded in the hypoglossal nerve in response to stretch (Cooper, 1954; Blom, 1960; Hanson and Widén, 1970; Morimoto and Kawamura, 1971).

Clinical Features of Hypoglossal Nerve Lesions

A unilateral lesion of the nerve does not interfere with speech, but bilateral involvement causes dysarthria and difficulty in swallowing. The signs of a lesion of the hypoglossal nerve are wasting of the ipsilateral half of the tongue, which may show excessive furring. Deviation toward the side of the paralysis occurs when the tongue is protruded, although there are occasional exceptions to this (Weber and Odom, 1969). With bilateral lesions, there is difficulty in tongue protrusion. Lesions involving the hypoglossal nucleus usually cause fibrillation of the tongue.

Lesions of the Hypoglossal Nerve

Congenital atrophy of the tongue is usually due to deficiency of the nerve. The neurons constituting the hypoglossal nucleus may be affected by the same diseases that attack anterior horn cells in the spinal cord, notably motor neuron disease and poliomyelitis. The nucleus and the intramedullary portion of the nerves may also be involved by structural lesions in the lower brain stem such as infarction, neoplasm, and syringobulbia. If the lesion is confined to one half of the medulla, ipsilateral hypoglossal paralysis may be associated with crossed hemiplegia.

Extrinsic lesions of the nerve in its intracranial portion may in rare instances be due to a primary tumor of the nerve (Williams and Fox, 1962; Ignelzi and Bucy, 1967; Arumugasamay, Sarvananthan, Rudralingan and Pillay, 1972). Selective involvement of one nerve has been described as the first sign of intracranial metastasis in patients with bronchial carcinoma, lymphoma, or leukemia (Rubinstein, 1969). Basal meningitis and vertebral artery aneurysms occasionally interfere with twelfth nerve function, but other cranial nerves are usually also implicated.

At the level of the hypoglossal canal, the nerve can be involved by glomus jugulare tumors, meningiomas, cordomas, and cholesteatomas. Occasionally the nerve may be damaged as a consequence of head injury or, in the neck, as the result of a penetrating wound.

GLOSSODYNIA

Glossodynia describes the syndrome of burning pain experienced in the tongue and often also throughout the oral mucosa. It occurs usually in the middle aged and elderly and more frequently in females than in males. Deficiency of the B vitamins including B_{12} has been named as a cause by Elfenbaum (1969), but in the majority of patients the symptom seems to be psychogenic in origin. In a series of 54 patients described by Quinn (1965), for example, 19 had cancerophobia.

REFERENCES

Aagenaes, Ö.: Neurovascular examinations on the lower extremities in young diabetics, with special reference to the autonomic neuropathy. Copenhagen, C. Hamburgers Bogtrykkeri, 1962.

Alexander, S., and Ping, W. C.: Fatal ventricular fibrillation during carotid sinus stimulation. Am. J. Cardiol., 18:289, 1966.

Arumugasamay, N., Sarvananthan, K., Rudralingan, V., and Pillay, D. R. P.: Intracranial hypoglossal neurinomas—a report of two cases. Med. J. Malaya, 26:168, 1972.

Ballantyne, J.: Neurological affections of the larynx. In Ballantyne, J., and Groves, J. (eds.): Diseases of the Ear, Nose and Throat. 3rd Edition. London, Butterworths, 1971.

Bateman, J. E.: Nerve injuries about the shoulder in sports. J. Bone Joint Surg., 49A:785, 1967.

Bell, D. S.: Pressure palsy of the accessory nerve. Br. Med. J., 1:1483, 1964.

Biscoe, T. J.: Carotid body: structure and function. Physiol. Rev., 51:437, 1971.

Blackburn, G., and Salmon, L. F.: Cord movements after thyroidectomy. Br. J. Surg., 48:371, 1961.

Blau, J. N., and Kapadia, R.: Idiopathic palsy of the recurrent laryngeal nerve: a transient cranial mononeuropathy. Br. Med. J., 4:259, 1972.

Blom, S.: Afferent influences on tongue activity. Acta Physiol. Scand., 49:Suppl. 170, 1960.

Bohm, E., and Strang, R. R.: Glossopharyngeal neuralgia. Brain, 85:371, 1962.

Bowden, R. E. M.: The surgery of the recurrent laryngeal nerve. Proc. R. Soc. Med., 48:437, 1955.

Bowden, R. E. M.: Innervation of intrinsic laryngeal muscles. In Wyke, B. (ed.): Symposium on the Larynx. London, Oxford University Press, in press.

Bowden, R. E. M., and Scheuer, J. L.: Weights of abductor and adductor muscles of the human larynx. J. Laryngol. Otol. 74:971, 1960.

Bowman, J. P., and Combs, C. M.: The cerebrocortical projection of hypoglossal afferents. Exp. Neurol., 23:291, 1969.

Brodal, A.: Central course of afferent fibers for pain in facial, glossopharyngeal and vagus nerves. Arch. Neurol. Psychiatry, 57:292, 1947.

Brodie, R. E., and Dow, R. S.: Studies in carotid compression and carotid sinus sensitivity. Neurology (Minneap.), 18:1047, 1968.

Bues, E.: The anterior zone of the ear in the diagnosis and treatment of glossopharyngeal neuralgia. Dtsch. Z. Nervheilkd., 185:471, 1963.

Cannon, W. B.: Law of denervation. Am. J. Med. Sci., 198:737, 1939.

Cannon, W. B., and Rosenblueth, A.: The Supersensitivity of Denervated Structures: a Law of Denervation. New York, Macmillan, Inc., 1949.

Chawla, J. C., and Falconer, M. A.: Glossopharyngeal and vagal neuralgia. Br. Med. J., 3:529, 1967.

Cherington, M.: Accessory nerve: conduction studies. Arch. Neurol., 18:708, 1968.

Coleman, C. C., and Walker, J. C.: Technic of anastomosis of the branches of the facial nerve with the spinal accessory for facial paralysis. Ann. Surg., 131:960, 1950.

Cooper, S.: Muscle spindles in the intrinsic muscles of the human tongue. J. Physiol. (Lond.), 122:193, 1953.

Cooper, S.: Afferent impulses in the hypoglossal nerve on stretching the cat's tongue. J. Physiol. (Lond.), 126:32P, 1954.

Corbin, K. B., and Harrison, F.: The sensory innervation of the spinal accessory and tongue musculature in the rhesus monkey. Brain, 62:191, 1939.

Cottle, M. K.: Degeneration studies of primary afferents of IXth and Xth cranial nerves in the cat. J. Comp. Neurol., 122:329, 1964.

Dandy, W. E.: Glossopharyngeal neuralgia (tic douloureux); its diagnosis and treatment. Arch. Surg., 15:190 and 198, 1927.

Davie, J. C., and Bourke, R. S.: Confirmation of atypical parasympathetic innervation of the parotid gland. Atypical distribution of ninth nerve. Arch. Neurol., 16:599, 1967.

Dejours, P.: Chemoreflexes in breathing. Physiol. Rev., 42:335, 1962.

Downman, C. B. B.: Afferent fibres of the hypoglossal nerve. J. Anat., 73:387, 1939.

DuBois, F. S., and Foley, J. O.: Quantitative studies of the vagus nerve in the cat. II. The ratio of jugular to nodose fibers. J. Comp. Neurol., 67:69, 1937.

Egel, R. T., Bowman, J. P., and Combs, C. M.: Caliber spectra of the lingual and hypoglossal nerves of the rhesus monkey. J. Comp. Neurol., 134:163, 1968.

Eisen, A., and Bertrand, G.: Isolated accessory nerve palsy of spontaneous origin. A clinical and electromyographic study. Arch. Neurol., 27:496, 1972.

Ekbom, K. A., and Westerberg, C. E.: Carbamazepine in glossopharyngeal neuralgia. Arch. Neurol., 14:595, 1966.

Elfenbaum, A.: Burning tongue in older patients. J. Can. Dent. Assoc., 35:533, 1969.

Ellis, M.: Laryngeal paralysis. In Ellis, M. (ed.): Modern Trends in Diseases of the Ear, Nose and Throat. London, Butterworths, 1954, p. 327.

Evans, R. J. C., Benson, M. K., and Hughes, D. T. D.: Abnormal chemoreceptor response to hypoxia in patients with tabes dorsalis. Br. Med. J., 1:530, 1971.

Ferreira-Santos, R.: Megacolon and megarectum in Chagas' disease. Proc. R. Soc. Med., 54:1047, 1961.

Foley, J. M.: The cranial mononeuropathies. N. Engl. J. Med., 281:905, 1969.

Gardner, W. J.: Crosstalk—the paradoxical transmission of a nerve impulse. Arch. Neurol., 14:149, 1966.

Garretson, H. D., and Elvidge, A. R.: Glossopharyngeal neuralgia with asystole and seizures. Arch. Neurol., 8:26, 1963.

Gejrot, T.: Jugular syndrome. Acta Otolaryngol. (Stockh.) 57:450, 1964.

Glaister, D. H., Hearnshaw, J. R., Heffron, P. F., and Peck, A. W.: The mechanisms of post-parotidectomy gustatory sweating. Br. Med. J., 2:942, 1958.

Guz, A., and Widdicombe, J. G.: Pattern of breathing during hypercapnia before and after vagal blockade in man. In Breathing. Ciba Foundation Symposium. London, J. & A. Churchill [Baltimore, Williams & Wilkins Co.], 1970, p. 41.

Guz, A., Noble, M. I. M., Eisele, J. H., and Trenchard, D.: The role of vagal inflation reflexes in man and other animals. In Breathing. Ciba Foundation Symposium. London, J. & A. Churchill [Baltimore, Williams & Wilkins Co.], 1970, p. 1.

Hanson, J., and Widén, L.: Afferent fibers in the hypoglossal nerve of cat. Acta Physiol. Scand., 79:24, 1970.

Harris, W.: Persistent pain in lesions of the peripheral and central nervous system. Br. Med. J., 2:896, 1921.

Hawe, P., and Lothian, K. R.: Recurrent laryngeal nerve injury during thyroidectomy. Surg. Gynecol. Obstet., 110:488, 1960.

Herxheimer, A.: Gustatory sweating and pilomotion. Br. Med. J., 1:688, 1958.

Hollander, F.: Insulin test for presence of intact nerve fibers after vagal operation for peptic ulcer. Gastroenterology, 7:607, 1946.

Humphreys, J.: A hazard of thyroidectomy. Proc. R. Soc. Med. 65:169, 1972.

Huppler, E. G., Schmidt, H. W., Devine, K. D., and Gage, R. P.: Ultimate outcome of patients with vocal-cord paralysis of undetermined cause. Am. Rev. Tuberc. Pulm. Dis., 73:52, 1956.

Ignelzi, R. J., and Bucy, P. C.: Intracranial hypoglossal neurofibroma—case report. J. Neurosurg., 26:352, 1967.

Kecht, B.: "Idiopathische" Stimmbandlämungen. Wien. Med. Wochenschr., 115:511, 1965.

Kerr, F. W. L.: Facial, vagal and glossopharyngeal nerves in the cat. Arch. Neurol., 6:264, 1962.

Koberle, F.: Zur Frage der Entstehung sogennanter "Idiopathischer Dilatation" muskulärer Hohlorgane. Virchows Arch. Pathol. Anat. Physiol., 329:337, 1956.

Koberle, F.: Megaesophagus. Gastroenterology, 34:460, 1958.

Kramer, P., and Ingelfinger, F. J.: Esophageal sensitivity of Mecholyl in cardiospasm. Gastroenterology, 19:242, 1951.

Kunč, Z.: Treatment of essential neuralgia of the ninth nerve by selective tractotomy. J. Neurosurg., 23:494, 1965.

Laage-Hellman, J. E.: Gustatory sweating and flushing after conservative parotidectomy. Acta Otolaryngol. (Stockh.), 48:234, 1957.

Lawn, A. M.: The localisation, in the nucleus ambiguus of the rabbit, of the cells of origin of motor nerve fibers in the glossopharyngeal nerve and various branches of the vagus nerve by means of retrograde degeneration. J. Comp. Neurol., 127:293, 1966.

Levin, B., Posner, J. B.: Swallow syncope. Neurology (Minneap.), 22:1086, 1972.

Lindquist, C., and Mårtensson, A.: Reflex responses induced by stimulation of hypoglossal afferents. Acta Physiol. Scand., 77:234, 1969.

Lucas Keene, M. F.: Muscle spindles in human laryngeal muscles. J. Anat., 95:25, 1961.

Maur, K. von, Nelson, E. W., Holsinger, J. W., and Eliot, R. S.: Hypersensitive carotid sinus syncope treated by implantable demand cardiac pacemaker. Am. J. Cardiol., 29:109, 1972.

Melerovich, A. E., and Liande, V. S.: Porazheniia gortani pri siringomielobul'bii. Vestn. Otorinolaryngol., 19:89, 1957.

Mills, J. E., Sellick, H., and Widdicombe, J. G.: Epithelial irritant receptors in the lungs. In Breathing. Ciba Foundation Symposium. London, J. & A. Churchill [Baltimore, Williams & Wilkins Co.], 1970, p. 77.

Mitchell, G. A. G.: Anatomy of the Autonomic Nervous System. London, E. & S. Livingstone, 1953.

Mitchell, G. A. G., and Warwick, R.: The dorsal vagal nucleus. Acta Anat., 25:371, 1955.

Miura, M., and Reis, D. J.: Termination and secondary projections of carotid sinus nerve in the cat brain stem. Am. J. Physiol., 217:142, 1969.

Morimoto, T., and Kawamura, Y.: Discharge patterns of hypoglossal afferents in a cat. Brain Res., 35:539, 1971.

Naunton, R. F., Proctor, L., and Elpern, B. S.: The audiologic signs of ninth nerve neurinoma. Arch. Otolaryngol., 87:222, 1968.

Nelson, D. A., and Mahru, M. M.: Death following digital carotid artery occlusion. Arch. Neurol., 8:640, 1963.

Palmer, E. D.: Achalasia: response to treatment in long-term effect. Am. Practnr. Dig. Treat., 8:1595, 1957.

Palmer, R. A.: The treatment of carotid sinus syncope with propantheline. Can. Med. Assoc. J., 104:923, 1971.

Pearson, A. A.: The spinal accessory nerve in human embryos. J. Comp. Neurol., 68:243, 1938.

Pickering, G. W., Sleight, P., and Smyth, H. S.: The reflex regulation of arterial pressure during sleep in man. J. Physiol. (Lond.), 194:46P, 1968.

Quinn, J. H.: Glossodynia. J. Am. Dent. Assoc., 70:1418, 1965.

Rexed, B.: Contributions to the knowledge of the postnatal development of the peripheral nervous system in man. Acta Psychiatr. Neurol. Scand., Suppl. 33, 1944.

Rhoton, A. L., O'Leary, J. L., and Ferguson, J. P.: The trigeminal, facial, vagal and glossopharyngeal nerves in the monkey. Arch. Neurol., 14:530, 1966.

Rubinstein, M. K.: Cranial mononeuropathy as the first sign of intracranial metastases. Ann. Intern. Med., 70:49, 1969.

Scheuer, J. L.: Fibre size frequency distribution in human laryngeal nerves. J. Anat., 98:99, 1964.

Schneck, S. A.: Peripheral and cranial nerve injuries resulting from general surgical procedures. A.M.A. Arch. Surg., 81:855, 1960.

Sharpey-Schafer, E. P.: Circulatory reflexes in chronic disease of the afferent nervous system. J. Physiol. (Lond.), 134:1, 1956.

Sharpey-Schafer, E. P., and Taylor, P. J.: Absent circulatory reflexes in diabetic neuritis. Lancet, 1:559, 1960.

Smith, B.: Neuropathology of the Alimentary Tract. London, Edward Arnold [Baltimore, Williams & Wilkins Co.], 1972.

Sunderland, S., and Swaney, W. E.: The intraneural topography of the recurrent laryngeal nerve in man. Anat. Rec., 114:411, 1952.

Szentágothai, J.: Die Lokalization der Kehlkopfmuskulatur in den Vaguskernen. Z. Anat. Entwicklungsgesch., 112:704, 1943.

Thomas, J. E.: Hyperactive carotid sinus reflex and carotid sinus syncope. Mayo Clin. Proc., 44:127, 1969.

Walker, L. B., and Rajagopal, M. D.: Neuromuscular

spindles in the human tongue. Anat. Rec., *133*:438, 1959.

Watkins, P. J.: Facial sweating after food: a new sign of diabetic autonomic neuropathy. Br. Med. J., *1*:583, 1973.

Weber, E. L., and Odom, G. L.: Paradoxical response to peripheral hypoglossal nerve section. J. Neurosurg., *30*:186, 1969.

Weisenburg, T. H.: Cerebellopontile tumor diagnosed for six years as tic douloureux: the symptoms of irritation of the ninth and twelfth cranial nerves. J.A.M.A., *54*:1600, 1910.

Weiss, S., and Baker, J. P.: The carotid sinus reflex in health and disease. Medicine (Baltimore), *12*:297, 1933.

Whisler, W. W., and Voris, H. C.: Effect of bilateral glossopharyngeal nerve section on blood pressure. J. Neurosurg., *23*:79, 1965.

White, J. C., and Sweet, W. H.: Pain and the Neurosurgeon. Springfield, Ill., Charles C Thomas, 1969, p. 265.

Whitwam, J. G., Kidd, C., and Fussey, I. F.: Brain Res., *14*:756, 1969.

Widdicombe, J. G.: Regulation of tracheobronchial smooth muscle. Physiol. Rev., *43*:1, 1963.

Williams, A. F.: Recurrent laryngeal nerve and thyroid gland. J. Laryngol. Otol., *68*:719, 1954.

Williams, A. F.: Recurrent laryngeal nerve lesions during thyroidectomy. Surgery, *43*:435, 1958.

Williams, J. M., and Fox, J. L.: Neurinoma of the intracranial portion of the hypoglossal nerve. Review and case report. J. Neurosurg., *19*:248, 1962.

Williams, R. G.: Idiopathic recurrent laryngeal paralysis. J. Laryngol. Otol., *73*:161, 1959.

Windle, W. F.: The sensory component of the spinal accessory nerve. J. Comp. Neurol., *53*:115, 1931.

Wózniak, W., and Young, P. A.: Nerve cells in the extracranial portion of the hypoglossal nerve in human fetuses. Anat. Rec., *162*:517, 1968.

Yee, J., Harrison, F., and Corbin, K. B.: The sensory innervation of the spinal accessory and tongue musculature in the rabbit. J. Comp. Neurol., *70*:305, 1939.

PART C
Diseases of Spinal Cord, Spinal Roots, and Limb Girdle Plexuses

Chapter 30

MYELOPATHIES AFFECTING ANTERIOR HORN CELLS

Walter G. Bradley

The anterior horn cell, as the cell body of the lower motor neuron, has the greater portion of its axon in the peripheral nervous system. Its cell body, however, lies in the central nervous system, and the intramedullary part of the motor axon has myelin of central nervous origin (Peters, 1968; Maxwell et al., 1969; Steer, 1971). Similarly, the central part of the first sensory neuron lies in the spinal cord, and has myelin provided by neuroglia. Primary degeneration of the anterior horn cell or of the dorsal root ganglion neuron therefore results in degeneration of the parts that lie within the central nervous system, though this degeneration usually is of little significance in itself. In the reverse situation, primary damage of the central nervous system produces damage to those parts of the lower motor neurons and first sensory neurons lying within it. Recognition that the lesion in a particular patient lies within the central nervous system rather than in the more peripheral parts of the peripheral nervous system is of more than academic interest. It indicates that a significant degree of recovery cannot be expected, since from a functional point of view regeneration does not occur in structures lying within the central nervous system.

In this chapter, consideration is restricted to the spinal cord, though similar processes occur in the parts of the cranial peripheral nervous system lying within the brain stem, and deals with diagnostic features of myelopathies and with the individual diseases. A number of conditions in which combined central and peripheral nervous degeneration occurs are considered in other chapters. These include system degenerations such as Friedreich's ataxia, motor neuron disease, vitamin B_{12} deficiency, and toxic conditions. An excellent general review of spinal cord disease is given by Hughes (1966).

DIAGNOSTIC FEATURES OF SPINAL CORD DISEASE

A number of disease processes within the spinal canal may damage both the spinal cord and spinal roots. It is therefore not always easy to decide the site and level and the lesion. This problem is discussed in greater detail in Chapter 31. Diagnostic features indicating spinal cord involvement rest upon the presence of signs of upper motor neuron damage, and upon a distribution of sensory loss in keeping with the known pattern of fiber pathways within the spinal cord. At times, the involvement of other structures, particularly the nerve roots, may obscure the picture, but

628

it is usually still possible to distinguish some signs of spinal cord involvement.

Upper Motor Neuron Lesions

Signs of an established upper motor neuron lesion are well known. They consist essentially of the release of a number of primitive reflexes inhibited by the corticospinal tract and loss of a number of fine movements associated with this tract. Such signs include the increased tone due to release of the servo-loop of α and γ motor neurons, the muscle spindles, and spindle afferent fibers. Similarly, the tendon reflexes are exaggerated, and spread occurs between segments. The primitive flexor withdrawal as shown by extension of the toe in the plantar response (Babinski sign) supplants the more advanced stepping reflex with flexion of the toe in the plantar response.

Spinal cord lesions in the cervical and upper thoracic region are associated with loss of the superficial abdominal and cremasteric reflexes. In the initial stages of a spinal cord lesion all spinal cord function may be abolished. This period of "spinal shock" may last for several weeks in man. The presence of an upper level above which corticospinal tract function is normal indicates the spinal localization of the lesion, though a parasagittal cerebral lesion is always a diagnostic pitfall. There is still some argument about the exact function of the corticospinal tract (Lawrence and Kuypers, 1968a, 1968b) and of the posterior columns (Schwartzman and Bogdonoff, 1969; Wall, 1970), though the foregoing outline usually holds true from the clinical point of view.

Spinal Cord Sensory Lesions

Loss of the modalities of sensation conveyed by the large myelinated nerve fibers, viz. classically joint position and vibration sensation, may result from the death of the terminals of the largest and longest nerve fibers (the "dying back" phenomenon of Cavanagh, 1964), from degeneration of the largest dorsal root ganglion neurons, or from lesions of the posterior columns. The presence of an upper border to such sensory loss on the trunk, or of a distribution corresponding with the known lamination of fibers in the posterior columns, points to a lesion in the spinal cord. Thus the loss of these modalities in one arm and one leg, or the progressive spread of such loss from one leg to the other, occurs in such lesions as a spinal cord tumor or a plaque of demyelination. Similarly, loss of the modalities of sensation conveyed by unmyelinated and small myelinated nerve fibers, viz. pain and temperature sensation, may result from peripheral nerve damage as reported in amyloidosis by Dyck and Lambert (1969), from dorsal root ganglion degeneration as in certain hereditary neuropathies described by Denny-Brown (1951) and Turkington and Stiefel (1965), or from damage to the fibers crossing in the anterior white commissures of the spinal cord before joining the spinothalamic tract or to the spinothalamic tract itself. Involvement of the latter may be indicated by an upper boundary of the loss of these modalities of sensation, by its unilateral nature, or by a deficit consistent with the lamination of the spinothalamic tract. Thus an intrinsic spinal cord tumor classically spares the more superficial parts of the tract related to the sacral dermatomes. The loss below a certain level of posterior column modalities, together with upper motor neuron signs on one side and the loss of spinothalamic modalities on the other side, is diagnostic of a lesion of one half of the spinal cord (the Brown-Séquard syndrome).

Investigations

Physiologic investigations may sometimes be of assistance in showing that a central nervous system lesion is present. The finding of preserved sensory nerve action potentials in an area of sensory loss indicates that the lesion is proximal to the dorsal root ganglion neuron (Warren et al., 1969). Similarly the presence of a normal evoked motor action potential in a paralyzed muscle shows that the cause of the paralysis is proximal to the anterior horn cell. Depression of the normal potentiation of the H reflex by a maximum voluntary contraction, which occurs on the side of an upper motor neuron lesion, may also be helpful (Sica et al., 1972). Generally, however, the diagnosis of the cause of the neurologic deficit rests upon the direct visualization of the area indicated by the clinical signs by myelography or, if necessary, surgical exploration. This is discussed more fully in the following sections.

MYELOPATHIES AFFECTING ANTERIOR HORN CELL AND PRIMARY SENSORY NEURON

Vascular Myelopathies

ARTERIAL DISEASE

The spinal cord receives its blood supply via a plexus of arteries derived from several major feeding vessels. The plexus consists of a single anterior spinal artery, running longitudinally in the anterior fissure, and a pair of posterior spinal arteries running longitudinally in relation to the dorsal roots. All three vessels are connected by circumflex arteries, which send deep penetrating arteries into the spinal cord substance. In addition, paired anterior sulcal arteries run from the anterior spinal artery posteriorly to supply the major part of the anterocentral part of the spinal cord. The longitudinal system receives a major supply from above via a pair of vessels derived from the vertebral arteries, and a segmental supply in the thoracic and lumbar regions from each radicular artery. The latter arise from intercostal or lumbar arteries and run with the mixed spinal nerve in the intervertebral foramen. In fact the major part of the supply of the lower spinal cord is provided by one such artery (arteria magna or artery of Adamkiewicz), which has a variable origin from the lower intercostal or lumbar arteries. A relative watershed is present at about the T4 segment in the spinal cord where the major supplies from above and below meet. Infarction may occur at this watershed during prolonged hypoxia or hypotension. For additional useful reviews the reader is referred to Hughes (1966) and Henson and Parsons (1967).

Causes. Arteriosclerotic vascular disease is the commonest cause of vascular myelopathies producing either thrombosis of one of the feeding arteries or embolism of the artery by platelet aggregates or cholesterol (Hughes and Brownell, 1966; Wolman and Bradshaw, 1967). Arteriosclerotic spinal cord disease is certainly more common than was once believed (Jellinger, 1967). Retrograde perfusion of the aorta in cardiac bypass operations is particularly likely to cause cholesterol emboli (Price and Harris, 1970). Ligation of one of the major feeding vessels, such as the arteria magna in surgical operations in the renal area, or the occlusion of several vessels by an aortic dissecting aneurysm will produce extensive spinal cord infarction.

In addition, many processes to be considered later cause spinal cord damage in part at least by ischemia. Chronic meningitides such as those due to tuberculosis and fungi, meningovascular syphilis, and chronic compressive lesions such as those of cervical spondylosis fall into this category.

Clinical Features. The patient may awake with an established defect, or the defect may develop progressively, heralded by pain and dysesthesia at the level of the eventual infarct. Usually this is relatively localized, though the neurologic deficit may be extensive because of the concentration of fibers within the spinal cord. An infarct in the territory of the anterior spinal artery is the commonest lesion, with loss of spinothalamic sensation and signs of upper motor neuron damage below the level of the lesion. Involvement of anterior horn cells in a localized segmental infarct in the thoracic region is relatively insignificant, but in the cervical and lumbosacral enlargements, where there are large concentrations of anterior horn cells, a localized infarct will produce a marked deficit. For instance, an infarct of the anterior horn at the C8 to T1 level will produce paralysis and atrophy of all the small muscles of the hand on that side.

A condition akin to intermittent ischemia of the calf muscles due to peripheral vascular disease of the legs may occasionally occur when the spinal cord arterial supply is restricted but not totally abolished. This is usually the result of arteriosclerosis, though compressive lesions of the spinal cord, and even spastic parapareses of various types may at times be responsible. In this condition, first described in Dejerine's clinic, the patient progressively develops pain in the legs and neurologic symptoms of weakness, numbness, and sometimes sphincter impairment as he walks (Dejerine, 1906). The pain may last 10 or more minutes after the cessation of exercise, while typical intermittent claudication due to ischemia of the calf muscles is immediately relieved by rest. The basis of the condition may be the combination of the increased metabolic demands of the neural activity involved in walking and a limited arterial blood supply. Functional ischemia of the spinal cord thereby produces a temporary neurologic deficit as well as pain. The delayed recovery is perhaps due to both the inherently greater vulnerability of the central nervous structures compared with muscle and the much greater decrease in metabolic demand occurring when a muscle relaxes than when a neuron becomes inactive.

A syndrome superficially resembling progressive muscular atrophy in the lower limbs resulting from progressive ischemic loss of anterior horn cells has been described by Skinhøj (1954). Fieschi, Gottlieb, and de Carolis (1970) found asymptomatic spinal cord infarcts in 5 of 10 elderly arteriosclerotic patients. These infarcts were mainly in the spinal gray matter and produced damage to anterior horn cells.

Pathology. In an infarct in the territory of the anterior spinal artery most of the anterior part of the cord is damaged, including the anterior gray horns. In the cervical and lumbosacral enlargements, extensive loss of anterior horn cells results. There is also damage to the spinothalamic and corticospinal tracts, but the posterior columns are usually spared. The infarct may involve only one of the pair of anterior sulcal arteries at any level and thus be unilateral. A spinal infarct in the cervical region is usually due to vertebral artery disease, and there may be associated medullary damage.

Treatment. As in most infarcts of the central nervous system, unless there is significant recovery within the first few hours, the lesion is likely to be permanent and recovery slow and incomplete. Because edema around an infarct may perhaps cause secondary damage to otherwise healthy tissue, treatment in the acute phase with large doses of corticosteroids like dexamethasone may be beneficial. In intermittent ischemia of the spinal cord, glyceryl trinitrate may occasionally be of benefit, though usually the patient becomes progressively more incapacitated by the advancing disease despite treatment.

VENOUS DISEASE

Venous infarcts of the spinal cord affect predominantly the posterior and central parts, the lesions lying in the posterior white columns and central gray matter (Hughes, 1966, 1971; Henson and Parsons, 1967). The hemorrhagic infarct may extend over many segments. Anterior horn cell damage is relatively slight, the clinical signs being mainly paraplegia and loss of posterior column sensation.

ARTERIOVENOUS MALFORMATIONS

The spinal cord may occasionally be the site of an angioma or arteriovenous malformation. This may remain symptomless throughout life, but on the other hand may be responsible for catastrophic spinal cord damage as a result either of infarction resulting from thrombosis of one of the major feeding vessels or of hemorrhage into the cord. Alternatively it may produce a state of chronic ischemia of the spinal cord thereby leading to the problems outlined in the discussion of arterial myelopathies. Rarely, enlargement of the mass of blood vessels may produce a compressive effect on the spinal cord as is described later.

Pathology. The structure of the spinal cord angioma or arteriovenous malformation is very similar to that in other sites. It consists of large blood vessels, some of which are thick-walled while others are abnormally thin-walled. Blood passes directly through them from artery to vein, and may therefore be "stolen" from the spinal cord, producing all the pathologic changes of ischemia.

Clinical Features. The most common presentation is with an insidiously progressive picture of spinal cord damage that may have a stuttering course related to minor additional infarcts or hemorrhages. These anomalies were comprehensively reviewed by Djindjian, Hurth, and Houdart (1969). Since the angioma is frequently extensive, the number of segments involved, particularly in terms of anterior horn cell damage, is often large. All parts of the cord may be damaged, depending upon the position of the malformation. Another presentation is with the sudden onset of a spinal cord lesion that may be difficult to distinguish from an infarct due to arteriosclerosis, or from transverse myelitis. A bruit over the spine is a useful but rare sign.

Investigation. These malformations may be seen on the myelogram as a series of sinusoidal filling defects, often with evidence of enlarged vessels on the adjacent roots. They may most elegantly be demonstrated by selective spinal cord angiography (Djindjian and Houdart, 1970).

Treatment. In some cases the malformation may be totally or partly removed without producing an increased neurologic deficit, though always there is the risk of producing infarction of the underlying cord. When the damage is already profound, nothing is to be gained by operating, but when the picture is slowly progressive then surgery stands a chance of preventing further deterioration. Radiotherapy has been used to thrombose the malformation, though radiation myelopathy (discussed later) and spinal cord infarction are hazards of this form of treatment.

SUBACUTE NECROTIZING MYELITIS OF FOIX AND ALAJOUANINE

In 1926, Foix and Alajouanine described in detail two patients suffering from paraplegia that gradually ascended from the lumbar to the cervical region, was at first spastic but later became flaccid, and was associated with marked muscular atrophy and the later development of sensory loss. Since that time a number of similar cases have been reported. The course is usually insidious, with death in one to two years. More males than females are affected, and the condition is more common in the older age groups and is often associated with cor pulmonale (Wirth et al., 1970; Gillilan, 1970; Hughes, 1971). The spinal cord in these cases showed ischemic necrosis, and all have remarked on the prominent thick-walled extramedullary and intramedullary veins usually affected with thrombophlebitis. Many now feel that this condition results from an underlying arteriovenous malformation (Wirth et al., 1970). Some, however, consider it to be the result of progressive spinal thrombophlebitis (Blackwood, 1963).

Traumatic Myelopathies

ACUTE INJURIES

The spinal cord may be injured in fractures of the spine or in penetrating injuries (Brock, 1960). Such lesions produce localized partial or complete transection with its accompanying neurologic deficit. The anterior horn cell damage is usually localized to one or two segments, and may be insignificant unless the lesion is in either the cervical or lumbar enlargements. The clinical picture and prognosis depend entirely upon the extent of the damage. Frequently following the injury, edema of the surrounding cord leads to ischemia and enlargement of the area of damage. Decompression by laminectomy, which was once advocated, has been replaced by high-dosage corticosteroid therapy. An acute intervertebral disk prolapse may result

from the trauma, particularly in the cervical region. The picture here is one of spinal cord compression and is considered later.

HEMATOMYELIA

A few patients with acute spinal trauma develop a central cord hematoma rather than focal transection. The clinical deficit is similar to that in syringomyelia, which is discussed later.

Pathology. The hemorrhage within the central part of the spinal cord usually ascends from the site of the lesion, in a path similar to that of the syrinx in syringomyelia. This has at times given rise to argument whether there was an underlying previously symptomless syrinx or angioma in that area (Perot et al., 1966).

Treatment. Symptomatic treatment is all that is indicated. The central cord tissue has been destroyed by the hemorrhage, and little recovery can be expected.

LATE EFFECTS

A late effect of spinal cord trauma, which may cause confusion, is the progressive central cavitation that may develop a number of years after the paraplegia. The patient, whose condition had previously been stable, develops pain and a gradually ascending deficit similar to syringomyelia with wasting, loss of reflexes, and a level of loss of pain and temperature sensation. The spinal cord shows a central necrotic cavity with surrounding ischemic change ascending from the level of the cord destruction, sometimes for six or more segments (Zellinger, 1964; Barnett et al., 1966). The cause is uncertain; perhaps chronic compression or local arachnoiditis at the site of the original lesion impairs the vascular supply, either arterial or venous, above the original level and produces central cord infarction and cyst formation. Surgical decompression of the "syrinx" has been advocated (Rossier et al., 1968).

Cervical spondylotic myelopathy is considered in a following section.

Compressive Myelopathies

The spinal cord may be damaged by compression from without. The effects of trauma have already been mentioned; in addition a number of other processes commencing either extradurally or between the dura and the spinal cord may chronically press upon the cord. Usually the nerve roots are also compressed, causing pain and sensory and motor loss in a radicular distribution (see Chapter 31). With a neurofibroma of a nerve root radicular symptoms and signs are likely to occur early (Russell and Rubinstein, 1963). The most common extradural compressive lesion is a secondary carcinoma (Brice and McKissock, 1965). Other conditions include a chordoma, which arises from notochordal rests, particularly in the sacral region but also at other levels (Kamrin et al., 1964); an acute or chronic intervertebral disk protrusion; an extradural reticulosis; an extradural or subdural abscess, which is usually caused by *Staphylococcus aureus* (Hirson, 1965); and granulation tissue from spinal tuberculosis (Pott's paraplegia). Extramedullary hematopoietic tissue in thalassemia may produce cord compression. Chronic disk degeneration in the cervical region is described later. In the thoracic region, a single chronic disk protrusion may cause spinal cord compression many years after the initial injury (Carson et al., 1971). Calcification of the disk space is often seen in such cases, but only calcification of the chronically prolapsed disk material lying within the spinal canal is diagnostic of the condition.

Intradural extramedullary cord compression is not as common as extradural compression. It may be caused by meningiomas, which are most common in the thoracic region, in females, and in middle life (Russell and Rubinstein, 1963). Other causes are arachnoid cysts, lipomas, and dermoid cysts, which are usually found in the lumbosacral areas but may at times press upon the conus medullaris (James and Lassman, 1972).

Pathology. The changes in the spinal cord are related both to displacement and to ischemia (Tarlov, 1957). The proportion of these two depends upon the size, distribution, nature, and rate of enlargement of the underlying lesion. When there is rapid development, as in acute disk prolapse, the former predominates. When there is slowly increasing compression, extensive displacement and thinning of the cord are combined with the effects of ischemia. When there is inflammation, as in an extradural abscess, endarteritic infarction may be the major process.

Clinical Features. Cord compression injures the spinal tracts, producing upper motor neuron damage and sensory loss gradually ascending from the lower limbs to the level of the compression. Anterior horn cells are damaged by both direct pressure and ischemia. If the lesion is at the level of the cervical or lumbosacral enlargement, the resultant amyotrophy may be extensive. Bladder involvement occurs relatively later than with intramedullary lesions.

Investigation. Radiology and surgical exploration are the most helpful methods of investigation. Plain radiographs of the spine may show vertebral erosion or collapse due to carcinomatous metastases, or widening of the spinal canal with thinning of the pedicles from a slow-growing tumor. An enlarged intervertebral foramen with an extraspinal mass indicates a neurofibroma of the nerve root. Myelography will help define the level and will indicate whether the mass is extradural or intradural and extramedullary (Banna and Gryspeerdt, 1971).

Treatment. Usually the treatment of choice is surgical decompression. Occasionally medical decompression is possible. Thus in Pott's paraplegia chemotherapy may be effective; in thalassemia blood transfusion may suppress the hematopoietic tissue; and in extradural reticuloses radiotherapy may be used.

Spinal Cord Tumors

Intrinsic tumors of the spinal cord are usually primary and of glial origin; secondary deposits are rare. Ependymomas are twice as frequent as astrocytomas (Slooff et al., 1964). Both are relatively slow-growing tumors and may involve many cord segments.

Clinical Features. The patient presents with a slowly developing picture of spinal cord damage affecting white matter more than gray. Damage to the long spinal tracts causes spastic paraparesis and spinal cord sensory loss, as already described, and early bladder involvement. There is frequently areflexia at he level of the tumor owing to dorsal horn damage. Amyotrophy is insignificant in dorsal tumors, but may be marked when the lumbar or cervical enlargements are damaged. Astrocytomas frequently infiltrate rather than destroy the gray matter, and amyotrophy may be slight with this tumor. Pain from radicular or vertebral compression may be a feature. When the tumor is in the central area of the spinal cord the clinical picture may be indistinguishable from syringomyelia.

Pathology. The spinal cord is enlarged. This may compress the normal cord tissue within the narrow spinal canal, leading to ischemic damage. Ependymomas are often centrally placed, thereby damaging anterior horn cells early. Astrocytomas usually infiltrate diffusely and cause less anterior horn cell damage, though they are sometimes associated with a cyst containing yellow proteinaceous fluid. Histologic examination permits the nature of the tumor to be recognized clearly (Russell and Rubinstein, 1963).

Treatment. Surgery should be undertaken to exclude extramedullary lesions, since myelography may at times be misleading. A partial removal of an intrinsic tumor is sometimes possible; ependymomas may "shell out" from the cord. Even a biopsy may increase the neurologic deficit, however, though it aids the prognosis concerning rate of growth and radiosensitivity. Ependymomas are more radiosensitive, and a full course of x-ray therapy is indicated.

Cervical Spondylotic Myelopathy

The normal spinal canal and intervertebral foramina, as well as the spinal cord and roots, undergo considerable changes in dimensions with movement of the neck. In a study of the normal cervical spinal canal, Breig (1960) and Breig and El-Nadi (1966) showed that movement from flexion to extension shortened the posterior dimension of the cervical spinal canal by 4.2 cm and the anterior contour of the canal by 0.9 cm. At the same time, the cervical spinal cord shortens during extension, becomes consequently thicker, and moves forward in the spinal canal. These movements have been confirmed by Adams and Logue (1971a, 1971b).

Degenerative disease of the cervical spine is almost universal after the age of 60 years, particularly in the male and in those whose occupation involves a great deal of neck movement, head and neck trauma, or the carrying of weights on the head (Irvine et al., 1965). This degenerative disease comes into the category of osteoarthritis (perhaps better termed osteoarthrosis), but is usually described as cervical spondylosis. The brunt of the disease falls upon the intervertebral disks and the zygoapophyseal joints (Brain and Wilkinson, 1967). The intervertebral disk becomes narrower in the axial direction, and splayed

in the anteroposterior direction. The parts of the disks that splay outside the limits of the vertebral bodies become ossified as osteophytes, the posterior of which impinge upon the lumen of the cervical canal. Similar osteophytes impinge upon the intervertebral foramina, compromising the mixed spinal nerve lying therein. The overall shortening of the cervical canal leads to buckling of the ligamenta flava posterior to the spinal canal. Both the osteophytes and buckled ligamenta flava compromise the cervical canal. Thus in the patient with marked cervical spondylosis, any movement of the neck away from the midposition is potentially hazardous. Extension of the neck makes the cord shorten and become thicker, while the increased buckling of the ligamenta flava thrusts it forward against the anterior osteophytic bars. Flexion pulls the cord forward, angulating it over the osteophytic bars. Both maneuvers therefore apply mechanical trauma to the cervical cord. In addition, extension narrows the intervertebral foramina, compressing not only the spinal nerves but also the radicular arteries supplying the spinal cord.

As might be expected, patients born with an unusually narrow spinal canal are inherently more susceptible to the compromising effects of cervical spondylosis. Cervical spondylotic myelopathy is mainly seen in those with congenitally narrow spinal canals (less than 14 mm anteroposterior diameter) (Pallis, Jones, and Spillane, 1954; Payne and Spillane, 1957; Burrows, 1963). The spinal cord in the midcervical region has an anteroposterior diameter of about 10 mm; an osteophytic bar of 2 to 3 mm, combined with buckling of the ligamenta flava, may reduce the canal to 8 or 9 mm diameter, markedly compressing the spinal cord. Flexion and extension, particularly if they are acute and excessive as in whiplash injuries, may produce disastrous damage.

The most common sites of spondylotic degeneration are at the C4–C5 and C5–C6 interspaces; changes at C3–C4 and C6–C7 are next in frequency, marked degeneration at other levels being relatively less frequent (Brain and Wilkinson, 1967).

For full reviews of the mechanics of the normal and the diseased cervical spine and the clinical effects of pathologic changes the reader is referred to Breig (1960), Breig and El-Nadi (1966), Hughes (1966), Brain and Wilkinson (1967), Walz (1967), Wilkinson (1971), and Adams and Logue (1971a, 1971b).

Pathology. At autopsy, the spinal cord of the patient with cervical spondylotic myelopathy is found to be grossly flattened and indented anteriorly by osteophytes and posteriorly by bulging ligamenta flava (Hughes, 1966). Laminectomy on similar patients demonstrates similar indentation of the cord, which is therefore not an artifact of death. Throughout the cervical part of the spinal cord there is atrophy resulting from loss of axons and, to a lesser extent, of gray matter. Above and below the C3 to C6 area, tract degeneration is usually apparent, that of the corticospinal tract being from C5 downward and that of the posterior columns and anterior and lateral spinothalamic tracts from C5 upward.

The anterior gray horns frequently show severe damage with atrophy and gliosis. There may be physical disruption of the gray matter with cavitation, but more commonly the overall structure is preserved though anterior horn cells are damaged (Hughes, 1966; Brain and Wilkinson, 1967). Signs of active degeneration of anterior horn cells with pyknosis and neuronophagia are relatively uncommon, though chromatolysis from radicular damage may be seen. A reactive arachnoiditis is common at the level of the major compression.

The pathogenesis of these changes has excited considerable discussion. The simplest explanation is that the spinal cord is compressed, particularly during movement, with consequent damage. The clinical pattern of stepwise deterioration, however, suggests a possible vascular etiology. This argument has been strongly advanced by Mair and Druckman (1953) and Taylor (1964) to explain both the clinical pattern and the fact that at operation the cord is often not apparently severely compressed and the damage is predominantly in the anterior spinal artery territory. Compression of the anterior spinal artery against osteophytes and of the radicular arteries in the intervertebral foramina has been supposed to be responsible for the ischemia. As explained later, the exact pathogenesis of the myelopathy in cervical spondylosis is of great importance in deciding the correct therapy.

Clinical Features. Patients with cervical spondylosis frequently have no symptoms whatsoever, though a history of neck pain, creaking, and radicular pain is not infrequent (Irvine et al., 1965). A few patients, however, develop significant neurologic disease, either myelopathy or radiculopathy, or vertebrobasilar ischemia from compression of the vertebral arteries in the canal within the transverse processes of the vertebrae.

The commonest presentation of cervical spondylosis, after the radiculopathies described in Chapter 31, is as a progressive myelopathy (Brain and Wilkinson, 1967). Sometimes this is shown by relatively pure spastic paraparesis with little or no sensory change. More often, however, there are signs suggesting impairment of one or more cervical nerves or nerve roots, combined with the spastic paraparesis. Wasting and weakness of certain of the muscles supplied by the cervical roots, together with loss of reflexes, may be due to damage to both the anterior horn cells and the motor roots, and it is often not easy to separate the two.

A very typical story is of a patient who complains of stiffness in one leg and who is found to have asymmetrical spastic paraparesis with bilateral Babinski signs and slight weakness of the biceps and brachioradialis muscles. The biceps reflex is absent, and the brachioradialis reflex inverted (viz., there is loss of the C5 and C6 brachioradialis reflex with spread to the C7 and C8 finger flexor reflex owing to myelopathy at C5). Lesions at other levels affect the appropriate muscles and reflexes. Isolated wasting of the small muscles of the hands is rarely due to cervical spondylosis since degenerative vertebral changes are rare at C7 and T1, and almost unknown at T1 and T2. When wasting of the small muscles of the hands is ascribed to this condition, the diagnosis is usually incorrect.

The myelopathy usually progresses in a stepwise manner with relatively rapid deterioration followed by a plateau during which symptoms often improve, though the signs remain relatively unchanged (Lees and Turner, 1963). There is then a further deterioration and plateau. This variable course and the variation between patients make it difficult to arrive at conclusions about the best form of treatment.

Investigations. Plain x-rays of the cervical spine, taken in the posteroanterior and lateral position, with flexion and extension in the latter, and oblique views to delineate the intervertebral foramina, are required to show the extent of the spondylosis. Myelography, both prone and supine, with the head in flexion and extension, will demonstrate the extent of compromise of the spinal canal and spinal cord by the degenerative changes

(Young, 1967). Electromyography, searching for the changes of denervation, may be of help in defining the roots and anterior horns involved.

Treatment. Attempts to treat the cervical spondylotic myelopathy have proceeded along logical lines, though the result has not always been what might be expected. The neck and arm pain of cervical spondylosis is usually relieved by immobilization of the neck in a cervical collar or by traction (see Chapter 31). These methods have been applied to treatment of cervical spondylotic myelopathy, with improvement in about a third of the patients, no change in a third, and continued deterioration in a third (Roberts, 1966). Since many such patients are seen by neuro-surgeons, and have definite compression or compromise of the spinal cord, posterior laminectomy has often been performed (Northfield, 1955; Bradshaw, 1957; Northfield and Osmond-Clarke, 1967; Symon and Lavender, 1967; Bishara, 1971). The overall result of many series is that about half the patients are improved, the remainder being unaffected or occasionally being severely worsened by the operation. Removal of laminae, when the spinal cord is compressed, may at times be hazardous for the cord. Many other operations have been devised, including anterior operations to remove the disk and osteophyte and fuse the vertebrae, and foraminotomies to decompress the nerve roots and radicular arteries. Insufficient series have been reported to assess the outcome of these newer operations clearly.

To be set against these reports indicating "improvement" with a particular form of treatment is the report of the natural history of cervical spondylosis by Lees and Turner (1963). The stepwise progression, arrest, and frequent symptomatic improvement is similar to that for many patients receiving either medical or surgical treatment. If the major pathologic process is ischemia, then such treatments are really only prophylactic. A carefully controlled trial of treatment in this condition is urgently required.

Myelopathies Due to Meningitis and Arachnoiditis

As previously indicated, many conditions within the spinal subarachnoid space may produce arachnoiditis or meningitis that damages the spinal cord, although the spinal roots are usually involved to a greater extent. The cord damage may extend over many segments, and the consequent mainly ischemic anterior horn cell damage and amyotrophy may be extensive.

The list of such conditions is long (Lombardi et al., 1962). Any meningitis if present for more than a few days may produce endarteritis of the blood vessels of the cord, causing infarction. Tuberculosis and fungal infections such as cryptococcosis should be particularly considered, though a low-grade or inadequately treated acute infection such as pneumococcal meningitis may also be responsible. Meningovascular syphilis causes an inflammatory arachnoiditis of the cord and roots and endarteritic infarction.

The injection of any toxic substance into the spinal subarachnoid space will damage the cord. Penicillin may produce profound necrosis of the cord if the dose is accidentally of the order of 500,000 I.U. Phenol and alcohol, which are used to damage the spinal roots to control intractable pain or flexion spasm in the lower limbs, as described in Chapter 31, may cause myelopathy if allowed to impinge upon the cord. A number of dis-stressing outbreaks of radiculomyelopathy or arachnoiditis have probably resulted from contamination of spinal anesthetics with detergents or preservatives (Winkleman et al., 1953; Hurst, 1955). Myelography for the demonstration of intraspinal disease has had a checkered history in this respect. One substance originally used was thorium dioxide, which was taken up by macrophages and remained for many years within the spinal subarachnoid space. The radioactive emissions of the thorium have been responsible for a number of cases of chronic radiculo-myelopathy (Dale and Love, 1967). Lipiodol, which was later used quite frequently, produced irritative reactions, sometimes followed by permanent damage. A rare group of conditions, the uveomeningoencephalitic syndromes, which include sarcoidosis, Behçet's disease, and the Vogt-Koyanagi-Harada syndrome, produces an ischemic and inflammatory myelopathy (Reed et al., 1958; Pattison, 1965; Riehl and Andrews, 1966). The co-existing presence of uveitis and central nervous system damage gives the clue to these conditions.

When all these causes of arachnoidal inflammation have been excluded, a number of cases remain to which the term "idiopathic adhesive spinal arachnoiditis" is given. The myelographic picture is characteristic, with pocketing of the contrast medium and arrest of the free flow by adhesions within the subarachnoid space. Radiotherapy and the surgical removal of adhesions have been advocated (Feder and Smith, 1962; Teng and Papatheodorou, 1967), though usually there is little effect or the patient is worsened by these procedures. The intrathecal and systemic administration of corticosteroids may be of value. Full investigation to the stage of surgical inspection and biopsy are always worthwhile, since in occasional cases a treatable cause may be found (Davidson, 1968).

Plaques of white calcified tissue arising in the arachnoid and attached to the spinal cord, frequently found at operation and at autopsy, are usually without symptoms. They probably result from simple degeneration of the arachnoid cells with secondary calcification. Occasionally this progresses to bone formation, and at times a myelopathy has been ascribed to them (Wise and Smith, 1965; Nizzoli and Testa, 1968).

Syringomyelia and Hydromyelia

Clinical Features. In an advanced case of syringomyelia, the myelopathy is extensive and the neurologic deficit characteristic (Barnett et al., 1973). There are signs of damage to the central part of the spinal cord with anterior horn cell degeneration producing extensive amyotrophy, damage to the crossing fibers of the secondary sensory neuron in the anterior white commissures producing the characteristic loss of pain and temperature sensation with an upper and lower border (suspended dissociated sensory loss), together with some degree of corticospinal tract damage. The sensory and lower motor neuron deficit is usually maximal in the upper limbs. Occasionally, wasting of the small muscles of the hands may be the sole deficit for a number of years.

Pathology. A large central sac, containing fluid of the same constitution as cerebrospinal fluid, is present in the spinal cord. This sac or syrinx was originally thought to be a degenerative cyst with surrounding, perhaps aberrant, glial tissue. The analogy was drawn to a similar cystic degeneration of a spinal cord astrocytoma causing a comparable picture (secondary syringomyelia). The astrocytoma cyst fluid is, however, yellow from its high protein content, and thus differs from that in syringomyelia.

Following the recognition that many such cases have an abnormality of the craniocervical junction, particularly the Chiari abnormality with prolapsed cerebellar tonsils, it became recognized that most syrinxes were lined with remnants of the ependyma (Gardner et al., 1957; Gardner and Angel, 1958; Appleby et al., 1968). They thus probably arise by dilatation of and the formation of diverticulae from a dilated central canal. For this reason hydromyelia is the term preferred by some. The exact mechanism of the formation of this hydromyelic cavity is still not clear, but it is suggested that some degree of obstruction of the foramen magnum is caused by the low brain stem and cerebellar tonsils, which impede the outflow of cerebrospinal fluid from the fourth ventricle. There may be outflow obstruction to the bulk of cerebrospinal fluid, or more likely to pressure waves passing from the ventricle and the cranium into the spinal canal (Gardner, 1965; Williams, 1969, 1970; Ellertsson and Greitz, 1970). The cerebrospinal fluid is thus forced down the spinal central canal, causing the dilatation. The finding of syringomyelia in patients with meningiomas, arachnoiditis, and other lesions of the foramen magnum region adds weight to this theory (Kosary et al., 1969; Appleby et al., 1969).

Investigation. Plain radiographs often show the cervical canal to be enlarged over its whole length from long-standing expansion of the spinal cord. Myelography will confirm this diffuse swelling of the spinal cord, especially in the cervical region. Supine myelography is the crucial investigation, showing a variety of abnormalities of the foramen magnum. In the Chiari abnormality, the tip of the cerebellar tonsils may lie as low as the second or third cervical vertebra. These changes are seen in about 90 per cent of patients with syringomyelia (Barnett et al., 1973).

Treatment. Originally little was available in the way of therapy. The chronic pain sometimes required medullary tractotomy or prefrontal leukotomy. Radiotherapy was given with the object of suppressing the supposed hypersecretion of fluid and the aberrant glia believed to underlie the process, and at times was effective in reducing the pain. Surgical decompression of the spinal canal was at times attempted without much benefit. Puncture and various drainage procedures of the cyst were, however, occasionally effective in altering the progress of the condition.

With the recognition of the importance of craniocervical abnormalities, surgical decompression of this region was undertaken (Gardner, 1965; Appleby et al., 1968). If the cerebellar tonsils are herniated, removal of the arch of the atlas and posterior lip of the foramen magnum appears sufficient to relieve the condition. Only when there is indication of posterior fossa arachnoiditis is decompression contraindicated (Appleby et al., 1969).

Dysrhaphism

The spinal cord is formed by rolling of the neural plate into a neural tube. Various congenital defects, ranging in severity from a defect in the laminae of one vertebra to anencephaly, may arise from impairment of this process. In the spine, the most common major lesion is spina bifida cystica, with failure of closure in the lumbosacral region producing either a simple meningocele or a myelomeningocele in which the spinal cord also is involved (Nash, 1968). The nerve roots are also frequently damaged in the process. There may be no neurologic deficit with a simple meningocele, but with a myelomeningocele the deficit may extend to total loss of lower spinal cord function with anesthesia, lower motor neuron paralysis, and total loss of sphincter control. Infection frequently enters the neural defect, causing meningitis and hydrocephalus, and many such babies die soon after birth. Heroic measures have been made in the past to salvage such children with early closure of the defect, the construction of ileal bladders, insertions of shunts to relieve the hydrocephalus, and the application of all appliances and help required for the life of a paraplegic. Ethical problems arise as to whether the quality of life is worth the pain and disabilities and the great expenditure of medical and surgical resources (Lightowler, 1971).

Less overt defects of closure of the neural tube are termed spina bifida occulta (James and Lassman, 1960, 1962, 1972; Lassman and James, 1964). Here there are a variety of abnormalities that may damage the spinal cord and cauda equina, including the dermoid cysts and lipomas described earlier, various

lesions causing tethering of and traction on the conus of the spinal cord, and diastematomyelia. In the latter the spinal cord is divided by a fibrous or bony septum, frequently in the midthoracic region. This may remain asymptomatic until growth, attempting to produce upward movement of the spinal cord within the spinal canal, causes pressure of the spur on the lower part of the bifurcation of the cord. This may damage both the anterior horn cells and other parts of the cord and produce a wide range of neurologic deficit. Deficient growth and wasting of one leg, progressive equinovarus deformities of the foot, trophic ulceration from anesthesia produced by the lesion, and incontinence are common sequelae (James and Lassman, 1964). In all cases in which spina bifida occulta is suspected, plain radiographs and myelography will help to resolve the diagnosis, and to decide whether surgical intervention should be undertaken.

Virus-Induced Spinal Cord Damage

Three neurotropic viruses in particular must be considered in a review of diseases affecting the anterior horn cell, namely those of poliomyelitis, rabies, and herpes zoster. In addition ECHO and Coxsackie viruses may rarely be responsible for an attack of lower motor neuron paralysis that is indistinguishable from acute poliomyelitis. Many other viruses, including those of mumps, measles, vaccinia, and varicella, may induce postinfectious encephalomyelitis. The predominant pathologic change in this is disseminated demyelination with little neuronal damage.

POLIOMYELITIS

This disease, until recently the scourge of all countries, has almost disappeared in immunized populations following the introduction of effective vaccines (Paul, 1971). It is due to one of the enteroviruses, and three distinct strains have been recognized. Type 1 (Brunhilde) is the most common, and like type 3 (Leon) causes severe paralytic disease; type 2 (Lansing) is pathogenic for rodents, but may cause a milder disease in man. Infection is transmitted by fecal contamination of hands or food, the latter either as a result of faulty sanitation, inadequate hygiene, or transmission of the virus by houseflies.

In poorer countries, prior to the development of effective immunization, the incidence of paralytic poliomyelitis was lower than in developed countries. This was probably because the infection was acquired in early infancy in such poor countries, at a time when the child was still partly protected by antibodies received from the mother; in more developed countries, exposure frequently did not occur until the second or third decade, when the full paralytic effect of the virus manifested itself (Paul et al., 1952). Poliomyelitis therefore tended to produce disastrous paralysis in juveniles and young adults, and frequently occurred in epidemics.

Studies of the development of antibodies against the prevalent virus strain showed that more than 100 persons became infected with the virus for every one who developed symptoms (Melnick and Ledinko, 1953). Of those who developed symptoms, only a proportion, varying from 30 to 60 per cent in different epidemics, developed paralysis. The remainder had a nonparalytic illness, which might be either diarrhea or a pyrexial episode. It was possible to isolate the responsible virus from both symptomatic and asymptomatic persons. Pharyngeal secretions contained the virus in the first few days of symptoms, while virus could be isolated from the feces of both symptomatic and asymptomatic persons for three or more weeks. This, combined with the fact that nasal instillation of virus induced the disease in monkeys, led to the belief that the virus entered the nervous system via the olfactory nerves. Only when a transient viremia was demonstrated in the preparalytic phase was it realized that infection of the nervous system occurred via the blood (Horstmann et al., 1954). For those interested in the historical developments of ideas of the etiology and pathogenesis of poliomyelitis, Paul (1971) provides a full account. Russell (1956), Van Bogaert (1958), and Bodian (1959) have fully reviewed the clinical and pathologic aspects of this now very fully understood disease.

Poliomyelitis is an acute monophasic illness, producing rapid paralysis in those affected, with later at least partial or sometimes complete recovery. The possibility has been advanced, however, that the virus may remain in previously infected anterior horn cells, in the form of a "slow virus," later to become activated and cause delayed cell death. This suggestion derives from the finding that the incidence of previous attacks of poliomyelitis is greater in patients with motor neuron disease than in the general population (Campbell et al., 1969). The increased branching of motor nerve fibers in patients who have suffered an attack of paralytic poliomyelitis may, however, put an added strain on the protein synthetic machinery of the perikarya, which subserves axoplasmic flow, and thereby predispose to metabolic failure, with delayed cell death.

Clinical Features. The full illness shows two phases (Russell, 1956). The preparalytic "minor illness" consists of fever, malaise, headache, and some gastrointestinal disturbance, which may last for one or two days. This phase is associated with the viremia (Horstmann et al., 1954). This is followed by a temporary improvement for two to five days during which the patient may be perfectly well before the development of the "major illness," with fever and severe headache, pain in the back and limbs, neck stiffness, and at times delirium. The cerebrospinal fluid white cell count may reach to 250 per cubic millimeter, the cells being both polymorphs and lymphocytes early in the illness, and lymphocytes later. The protein concentration rises in the second week to about 200 mg per 100 ml. In 30 to 60 per cent of cases developing the "major illness," paralysis develops, heralded by widespread fasciculation, and may be asymmetrical and focal. Paralysis appears on the first to the fifth day of the "major illness," and progresses for one to three days. In mild cases improvement may appear within a week, but in a few severe cases the first signs of recovery may not be seen for a month. Physical exertion during the early phase of the "major illness" leads to a gross increase in the severity of paralysis. Paralysis is accompanied by rapid wasting of the involved muscles, which show classic denervation atrophy. The bulbar and respiratory musculature is frequently involved owing to invasion of the brain stem and phrenic and thoracic motor neurons by the virus, and without special treatment the patient will die. The disease is almost entirely restricted to the lower motor neuron, but rarely the inflammatory reaction and edema resulting from widespread neuronal involvement may lead to more diffuse damage of the spinal cord with some signs of sensory disturbance. Recovery of function may begin within one to three weeks after the peak of paralysis and continue for several years.

Recovery is partly due to restoration of function of neurons that are not irreversibly damaged, and partly due to the reinnervation of denervated muscle fibers by collateral sprouting from surviving axons.

Pathology. The primary change is damage to the neurons with nuclear pyknosis, cytolysis, and neuronophagia. Less severely damaged neurons show chromatolysis. Infiltration of gray matter with microglial cells and proliferation of astrocytes are prominent. Engorgement of blood vessels is widespread, and there are often hemorrhage in the surrounding gray matter and perivascular inflammatory cell infiltrates. The anterior roots and peripheral nerves show consequent axonal degeneration and loss, and the skeletal muscle undergoes profound denervation atrophy. When some degree of recovery occurs, marked enlargement of the motor units within the muscles develops owing to branching of the motor nerve fibers.

In man, an inflammatory reaction remains in the spinal cord for several weeks. In man and the monkey, Bodian (1949) showed that up to a third of the motor neurons in a nucleus may be destroyed without there being detectable weakness. In severe cases of paralysis, more than two thirds of the cells may be lost.

Treatment. The important form of treatment is prophylaxis, for once the disease is established only symptomatic therapy is possible. Two major classes of vaccine have been developed (Paul, 1971). Those derived from killed virus (Salk and British vaccines), which must be injected, have largely been replaced by oral live attenuated virus (Sabin vaccine). The latter has the advantage of convenience of administration as well as the theoretical advantage of the production of specific intestinal mucosal cell immunity. There is no evidence of reversion of the attenuated virus to the wild type, nor of significant passage from person to person. All children should receive this vaccine in early childhood as part of their routine immunization.

Treatment of the established case involves isolation, symptomatic analgesics, treatment of the fever, and passive movements of the affected limbs (Russell, 1956). When there are respiratory and bulbar symptoms, artificial respiration and tracheostomy are required. There is still a small number of individuals in the world living with the help of respirators following previous outbreaks of poliomyelitis.

RABIES

Rabies is an endemic disease of carnivores, particularly dogs, wolves, and vampire bats. The virus resides in the salivary glands; it is transmitted by biting and, in man, may produce fatal encephalomyelitis. There is evidence that the virus reaches the nervous system by retrograde passage along the axons from the site of the wound to the spinal cord and thence to the brain, since the incubation period for the development of the encephalitis is longer the further from the brain the bite happens to be.

Clinical Features. The interval between the bite and the appearance of the symptoms varies from 25 to 70 days, depending on the proximity to the head. Local changes at the bite give no indication of whether rabies virus has been inoculated or not, and during the latent period there are no symptoms. In the typical disease, the first generalized symptom is depression and sleeplessness, followed by the development first of painful pharyngeal spasms. These rapidly spread to involve all muscles of swallowing and respiration, and later the whole skeletal musculature. They are induced by any sound, and particularly by attempts to or even the thought of drinking, which is why the disease is termed "hydrophobia." Death is usually due to dehydration, pneumonia, or exhaustion. In a few cases the changes are confined to the spinal cord with consequent lower motor neuron paralysis.

Pathology. The damage is widespread throughout the central nervous system and also involves the dorsal root and sympathetic ganglia and peripheral nerves (Hurst and Pawan, 1931, 1932; Sükrü-Aksel, 1958; Tangchai and Vejjajiva, 1971). Endothelial damage, necrosis of the nervous tissue, and extensive inflammatory cell infiltration occur. Neurons throughout the central nervous system develop characteristic Negri bodies, eosinophilic round inclusions 5 to 10 μm in diameter containing basophilic granules. There are also extensive neuronophagia and glial proliferation. In the spinal cord the anterior and posterior horns are equally affected.

Investigations. In the countries where the

disease is endemic, every effort should be made to catch the animal that has bitten a person, to observe whether it develops signs of rabies, and to examine the central nervous system for evidence of the virus.

Treatment. In most cases, despite symptomatic measures, rabies proves fatal. Only rare patients survive (Hattwick et al., 1972). Immunization with a vaccine prepared from the nervous system of rabid rabbits has been available for many years, but unfortunately the presence of the foreign brain protein causes a relatively high rate of incidence of allergic encephalomyelitis in patients who receive it. A vaccine derived from virus grown on duck embryos has proved to be neither effective nor totally free of risk, and current efforts are being devoted to produce a vaccine by growing the virus in tissue culture (*Lancet*, 1972). Moreover, unless immunization is undertaken very early in the incubation period it is ineffective.

As a result of the control of wild life populations and the eradication of infected animals, rabies has become rare in Western Europe. Great Britain has eliminated the disease by strict quarantine regulations governing the importation of any potentially infected animal.

HERPES ZOSTER

Shingles is primarily a disease of dorsal root ganglia caused by the varicella virus, with inflammation, hemorrhage and infarction. Herpes zoster appears to be due to reactivation of the varicella virus that has lain dormant in the dorsal root ganglion neurons since childhood infection with chickenpox. It is particularly common in older people and in those with a debilitating condition such as Hodgkin's disease.

Though the major damage is in the dorsal root ganglion, in many cases the disease spreads to the same segment of the spinal cord, with inflammation mainly in the posterior and anterior horns and some degree of destruction of the anterior horn cells with consequent lower motor neuron paralysis (*British Medical Journal*, 1970). In the abdominal wall, this may be seen as an area of paradoxical movement of the muscles. Long-tract damage sometimes amounting to transverse myelitis may occasionally occur (Gordon and

Tucker, 1945). Clinical signs of such cord damage are not common. The lesions are usually permanent, though some reinnervation of paralyzed muscles may occur from adjacent myotomes.

Radiation Myelopathy

The adult central nervous system is relatively resistant to the effects of x-irradiation since there are almost no dividing cells. If the spinal cord is exposed to more than 3500 rads, however, late damage may occur (Gangloff and Hug, 1965; Haymaker, 1969). Such irradiation is inevitable when treating an intraspinal lesion such as ependymoma, but more commonly and tragically happens as an accident of proximity during the radiotherapy of thoracic or cervical neoplasms (Hughes, 1966; Kristensson et al., 1967; Reagan et al., 1968). The damage is usually dose dependent, though some instances suggest unusual individual susceptibility. The myelopathy presents three months to three or more years after exposure with dysesthesias, spastic paraparesis and sphincter impairment below the level of long-tract damage, and some degree of local paralysis from anterior horn cell damage. It is slowly progressive, and the signs indicate that the whole spinal cord is involved. Less commonly the onset is sudden and the distribution indicates the occurrence of a vascular lesion. Pathologically, the cord shows areas of infarction, diffuse spongy degeneration of the white matter, and neuronal damage. There is endarteritis of blood vessels, often with extensive new vessel formation. Once irradiation has occurred, there is no known way to prevent the process from developing. Clinically it may be difficult to separate radiation myelopathy from a spinal tumor, but the myelogram is normal, and the cerebrospinal fluid may only show a slight increase in protein.

Damage of the spinal cord may occur when a patient is struck by lightning or electrocuted (Panse, 1970). Cerebral damage is frequently the most obvious, but when the current flows from one hand to the ground through the spine, damage due to direct dissipation of energy within the cord is not uncommon. There may be immediate paralysis, sensory loss, and bladder disturbance, but one of the striking features is that some patients develop lower motor neuron paralysis from degeneration of anterior horn cells in the area of the electrical injury only after some months (see Chapter 36).

CONCLUDING REMARKS

The spinal cord as part of the central nervous system is heir to many diseases. The anterior horn cell and primary sensory neuron as part of the peripheral nervous system suffer from many others. Not infrequently damage to one may affect the other. At times it may be difficult clinically to distinguish whether the central or peripheral nervous elements are predominantly involved, and recourse must be made to a number of special investigations. Accurate diagnosis is of the utmost importance since many of the conditions discussed in this chapter are susceptible to treatment.

Acknowledgment: I am grateful to Mrs. E. Mooney for unfailing secretarial services.

REFERENCES

Adams, C. B. T., and Logue, V.: Studies in cervical spondylotic myelopathy. I. Movement of the cervical roots, dura and cord, and their relation to the course taken by the extrathecal roots. Brain, *94*:557, 1971a.

Adams, C. B. T., and Logue, V.: Studies in cervical spondylotic myelopathy. II. Observations on the movement and contour of the cervical spine in relation to the neural complications of cervical spondylosis. Brain, *94*:569, 1971b.

Appleby, A., Foster, J. B., Hankinson, J., and Hudgson, P.: The diagnosis and management of the Chiari anomalies in adult life. Brain, *91*:131, 1968.

Appleby, A., Bradley, W. B., Foster, J. B., Hankinson, J., and Hudgson, P.: Syringomyelia due to chronic arachnoiditis at the foramen magnum. J. Neurol. Sci., *8*:451, 1969.

Banna, M., and Gryspeerdt, G. L.: Review article: intraspinal tumors in children (excluding dysraphism). Clin. Radiol., *22*:17, 1971.

Barnett, H. J. M., Foster, J. B., and Hudgson, P.: Syringomyelia. London, W. B. Saunders Co., 1973.

Barnett, H. J. M., Botterell, E. H., Jousse, A. T., and Wynne-Jones, M.: Progressive myelopathy as a sequel to traumatic paraplegia. Brain, *89*:159, 1966.

Bishara, S. N.: Posterior operation in the treatment of cervical spondylosis with myelopathy. J. Neurol. Neurosurg. Psychiatry, *34*:393, 1971.

Blackwood, W.: Vascular disease of the central nervous system. *In* Blackwood, W., McMenemey, W. H., Meyer, A., Norman, R. M., and Russell, D. S. (eds.): Greenfield's Neuropathology. 2nd Edition. London,

Edward Arnold Ltd. [Baltimore, Williams & Wilkins Co.] 1963, p. 71.

Bodian, D.: *In* Poliomyelitis: Papers and Discussions Presented at the First International Poliomyelitis Conference. Philadelphia, J. B. Lippincott Co., 1949.

Bodian, D.: *In* Rivers, T., and Horsfall, F. L., (eds.): Viral and Rickettsial Infections in Man. 3rd Edition. Philadelphia, J. B. Lippincott Co., 1959, p. 479.

Bradshaw, P.: Some aspects of cervical spondylosis. Quart. J. Med., *26*:177, 1957.

Brain, Lord, and Wilkinson, M.: Cervical Spondylosis. London, William Heinemann Ltd. [Philadelphia, W. B. Saunders Co.], 1967.

Breig, A.: Biomechanics of the Central Nervous System. Some Basic Normal and Pathologic Phenomena. Stockholm, Almquist & Wiksell, 1960.

Breig, A., and El-Nadi, A. F.: Biomechanics of the cervical spinal cord. Acta Radiol. Scand. [Diagn.] (Stockh.), *4*:602, 1966.

Brice, J., and McKissock, W.: Surgical treatment of malignant extradural spinal tumours. Br. Med. J., *1*:1341, 1965.

British Medical Journal: Leading article: Paralysis in herpes zoster. *2*:ii, 379, 1970.

Brock, S.: Injuries of Brain and Spinal Cord and Their Coverings. 4th Edition. New York, Springer Publishing Co., 1960.

Burrows, E. H.: Sagittal diameter of the spinal canal in cervical spondylosis. Clin. Radiol., *14*:77, 1963.

Campbell, A. M. G., Williams, E. R., and Pearce, J.: Late motor neuron degeneration following poliomyelitis. Neurology (Minneap.), *19*:1101, 1969.

Carson, J., Gumpert, J., and Jefferson, A.: Diagnosis and treatment of thoracic intervertebral disc protrusions. J. Neurol. Neurosurg. Psychiatry, *34*:68, 1971.

Cavanagh, J. B.: The significance of the "dying back" process in experimental and human neurological disease. Int. Rev. Exp. Pathol., *3*:219, 1964.

Dale, A. J. D., and Love, J. G.: Thorium dioxide myelopathy. J.A.M.A., *199*:606, 1967.

Davidson, S.: Cryptococcal spinal arachnoiditis. J. Neurol. Neurosurg. Psychiatry, *31*:76, 1968.

Dejerine, J.: Sur la claudication intermittente de la moelle épinière. Rev. Neurol. (Paris), *8*:341, 1906.

Denny-Brown, D.: Hereditary sensory radicular neuropathy. J. Neurol. Neurosurg. Psychiatry, *14*:237, 1951.

Djindjian, R., and Houdart, M.: L'arteriographie de la moelle épinière. Paris, Masson & Cie, 1970.

Djindjian, R., Hurth, M., and Houdart, R.: Los angiomes médullaires. Paris, Sandoz, 1969.

Dyck, P. J., and Lambert, E. H.: Dissociated sensation in amyloidosis. Arch. Neurol., *20*:490, 1969.

Ellertsson, A. B., and Greitz, T.: The distending force in the production of communicating syringomyelia. Lancet, *1*:1234, 1970.

Feder, B. H., and Smith, J. L.: Roentgenologic therapy in chronic spinal arachnoiditis. Radiology, *78*:192, 1962.

Fieschi, C., Gottlieb, A., and de Carolis, V.: Ischaemic lacunae in the spinal cord of arteriosclerotic subjects. J. Neurol. Neurosurg. Psychiatry, *33*:138, 1970.

Foix, C., and Alajouanine, T.: La myélite nécrotique subaigue. Rev. Neurol. (Paris), *2*:1, 1926.

Gangloff, H., and Hug, O.: Effects of ionizing radiation on the nervous system. Adv. Biol. Med. Phys., *10*:1, 1965.

Gardner, W. J.: Hydrodynamic mechanism of syringomyelia: its relationship to myelocele. J. Neurol. Neurosurg. Psychiatry, *28*:247, 1965.

Gardner, W. J., and Angel, J.: The cause of syringomyelia

and its surgical treatment. Cleveland Clin. Q., *25*:4, 1958.

Gardner, W. J., Abdullah, A. F., and McCormack, L. J.: The varying expressions of embryonal atresis of the fourth ventricle in adults. J. Neurosurg., *14*:591, 1957.

Gillilan, L. A.: Veins of the spinal cord. Anatomic details; suggested clinical applications. Neurology (Minneap.), *20*:860, 1970.

Gordon, I. R. S., and Tucker, J. F.: Lesions of the central nervous system in herpes zoster. J. Neurol. Neurosurg. Psychiatry, *8*:40, 1945.

Hattwick, M. A. W., Weis, T. T., Stechschulte, C. J., Baer, G. M., and Gregg, M. B.: Recovery from rabies. Ann. Intern. Med., *76*:931, 1972.

Haymaker, W.: The effect of ionizing radiation on the nervous system. *In* Bourne, G. H. (ed.): The structure and function of nervous tissue. Vol. III. New York, Academic Press, 1969, p. 441.

Henson, R. A., and Parsons, M.: Ischaemic lesions of the spinal cord: an illustrated review. Q. J. Med., *36*:205, 1967.

Hirson, C.: Spinal subdural abscess. Lancet, *2*:1215, 1965.

Horstmann, D. M., McCollum, R. W., and Mascola, A. D.: Viremia in human poliomyelitis. J. Exp. Med., *99*:355, 1954.

Hughes, J. T.: Pathology of the Spinal Cord. London, Lloyd-Luke, Ltd., 1966.

Hughes, J. T.: Venous infarction of the spinal cord. Neurology (Minneap.), *21*:794, 1971.

Hughes, J. T., and Brownell, B.: Spinal cord ischemia due to arteriosclerosis. Arch. Neurol., *15*:189, 1966.

Hurst, E. W.: Adhesive arachnoiditis and vascular blockage caused by detergents and other chemical irritants: experimental study. J. Pathol. Bacteriol., *70*:167, 1955.

Hurst, E. W., and Pawan, J. L.: An outbreak of rabies in Trinidad. Lancet, *2*:622, 1931.

Hurst, E. W., and Pawan, J. L.: A further account of the Trinidad outbreak of acute rabic myelitis. J. Pathol. Bacteriol., *35*:301, 1932.

Irvine, D. H., Foster, J. B., Newell, D. J., and Klukvin, B. N.: Prevalence of cervical spondylosis in a general practice. Lancet, *1*:1089, 1965.

James, C. C. M., and Lassman, L. P.: Spinal dysraphism. Arch. Dis. Child., *35*:315, 1960.

James, C. C. M., and Lassman, L. P.: Spinal dysraphism. The diagnosis and treatment of progressive lesions in spina bifida occulta. J. Bone Joint Surg., *44B*:828, 1962.

James, C. C. M., and Lassman, L. P.: Diastematomyelia. Arch. Dis. Child., *39*:125, 1964.

James. C. C. M., and Lassman, L. P.: Spinal dysraphism: spina bifida occulta. London, Butterworth & Co., Ltd., 1972.

Jellinger, K.: Spinal cord arteriosclerosis and progressive vascular myelopathy. J. Neurol. Neurosurg. Psychiatry, *30*:195, 1967.

Kamrin, R. P., Potanos, J. N., and Pool, J. L.: An evaluation of the diagnosis and treatment of chordoma. J. Neurol. Neurosurg. Psychiatry, *27*:157, 1964.

Kosary, I. Z., Braham, J., Shaked, I., and Tadmor, R.: Cervical syringomyelia associated with occipital meningioma. Neurology (Minneap.), *19*:1128, 1969.

Kristensson, K., Molin, B., and Sourander, P.: Delayed radiation lesions of human spinal cord. Report of five cases. Acta Neuropathol. (Berl.), *9*:34, 1967.

Lancet: Newer rabies vaccines. *1*:132, 1972.

Lassman, L. P., and James, C. C. M.: Spina bifida cystica and occulta. Some aspects of spinal dysraphism. Paraplegia, *2*:96, 1964.

Lawrence, D. G., and Kuypers, H. G. J. M.: The functional organization of the motor system in the monkey. I. The effects of bilateral pyramidal lesions. Brain, *91*:1, 1968a.

Lawrence, D. G., and Kuypers, H. G. J. M.: II. The effects of lesions of the descending brain stem pathways. Brain, *91*:15, 1968b.

Lees, F., and Turner, J. W.: Natural history and prognosis of cervical spondylosis. Br. Med. J., *2*:1607, 1963.

Lightowler, C. D. R.: Meningomyelocele: the price of treatment. Br. Med. J., *2*:385, 1971.

Lombardi, G., Passerini, A., and Migliavacca, F.: Spinal arachnoiditis. Br. J. Radiol., *35*:314, 1962.

Mair, W. G. P., and Druckman, R.: Pathology of spinal cord lesions and their relationship to clinical features in protrusion of cervical intervertebral discs. Brain, *76*:70, 1953.

Maxwell, D. S., Kruger, L., and Pineda, A.: The trigeminal root with special reference to the central-peripheral transition zone: an electron microscopic study in the Macaque. Anat. Rec., *164*:113, 1969.

Melnick, J. L., and Ledinko, N.: Development of neutralizing antibodies against three types of poliomyelitis virus during an epidemic period. Am. J. Hyg., *58*:207, 1953.

Nash, D. F. E.: Spina bifida and allied disorders. Hospital Medicine, 439, 1968.

Nizzoli, V., and Testa, C.: A case of calcification in the spinal arachnoid giving spinal cord compression. J. Neurol. Sci., *7*:381, 1968.

Northfield, D. W. C.: Diagnosis and treatment of myelopathy due to cervical spondylosis. Brit. Med. J., *2*:1474, 1955.

Northfield, D. W. C., and Osmond-Clarke, H.: Surgical treatment. *In* Brain, Lord, and Wilkinson, M. (eds.): Cervical Spondylosis. London, William Heinemann Ltd. [Philadelphia, W. B. Saunders Co.], 1967, p. 207.

Pallis, C., Jones, A. M., and Spillane, J. D.: Cervical spondylosis. Incidence and implications. Brain, *77*:274, 1954.

Panse, F.: Electrical lesions of the nervous system. *In* Vinken, P. J., and Bruyn, G. W. (eds.): Handbook of Clinical Neurology. Vol. 7. Diseases of Nerve, Part I. Amsterdam, North-Holland Publishing Co., 1970, p. 344.

Pattison, E. M.: Uveomeningoencephalitic syndrome (Vogt-Koyanagi-Harada syndrome). Arch. Neurol., *12*:197, 1965.

Paul, J. R.: A History of Poliomyelitis. New York, Yale University Press, 1971.

Paul, J. R., Melnick, J. L., Barnett, V. H., and Goldblom, N.: A survey of neutralizing antibodies to poliomyelitis in Cairo, Egypt. Am. J. Hyg., *55*:402, 1952.

Payne, E. E., and Spillane, J. D.: The cervical spine. An anatomico-pathological study of seventy specimens with particular reference to the problem of cervical spondylosis. Brain, *80*:571, 1957.

Perot, P., Feindel, W., and Lloyd-Smith, D.: Hematomyelia as a complication of syringomyelia: Gowers' syringal hemorrhage. J. Neurosurg., *25*:447, 1966.

Peters, A.: The morphology of axons of the central nervous system. *In* Bourne, G. H. (ed.): The Structure and Function of Nervous Tissue. New York, Academic Press, 1968, p. 141.

Price, D. L., and Harris, J.: Cholesterol emboli in cerebral arteries as a complication of retrograde aortic perfusion during cardiac surgery. Neurology (Minneap.), *20*:1209, 1970.

Reagan, T. J., Thomas, J. E., and Colby, M. Y.: Chronic progressive radiation myelopathy. J.A.M.A., *203*: 106, 1968.

Reed, H., Lindsay, A., Silversides, J. L., Speakman, J., Monckton, G., and Rees, D. L.: The uveoencephalitic syndrome or Vogt-Koyanagi-Harada disease. Can. Med. Assoc. J., *79*:451, 1958.

Riehl, J.-L., and Andrews, J. M.: The uveomeningo-encephalitic syndrome. Neurology (Minneap.), *16*: 603, 1966.

Roberts, A. H.: Myelopathy due to cervical spondylosis treated by collar immobilization. Neurology (Minneap.), *66*:951, 1966.

Rossier, A. B., Werner, A., Wildi, E., and Berney, J.: Contribution to the study of late cervical syringomyelic syndrome after dorsal and lumbar traumatic paraplegia. J. Neurol. Neurosurg. Psychiatry, *31*:99, 1968.

Russell, D. S., and Rubinstein, L. J.: Pathology of Tumours of the Nervous System. 2nd Edition. London, Edward Arnold Ltd. [Baltimore, Williams & Wilkins Co.], 1963.

Russell, W. R.: Poliomyelitis. 2nd Edition. London, Edward Arnold Ltd. [Baltimore, Williams and Wilkins Co.], 1956.

Schwartzman, R. J., and Bogdonoff, M. D.: Proprioception and vibration sensibility discrimination in the absence of posterior columns. Arch. Neurol., *20*:349, 1969.

Sica, R. E. P., McComas, A. J., and Upton, A. R. M.: Impaired potentiation of H-reflexes in patients with upper motoneurone lesions. J. Neurol. Neurosurg. Psychiatry, *34*:712, 1972.

Skinhøj, E.: Arteriosclerosis of the spinal cord. Three cases of pure "syndrome of the anterior spinal artery." Acta Psychr. Neurol. (Scand.), *29*:139, 1954.

Slooff. J. L., Kernohan, J. W., and MacCarty, C. S.: Primary Intramedullary Tumors of the Spinal Cord and Filum Terminale. Philadelphia, W. B. Saunders Co., 1964.

Steer, J. M.: Some observations on the fine structure of the rat dorsal spinal nerve roots. J. Anat., *109*:467, 1971.

Sükrü-Aksel, I.: Pathologische Anatomie der Lyssa. *In* Scholz, W. (ed.): Handbuch der Speziellen Pathologischen Anatomie und Histologie. Vol. XIII, 2A. Berlin, Springer-Verlag, 1958, p. 417.

Symon, L., and Lavender, P.: Surgical treatment of cervical spondylotic myelopathy. Neurology (Minneap.), *17*:117, 1967.

Tangchai, P., and Vejjajiva, A.: Pathology of the peripheral nervous system in human rabies. A study of nine autopsy cases. Brain, *94*:299, 1971.

Tarlov, I. M.: Spinal cord compression: mechanisms of paralysis and treatment. Springfield, Ill., Charles C Thomas, 1957.

Taylor, A. R.: Vascular factors in the myelopathy of cervical spondylosis. Neurology (Minneap.), *14*: 62, 1964.

Teng, P., and Papatheodorou, C.: Myelographic findings in adhesive spinal arachnoiditis (with a brief surgical note). Br. J. Radiol., *40*:201, 1967.

Turkington, R. W., and Stiefel, J. W.: Sensory radicular neuropathy. Arch. Neurol., *12*:19, 1965.

Van Bogaert, L.: Poliomyelite anterieure aiguë. (Maladi de Heine-Medin). *In* Scholz, W. (ed.): Handbuch der Speziellen pathologischen Anatomie und Histologie. Vol. XIII, 2A. Berlin, Springer-Verlag, 1958, p. 244.

Wall, P. D.: The sensory and motor role of impulses travelling in the dorsal columns towards the cerebral cortex. Brain, *93*:505, 1970.

Waltz, T. A.: Physical factors in the production of the myelopathy of cervical spondylosis. Brain, *90*:395, 1967.

Warren, J., Gutmann, L., Figueroa, A. F., and Bloor, B. M.: E.M.G. changes of brachial plexus root avulsions. J. Neurosurg., *31*:137, 1969.

Wilkinson, M. (ed.): Cervical Spondylosis. Its Early Diagnosis and Treatment. London, William Heinemann, Ltd. [Philadelphia, W. B. Saunders Co.], 1971.

Williams, B.: The distending force in the production of "communicating syringomyelia." Lancet, *2*:189, 1969.

Williams, B.: Current concepts of syringomyelia. Br. Med. J., *4*:331, 1970.

Winkleman, N. W., Gotten, N., and Scheibert, D.: Localized adhesive spinal arachnoiditis. A study of 25 cases with reference to etiology. Trans. Am. Neurol. Assoc., *78*:15, 1953.

Wirth, F. P., Jr., Post, K. D., Di Chiro, G., Doppman, J. L., and Ommaya, A. K.: Foix-Alajouanine disease. Spontaneous thrombosis of a spinal cord arteriovenous malformation: a case report. Neurology (Minneap.), *20*:1114, 1970.

Wise, B. L., and Smith, M.: Spinal arachnoiditis ossificans. Arch. Neurol., *13*:391, 1965.

Wolman, L., and Bradshaw, P.: Spinal cord embolism. J. Neurol. Neurosurg. Psychiatry, *30*:446, 1967.

Young, A. C.: Radiology of cervical spondylosis. *In* Brain, Lord, and Wilkinson, M. (eds.): Cervical Spondylosis. London, William Heinemann, Ltd. [Philadelphia, W. B. Saunders Co., 1967, p. 133.

Zellinger, K.: Zur Morphologie und Pathogenese spinaler Läsionen bei Verletzungen der Halswirbelsaule. Acta Neuropathol. (Berl.), *3*:451, 1964.

Chapter 31

DISEASES OF THE SPINAL ROOTS

Walter G. Bradley

The spinal nerve roots may be damaged because of their site in the spinal canal, or because of their inherent susceptibility to certain diseases. An example of the former is compression of the root by a prolapsed intervertebral disk, and consideration of this and other conditions forms the main part of this chapter. Certain diseases show a predisposition for the spinal roots, including the Guillain-Barré syndrome, as reported by Haymaker and Kernohan (1949) and Asbury, Arnason, and Adams (1969), and diphtheritic neuropathy (Waksman et al., 1957). These conditions are considered respectively in Chapter 56 and Chapter 63. Hypertrophic neuropathies, though usually diffuse, may sometimes predominantly affect the spinal roots (see Chapters 41 and 42). Thickening of the roots may occasionally cause spinal cord compression (Symonds and Blackwood, 1962). Since these conditions are considered elsewhere, they are not discussed further in this chapter. It is, however, interesting to speculate why the roots are particularly involved in these diseases. It is perhaps owing to the absence of a blood-nerve barrier in the roots, unlike the remainder of the nervous system, allowing easier access of toxins and antibodies to the roots (Waksman, 1961; Olsson, 1968).

Tumors of the spinal roots are discussed in Chapters 66, 67, and 68. The spinal nerve roots are damaged to a varying extent in many of the diseases of the peripheral nervous system discussed in Section V of this book, and they also show secondary degeneration following damage to the anterior horn cells and dorsal root ganglia. These processes also are outside the scope of this chapter, in which consideration is restricted to the spinal nerve roots, though many of the processes affecting the cranial nerves are similar.

ANATOMICAL CONSIDERATIONS

A disease process damaging both the motor and sensory roots, particularly if several such roots are affected, may be difficult to separate from disease of the more distal parts of the peripheral nerves. Careful clinical examination is required to define the neurologic deficit exactly.

Aids to Diagnosis of the Site of the Lesion

In typical cases, application of a little anatomical and physiologic knowledge makes the identification of the site of the lesion easy. Thus, if the sensory or motor loss follows a dermatomal or myotomal distribution, the lesion lies in the dorsal or ventral root. If there is pure motor or pure sensory loss, the lesion is either in the root or the neuronal cell body. At times the sensory loss involves only one group of modalities of sensation, either pain and temperature or joint position and vibration. This may be the result of the specific degeneration of one type of primary sensory neuron. For instance, tabes dorsalis and a number of toxic neuropathies begin with damage to the large neurons and axons carrying joint position and vibration sensation.

On the other hand, in hereditary sensory neuropathies and amyloidosis, the damage falls on the smaller neurons and axons, producing loss of pain and temperature sensation. Such a loss may also be due to damage to specific sensory tracts in the spinal cord (see Chapter 30). Sensory and motor loss restricted to ·the lower parts of the body indicate a lesion of the spinal cord. If only the legs are involved, without signs of an upper motor neuron lesion, damage to the cauda equina or the lumbosacral plexus may be responsible.

Investigations

At times it is difficult to define the site of the lesion without a number of specialized investigations. Arachnoiditis may produce a sensorimotor deficit that is difficult to separate from mixed sensorimotor neuropathies such as that associated with a carcinoma, though myelography will be diagnostic (Croft et al., 1967; Croft and Wilkinson, 1969; Trojaborg et al., 1969). A neurofibroma of one thoracic root may produce signs limited to the spinal cord, the radicular sensory signs being insignificant owing to overlap of dermatomal supply. Again myelography will be diagnostic. Lesions of the dorsal roots may be difficult to distinguish from a dorsal root ganglion neuronal degeneration or a diffuse sensory neuropathy. The triple response to skin injury or intradermal histamine, and the sensory nerve action potentials may help resolve this problem. The triple response consists of local vasodilatation, edema, and the surrounding vasodilatation produced by an axon reflex, termed the flare. Impulses passing from the damaged area in the sensory nerves travel in a retrograde fashion down a branch of the fiber to the adjacent undamaged skin, where they release substances that cause vasodilatation. The sensory nerve action potential depends on the presence of peripheral sensory branches (Warren et al., 1969). When the flare and sensory nerve action potential are lost, the peripheral sensory nerves have degenerated. On the other hand, when they are present in an anesthetic area, the cause of the sensory loss lies proximal to the dorsal root ganglion. The finding of denervation changes in axial muscles indicates a very proximal lesion (Zverina and Skorpil, 1969).

The site of the lesion causing axonal degeneration remains undecided, though its elucidation is important in the understanding of pathogenetic mechanisms. The argument, which centers around whether the damage is primarily of the axon or the perikaryon, is made more complex by the interplay between these two parts of the neuron. Thus death of the perikaryon causes degeneration of the peripheral axons, while a focal lesion of the peripheral nerve causes central chromatolysis of the perikaryon. If the axonal lesion is very proximal, it may lead to death of the cell body. The distal degeneration of axons ("dying back" neuropathy) may result from metabolic change in the perikaryon (Cavanagh and Chen, 1971). Finally there is the possibility that an agent such as a toxin damages both the perikaryon and the peripheral axon.

Because of the anatomical arrangement of the cauda equina, it may be difficult to define the site of a lesion in this area without myelography. A focal lesion such as a large intervertebral disk prolapse will damage the roots of many lumbosacral segments, and the clinical picture may be indistinguishable from that of an extensive tumor such as an ependymoma in this region. Similarly a central disk prolapse in the upper lumbar areas may damage only the lower sacral roots as they run down from the conus medullaris.

PATHOLOGIC CONSIDERATIONS

The nerve root, like the peripheral nerve fiber in general, has a rather limited repertoire of pathologic reactions, though these can be evoked by a large number of mechanisms. Minor forms of damage, whether compressive or ischemic or toxic, may simply damage the Schwann cells, producing segmental demyelination. This may block nerve conduction, with relatively rapid recovery when the noxious agent is removed. More severe injury causes axonal degeneration and retrograde changes in the neuronal perikaryon. Even if this does not lead to cell death, the distance for regeneration from the roots is so long that permanent muscular denervation is common. Functional regeneration of the primary sensory neuron into the spinal cord does not occur. Thus if the damage to the nerve root is sufficiently severe to cause axonal degeneration, it is usually permanent.

VARIOUS RADICULOPATHIES

Trauma

ACUTE INTERVERTEBRAL DISK PROLAPSE

The cervical and lumbar regions are the most prone to suffer intervertebral disk degeneration, being the most mobile parts of the spine. The frequency of disk prolapse is greatest in the lumbar region because of the greater forces there. All movements of the spine impose deformational changes on the intervertebral disks, and if excessive, or if degenerative changes are present in the disk, the anulus fibrosus may rupture, allowing partial or total prolapse of the softer central nucleus pulposus into the spinal canal. This is more frequently lateral than central, and thus the spinal roots are more often compressed than the cord in the cervical region, and root pain is more usually unilateral than bilateral in the lumbar region. For a brief review the reader is referred to Greenfield (1963b).

Clinical Features. As a result of an excessive or sudden movement, the patient feels a sudden click and pain in the neck or lumbar region, the pain developing in a radicular distribution. The most common disk prolapse in the cervical region is at the C5–C6 interspace, and therefore pain is most frequently down the shoulder and outside of the arm. Characteristically, movement worsens the pain. If the compression is mild, paresthesias and loss of tendon reflexes in the affected spinal segments may be the only result. If it is severe, then sensory loss and muscle weakness occurs in the appropriate segments. The commonest signs are of a C5 lesion with weakness of the deltoids, biceps, and brachioradialis muscles, and loss of the tendon reflexes in the latter. There is often mild corticospinal tract damage at C5 with resultant hyperreflexia in the C7 and C8–innervated finger flexors on percussion over the radial tubercle, the so-called "inverted radial jerk." The clinical picture does, of course, differ when the prolapse is at a different level. A high cervical disk prolapse may impinge on the first and second cervical roots, causing occipital and frontal headache.

In the lumbar region the most common disk prolapse is in the L5–S1 interspace, producing pain in the back and down the back of the leg on that side. Major sensory and motor signs are relatively uncommon, but depression of the ankle jerk and a small area of impairment of pinprick sensation under the lateral malleolus may often be found. As a result of nerve root compression, stretching the root by straight leg raising causes pain. A high lumbar disk lesion (L2–L3) causes pain radiating to the thigh and knee, and loss of the knee jerk. In this instance pain is elicited by having the patient lie prone and hyperextending the leg with the knee flexed. An L4–L5 disk prolapse may produce pain in a sciatic distribution, and the only physical sign may be weakness of dorsiflexion of the big toe.

Investigations. The signs are often sufficient to define the level of the lesion, though plain radiography and myelography are occasionally required. The myelogram, however, may be normal despite a large lumbar disk prolapse. Signs of denervation may be revealed electromyographically, though there will be no loss of sensory nerve action potentials in the affected segments. Pain resulting from lesions of the vertebral articular joints may cause difficulty in the differential diagnosis. This pain may be dermatomal in distribution, though there are no neurologic signs. The electrophysiologic and myelographic findings are negative.

Treatment. The pain may be so severe that opiates are required to control it, and a frozen shoulder or the shoulder-hand syndrome may develop (Abbott and Mitts, 1970). In other cases the pain may be mild, and spontaneously remit after one or two weeks. Restriction of neck or lumbar movements (often erroneously termed "immobilization") in a cervical collar or lumbar corset aids the resolution of the condition, perhaps by ensuring that further disk prolapse does not occur and that edema of the damaged root is allowed to settle. Radiant heat therapy is also often helpful.

In cases in which symptoms and signs of root compression are severe, traction should be applied, either intermittently or continuously. In the lumbar region this is applied by traction on the iliac crests, and in the cervical region with a chin collar; weights are attached and allowed to hang over the edge of the bed. Traction is often rapidly effective in relieving the pain. It is difficult to conceive of nucleus pulposus being "aspirated" back into the intervertebral space, and it seems more likely that traction works both by preventing the bulging of the annulus fibrosus and by restricting movements. When the pain and neurologic signs are not relieved, surgical removal of the disk prolapse is required. If the motor and sensory roots are severely compressed, then the lesion is likely to be permanent and recovery dependent upon sprouting from fibers of the adjacent motor and sensory segments.

ROOT AVULSION

Injuries leading to the distraction of the head from one shoulder produce traction on the nerves and nerve roots running from the cervical cord to that arm. A typical instance is of a motor cyclist falling from his machine and hitting his shoulder on an obstruction. This may cause avulsion of the nerve roots from the cervical cord or rupture of the nerves in the brachial plexus (Taylor, 1962). Both produce profound paralysis and sensory loss, usually extending over several segments. The prognosis for recovery is different in the two lesions. As indicated earlier, no recovery occurs with a severe lesion such as root avulsion. When the site of nerve rupture (neurotmesis) is in the brachial plexus, regeneration of both motor and sensory nerves is possible, though the extent is proportional to the degree of the disruption of the nerves and to the distance of the site of rupture from the innervated structures. The rate of growth of axons is approximately 1 to 3 mm per day, and when the endoneurial tubes remain without nerve fibers for a prolonged period irreversable fibrosis may occur. Nevertheless, some reinnervation may continue for up to three years after a proximal lesion (Sunderland, 1968).

Knowledge of the site of the lesion helps in advising on the prognosis. When the roots are avulsed, there is usually rupture of the root sleeve producing the appearance on the myelogram of gross dilatation and elongation of the root sleeves (Taylor, 1962). This finding indicates that no recovery in the signs can be expected. As already described, the presence of an axon flare or of a sensory nerve action potential in an anesthetic area indicates that there is a lesion of the nerve roots with no likelihood of recovery in those segments. The converse does not apply, however. Proximal to a plexus lesion producing loss of axon flare and sensory nerve action potentials there may be avulsed nerve roots.

Compression

INTRASPINAL TUMORS

Any expanding lesion within the spinal canal will compress the nerve roots and the spinal cord, if present, at that level. Due to condensation of the tracts within the spinal cord, compression of the latter usually produces a far more dramatic picture than the root compression. This is considered more fully in Chapter 30.

Pathology. The effect of chronic compression is both mechanical, causing stretching and distortion, and ischemic (Tarlov, 1957). As in compressive neuropathies of the peripheral nerves elsewhere, initially there is segmental demyelination, which may block conduction but allow relatively rapid recovery (see Chapters 34 and 35). More advanced lesions cause axonal degeneration with little recovery.

Clinical Features. The pain of an intramedullary spinal cord tumor such as an astrocytoma or ependymoma may be due to root compression, but signs of damage to the lower motor neuron and primary sensory neuron are probably due to intramedullary rather than root damage. Intradural extramedullary compression of the nerve roots may be due to a meningioma, discussed by Russell and Rubinstein (1963), or a schwannoma (neurofibroma or neurinoma). The latter, considered in Chapters 67 and 68, usually causes compression of only one root with relatively little sensory or motor disturbance other than pain unless that root innervates the arm or leg. In von Recklinghausen's disease (generalized neurofibromatosis), multiple neurofibromas may occur with consequently complex physical signs. Meningiomas are most common in the dorsal region and in middle-aged women, and may compress more than one nerve root. Lipomas and dermoid cysts are associated with spina bifida occulta, and are considered in a following section. Extradural compression due to carcinoma is usually restricted, and radicular signs and symptoms are mild. The local pain is due both to bone involvement and to radicular compression. Extradural reticuloses and abscesses produce more extensive damage to nerve roots and the mixed spinal nerve as it runs through the extradural space. In the case of an extradural abscess, widespread direct toxic damage and endarteritis make damage to the initial part of the mixed spinal nerve a prominent part of the syndrome, in addition to the signs of infection with fever and leukocytosis (Abrahamson et al., 1934; Hirson, 1965).

The anatomical arrangements of the cauda equina make this a region for special consideration (see earlier discussion of anatomical considerations). The primary symptom of cauda equina compression is pain in a radicular distribution. More severe lesions also cause weakness and numbness in the sacral segments. Sphincter impairment is an early symptom. The loss of the anal and bulbocavernosus reflexes as well as loss of knee and ankle jerks are useful diagnostic signs. The commonest intradural lesion responsible is an ependymoma of the filum terminale or conus medullaris (Mabon et al., 1949). Intradermal lipomas or dermoid cysts may be associated with dysrhaphism, as described in a later section. An implantation dermoid is a rare complication of a previous lumbar puncture carried out without a stylet so that a small piece of the malpighian layer of the skin is carried with the needle into the subarachnoid space (Choremis et al., 1956; Blockey and Schorstein, 1961). This may slowly grow and compress the cauda equina. Extradural compression of the cauda equina may be due to intervertebral disk degeneration, carcinoma, or chordoma in that order of frequency. The latter tumors are derived from notochordal rests and are particularly common in the base of the skull and the sacrum (Sensenig, 1956; Kamrin et al., 1964).

Investigations. Plain radiographs may be helpful in showing vertebral erosion or collapse in carcinoma or tuberculosis or chordoma, expansion of the canal by a long-standing space-occupying lesion, or enlargement of the intervertebral foramen with an extraspinal mass in a schwannoma (neurinoma) of the nerve roots. There may be spina bifida occulta. Myelography is helpful in defining the level of the lesion, and may indicate its nature (see Chapter 30). In the investigation of cauda equina lesions, however, lumbar puncture in the region of the suspected tumor is unwise. This also applies if an extradural abscess is suspected because of the danger of producing meningitis. In both instances, cisternal myelography is the investigation of choice.

Treatment. Surgical decompression with the removal of the compressive lesion should be undertaken whenever possible and is often required to make the exact diagnosis. Radiotherapy is sometimes recommended as the initial treatment when the diagnosis of carcinomatous compression is clear on clinical grounds or operation is impossible, and it may be remarkably effective if the lesion is radiosensitive. It is also indicated following the removal of an ependymoma. Chordomas are usually believed to be insensitive to radiotherapy, though some benefit has been demonstrated (Zoltan and Fenyes, 1960; Kamrin et al., 1964).

CHRONIC INTERVERTEBRAL DISK DEGENERATION (SPONDYLOSIS)

As already outlined, continual bending and twisting of the intervertebral disk may produce rupture of the anulus fibrosus with acute prolapse of the nucleus pulposus. In the chronic phase there may be gradual splaying of the fibrocartilaginous disk, which may bulge into the spinal canal and intervertebral foramina. Secondary calcification of the junction of the bulge with the vertebrae produces a bony osteophyte on each side of the disk. The consequent narrowing of the intervertebral disk space shortens the spinal canal, thereby tending to produce thickening of the spinal cord and roots and backward bulging of the ligamenta flava, at the same time as the canal and intervertebral foramen are being narrowed by osteophytes and chronic disk protrusion (Breig, 1960; Breig and El-Nadi, 1966; Hughes, 1966; Waltz, 1967; Adams and Logue, 1971a, 1971b). The effect of this on the spinal cord is discussed in Chapter 30. For a review of cervical spondylosis the reader is referred to Wilkinson (1971). Individuals with a congenitally narrow spinal canal, including those with achondroplasia, are particularly liable to suffer neurologic damage from disk degeneration (Pallis et al., 1954; Epstein and Malis, 1955; Duvoisin and Yahr, 1962).

Clinical Features. The degenerative changes of cervical spondylosis compress the spinal roots and nerves predominantly in the intervertebral foramina rather than within the spinal canal. As in other radicular compressions and many nerve entrapments elsewhere in the body, pain is one of the most prominent features (British Association of

Physical Medicine, 1966). This may occur spontaneously, or develop after a neck injury such as a whiplash. The pain is radicular in distribution, and since C4–C5 and C5–C6 degeneration is the most common, the shoulder and arm are the most common sites for the referral of pain.

There may be sensory symptoms including subjective impairment of touch sensation and paraesthesias, though rarely does clinical testing reveal gross sensory loss. Refined testing methods might perhaps prove more helpful (Dyck et al., 1971, 1972). Motor weakness is uncommon, though movements are often inhibited by pain, but reflex loss is quite frequent. Patients with osteophytic compression at C5–C6 often have depressed biceps and brachioradialis reflexes. As outlined in Chapter 30, signs of myelopathy below this level are not uncommon. When the spondylosis is long-standing and severe, mild amyotrophy is not uncommon. It is, however, not easy to know whether this results from the myelopathy with consequent anterior horn cell degeneration, or from the radiculopathy.

One peculiar clinical syndrome, which most commonly results from lumbar spondylosis combined with a congenital narrowing of the lumbar canal, is intermittent ischemia of the cauda equina. There is usually degeneration with osteophyte formation, and marked sclerosis and hypertrophy of the lumbar laminae posteriorly (Verbiest, 1954, 1955; Joffe et al., 1966). As outlined in Chapter 30, patients have symptoms similar to intermittent claudication from ischemia of the calves with pain in the legs on exertion, relieved by rest. Two features aid in the recognition of this syndrome: first, the development of neurologic symptoms and signs at the time of the pain, often with loss of reflexes and power; and second, the interval between cessation of exertion and relief of the pain. In intermittent claudication from ischemia of the calves, relief occurs within a minute of cessation of exercise, but in intermittent ischemia of the cauda equina up to 5 or 10 minutes may be required. This syndrome may arise from other causes of compression of the cauda equina, including tumors such as ependymomas, and also from ischemia of the roots due to peripheral vascular disease.

Pathology. In addition to mechanical compression of the nerve fibers, the effects of restriction of the arterial supply by pressure on the radicular arteries within the inter-vertebral foramina are important. Changes in the nerve fibers are presumed to be similar to those seen in entrapment neuropathies elsewhere, with focal demyelination and a decreased diameter of the axons distal to the lesion (Thomas and Fullerton, 1963; see also Chapter 34). Wallerian degeneration occurs when the lesion is more severe.

Investigations. Plain spinal x-rays will reveal disk degeneration. On the lateral radiographs osteophytes can be seen encroaching posteriorly into the spinal canal, and on the oblique radiographs in the cervical region they can be seen in the intervertebral foramina. These changes are so frequently present in persons over the age of 50 that it is important to remember that they may be coincidental, some other process being responsible for the syndrome. Myelography will aid by excluding a compressive tumor and showing typical disk degeneration. In lumbar canal stenosis the typical myelographic picture is of an hourglass deformity of the lumbar theca (Joffe et al., 1966).

Treatment. Clinical symptoms of both lumbar and cervical spondylotic radiculopathy quite frequently show a relapsing and remitting course, making assessment of the efficacy of treatment difficult (Lees and Turner, 1963). Restriction of movements by a collar or corset often helps, as does heat therapy (British Association of Physical Medicine, 1966). It is important that the cervical collar should maintain the neck in mid-position for both excessive flexion and extension produce greater compression of the roots (Breig, 1960; Breig and El-Nadi, 1966). Continuous traction for a week or 10 days may sometimes be of use by maintaining immobility rather than as a result of a specific effect. Occasionally surgical decompression is required for unremitting pain or neurologic signs, particularly in the syndrome of intermittent claudication from lesions of the cauda equina. In the lumbar region, laminectomy is all that is required, though this is often difficult owing to hemorrhage from hypertrophic bone. In the cervical region laminectomy may also be effective, but may need to be combined with decompression of the intervertebral foramina. An anterolateral surgical approach for removal of the intervertebral disks and osteophytes and the insertion of a bony dowel to separate and fuse the vertebrae has also achieved some success. For a review of the surgical treatment of cervical spondylosis the reader is referred to Northfield and Osmond-Clarke (1967). No controlled trial of the effect of conservative medical and operative surgical treatment is available.

OTHER CAUSES OF SPINAL ROOT COMPRESSION

Tarlov (1938, 1970) has called attention to perineurial cysts that may compress the first part of the mixed spinal nerve. These are particularly to be found in the sacral region, but similar cysts are occasionally seen on the cervical or thoracic roots (Holt and Yates, 1964). These cysts arise as focal outpouchings of the dural root sleeve, the nerve constituting part of the wall. Their lumen is in partial but not free communication with the subarachnoid space. Patients usually present with symptoms and signs indistinguishable from the radiculopathy of a chronic disk protrusion. Myelography may show no abnormality at the initial screening since the cysts fill slowly, but they can usually be seen as bulbous outpouchings of the root sleeve on radiographs taken 24 hours later. Tarlov (1970) recommends surgical excision of the affected root, and plication of the dura. Excision of the dome of the cyst, sparing the root, is perhaps worthy of trial in the first instance, though recurrence is more frequent than with the more radical procedure.

Chou and Fakadej (1971) noted a peculiar abnormality of the anterior roots in two patients with infantile spinal muscular atrophy (Werdnig-Hoffmann disease), consisting of large masses of glial processes full of glial fibrils. This produced an appearance of hypertrophy of the nerve roots. He suggested that the aberrant glial tissue compressed the motor axons in the anterior roots, causing denervation and also retrograde neuronal death. This interesting possibility remains to be confirmed.

Dysrhaphism

The spinal cord and brain are formed by the rolling of the neural plate into the neural tube. Defects of closure of the tube, which may occur particularly at the two ends, have been mentioned in Chapter 30. In fetal development, the vertebrae arise in relation to the neural tube; in a similar manner, defects in

fusion of the vertebral laminae may also occur. This situation is termed spina bifida, and if no major external abnormality is visible, the term spina bifida occulta is applied (James and Lassman, 1972). Occasionally a small dimple, tag of hair, nevus, or subcutaneous lipoma over the sacral or lumbar region may give a clue to the underlying spina bifida occulta.

Various abnormalities associated with dysrhaphism may be associated with damage to the cauda equina. Myelomeningocele constitutes a major defect in which the spinal cord opens onto the surface in the lumbosacral region (see Chapter 30). Sometimes only the nerve roots are involved in the wall of such a sac, though damage may still be profound. A meningocele may arise without damage to the nervous tissue, though secondary infection is a hazard and immediate postnatal closure is recommended. Another associated developmental abnormality is an abnormally low conus, perhaps produced by "tethering" of the filum terminale and causing varying degrees of conus and cauda equina dysfunction.

There may be mesenchymal rests within the lumbosacral spinal cord that slowly grow into lipomas. There may also be a small dermal sinus leading to a dermoid cyst in a similar position (List, 1941). Both will slowly compress the cauda equina, producing pain, weakness and numbness of the lower limbs, and early sphincter impairment. Recurrent bouts of infection may occur in dermoid cysts.

Meningeal diverticula may be present in the lumbosacral region with no surface abnormality. Their size may range from a large meningocele passing into the axial musculature to a minor outpouching of the meninges or the nerve root sheath (Tarlov, 1970). Roots of the cauda equina may become trapped in these diverticula, causing symptoms and signs of root damage. These diverticula may become cysts if the neck is pinched off, and may thereby compress the cauda equina generally. In all instances in which signs indicate a cauda equina lesion, plain radiology and myelography are indicated, followed by surgical correction of the defect in most instances.

Toxic Radiculopathies

The nerve roots are affected by many of the conditions that damage the peripheral nervous system in general. For instance, in acrylamide neuropathy, which is predominantly of the "dying back" type, degenerating fibers can be found in the dorsal roots of experimental animals (Bradley and Williams, 1972). They are also specifically damaged by toxins injected into the subarachnoid space, either by accident or by design. The use of intrathecal alcohol to destroy the roots to relieve intractable pain due to carcinomatous infiltration of the pelvic plexus was introduced by Dogliotti (1931). Phenol was later used for the same purpose and for the relief of flexor spasms (Maher, 1955; Nathan, 1959; Kelly and Gautier-Smith, 1959). Use is made of the difference between the specific gravity of the therapeutic agent and of cerebrospinal fluid, absolute alcohol being lighter and phenol dissolved in glycerin or iophendylate (Myodil) heavier. For alcohol injection, the patient lies on his side with the roots to be destroyed at the highest point and the head downward. The position is reversed with phenol in glycerin. With the latter, the correct position can easily be obtained by making use of the warm sensation induced in the distribution of the roots being affected by the toxin. The use of phenol dissolved in radiopaque iophendylate allows additional radiographic control.

It is usual to administer about 0.3 to 1.0 ml of a 5 or 10 per cent solution of phenol for this purpose. The action of the solution is terminated in about 20 minutes by the dissolution of the phenol into the larger volume of cerebrospinal fluid. Troublesome flexion spasms and contractures in patients with severe paraplegia may be relieved by similar means, though the approach is generally more cautious, using 2.5 or 5 per cent phenol solution and multiple administrations of small volumes (Nathan, 1959, 1965; Kelly and Gautier-Smith, 1959). The danger of both procedures is severe sensory denervation of the skin and denervation atrophy of the muscles, with consequent marked predisposition to decubitis (pressure) ulcers. Though it was suggested by Maher (1955) and Nathan and Sears (1960) that the unmyelinated and small myelinated pain-carrying fibers were specifically damaged by phenol, it is now clear that fibers of all diameters are in fact equally affected (Berry and Olszewski, 1963; Hughes, 1966; Schaumberg et al., 1970). The phenol and alcohol damage both the axons and the Schwann cells of the nerve fibers, with consequent axonal degeneration.

Other substances accidentally allowed to contaminate the cerebrospinal fluid may also damage the roots and often the spinal cord in addition. Outbreaks of radiculopathy and arachnoiditis, probably from contamination of the spinal anesthetic with detergents or preservatives have been reported from time to time (Winkleman et al., 1953; Hurst, 1955). Occasionally disastrous reactions arise from the administration of the incorrect dose of penicillin intrathecally. A dose of 10,000 I.U. is tolerated, but if amounts of the order of 500,000 I.U. are administered there is immediate radicular pain in the distribution of the cauda equina, and often an encephalopathy with unconsciousness, seizures, and irreversible cerebral damage. The repeated daily instillation of streptomycin in the treatment of tuberculous meningitis may produce a mild chronic radiculopathy with pain and areflexia in the lower limbs (Smith, 1964).

Contrast media used for myelography may damage the nerve roots (see Chapter 30). Thorium dioxide, reported by Dale and Love (1967), and Lipiodol have now been abandoned. Even iophendylate, which is in current use, often produces pain in a sciatic distribution that may last for days or weeks. Though cases of significant radiculomyelopathy following the use of iophendylate are rare, it is the practice in the United States to remove the contrast agent after myelography.

Chronic Meningitis and Arachnoiditis

The nerve roots are prey not only to toxic damage as just described, but also to any infective, inflammatory, or neoplastic process affecting the cerebrospinal fluid. The diagnosis of these conditions is not easy and requires that each cause be considered and appropriately investigated. The roots may be subject to injury by "toxins" produced by such processes, as well as to varying degrees of compression and vascular damage. The spinal cord is often similarly involved adding to the diagnostic difficulty (see Chapter 30).

CHRONIC INFECTIVE MENINGITIS

Bacterial infections of the cerebrospinal fluid usually produce acute meningitis. The signs of meningitis include neck stiffness and pain on flexion of the leg onto the trunk due to inflammation of the nerve roots and cord that renders them more sensitive to stretching. Any bacterial meningitis may enter a chronic phase if there is inadequate reaction on the part of the body, or if treatment is too little or too late. Also tubercle bacilli and fungi such as cryptococci characteristically produce a more indolent process (Smith and Daniel, 1947). The damage to nerve roots is proportionately more severe in these chronic meningitides. Cranial nerve palsies not infrequently result from basal meningitis, and similarly a severe diffuse radiculopathy of the cauda equina may occur. The diagnosis rests on the isolation of organisms from the cerebrospinal fluid. Treatment consists of the appropriate antibiotic, which in such instances may best be administered intrathecally until the condition is well under control (Smith, 1964).

SYPHILIS

Syphilis may damage the nerve roots in three main ways (Brain and Walton, 1969). The most common form, meningovascular syphilis, produces a chronic diffuse inflammatory meningitis with endarteritis and thrombosis of the small arteries. The spinal cord is particularly involved, the radiculopathy often being indicated only by areflexia. Tabes dorsalis is the clinical syndrome resulting from loss of joint position and deep pain sensation. Superficial pain and temperature sensation over most of the body is preserved, though classically there is either loss or profound delay of perception of superficial pain over the bridge of the nose, the front of the chest, the inside of the arms, the outside of the leg, and the perianal area. Though posterior column degeneration in the spinal cord is most striking, and gave rise to the name of the syndrome, it is unlikely that this is primary, since degeneration of the dorsal roots is often found. The site of the lesion affecting the large nerve fibers carrying joint position sense has given rise to much dispute (Greenfield, 1963a; Hughes, 1966). Obersteiner and Redlich (1894–1895) believed the site of damage to be the root entry zone, while Nageotte (1903) believed that it lay in the dorsal root itself. Both theories have difficulty in explaining why only the larger fibers are damaged, and the hypothesis of a lesion of

the larger dorsal root ganglion neurons might be more attractive. Only minor changes are found in the ganglia, however, while significant inflammation and degeneration of the dorsal root make this the most likely site of damage. Large gummas of the meninges, which are rare, compress the nerve roots as any other space-occupying lesion, and also produce ischemia due to endarteritis.

UVEOMENINGITIC SYNDROMES

Sarcoidosis is the most common disease in this category (Colover, 1948; Jefferson, 1952, 1957; Camp and Frierson, 1962; Matthews, 1965; Silverstein et al., 1965). Uveitis, damage to the facial nerve in the parotid gland, and a diffuse polyneuropathy are the most frequent neurologic complications of this disease. A few patients develop symptoms from granulomas in the meninges, or less commonly in the brain substance. A basal arachnoiditis with damage to the pituitary gland and hypothalamus, and obstructive hydrocephalus are the most common complications in these patients. Occasionally a cranial nerve palsy or a single radiculopathy point to a focal lesion due to meningeal granulomas, though a diffuse radiculopathy is difficult to distinguish from a polyneuropathy. Most such patients have one or more peripheral manifestations of sarcoidosis such as lung or skin or bone changes, lymphadenopathy, or hypercalcemia. Rarely a patient may be encountered with no systemic evidence of sarcoidosis, who nevertheless has the typical sarcoid granulomas in the meninges. Some would not accept these as cases of true sarcoidosis, but until such time as they are shown to have a clinical course or a cause different from that of disseminated sarcoidosis, it seems to the author simplest to include them in this category.

Behcet's disease is another condition in this group (Wolf et al., 1965). The diagnostic features are recurrent attacks of uveitis associated with oral and genital ulceration and frequently thrombophlebitis. Occasionally viruses have been isolated in such cases (Evans et al., 1957; Noyan et al., 1969). The nervous system may be involved, predominantly with a relapsing encephalomyelitis, as reported by Herring and Urich (1969), though occasionally a radiculopathy or neuropathy is associated (O'Duffy et al., 1971; Lobo-Antunes,

1972). The uveoencephalomeningitic (Vogt-Koyanagi-Harada) syndromes should also be considered (Reed et al., 1958; Pattison, 1965; Riehl and Andrews, 1966).

NEOPLASTIC RADICULOPATHY

Tumors disseminated within the cerebrospinal fluid pathways will often settle under gravity to the lower part of the spinal canal with consequent growth and metastases on the nerve roots and around the spinal cord. Medulloblastomas seed throughout the central nervous system, and one of the early symptoms may be backache from such metastases (Russell and Rubinstein, 1963). Carcinomatous meningitis is a rare form of dissemination, usually from primary tumors in the bronchus, breast, or gastrointestinal tract, again with the same symptoms and signs (Russell and Rubinstein, 1963). In both conditions, myelography may show multiple rounded filling defects on the roots or granular irregularities, neoplastic cells may be found in the cerebrospinal fluid, and the cerebrospinal fluid sugar may be decreased (McMillan, 1962; Love et al., 1970). The carcinoma cells, however, often form a tight sheet around the affected roots, without free cells in the cerebrospinal fluid, and even on macroscopic examination, may appear normal. Though most patients with this condition die fairly quickly, in a few the progress is slow and painful, and the diagnosis extremely difficult without surgical exploration and biopsy.

With a radiosensitive neoplasm such as medulloblastoma, neuraxis x-ray therapy can be remarkably effective. Systemic cytotoxic agents may also be effective (Lassman et al., 1965; 1966). Carcinomatous meningitis is more difficult to treat because it is less radiosensitive. Cytotoxic agents may be tried, even administered intrathecally. Even methotrexate, however, which is the best tolerated of this group of drugs, is not without its dangers by the subarachnoid route (Back, 1969; Duttera et al., 1972).

RADICULOPATHY DUE TO ENDOGENOUS TOXINS

Endogenous intoxication within the subarachnoid space occurs in two conditions. In both cases intensive search for the underlying lesion is indicated, since otherwise the condition gradually progresses to a fatal outcome.

A dermoid cyst may leak into the subarachnoid space either spontaneously or postoperatively, to produce a severe granulomatous, inflammatory reaction (Cantu and Wright, 1968). Cholesterol crystals are probably the agent responsible. Corticosteroids may be dramatically beneficial in the acute phase (Cantu and Ojeman, 1968). The clinical signs and symptoms are indistinguishable from acute or chronic meningitis, though the diagnosis can be made by the recognition of cholesterol crystals and squames in the cerebrospinal fluid. Occasionally the picture is more indolent, with progressive encephalopathy and deafness, cranial nerve signs, and areflexia indicating radicular damage (Tomlinson and Walton, 1967).

The leakage of blood into the cerebrospinal fluid produces a similar picture. Acute subarachnoid hemorrhage almost invariably produces signs of meningeal irritation. Chronic subarachnoid leakage of blood may produce the syndrome of superficial hemosiderosis of the central nervous system in which the deposition of iron pigment in the meninges and subjacent nervous tissue damages the brain, cranial nerves, and nerve roots (Tomlinson and Walton, 1964; Hughes and Oppenheimer, 1969). This may occur with repeated small hemorrhages from an arteriovenous malformation, an aneurysm, or a vascular tumor such as an ependymoma or choroid plexus papilloma. Hemosiderin-laden macrophages in the cerebrospinal fluid will confirm the diagnosis.

CHRONIC IDIOPATHIC ADHESIVE ARACHNOIDITIS

Damage to the nerve root of any cause, from syphilis and disk prolapse to intrathecal phenol, induces secondary inflammation and thickening of the adjacent arachnoid. When all known causes of inflammation of the arachnoid are excluded, however, a group of patients remains to whose disease the label of chronic idiopathic adhesive arachnoiditis is applied. The fullest investigation of all such patients, including surgical exploration and biopsy, is indicated since an occasionally treatable cause may yet be brought to light (Davidson, 1968). Damage to the nerve roots is frequently extensive, pain in a radicular distribution being the most usual symptom. Spinal cord involvement often dominates the picture, and the investigation and treatment are discussed in Chapter 30.

Radiation Radiculopathy

The peripheral nerves including the nerve roots are probably somewhat more resistant to radiation damage than the central nervous system, as reported by Kristensson, Molin and Sourander (1967), but nevertheless they may degenerate following deep x-ray therapy (Innes and Carsten, 1961; Stoll and Andrews, 1966). It may be difficult to distinguish spinal root damage from that of the limb girdle plexuses, which lie adjacent to the spine, and when the spinal cord is irradiated, symptoms and signs of the myelopathy usually dominate the picture (see Chapter 30). A dose of more than 5000 rads is liable to cause a progressive syndrome of paresthesias, muscle weakness, and atrophy. Occasionally as in radiation myelopathy, the onset may be sudden, indicating infarction due to radiation-induced endarteritis. The latent interval between irradiation and the onset of the syndrome is usually three months to three or more years, and the pathologic changes are predominantly loss of nerve fibers with fibrosis and endarteritis. No treatment is of avail once the irradiation has occurred, and the object of radiotherapists is to keep the dose below threshold. It may be extremely difficult to separate a progressive radiation radiculopathy from further compression of the nerve roots by recurrent tumor. This is particularly so following x-ray therapy given for ependymoma of the filum terminale. All cases should be subjected to investigation prior to acceptance of the diagnosis of radiation neuropathy.

CONCLUDING REMARKS

The spinal nerve roots constitute the part of the peripheral sensory and motor nerves that happen to lie within the spinal canal. They are liable to most diseases that affect the peripheral nervous system. Certain generalized diseases of the peripheral nervous system have a predilection for the roots, perhaps because of the absence of the blood-nerve barrier in the roots. In addition, the roots are vulnerable to every disease occurring within the spinal canal. Signs of root involvement may not be obvious when spinal cord damage predominates, and it is really only in the cauda equina that they are seen in their purest form. Because of the proximity to the nerve cell body and the great distance from the innervated structures, regeneration is slight once axonal interruption has occurred in the spinal roots. The pain of radicular involvement is, however, relieved by removing the offending disease process, and some degree of recovery can be expected by peripheral reinnervation from adjacent segments. When the injury is less severe and segmental demyelination is the predominant lesion, recovery may be relatively rapid following the removal of the underlying disease. Early diagnosis, careful investigation, and effective therapy are thus of great importance.

Acknowledgment: I am grateful to Mrs. E. Mooney for unfailing secretarial services.

REFERENCES

Abbott, K. H., and Mitts, M. G.: Reflex neurovascular syndromes. *In* Vinken, P. J., and Bruyn, G. W. (eds.): Handbook of Clinical Neurology. Vol. 8. Amsterdam, North-Holland Publishing Co., 1970, p. 321.

Abrahamson, L., McConnell, A. A., and Wilson, G. R.: Acute epidural spinal abscess. Br. Med. J., *1*:1114, 1934.

Adams, C. B. T., and Logue, V.: Studies in cervical spondylotic myelopathy. I. Movement of the cervical roots, dura and cord, and their relation to the course taken by the extrathecal roots. Brain, *94*:557, 1971a.

Adams, C. B. T., and Logue, V.: Studies in cervical spondylotic myelopathy. II. Observations on the movement and contour of the cervical spine in relation to the neural complications of cervical spondylosis. Brain, *94*:569, 1971b.

Asbury, A. K., Arnason, B. G., and Adams, R. D.: The inflammatory lesion in idiopathic polyneuritis. Its role in pathogenesis. Medicine (Baltimore), *48*:173, 1969.

Back, E. H.: Death after intrathecal methotrexate. Lancet, 2:1005, 1969.

Berry, K., and Olszewski, J.: Pathology of intrathecal phenol injection in man. Neurology (Minneap.), *13*:152, 1963.

Blockey, N. J., and Schorstein, J.: Intraspinal epidermoid tumours in the lumbar region of children. J. Bone Joint Surg., *43B*:556, 1961.

Bradley, W. G., and Williams, M. H.: Unpublished observations, 1972.

Brain, Lord and Walton, J. N.: Brain's Diseases of the Nervous System. 7th Edition. London, Oxford University Press, 1969.

Breig, A.: Biomechanics of the Central Nervous System. Some Basic Normal and Pathologic Phenomena. Stockholm, Almquist & Wiksell, 1960.

Breig, A., and El-Nadi, A. F.: Biomechanics of the cervical spinal cord. Acta Radiol. [Diagn.] (Stockh.), 4:602, 1966.

British Association of Physical Medicine: Pain in the neck and arm: a multicentre trial of the effects of physiotherapy. Br. Med. J., 1:253, 1966.

Camp, W. A., and Frierson, J. G.: Sarcoidosis of the central nervous system. A case with post-mortem studies. Arch. Neurol., 7:432, 1962.

Cantu, R. C., and Ojeman, R. D.: Glucosteroid treatment of keratin meningitis following the removal of a fourth ventricle epidermoid tumour. J. Neurol. Neurosurg. Psychiatry, 31:73, 1968.

Cantu, R. C., and Wright, R. L.: Aseptic meningitic syndrome with cauda equina epidermoid tumor. J. Pediatr., 73:114, 1968.

Cavanagh, J. B., and Chen, F. C. K.: Amino acid incorporation in protein during the "silent phase" before organomercury and p-bromophenylacetylurea neuropathy in the rat. Acta Neuropathol., (Berl.), 19:216, 1971.

Cavanagh, J. B., and Mellick, R. S.: On the nature of the peripheral nerve lesions associated with acute intermittent porphyria. J. Neurol. Neurosurg. Psychiatry, 28:320, 1965.

Cavanagh, J. B., and Ridley, A. R.: The nature of the neuropathy complicating acute intermittent porphyria. Lancet, 2:1023, 1967.

Choremis, C., Economos, D., Papadatos, C., and Gargoulas, A.: Intraspinal epidermoid tumours (Cholesteatomas) in patients treated for tuberculous meningitis. Lancet, 2:437, 1956.

Chou, S. M., and Fakadej, A. V.: Ultrastructure of chromatolytic motoneurons and anterior spinal roots in a case of Werdnig-Hoffmann disease. J. Neuropathol. Exp. Neurol., 30:368, 1971.

Colover, J.: Sarcoidosis with involvement of the nervous system. Brain, 71:451, 1948.

Croft, P. B., and Wilkinson, M.: The course and progress of some types of carcinomatous neuromyopathy. Brain, 92:1, 1969.

Croft, P. B., Urich, H., and Wilkinson, M.: Peripheral neuropathy of sensorimotor type associated with malignant disease. Brain, 90:31, 1967.

Dale, A. J. D., and Love, J. G.: Thorium dioxide myelopathy. J.A.M.A., 199:606, 1967.

Davidson, S.: Cryptococcal spinal arachnoiditis. J. Neurol. Neurosurg. Psychiatry, 31:76, 1968.

Dogliotti, A. M.: Traitment des syndromes douloureux de la périphérie par l'alcoolisation sub-arachnoidienne des racines postérieures à leur émergence de la moelle épinière. Presse Méd., 1249, 1931.

Duttera, J. M., Gallelli, J. F., Kleinman, L. M., Tangrea, J. A., and Wittgrove, A. C.: Intrathecal methotrexate. Lancet, 1:540, 1972.

Duvoisin, R. C., and Yahr, M. D.: Compressive spinal cord and root syndromes in achondroplastic dwarfs. Neurology (Minneap.), 12:202, 1962.

Dyck, P. J., Lambert, E. H., and Nichols, P. C.: Quantitative measurement of sensation related to compound action potential and number and sizes of myelinated and unmyelinated fibers of sural nerve in health, Friedreich's ataxia, hereditary sensory neuropathy and tabes dorsalis. Electroencephalogr. Clin. Neurophysiol., 9:9, 1971.

Dyck, P. J., Shultz, P. W., and O'Brien, P. C.: Quantitation

of touch-pressure sensation. Arch. Neurol., 26:465, 1972.

Epstein, J. A., and Malis, L. I.: Compression of spinal cord and cauda equina in achondroplastic dwarfs. Neurology (Minneap.), 5:875, 1955.

Evans, A. D., Pallis, C. A., and Spillane, J. D.: Involvement of the nervous system in Behçet's syndrome. Report of three cases and isolation of the virus. Lancet, 2:349, 1957.

Fisher, C. M., and Adams, R. D.: Diphtheritic polyneuritis—a pathological study. J. Neuropathol. Exp. Neurol., 15:243, 1955.

Greenfield, J. G.: Infectious diseases of the central nervous system. In Blackwood, W., McMenemey, W. H., Meyer, A., Norman, R. M., and Russell, D. S. (eds.): Greenfield's Neuropathology. London, Edward Arnold Ltd. [Baltimore, Williams & Wilkins Co.], 1963a, p. 138.

Greenfield, J. G.: Lesions of the nervous system associated with disease or malformations of the cranium and spinal column. In Blackwood, W., McMenemey, W. H., Meyer, A., Norman, R. M., and Russell, D. S. (eds.): Greenfield's Neuropathology. London, Edward Arnold Ltd. [Baltimore, Williams & Wilkins Co.], 1963b.

Haymaker, W., and Kernohan, J. W.: The Landry-Guillain-Barré syndrome. Medicine (Baltimore), 28:59, 1949.

Herring, A. B., and Urich, H.: Sarcoidosis of the central nervous system. J. Neurol. Sci., 9:405, 1969.

Hirson, C.: Spinal subdural abscess. Lancet, 2:1215, 1965.

Holt, S., and Yates, P. O.: Cervical nerve root "cysts." Brain, 87:481, 1964.

Hughes, J. T.: Pathology of the Spinal Cord. London, Lloyd-Luke Ltd. [Philadelphia, J. B. Lippincott Co.], 1966.

Hughes, J. T., and Oppenheimer, D. R.: Superficial siderosis of the central nervous system. Acta Neuropathol. (Berl.), 13:56, 1969.

Hurst, E. W.: Adhesive arachnoiditis and vascular blockage caused by detergents and other chemical irritants: experimental study. J. Pathol. Bacteriol., 70:167, 1955.

Innes, J. R. M., and Carsten, A.: Delayed effects of localized x-irradiation of the nervous system of experimental rats and monkeys. In "Fundamental Aspects of Radiosensitivity." Brookhaven Symp. Biol., 14:200, 1961.

James, C. C. M., and Lassman, L. P.: Spinal Dysraphism: Spina Bifida Occulta. London, Butterworth & Co. Ltd., 1972.

Jefferson, M.: Nervous signs in sarcoidosis. Br. Med. J., 2:916, 1952.

Jefferson, M.: Sarcoidosis of the nervous system. Brain, 80:540, 1957.

Joffe, R., Appleby, A., and Arjona, V.: 'Intermittent ischaemia' of the cauda equina due to stenosis of the lumbar canal. J. Neurol. Neurosurg. Psychiatry, 29:315, 1966.

Kamrin, R. P., Potanos, J. N., and Pool, J. L.: An evaluation of the diagnosis and treatment of chordoma. J. Neurol. Neurosurg. Psychiatry, 27:157, 1964.

Kawakita, H., Nishimura, M., Satoh, Y., and Shiba, N.: Neurological aspects of Behçet's disease. A case report and clinico-pathological review of the literature in Japan. J. Neurol. Sci., 5:417, 1967.

Kelly, R. E., and Gautier-Smith, P. C.: Intrathecal phenol in the treatment of reflex spasms and spasticity. Lancet, 2:1102, 1959.

Kristensson, K., Molin, B., and Sourander, P.: Delayed radiation lesions of human spinal cord. Report of five cases. Acta Neuropathol. (Berl.), 9:34, 1967.

Lassman, L. P., Pearce, G. W., and Gang, J.: Sensitivity of intracranial gliomas to vincristine sulphate. Lancet, 1:296, 1965.

Lassman, L. P., Pearce, G. W., and Gang, J.: Effect of vincristine sulphate on the intracranial gliomata of childhood. Br. J. Surg., 53:774, 1966.

Lees, F., and Turner, J. W.: Natural history and prognosis of cervical spondylosis. Br. Med. J., 5373:1607, 1963.

List, C. F.: Intraspinal epidermoids, dermoids and dermal sinuses. Surg. Gynecol. Obstet., 37:525, 1941.

Lobo-Artunes, J.: Behçet's disease. Ann. Intern. Med., 76:332, 1972.

Love, J. G., Kao, C. C., and Baker, H. L., Jr.: Painless intraspinal leptomeningeal carcinomatosis. A myelographic demonstration. J. Neurosurg., 32:108, 1970.

Mabon, R. F., Svien, H. J., Kernohan, J. W., and Craig, W. M.: Ependymomas. Mayo Clin. Proc., 24:65, 1949.

McMillan, J. A.: Meningitis due to carcinomatosis. Case with free carcinoma cells in cerebrospinal fluid. Br. Med. J., 1:1452, 1962.

Maher, R. M.: Relief of pain in incurable cancer. Lancet, 1:18, 1955.

Matthews, W. B.: Sarcoidosis of the nervous system. J. Neurol. Neurosurg. Psychiatry, 28:23, 1965.

Nageotte, J.: Pathogenie du Tabes Dorsal. Paris, Naud, 1903.

Nathan, P. W.: Intrathecal phenol to relieve spasticity in paraplegia. Lancet, 2:1099, 1959.

Nathan, P. W.: Chemical rhizotomy for relief of spasticity in ambulant patients. Br. Med. J., 1:1096, 1965.

Nathan, P. W., and Sears, T. A.: Effects of phenol on nervous conduction. J. Physiol. (Lond.), 150:565, 1960.

Northfield, D. W. C., and Osmond-Clarke, H.: Surgical treatment. In Brain, Lord, and Wilkinson, M. (eds.): Cervical Spondylosis. London, William Heinemann Ltd. [Philadelphia, W. B. Saunders Co.], 1967.

Noyan, B., Gürsoy, G., and Aktin, E.: Inoculationsversuchs bei Maüsen mit dem Liquor eines Falles von Neuro-Behçetscher Krankheit. Acta Neuropathol. (Berl.), 12:195, 1969.

Obersteiner, H., and Redlich, E. (1894–1895): Quoted by Greenfield, J. G.: Infectious diseases of the central nervous system. In Blackwood, W., McMenemey, W. H., Meyer, A., Norman, R. M., and Russell, D. S. (eds.): Greenfield's Neuropathology. 2nd Edition. London, Edward Arnold Ltd. [Baltimore, Williams & Wilkins Co.], 1963.

O'Duffy, J. D., Carney, J. A., and Deodhar, S.: Behçet's disease. Report of ten cases, three with new manifestations. Ann. Intern. Med., 75:561, 1971.

Olsson, Y.: Topographical differences in the vascular permeability of the peripheral nervous system. Acta Neuropathol. (Berl.), 10:26, 1968.

Pallis, C., Jones, A. M., and Spillane, J. D.: Cervical spondylosis. Incidence and implications. Brain, 77:274, 1954.

Pattison, E. M.: Uveomeningoencephalitic syndrome (Vogt-Koyanagi-Harada syndrome). Arch. Neurol., 12:197, 1965.

Payne, E. E., and Spillane, J. D.: The cervical spine. An anatomicopathological study of seventy specimens with particular reference to the problem of cervical spondylosis. Brain, 80:571, 1957.

Reed, H., Lindsay, A., Silversides, J. L., Speakman, J.,

Monckton, G., and Rees, D. L.: The uveoencephalitic syndrome or Vogt-Koyanagi-Harada disease. Can. Med. Assoc. J., 79:451, 1958.

Riehl, J.-L. and Andrews, J. M.: The uveomeningoencephalitic syndrome. Neurology (Minneap.), 16:603, 1966.

Russell, D. S., and Rubinstein, L. J.: Pathology of tumors of the Nervous System. 2nd Edition. London, Edward Arnold Ltd. [Baltimore, Williams & Wilkins Co.], 1963.

Schaumberg, H. H., Byck, R., and Weller, R. O.: The effect of phenol on peripheral nerve. A histological and electrophysiological study. J. Neuropathol. Exp. Neurol., 29:615, 1970.

Sensenig, E. C.: Adhesions of notochord and neural tube in the formation of chordomas. Am. J. Anat., 98:357, 1956.

Silverstein, A., Feuer, M. M., and Siltzbach, L. E.: Neurologic sarcoidosis. Study of 18 cases. Arch. Neurol., 12:1, 1965.

Smith, H. V.: Tuberculous meningitis. Int. J. Neurol., 4:134, 1964.

Smith, H. V., and Daniel, P.: Some clinical and pathological aspects of tuberculosis of the central nervous system. Tubercle, 28:64, 1947.

Stoll, B. A., and Andrew, J. T.: Radiation-induced peripheral neuropathy. Br. Med. J., 2:834, 1966.

Sunderland, S.: Nerves and Nerve Injuries. Edinburgh, E. & S. Livingstone Ltd. [Baltimore, Williams & Wilkins Co.], 1968.

Symonds, C. P., and Blackwood, W.: Spinal cord compression in hypertrophic neuritis. Brain, 85:251, 1962.

Tarlov, I. M.: Perineurial cysts of the spinal nerve roots. Arch. Neurol. Psychiatry, 40:1067, 1938.

Tarlov, I. M.: Spinal cord compression: mechanisms of paralysis and treatment. Springfield, Ill., Charles C Thomas, 1957.

Tarlov, I. M.: Spinal perineurial and meningeal cysts. J. Neurol. Neurosurg. Psychiatry, 33:833, 1970.

Taylor, P. E.: Traumatic intradural avulsion of the nerve roots of the brachial plexus. Brain, 85:579, 1962.

Thomas, P. K., and Fullerton, P. M.: Nerve fibre size in the carpal tunnel syndrome. J. Neurol. Neurosurg. Psychiatry, 26:520, 1963.

Tomlinson, B. E., and Walton, J. N.: Superficial haemosiderosis of the central nervous system. J. Neurol. Neurosurg. Psychiatry, 27:332, 1964.

Tomlinson, B. E., and Walton, J. N.: Granulomatous meningitis and diffuse parenchymatous degeneration of the nervous system due to an intracranial epidermoid cyst. J. Neurol. Neurosurg. Psychiatry, 30:341, 1967.

Trojaborg, W., Frantzen, E., and Andersen, I.: Peripheral neuropathies and myopathies associated with carcinoma of the lung. Brain, 92:71, 1969.

Verbiest, H.: Radicular syndrome from developmental narrowing of the lumbar vertebral canal. J. Bone Joint Surg., 36B:230, 1954.

Verbiest, H.: Further experience on the pathological influence of developmental narrowness of the bony lumbar vertebral canal. J. Bone Joint Surg., 37B:576, 1955.

Waksman, B. H.: Experimental study of diphtheritic polyneuritis in the rabbit and guinea pig. III The blood-nerve barrier in the rabbit. J. Neuropathol. Exp. Neurol., 20:35, 1961.

Waksman, B. H., Adams, R. D. A., and Mansman, H. C.,

Jr.: Experimental study of diphtheritic polyneuritis in the rabbit and guinea pig. I. Immunologic and histopathologic observations. J. Exp. Med., *105*: 591, 1957.

Waltz, T. A.: Physical factors in the production of the myelopathy of cervical spondylosis. Brain, *90*:395, 1967.

Warren, J., Gutmann, L., Figueroa, A. F., and Bloor, B. M.: E.M.G. changes of brachial plexus root avulsions. J. Neurosurg., *31*:137, 1969.

Wilkinson, M. (ed.): Cervical spondylosis. Its early diagnosis and treatment. London, William Heinemann Ltd. [Philadelphia, W. B. Saunders Co.], 1971.

Winkleman, N. W., Gotten, N., and Scheibert, D.: Localized adhesive spinal arachnoiditis. A study of 25 cases with reference to etiology. Trans. Am. Neurol. Assoc., *78*:15, 1953.

Wolf, S. M., Schotland, D. L., and Phillips, L. L.: Involvement of the nervous system in Behçet's syndrome. Arch. Neurol., *12*:315, 1965.

Zverina, E., and Skorpil, V.: Possibilities of the electromyographic diagnosis of brachial plexus injury. Electroencephalogr. Clin. Neurophysiol., *26*:233, 1969.

Zoltan, L., and Fenyes, I.: Stereotactic diagnosis and radioactive treatment on a case of speno-occipital chordoma. J. Neurosurg., *17*:888, 1960.

Chapter 32

BRACHIAL PLEXUS NEUROPATHIES

Peter Tsairis

Brachial plexus neuropathies are often perplexing problems, not only for the patient, but also for the physician. These neuropathies may occur suddenly without apparent cause or may result from direct compression by adjacent skeletal anomalies, tumors, or congenital fascial bands or from various forms of trauma. The trauma may be direct, such as that from perforating wounds, or indirect from humeral or rib fractures and dislocations of the shoulder. Difficult births and sudden traction applied to the arm or neck or both may also injure the brachial plexus. Complete or partial plexus involvement may follow a parenteral injection of foreign serum or vaccine, or accompany certain systemic illnesses or toxic metabolic states. Cryptogenic brachial plexus neuropathy, sometimes called neuralgic amyotrophy or paralytic brachial neuritis is a distinct nosologic entity that is often confused with more common causes of brachial pain and weakness. Familial cases of this type of plexus neuropathy are well documented. Table 32–1 summarizes the different types of brachial plexus neuropathy on an etiologic basis.

ANATOMICAL ASPECTS OF CLINICAL IMPORTANCE

The anatomical design of the brachial plexus is complex (Figs. 32–1 and 32–2). An understanding of the relationship between the plexus, the blood vessels, and the adjacent bony structures is essential in understanding the various types of clinical plexus lesions.

The anterior primary rami of the fifth, sixth, seventh, and eighth cervical roots and the first thoracic root are constant contributors to the plexus. These roots are interwoven and sorted to emerge from the axilla as peripheral nerves of the upper extremity. Occasionally, when the fourth cervical root contributes significantly to the plexus, it is called prefixed; while a contribution by the second thoracic root produces a postfixed plexus (Harris, 1939). As shown in Figure 32–1, the fifth and sixth cervical roots combine to form the upper trunk; the seventh cervical root emerges singly as the middle trunk; and the eighth cervical and first thoracic roots unite to form the lower trunk. Two clinically important peripheral nerves originate from the anterior primary rami of the fifth and sixth cervical roots near the vertebral column; the dorsal scapular nerve serving the rhomboid and levator scapulae muscles and the long thoracic nerve, which innervates the serratus anterior muscle. Clinical evaluation of these muscles may be helpful in localizing the level of a plexus lesion. In the supraclavicular fossa, the trunks become quite superficial, protected only by the skin, subcutaneous tissues, and investing fascia. While in the supraclavicular fossa they come into close relationship to the subclavian artery, the lower trunk going immediately behind it and the middle and upper trunks going dorsal and lateral to it, respectively (see Fig. 32–2). In the supraclavicular fossa, the plexus, especially the lower trunk, and subclavian artery are close to the pulmonary apex. At the level of the clavicle, the trunks divide into anterior and posterior divisions. These divisions pass beneath the middle third of the

659

TABLE 32–1 ETIOLOGIC CLASSIFICATION OF BRACHIAL PLEXUS NEUROPATHY (BPN)

I. BPN of systemic illness, infections, and toxins	
Local septic infections	Direct extension to plexus
Systemic infections	Dysentery, typhoid fever, gonorrhea, parotitis, infectious mononucleosis, toxoplasmosis (? hypersensitivity)
Systemic illness	? Diabetes mellitus, polyarteritis nodosa
Toxins	Heroin addiction (? direct toxic effect)
II. Cryptogenic BPN (neuralgia amyotrophy, paralytic branchial neuritis)	
Antecedent infection or illness, convalescence from surgery	? Allergic-vascular disturbance
Epidemic form	? Viral etiology
Serum and vaccine induced	? Allergic reaction
III. Heredofamilial BPN	Genetic susceptibility to pathogenetic factors in II
IV. Traumatic plexus neuropathies	
Open wound injury	Penetrating missiles, lacerations, stab wounds
Closed injuries	Fracture-dislocation of shoulder
	Traction-compression lesions (vehicular injuries, postoperative or postanesthesia BPN, "rucksack paralysis," "pallbearer's palsy," hematomas from anticoagulant therapy and axillary percutaneous catheterization)
	Avulsion injury
Birth injury	Traction or stretching (? direct trauma)
V. Isolated mononeuropathies	
Long thoracic, suprascapular musculocutaneous, axillary nerves	Systemic infections, trauma
VI. BPN of thoracic outlet obstruction	
Congenital anomalies	Compression from cervical rib, first rib anomalies, abnormal scalene muscles, fibrous fascial bands, flat clavicle, subclavian vessel anomalies
Secondary anatomic changes	Postoperative sagging and drooping of shoulder, chest trauma
VII. BPN due to physical agents	
Irradiation	Direct injury to nerves
Electrical injury	
VIII. Neoplasms of the brachial plexus	
Primary tumors	Neurilemmoma, neurofibroma (solitary or multiple von Recklinghausen's disease)
	Ganglioneuroma, amputation neuroma
Secondary tumors	Fibrous dysplasia and bone cysts of clavicle, metastatic breast and lung cancer (superior sulcus tumor), lymphoma

clavicle and on top of the first rib. At this junction, the plexus is in the infraclavicular fossa, and the divisions extend to a point just beyond the lateral border of the first rib. The anterior divisions unite to form the lateral and medial cords, and the posterior divisions form the posterior cord. These cords then pass into the upper part of the axilla adjacent to the axillary artery. Here they come to lie close to the first and second parts of the axillary artery; the third part of the artery is contiguous with the terminal branches of the cords. In the axilla, both the cords and blood vessels are surrounded by a thick pad of fat and connective tissue, which permits unrestricted movement during use of the upper extremity.

Tension or traction on the upper cervical roots or trunk of the plexus occurs when the shoulder is forcibly depressed or when the arm is abducted with the head tilted toward the opposite side. Apical pulmonary lesions and skeletal anomalies in the infraclavicular fossa and axilla may compress the brachial plexus and subclavian vessels to produce the various syndromes of thoracic outlet obstruction. High in the supraclavicular fossa, the fascia and scalene muscles protect the plexus.

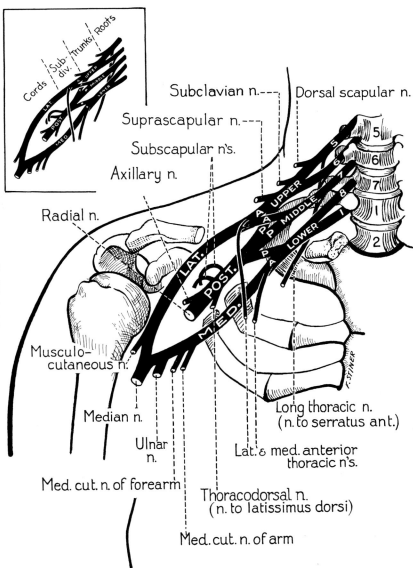

Figure 32–1 Diagram of the brachial plexus. (From Haymaker, W., and Woodhall, B.: Peripheral Nerve Injuries. 2nd Edition. Philadelphia and London, W. B. Saunders Co., 1953. Reprinted by permission.)

Damage to the nerves in this area must result either from direct rupture of these muscles or from avulsion of the nerves from their attachments in the intervertebral foramina or cord.

The plexus may be divided into an anterior (flexor) and posterior (extensor) portion corresponding to the flexor and extensor limb muscles. The medial and lateral cords of the plexus form the anterior portion and supply the muscles of the pectoral region and all the muscles on the anterior (volar) aspects of the arm, forearm, and hand. The posterior cord supplies most of the muscles of the shoulder and all the posterior (extensor) muscles in the arm and forearm. In the supraclavicular region, nerve fibers are arranged segmentally; lesions in this area usually produce dermatomal or sensory root deficits. Infraclavicular lesions produce complex motor and sensory deficits in either a cord or peripheral nerve distribution. Sympathetic fibers to sweat glands accompany the sensory nerves, so that defects of sweating correspond to areas of cutaneous sensory loss. Preganglionic sympathetic fibers of the first and second thoracic roots pass through the sympathetic chain to reach the superior cervical ganglion, therefore lesions of the lower portions of the plexus may cause a Horner's syndrome.

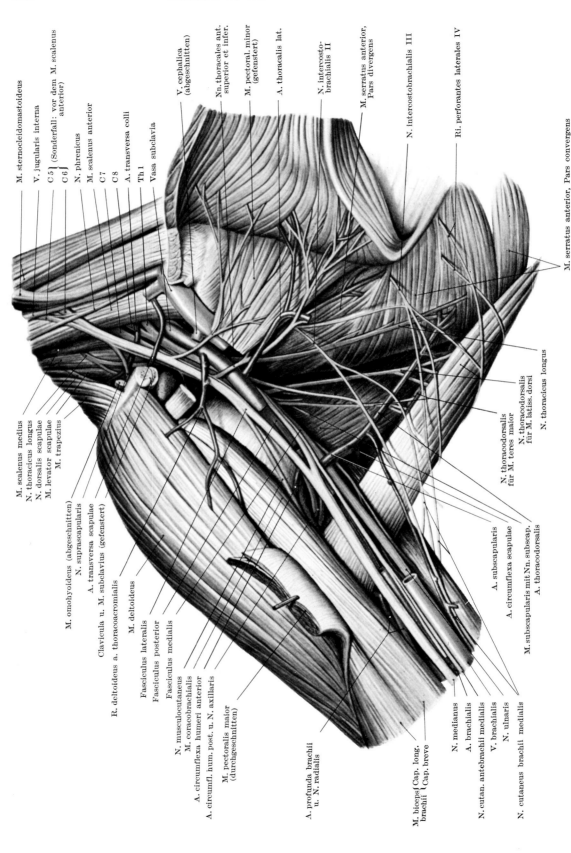

Figure 32–2 Relationship of the plexus components to surrounding vessels and bony structures. (From von Lantz, T., and Wachsmuth, W.: Praktische Anatomie. Berlin, Springer-Verlag, 1935. Reprinted by permission.)

M. sternocleidomastoideus

V. jugularis interna

C 5 } (Sonderfall: vor dem M. scalenus
C 6 } anterior)

N. phrenicus

M. scalenus anterior

C7

C8

A. transversa colli

Th 1

Vasa subclavia

V. cephalica (abgeschnitten)

Nn. thoracales ant. superior et infer.

M. pectoral. minor (gefenstert)

A. thoracalis lat.

N. interostobrachialis II

M. serratus anterior, Pars divergens

N. interostobrachialis III

Rl. perforantes laterales IV

M. serratus anterior, Pars convergens

N. thoracicus longus

N. thoracodorsalis für M. latiss. dorsi

N. thoracodorsalis für M. teres major

M. subscapularis mit Nn. subscap.

A. circumflexa scapulae

A. thoracodorsalis

A. subscapularis

N. cutaneus brachii medialis

N. ulnaris

V. brachialis

N. cutan. antebrachii medialis

A. brachialis

N. medianus

M. biceps { Cap. long.
brachii { Cap. breve

A. profunda brachii u. N. radialis

M. pectoralis maior (durchgeschnitten)

A. circumfl. hum. post. u. N. axillaris

A. circumflexa humeri anterior

M. coracobrachialis

N. musculocutaneus

Fasciculus medialis

Fasciculus posterior

Fasciculus lateralis

M. deltoideus

R. deltoideus a. thoracoacromialis

Clavicula u. M. subclavius (gefenstert)

A. transversa scapulae

N. suprascapularis

M. omohyoideus (abgeschnitten)

M. trapezius

M. levator scapulae

N. dorsalis scapulae

N. thoracicus longus

M. scalenus medius

CLINICAL FEATURES AND DIAGNOSIS OF PLEXUS LESIONS

Plexus lesions are most often incomplete. They are characterized by combinations of weakness, muscle atrophy, abnormalities of stretch reflexes, sensory changes, and less often, sympathetic nerve dysfunction. The brachial pain is usually constant, rarely intermittent, quite severe, and most often localized above the elbow. In most patients it is aggravated by arm movement and accompanied by a variable degree of weakness. Occasionally, weakness without pain or other sensory disturbance is the presenting manifestation of plexus involvement, especially that due to tumor or following inoculations. Sensory impairment is often patchy and incomplete; partial lesions may be associated with hyperesthesia or dysesthesia. Sympathetic function is usually preserved unless injury extends to the thoracic roots. Muscle atrophy may occur rapidly following acute plexus injury. Fasciculations are uncommon and may occur late in the clinical course. If the injury is severe enough to produce scarring, traumatic neuromas may form in the region of injury. Uncommonly, phantom limb pain may develop after severe trauma to the plexus. Long-term complications of plexus lesions may include skin ulcers, blisters, and secondary infection; joint contractures; osteoporosis and sympathetic reflex dystrophy or causalgia. Causalgic pain, characterized as a burning, throbbing, squeezing pain with associated hyperesthesia of the affected area, may occur at a variable time after nerve damage. The severity of the lesion will determine the duration of symptoms, the proportions of neurologic dysfunction, and the extent of recovery. Severity may be difficult to assess either by examination or after surgical exploration.

Upper Plexus Lesion

This lesion follows damage to the fifth and sixth cervical roots or upper trunk. It is the most common type of plexus involvement from any cause and is usually incomplete. The involved muscles include the deltoid, biceps, brachioradialis, brachialis, and less frequently the infraspinatus, supraspinatus, and sub-scapularis. The resulting dysfunction may be a "policeman's or porter's tip position" of the arm. Impaired functions include abduction of the shoulder, external rotation of the arm, elbow flexion, and supination of the forearm. Paralysis of the rhomboid, levator scapulae, serratus anterior, and scalenus muscles occurs with avulsion of the roots proximal to the origin of the dorsal scapula and long thoracic nerves. In lesions of a prefixed plexus there may be phrenic nerve paralysis. In most upper plexus lesions sensation is often unaffected; occasionally, there may be mild sensory loss involving the lateral aspect of the shoulder or upper part of the arm (circumflex nerve) or the thumb and index finger (median nerve) or both.

Middle Plexus Lesion

This lesion is characterized by paralysis of the triceps muscle and the extensor muscles supplied by the middle trunk or the corresponding undivided anterior primary ramus of the seventh cervical root, and involves chiefly the fibers extending to the radial nerve. The brachioradialis muscle is not weakened because it is supplied chiefly by the sixth cervical root. There may be sensory deficit on the back of the forearm or radial aspect of the dorsum of the hand, but this is usually minor and very restricted. Isolated lesions of this part of the plexus are rare except in penetrating wounds.

Lower Plexus Lesion

Lesions of the eighth cervical and first thoracic roots or the lower trunk of the plexus result in paralysis and atrophy of the flexors of the forearm and intrinsic hand muscles, as in combined median and ulnar nerve palsy. Extensors of the forearm and thumb may be minimally involved. Sensation may be normal or there may be a deficit along the postero-medial arm, midforearm, and ulnar aspect of the hand. If the first thoracic root is damaged a Horner's syndrome will result. This type of lesion produces a paralyzed hand. It is most often encountered as a result of sudden upward pull on the shoulder and may occur in adults consequent to being dragged by the arm. Recovery is poor.

Lesion of the Whole Plexus

These lesions may be complete or incomplete; when complete, the entire arm is paralyzed and dangles lifelessly. All limb muscles may undergo rapid atrophy. The sensory deficit varies; usually there is total anesthesia of the entire upper extremity below a line beginning at the shoulder and extending diagonally downward and medially to the middle third of the upper arm. A fall from a rapidly moving vehicle is the most common cause, but total plexus involvement may occur infrequently in the cryptogenic nontraumatic type of brachial plexus neuropathy.

Lesions of the Cords

A lesion of the lateral cord causes weakness of muscles innervated by the musculocutaneous nerve and the lateral head of the median nerve; the latter supplies all median innervated muscles except for the intrinsic muscles of the hand. This type of injury manifests itself chiefly as weakness of flexion and pronation of the forearm. Sensory deficit is usually mild and restricted to a small area on the radial aspect of the forearm.

A lesion of the medial cord produces weakness of muscles innervated by the ulnar nerve and medial head of the median nerve and results in severe disability of the hand. Sensory loss results from dysfunction of the medial cutaneous nerve of the arm and forearm. This lesion simulates a combined median and ulnar nerve lesion.

A posterior cord lesion produces weakness of the deltoid and the extensors of the wrist and fingers due to dysfunction of the axillary and radial nerves and sensory loss in the upper outer region of the arm. Less frequently, the subscapular and thoracodorsal nerves may be involved. All cords of the plexus (mainly the posterior cord) may be injured in a dislocation of the humerus or direct injury to the axilla. These injuries usually result in mixed patterns of motor and sensory loss. Hemorrhage from adjacent vessels may accompany these lesions and lead to further compression and ischemia of the neural structures.

CRYPTOGENIC BRACHIAL PLEXUS NEUROPATHY

The number of different names designating this disorder reveals our lack of knowledge regarding its pathogenesis. Surprisingly, there is little mention of this entity in sections on peripheral neurology in standard neurologic texts and yet it is a relatively common disorder (Tsairis et al., 1972). This type of neuropathy first became widely known in the 1940's among military personnel. Although it has been described previously as "multiple neuritis" or "localized neuritis of the shoulder girdle" by Burnard and Fox (1942) and Spillane (1943), "acute brachial radiculitis" by Turner (1944) and Dixon and Dick (1945), "localized non-traumatic neuropathy in military personnel" by Weinstein (1947), "neuralgic amyotrophy" (shoulder girdle syndrome) by Parsonage and Turner (1948), "acute shoulder neuritis" by Hook (1950), and "paralytic brachial neuritis" by Turner and Parsonage (1957) and Magee and DeJong (1960) and Weikers and Mattson (1969), the term "brachial plexus neuropathy" is preferred because it has not been established that this disease is inflammatory or infectious, always restricted to the shoulder girdle, or always paralytic. The upper, lower, or entire plexus may become either completely or partially involved on one side or on both. The lower plexus is rarely affected alone. Despite lack of unanimity as to the name of this disorder, it is a well-defined clinical entity with a fairly typical pattern of signs and symptoms that usually can be differentiated from acute cervical root disease, spinal cord tumors, diffuse polyneuropathies, or the more severe anterior horn cell disorders, including poliomyelitis.

Signs and Symptoms

In a recent study of 99 patients, the majority of those affected were distributed fairly evenly between the third and seventh decades, and males predominated in a ratio of 2.4 to 1 (Tsairis et al., 1972). The most striking feature in this group and in the other series, reported by Magee and De Jong (1960), was the rapid onset of sudden, severe, often nocturnal pain either accompanied simultaneously or followed, in most cases, within the first two weeks, by muscle weakness or paralysis (Table 32–2). Occasionally, a patient may not have pain or paresthesias prior to the onset of weakness. Pain is not necessarily restricted to the shoulder girdle; various combinations of scapular, trapezius ridge, shoulder, arm, forearm, and hand pain may occur

TABLE 32–2 INTERVAL BETWEEN PAIN AND WEAKNESS IN BRACHIAL PLEXUS NEUROPATHY*

Interval (days)	Patients	Total
0 (Simultaneous)	8	
1	2	
1–3	13	
3–5	3	
5–7	8†	
7–10	25	
10–14	5	68
14–21	8	
21–28	10	
7–28	3	
Uncertain	8	29
		97‡

*From Tsairis, P., Dyck, P. J., and Mulder, D. W.: Natural history of brachial plexus neuropathy; report on 99 patients. Arch. Neurol., 27:109, 1972. Copyright 1972, American Medical Association. Reprinted by permission.

†Two with paresthesias at onset.

‡Two had no pain prior to weakness.

during the acute stage of this illness. In predominantly upper plexus lesions the pain rarely extends below the elbow. Patients often complain of pain with arm movement and elbow flexion, and thus keep the arm at the side in a flexed position. Neck traction usually aggravates symptoms. In most, pain remains continuous for several days to weeks and then gradually subsides as the weakness appears. Less commonly the pain may be intermittent for up to one year after the appearance of the weakness. Weakness is confined to the shoulder girdle in about 50 per cent of patients. The axillary and suprascapular nerves are the ones most commonly affected. Complete unilateral limb paralysis is rarely seen; it was noted in only 4 of 99 patients in the most recent report (Tsairis et al., 1972). Although most have unilateral plexus involvement, there may be electromyographic evidence of plexus or isolated peripheral nerve involvement in the unaffected limb. In the bilateral cases the plexus involvement is never complete and rarely symmetrical; some patients may have unilateral proximal weakness with contralateral isolated mononeuropathy. Diaphragmatic paresis or paralysis may be an associated finding both in patients who have and in those who have not received prior innoculations (Comroe et al., 1951; Smith and Smith, 1955; Cape and Fincham, 1965; Tsairis et al., 1972).

Weikers and Mattson (1969) found evidence of widespread slowing of motor conduction velocity in five of seven of their cases of "acute paralytic brachial neuritis" and suggested that the plexus involvement might be a localized form of a diffuse polyneuropathy. No further evidence to support this view has been reported (Tsairis et al., 1972). Such cases would not, however, be unexpected following immunizations.

The anatomical involvement appears to be restricted to the brachial plexus. The lack of radicular features of the pain pattern, the diffuse nonsegmental signs and symptoms, and the normal cerebrospinal fluid findings suggest an absence of root involvement (Magee and De Jong, 1960; Tsairis et al., 1972).

Laboratory Data

Cerebrospinal fluid protein and cell counts in the acute and chronic stages are invariably normal. Immunologic studies of blood and cerebrospinal fluid have not been rewarding. The sedimentation rate may be normal or minimally elevated in the acute stages; results of other hematologic studies are normal. In two patients reported by Tsairis, Dyck, and Mulder (1972), biopsy of a cutaneous branch of the radial nerve showed profound axonal degeneration.

Pathogenesis

There is no evidence that this disease is either a manifestation of a systemic infection, presumably viral, or an allergic reaction to an infectious process or toxin. More than 50 per cent of patients had no history of antecedent illness or exposure to toxic substances, and for only 25 per cent could a history of an antecedent upper respiratory illness be obtained (Tsairis et al., 1972).

In an epidemiologic study of a "brachial plexus neuritis" outbreak in Czechoslovakia, it was suggested that a Coxsackie virus could be the etiologic agent and that the disease could be contagious (Bárdos and Somodskà, 1961). Some of the other epidemic forms of brachial neuritis also raised the question of a viral cause (Wyburn-Mason, 1941; Rektor and Libikova, 1953). Naturally the idea of a virus infection is attractive, but symptoms of an extensive nature have not been observed in most patients, nor has a virus been cultured to date. Although the serum- or vaccine-induced plexus neuropathy is clinically similar to the nonimmune form, there has been no conclusive evidence to even support an allergic hypersensitivity pathogenesis. Although Magee and DeJong (1960) maintain that the essential factor in pathogenesis is a generalized reduction in body resistance, many patients have no such history. In the author's experience many healthy athletes have been similarly affected. In summary, the statement by Plum and Druckemiller (1952), "the etiology of this acute multiple brachial neuropathy is unknown, but in its pathogenesis the relationship to diverse apparently unrelated antecedent illness (and factors) is striking," best explains our ignorance regarding pathogenesis.

Differential Diagnosis

Brachialgia, or pain in the upper extremity, may simulate the pain of brachial plexus involvement. The brachial pain caused by local conditions, such as the periarthritides of the shoulder joint, or referred pain from disturbances of the gallbladder, the heart, or the liver or from a subphrenic abscess can often be difficult to distinguish in the acute stages from the pain of brachial plexus involvement. Shoulder affections, however, are often attended by local tenderness and painful arm movements; the patient may not move the arm because of pain and limitation, thus appearing to have weakness. Weakness and other objective neurologic findings often dominate early in the course of these brachial plexus neuropathies and thus are key differential signs. The pain occurring with acute poliomyelitis can sometimes present a difficult diagnostic problem. The history (prodrome) and cerebrospinal fluid findings differentiate the two conditions. In elderly people cervical disk disease may cause pain and weakness in the fifth and sixth cervical root distribution; electrodiagnostic studies and a cervical myelogram are often necessary to differentiate these cases. In some cases of brachialgia there are no abnormal objective findings. If the pain is intermittent and positional or associated with sympathetic nerve dysfunction (cold hands, Raynaud's phenomenon, or discoloration of the fingers), a neurovascular compression syndrome of the brachial plexus due to thoracic outlet obstruction should be considered. Brachialgia statica paresthetica is a condition that was described in debilitated women who developed transient dysesthesias during recumbency (Wartenberg, 1944). This is presumed to be another form of thoracic outlet obstruction.

Serum- and Vaccine-Induced Brachial Plexus Neuropathy

Brachial plexus involvement may be one of several complications or the only complication following injection of foreign sera or vaccines. This type of plexus neuropathy is on the decline because more effective treatments are now available against most microorganisms. Fewer cases have been reported following administration of vaccines than of heterologous immune sera. It is of interest that most of these patients do not have generalized manifestations of serum sickness, especially those with vaccine-induced neuropathies. It has been postulated that an allergic vascular disturbance with edema of the neural structures is the basis for the underlying pathologic changes and consequent neurologic complications (Gathier and Bruyn, 1968).

Prophylactic administration of tetanus antitoxin in casualties accounts for the majority of these types of plexus neuropathy. Since the initial report by Lhermitte (1919) of three such cases, there have been a number of other reports following administration of antiserum against diphtheria, scarlet fever, streptococci, pneumococci, gonococci, anthrax, and gas gangrene (see Gathier and Bruyn, 1970). Severe pain, weakness, and wasting (particularly in the distribution of the upper trunk of the plexus), and isolated mononeuropathies (axillary, suprascapular, musculocutaneous, and long thoracic nerve) are characteristic findings. The pattern of involvement (either unilateral or bilateral) and the severity are similar to the cryptogenic plexus neuropathies of nonimmune origin. No correlation can be made between right- or left-sided localization and site of administration of sera or vaccine. Occasionally mild increase of cerebrospinal fluid protein occurs in the acute stage.

Plexus neuropathies following administration of vaccines may occur after the first injection, or more frequently, after the second or third injection. They have been reported to follow administration of typhoid (paratyphoid A and B) vaccine (Peacher and Robinson, 1945); rarely, smallpox vaccine (Winkelman, 1949) and tetanus toxoid (Woolling and Rushton, 1950; Tsairis et al., 1972); triple vaccine (pertussis, diphtheria, and tetanus toxoid) (Tsairis et al., 1972) or diphtheria vaccine only (Gathier and Bruyn, 1970); and more recently, influenza vaccines (Tsairis et al., 1972). There are no reported cases following whooping cough vaccination. From the reports in the literature, it appears that complications of the central nervous system related to vaccination are more common than those of the peripheral nervous system and that diffuse neuropathies or polyradiculopathies occur more often after administration of these vaccines.

Rarely, unilateral or bilateral paralysis of the diaphragm occurs with the immune forms of brachial plexus neuropathy. Comroe and associates (1951) reported a combination of partial paralysis of the diaphragm with complete paralysis of the thoracic respiratory muscles following injection of tetanus antitoxin. In some patients diaphragmatic paralysis was first discovered by chest fluoroscopy later in the clinical course; it may also occur without respiratory difficulty (Dyke, 1918; Smith and Smith, 1955; Tsairis, et al., 1972). Diaphragmatic involvement has occurred mainly after administration of tetanus antitoxin. Although cases of isolated mononeuropathies following serum treatment were reported by Gordon (1928), closer inspection of many of these patients reveals paresis of shoulder girdle muscles in other peripheral nerve distributions. Despite the generally assumed clinical similarity of the immune to the nonimmune form of plexus neuropathy, the interval between pain and onset of weakness is much less constant and frequently is significantly longer in the nonimmune cases (Turner and Parsonage, 1957; Gathier and Bruyn, 1970; and Tsairis et al., 1972).

Therapeutic Aspects

There is no specific therapy for these plexus neuropathies. Treatment is largely symptomatic and tailored to the individual's needs. In many patients the use of oral steroids or ACTH early in the course may reduce the pain (Smith and Smith, 1955; Tyler et al., 1958; Tsairis et al., 1972). There is no con-crete evidence from any series, however, that early treatment with steroids alters the course of this disease, although Fetter (1953) reported that steroids promoted recovery in some of his immune cases. Strong analgesics or narcotics may be required in the management of the acute stage of the illness, but they are not always helpful and narcotics are better avoided because of the likelihood of long-term pain and discomfort in some cases.

During the acute illness complete rest of the arm is recommended. Subsequently, physical therapy in the form of appropriate range of motion exercises should be instituted with or without massage and heat treatment. This treatment is strongly advised for the severely disabled individual as a preventive measure against muscle atrophy and joint contractures. Splints may be used when there is total deltoid paralysis or wrist drop. Physical therapy is not an absolute requirement; some patients with mild to moderate plexus involvement recover completely without therapy. Although physical therapy may theoretically enhance the speed of recovery this cannot be judged satisfactorily from the reported series. Exploration of the plexus or reconstructive operations on muscles, tendons, or joints are not advisable even in severe cases with flail limbs, since all patients can be expected to regain adequate function if given time (Tsairis et al., 1972).

Prognosis

Since it is virtually impossible to be certain of the degree of injury, the extent of the lesion, and the rate of regeneration of nerve fibers, the prognosis for these nontraumatic brachial plexus lesions has usually been uncertain. This form of plexus neuropathy, however, carries an excellent prognosis. Accurate diagnosis is essential because patients with severe muscle weakness and atrophy, or with a flail limb, may recover completely. Favorable recoveries have been reported by several authors (Dixon and Dick, 1945; Turner and Parsonage, 1957; Kennedy and Resch, 1966; Evans, 1965). In the series reported by Tsairis, Dyck, and Mulder (1972) more than 80 per cent of the patients recovered within two years after onset of symptoms and nearly 90 per cent were expected to recover by the end of three years regardless of the duration of the acute course and the location and severity of the plexus lesions (Fig. 32-3). Patients with uni-

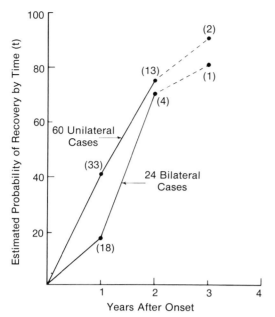

Figure 32–3 Recovery rates with unilateral and bilateral involvement. Numbers in parentheses indicate number of patients who had not recovered and were still under observation. (From Tsairis, P., Dyck, P. J., and Mulder, D. W. : Natural history of brachial plexus neuropathy; report on 99 patients. Arch. Neurol., 27:109, 1972. Copyright 1972, American Medical Association. Reprinted by permission.)

lateral involvement appear to recover at a faster rate during the first year than those with bilateral involvement, 41 per cent versus 81 per cent respectively, although this difference is of borderline statistical significance (Tsairis et al., 1972). In this series there was essentially no difference in recovery rates between unilateral and bilateral cases by the end of two years, at which time 75 per cent of the patients had reached full functional recovery. There are no striking differences in the clinical course and recovery rates between the nonimmunized and immunized cases or between male and female patients. Factors suggesting a poor recovery rate are (1) severe and prolonged pain or recurrences of pain, (2) lack of any signs of improvement in three months, and (3) complete plexus or lower plexus lesions. Residual deficits are minimal. None of these patients develop progressive neurologic disease. Recurrences are rare and usually less severe; they occurred in only 4 of 84 patients seen in follow-up by Tsairis, Dyck, and Mulder (1972). Recurrences have also

been described in other series (Turner and Parsonage, 1957; Magee and De Jong, 1960).

PLEXUS NEUROPATHY WITH INFECTIONS, SYSTEMIC ILLNESS, AND TOXINS

Plexus involvement resulting from direct extension to the plexus from a septic focus in the hand or nearby area occurs rarely. That occurring during the course of organ infection elsewhere, e.g., in the gallbladder, tonsils, teeth, or pelvis, or as part of a generalized infection, such as seen in syphilis, tuberculosis, and infectious mononucleosis, are more common. Diffuse plexus involvement or isolated lesions of the long thoracic nerve have been reported in infectious mononucleosis (Saksena, 1943; Richardson, 1942; Schnell et al., 1966; Tsairis et al., 1972). These cases probably fall within the spectrum of cryptogenic brachial plexus neuropathy.

In tuberculous and syphilitic infections, brachial monoplegia associated with edema of the arm may result from pressure of a thrombosed subclavian vein (Archer, 1887); the weakness and sensory loss in the arm may be insidious, leading one to believe it is of cortical or of subcortical origin. Obviously, the pathogenetic mechanisms in these rare cases are different. Bilateral brachial plexus involvement has also been reported in adult toxoplasmosis (Tejero Lamarca et al., 1970).

Neuritis of the circumflex (axillary) nerve has been reported in diabetes mellitus (Althaus, 1890). It has been my experience that partial or diffuse brachial plexus involvement does not occur in diabetes mellitus. Polyarteritis nodosa may cause a mononeuritis multiplex in one upper extremity, which may simulate a plexus lesion, but this is very uncommon.

Unilateral brachial plexus involvement has been described in heroin addicts following intravenous administration of heroin-adulterant mixtures (Challenor et al., 1973). These patients developed painless monoparesis, affecting muscles supplied chiefly by the posterior and medial cords; thus their neuropathy was clinically different from the cryptogenic and vaccine-induced types of plexus involvement. It was not possible to be sure of the pathogenesis, but it was speculated that the effects were due to direct toxic or hypersensitivity phenomena.

HEREDOFAMILIAL BRACHIAL PLEXUS NEUROPATHY

Since Dreschfeld's report (1886) of two sisters with this neuropathy there have been 46 additional cases reported in several families up to 1973 (in Smith et al., 1971, and Guillozet and Mercer, 1973). Almost all these families have been described in England, and all those affected have been members of unrelated families with no known consanguinity. Taylor (1960) reported on 24 members of a family of 119 individuals covering five generations who had single or multiple attacks (up to seven) of acute brachial neuropathy characterized by excruciating shoulder pain, severe weakness and atrophy, and incomplete sensory loss that was either unilateral or, less commonly, bilateral. Taylor felt that the familial influence was genetic rather than environmental. The putative genetic influence would appear to be a contributing factor rather than a sufficient cause of the disease.

There are other features of this disorder that make it quite distinct from the cryptogenic or immune types of plexus neuropathy. In some of Taylor's cases, there were lower cranial nerve involvement and isolated mononeuropathies in other extremities. In other families, affected members had a peculiar physiognomy (deep and close set eyes) syndactyly, and dwarfism (Gardner and Maloney, 1968). Others had involvement of either the lumbosacral plexus, lower cranial nerves, or recurrent laryngeal nerves (Jacob et al., 1960; Poffenbarger, 1968). Single and recurrent attacks, some associated with pregnancy or during the puerperium, also occurred in some families (Ungley, 1933; Poffenbarger, 1968; and Taylor, 1960); this in contrast to the cryptogenic form, which rarely recurs or is associated with pregnancy.

Jacob and co-workers and Taylor suggested that the inheritance in these families was due to an autosomal dominant gene with high penetrance. In both the familial and nonfamilial forms the same pathogenetic factors may be operable, with the familial form involving an underlying genetically based vulnerability rather than the genetic factors being the cause of the neuropathy.

As a rule, the course of the heredofamilial brachial neuropathy is benign and self-limiting with full functional recovery after many months. Partial recovery occurred in some patients and long-standing mild residual deficits were reported by Taylor. In Poffenbarger's series of seven patients complete or nearly complete recovery occurred within four to eight months, and in the acute stage, oral steroids helped to relieve the pain without affecting the rate of recovery.

TRAUMATIC BRACHIAL PLEXUS NEUROPATHIES

Trauma accounts for an estimated 50 per cent of all lesions of the brachial plexus. Plexus injury occurs as a result of direct violence through an open wound (lacerations and penetrating missiles), or is due to closed injuries (bony displacement, traction, stretch, or compression). In either open or closed injuries the entire plexus may suffer or the lesion may be confined to a portion of it. Traumatic plexus lesions are seldom uniform; some parts of the plexus suffers more severely than others. The traction or stretch injuries are the most common type, especially in peacetime. Anomalies in the region of the plexus may make the individual more susceptible to the effects of trauma.

Open Wounds

These lesions occur most frequently during wartime and are due to high-velocity penetrating missiles or shell fragments. In civilian life, stab wounds and other penetrating injuries may injure the plexus, the supraclavicular being the most vulnerable portion.

The position of a missile track usually gives some indication of what portion of the plexus is likely to have been injured. Lesions above the clavicle that involve the upper and middle trunks and their emergent nerves (supraclavicular, dorsal scapular) are the most common (Brooks, 1954). Wounds below the clavicle or in the axilla are most likely to damage either the lower trunk of the plexus or the cords are their emergent nerves (axillary, thoracodorsal). Lesions of the lower plexus are likely to be more serious and possibly fatal because of concomitant damage to the lung and great vessels at the base of the neck. Axillary wounds are more likely to damage blood vessels, causing hemorrhage and compression of nerves emerging from the axillary plexus (Sunderland, 1968).

The explosive force of a missile may temporarily affect all components of the plexus although the missile may have actually penetrated only one component. Sometimes it is necessary to wait one to three weeks before assessing the true injury to the plexus. In open wound injuries it is also important to examine the bones, joints, and blood vessels because injuries to these structures may interfere with the performance of arm movement, making it difficult to assess the degree of neural damage. With injury to blood vessels there is a likelihood of subsequent development of gangrene, arterial aneurysm, or arteriovenous fistulas.

TREATMENT AND PROGNOSIS

Management of these injuries should be individualized. There is some controversy whether open penetrating wounds should be explored. Major surgical experience with open wounds of the plexus has been gained chiefly in battle casualties. Most surgeons feel that any injury to vessels should be immediately repaired; few, however, support the view that any break in the continuity of the plexus components should be repaired. Neurolysis of intact nerve elements in chronic lesions has not been proved very beneficial. Björkesten (1947) found no difference in recovery between those of his cases that were operated on and those that were not. Brooks (1954) explored the plexus in 54 of 820 patients with open wounds. He found severed nerve tissue in only 16 and that massive scar tissue prevented repair in all but 11. In Brooks's series damage to the medial and posterior cords was usually permanent; Horner's syndrome associated with total or lower plexus injury had a poor outlook; recovery of hand muscle function had a poor prognosis even with surgical neurolysis; and significant recovery did occur after upper plexus injuries. His data support the contention that recovery from upper plexus lesions is potentially better because regenerating axons have a shorter distance to grow. He concluded, and most will agree today, that "routine exploration of open wounds of the brachial plexus is rarely profitable or justifiable." As a rule, if there are no signs of recovery of proximal muscle function within a year, the outlook is generally poor.

Closed Injuries

In this group traction injuries are the most common cause of paralysis or weakness of the upper extremity. Figure 32–4 is a diagrammatic representation of the types of traction injury suffered by the different components of the brachial plexus. There may be either a transitory physiologic loss of motor and sensory conduction (neurapraxia), or axonal degeneration (axonotmesis), or severence of the nerve root (neurotmesis). Neural damage is seldom uniform, i.e., there may be severance and degeneration of nerve fibers due to stretching and a physiologic conduction block in other fibers. When one root is avulsed, another may be stretched. With severe injuries, hemorrhage may occur in the soft tissues, leading to edema and scar formation and thus additional problems.

FRACTURE-DISLOCATION INJURIES

Direct injuries to the plexus occasionally result from a dislocation or fracture about the shoulder joint. The plexus may be stretched, compressed, contused, or lacerated (Leffert and Seddon, 1965). Almost all these injuries affect the infraclavicular components of the plexus. Dislocation of a fractured greater tuberosity accounts for the majority. Most injuries result from a fall from a moving vehicle or while walking. In 50 per cent of Leffert and Seddon's series all three cords of the plexus were affected either partially or completely. The posterior cord for anatomical reasons was more liable to damage than the other two. This cord along with its radial and axillary nerves may be stretched across the head of the humerus in a fall on an arm that is abducted and externally rotated or in a dislocation of the head of the humerus. The axillary nerve may be either ruptured or avulsed in such situations.

These lesions are usually mild and thus should be kept under observation. In treatment the most important aspect is prevention of joint stiffness and muscle atrophy. Functional recovery may take up to six months. If there is injury to supraclavicular branches, for example, to the dorsal scapular, suprascapular, and long thoracic nerves, full functional recovery is not likely. Swelling, induration, or tenderness in the supraclavicular fossa are features suggestive of associated supraclavicular plexus injury. Exploration should

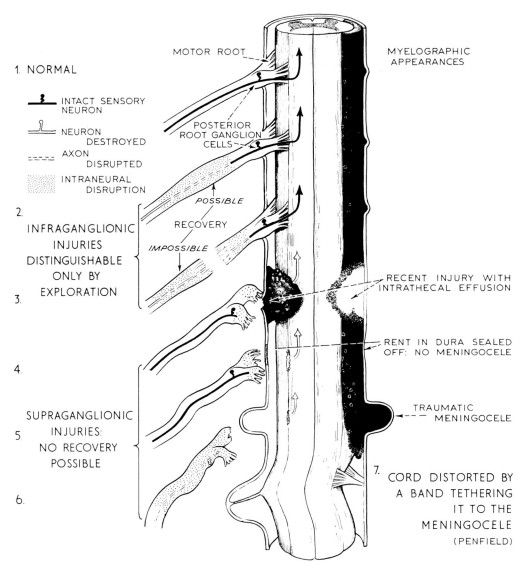

Figure 32–4 Types of traction injury suffered by nerve components of the brachial plexus. (From Seddon, H. J.: Surgical Disorders of the Peripheral Nerves. Edinburgh, Churchill Livingstone, 1972. Reprinted by permission.)

be deferred for at least six months until any regeneration of nerve fibers is well advanced and the limits of the permanent damage to the plexus can be clearly assessed. Except for isolated axillary nerve injuries, prognosis is generally good regardless of which part of the infraclavicular plexus is damaged (Leffert and Seddon, 1965).

TRACTION AND COMPRESSION INJURIES

Most closed traction injuries are the result of high-speed vehicular traffic accidents, par-

ticularly in England and America where motorcycles are popular (Bonney, 1959; Yeoman and Seddon, 1961). Other severe traction injuries may result from falling from a height or striking a tree while sledding or skiing. Mild stretch injuries of the plexus may occur from lifting or pulling on heavy objects, or during unaccustomed exertion such as throwing a ball or annual house cleaning. A vigorous downward thrust on the shoulder, especially if the neck is pushed to the opposite side, puts traction on the upper plexus or roots (Hornsley, 1899). Lateral flexion injuries of the cervical spine are well-documented causes of plexus injury (Roaf, 1963). Similarily, carrying heavy weights on the shoulder (as done by coal miners or soldiers) or heavy objects falling on the same area may result in plexus injury due to separation of the head and shoulder.

Severe traction injuries may also avulse the entire plexus. Upward pull on the lower plexus or roots may occur when the arm is outstretched or jerked upward by a moving belt (Adson, 1922). If the injury is severe enough the lower roots may be avulsed from the spinal cord (Taylor, 1962). With either a downward thrust or an upward pull of the shoulder and arm there may be complicating injuries to the muscles and tendons or fracture-dislocation of the arm and shoulder.

Prolonged abduction of the arm during sleep or while the patient is under anesthesia may stretch the cords or emerging nerves in the axilla. Particularly vulnerable is the posterior cord, which may be stretched across the head of the humerus by prolonged hyperabduction and extension of the limb. Similar damage may occur during reduction of a dislocated shoulder or during manipulation of a frozen shoulder. In patients in whom pain in the shoulder prevents adequate examination of muscles prior to a closed reduction procedure it is sometimes impossible to know whether the injury to nerves occurred before or during such manipulation.

Compressive plexus injuries occur when external pressure is directly applied to the plexus either in the supraclavicular fossa or in the axilla. These types of plexus neuropathy may occur following transient severe compression or during prolonged mild compression. Supraclavicular plexus injury may occur following the sudden recoil of a gun or from carrying heavy objects on the shoulder. "Pallbearer's palsy" is an upper plexus neuropathy that resulted in two soldiers who carried a heavy coffin on their shoulders in a military funeral (Coni, 1966). The constant pressure of shoulder straps of an army pack or pressure of a cast may cause similar injury. A shoulder rest may compress the brachial plexus during an operation. Axillary plexus injuries may result from using crutches, from the pressure of casts or tourniquets or splints, and from carrying baggage under the arm with the arm hyperabducted. By and large, the compressive injuries are not associated with avulsion of the nerve roots.

POSTOPERATIVE AND POSTANESTHESIA BRACHIAL PLEXUS NEUROPATHY

This plexus neuropathy is a well-recognized complication following general anesthesia and operations. Although it was noted only 11 times after 30,000 anesthestics in one series of patients reported by Dhuner (1950), it probably occurs more frequently than reports in the literature would suggest. Upper plexus neuropathy following a gynecologic operation in the Trendelenberg position is well known. This is not as frequently encountered today because of improvement in positioning the patient on the operating table. The mechanism of such an injury is felt to be stretching or compression of the plexus during the course of an operative procedure, but it may follow almost any type of procedure, cardiac catheterization and long operations being the most common (Jackson and Keats, 1965; Kwaan and Rappaport, 1970). It is felt that injury to the plexus occurs when the arm is maintained in a hyperabducted and externally rotated position for more than 40 minutes on the operating table. The most frequently encountered pattern of involvement is one affecting the upper trunk and suprascapular nerve (see Kwaan and Rappaport, 1970). Loss of function may be unilateral or, rarely, bilateral. There has been no report of permanent injury, and most patients recover within six months (Ewing, 1950; Woodsmith, 1952; Clausen, 1942). Obviously, the best therapy for this type of plexus injury is its prevention. In rare instances, local anesthetic block of the brachial plexus in the axilla causes pain and weakness, which may persist if hemorrhagic compression and nerve injury result from trauma from the needle.

RUCKSACK PARALYSIS

Incomplete paralysis of the upper extremity may occur in soldiers wearing heavy back packs or rucksacks (Daube, 1969). Daube described 17 cases in United States Army personnel. The diagnosis of this type of paralysis can be made by obtaining a history of sustained compression of the shoulder from a soldier or hiker who presents with shoulder weakness. The weakness is felt to result from damage to the upper trunk. The differentiation between this neuropathy and that resulting from immunization may sometimes be difficult, especially when the weakness develops after both intermittent pack bearing and prophylactic vaccinations. Severe pain is usually associated with the serum- or vaccine-induced plexus neuropathy. In Daube's series most patients who had mild to moderate plexus involvement gradually recovered in one to three months. Similar neuropathies may occur in the civilian population as a result of the growing interest in camping, hiking, and mountain climbing in which back packs are used.

MISCELLANEOUS TYPES OF COMPRESSIVE PLEXUS INJURY

Hemorrhage into the plexus can produce compression and subsequent acute limb paralysis. Cord lesions may occur after percutaneous puncture of the axillary artery for angiographic procedures (Staal et al., 1966; Dudrick, 1967). Hemophiliacs who use crutches for an episode of hemarthrosis in the leg and patients who are taking anticoagulants and who use crutches improperly may suffer such a plexus lesion (see case report by Salam, 1972).

AVULSION INJURY

An attempt to determine whether trauma has involved the plexus proper or has resulted in avulsion of the cervical roots is of great prognostic importance. Regeneration cannot occur if the rootlets are avulsed (see Fig. 32–4). Avulsion may be suspected from the type of trauma or from such ominous signs as paralysis of the rhomboid, levator scapulae, or serratus anterior muscles and diaphragm, or evidence of spinal cord damage. Following partial or complete avulsion, the rootlets may be pulled intradurally without damage to the cord, leading to development of meningoceles. The upper cervical roots are more commonly involved than the lower ones. When the plexus is avulsed from below upward, Horner's syndrome is a likely result. Complete avulsion of all roots is rare; when it does occur the paralyzed arm rapidly atrophies and becomes useless. Coran and co-workers (1968) reported two cases of complete avulsion in which the patient's arm was amputated at the mid-humeral level (not the shoulder) in order to

provide support for a prosthesis. The severe injuries are often associated with other injuries such as cerebral trauma. The latter requires immediate therapy and can mask the trauma to the brachial plexus.

The best evidence of root avulsion is myelographic demonstration of the traumatic meningoceles in the region of the affected roots (Murphey et al., 1947; Taylor, 1962). Myelography is of considerable help in establishing a diagnosis and prognosis, but occasionally, these lesions may not be demonstrated. In such instances, when avulsion is still suspected, the axon reflex test may be helpful in determining whether the lesion is located distal or proximal to the dorsal root ganglion (Bonney, 1954, 1959). Bonney (1959) employed the intradermal injection of 1 per cent histamine to produce a cutaneous wheal and flare response. If the lesion is postganglionic, there will be no cutaneous flare response, indicating degeneration of axons. Such a negative response usually occurs within three to six weeks after injury. Some surgeons accept such data as justification for exploration of the plexus with the view of repairing discontinuity of nerve components. If the lesion is preganglionic (root avulsion) the axon reflex will be preserved. If the findings indicate damage to more than one dorsal root, prognosis is poor and surgery is definitely not indicated. Differing types of lesions may coexist; e.g., avulsion of the ventral roots may occur with only traction on the dorsal roots, or avulsion of the upper roots may be associated with a traction injury of the lower roots (Taylor, 1962). Therefore evaluation of the axon reflex test and a patient's prognosis must be guarded at all times.

Needle electromyography may be a valuable adjunct in such injuries. This study has its limitations, especially in the acute stages when decisions regarding exploration have to be made. Bufalini and Pescatori (1969) claim that electromyography of the posterior cervical muscles can be helpful in identifying the affected roots or determining whether the lesion is distal or proximal to the foramina. If motor unit action potentials are absent or if only fibrillations (implying denervation) are recordable, they state, damage is close to the spinal cord and prognosis is poor. This simplistic explanation is probably inadequate because of the overlapping nerve supply to and the variable anatomy of the paracervical muscles.

MANAGEMENT AND PROGNOSIS OF CLOSED INJURIES

In all plexus injuries the crux of the problem is to determine the severity and extent of the plexus lesion. In mild acute traction injuries, the plexus usually recovers if given enough time; therefore, exploration should not be undertaken. Early initiation of physical therapy is of the utmost importance in order to prevent muscle atrophy and contractures. In blunt injuries or mild compression of the plexus, continuity of the nerves is preserved and complete or nearly complete recovery should also be expected. This type of plexus injury is exemplified by the upper trunk lesion following a gynecologic operation in the Trendelenburg position or a blow to the base of the neck.

The greatest problem occurs when there is severe stretching or compression of the plexus. During the acute state, the myelogram and the cutaneous axon reflex response are helpful in determining if there is an avulsion. These lesions have the poorest prognosis. Reconstructive procedures, such as tendon transfers, may be of benefit to the patient by restoring added function in the incomplete avulsive lesion. Experience accumulated over the years has demonstrated that recovery following supraclavicular traction injuries is generally mediocre or unsatisfactory. In 1959, Bonney exhaustively studied 29 patients with severe supraclavicular traction lesions. There were no complete recoveries and surgical treatment was of little or no benefit.

Infraclavicular lesions from any cause merit separate consideration because they have fared better, especially those associated with shoulder injuries (Leffert and Seddon, 1965). In this group the axillary nerve lesion has the poorest prognosis. Exploration is not indicated unless there is a concomitant vascular lesion. Again, physical therapy is important.

Surgical exploration of a severe plexus injury is a controversial issue. Some surgeons recommend early exploration of the plexus, as soon as the acute effects of injury have subsided in order to assess continuity of nerves and thus determine prognosis. Discontinuity of the postganglionic axons is considered as irreversible as root avulsion. It is wise to delay exploration until the prospects of any natural recovery can be determined. Lesions that fail to show signs of recovery in six months are considered almost certainly beyond surgical repair.

In some patients with supraclavicular lesions neurolysis resulted in mild improvement of motor function and relief of persistent pain. Autografting has given variable results. Seddon (1947) reported that the use of autogenous grafts to close large gaps in nerves was unsound. Recently, promising technical advances in surgical nerve repair have been reported. Millesi and co-workers (1971, 1972) described a microsurgical technique for interfascicular nerve grafting with sural autografts. This technique was tried on 126 patients with various types of peripheral nerve lesions including those in the brachial plexus. Overall, they reported a 93 per cent incidence of some functional return. Such improvements in nerve grafting are noteworthy and will undoubtedly have an immense impact on the surgical treatment of plexus as well as other peripheral nerve lesions. Reconstructive surgery in severe brachial plexus lesions is reviewed by Yeoman and Seddon (1961).

Birth Injuries

Brachial plexus injuries in newborn infants have been of considerable interest in the annals of obstetrical history. Although the number of cases of obstetrical paralysis has decreased in recent years owing to better methods of delivery, these lesions nevertheless are still with us. Factors predisposing to such injuries include disproportion between the size of the baby and the birth canal, the use of instruments, breech delivery, and difficult labor (Rubin, 1964). Traction on the plexus is the most frequent cause of the lesions. The plexus may be subjected to either downward or upward traction. The most common area of injury is at Erb's point, the junction of the C5 and C6 roots where the suprascapular nerve emerges.

In most babies, complete paralysis or weakness is immediately evident after birth. Most lesions are unilateral. Bilateral involvement occurs rarely and must be differentiated from bilateral arm paralysis caused by central infarction of the cervical cord resulting from circulatory disorders (Adams and Cameron, 1965). Lesions of the upper trunk account for the majority of cases and are usually the least severe of all plexus injuries (Gjorup, 1966). After the upper plexus, the entire plexus is most frequently involved, and the lower plexus is least often involved. Horner's syndrome is extremely rare in the latter lesions. Electromyography is useful to confirm the diagnosis, to delineate the extent of injury, and to determine the prognosis.

Early recognition of these lesions is extremely important in order to prevent muscle atrophy and joint contractures. Electrotherapy to prevent fibrosis of denervated muscles is recommended, although this is controversial. Prognosis of mild upper plexus lesions is favorable providing joint contractures are averted. Diffuse and lower plexus lesions carry a less favorable prognosis. In the severe injuries with very little return of function there may be a delay in bone growth, dislocation of the shoulder, and peculiar posturing of the arm despite active physical therapy with or without electrotherapy (Eng, 1971). In Gjorup's (1966) series of 100 cases, full recovery occurred in almost 40 per cent and about one third did poorly.

Surgical intervention has been of no value. If there is no significant return of function, then reconstructive procedures may be planned at a later date when the child is more cooperative. Arthrodesis should not be performed before completion of epiphysial growth. Eng's (1971) account of long-term experience with 25 babies with varying degrees of plexus involvement presents a thorough evaluation of the problem.

ISOLATED MONONEUROPATHIES OF THE PLEXUS

Involvement of the individual peripheral nerves from proximal parts of the plexus have been reported following various types of closed injuries and during or following systemic illness. Occasionally, they occur de novo.

The long thoracic nerve of Bell, which supplies the serratus anterior muscle, lies superficially and thus may be pressed upon by a weight such as a knapsack carried on the shoulder, as reported by Ilfield and Holder (1942), or by strapping the shoulder on the operating table. It may be stretched in occupations requiring prolonged elevation of the arms or pushing movements and injured in radical mastectomies for breast cancer. It may be affected singly by serum injections or during systemic infections such as measles, diph-

theritic pneumonia, typhoid fever, and influenza (Tournay and Krans, 1924; Richardson, 1942). Winging of the scapula presumably due to involvement of the long thoracic nerve is a fairly common residual deficit in nontraumatic cryptogenic brachial plexus neuropathies (Tsairis et al., 1972). Clinically, the scapula moves upward and laterally with forward flexion of the arm or with pressure on the hyperextended arm. In partial injury, the scapular winging may go unnoticed until discovered as part of a routine examination.

Several cases of neuritis of the suprascapular nerve are on record (Haymaker and Woodhall, 1953). This mononeuropathy may be complete, resulting in almost total paralysis of external rotation of the arm despite the assistance of the teres minor muscle. Atrophy of the supraspinatus and infraspinatus muscles above and below the scapula may be seen and palpated. These lesions have occurred in gymnasts and during both obscure and known infections such as malaria (Wartenburg, 1958). In the cryptogenic form of plexus neuropathy, this nerve is often involved in combination with the other individual nerves of the plexus (Turner, 1944; Tsairis et al., 1972).

The musculocutaneous nerve emerges from the lateral cord of the plexus. Involvement of this nerve results in weakness and atrophy of the biceps brachii, coracobrachialis, and brachialis muscles, and flattening of the contours of the flexor surface of the upper arm. Sensation may be partially or totally impaired along the radial and volar aspects of the forearm (lateral cutaneous nerve of the forearm). Musculocutaneous nerve lesions occur mainly with fractures of the humerus (Seddon, 1972); they have also been reported, on rare occasions, following systemic illness such as pneumonia, influenza, tuberculosis, and malaria (Wartenburg, 1958).

The axillary nerve emerges from the posterior cord of the plexus and innervates the deltoid and teres minor muscles. Wartenburg (1958) cites several cases of isolated axillary nerve lesions following smallpox vaccination, dysentery, malaria, and barbiturate and carbon monoxide poisoning reported in the French and German literature. The axillary nerve is also affected singly during the course of "acute brachial neuropathy" (Turner, 1944). Traction or compressive injury to this nerve occurs in dislocations of the shoulder joint (most commonly subcoracoid) and in fractures of the surgical neck of the humerus and scapula. It may also be injured by violent upward jerking of the arm (Seddon, 1972). Weakness of the deltoid muscle results in inability to abduct the arm to the horizontal, whereas teres minor weakness produces little impairment of external rotation of the arm providing the infraspinatus muscle is intact. If the sensory (circumflex) branch is also involved, loss of sensation to pinprick and light touch will occur over the lateral and upper aspects of the arm. Recovery from traction-compression injuries to this nerve is variable but generally poor. The best functional recovery occurs following a closed reduction of a shoulder dislocation.

Isolated lesions of the dorsal scapular nerve, subscapular nerves, and thoracodorsal nerve have not been reported. Subscapular nerve involvement usually occurs in association with involvement of the more proximal part of the posterior cord. The patient may find it difficult to scratch the low back because of weakness of medial rotation of the arm at the shoulder. Similarly, involvement of the thoracodorsal nerve (innervating the latissimus dorsi muscle) also occurs with lesions of the posterior cord and results in some limitation of adduction of the arm. Because dorsal scapular nerve lesions impair it, function of the rhomboid and levator scapulae muscles is important in the assessment of proximal plexus lesions.

THORACIC OUTLET OBSTRUCTION SYNDROMES

Brachial plexus involvement in these syndromes is often associated with compression of the subclavian vessels at the superior aperture of the thorax. They may, therefore, be more appropriately grouped under the term "neurovascular compression of the shoulder girdle" (Rob and Standoven, 1958). The most convincing of them occur when there is a congenital anomaly such as a cervical rib, a demonstrable abnormal first thoracic rib, or a fibrous fascial band extending from the seventh cervical transverse process. Abnormal insertion or disposition of the scalene muscles may also be important compression factors, but these findings are not easily demonstrable preoperatively. Accessory cervical ribs are said to occur in 0.5 per cent of the population, and about 75 per cent of them are bilateral

(Mayfield, 1970). In the absence of the congenital anomalies, the specific compression mechanism in these syndromes is difficult to identify.*

Signs and Symptoms

The symptomatology of the thoracic outlet syndrome depends on whether the plexus or blood vessels or both are compressed. In one series of 138 patients, sensory symptoms of neural compression were observed in the C8 and T1 segments in all but six patients, and weakness occurred in only 28 patients (Urschel et al., 1971). In general the lower trunk of the plexus is consistently affected, although some middle trunk fibers may also be involved. Pain in the majority of these patients has an insidious onset, is intermittent, and commonly involves the neck, shoulder, upper arm, and hand, with radiation into the anterior chest and parascapular area in some. Unfortunately, subjective complaints of pain and paresthesias outnumber objective findings. In some patients with significant compression, there may be cyanosis, swelling, and severe weakness of the hand and, rarely, Raynaud's phenomena or digital gangrene (Beyer and Wright, 1951; Urschel et al., 1971). The vascular symptoms have been attributed by some to irritation (stretch or angulation) of the vasomotor fibers in the lower plexus. Auscultation of the supraclavicular and infraclavicular areas or axilla for a bruit should be performed routinely, especially during hyperabduction of the arm. This maneuver will diminish or obliterate the radial pulse in affected individuals but may also do so in a number of healthy individuals. The distal portion of the subclavian artery may be compressed when it is tense and bowed beneath the coracoid process and the pectoralis muscle during hyperabduction in normal as well as affected individuals. Compression of the subclavian vein is not as common; if it is present there may be edema, venous distention with prominence of chest veins as a sign of collateral circulation, and discoloration of the arm (Sampson et al., 1940).

---

*Secondary anatomical changes of the thoracic outlet can occur as a result of trauma and surgery. The loss of tone in suspensory muscles of the anterior chest and shoulder girdle, namely, the trapezius, levator scapulae and rhomboid muscles, may result in sagging of the shoulder and secondary mechanical compression of the neurovascular structures in the cervicobrachial area.

Laboratory Data

Positional axillary arteriography or venography has been shown to be helpful in establishing a diagnosis of subclavian vessel compression or thrombosis (Rosenberg, 1966; Adams et al., 1968). During angiography many normal individuals may have "kinking" of the subclavian vessels during positioning of the arm, and thus one may question the justification of such a procedure. If the patient has a loud bruit or shows signs of significant arterial or venous compression, an angiogram should be performed.

Measurements of motor conduction velocities across the brachial plexus have been reported to be of value in recognition of these syndromes, particularly in those patients with predominantly neural symptoms (Caldwell et al., 1971; Urschel et al., 1971). Motor conduction velocities over proximal and distal segments of the ulnar nerve are determined by recording the evoked muscle action potential from the hypothenar eminence. Normally the motor conduction velocity in the proximal segment of the ulnar nerve (above the elbow) should be faster than that in the distal segment (below the elbow) because myelinated nerve fibers are larger in diameter in proximal portions of peripheral nerves. In a series of 95 extremities studied prior to operation, Urschel and coworkers reported that the ulnar motor conduction velocity across the proximal segment was reduced from his normal average value of 72 m per second to 53 m per second, the range being between 32 and 65 m per second. In my experience exact measurements of the distance along the proximal segment of the ulnar nerve may be inconsistent from patient to patient and thus lead to an incorrect value for the motor conduction velocity. More important data may be obtained by comparing the values of proximal ulnar motor conduction velocity in both upper extremities to ascertain if there is a difference between the symptomatic and nonsymptomatic sides. Distal ulnar and median sensory conduction times are often also a helpful determination. The distal ulnar sensory latency may be slowed because of a proximal lesion (presumably a result of "dying back" of the distal sensory nerve fibers).

The laboratory data may be normal and thus are not absolute criteria for diagnosis; the history and clinical examination remain most important.

Treatment and Prognosis

In the absence of a cervical rib most authors would agree that conservative measures should be tried first unless serious vascular or neurologic signs are present. Most patients respond favorably to proper physical therapy: moist heat and massage, exercises such as strengthening of the upper trapezius and pectoral muscles, scalene muscle stretching, swimming, and postural instruction are recommended (Rosati and Lord, 1961). Patients with severe symptoms even without significant neurologic or vascular findings may not tolerate or benefit from physical therapy. As long as therapy offers relief it should be continued. When it makes the patient worse, it should be discontinued.

In intractable cases surgical treatment is advised. Resection of the first thoracic rib either through a posterior approach (Clagett, 1962) or the transaxillary approach (Roos, 1971) is the operation of choice and provides the most beneficial results. In the series of Urschel and associates (1971) the first rib was resected to relieve compression in 128 extremities of 112 patients; 96 per cent showed complete remission or improvement. Removal of the first rib was superior to scalenotomy alone or to a scalenotomy in combination with excision of a cervical rib.

BRACHIAL PLEXUS INJURY FOLLOWING RADIATION

Delayed involvement of the brain and spinal cord following radiotherapy of neighboring structures are well-known pathologic entities. Radiation damage to the brachial plexus is not common but may occur in patients receiving radiotherapy for breast cancer or head and neck tumors (Mumenthaler, 1964, 1969; Nisce and Chu, 1968). In all these lesions there may be either a delay of several months or, in most instances, several years following irradiation before the onset of symptoms and signs. Haymaker and Lindgren (1970) reported that objective signs in the distribution of the plexus occurred between two and six years postexposure and, in one patient, some nine years after irradiation to the mammary and axillary areas.

Mumenthaler (1969) reported that brachial pain was usually the first symptom. This was followed by progressive weakness, atrophy, and sensory loss over months or years. His patients also showed marked skin discoloration and subcutaneous induration in the irradiated field. If symptoms involved the hand, then recovery was either delayed or did not occur. The irradiation dose may or may not exceed the usual range used for treatment (Mumenthaler, 1969; Haymaker and Lindgren, 1970).

In histopathologic specimens of the brain and spinal cord, marked degenerative lesions of small blood vessels that narrow the lumina are regularly described features (Pallis et al., 1961; Pennybacker and Russell, 1948). In cases with central nervous system damage, a local circulatory disorder, presumably a late sequel of slowly progressive vascular damage initiated at the time of the radiotherapy, is considered to be the principal cause of the clinical pattern of involvement. Direct radiation injury of the neural elements is felt to be the primary cause in the peripheral nerve lesions (John, 1946; see also Haymaker and Lindgren, 1970). Proliferation of connective tissue as a reaction to a metastasis to lymph nodes could damage the plexus, but according to Haymaker and Lindgren (1970), not to the extent observed following radiation exposure.

Surgical neurolysis of the plexus has been reported to be of minimal benefit to these patients. In the cases that were operated on, Mumemthaler (1969) found masses of induration that he felt were causing compression of the plexus components. In Bateman's (1962) experience with neurolysis, pain and sensory loss were more responsive than motor loss. There have been no documented cases in which there was a remission of symptoms or a spontaneous improvement with or without neurolysis.

Brachial plexus involvement following electrical injuries are uncommon because most of the patients do not survive. Rarely, the patient may recover, and atrophic paralysis of an upper extremity may ensue as a late manifestation of the electrical injury. The injury to the plexus is considered to be caused by the direct effect of the current. This is in contrast to the lesions reported in the central nervous system, which are felt to be due to

either damage to blood vessels or cerebral anoxia. If the patient survives the acute episode, the treatment of the neurologic residua is the same as for similar defects due to other causes (Silversides, 1964).

NEOPLASMS OF THE BRACHIAL PLEXUS

Primary tumors of the brachial plexus are rare, usually benign, and may arise either from the Schwann cell of the neural sheath (neurilemomas, neurofibromas) or from the nerve fibers (ganglioneuroma or amputation neuroma). The isolated, benign, encapsulated neurilemomas (also called perineurial fibroblastomas) constitute the majority of these primary tumors (Fisher and Tate, 1970).

Most patients with the Schwann cell tumors present with a lump but have a paucity of neurologic symptoms or objective findings. Fisher and Tate (1970) reported four patients with neurilemomas and reviewed 33 previously reported cases. These tumors are firm, rarely cystic, vary greatly in size, and arise anywhere in the plexus. Some may be quite massive and adherent to surrounding vessels. A benign neurilemoma can be enucleated without sacrifice of the nerve segment (Godwin, 1957). With massive tumors the nerves often have to be sacrificed, leading to permanent neurologic deficit. Occasionally, these tumors may coexist with a neurofibroma or a neurilemoma in the intervertebral foramen.

There is no alternative to wide excision when confronted with neurofibromas, since these tumors are prone to recur after surgical removal. There is some debate, however, whether a solitary neurofibroma without associated symptoms should be removed, since this is almost certain to produce major neurologic deficit. In some of these tumors a conservative approach would seem best, providing the clinical course is relatively benign (Woodhall, 1954).

Metastatic tumors to the brachial plexus may present with acute signs and symptoms that are similar to those seen with the nontraumatic cryptogenic plexus neuropathies. The most common tumors in this category are those extending from the breast (Castaigne, 1969) or from the lung, namely, the superior sulcus adenocarcinomas. Malignant lymphomas may also compress the brachial plexus. Pain may be unbearable with these malignant lesions. In these situations, the patient may obtain relief following high cervical cordotomy at the C2 root level or ipsilateral section of upper cervical sensory roots; radiation therapy is rarely helpful in aborting the process and often results in late complications. I have seen a few patients with a flail arm due to metastatic breast cancer recover arm function almost fully following radiotherapy.

Solitary foci of fibrous dysplasia or aneurysmal bone cysts of the clavicle or first rib are rare but may cause compression of the neurovascular structures and should be resected (Harris et al., 1962; Jaffe, 1950). Rarely, excess callus formation at the site of a fractured clavicle may also compress the neurovascular components in the thoracic outlet. In chronic cases, excision of a portion of the clavicle may have to be supplemented by lysis of the neural elements.

REFERENCES

Adams, J. H., and Cameron, H. M.: Obstetric paralysis due to ischemia of the spinal cord. Arch. Dis. Child., 40:93, 1965.

Adams, J. T., De Weese, J. A., Mahoney, E. B., and Rob, C. G.: Intermittent subclavian vein obstruction without thrombosis. Surgery, 63:147, 1968.

Adson, A. W.: The gross pathology of brachial plexus injuries. Surg. Gynecol. Obstet., 34:351, 1922.

Althaus, J.: Neuritis of the circumflex nerve in diabetes. Lancet, 1:455, 1890.

Archer, R. S.: Brachialmonoplegia complicating a case of enteric fever. Br. Med. J., 1:727, 1887.

Bárdos, V., and Somodskà, V.: Epidemiologic study of a brachial plexus neuritis outbreak in northeast Czechoslovakia. World Neurol., 2:973, 1961.

Bateman, J. E.: Trauma to Nerves in Limbs. Philadelphia, W. B. Saunders Co., 1962, p. 107.

Beyer, J. A., and Wright, I. S.: The hyperabduction syndrome with special reference to its relationship to Raynaud's syndrome. Circulation, 4:161, 1951.

Björkesten, G.: Suture of war injuries to peripheral nerves. Clinical studies of results. Acta. Chir. Scand., 95, Suppl. 119:1, 1947.

Bonney, C.: The value of axon responses in determining the site of lesion in traction injuries of the brachial plexus. Brain, 77:588, 1954.

Bonney, G.: Prognosis in traction lesions of the brachial plexus. J. Bone Joint Surg., 41B:4, 1959.

Brooks, D. M.: Open wounds of the brachial plexus. In Seddon, H. J. (ed.): Peripheral Nerve Injuries. Spec. Rep. Ser. Med. Res. Coun., No. 282. London, Her Magesty's Stationery Office, 1954.

Bufalini, C., and Pescatori, G.: Posterior cervical electromyography in the diagnosis and prognosis of brachial plexus injuries. J. Bone Joint Surg., 51B:627, 1969.

Burnard, E. D., and Fox, T. G.: Multiple neuritis of the shoulder girdle; report of nine cases occurring in Second New Zealand Expeditionary Force. N. Z. Med. J., 41:243, 1942.

Caldwell, J. W., Crane, C. R., and Krusen, U. L.: Nerve conduction studies in diagnosis of the thoracic outlet syndrome. South. Med. J., 64:210, 1971.

Cape, C. A., Fincham, R. W.: Paralytic brachial neuritis with diaphragmatic paralysis. Contralateral recurrence. Neurology (Minneap.), 15:191, 1965.

Castaigne, P.: Paralysis of the brachial plexus in breast cancer. Presse Méd., 77:1801, 1969.

Challenor, Y., Richter, R. W., Brunn, B., and Pearson, J.: Nontraumatic plexitis and heroin addiction. J.A.M.A., 225:958, 1973.

Clagett, D. T.: Presidential address: research and prosearch. J. Thorac. Cardiovas. Surg., 44:153, 1962.

Clausen, E. G.: Postoperative (anesthetic) paralysis of brachial plexus: review of literature and report of nine cases. Surgery, 12:933, 1942.

Comroe, J. H., Jr., Wood, F. C., Kay, C. F., and Spoont, E. M.: Motor neuritis after tetanus antitoxin with involvement of the muscles of respiration. Am. J. Med., 10:786, 1951.

Coni, N. K.: Pall-bearer's palsy. Br. Med. J., 2:808, 1966.

Coran, A. G., Simon, A., Heimberg, F., and Beberman, N.: Avulsion injury of the brachial plexus. Am. J. Surg., 115:840, 1968.

Daube, J. R.: Rucksack paralysis. J.A.M.A., 208:2447, 1969.

Dhuner, K. G.: Nerve injuries following operations; a survey of cases occurring during a six year period. Anesthesiology, 11:289, 1950.

Dixon, G. J., and Dick, T. B. S.: Acute brachial radiculitis: course and prognosis. Lancet 2:707, 1945.

Dreschfeld, J.: On some of the rarer forms of muscular atrophies. Brain, 9:178, 1886.

Dudrick, S.: Brachial plexus paralysis after axillary artery puncture. Radiology, 88:271, 1967.

Dyke, S. C.: Peripheral nerve lesions after antitetanic serum. Lancet, 1:570, 1918.

Eng, G. D.: Brachial plexus palsy in newborn infants. Pediatrics, 48:18, 1971.

Evans, H. W.: Paralytic brachial neuritis. N.Y. State J. Med., 65:2926, 1965.

Ewing, M. R.: Posteroperative paralysis in upper extremity (Role of Trendelenburg position): report of five cases. Lancet, 1:103, 1950.

Fetter, F.: Peripheral neuritis from tetanus antitoxin J.A.M.A., 14:137, 1953.

Fisher, R. G., and Tate, H. B.: Isolated neurilemomas of the brachial plexus. J. Neurosurg., 32:463, 1970.

Gardner, J. H., and Maloney, W.: Hereditary brachial and cranial neuritis genetically linked with ocular hypotelorism and syndactyly. Neurology, 18:278, 1968.

Gathier, J. W., and Bruyn, G. W.: Peripheral neuropathies following the administration of immune sera. A critical evaluation. Psychiatr. Neurol. Neurochir., 71:351, 1968.

Gathier, J. C., and Bruyn, G. W.: The serogenetic peripheral neuropathies. In Vinken, P. J., and Bruyn, G. W. (eds.): Handbook of Clinical Neurology. Vol. 8. Amsterdam, North-Holland Publishing Co., 1970, pp. 95–111.

Gjorup, L.: Obstetrical lesion of the brachial plexus. Acta. Neurol. Scand., 42:Suppl. 18:9, 1966.

Godwin, J. T.: Encapsulated neurilemmoma (schwannoma) of the brachial plexus: report of 11 cases. Cancer (N.Y.), 5:708, 1952.

Gordon, A.: Motor paralysis of individual nerve trunks

following administration of prophylactic serum. Med. J. Rec., *127*:530, 1928.

Guillozet, N., and Mercer, R. D.: Hereditary recurrent brachial neuropathy. Am. J. Dis. Child., *125*:884, 1973.

Harris, W.: The Morphology of the Brachial Plexus. London, Oxford University Press, 1939.

Harris, W. H., Dudley, H. R., Jr., and Barry, R. J.: The natural history of fibrous dysplasia. J. Bone Joint Surg., *44A*:207, 1962.

Haymaker, W., and Lindgren, M.: Nerve disturbances following exposure to ionizing radiation. *In* Vinken, P. J., and Bruyn, G. W. (eds.): Handbook of Clinical Neurology. Vol. 7. Amsterdam, North-Holland Publishing Co., 1970.

Haymaker, W., and Woodhall, B.: Injuries of peripheral nerves derived from the brachial plexus. *In* Haymaker, W., and Woodhall, B. (eds.): Peripheral Nerve Injuries. Philadelphia and London, W. B. Saunders Co., 1953.

Hook, O.: Acute shoulder neuritis: a syndrome characterized by pain, paralysis and muscular atrophy. Acta. Psychiatr. Neurol., *25*:209, 1950.

Hornsley, V.: On injuries to peripheral nerves. Practitioner, *63*:131, 1899.

Ilfield, F., and Holder, H.: Winged scapula: a case occurring in a soldier from knapsack. J.A.M.A., *120*:448, 1942.

Jackson, L., and Keats, A. S.: Mechanism of brachial plexus plasy following anesthesia. Anesthesiology, *26*:190, 1965.

Jacob, J. C., Andermann, F., and Robb, J. P.: Heredofamilial neuritis with brachial predilection. Neurology, *11*:1025, 1960.

Jaffe, H. L.: Aneurysmal bone cyst. Bull. Hosp. Joint Dis., *11*:3, 1950.

John, F.: Röntgenspätschäden der Haut und neurvoses Terminalreticulum. Strahlentherapie, *76*:271, 1946.

Kennedy, W. R., and Resch, J. A.: Paralytic brachial neuritis. J. Lancet, *86*:459, 1966.

Kwaan, J. H. M., and Rappaport, I.: Postoperative brachial plexus palsy; a study on the mechanism. Arch. Surg., *101*:612, 1970.

Leffert, R. D., and Seddon, H. J.: Infraclavicular brachial plexus injuries. J. Bone Joint Surg., *47B*:9, 1965.

Lhermitte, J.: Paralysies amyotrophiques dissociées du plexus brachial à type superieur consecutives à la serotherapie antititanique. Rev. Neurol., *26*:894, 1919.

Magee, K. R., and DeJong, R. N.: Paralytic brachial neuritis. J.A.M.A., *174*:1258, 1960.

Mayfield, F. H.: Neural and vascular compression syndromes of the shoulder girdles and arms. *In* Vinken, P. J., and Bruyn, G. W. (eds.): Handbook of Clinical Neurology. Vol. 7. Amsterdam, North-Holland Publishing Co., 1970.

Millesi, H.: The interfascicular nerve graft. J. Bone Joint Surg., *53A*:813, 1971.

Millesi, H., Meissl, G., and Berger, A.: The interfascicular nerve-grafting of median and ulnar nerves. J. Bone Joint Surg., *54A*:727, 1972.

Mumenthaler, M.: Armplexusparesen in Anschlussan Röntgenbestrahlung. Mitteilung von 8 eigenen Beobachtungen. Schweiz. Med. Wochenschr., *94*:1069, 1964.

Mumenthaler, M.: Some clinical aspects of peripheral nerve lesions. Eur. Neurol., 2:257, 1969.

Murphey, F., Hartung, W., and Kirklin, J. W.: Myelographic demonstration of avulsing injury of the brachial plexus. Am. J. Roentgenol. Radium Ther., *58*:102, 1947.

Nisce, L. Z., and Chu, F. C. H.: Radiotherapy of the brachial plexus syndrome for breast cancer. Radiology, *91*:1022, 1968.

Pallis, C., Louis, S., and Morgan, R. L.: Radiation myelopathy. Brain, *84*:460, 1961.

Pennybacker, J., and Russell, D. S.: Necrosis of the brain due to radiation therapy. Clinical and pathological observations. J. Neurol. Neurosurg. Psychiatry, *11*:183, 1948.

Parsonage, M. J., and Turner, J. W. A.: Neuralgic amyotrophy: the shoulder-girdle syndrome. Lancet, *1*:973, 1948.

Peacher, W. G., Robinson, R. C. L.: Neurological complications following the use of typhoid vaccine. J. Nerv. Ment. Dis., *101*:515, 1945.

Plum, F., and Druckemiller, W. H.: Acute multiple neuropathy of the shoulder girdle following antecedent illness. Trans. Am. Neurol. Assoc., *77*:250, 1952.

Poffenbarger, A. L.: Heredofamilial neuritis with brachial predilection. W. Va. Med. J., *64*:425, 1968.

Rektor, L., and Libikova, H.: Hromadny vyskyt neuritid plexus brachialis na severnom slavensku. Bratisl. Lek. Listy, *33*:293, 1953.

Richardson, J. S.: Serratus magnus palsy. Lancet, *1*:618, 1942.

Roaf, R.: Lateral flexion injuries of the cervical spine. J. Bone Joint Surg., *45B*:36, 1963.

Rob, C. G., and Standoven, A.: Arterial occlusion complicating thoracic outlet obstruction. Br. Med. J., 2:709, 1958.

Roos, D. B.: Experience with first rib resection for thoracic outlet syndrome. Ann. Surg., *173*:429, 1971.

Rosati, L. M., and Lord, J. W.: Neurovascular Compression Syndromes of the Shoulder Girdle. Modern Surgical Monographs. New York, Grune & Stratton, 1961.

Rosenberg, J. C.: Arteriographic demonstration of compression syndromes of the thoracic outlet. South. Med. J., *59*:400, 1966.

Rubin, A.: Birth injuries: incidence, mechanism and end-results. Obstet. Gynecol., *23*:218, 1964.

Saksena, A. C.: Paralysis of the serratus anterior following glandular fever. Br. Med. J., 2:267, 1943.

Salam, A. A.: Brachial plexus paralysis; an unusual complication of anticoagulant therapy. Am. Surg., *38*:454, 1972.

Sampson, J. J., Saunders, J. B. De C. M., and Capp, C. S.: Compression of the subclavian vein by the first rib and clavicle, with special reference to the prominence of the chest veins as a sign of collateral circulation. Am. Heart J., *19*:292, 1940.

Schnell, R. G., Dyck, P. J., Bowie, E. J., et al.: Infectious mononucleosis: neurologic and EEG findings. Medicine, *45*:51, 1966.

Seddon, H. J.: The use of autogenous grafts for repair of large gaps in peripheral nerves. Br. J. Surg., *35*: 151, 1947.

Seddon, H. J.: Lesions of individual nerves: upper limb. *In* Surgical Disorders of the Peripheral Nerves. Baltimore, Md., Williams & Wilkins Co., 1972.

Silversides, J.: The neurological sequelae of electrical injury. Can. Med. Assoc. J., *91*:195, 1964.

Smith, B. H., Ramakrishna, T., and Schlagenhauf, R. E.: Familial brachial neuropathy; two case reports with discussion. Neurology, *21*:941, 1971.

Smith, H. P., and Smith, H. P., Jr.: Phrenic paralysis due to serum neuritis. Am. J. Med., *19*:808, 1955.

Spillane, J. D.: Localised neuritis of the shoulder girdle: a report of 46 cases in MEF. Lancet, *2*:532, 1943.

Staal, A., van Voorthuisen, A. E., and van Diijk, L. M.: Neurological complication following arterial catheterization by the axillary approach. Br. J. Radiol., *39*:115, 1966.

Sunderland, S.: Brachial plexus lesions due to compression, stretch and penetrating injuries. *In* Nerves and Nerve Injuries. Baltimore, Williams & Wilkins Co. 1968.

Taylor, P. E.: Traumatic intradural avulsion of the nerve roots of the brachial plexus. Brain, *85*:579, 1962.

Taylor, R. A.: Heredofamilial mononeuritis multiplex with brachial predilection. Brain, *83*:113, 1960.

Tejero Lamarco, J., and Souto Crespo, J. M.: Adult toxoplasmosis; considerations on a case with associated bilateral brachial plexitis. Rev. Clin. Esp., *119*:445, 1970.

Tournay, A., and Kraus, W. M.: Postinfections and isolated paralysis of the serratus magnus. J. Neurol. Psychopathol., *5*:115, 1924.

Tsairis, P., Dyck, P. J., and Mulder, D. W.; Natural history of brachial plexus neuropathy; report on 99 patients. Arch. Neurol., *27*:109, 1972.

Turner, J. W. A.: Acute brachial radiculitis. Br. Med. J., *2*:592, 1944.

Turner, J. W. A., and Parsonage, M. J.: Neuralgic amyotrophy (paralytic brachial neuritis). Lancet, *2*:209, 1957.

Tyler, L. T., Kaplan, I. W., and Levy, R. Q.: Brachial plexus paralysis following administration of tetanus antitoxin. Am. J. Surg., *95*:668, 1958.

Ungley, C. C.: Recurrent polyneuritis in pregnancy and puerperium affecting three members in a family. J. Neurol. Psychopathol., *14*:15, 1933.

Urschel, H. G., Razzuk, M. A., Wood, R. E., Parekh, M., and Paulson, D. L.: Objective diagnosis (ulnar) nerve conduction velocity and current therapy of the thoracic outlet syndrome. Ann. Thorac. Surg., *12*: 608, 1971.

Wartenberg, R.: Brachialgia statica paresthetica (nocturnal arm dysesthesias). J. Nerv. Ment. Dis., *99*:877, 1944.

Wartenberg, R.: Neuritis of the cervical and brachial plexus. *In* Neuritis Sensory Neuritis Neuralgia. London, Oxford University Press, 1958.

Weikers, N. J., and Mattson, R. H.: Acute paralytic brachial neuritis. Neurology, *19*:1153, 1969.

Weinstein, E. A.: Localized nontraumatic neuropathy in military personnel. Arch. Neurol. Psychiatry, *57*: 369, 1947.

Winkelman, N. W.: Peripheral nerve and root disturbances following vaccination against smallpox. Arch. Neurol. Psychiatry, *62*:421, 1949.

Woodhall, B.: Peripheral nerve tumors. Surg. Clin. North Am., *34*:1167, 1954.

Woodsmith, F. G.: Post-operative brachial plexus paralysis. Brit. Med. J., *1*:1115, 1952.

Woolling, K. R., and Rushton, J. G.: Serum neuritis: report of two cases and brief review of the syndrome. Arch. Neurol. Psychiatry, *64*:568, 1950.

Wyburn-Mason, R.: Brachial neuritis occurring in epidemic form. Lancet, *2*:662, 1941.

Yeoman, P. M., and Seddon, H. J.: Brachial plexus injuries; treatment of the flail arm. J. Bone Joint Surg., *43B*:493, 1961.

Chapter 33

LUMBOSACRAL PLEXUS LESIONS

John R. Calverley

The lumbosacral plexus extends from the upper lumbar area to the lower portion of the sacrum and lies adjacent to most of the organs of the lower part of the abdomen and pelvis. This length and location leave the divisions and branches of the plexus vulnerable to damage of many different types. The inaccessibility of the fibers to direct examination may make the precise cause of a plexus neuropathy frustratingly difficult to determine. Lesions of the plexus are common, yet such neuropathies are usually not related to a fatal illness, and knowledge of their cause is based upon remarkably few necropsy studies.

Localization of a lesion to a part of the plexus is nearly always based upon the clinical examination and electromyography, but it is sometimes difficult to determine whether the site of the pathologic process is in the plexus or in the cauda equina, the nerve root, or the proximal portion of a peripheral nerve. Plexus neuropathy characteristically causes unilateral muscle weakness, sensory alteration, and reflex changes that are not confined to the structures supplied by a single root or peripheral nerve. It is my opinion that mechanical stretching, such as occurs with straight-leg raising, may accentuate pain that is present, but maneuvers that increase intraspinal pressure, such as coughing and sneezing, do not. With plexus disease, pain caused in this way implies additional involvement of nerve roots. While there are sometimes problems in localizing the lesion to an anatomical level, several distinct types of neurologic dysfunction occur in patients with lesions of the lumbosacral plexus. Those whose site of neuropathy is in the upper or lumbar portion usually have involvement of the structures supplied by the femoral nerve. While isolated neuropathies of that nerve may occur, many of the patients reported to have "femoral neuropathy" have had weakness of the iliopsoas and even the thigh adductor muscles that has almost certainly reflected a lesion in the upper plexus rather than in the femoral nerve itself.

When the entire lumbosacral plexus is destroyed, complete paralysis of the lower extremity ensues. More commonly, disease affecting both the lumbar and sacral plexuses is incomplete so that weakness and sensory loss do not conform to any radicular or peripheral nerve distribution. Dysfunction will be found in both the proximal and distal portions of the limb. A neuropathy may involve only the lower sacral plexus and cause abnormalities in the distribution of the sciatic or even solely in the tibial or peroneal nerve territory.

TRAUMA

Unlike the vulnerable brachial plexus, the fibers of the lumbosacral plexus are rarely subject to isolated injury. Traffic and industrial accidents, war wounds, and other injuries to this well-protected group of fibers almost invariably also produce gross trauma to major vessels, the ureters, the urinary bladder, or the gastrointestinal tract, or massive fractures are present. Such wounds are either fatal or so life-threatening that the lumbosacral plexus damage is overlooked. Yedinak (1971) reported upon a survivor of a spectacular highway accident who was impaled upon a long 8 by 10 cm timber. To the surprise of that physician, the only residual deficit was weakness in the muscles supplied by the upper lumbar plexus.

Fractures of the pelvic bones, and particularly the sacrum, may produce damage to the sacral portion of the plexus and result in weakness and sensory loss in the distribution of the sciatic nerve and particularly in structures supplied by the common peroneal portion of the sciatic. Those branches of the plexus that travel within the psoas muscle and form the femoral nerve may be damaged by lifting heavy objects while in a squatting position.

Surgical procedures may result in lesions of the lumbosacral plexus and its branches, and the etiology of such neuropathies sometimes may be quite obscure. Hysterectomy has been associated with weakness of the structures supplied by the femoral nerve in an unusually large number of patients, and two distinctly different mechanisms seem responsible. Investigating the forces acting on this branch of the lumbosacral plexus during abdominal hysterectomy, Rosenbloom, Scheartz, and Bendler (1966) showed that retractors, and particularly self-retaining retractors, may cause prolonged pressure against the psoas muscle and upper plexus fibers and produce a neuropathy. Care in placing retractors and palpation of the pulse of the adjacent femoral artery as an index of the degree of pressure on the vulnerable nerve should prevent such complications. Vaginal hysterectomies, on the other hand, produce femoral lesions by an entirely different mechanism. Autopsy studies by Sinclair and Pratt (1972) have shown that when the patient is positioned so that her thighs are flexed, abducted, and externally rotated, hand-held or self-retaining retractors cannot be brought to bear against the femoral nerve. Rather, the nerve is forcibly pressed against the rigid inguinal ligament, and damage occurs distal to the fibers innervating the psoas muscle. This pressure is continuous while the lithotomy posture is maintained, and it seems likely that the duration of the operation and the vigor with which the thighs are flexed and externally rotated are factors in producing these symptoms. In nearly all reported instances of such injury, recovery has occurred in three months to two years.

COMPRESSION OF PLEXUS

Sciatica of rapid onset associated with a Lasègue sign and with weakness of the dorsiflexors of the foot may be due to other pathologic changes than a herniated intervertebral disk. Exactly these symptoms may be produced by pressure on the lumbosacral plexus by aneurysms of the hypogastric and common iliac arteries (Chapman et al., 1964). The symptoms may closely resemble nerve root compression from a ruptured intervertebral disk, but a pulsating mass palpable on rectal examination and demonstration of calcification in the wall of the aneurysm by radiography of the pelvis should confirm the diagnosis of this rare cause of plexus neuropathy.

Compression of the lumbar portion of the plexus by an aortic aneurysm produces a somewhat different picture (Razzuk et al., 1967). Severe back pain that radiates to the hip, flank, anterior thigh, and leg may accompany decreased sensation in the thigh and weakness of the iliopsoas and quadriceps muscles. Extension of the thigh on the pelvis markedly aggravates the pain, and a pulsating mass may be palpable in the abdomen. In each patient described by Razzuk and his associates, the aneurysm had ruptured and formed a secondary false aneurysm that dissected into the substance of the iliopsoas muscle and down into the pelvis.

Spontaneous bleeding into the psoas muscle may occur in patients with hemophilia and other defects of coagulation and is a frequent cause of disability in hemophiliacs. Such bleeding may also occur in patients receiving anticoagulant therapy. It usually produces the abrupt onset of severe pain in the groin, anterior thigh, and hip. Weakness of the quadriceps, of the iliopsoas, and occasionally of the thigh adductor muscles develops. There is often decreased appreciation of cutaneous sensation of the anterior thigh and medial aspect of the leg, and the patellar reflex is absent. The hematoma responsible for the pressure is usually in the iliopsoas muscle and occasionally is large enough to be palpable. Some surgeons recommend surgical drainage of the hematoma if the patient's coagulation defect is correctable.

Abscesses in the psoas muscle and surrounding tissues, which were common when tuberculosis was more prevalent, are now rare causes of compression of the upper fibers of the plexus. Such an abscess may mimic a femoral nerve lesion, although the nerve fibers to the iliopsoas muscle are usually involved. Abscesses producing sciatic dysfunction are distinctly rare.

TUMORS

The length of the lumbosacral plexus, its proximity to the sacrum and the pelvic wall, to urinary and genital and gastrointestinal structures, and to lymph nodes, make it particularly vulnerable to compression or invasion by tumors. Direct extension from malignant neoplasms of the prostate, genital tract, and rectum may produce damage in any portion of the plexus. The dysfunction usually is not limited to the distribution of a single nerve or nerve root, but results from patchy involvement of the plexus. A patient with such a neuropathy may present a difficult diagnostic problem, particularly if the plexus lesion is the first manifestation of an undiagnosed malignant tumor. The pain, weakness, and sensory changes are usually insidious in their onset, relentlessly progressive, and confined to one side. Radiographs of the sacrum, lumbar portion of the spinal column, and potential primary sites of tumor often are unrevealing. Very careful rectal or pelvic examinations do not always disclose the presence of an infiltrative scirrhous growth in the plexus, and surgical exploration of this area is sometimes necessary before a proper diagnosis can be made. Diabetic lumbosacral plexus neuropathy, described later, may be particularly hard to differentiate from an infiltrative malignant process.

PUERPERAL PLEXUS LESIONS

Injury to the upper portion of the lumbosacral plexus by prolonged hyperabduction and flexion of the thighs, as might occur during a long delivery, is analogous to the previously described injury during hysterectomy. Along with others, we have encountered several patients with another type of injury to the lower fibers of the lumbosacral plexus related to childbirth (cf. Schaafsma, 1970). Some patients complained of paresthesias and mild pains in both legs in the last several weeks of pregnancy. During labor each patient

felt sharp pains in the posterior aspect of one or both thighs. After delivery, they had numbness, weakness, and decreased ankle jerks, usually in both lower extremities but more severe on one side. The weakness was diffuse and most severe distally, but not limited to the distribution of the peroneal nerve. While recovery is the rule for such injuries, some patients have been reported to have thigh pain for several months and residual weakness for a year or more.

The precise cause for this obstetrical complication is not entirely clear. It most often occurs in the primiparous, although we have seen such a symptom complex in one patient in each of her three pregnancies. It has been attributed to pressure on the sacral portion of the plexus by the fetal head or by forceps, although it has been described in patients whose deliveries were without use of forceps, and symptoms sometimes begin before labor is in progress. A large fetus seems to predispose to the problem, and cephalopelvic disproportion may be present.

VASCULAR LESIONS

Both the upper and lower portions of the lumbosacral plexus receive their blood supply from segmental arteries, and collateral circulation in this region is very extensive. Despite this, the plexus may undergo infarction if an insult to its supply is sufficiently severe. Usubiaga, Kolodny, and Usubiaga (1970) described a patient with an aortic aneurysm that involved the proximal iliac arteries. This was resected and replaced with a graft. After the operation the patient had profound weakness of the distal muscles of the left lower limb and paresis of the quadriceps and hamstring groups. All reflexes were absent and there was severe diffuse sensory loss in that extremity. The other lower limb was not involved. The patient died, and an autopsy showed infarction of the left iliopsoas muscle and of the entire lumbosacral plexus. The spinal cord was entirely normal.

Except in such rare patients, occlusion of a major vessel, such as an iliac artery, usually produces remarkably little plexus neuropathy, while small-vessel disease seems much more likely to do so. Diabetes mellitus is regarded as the most common cause of such small-vessel disease and the most common cause of spontaneous lumbosacral plexus dysfunction.

DIABETIC PLEXUS NEUROPATHY

The precise pathogenesis of the lumbosacral plexopathy seen in diabetes is still uncertain. Since Bruns (1890) described three patients with mild diabetes mellitus who developed hip pain followed by asymmetrical weakness and wasting of their thigh muscles, there have been a number of similar reports. Garland and Taverner (1953) described five such patients, three of whom had unequivocal extensor plantar responses. They felt at that time that the responsible lesion was in the spinal cord. "Diabetic anterior neuronopathy" was the name used by Alderman (1938) to describe these same symptoms. An autopsy of one of his patients showed atrophy of the lower portion of the spinal cord and microscopic evidence of anterior horn cell degeneration and also degenerative changes in the cauda equina and anterior roots. Others have examined spinal cords from very similar patients and found little myelopathy. Skanse and Gydell (1956) found no remarkable cord changes but noted myelin degeneration in peripheral nerves. After analysis of the findings in 27 cases in which the symptoms were the same as those he had described earlier, Garland (1961) concluded that weakness and wasting of the muscles were perhaps the only constant features of this diabetic disorder and that only rare patients had extensor plantar responses. He thereafter called this symptom complex "diabetic amyotrophy."

Diabetic plexus neuropathy commonly presents as either of two quite separate clinical syndromes. The first results from lesions in the fibers of the lumbar portion of the plexus and produces symptoms that most often occur in middle-aged or elderly patients with mild adult-onset diabetes. The symptoms characteristically begin abruptly with severe pain in the hip, anterior thigh, knee, and occasionally the medial aspect of the calf. Accompanying this pain, there is weakness of the quadriceps muscle and often weakness of the iliopsoas and even of the adductors of the thigh. The quadriceps reflex is lost, and there may be decreased sensation in the anterior and medial aspect of the thigh and the medial aspect of the lower leg. The pain resolves gradually over several weeks in these very disabled patients; the weakness subsides only after many weeks or months.

These patients have been described as having "femoral neuropathy," although it is recognized that the neuropathy is probably in the superior portion of the plexus. Fourteen of nineteen patients previously described by Calverley and Mulder (1960) had diabetes mellitus, and 8 of the 14 had the abrupt onset of pain, weakness, and loss of sensation without any preceding symptoms of a neurologic nature. Such an abrupt onset strongly suggested acutely impaired blood supply to the superior fibers of the plexus. Diabetic mononeuropathy of the oculomotor nerve also has an abrupt, painful onset with very gradual resolution. A detailed pathologic study of such a case by Dreyfus, Hakim, and Adams (1957) revealed enlargement of an intracavernous segment of the involved nerve with demyelination and axis cylinder damage, particularly in the center of the nerve. These findings suggested that infarction of the nerve was very likely responsible for the oculomotor palsy. The similarity between the onset of this ischemic oculomotor palsy and the superior lumbosacral plexus lesions is apparent. The abrupt onset noted in many of our patients has been subsequently reported by others and is distinctly different from the experience of Garland (1961), who stated that the weakness was never of sudden onset.

The second type of diabetic plexus neuropathy also is seen in middle-aged or elderly patients with mild, recently discovered diabetes. This is often a devastating and debilitating disorder that begins insidiously with deep aching and burning pain in the hip, buttocks, and thigh. Steadily progressive weakness accompanies this pain and spreads to involve both proximal and distal muscles. Sensory loss is usually only a minor finding. The patients are frequently bedfast, and their cachexia, pain, and widespread weakness suggest that an infiltrating malignant process is responsible for their neuropathy.

The pain may intensify and the weakness worsen for weeks or even several months before very gradual resolution occurs. Frequently, similar symptoms develop in the opposite extremity during the course of the neuropathy in the first limb (or later), and a similar, but milder neuropathy may occur simultaneously in the upper limbs. These patients clearly have damage to many areas of the lumbosacral plexus, and the damage may be secondary to vascular disease. Raff and his associates (1968) evaluated such a patient who died of an unrelated cause. Numerous small areas of infarction were seen in the plexus and in involved peripheral nerves, particularly in bridging interfascicular nerve bundles. Those investigators made serial cross sections of long segments of two nerves and found only one occluded vessel. Despite the widespread evidence of infarction, all the other vessels were patent, but many of the arterioles and capillaries around the nerve infarcts showed endothelial and parathelial thickening. That thickening may have represented diabetic vasculitis and played a part in producing the infarction, or may have been a secondary change that occurred after the infarction. The authors felt that the neurologic deficits demonstrated by their patient should be called "ischemic mononeuropathy multiplex."

Diseases other than diabetes may cause plexus neuropathies of vascular nature. Polyarteritis nodosa characteristically produces a mononeuritis multiplex and in my opinion may result in multiple and widespread areas of ischemia throughout the lumbosacral plexus. The clinical manifestations may very closely resemble a diabetic plexopathy that involves the entire plexus, and the diagnosis of a collagen vascular disease may rest on finding evidence of the characteristic necrotizing angiopathy in other organs.

The role of atherosclerosis in the production of ischemia in the plexus is much less clear. Hutchinson and Liversedge (1956) examined 32 patients without diabetes who had severe peripheral vascular disease and found that 28 of them had evidence of peripheral neuropathy. There were no examples of plexus involvement. Apparently, the extensive collateral blood supply of the plexus protects those fibers from occlusive disease of major vessels, and ischemia of plexus fibers occurs only when small-vessel disease is present.

I have evaluated a large number of patients with lumbosacral plexus lesions and only a few have not eventually been classifiable in one of the previous categories. My experience does not parallel that of Biemond (1970) who felt that 18 of the 50 patients he described had "idiopathic femoral neuropathy." All his patients were middle-aged or older, and it is not clear how extensive was his search for diabetes mellitus or other angiopathic causes of the neuropathy.

Sciatic pain that either begins abruptly or starts slowly and gradually worsens is the presenting problem in another group of patients who may also have vascular disease of the lower plexus. Many of these patients have weakness, sensory findings, and reflex changes strongly suggesting a herniated intervertebral disk, and electromyography discloses denervation in appropriate muscles, but myelography has shown no defect. Some of these patients have undergone laminectomy in which the findings were totally negative. Many were middle-aged or elderly, and it is attractive to surmise that they have had infarction in the sacral portion of the lumbosacral plexus, but necropsy proof of such a cause is not available.

Herpes zoster may produce the well-known burning dysesthetic neuralgia that accompanies the vesicular eruption and that may also be associated with pronounced motor weakness. The roots that make up the lumbosacral plexus may be involved, with resulting pain and weakness of the muscles supplied by both the upper and lower plexus fibers.

Injections and immunizations have been held responsible for some cases of "neuralgic amyotrophy" of the brachial plexus. A similar neuropathy of the lumbosacral plexus may follow immunizations, especially with tetanus toxoid. Rabies vaccine prepared from rabbit nervous tissue may cause lumbosacral plexus disease, but currently available vaccine prepared in duck embryo medium is much less likely to produce such a neuropathy.

Leg pain for several hours each morning, a limp, and slowed peripheral nerve conduction accompany a myeloradiculoneuritis that follows rubella vaccination (Gilmartin et al., 1972). These children develop the symptoms approximately six weeks following vaccination and characteristically walk on their toes with their knees flexed and complain of pain in the backs of the thighs. Straight-leg raising is painful. The symptoms may persist for many weeks and disappear spontaneously.

REFERENCES

Alderman, J. E.: Diabetic anterior neuronopathy—clinical and pathological observations. J. Mt. Sinai Hosp. N.Y., 5:396–402, 1938.

Biemond, A.: Femoral neuropathy. *In* Handbook of Clinical Neurology. Vol. 8, Part II. Amsterdam, North-Holland Publishing Co., 1970, pp. 303–310.

Bruns, L.: Über neuritische Lahmungen beim Diabetes Mellitus. Berl. Klin. Wochenschr., 27:509–515, 1890.

Calverley, J. R., and Mulder, D. W.: Femoral neuropathy. Neurology, 10:963–967, 1960.

Chapman, E. M., Shaw, R. S., and Kubik, C. S.: Sciatic

pain from arteriosclerotic aneurysm of pelvic arteries. N. Engl. J. Med., *271*:1410–1411, 1964.

Dreyfus, P. M., Hakim, S., and Adams, R. D.: Diabetic ophthalmoplegia. Arch. Neurol. Psychiatry, *77*:337–349, 1957.

Garland, H.: Diabetic amyotrophy. Br. J. Clin. Prac., *15*:9–13, 1961.

Garland, H., and Taverner, D.: Diabetic myelopathy. Br. Med. J., *1*:1405–1408, 1953.

Gilmartin, R. C., Jabbour, J. T., and Duenas, D. A.: Rubella vaccine myeloradiculoneuritis. J. Pediatr., *80*:406–412, 1972.

Hutchinson, E. C., and Liversedge, L. A.: Neuropathy in peripheral vascular disease; its bearing on diabetic neuropathy. Q. J. Med., *25*:267–274, 1956.

Raff, M. C., Sangalang, V., and Asbury, A. K.: Ischemic mononeuropathy multiplex associated with diabetes mellitus. Arch. Neurol., *18*:487–499, 1968.

Razzuk, M. A., Linton, R. R., and Darling, R. C.: Femoral neuropathy secondary to ruptured abdominal aortic aneurysms with false aneurysms. J.A.M.A., *201*:817–818, 1967.

Rosenblum, J., Scheartz, G. A., and Bendler, E.: Femoral neuropathy—a neurological complication of hysterectomy. J.A.M.A., *195*:409–410, 1966.

Schaafsma, S. J.: Plexus Injuries. *In* Vinken, P. J., and Bruyn, G. W. (eds.): Handbook of Clinical Neurology. Vol. 7, Part I. Amsterdam, North-Holland Publishing Co., 1970, pp. 402–429.

Sinclair, R. H., and Pratt, J. H.: Femoral neuropathy after pelvic operation. Am. J. Obstet. Gynecol., *112*:404–407, 1972.

Skanse, B., and Gydell, K.: A rare type of femoral-sciatic neuropathy in diabetes mellitus. Acta Med. Scand., *155*:463–468, 1956.

Usubiaga, J. E., Kolodny, J., and Usubiaga, L. E.: Neurological complications of prevertebral surgery under regional anesthesia. Surgery, *68*:304–309, 1970.

Yedinak, P. R.: An unusual foreign body. Rocky Mt. Med. J., *68*:13–14, 1971.

PART D

Neuropathy Due to Ischemia and Physical Agents

Chapter 34

NEUROPATHY DUE TO COMPRESSION AND ENTRAPMENT

Albert J. Aguayo

Many peripheral nerves, because of their long and superficial course, are vulnerable to mechanical injury. Accordingly, compression neuropathies are characterized by involvement of single nerves at sites where they are anatomically most exposed to pressure. In such neuropathies, the degree of damage is determined by a combination of factors, the most important of which are the magnitude and duration of the injurious force and the composition and anatomical relationships of the particular nerve. Narrowing of anatomical passageways, habitual or occupational exposure to repeated trauma, and an excessive susceptibility to pressure injury are factors that commonly contribute to the development of compression neuropathies.

This chapter deals with mechanisms of injury, pathologic changes and specific clinical syndromes that result from compression of peripheral nerves in the extremities. Chronic types of compression injury, rather than acute damage, are emphasized.

PATHOPHYSIOLOGY OF PERIPHERAL NERVE COMPRESSION

The degree of functional and structural change caused by compression in large part reflects the anatomical composition of peripheral nerves. Since nerves are made up of fascicles of fibers surrounded and separated by connective tissue, the interfascicular spaces and relatively elastic connective tissue provide a degree of protective cushioning from compression. In addition, superficially located nerve fibers presumably protect more deeply situated fibers. Such factors may explain the patchy cross sectional damage produced by constriction of peripheral nerves (Fig. 34–1*A*) (Aguayo et al., 1971). On the other hand, when external mechanical forces act tangentially, or when circumscribed injury is caused by friction of nerve trunks against hard bony surfaces, some fascicles may be affected while others are spared (Fig. 34–1*B*). This differential involvement reflects the intraneural topography of nerve fascicles and their relation to the damaging forces. The position of sensory and motor fascicles within mixed nerves has been outlined by Sunderland (1968). This anatomical knowledge is helpful in understanding clinical findings in pressure and other neuropathies that result in partial fascicular damage within nerve trunks (Trojaborg, 1970).

Clinical studies have suggested that nerves supplying muscles are more susceptible than cutaneous nerves to the effects of compression (Erb, 1876; Denny-Brown and Brenner, 1944; Sunderland, 1945). The incidence of such

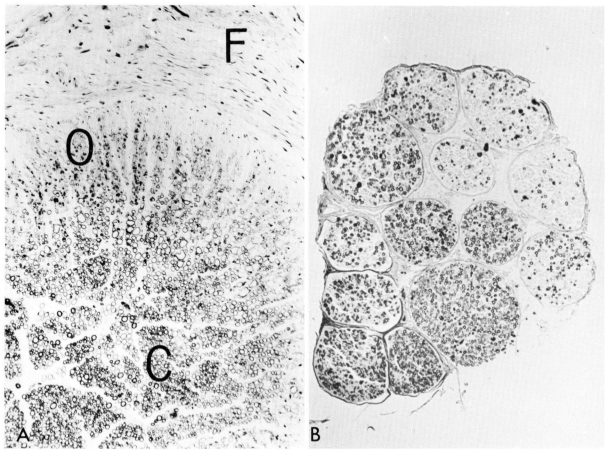

Figure 34–1   *A.* Partial representation of the transverse section of a constricted rabbit sciatic nerve demonstrating extensive damage of outer myelinated fibers (O) while fibers in the center (C) are better preserved. Reactive fibrous tissue (F) surrounds the nerve. (From Aguayo, A., Nair, C. P. V., and Midgley, R.: Experimental progressive compression neuropathy in the rabbit. Arch. Neurol., *24*:358–364, 1971. Copyright 1971, American Medical Association. Reprinted by permission.) *B.* Differences in the extent of fiber damage among 13 nerve fascicles of injured rabbit posterior tibial nerve (transverse section at the ankle level six weeks after partial crush injury of the sciatic nerve in the thigh).

differential effects cannot easily be determined in mixed peripheral nerves, but it is likely that they reflect differences in biochemical properties (Brody, 1966) and fiber composition known to exist between muscular and cutaneous nerves. The importance of nerve fiber composition is suggested by the observation that thick myelinated fibers are less resistant to pressure than thin fibers (Gasser and Erlanger, 1929). Correspondingly a greater involvement of thick fibers has been shown in both human (Thomas and Fullerton, 1963) and experimental compression neuropathies (Duncan, 1948; Fullerton and Gilliatt, 1967a, 1967b; Anderson et al., 1970; Ochoa et al., 1971). Myelinated fiber damage associated with relative sparing of unmyelinated nerve fibers has also been demonstrated in experimental lesions produced by ligatures inserted through rat peripheral nerves (Lehman and Pretschner, 1966). Although the thickest myelinated fibers in peripheral nerve are sensory (Ia and Ib afferents), there is a numerical predominance of thick myelinated fibers in muscular nerves. Conversely, in cutaneous nerves 75 per cent of fibers are unmyelinated (Ochoa and Mair, 1969). Such differences in composition and susceptibility to pressure may thus influence the overall effects of pressure on muscular and cutaneous nerves.

Both the magnitude and duration of compression also affect the nature and extent of nerve damage. Thus, pressures of 120 mm of mercury applied to cat sciatic nerve within a chamber for approximately three hours produced only moderate impairment of nerve

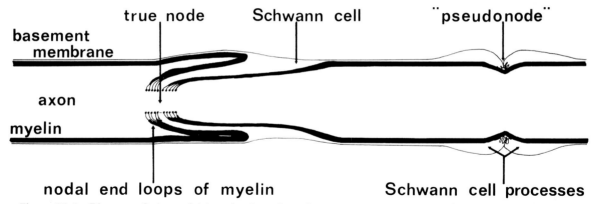

Figure 34–2 Diagram of paranodal invagination of myelin after experimental tourniquet paralysis. The node of Ranvier has been displaced from the site of compression (right to left) and is covered by myelin folds. This results in obliteration of the nodal gap. The original site of the node (true node) is labeled "pseudonode." (From Ochoa, J., Fowler, T. J., and Gilliatt, R. W.: Changes produced by a pneumatic tourniquet. *In* Desmedt, J. (ed.): New Developments in Electromyography and Clinical Neurophysiology. Vol. 2. Basel, S. Karger, 1973. Reprinted by permission.)

conduction, whereas pressures between 130 and 200 mm of mercury applied for the same period blocked conduction completely (Bentley and Schlapp, 1943). In baboons, pneumatic cuff compression of the lower limb at pressures of 1000 mm of mercury for one to three hours produced segmental conduction block in the medial popliteal nerve directly under the cuff, while conduction was preserved distally (Danta et al., 1971). Histologic examination of such nerves revealed paranodal invagination of compressed fibers, as is described later. This is presumably due to longitudinal displacement of myelin and consequent obliteration of the nodes of Ranvier (Fig. 34–2). Paranodal invagination could result from differential pressure gradients between the compressed and adjacent uncompressed portions of nerve fibers. The occurrence of paranodal invagination as early as 24 hours after tourniquet application suggests that early functional changes could result from nodal occlusion. Ischemia has also been thought responsible for tourniquet paralysis (Denny-Brown and Brenner, 1944; Mayer and Denny-Brown, 1964; Martin and Paletta, 1966). Since it has been impossible in experimental nerve compression clearly to separate ischemia from purely mechanical factors, the precise pathogenesis of the disordered nerve function remains a matter of conjecture.

Effects of Pressure on Schwann Cells

The Schwann cells of myelinated nerve fibers are particularly susceptible to the effects

of pressure. In the early stages of tourniquet paralysis, the nodes of Ranvier at the edges of the compressed portions of fibers are obliterated by the paranodal invagination of myelin. These changes extend from 200 to 300 μm on either side of the nodes while the rest of the internodal segment of the fiber shows no visible alteration. In later stages, however, the whole of the internodal myelin sheath may be thinned or completely lost. In contrast, even over a wide range of tourniquet pressures, the myelin sheath of nerve segments farthest from the compression site remains intact.

Once the compression is released there is a repair of demyelinated segments. When remyelination eventually occurs, it results in the formation of internodes of varying lengths. In addition, when repeated demyelination is experimentally induced by multiple tourniquet applications to rat sciatic nerve, remyelination is accompanied by hypertrophic changes resulting from concentric rearrangement of Schwann cells (Dyck, 1969).

Effects of Pressure on Axons

Although it is the myelin sheath that is primarily affected by nerve compression, axonal damage may occur and be severe enough to result in wallerian degeneration distal to the site of injury. Axonal enlargement and an accumulation of organelles and enzymes normally found within the axon have been demonstrated to occur proximal to nerve constrictions and affect both myelinated and unmyelinated axons (Kapeller and Mayor, 1969a; Lubińska et al., 1964). Enzyme accumulation may result from local synthesis or from relocation within damaged axons. The significance of axonal enlargements remains unclear. Weiss and Hiscoe (1948), suggested that they are due to the damming of centrifugal axoplasmic flow, but this concept has recently been questioned (Spencer, 1972). Interestingly, there are also axonal dilatations just distal to the site of compression, presumably as a consequence of impaired centripetal axonal flow (Dahlström and Haggendal, 1966; Kapeller and Mayor, 1969b).

During compression, the limits of axonal membrane resistance to stretch and distortion may be surpassed, thereby leading to breakdown of the peripheral portion of damaged fibers. Indeed, axonal degeneration has been demonstrated in human entrapment neuropathies by Thomas and Fullerton (1963), in animal nerves subjected to experimental chronic progressive constriction by Aguayo, Nair, and Midgley (1971), and in naturally occurring pressure neuropathies involving foot nerves of guinea pigs by Fullerton and Gilliatt (1967a). There are also retrograde changes in fibers of injured nerves (Aitken and Thomas, 1962; Anderson et al., 1970). These retrograde changes may result in neuronal loss when damage occurs close to the nerve cell body. Retrograde structural changes presumably explain the reduction in nerve conduction velocity found proximal to the site of peripheral nerve injury (Kiraly and Krnjević, 1959; Cragg and Thomas, 1961).

Following axonal injury, regeneration may lead to the formation of multiple closely packed axonal sprouts (Ramón y Cajal, 1928). There is as yet no direct evidence concerning the functional alterations that result from the growth of closely packed immature axons, but it has been suggested that sprouts that are not separated by Schwann cell processes could interact electrically (Ruska and Ruska, 1961). Fullerton and Gilliatt (1965) postulated that axonal branching after regeneration from circumscribed nerve lesions might account for the electrophysiologic findings of reflex responses with latencies too short to be explained as spinal reflexes or antidromic discharges of motor neurons. Such short latency reflex responses could be accounted for if impulses were propagated in a proximal direction up to the point of axonal branching, from where they would orthodromically generate a motor response.

HUMAN PRESSURE NEUROPATHIES

In man, pressure neuropathies usually result from prolonged or repeated trauma at sites where nerves are anatomically exposed to external mechanical forces. In such circumstances, the nerve is compressed against structures within the limb (Mulder et al., 1960). Certain circumstances commonly predispose to such disorders. One of the most common is the habitual adoption of certain postures such as leaning on the elbows, causing compression of the ulnar nerve, and repeated and prolonged leg crossing, causing peroneal palsy. Slender individuals are particularly prone to pressure neuropathies since their nerves are less well protected than those of the rest of the population. Working methods may also lead to pressure palsies, a common variety being damage to the palmar motor branch of the ulnar nerve in workmen using pneumatic drills (Spaans, 1970). Finally, pressure neuropathies often result from the adoption of unusual positions during sleep, particularly sleep deepened by alcohol or sedatives, and may complicate the recovery of patients who have been anesthetized or are in coma (Britt and Gordon, 1964).

In this section, a general introduction to pressure and entrapment neuropathies, symptomatology, and diagnostic aids is followed by a detailed discussion of specific clinical entities.

Increased Susceptibility of Nerves to Pressure Injuries

Once damaged by disease, peripheral nerves become even more sensitive to the effects of pressure. Thus in patients suffering from malnutrition (Denny-Brown, 1947), alcoholism, diabetes (Mulder et al., 1961; Gilliatt and Willison, 1962), renal failure (Preswick and Jeremy, 1964), or the Guillain-Barré syndrome (Lambert and Mulder, 1964), pressure neuropathies are a common complication. Such disorders usually appear in nerves that are naturally exposed to pressure. The cause of the increased susceptibility remains unknown. It is noteworthy, however, that in guinea pigs with experimentally induced diphtheritic polyneuropathy that are housed in cages with hard floors, severe histologic changes appear in the plantar nerves (Hopkins and Morgan-Hughes, 1969). Since such changes do not occur in nerves that are naturally protected from pressure, nor in plantar nerves of animals suspended above the cage floor, the histologic lesions would seem to result from the combined action of the diphtheria toxin and pressure.

In addition to disease, genetic factors also predispose to pressure neuropathy. A familial form of multiple mononeuropathy, precipitated by minor pressure or traction, has been described by Davies (1954). Family members gave a history of recurrent weakness and sensory symptoms in the distribution of peripheral nerves that were exposed to minor forms of compression. Although most of these neuropathies were transient, some resulted in persistent deficits. In some instances in which there was a similar family history, electrophysiologic abnormalities were found in non-symptomatic members (Earl et al., 1964; Behse et al., 1972). In addition, in some affected members of these families, sural nerve biopsies have shown irregular thickening of the myelin sheath and demyelination (Behse et al., 1972).

Entrapment Neuropathies

Entrapment neuropathies are specific forms of pressure neuropathy in which nerve injury results from compression by neighboring anatomical structures (Kopell and Thompson, 1963; Staal, 1970). In nerves normally confined to narrow anatomical passageways, injury may be due to the effect of local pathologic changes such as inflammation or scarring of surrounding tissues. In addition, compression may result from bony, vascular, or muscular structures that alter the normal contour or reduce the size of these anatomical passageways. In the limbs, many entrapments occur in relation to joints, presumably because here nerves are subject to repeated stretching and relaxation during movement. If such nerves become pathologically anchored by the entrapment process so that excessive stretching occurs, further damage will ensue.

A favorable ground for the development of nerve entrapments is provided by a variety of conditions; congenital or posttraumatic bone deformities, soft tissue swellings such as occur in pregnancy, hypothyroidism or acromegaly, and inflammatory joint diseases, particularly

rheumatoid arthritis. In addition, vascular malformations, tumors, or the fibrous edges of normally or abnormally located muscles may also lead to nerve compression. Familial disorders of metabolism that produce soft tissue or bone changes may in turn lead to neural entrapments. Such a mechanism has been described by McKusick and co-workers (1965) in mucopolysaccharidosis V (Scheie syndrome) in which compression of the median nerve in the carpal tunnel is a common complication. Karpati and associates (1973) have described clinical and electrophysiologic findings in three brothers who presented with multiple nerve entrapments. In one of the brothers a sural nerve biopsy was performed, and although clinically normal, the nerve showed axonal degeneration and numerous "Renaut corpuscles" (see Chapter 15). Vacuolated fibroblasts were present in the epineurium as well as in the endomysium of muscle biopsy material, and during surgical decompression of the median nerve at the wrist, the flexor retinaculum was found to be unusually thickened and to contain fibrocartilage. The urine of one of the brothers contained large quantities of mucopolysaccharides; however, none of the brothers showed the corneal clouding or skeletal abnormalities that occur in most mucopolysaccharidoses.

SYMPTOMATOLOGY

Acute injury of peripheral nerves usually produces an immediate impairment of sensory and motor function. In contrast, the symptoms of compression and entrapment neuropathies usually develop gradually. Indeed, in the initial stages, physical signs may be minimal or entirely lacking. Since the impairment of nerve function is usually reversible, particularly in the early stages, early diagnosis is of obvious importance to successful management.

The first essential step in the diagnosis of pressure neuropathies consists of obtaining an accurate description of symptoms from the patient. In entrapment neuropathies, pain is one of the most common complaints and it very often occurs at rest. An outstanding example of this phenomenon occurs in the carpal tunnel syndrome in which pain is experienced at its worst in the early hours of the morning after a period of sleep. The pain is usually felt at the site of compression, but it may radiate or be referred to sites at a considerable distance. Tingling, prickling, numbness, burning of the skin, coldness, and other distorted sensations are other prominent complaints. Percussion of the nerve trunk at or near the site of compression often causes acute pain and tingling (Tinel's sign) (Wilkins and Brody, 1971). In addition, symptoms may be reproduced by certain postures or movements that lead to further nerve compression or stretching. Since compression neuropathies, whether unilateral or bilateral, tend to occur in the distribution of single peripheral nerves, it is important to determine whether the symptoms and signs correspond to the distribution of the nerve or branches of the nerve in question. In addition since most compression and entrapment neuropathies affect nerves distally in the limbs, changes in light touch, pain and temperature sensibility, and appreciation of texture are more prominent than alterations in deep sensory modalities such as vibration and joint position sense. For the same reason deep tendon reflexes are not usually altered in these neuropathies.

Impairment of muscle strength varies greatly. Patients either do not complain of weakness or notice difficulty only in performing specific movements. An inability to open jars or the noticeable slapping of the foot against the floor while walking are presenting complaints in patients with median or peroneal nerve lesions respectively. There may also be clear loss of muscle bulk, but more commonly the loss is so subtle as to be revealed only by careful inspection and palpation.

Careful scrutiny along the course of nerves suspected of being compressed can be rewarding. This simple maneuver may reveal a pulsatile mass due to a vascular malformation, abnormal angulation of joints resulting from congenital defects or trauma, as well as synovial ganglia or lipomas. Furthermore, at sites of repeated compression injury, there is frequently a circumscribed thickening of the affected nerve trunk.

DIAGNOSTIC AIDS

The most important anciliary method in the diagnosis and management of pressure neuropathies is the electrophysiologic measurement of the velocity of nerve conduction. Although the initial studies reported by Simpson (1956) dealt with changes in motor conduction, determination of the amplitude and velocity of sensory nerve action potentials is now recognized as a source of valuable additional information (Buchthal and Rosenfalck, 1966).

Since pressure is known to affect the fastest conducting peripheral nerve fibers, it is not surprising that slowing of conduction is found very commonly in neuropathies due to localized compression or entrapment. In these circumstances, however, the slowing of nervous impulses is restricted to, or more pronounced at, the site of pressure. The focal character of the impairment helps to differentiate these disorders from the more diffuse conduction changes seen in polyneuropathy. Conversely, in patients with compression neuropathy who are suspected of having an underlying disease that renders nerves susceptible to pressure, diagnosis is aided by the demonstration of diffusely impaired nerve conduction even in the absence of clinical signs of polyneuropathy (Preswick and Jeremy, 1964).

In nerves whose function is impaired by disease and that are subjected to compression by a sphygmomanometer cuff inflated around a limb to above systolic arterial pressure, changes in nerve conduction appear earlier and are more pronounced than those that occur when normal nerves are similarly compressed (Gilliatt and Wilson, 1953; Fullerton, 1963). In addition, the responses induced in compressed nerves are different depending upon whether the intensity of stimulating current is threshold or supramaximal. As an example, in a group of patients with mild forms of carpal tunnel entrapment, Preswick (1963) found abnormal responses in 50 per cent when supramaximal stimulation was used, but in 80 per cent when threshold current was employed.

Needle electromyography and nerve conduction determinations can be of assistance in differentiating between peripheral nerve compression and lesions of nerve roots. Normal motor nerve conduction, combined with evidence of denervation in muscles that have the same segmental innervation (myotomes) but that are not supplied by the same peripheral nerve, is evidence in favor of a radiculopathy. On the other hand, slowing of motor and sensory nerve conduction and evidence of muscle denervation confined to a single nerve distribution are indicative of a peripheral nerve lesion. Since most compressive radicular lesions spare the dorsal root ganglion cells, the axons of peripheral sensory fibers remain intact. Thus, in root lesions sensory action potentials may be normal even in the presence of profound sensory impairment (Bonney and Gilliatt, 1958). For the same reason, electrical skin resistance and the histamine mediated axonal reflex are altered in patients with neuropathies, whereas they are normal in patients with root lesions (Bonney, 1954).

In addition to these methods of investigation, radiologic examination may be of assistance in explaining otherwise obscure compressive nerve injuries. This is especially the case where nerves are encroached upon by bony spurs, osteomas, ectopic calcifications, or deformities that ensue upon trauma.

PRESSURE SYNDROMES OF THE UPPER LIMB

Median Nerve

ANATOMY AND COMMON SITES OF COMPRESSION

The median nerve is formed at the level of the pectoralis minor muscle by union of branches from the lateral and medial cords of the brachial plexus. Radicular contributions to this nerve derive from the fifth cervical to the first thoracic spinal segments. The median nerve gives off no important branches in the arm, but in the upper forearm it supplies the pronator teres and most muscles responsible for wrist and finger flexion. The anterior interosseous nerve, which innervates the flexor digitorum profundus to the index and middle fingers, the flexor pollicis longus, and the pronator quadratus muscles, is a purely motor nerve branch that arises from the median nerve just after it passes between the two heads of the pronator teres muscle. At the wrist, the median nerve runs under the transverse carpal ligament (carpal tunnel), and once in the hand, it innervates the thenar muscles and supplies palmar digital nerves to the thumb, index, and middle fingers, and to half of the ring finger (Fig. 34–3). The motor nerve branches innervate the abductor pollicis brevis, the opponens pollicis, and the first two lumbricals.

As shown in Figure 34–3, the median nerve may be compressed high in the forearm (A) or at the wrist (B). In addition, median digital nerves (C) and branches to the thenar muscles

(D) may be damaged within the hand. At all three levels, the nerve is compressed while passing through narrow anatomical passageways. In the hand, direct trauma and traction are additional causes of nerve damage.

LESIONS IN THE UPPER FOREARM

In the upper forearm the median nerve is usually compressed at the level of the pronator teres muscle (pronator teres syndrome). The whole nerve may be involved or there may be isolated compression of the anterior interosseous nerve. The main complaint of patients with compression injury of the median nerve at this level is pain in the hollow of the upper forearm (Kopell and Thompson, 1958). The pain may radiate toward the hand or reach the shoulder and neck. Repeated gripping or pronating movements or both lead to muscle aching, and the upper forearm muscles may become firm and tender to palpation (Seyffarth, 1951). In such circumstances, patients may complain of inability to straighten their fingers or of difficulty in making flexion movements of the distal phalanx of the thumb and index finger. In the pronator teres syndrome it is unusual to find marked muscle weakness or wasting. Numbness and tingling occur either at rest or after exertion and are felt in the palm and first three fingers. Since the palmar cutaneous branch of the median nerve usually arises above the wrist, lesions within the forearm generally impair sensation in the palm to a greater extent than do lesions at the wrist (see Fig. 34–3). When the anterior interosseous nerve alone is compressed, there is no weakness of the thenar muscles in the hand and, since this is a purely motor nerve, there is no sensory loss (O'Brien and Upton, 1972).

Entrapments of the median nerve in the upper forearm are rare, but they should be suspected when local symptoms are prominent or when pressure, scars, ischemic contracture (Volkmann's), or other focal pathologic changes provide favorable conditions for nerve compression. Differentiation, on the basis of symptoms, between entrapment in the upper forearm or in the carpal tunnel can be difficult. A careful analysis of the history and signs, the response to local injection of anesthetic or antiinflammatory drugs, and adequate electrophysiologic testing will, however, usually ensure that the correct diagnosis is made.

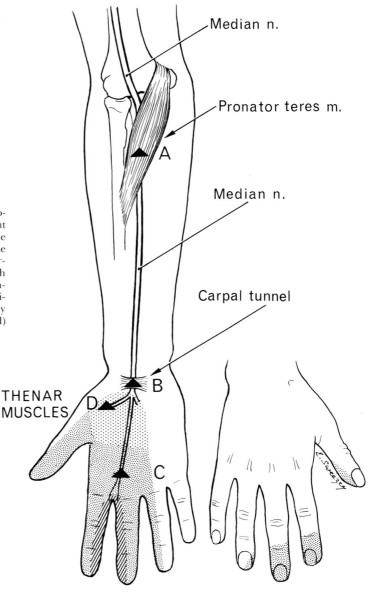

Figure 34–3 Median nerve: schematic representation of its course and clinically relevant anatomical relations. Common sites of nerve compression are: the pronator teres muscle (A), carpal tunnel (B), and transverse intermetacarpal ligaments (C). The motor branch to the thenar muscles (D), cutaneous innervation to the hand (heavily stippled), and distribution of the palmar cutaneous branch (lightly stippled) and of an interdigital nerve (hatched) are indicated.

The treatment of median nerve compression in the upper forearm depends on the severity and mechanism of the injury. When avoidance of undue exertion by forearm muscles and prevention of external trauma is unsuccessful and there are signs of progressive dysfunction of the median nerve, surgical treatment is necessary (Spinner, 1970).

LESIONS AT THE WRIST

The carpal tunnel is the site of the most common form of entrapment in the upper limb. Here the median nerve is rendered particularly vulnerable to compression as it passes into the hand between the carpal bones and the transverse carpal ligament (see Fig. 34–3B).

The carpal tunnel syndrome is characterized by bouts of pain and paresthesias in the wrist and hand that are very often most severe and troublesome in the hours of sleep. Indeed, many patients complain bitterly of sleeplessness due to recurrent nocturnal pain. In these circumstances, some relief is obtained by rising and shaking or rubbing the hands, or by letting them hang over the bedside. Pain is felt at the wrist, but may spread toward the fingers or upward into the forearm. Paresthesias are commonly localized to the palmar aspects of the fingers and may include numbness or a sense of swelling of the digits. Many patients are uncertain whether the paresthesias spare the ulnar innervated ring and little fingers. There may be clumsiness and difficulty in performing certain tasks, such as unscrewing bottle tops, turning a key, crocheting, or knitting. These symptoms are made worse by typing, kneading, wringing clothes, and other activities that demand repeated wrist and finger flexion and extension.

Flattening of the lateral portion of the thenar eminence was formerly a common sign of median neuropathy. Now, however, in view of the greater awareness of entrapment neuropathies, cases of carpal tunnel syndrome with marked thenar wasting are seldom seen. This serves to emphasize that severe, distressing sensory symptoms may long precede any sign of muscle wasting or weakness. A revealing sign, when present, is a mild weakness of the abductor pollicis brevis or of the opponens pollicis muscle. The former, which abducts the thumb at right angles to the palm, is usually innervated by the median nerve. The opponens pollicis, however, may be anomalously supplied by the ulnar nerve and is thus not as reliable an index of median nerve impairment. Sensory signs within the median distribution are best sought for in the finger tips, where impairment is as a rule more pronounced. Occasionally, however, in place of hypesthesia and hypalgesia there is an overreaction to cutaneous or painful stimuli. Isolated thenar wasting or sensory impairment in the distribution of individual digital nerves may be the presenting feature of median nerve lesions at the wrist. Such peculiar signs presumably result from entrapment of the recurrent motor branch as it crosses over the transverse carpal ligament or the predominant involvement of only some nerve fascicles of the median nerve at the wrist. Manual pressure over the flexor aspect of the wrist or prolonged hyperextension or hyperflexion of this joint may reproduce sensory symptoms. A Tinel sign, consisting of shocklike pain and tingling elicited by percussion of the median nerve at the wrist, is less common a finding than often thought.

Although carpal tunnel entrapments are bilateral in more than half the cases (Cseuz et al., 1966), symptoms usually first appear and are more severe in the dominant hand, likely as a result of greater use.

Obesity, rheumatoid arthritis (Phalen and Kendrick, 1957), hypothyroidism (Purnell et al., 1961), pregnancy (Soferman et al., 1964), acromegaly (Schiller and Kolb, 1954), multiple myeloma (Grokoest and Demartini, 1954), and trauma to the carpal bones (Short, 1951) are among the more common disorders associated with entrapment of the median nerve at the wrist. More often than not, however, there is no evident associated primary disorder; indeed, a large proportion of these entrapments occur in otherwise healthy, middle-aged individuals.

DIAGNOSIS

The complaint of nocturnal pain or paresthesias in the hand should always raise the suspicion of a carpal tunnel syndrome, for it is an almost universal symptom of this disorder. The distribution of distal sensory symptoms and proximal radiation of pain may suggest the diagnosis of a C6 or C7 root compression. The difficulty in differential diagnosis is compounded if x-rays show the presence of osteoarthritic changes in the spine, a common finding in the age group most often afflicted by median nerve compression. In radiculopathy, however, the symptoms are usually relieved by rest and worsened by straining or by movement of the neck. Furthermore, in place of the predominantly palmar location of symptoms in median nerve lesions, the sensory impairment in isolated root compression is found over the dorsal and palmar aspects of the thumb (C6) or of the first two fingers (C7). Furthermore, in C6 and C7 root lesions there is often weakness of muscles within the arm as well as the forearm, and the brachioradialis or triceps jerks may be impaired.

Wasting of the muscles of the hand may result from a cervical rib or from a band compressing the brachial plexus. When the signs predominate in the thenar muscles, differentiation from the carpal tunnel syndrome is necessary (Gilliatt et al., 1970). Conversely, loss of bulk or strength in hand muscles other than the thenar, together with sensory findings on the inner side of the hand or forearm, in a patient suspected of suffering from an entrapment of the median nerve suggests the alternative diagnosis of a thoracic outlet syndrome.

Sensory and, to a lesser extent, motor

nerve conduction studies have proved useful in the diagnosis of median nerve lesions at the carpal tunnel. Cseuz and co-workers (1966) found abnormalities of nerve conduction in 85 per cent of 351 entrapped median nerves; of these, motor nerve conduction was abnormal in only 69 per cent. In those instances in which sensory and motor nerve conduction velocities are normal when tested by standard procedures, slowing may be demonstrated either for mechanically evoked sensory responses (McLeod, 1966) or by the analysis of differences in velocities recorded between digit to palm and palm to wrist (Buchthal and Rosenfalck, 1971). The evaluation of changes in the speed and amplitude of sensory and motor electrical responses during ischemia, reported by Gilliatt and Wilson (1953) and Fullerton (1963), and in relation to threshold and supramaximal stimulating currents, described by Preswick (1963), may also be helpful. Finally, electrophysiologic investigations are of use in documenting recovery after treatment (Goodman and Gilliatt, 1961).

TREATMENT

In mild cases of carpal tunnel syndrome or when the condition can be assumed to be self-limited (pregnancy) or medically treatable (hypothyroidism), immobilization of the wrist in the neutral position as well as local wrist injections of hydrocortisone are justified (Foster, 1960). In most instances, however, pain and discomfort are so persistent as to interfere with normal activity and sleep. In such cases surgical decompression is necessary. Recovery is prompt after surgery, with relief from pain and paresthesias being almost immediate (Thomas et al., 1967). Sensory loss and motor signs, however, take longer to disappear. Failure to improve following operative treatment suggests either an incomplete section of the transverse carpal ligament or, one must hope rarely, an erroneous diagnosis.

Ulnar Nerve

ANATOMY

The ulnar nerve receives contributions from the C7, C8, and T1 roots and arises in the axilla as a branch of the medial cord of the brachial plexus. In the upper arm it maintains a medial position and gives off no branches. It lies superficially until it reaches the middle of the arm, where it pierces the intermuscular septum to reach the condylar groove behind the medial epicondyle. As the nerve enters the forearm it lies in the cubital tunnel, of which the floor is formed by the medial ligament of the elbow joint and the roof by an aponeurosis between the olecranon and medial epicondyle (Fig. 34–4). The nerve then passes between the two heads of the flexor carpi ulnaris and descends on the surface of the flexor digitorum profundus; it innervates the flexor carpi ulnaris and the medial half of the flexor digitorum profundus. The palmar cutaneous branch arises in the middle of the forearm and supplies the skin overlying the hypothenar eminence (Fig. 34–5). The dorsal cutaneous branch winds around the ulna above the wrist and supplies the dorsum of the medial half of the hand and all of the little and half of the ring fingers. The rest of the nerve enters the hand volar to the transverse carpal ligament and divides into two terminal branches: the cutaneous branch to the remainder of the palm and to the ulnar-supplied fingers, and the muscle branch, which passes between the pisiform bone and the hook of the hamate (the tunnel of Guyon). The latter branch innervates the hypothenar muscles, the third and fourth lumbricals, and all the interossei.

LESIONS AT THE ELBOW

Ulnar nerve lesions are rare in the arm, but at the elbow the nerve is more vulnerable to pressure than anywhere else along its course. The neuropathy that results from pressure at this level is often manifested by numbness and tingling in the two ulnar-innervated fingers. These symptoms may be associated with pain in the hand, forearm, or elbow, and with clumsiness. In addition, muscle wasting may occur and appear as hollowing between the metacarpal bones, especially in the space between the thumb and index finger. In many cases, however, nerve injury at the elbow is only partial, some nerve fascicles being spared; this is reflected in a corresponding variation in symptoms and signs.

Complete nerve injuries cause weakness of all ulnar-innervated muscles in the forearm and hand. As a result of involvement of the motor supply to the flexor carpi ulnaris, the hand deviates radially when the wrist is flexed

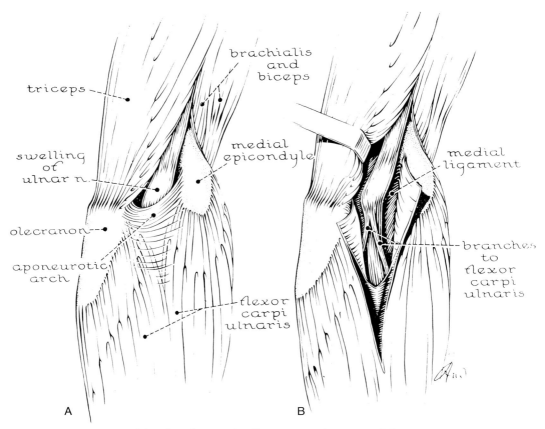

Figure 34–4 Compression of the ulnar nerve at the elbow. *A.* Posterior aspect of elbow illustrating anatomical relations at the cubital tunnel. *B.* The tunnel has been opened to show the compressed nerve. Note position of branches to flexor carpi ulnaris muscle. (From Feindel, W., and Stratford, J.: The role of the cubital tunnel in tardy ulnar palsy. Can. J. Surg., *1*:287–300, 1958. Reprinted by permission.)

against resistance. When the flexor digitorum profundus is affected, bending of the ring and little fingers at the terminal interphalangeal joint is also weak. Wasting of these two muscles causes a loss of the normally convex contour of the medial border of the forearm. Since the flexor carpi ulnaris and the flexor digitorum profundus receive their innervation approximately one inch below the elbow, weakness of these muscles indicates that the lesion is proximal to this level. Unfortunately, weakness may be difficult to determine, since the action of these muscles can be compensated for to a considerable extent by the action of muscles supplied by the median nerve. In such circumstances, electromyographic evidence of denervation may be of localizing value.

In the hand there is loss of strength in the hypothenar muscles with impaired abduction and opposition of the little finger. Weakness of the two medial lumbricals leads to impaired flexion of the medial two fingers at the metacarpophalangeal joints, while weakness of the

interossei leads to impaired abduction and adduction of all digits. Adduction movements should be tested with the outstretched hand lying prone against a hard surface; this is necessary in order to avoid the adducting action of the long finger flexors. Since the lumbrical and interosseous muscles acting together extend the interphalangeal joints of the ring and little fingers, weakness of these muscles leaves unopposed the action of the flexors and extensors in the forearm that are innervated by the radial and median nerves. This results in a characteristic claw hand deformity. Finally, in ulnar nerve lesions the index finger and thumb cannot be pressed firmly against each other because of weakness of the adductor pollicis and first dorsal interosseus muscles. Weakness of the latter is also reflected in flexion of the distal phalanx of the thumb, the result of the unopposed action of the flexor pollicis longus (Froment sign).

The sensory findings resulting from ulnar neuropathies at the elbow vary with the sever-

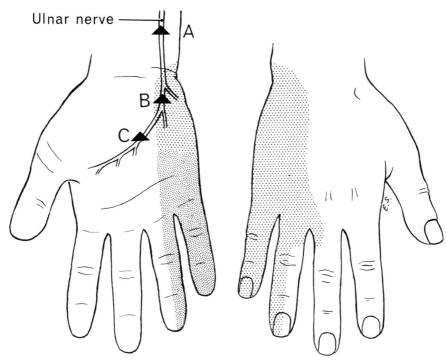

Figure 34–5 Ulnar nerve: cutaneous innervation (stippled) with indication of distribution of palmar and dorsal branches (lightly stippled). Common compression sites are: the wrist (A), the pisohamate tunnel (B), and within the palm (C).

ity of the nerve compression. Thus, there may be complete sensory loss in the whole ulnar distribution or only subtle changes in the finger tips.

In patients with ulnar compression at the elbow, the nerve is often found to be tender and enlarged when palpated at the condylar groove and may be displaced from the groove during flexion movements. The nerve is particularly in jeopardy when the normal carrying angle of the elbow (170 degrees) is exceeded. Congenital or posttraumatic deformities, osteophytic formation, and Charcot arthropathy of the elbow are disorders known to be capable of producing such an abnormal joint angle. In such persons, flexion of the elbow may cause harmful stretching of the nerve.

Other ulnar nerve lesions result from entrapment at the cubital tunnel. Compression is caused by narrowing of the tunnel during movement. This may be produced by an abnormal thickening of the aponeurosis that joins the two heads of the flexor carpi ulnaris or as a result of bulging of the ligamentous floor of the tunnel during flexion (Feindel and Stratford, 1958). Flexion at the wrist, when associated with elbow flexion, further adds to the compression because of the greater

tautness of the flexor carpi ulnaris. When the elbow is once again extended the aponeurosis of the flexor carpi ulnaris relaxes with the coming together of the attachment points to the olecranon and medial epicondyle. Activities such as hammering, shoveling, and lifting, because they incorporate such movements, may result in ulnar nerve damage.

Treatment. In many cases improvement results simply from the careful avoidance of pressure on the elbows. When the pressure neuropathy is associated with a hypermobile or abnormally stretched nerve, surgical antecubital transposition is often of benefit (Harrison and Nurick, 1970). In entrapments at the cubital tunnel, nerve decompression and subperiostial excision of the medial epicondyle provide relief (Feindel and Stratford, 1958).

LESIONS IN THE HAND

From a clinical and anatomical standpoint, Ebeling, Gilliatt, and Thomas (1960) divide ulnar nerve lesions within the hand into three groups.

1. Compression distally along the terminal motor branch. This is accompanied by weak-

ness of the interossei, the medial two lumbricals, and the adductor pollicis. The hypothenar muscles and sensory fibers to the hand are spared. As in all ulnar nerve lesions in the hand, pain is common (see Fig. 34–5C).

2. Compression of the most proximal part of the terminal motor branch. In these cases all the ulnar innervated hand muscles are affected but there is no sensory impairment. Neuropathies due to compression at the pisohamate tunnel usually fall within this category (see Fig. 34–5B).

3. Compression of the nerve as it enters the hand (Fig. 34–5A). All the ulnar-innervated muscles are affected, but the sensory impairment is restricted to the distal palm and volar surface of the little and medial ring fingers. Sensation over the dorsum of the hand and proximal palmar region is spared because the corresponding branches arise in the forearm.

Mechanisms of Injury. Thickening of the pisohamate ligament may lead to entrapment of the ulnar motor branch, as reported by Nicolle and Woolhouse (1965), but most ulnar lesions within the hand are of traumatic origin. They result from such occupational hazards as the low-amplitude vibratory compression caused by using pneumatic drills or the repeated injury from using staplers, shears, pliers, a plane, or a shoemaker's knife. Other hazards include the inappropriate gripping of a cane or crutches, the banging of a typewriter carriage return lever with the palm (Ebeling et al., 1960), and the bicyclist's prolonged leaning of the base of the palm on the handle bars. Inflammatory processes within the hand, vascular malformations, fractures of the carpal bones, and lipomas and ganglia (Seddon, 1952) and other tumors have all been reported as causes of such compression.

Radial Nerve

ANATOMY

The radial nerve is a continuation of the posterior trunk of the brachial plexus and receives contributions from the fifth to the eighth cervical roots. After leaving the axilla, the nerve winds round the shaft of the humeral spiral groove in close relation to the bone. It reaches the lateral intermuscular septum immediately below the insertion of the deltoid muscle and, at this point, is superficial to and palpable against the humerus.

Subsequently, the nerve lies in a deep intermuscular position, dividing into two terminal branches: the deep motor branch (posterior interosseous nerve) and the superficial cutaneous branch. This bifurcation is usually situated in the upper forearm, but its position may vary from 4.5 cm above to 4 cm below the lateral epicondyle (Linell, 1921). The posterior interosseous nerve pierces the supinator muscle to reach the posterior aspect of the forearm in close relation to the interosseous membrane and the head of the radius. The terminal cutaneous branch becomes superficial approximately 10 cm above the wrist. It descends along the lateral border of the forearm and ends by supplying the skin on the dorsum of the hand, thumb, and lateral three fingers (Fig. 34–6). The important muscular and cutaneous branches given off by the radial nerve are summarized in Table 34–1. The number and location of these branches varies greatly (Sunderland, 1946).

LOCALIZATION AND CLINICAL SYMPTOMATOLOGY

High axillary lesions affect all of the sensory and motor innervation derived from the radial nerve. More commonly, however, the nerve is compressed either as it winds round the humerus or where it lies superficially on the lateral aspect of the arm (A and B in Figure 34–6; I and II in Table 34–1). Lesions of this segment of the radial nerve spare the branch to the triceps muscle, but the posterior cutaneous nerve of the forearm, a branch that frequently runs parallel to the radial trunk in the humeral spiral groove, is often damaged by compression at this level. Radial nerve injury at this level often results from prolonged hanging of the arm over the back of a chair, but may also follow compression resulting from improper positioning of the arm during anesthesia or sleep. Many cases of so called "sleep paralysis" result from improper positioning of the arm combined with the effects of intoxication with alcohol or hypnotic drugs. The careless application of a tourniquet may also be responsible for lesions at this level. Finally, irritation and compression of the nerve by callous bone may be a late complication of fractures of the shaft of the humerus.

Compression of that part of the nerve that lies between the lateral intermuscular septum and the point where the posterior interosseous

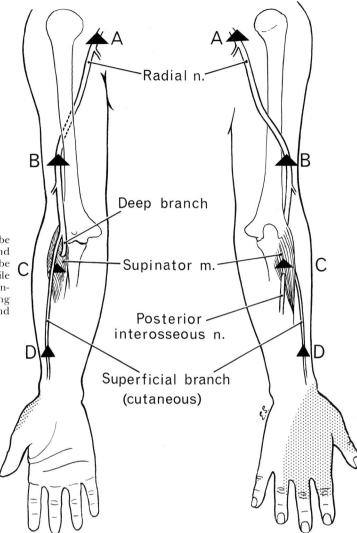

Figure 34–6 Radial nerve. This nerve can be compressed at the axilla (A) or as it winds round the humerus (B). Its deep motor branch may be entrapped at the supinator muscle (C), while the superficial cutaneous branch may be injured along the forearm or wrist (D), causing sensory symptoms over the dorsum of the hand (stippled).

branch pierces the supinator muscle always produces weakness of this muscle as well as of all the other muscles supplied by the posterior interosseous branch. The muscle branches to the brachioradialis and extensor carpi radialis longus and the terminal cutaneous branch may, however, be spared (Table 34–1 II to IV). Thus, patients with compression in this portion are unable to straighten their fingers or supinate the wrist but may not have wristdrop. Sensory impairment, if present, usually reflects a more proximal lesion.

Nerve compression distal to the supinator muscle (C in Figure 34–6 and IV in Table 34–1) not only spares this muscle but is also never associated with clinically or electrophysiologically demonstrable sensory abnor-

malities. Because the extensor carpi ulnaris is weak while both the extensor carpi radialis longus and brevis are unaffected, the wrist tends to deviate radially when the patient attempts to make a fist. There is localized wasting of the rest of the dorsal forearm muscles innervated by the posterior interosseous nerve but preservation and even compensatory hypertrophy of the unaffected brachioradialis, supinator, and radial wrist extensors situated in the posterolateral region of the upper forearm and lower arm. An early sign of compression at this level may be isolated weakness of extension of the index finger at the time when extension of other fingers is intact. Injury to the posterior interosseous nerve at the supinator muscle level may result from repeated supination of the forearm or from

TABLE 34–1　APPROXIMATE SITE OF ORIGIN OF RADIAL NERVE MAIN BRANCHES

I. Inferior axillary border	Triceps Cutaneous nerve of forearm
II. Between lateral inter- muscular septum and bifurcation into motor and terminal cutane- ous branches	Brachialis Brachioradialis Extensor carpi radialis longus
III. Between bifurcation and passage of motor branch through supinator mus- cle	Extensor carpi radialis Supinator
IV. Distal to supinator muscle	Extensor digitorum communis Extensor digiti quinti Extensor carpi ulnaris Extensor pollicis longus Extensor pollicis brevis Extensor indicis Abductor pollicis longus

compression by lipomas, other soft tissue tumors (Barber et al., 1962), or subluxation of the head of the radius (Kopell and Thompson, 1963).

Injury of the terminal cutaneous branch results in pain and distressing paresthesias located along the distal radial border and dorsum of the web between the thumb and index finger (Fig. 34–6C). Encroachment on this branch may be the aftermath of a fractured radius, or the nerve, since it lies in close proximity to the radial artery, may be compressed by the perivascular tissue reaction to indwelling catheters such as are used in hemodialysis of patients in renal failure. Less frequently this branch is compressed by tight bracelets or wrist watch bands and by roping the wrists together.

DIAGNOSIS AND TREATMENT

Difficulties in the exact clinical localization of the level of radial nerve compression result from the variability of the fascicular organization of sensory and motor fibers and from the inconsistency of the site of origin of branches (Trojaborg, 1970). In such circumstances, nerve conduction and electromyographic tests may provide valuable assistance toward an accurate anatomical diagnosis (Downie and Scott, 1967; Trojaborg, 1970).

If pressure is avoided, most types of radial nerve compression palsy recover within a few weeks or months. Encroachment on the nerve by bone or soft tissue as well as its entrapment at the supinator muscle usually requires operative treatment.

Digital and Interdigital Nerves

ANATOMY AND SYMPTOMATOLOGY

The digital nerves are the terminal cutaneous branches of the median and ulnar nerves. They originate at the level of the distal epiphysis of the metacarpals and, as interdigital nerves, pass distally between the deep and superficial transverse metacarpal ligaments. The two digital branches of each interdigital nerve supply the facing halves of contiguous fingers (C in Figure 34–3).

Injury to individual interdigital nerves causes sensory changes in two adjacent fingers. When a single digital nerve is damaged, the impairment is restricted to the corresponding half of the digit. The most common complaint of patients with interdigital or digital compression neuropathies is pain, tingling, and burning paresthesias localized in the digits. Symptoms are usually worse during sleep or after manual exertion. In interdigital neuropathies, pressure between the metacarpal heads of the suspected fingers produces localized pain, which at times radiates into the cutaneous projection of the digital nerves. In an isolated digital neuropathy, a Tinel sign may be elicited by the examiner's running his fingernail along the course of the nerve on the lateral aspect of the patient's finger.

MECHANISMS OF INJURY

Interdigital neuropathies may result from entrapment of the nerve within the tunnel formed by the intermetacarpal transverse ligaments. Narrowing of this space usually results from inflammation due to such diseases as rheumatoid arthritis but may also result from repeated trauma to the palm. The improper use of a screwdriver or a stapler may lead to direct damage of interdigital nerves within the palm. Sudden or repeated hyperextension of the fingers may also cause damage as the nerves are pulled against the taut transverse intermetacarpal ligaments (Kopell and Thompson, 1963). Within the fingers, individual digital nerves have been damaged by the repeated use of scissors, reported by Mumenthaler and Schliack (1965), and from bowling (bowler's thumb) (Marmor, 1966).

DIAGNOSIS AND TREATMENT

The restricted distribution of symptoms and the ready demonstration of localized pain are usually sufficient clues for the clinical diagnosis of these neuropathies. In some patients, particularly in those suffering from rheumatoid arthritis, compression of an interdigital nerve may coexist with carpal tunnel entrapment. The presence of the double lesion is only suspected when, after proper treatment of the entrapment at the wrist, symptoms in one or two fingers fail to improve.

Measurement of digital sensory nerve conduction may be of assistance in diagnosis (Buchthal and Rosenfalck, 1971). Aside from providing temporary relief, injections of local anesthetics or hydrocortisone often provide supportive evidence for the diagnosis.

The severity of symptoms and the mechanism of injury should dictate whether medical or surgical treatment is indicated. In most patients the symptoms improve simply by avoiding pressure on the hand.

PRESSURE SYNDROMES OF THE LOWER LIMB

Pressure neuropathies in the lower limb appear to be less common than those in the upper limb, although this may be but an impression resulting from a better knowledge of the clinical characteristics of lesions in the upper limb and the greater ease with which routine electrophysiologic methods can be applied to the upper limb.

Pressure syndromes in the lower limb are divided into those that involve mainly nerves to the thigh (lateral, anterior, and medial) because of compression of the lateral femoral cutaneous nerve, femoral nerve, or obturator nerve; those that affect nerves to the posterior thigh (sciatic nerve) and the leg (common peroneal, tibial nerve, and their branches); and those pressure syndromes arising from compression at the ankle (tarsal tunnel syndromes) and foot.

Nerve Compression Within the Thigh

LATERAL FEMORAL CUTANEOUS NERVE

The lateral femoral cutaneous nerve is formed by branches arising directly from the second and third lumbar nerves. After an initial intrapelvic course the nerve enters the thigh through an opening formed by the attachment of the inguinal ligament to the anterior superior iliac spine. Here the nerve lies in close relation not only to bone and ligament but also to the insertion of the sartorius muscle. This nerve is purely sensory and supplies the anterolateral and the lateral aspects of the thigh, reaching almost to the knee (Fig. 34–7).

Symptomatology. Compression of this nerve causes the characteristic burning pain on the outer side of the thigh known as meralgia paresthetica (Keegan and Holyoke, 1962). The pain is usually accompanied by prickling, numbness, and an increased sensitivity to such cutaneous stimuli as clothing and stockings. The symptoms are made worse by prolonged standing or walking or, at times, simply by sustained extension and adduction of the lower limb. Sitting or lying prone usually provides relief.

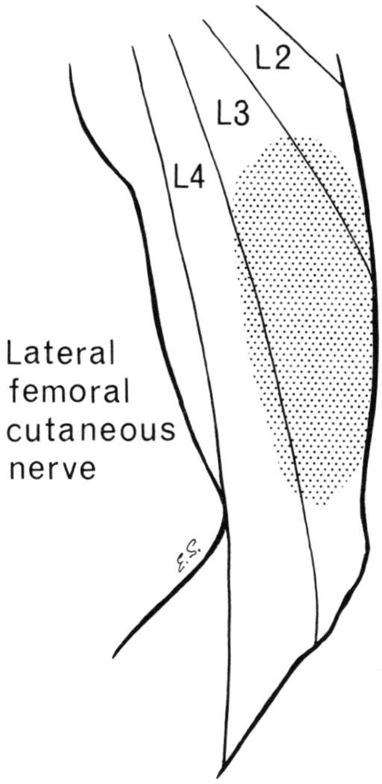

Figure 34–7 Outline of areas of the thigh where sensation is supplied by the lateral femoral cutaneous nerve (stippled) and lumbar roots. Note the partial overlap.

Examination often shows altered touch and pain sensation over the lateral aspect of the thigh; pressure medial to the superior iliac spine may elicit pain. As a rule, meralgia paresthetica is unilateral, but in approximately 20 per cent of cases the disorder is bilateral (Ecker and Woltman, 1938). Since the nerve is strictly sensory, there are no motor abnormalities.

Meralgia paresthetica often occurs in association with obesity or pregnancy (Rhodes, 1957; Pearson, 1957), but it may appear as a result of trauma to the pelvic bones or of scarring in the lateral inguinal region. The disorder is peculiarly prone to occur in diabetics, perhaps as a result of an increased susceptibility of nerve to compression injuries.

Mechanisms of Injury. The site of entrapment is where the nerve leaves the abdominal wall at the level of the anterior superior iliac spine. Standing, walking, and other leg movements, often in association with a lax abdominal wall, presumably cause sufficient repetitive traction and angulation of the nerve to produce symptoms.

Diagnosis. In patients in whom meralgia paresthetica is suspected, care should be taken not to overlook a femoral neuropathy or a lesion of the second or third lumbar roots. Lumbar root compression is usually associated with low back pain that radiates into the lower leg. In either femoral neuropathy or L2 or L3 root lesions, the sensory changes usually extend more anteromedially than in entrapments of the lateral femoral cutaneous nerve and there is almost always weakness of hip flexion or extension of the knee. In both femoral neuropathy and L3 root lesions, the knee jerk also is usually decreased or absent. Weakness and reflex changes never occur in meralgia paresthetica.

Treatment. This neuropathy tends to regress spontaneously, but recurrences are common. In obese patients, weight loss and exercises to strengthen the abdominal muscles are often of benefit. Hydrocortisone injections at the point where the nerve lies medial to the anterior superior iliac spine may provide temporary relief. The value of neurolysis or of nerve section or crush, surgical procedures used in more severe cases, has yet to be determined.

FEMORAL NERVE

Anatomy. The femoral nerve arises from the second, third, and fourth lumbar nerves.

Within the pelvis it courses along the lateral border of the psoas muscle before entering the thigh in close association with the femoral vessels and deep to the inguinal ligament. Just distal to the ligament, the nerve separates into anterior and posterior divisions. The anterior division supplies cutaneous sensation and muscular branches to the pectineus and sartorius muscles. The posterior division provides the major innervation of the quadriceps muscle and terminates as the saphenous nerve. The latter descends anterior to the femoral artery in the subsartorial canal and emerges from the canal just above the knee. From this point it is subcutaneous and supplies sensation to the skin of the medial aspect of the leg as far down as the medial malleolus (Fig. 34–8).

Symptomatology. Femoral neuropathy is manifested by wasting and weakness of the quadriceps muscle, diminution or absence of knee jerk, and sensory impairment over the anteromedial aspect of the thigh with occasional extension into the leg. When, in addition, there is marked weakness of hip flexion, it is likely that the site of the lesion is in the lumbar plexus. Compression of the femoral nerve often induces spontaneous pain in the groin, which is increased by extension of the thigh (inverted Lasègue sign). Curiously, however, sensory symptoms in the saphenous distribution are rare when the lesion involves the main trunk of the femoral nerve.

Mechanisms of Injury. Entrapment of the femoral nerve in the inguinal region is uncommon but may be associated with an inguinal hernia or result from scarring in the inguinal region. Deeply placed surgical sutures may injure the nerve during hernia repair. Lesions of the femoral nerve or lumbar plexus in the pelvis usually result from careless retraction during abdominal surgery (Johnson and Montgomery, 1958), from direct involvement by tumor, or from compression by a retroperitoneal hematoma. The latter may develop as a complication of hemophilia (Wilkinson et al., 1961) or in patients receiving anticoagulants (Groch et al., 1959).

Compression of the saphenous nerve against the distal condyle may occur when the leg is improperly suspended as in certain perineal operations or in childbirth (Britt and Gordon, 1964). Entrapment of the nerve in scar tissue may be a late consequence of the stripping of an adjacent varicose saphenous vein.

Diagnosis. The most common cause of femoral neuropathy is diabetes. Predomin-

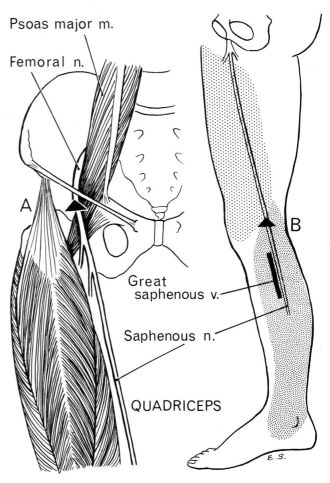

Figure 34–8 Femoral nerve. This nerve has a close anatomical relation with the psoas muscle and inguinal ligament (A). Compression at the groin may cause quadriceps weakness and sensory impairment in the nerve's distribution to the thigh (lightly stippled) and in that of its saphenous branch (heavily stippled). Pressure at the knee (B) or surgery to the saphenous veins may affect the saphenous nerve.

antly motor signs or a combination of pain in the thigh, weakness and sensory deficit can be manifestations of an isolated diabetic femoral neuropathy, although in such cases the involvement is commonly more widespread (Garland, 1955; Raff et al., 1968). Consequently, when the possibility of femoral nerve compression is considered, care should be taken to rule out diabetes as a cause or contributory factor of neuropathy. In the presence of wasting and weakness of the quadriceps muscle, an idiopathic form of femoral neuropathy, disuse atrophy and primary proximal myopathy may also enter the differential diagnosis (Biemond, 1970). Important clues in differentiating disuse atrophy and myopathies from femoral neuropathy are the lack of pain and sensory impairment in the former two. Furthermore, in disuse atrophy, there is the patient's history of immobilization and the knee jerk is usually preserved. Elevated serum enzyme levels and characteristic changes in muscle revealed by biopsy or by electromyography assist in the diagnosis of a proximal myopathy. When only pain and

paresthesias are prominent in the thigh, meralgia paresthetica should be ruled out, as discussed earlier.

Femoral and saphenous nerve conduction tests provide helpful tools for the diagnosis and localization of lesions affecting these two nerves (Lawrence and Locke, 1961; Gassel, 1963; Chopra and Hurwitz, 1968; Ertekin, 1969).

OBTURATOR NERVE

The obturator nerve originates in the lumbar plexus from fibers of the second, third, and fourth lumbar roots. It courses along the wall of the pelvis and passes through the obturator canal with the obturator vessels (Fig. 34–9). At this level the nerve divides into an anterior and posterior branch. These branches supply the skin of the inner side of the thigh, the obturator externus muscle, and the adductor longus and brevis muscles as well as the gracilis and adductor magnus muscles.

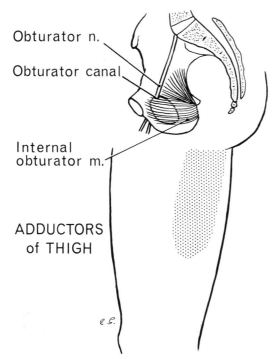

Figure 34–9 Obturator nerve. This nerve may be compressed along the wall of the pelvis or in the obturator canal. Nerve injury results in weakness of limb adduction and sensory impairment (stippled area).

Compression of this nerve causes pain in the groin and sensory impairment in its distribution, together with weakness for adduction and internal and external rotation of the thigh.

Pressure lesions of the obturator nerve are rare. They result from compression by an obturator hernia or from damage within the pelvis by tumors or inflammation. During difficult labor, pressure from the fetal head or by forceps may injure the obturator nerve.

SCIATIC, PERONEAL, AND TIBIAL NERVES

Anatomy. The sciatic nerve is the largest nerve in the body. It originates from the lumbosacral plexus (L4 to S3), leaving the pelvis through the sciatic notch after passing below and often through the pyriformis muscle. The inferior gluteal nerve, which supplies the gluteus maximus, and the superior gluteal nerve, which supplies the glutei minimus and medius, also originate from the lumbosacral plexus and accompany the sciatic nerve along its short intrapelvic course. In the buttock, the sciatic nerve lies

under cover of the gluteus maximus and descends between the greater trochanter and the ischial tuberosity. At the level of the gluteal fold it is relatively superficial, but within the thigh it again assumes a deep, sheltered course. The muscular branches of the sciatic nerve supply the hamstring muscles. The posterior cutaneous nerve of the thigh, which arises from sacral spinal nerves 1 to 3, accompanies the sciatic nerve in the upper part of its course within the thigh.

The common peroneal (lateral popliteal) and tibial (medial popliteal) nerves are the two terminal branches of the sciatic nerve. The bifurcation takes place at various levels within the thigh, often at the junction between the middle and distal thirds.

The common peroneal nerve, the lateral division of the sciatic nerve, passes behind the head of the fibula in close relationship to the tendon of the biceps femoris and divides into the superficial and deep peroneal nerves. It is about half the width of the tibial nerve. Two branches, the lateral cutaneous nerve of the leg and the sural communicating nerve, leave the common peroneal nerve within the popliteal fossa. In the leg the deep peroneal (anterior tibial) nerve supplies muscle branches to the tibialis anterior, extensor hallucis longus, extensor digitorum longus, and peroneus tertius; these muscles dorsiflex the foot and toes. In the foot the deep peroneal nerve supplies the extensor digitorum brevis and the second dorsal interosseous muscle. In as many as 28 per cent of people the extensor digitorum brevis is also innervated by the accessory deep peroneal nerve, a branch of the superficial peroneal nerve (Gutmann, 1970). A cutaneous branch supplies the skin between the hallux and second toe (Fig. 34–10). The superficial peroneal (musculocutaneous) nerve provides innervation to peroneus longus and brevis muscles that evert the foot and to the skin of the lateral distal portion of the lower leg and dorsum of the foot.

The tibial nerve is the largest terminal branch of the sciatic nerve. It descends along the back of the thigh and through the middle of the popliteal fossa until it reaches the popliteus muscle, where on entering the calf, it becomes the posterior tibial nerve. The posterior tibial nerve is well covered by the triceps surae muscle until the junction of the distal and middle thirds of the lower leg, where it becomes superficial. On the medial side of the ankle this nerve enters the tarsal

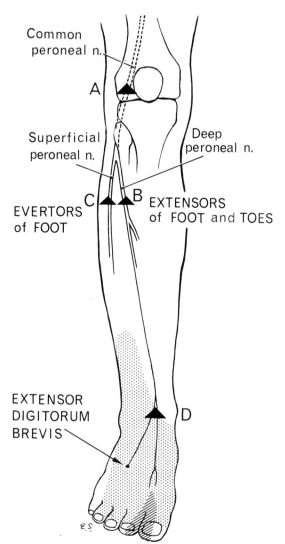

Figure 34-10 The common peroneal nerve may be compressed at the level of the knee (A). When only the deep peroneal branch (B) is injured, dorsiflexion of the foot and toes is weak and there is sensory loss between the first and second toes (hatched). Damage of the superficial peroneal branch causes weakness of the evertors and more extensive sensory impairment over the foot (stippled). In compression of the deep peroneal branch at the ankle (D) only the extensor digitorum brevis is weak and there is little sensory impairment (hatched area).

tunnel and divides into the medial and lateral plantar nerves (Fig. 34–11). The tibial nerve supplies the gastrocnemius, plantaris, soleus, and popliteus muscles, while the posterior tibial nerve innervates the rest of the muscles of the calf; all these muscles act to plantar flex the foot and toes. The sural nerve originates at the popliteal fossa level and, after piercing the deep fascia about the middle of

the back of the leg, is joined by the communicating branch from the common peroneal nerve and descends along the lateral margin of the Achilles tendon to supply the lateral aspect of the foot and little toe.

Common Sites of Compression. The sciatic nerve may be compressed by tumors within the pelvis or gluteal region or against the bone of the prominent sciatic notch. Tumors that have been reported to cause compression include sarcomas and lipomas. Compression against the sciatic notch may occur when sitting or may result from a fall onto the buttocks. Traction of the nerve due to prolonged periods of bending forward with the legs straight, as occurs in harvesting, has been known to cause sciatic nerve injury. Compression resulting from gluteal abscesses, wound scars, or anomalies of the pyriformis muscle has also been reported (Kopell and Thompson, 1963). Sciatic nerve compression rarely results from external pressure, presumably because of the thickness of the nerve and its protected position within the buttock and thigh.

Lesions involving the lumbosacral plexus may present with pain and other signs in a sciatic distribution. Weakness of the gluteal muscles and pain in the region of the sciatic notch suggest compression within the pelvis. Lesions just beyond the sciatic notch spare the gluteal muscles, but there is involvement of the hamstrings and of all the muscles in the lower leg. The presence of sensory impairment in the distribution of the posterior cutaneous nerve of the thigh is a helpful clue to diagnosis of high sciatic nerve compression. Radiologic examination of the sciatic notch and a search for electromyographic evidence of a neurogenic disorder in the gluteal muscles are helpful auxiliary aids in localizing compressive lesions at this level (Gassel and Trojaborg, 1964; Yap and Hirota, 1967).

Common peroneal nerve compression occurs mainly at the level of the fibular head, where the nerve is superficial, fixed, and angulated (Sunderland, 1953). Habitual sitting with one leg crossed over the other, as reported by Woltman (1929), Nagler and Rangell (1947) and Marwak (1964); pressure during sleep or while under the effects of anesthesia; and pressure by casts, tight high boots, garters, or obstetrical stirrups are among the most common causes of compression. Bone tumors, posttraumatic calluses,

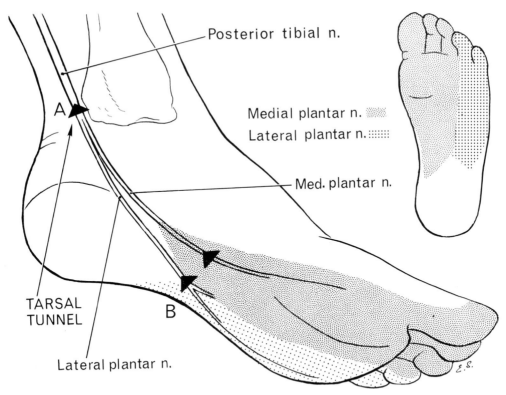

Figure 34–11 Compression of the posterior tibial nerve at the tarsal tunnel (A) or of the plantar nerves (B) causes sensory impairment in the sole of the foot and weakness of the intrinsic pedal musculature.

cysts (Stack et al., 1965), vascular malformations, and hematomas within the popliteal fossa or in the region of the fibular head may also produce peroneal nerve compression.

Compression of the common peroneal nerve leads to impaired dorsiflexion and eversion of the foot, to impaired extension of the toes, and frequently to wasting of the muscles of the anterolateral compartment of the leg and of the extensor digitorum brevis. Paralysis of the common peroneal nerve results in footdrop and a characteristic slapping gait. Although compression most usually affects the common peroneal nerve, selective involvement of the deep peroneal nerve or superficial peroneal nerves may occur. Damage to the deep peroneal nerve results in an inability to dorsiflex the foot and toes, while eversion is weak after selective injury to the superficial peroneal nerve. Since, when present, the accessory deep peroneal nerve originates from the superficial peroneal, injury to the latter may also result in partial denervation of the extensor digitorum brevis muscle. In addition to the differences in muscle weakness that result from involvement of these nerves, the cutaneous impairment is also

quite different, a larger area over the dorsal foot being affected in superficial peroneal nerve lesions (see Fig. 34–10D). Entrapment of the cutaneous branch of the superficial peroneal nerve may occur as the nerve pierces the deep fascia in the leg. This causes considerable pain and some sensory impairment, which may be relieved by local injections of hydrocortisone or surgical decompression of the nerve (Kopell and Thompson, 1963).

Tibial and posterior tibial nerve compression injuries are infrequent. A complete lesion of the tibial nerve results in paralysis of plantar flexion and adduction of the foot and toes. Sensory impairment may be confined to the sole of the foot or extend to its lateral border when the sural nerve is also affected. The ankle and plantar reflexes are abolished. The tibial nerve may be compressed in the popliteal fossa by vascular malformations, cysts, or hematomas. In its deep position beneath the soleus the posterior tibial nerve is subject to compression in Volkmann's ischemic contracture. The sural and posterior tibial nerves may also be damaged by tightly fitted high ski boots.

As in peroneal palsy, complete or partial

recovery is the rule when paralysis results from transient pressure. Treatment consists of physical therapy, the use of a foot brace, and careful avoidance of further compression. Electrophysiologic measurements of nerve conduction in the peroneal and posterior tibial nerves assist with the localization and management of these neuropathies (Thomas et al., 1959; Gilliatt et al., 1961; Mavor and Acheson, 1966; Buchthal and Rosenfalck, 1966).

Nerve Compression Within the Ankle or Foot

The following nerves supply cutaneous innervation to the foot and ankle: sural, saphenous, branches of the superficial and deep peroneal nerves, and plantar and calcaneal branches of the posterior tibial nerve. The intrinsic foot musculature is innervated by the medial and lateral plantar branches of the tibial nerve and by the deep peroneal nerve. Sensory symptoms in the foot may be due to injury of any of these. Symptoms in the distribution of the sural, saphenous, and superficial peroneal nerves are almost always due to compression within the leg or thigh, as described earlier. Compression of the tibial, deep peroneal, or plantar nerves either at the ankle or in the foot gives rise to well-defined clinical syndromes.

POSTERIOR TIBIAL NERVE AT THE ANKLE

Anatomy. Compression usually occurs in the medial tarsal tunnel, an osteofibrous passage roofed over by the flexor retinaculum as it descends from the medial ligament of the ankle to the calcaneus. Accompanying the tibial nerve in this tunnel are the tendons of the tibialis posterior, flexor digitorum longus, and flexor hallucis longus muscles and the posterior tibial vessels. The tibial nerve divides in the tunnel into the medial and lateral plantar nerves. The latter form the equivalents in the foot of the median and ulnar nerves in the hand. Thus, the medial plantar nerve innervates the abductor hallucis, flexor hallucis brevis, flexor digitorum brevis, and first lumbrical muscles. It also supplies plantar cutaneous sensation, which extends laterally to the axial line of the fourth toe. The lateral plantar nerve innervates the abductor, flexor, and opponens digiti minimi, the quadratus plantae, the three lateral lumbricals, and all the interossei. It also supplies cutaneous sensation to the rest of the sole. Calcaneal branches supply the heel (see Fig. 34–11).

Symptomatology. The most common complaints of patients with the tarsal tunnel syndrome are pain and burning and tingling paresthesias, usually confined to the sole of one foot. The disorder may, however, be bilateral (Lam, 1967). The symptoms usually appear on or are aggravated by prolonged standing or walking, but they may occur at rest. A lateral or medial predominance of the symptoms indicates a greater degree of involvement of the corresponding plantar nerve. Since calcaneal branches usually leave the tibial nerve before its entry into the tarsal tunnel, the symptoms do not usually involve the heel (Linscheid et al., 1970).

Patients seldom complain of any motor deficit, so this must be searched for by careful inspection and palpation of the small foot muscles. Particular note should be made of the bulk of the abductor hallucis as it lies along the medial longitudinal arch of the foot and of the strength of the flexors of the toes; there is no weakness of extension of the toes. Digital pressure applied below the medial malleolus may produce local pain and paresthesias, which may then radiate toward the toes.

Mechanisms of Injury. Narrowing of the tarsal tunnel is often caused by osteoarthritis or posttraumatic deformities. Chronic swelling of the ankles, tenosynovitis of the flexor tendons that accompany the nerve, and overpronation of the foot may also cause nerve compression at this level.

PLANTAR NERVES

Direct compression of one or both plantar nerves in the foot may result from poor foot posture, overpronation, or prolonged standing on the rungs of a ladder with little or no shoe protection. Because of close proximity of these nerves to plantar tendon sheaths, plantar nerve compression may result from tenosynovitis.

The interdigital nerves are the cutaneous branches of the plantar nerves and supply the distal tips and opposing surfaces of contiguous toes. They become the interdigital nerves as they cross over the deep transverse tarsal ligament that joins adjacent metatarsal heads. Compression of the nerves at this point may result from excessive hyperextension at the metatarsophalangeal joints such as occurs during deep squatting. Entrapment of these nerves may occur in inflammatory processes such as rheumatoid arthritis. Morton's neuroma results from recurrent compression of the interdigital nerve to the third and fourth toes (Kopell and Thompson, 1963).

Injury of isolated digital nerves, particularly the medial one to the big toe, may result from compression against the adjacent metatarsal heads. Most often this is a consequence of wearing ill-fitted shoes.

DEEP PERONEAL (ANTERIOR TIBIAL) NERVE AT THE ANKLE

Anatomy. Entrapments of this nerve usually occur in the anterior tarsal tunnel (Marinacci, 1968). This is a deep passage on the dorsum of the foot, roofed over by the inferior extensor retinaculum which extends from the lateral to the medial malleolus. After passing under the retinaculum and the tendon of the extensor hallucis longus, the deep peroneal nerve divides into a medial and a lateral branch. The medial branch innervates the first dorsal interosseous muscle and the skin between the first and second toes; the lateral branch innervates the extensor digitorum brevis and has no cutaneous distribution (see Fig. 34–10).

Symptomatology and Mechanisms of Injury. Compression neuropathy of the deep peroneal nerve at the ankle may be manifested only by wasting of the extensor digitorum brevis and impaired pinprick and touch sensation between the first and second toes. The same factors that produce nerve compression in the medial tarsal tunnel also operate to the same effect in the anterior tunnel.

DIAGNOSIS OF NERVE COMPRESSION AT THE ANKLE OR IN THE FOOT

Apart from peripheral vascular or joint diseases that cause local symptoms, nerve compression at the ankle or in the foot must, for the most part, be distinguished from root compression syndromes. Some signs of compression of the fifth lumbar root can mimic those arising from compression of the deep peroneal nerve or its branches. With L5 compression, however, the impaired cutaneous sensation is more extensive and there is usually weakness of the long extensors of the toes as well as of other leg muscles. With S1 compression, as with compression of the tibial or plantar nerves, there is impaired sensation over the sole of the foot. In addition, however, with a root lesion cutaneous sensation is impaired along the lateral border of the foot and the ankle jerk is diminished or abolished. The latter sign in particular serves to distinguish absolutely the root lesion from the peripheral nerve lesion.

It is likely that greater recognition of the subtle manifestations of pressure neuropathies of the distal leg will improve as clinical awareness of the presenting symptoms and understanding of the pathogenetic mechanisms involved becomes more widespread. Recent improvements in electrophysiologic methods have already led to more precise localization of nerve lesions within the foot (Thomas et al., 1959; Marinacci, 1957; Buchthal and Rosenfalck, 1966). It is hoped that these advances will in turn lead to improvement in management.

REFERENCES

Aguayo, A., Nair, C. P. V., and Midgley, R.: Experimental progressive compression neuropathy in the rabbit. Arch. Neurol., 24:358–364, 1971.

Aitken, J. T., and Thomas, P. K.: Retrograde changes in fibre size following nerve section. J. Anat., 96:121–129, 1962.

Anderson, M. H., Fullerton, P. M., Gilliatt, R. W., and Hern, J. E. C.: Changes in the forearm associated with median nerve compression at the wrist in the guinea-pig. J. Neurol. Neurosurg. Psychiatry, 33:70–79, 1970.

Barber, K. W., Bianco, A. J., Soule, E. H., and MacCarty, C. S.: Benign extra-neural soft tissue tumors of the extremities causing compression of nerves. J. Bone Joint Surg., 44A:98–104, 1962.

Behse, F., Buchthal, F., Carlsen, F., and Knappeis, G. G.: Hereditary neuropathy with liability to pressure palsies; electrophysiological and histopathological aspects. Brain, 95:777–794, 1972.

Biemond, A.: Femoral neuropathy. In Vinken, P. J., and Bruyn, G. W. (eds.): Handbook of Clinical Neurology. Vol. 8. Amsterdam, North-Holland Publishing Co., 1970, pp. 303–310.

Bentley, F. H., and Schlapp, W.: The effects of pressure on conduction in peripheral nerve. J. Physiol. (Lond.), 102:72–82, 1943.

Bonney, G.: The value of axon responses in determining the site of lesion in traction injuries of the brachial plexus. Brain, 77:588–609, 1954.

Bonney, G., and Gilliatt, R. W.: Sensory nerve conduction after traction lesion of the brachial plexus. Proc. R. Soc. Med., *51*:365–367, 1958.

Britt, B. A., and Gordon, R. A.: Peripheral nerve injuries associated with anesthesia. Can. Anaesth. Soc. J., *11*:514–536, 1964.

Brody, I. A.: Lactate dehydrogenase isoenzymes; a difference between cutaneous and muscular nerves. J. Neurochem., *13*:975–978, 1966.

Buchthal, F., and Rosenfalck, A.: Evoked action potentials and conduction velocity in human sensory nerves. Brain Res., *3*:1–122, 1966.

Buchthal, F., and Rosenfalck, A.: Sensory conduction from digit to palm and from palm to wrist in the carpal tunnel syndrome. J. Neurol. Neurosurg. Psychiatry, *34*:243–252, 1971.

Chopra, J. S., and Hurwitz, L. J.: Femoral nerve conduction in diabetes and chronic occlusive vascular disease. J. Neurol. Neurosurg. Psychiatry, *31*:28–33, 1968.

Cragg, B. G., and Thomas, P. K.: Changes in conduction velocity and fibre size proximal to peripheral nerve lesions. J. Physiol. (Lond.), *157*:315–327, 1961.

Cseuz, K. A., Thomas, J. E., Lambert, E. H., Graftonlove, J., and Lipscomb, P. R.: Long-term results of operation for carpal tunnel syndrome. Mayo Clin. Proc., *41*:232–241, 1966.

Dahlström, A., and Haggendal, J.: Studies on the transport and life span of amine storage granules in a peripheral adrenergic neuron system. Acta Physiol. Scand., *67*:278–288, 1966.

Danta, G., Fowler, T. J., and Gilliatt, R. W.: Conduction block after a pneumatic tourniquet. J. Physiol. (Lond.), *215*:50–52P, 1971.

Davies, D. M.: Recurrent peripheral nerve palsies in a family. Lancet, *2*:266–268, 1954.

Denny-Brown, D.: Neurological conditions resulting from prolonged and severe dietary restriction. Medicine (Baltimore), *26*:41–114, 1947.

Denny-Brown, D., and Brenner, C.: Paralysis of nerve induced by direct pressure and by tourniquet. Arch. Neurol. Psychiatry, *51*:1–26, 1944.

Downie, A. W., and Scott, T.: An improved technique for radial nerve conduction studies. J. Neurol. Neurosurg. Psychiatry, *30*:332–336, 1967.

Duncan, D.: Alterations in the structure of nerves caused by restricting their growth by ligatures. J. Neuropathol. Exp. Neurol., *7*:261–273, 1948.

Dyck, P. J.: Experimental hypertrophic neuropathy. Arch. Neurol., *21*:73–95, 1969.

Dyck, P. J., and Lambert, E. H.: Polyneuropathy associated with hypothyroidism. J. Neuropathol. Exp. Neurol., *29*:631–658, 1970.

Earl, C. J., Fullerton, P. M., Wakefield, G. S., and Schutta, H. S.: Hereditary neuropathy with liability to pressure palsies. Q. J. Med., *33*:481–497, 1964.

Ebeling, P., Gilliatt, R. W., and Thomas, P. K.: A clinical and electrical study of ulnar nerve lesions in the hand. J. Neurol. Neurosurg. Psychiatry, *23*:1–9, 1960.

Ecker, A. D., and Woltman, H. W.: Meralgia paresthetica: a report of one hundred and fifty cases. J.A.M.A., *110*:1650–1652, 1938.

Erb, W. M.: Diseases of the peripheral cerebrospinal nerves. *In* von Ziemssen, H. W. (ed.): Cyclopaedia of the Practice of Medicine. Vol. 2. New York, William Wood & Co., 1876.

Ertekin, C.: Saphenous nerve conduction in man. J. Neurol. Neurosurg. Psychiatry, *32*:530–540, 1969.

Feindel, W., and Stratford, J.: The role of the cubital tunnel in tardy ulnar palsy. Can. J. Surg., *1*:287–300, 1958.

Foster, J. B.: Hydrocortisone and the carpal tunnel syndrome. Lancet, *1*:454–456, 1960.

Fullerton, P. M.: The effect of ischaemia on nerve conduction in the carpal tunnel syndrome. J. Neurol. Neurosurg. Psychiatry, *26*:385–397, 1963.

Fullerton, P. M., and Gilliatt, R. W.: Axon reflex in human motor nerve fibres. J. Neurol. Neurosurg. Psychiatry, *28*:1–11, 1965.

Fullerton, P. M., and Gilliatt, R. W.: Median and ulnar neuropathy in the guinea pig. J. Neurol. Neurosurg. Psychiatry, *30*:393–402, 1967a.

Fullerton, P. M., and Gilliatt, R. W.: Pressure neuropathy in the hind foot of the guinea pig. N. Neurol. Neurosurg. Psychiatry, *30*:18–25, 1967b.

Garland, H.: Diabetic amyotrophy. Br. Med. J., *2*:1287–1290, 1955.

Gassel, M. M.: A study of femoral nerve conduction time. Arch. Neurol., *9*:607–614, 1963.

Gassel, M. M, and Trojaborg, W.: Clinical and electrophysiological study of the pattern of conduction times in the distribution of the sciatic nerve. J. Neurol. Neurosurg. Psychiatry, *27*:351–357, 1964.

Gasser, H. S., and Erlanger, J.: The role of fiber size in the establishment of a nerve block by pressure or cocaine. Am. J. Physiol., *88*:581–591, 1929.

Gilliatt, R. W., and Willison, R. G.: Peripheral nerve conduction in diabetic neuropathies. J. Neurol. Neurosurg. Psychiatry, *25*:11–18, 1962.

Gilliatt, R. W., and Wilson, T. G.: A pneumatic-tourniquet test in the carpal tunnel syndrome. Lancet, *2*:595–597, 1953.

Gilliatt, R. W., Goodman, H. V., and Willison, R. G.: The recording of lateral popliteal nerve action potentials in man. J. Neurol. Neurosurg. Psychiatry, *24*:305–318, 1961.

Gilliatt, R. W., LeQuesne, P. M., Logue, V., and Sumner, A. J.: Wasting of the hand associated with a cervical rib or band. J. Neurol. Neurosurg. Psychiatry, *33*:615–624, 1970.

Goodman, H. V., and Gilliatt, R. W.: The effect of treatment on median nerve conduction in patients with the carpal tunnel syndrome. Ann. Phys. Med., *6*:137–155, 1961.

Groch, S. N., Hurwitz, L. J., McDevitt, E., and Wright, I. S.: Problems of anticoagulant therapy in cerebrovascular diseases. Neurology, *9*:786–793, 1959.

Grokoest, A. W., and Demartini, F. E.: Systemic disease and the carpal tunnel syndrome. J.A.M.A., *155*:635–637, 1954.

Gutmann, L.: Atypical deep peroneal neuropathy. J. Neurol. Neurosurg. Psychiatry, *33*:453–456, 1970.

Harrison, M. J. G., and Nurick, S.: Results of anterior transposition of the ulnar nerve for ulnar neuritis. Br. Med. J., *1*:27–29, 1970.

Hopkins, A. P., and Morgan-Hughes, J. A.: The effect of local pressure in diphtheritic neuropathy. J. Neurol. Neurosurg. Psychiatry, *32*:614–623, 1969.

Johnson, D. A., and Montgomery, R. R.: Femoral neuropathy in abdominopelvic surgery. Med. Ann. D.C., *27*:513–514, 1958.

Kapeller, K., and Mayor, D.: An electron microscope study of the early changes proximal to a constriction in sympathetic nerves. Proc. R. Soc. Lond. [Biol.] *172*:39–51, 1969a.

Kapeller, L., and Mayor, D.: An electron microscope study of the early changes distal to a constriction in sympathetic nerves. Proc. R. Soc. Lond. [Biol.], *172*:53–63, 1969a.

Karpati, G., Carpenter, S., Eisen, A. A., and Feindel, W.: Familial multiple peripheral nerve entrapments. Trans. Am. Neurol. Assoc., *98*:267–269, 1973.

Keegan, J. J., and Holyoke, E. A.: Meralgia paresthetica. J. Neurosurg., 19:341–345, 1962.

Kiraly, J. K., and Krnjević, L.: Some retrograde changes in function of nerves after peripheral nerve section. Q. J. Exp. Physiol., 44:244–257, 1959.

Kopell, H. P., and Thompson, W. A. L.: Pronator syndrome. N. Eng. J. Med., 259:713–715, 1958.

Kopell, H. P., and Thompson, W. A. L.: Peripheral Entrapment Neuropathies. Baltimore, Williams & Wilkins Co., 1963.

Lam, S. J. S.: Tarsal tunnel syndrome. J. Bone Joint Surg., 49B:87–92, 1967.

Lambert, E. H., and Mulder, D. W.: Nerve function studies in experimental polyneuritis. Electroencephalogr. Clin. Neurophysiol., Suppl. 22:29–35, 1964.

Lawrence, D. G., and Locke, S.: Motor nerve conduction velocity in diabetes. Arch. Neurol., 5:483–489, 1961.

Lehmann, H. J., and Pretschner, D. P.: Experimentelle Untersuchungen zum Engpassyndrom peripherer Nerven. Dtsch. Z. Nervenheilkd., 188:308–330, 1966.

Linell, E. A.: The distribution of nerves in the upper limb with reference to variabilities and their clinical significance. J. Anat., 55:79–112, 1921.

Linscheid, R. L., Burton, R. C., and Fredericks: The tarsal tunnel syndrome. South. Med. J., 63:1313–1323, 1970.

Lubińska, L., Niemierko, S., and Oderfeld-Nowak, B.: Behaviour of acetylcholinesterase in isolated nerve segments. J. Neurochem., 11:493–503, 1964.

McKusick, V. A., Kaplan, D., Wise, D., Hanley, W. B., Suddarth, S. B., Sevick, M. E., and Maumenee, A. E.: The genetic mucopolysaccharidoses. Medicine (Baltimore), 44:445–483, 1965.

McLeod, J. G.: Digital nerve conduction in the carpal tunnel syndrome after mechanical stimulation of the finger. J. Neurol. Neurosurg. Psychiatry, 29:12–22, 1966.

Marinacci, A. A.: Clinical manifestations of plantar nerve disorders. Value of the electromyogram in correct evaluation of the lesion. Bull. Los Angeles Neurol. Soc., 22:171–176, 1957.

Marinacci, A. A.: Neurological syndromes of the tarsal tunnel. Bull. Los Angeles Neurol. Soc., 33:90–100, 1968.

Marmor, L.: Bowler's thumb. J. Trauma, 6:282–284, 1966.

Martin, F. R., and Paletta, F.: Tourniquet paralysis. A primary vascular phenomenon. South. Med. J., 59:951–953, 1966.

Marwak, V.: Compression of the lateral popliteal (common peroneal) nerve. Lancet, 2:1367–1369, 1964.

Mavor, H., and Atcheson, J. B.: Posterior tibial nerve conduction. Arch. Neurol., 14:661–669, 1966.

Mayer, R. F., and Denny-Brown, D.: Conduction velocity in peripheral nerve during experimental demyelination in the cat. Neurology, 14:714–726, 1964.

Mulder, D. W., Calverley, G. R., and Miller, R. H.: Autogenous mononeuropathy: diagnosis, treatment and clinical significance. Med. Clin. North Am., 44:989–999, 1960.

Mulder, D. W., Lambert, E. H., Bastron, J., and Sprague, R. G.: The neuropathies associated with diabetes mellitus. A clinical and electromyographic study of 103 unselected diabetic patients. Neurology, 11:275–284, 1961.

Mumenthaler, M., and Schliack, H.: Digital nerve injuries due to chronic pressure by scissors. In Läsionem peripherer Nerven. Stuttgart, Thieme, 1965.

Nagler, S. H., and Rangell, L.: Peroneal palsy caused by crossing legs. J.A.M.A., 133:755–761, 1947.

Nicolle, F. V., and Woolhouse, F. M.: Nerve compression syndromes of the upper limb. J. Trauma, 5:313–318, 1965.

O'Brien, M. D., and Upton, A. R. M.: Anterior interosseous nerve syndrome. J. Neurol. Neurosurg. Psychiatry, 35:531–536, 1972.

Ochoa, J., and Mair, W. G. P.: The normal sural nerve in man. I. Ultrastructure and numbers of fibres and cells. Acta Neuropathol., 13:197–216, 1969.

Ochoa, J., Danta, G., Fowler, T. J., and Gilliatt, R. W.: Nature of the nerve lesion caused by a pneumatic tourniquet. Nature (Lond.), 233:265–266, 1971.

Ochoa, J., Fowler, J. T., and Gilliatt, R. W.: Changes produced by a pneumatic tourniquet. In Desmedt, J. (ed.): New Developments in Electromyography and Clinical Neurophysiology. Vol. 2. Basel, S. Karger, 1973. pp. 88–91.

Pearson, M. G.: Meralgia paraesthetica. J. Obstet. Gynaecol. Br. Emp., 64:427–430, 1957.

Phalen, G. S., and Kendrick, J. I.: Compression neuropathy of the median nerve in the carpal tunnel. J.A.M.A., 164:524–530, 1957.

Preswick, G.: The effect of stimulus intensity on motor latency in the carpal tunnel syndrome. J. Neurol. Neurosurg. Psychiatry, 26:398–401, 1963.

Preswick, G., and Jeremy, D.: Subclinical polyneuropathy in renal insufficiency. Lancet, 2:731–732, 1964.

Purnell, D. C., Daly, D. D., and Lipscomb, P. R.: Carpal tunnel syndrome associated with myxedema. Arch. Intern. Med., 108:751–756, 1961.

Raff, M. C., Sangalang, V., and Asbury, A. K.: Ischemic mononeuropathy multiplex associated with diabetes mellitus. Arch. Neurol., 18:487–499, 1968.

Ramón y Cajal, S.: Degeneration and Regeneration in the Nervous System. Trans. by R. May. London, Oxford University Press, 1928.

Rhodes, P.: Meralgia paraesthetica in pregnancy. Lancet, 2:831, 1957.

Ruska, H., and Ruska, C.: Licht und Electronenmikroskopie peripheren neurovegetativen Systems in Hindblick auf die Funktion. Dtsch. Med. Wochenschr., 86:1697–1772, 1961.

Schiller, F., and Kolb, F. O.: Carpal tunnel syndrome in acromegaly. Neurology (Minneap.), 4:271–282, 1954.

Seddon, H. J.: Carpal ganglion as a cause of paralysis of the deep branch of the ulnar nerve. J. Bone Joint Surg., 34B:386–390, 1952.

Seyffarth, H.: Primary myoses in m. pronator teres as cause of a lesion of n. medianus (pronator syndrome). Acta Psychiatr. Neurol. Scand., Suppl. 74:251–254, 1951.

Short, D. W.: Tardy median nerve palsy following injury. Glasgow. Med. J., 32:315–320, 1951.

Simpson, J. A.: Electrical signs in the diagnosis of carpal tunnel and related syndromes. J. Neurol. Neurosurg. Psychiatry, 19:275–280, 1956.

Soferman, N., Weisman, S. L., and Hamov, M.: Acroparesthesia in pregnancy. Am. J. Obstet. Gynecol., 89:528–531, 1964.

Spaans, F.: Occupational nerve lesions. In Vinken, P. J., and Bruyn, G. W. (eds.): Handbook of Clinical Neurology. Amsterdam, North Holland Publishing Co., 1970, pp. 326–343.

Spencer, P. S.: Reappraisal of the model for "bulk axoplasmic flow." Nature [New Biol.], 240:283, 1972.

Spinner, M.: The anterior interosseous nerve syndrome. J. Bone Joint Surg., 52A:84–94, 1970.

Staal, A.: The entrapment neuropathies. *In* Vinken, P. J., and Bruyn, G. W. (eds.): Handbook of Clinical Neurology. Amsterdam, North Holland Publishing Co., 1970, pp. 285–325.

Stack, R. E., Bianco, A. J., and MacCarty, C. S.: Compression of the common peroneal nerve by ganglion cysts. J. Bone Joint Surg., *47-A*:733–778, 1965.

Sunderland, S.: Traumatic injuries of peripheral nerves. I. Simple compression injuries of the radial nerve. Brain, *68*:56–72, 1945.

Sunderland, S.: Metrical and non-metrical features of the muscular branches of the radial nerve. J. Comp. Neurol., *85*:93–111, 1946.

Sunderland, S.: The relative susceptibility to injury of the medial and lateral popliteal divisions of the sciatic nerve. Br. J. Surg., *41*:1–4, 1953.

Sunderland, S.: Nerves and Nerve Injuries. Edinburgh and London, E. & S. Livingstone Ltd., 1968, pp. 678–686.

Thomas, J. E., Lambert, E. H., and Cseuz, K. A.: Electrodiagnostic aspects of the carpal tunnel syndrome. Arch. Neurol., *16*:635–641, 1967.

Thomas, P. K., and Fullerton, P. M.: Nerve fibre size in the carpal tunnel syndrome. J. Neurol. Neurosurg. Psychiatry, *26*:520–527, 1963.

Thomas, P. K., Sears, T. A., and Gilliatt, R. W.: The range of conduction velocity in the normal motor nerve fibres to the small muscles of the hand and foot. J. Neurol. Neurosurg. Psychiatry, *22*:175–181, 1959.

Trojaborg, W.: Rate of recovery in motor and sensory fibres of the radial nerve: clinical and electrophysiological aspects. J. Neurol. Neurosurg. Psychiatry, *33*:625–638, 1970.

Weiss, P., and Hiscoe, H. B.: Experiments on the mechanism of nerve growth. J. Exp. Zool., *107*:315–395, 1948.

Wilkins, R. H., and Brody, I. A.: Tinel's sign. Arch. Neurol., *24*:573, 1971.

Wilkinson, J. F., Nour-Eldin, F., Israels, M. C. G., and Barrett, K. E.: Hemophilia syndromes. Lancet, *2*: 947–950, 1961.

Woltman, H. W.: Crossing the legs as a factor in the production of peroneal palsy. J.A.M.A., *93*:670–672, 1929.

Yap, C. B., and Hirota, T.: Sciatic nerve motor conduction velocity study. J. Neurol. Neurosurg. Psychiatry, *30*:233–239, 1967.

Chapter 35

NEUROPATHY DUE TO PERIPHERAL VASCULAR DISEASES

Jasper R. Daube *and* Peter James Dyck

The association between impaired circulation and peripheral nerve disorders has been recognized for many years (Lapinsky, 1899; Richards, 1951; Krücke, 1955; Sunderland, 1968; Asbury, 1970; Hutchinson, 1970). Such ischemic nerve disorders can be divided into those occurring with diseases affecting large arteries and those occurring with diseases affecting small arteries (Table 35–1). The former are discussed in this chapter; for a discussion of the latter see Chapter 57,

TABLE 35–1 NEUROPATHIES ASSOCIATED WITH ISCHEMIC NERVE DAMAGE

Mainly Affects	Neuropathy
Small arteries	Arteritis (polyarteritis, rheumatoid arthritis)
	Diabetes
	Amyloid
	Infectious diseases (typhus)
	Blood viscosity disorders (macroglobulinemia, cryoglobulinemia, sickle cell disease, polycythemia, thrombocytopenia)
	Clotting disorders (hemophilia, anticoagulation)
	Cold (trench foot, immersion foot)
Large arteries	Emboli (cardiac disease, subacute bacterial endocarditis, tumor, air)
	Compression (mass, trauma, tourniquet)
	Injections (antibiotics, addictive drugs, analeptics)
	Volkmann's ischemic contracture
	Thromboangiitis obliterans (Buerger's)
	Thrombosis (arteriosclerotic occlusive disease)
	Anterior tibial syndrome

Angiopathic Neuropathy in Connective Tissue Diseases, by Conn and Dyck; Chapter 9, Microscopic Anatomy and Function of the Connective Tissue Components of Peripheral Nerve, by Thomas and Olsson; Chapter 47, Diabetic Neuropathy, by Thomas and Eliasson; Chapter 53, Amyloid Neuropathy, by Cohen and Benson; and Chapter 10, Vascular Permeability in the Peripheral Nervous System, by Olsson.

The pathologic processes that affect large arteries and result in peripheral nerve disease may be further divided into acute and chronic disorders. Acute ischemia may develop from embolism, thrombosis, or compression or laceration of the aorta or major limb arteries. Chronic ischemia is usually the result of severe atherosclerosis of the aorta or limb arteries or both, or of thromboangiitis obliterans. The neuropathy associated with arteriosclerosis and thromboangiitis obliterans is commonly referred to as an "ischemic neuritis" or "ischemic neuropathy." Because ischemia of nerve is involved in necrotizing angiopathy and possibly in the other disorders listed in Table 35–1, we do not use the term "ischemic neuropathy."

ANATOMICAL AND PHYSIOLOGIC FACTORS IN ISCHEMIA OF NERVE

The axon of a peripheral nerve is an "excitable system poised with a reserve of energy trapped by a valve with an automatic shutoff" (Shanes, 1958). The "reserve of energy" is the ionic gradient of sodium and potassium across the membrane, and the "valve" is the configuration of the membrane that regulates ionic flow. This stored energy is manifested as the resting potential, which requires energy for its generation, maintenance, and restoration (Gerard, 1930). In normal nerve, which contains the enzyme systems for glycolysis, the Krebs cycle, and electron transport, this energy is derived from aerobic metabolism (Brobeck, 1973). The oxygen requirement of mammalian nerve is small, approximately 0.3 ml per 100 gm (Gerard, 1927). Even when increased by activity, the oxygen consumption remains much less than that of many other tissues (Gerard, 1932). At rest there is a continual leakage of charge across the membrane down the ionic concentration gradients. This leakage is increased during activity. The nerve must therefore continually utilize energy to restore and maintain the ionic gradients— 0.15 cal per hour per gram (Brobeck, 1973). Calcium decreases the leakage of charge across the membrane and thereby acts to conserve energy by "stabilizing" the membrane (Frankenhaeuser and Hodgkin, 1957).

The major function of nerve fibers is the transmission of information between the central nervous system and the periphery. This is accomplished by action potentials, transient depolarizations of limited portions of membrane, during which sodium and potassium diffuse down their concentration gradients. The ionic flow during the action potential decreases the energy stores. But, because it is stored energy that is utilized, immediate generation of energy is not required. Cessation of aerobic metabolism does not directly impair generation of action potentials, but it does result in uncompensated leakage of sodium and potassium across the membrane with a gradual decrease in the resting potential (Lorente de Nó, 1947; Hodgkin and Keynes, 1955). This decrease in resting potential can be partially overcome by glycolysis; it is lessened by membrane "stabilizers" such as calcium. Diffusion of potassium away from the axon also tends to maintain the resting potential and permit continued anaerobic activity (Shanes, 1951). Potassium diffusion is probably limited by three histologic features of nerve: the tightly applied cytoplasm of a Schwann cell surrounding each axon; the basement membrane that surrounds each Schwann

cell, described by Feng and Liu (1949) and Krnjević (1954); and the tight junctions of endothelial cells of endoneurial vessels (see Chapter 10). Alteration of any of these structures by disease might therefore alter the response of a nerve to ischemia.

In summary, peripheral nerve activity is relatively resistant to ischemia because of its small energy requirements, the presence of energy stores for continued activity in the absence of oxygen, the capability for some glycolysis, and the ability of potassium to be removed from the immediate extracellular environment. There is evidence that other peripheral nerve functions such as the steady-state level of sodium conductance (Schoepfle and Bloom, 1959) and fast axoplasmic transport (Ochs and Hollingsworth, 1971; see also Chapter 12) also may be dependent on aerobic metabolism. The significance of these activities for nerve function is not well defined. It has been suggested that ongoing protein metabolism of the axoplasmic membrane, synthesis of transmitter substances, and trophic functions of nerve in maintaining end organs may depend on fast axoplasmic transport (Ochs, Chapter 12). How impairment of these processes by anoxia would modify the electrophysiologic and morphologic characteristics of axons is unknown.

The metabolic needs of large nerves are met by the intraneural blood vessels, the vasa nervorum. Those of small nerves can be met by diffusion from the surrounding tissue. The major peripheral nerves receive blood from nutrient arteries that arise from nearby major arteries and enter nerve trunks at multiple levels. Points of entry are variable but are commonly at the level of joints. Long stretches of nerve may lack a nutrient artery. The nutrient arteries enter the epineurium via a mesoneurium, and branch to form a complex network of interfascicular arteries that course longitudinally in both directions and anastamose with similar arteries from other levels. These small arteries give rise to precapillaries that penetrate the perineurium to enter the endoneurium, where they divide to form a complex terminal mesh of capillaries. The extensive anastomosis, particularly of epineurial arteries, provides a generous blood supply even to segments of nerve some distance from nutrient arteries (Quénu and Lejars, 1892; Bartholdy, 1897; Tonkoff, 1898; Adams, 1942). The extensive longitudinal anastomoses preserve the intraneural blood supply, even when nutrient or epineurial arteries are occluded by disease or by surgical interruption, and thereby prevent nerve damage. The pattern of nutrient and epineurial vessels varies in different nerves, and some nerves, such as the lateral popliteal, sciatic, and median, may be more susceptible to ischemic damage than others (Sunderland 1945a, 1945b, 1968).

EXPERIMENTAL STUDIES OF NERVE ISCHEMIA

Physiologic Studies in Animals

Although recognized long ago by Fröhlich and Tait (1904), ischemic nerve dysfunction had to await elucidation until modern techniques for recording electrical activity were developed. In early experimental studies, transient physiologic dysfunction did not produce morphologic changes (or if it did, they were not recognized). These studies relied on experimental preparations in which the effects of ischemia could be occurring at a number of sites that were not readily differentiated. In a nerve-muscle preparation, for example, ischemia may produce impairment of the twitch response as a result of changes in the nerve, in the neuromuscular junction, or in the muscle. In studies of compound action potentials from nerve trunks, ischemia may affect either the excitability or the action potential, and it may do so to differing degrees in different axons. The action potential has a number of characteristics that may be altered by ischemia — for example, the amplitude, the afterpotential, the refractory period, and the conduction velocity. These depend on the characteristics of the axon membrane, ionic concentrations, myelin, and local metabolic activity, each of which may be altered by ischemia. In addition, a nerve trunk is made up of fibers that vary in size, myelination, physiologic characteristics, and function, all features that may be altered selectively by ischemia. Because a nerve trunk contains different classes of axons, changes in the amplitude of the compound action potential, in excitability, in conduction rate, or in other measurable aspects may result from either selective alteration in one group of fibers or from alterations in all fibers (Paintal, 1965). All these must be considered in studies of the effects of ischemia on peripheral nerve function.

In vitro studies of peripheral nerve action potentials probably provide the most reliable information on the response of nerve to anoxia. Heinbecker (1929) showed the dependence of the electrical activity of peripheral nerve on oxygenation in nonmammalian species. Under anoxic conditions, compound action potentials of nerve trunks showed a decreased amplitude, a slowed conduction rate, an increased refractory period, and an increased threshold. The changes occurred over a two hour period, and recovery was rapid. Anoxia appeared to affect the small myelinated fibers before the large fibers, although this could have resulted from an artifact of the recording technique.

Gerard (1930) confirmed these findings in mammalian nerves, noting that the changes occurred more rapidly in nerves from higher animals, especially at higher temperatures or with faster rates of stimulation. He also noted the resistance of unmyelinated fibers to anoxia, which was confirmed by Clark, Hughes, and Gasser in 1935. Lehmann (1937) described a transient early decrease and a later increase in threshold as the effect of anoxia on cat sciatic nerve. He also found that the afterpotentials changed more rapidly and took longer to recover than did the remainder of the action potential. This observation is in accord with the evidence that the afterpotential represents the restoring of the ionic gradients by metabolically dependent active transport of ions. He speculated that these changes might be based on the accumulation of lactic acid, pH changes, potassium accumulation, or changes in calcium concentration.

Wright (1946; 1947) made comparative studies of the response of nerve action potentials to anoxia in different animals and with different experimental methods. He found that all agents that blocked aerobic metabolism had similar effects and that the severity of the change was dependent on the temperature and the metabolic rate of the nerve. Nerves with higher rates of oxygen consumption showed more rapid loss of action potential in anoxic conditions. He also demonstrated that the decrease in the compound action potential was due to a combination of a block of conduction in some fibers and a decrease in amplitude of the action potential in other fibers. In mammalian nerves, asphyxia for one to two hours delayed recovery by approximately 10 minutes, and in some fibers recovery did not occur.

A detailed description of the changes occurring in single fibers during anoxia was provided by Maruhashi and Wright (1967), who made recordings from single nodes of Ranvier in rat sciatic nerve. During the first 5 to 15 minutes there was a slow decrease in resting potential and action potential with a slight decrease in membrane resistance. At 10 to 15 minutes there was a rapid decrease in action potential, and conduction was blocked although a local graded response remained. The resting potential decreased further at this time. There was an early decrease in threshold in association with the decrease in resting potential, followed by a loss of excitability. Recovery began 1 to 2 minutes after oxygenation was restored and was complete in 10 minutes. The changes occurring with anoxia could be reproduced with cyanide or hypocalcemia, and local hyperpolarization could restore the action potential after a block.

These results all are consistent with the hypothesis that the effect of ischemia is impairment of the metabolic processes that maintain the ionic gradient and the production of local potassium accumulation with depolarization. The resistance of unmyelinated fibers to ischemia results from their smaller metabolic requirements and better local diffusion. The apparent greater susceptibility of the small myelinated fibers noted by Lehmann (1937) and Gelfan and Tarlov (1956) may be an artifact of recording, as was demonstrated in the single-fiber studies of Paintal (1965). He found an apparent loss of the Aδ potential while these axons were still conducting. They were no longer recognized in the compound action potential because of their relative dispersion.

In addition to these changes in the nerve trunk, recent studies have shown that anoxia also impairs function of nerve terminals, the neuromuscular junction, and muscle fibers. Calkins, Taylor, and Hastings (1954) reviewed the evidence that the membrane in muscle fibers is affected in a manner similar to that described for nerve. Paul (1961) has, however, shown that muscle is more resistant than nerve or neuromuscular junctions to anoxia although it is depolarized by anoxia (Creese et al., 1958); anoxic block of neuromuscular transmission occurs while the muscle still can be excited directly. Their findings also suggested that neuromuscular transmission is impaired before nerve function. This was confirmed by Hubbard and Løyning (1966) in microelectrode studies of neuromuscular transmission. They found that the amplitude of the endplate potential decreased to below threshold while the nerve terminals were still conducting. The characteristics of the neuro-

muscular block, including its rapid reversal, suggested that it was due to nerve terminal depolarization rather than to impaired acetylcholine production. Block of nerve terminal conduction did occur soon after the block of neuromuscular transmission, and they concluded, as had Krnjević and Miledi (1958; 1959), that the block of nerve conduction with anoxia was probably occurring at branch points in the distal part of the axon. There is no in vitro evidence of a differential susceptibility along the length of the nerve before the terminal branching.

The in vitro studies of peripheral nerve thus demonstrate electrophysiologic abnormalities with anoxia. In vivo studies are, however, needed to determine whether these abnormalities are the same in the living animal. The earliest of the in vivo studies is that of Koch (1926) who demonstrated a decrease in the injury current of whole nerve after aortic occlusion in rabbits. More specific information about these changes was provided by Clark and co-workers (1935), who studied the effect of anoxia and pressure on the nerve action potential in cat saphenous nerve. They found that the potential could be obliterated if a blood pressure cuff was applied proximally to the region being studied. They noted that, in contrast to the A potential, the C potential was quite resistant to the anoxia. Other authors also used a blood pressure cuff to produce anoxia but did not distinguish effects peripheral to the cuff from those under the cuff, as Clark's group had. The difference between the effects of local compression and vascular occlusion was suggested early by the studies of Allen (1938a), who compared the effects of hind leg ligation with those of abdominal aortic occlusion in rats. The latter produced paralysis and anesthesia that was transient and less severe. This observation and the work of Bülbring and Burn (1939) provide convincing evidence that normal function of peripheral nerve in vivo does depend on an adequate blood supply to the limb. Bülbring and Burn perfused the femoral artery of dogs after clamping the aorta and found a block of conduction in the sciatic nerve in the thigh. They demonstrated that this was due to anoxia of the tissues of the thigh, which were not perfused in this technique.

Bentley and Schlapp (1943) used recordings of nerve action potentials to analyze the effects of impairment of the vascular supply to the cat sciatic nerve. They demonstrated that nerve conduction is lost within 30 minutes if the nerve is truly ischemic. A minimal blood supply can, however, significantly delay or abolish this impairment (such a minimal blood supply may come through the intraneural plexuses even when all major vessels entering the limb are occluded). They also demonstrated the importance of diffusion from surrounding tissues. Placing the nerve in a rubber sheath in an ischemic limb produced a much more rapid loss of action potential. Initial experiments had suggested that the distal response was lost earlier than the proximal, but this was shown to be a function of local diffusion because, when the distal portion of the nerve was placed next to the proximal, the survival times of the responses were equal. In studies on the effect of ischemia on the peroneal nerve, Porter and Wharton (1949) showed, in addition, that ligation of nutrient arteries could impair function locally if the adjacent nutrient vessels were some distance away. Neither of these studies separated the effects on threshold (both found an early decrease) from those on action potential amplitude, generation, and conduction.

Causey and co-workers (1951; 1953) looked more carefully at the apparent absence of abnormality after partial obliteration of the vascular supply. They found that, although conduction of single responses was normal after damage to the major nutrient arteries or the epineurial vessels, the response to stimulation at rapid rates was much decreased. Thus, while the nerve could maintain limited function, vascular supply was insufficient to keep up with much more than the resting energy demands. The effects were much more prominent if the loss of nutrient arteries was combined with damage to the intraneurial vessels at one end of the nerve or the other. Groat and Koenig (1946) reported that function was lost earlier in the proximal portion of the nerve and that the Aδ component was lost before the Aα. They did not, however, consider the effect of varying the length of nerve between stimulating and recording eletrodes, the effect of dispersion of the Aδ potential reported by Paintal (1965), or the effect of diffusion of oxygen from surrounding tissues or from room air. Frankenhaeuser (1949) has shown that these can be of major significance. With these factors controlled, he found no difference in susceptibility of proximal and distal segments. More recent studies have not adequately controlled the multitude of factors that may influence the response of a nerve to ischemia in vivo (Fox and Kenmore, 1967).

Most in vitro and in vivo studies have been of the effects of ischemia on electrical function. A few studies have examined the effects of anoxia on other aspects. Blunt and Stratton (1956a, 1956b) showed that the regional blood supply provides a major pathway for clearance of radioactive sodium from rabbit sciatic nerve and that occlusion of the nutrient arteries could decrease this clearance significantly. Of particular importance was the rapid recovery of clearance rates after nerve damage: new vessels developed rapidly, and clearance returned to normal within 10 days.

Fast axoplasmic transport also depends on an adequate blood supply (Ochs and Hollingsworth, 1971; see also Chapter 12). This transport of material in the axon is impaired by ischemia at about the same time as the conduction is impaired, suggesting that both depend on the same sources of energy. The block of fast axoplasmic transport becomes irreversible after five to six hours of ischemia, a point that most electrophysiologic studies do not investigate. The permeability of endoneurial vessels during ischemia also is not impaired for 9 to 10 hours (see Chapter 10). Apparently, ischemia of many hours is needed before irreversible changes occur in nerve.

These in vivo studies confirm that function of peripheral nerve can be impaired in a transient and physiologic manner if ischemia is mild or of short duration, or permanently if ischemia is severe or prolonged. The relatively slight metabolic needs allow nerve to survive with minimal blood supply or, in some cases, by diffusion of nutrients from surrounding tissues. Acute ischemia may be compensated for by these mechanisms and by growth of new vessels. If these mechanisms are inadequate, or if ischemia is sufficiently prolonged, histologic changes will occur in peripheral nerve.

Morphologic Studies in Animals

Okada (1905) ligated the inferior gluteal artery to the sciatic nerve in rabbits and produced clinical and histologic evidence of nerve damage. A number of subsequent studies have, however, demonstrated the difficulty of producing histologic evidence of peripheral nerve damage by occlusion of nutrient arteries. Modifying the techniques of Okada, Adams (1943) repeated and extended these studies but was unable to produce nerve degeneration by ligation of the inferior gluteal artery alone. If other nutrient arteries to the sciatic nerve also were occluded, histologic changes sometimes occurred. That nutrient arteries can be occluded without production of nerve fiber damage was confirmed by Durward (1948). He also demonstrated that placing a ligature on a nerve might result in nerve damage proximal to the ligature, from occlusion of anastomotic arterioles; stripping the nerve of superficial epineurial vessels also resulted in nerve damage. Roberts (1948) demonstrated that occlusion of the interfascicular arteries of the nerves of dog by stretch or by small emboli produced clinical neuropathic signs; occlusion of nutrient arteries produced lesser signs. Blunt (1960) showed that diffusion of oxygen from surrounding tissues may prevent nerve fiber damage during ischemia. Ligation of regional arteries and mobilization of the nerve was not associated with fiber degeneration or clinical deficit unless the nerve trunk was ensheathed in polyethylene.

Nerve regeneration may or may not be impeded by a poor blood supply. Shumacker and Stokes (1950) found that there was a greater deficit and that recovery was delayed after nerve crush in rats when the femoral artery was clamped. In later studies, Shumacker, Boone, and Kunkler (1953) found no difference in regeneration of cat sciatic with iliac artery ligation. Gutmann (1942) found no impairment of nerve regeneration in rabbits after major vessel occlusion. This was confirmed by Bacsich and Wyburn (1945a, 1945b). These authors also noted that at the cut end of nerve the new vessels arise from intraneurial vessels; this formation of new vessels may be impaired if longitudinal anastomotic arteries are occluded. Kline and co-workers (1972) reached the same conclusion on the basis of clinical and electrophysiologic studies of nerve function. Allbrook and Aitken (1951) showed that nerve regeneration lags behind revascularization during repair of muscle after infarction.

The duration of anoxia necessary to produce structural changes in nerve has not been adequately defined. It may be 30 minutes or more in retina, according to Webster and Ames (1965), but may be hours in other nerves (see preceding section). If ischemia is sufficiently prolonged, however, it will produce not only wallerian degeneration of fibers but also paranodal demyelination and segmental demyelination as early as 24 hours after major vessel occlusion (Hess, 1969). Axonal damage occurs later and to a lesser extent, and Schwann cell abnormalities are not seen. The mechanism by which these destructive changes

occur has not been defined but is most likely impaired respiration and protein metabolism in the axon and the Schwann cell. Prolonged ischemia may be associated with a variable endoneurial collagenosis (Blackwood and Holmes, 1954); this may be due to the variable collateral blood supply to the nerves in the ischemic limbs, demonstrated arteriographically after femoral and iliac occlusion in the rabbit.

These animal studies indicate that damage to single nutrient arteries is unlikely to produce any histologic damage, that destruction of epineurial vessels may produce local and variable damage, and that occlusion of major vessels produces damage primarily distally and varying with the extent of collateral supply and diffusion from surrounding tissues. If damage occurs, wallerian degeneration and local demyelination are found; if ischemia is prolonged, fibrosis of the nerve may develop.

Studies in Man

A single experimental morphologic study in man by Smith (1966a, 1966b) suggested that occlusion of nutrient arteries might produce relative nerve ischemia. Using postmortem injections, he demonstrated the entry of nutrient vessels into the nerve via the "mesoneurium." If vessels were destroyed by isolating a long segment of nerve, some intraneurial blood vessels remained unfilled after injection, while those distal to the region of isolation filled well. Thus, in the longer nerves in man the nutrient vessels may be of greater importance. In addition, the larger diameter of the nerves in man would make local diffusion a less effective process than it is in small animals.

Many experimental studies in man have been attempted in an effort to define the effect of ischemia on peripheral nerves, with goals varying from elucidation of the pathophysiology of localized nerve lesions to determination of the source of the paresthesias that occur with vascular occlusion. In virtually all such studies, however, the blood supply was occluded by means of a blood pressure cuff. Such an occlusion may damage nerves in two ways: (1) directly by pressure and (2) secondarily by occluding either their instrinsic blood vessels or the major vessels of supply. In addition, the ischemic effects may occur locally under the cuff, distal to the cuff, or at both sites. The complexity of this experimental method has resulted in an unsettled controversy over the relative effects of the ischemia and the pressure in producing impaired nerve function. The effects of compression on nerves is discussed by Aguayo in Chapter 34. In this section, only the short-term experimental studies in man that rely on measurement of nerve function distal to an occluding cuff are reviewed. The findings in such experiments can be reliably attributed to ischemia.

Studies of the threshold changes with ischemia were first reported by Thompson and Kimball (1936) and Kugelberg (1944). They demonstrated an initial increase in excitability after the first few (1 to 6) minutes of ischemia, followed by an increase in threshold until the nerve was blocked at 20 to 30 minutes. The time course of these changes is similar to that seen in animal studies. The effects of ischemia on the threshold of the medium-sized sensory fibers in distal portions of ischemic extremities were demonstrated with recordings of nerve action potentials by Seneviratne and Peiris (1968). They found the same early decrease in threshold, followed by block; also, they showed an earlier effect on large fibers.

Magladery, McDougal, and Stoll (1950) were the earliest to define accurately the changes in latency and conduction velocity in nerves distal to an occluding cuff. There was an increase in latency associated with a decrease in action potential amplitude for motor and sensory fibers, with an apparently greater effect on the proximal portions of the fibers although changes were seen along the entire length of the nerve. Abramson and associates (1970a, 1970b, 1971) and Cathala and Scherrer (1963) reported similar changes but did not include data on amplitude. The former authors showed a greater effect at lower temperatures. In studies of sensory nerve action potentials in normal subjects, Caruso and co-workers (1973) found a correlation of the degree of latency, amplitude, or conduction velocity change with the subject's age: the percentage changes were greater in younger subjects for all three measurements. The maximal slowing, however, was 20 m per second, and the values in young persons never were significantly below those of the elderly persons. These electrophysiologic changes could be due to the smaller number of large fibers in the elderly combined with a greater susceptibility of large fibers to ischemia.

Other recent studies have attempted to define the relative susceptibility of small and large fibers to ischemia by comparing the changes in conduction velocity of the fast- and slow-conducting fibers, using a method of antidromic blocking (Hershey and Wagman, 1966; Ruskin et al., 1967). They confirmed the decrease in amplitude and increase in latency during ischemia but did not provide convincing evidence of a differential effect on the large and small fibers.

The site of the effect of the ischemia in motor axons was studied in detail by Dahlbäck and associates (1970) by using single-fiber electromyography to record the jitter in pairs of muscle fibers in a single motor unit during ischemia in normal men. The occurrence of the block was dependent on the number of times the fibers had discharged, suggesting that the presynaptic block may be due to an impairment of acetylcholine synthesis. The patterns of nerve blocking that they found were attributed to changes in nerve terminals and in afferent fibers from muscle spindles.

ACUTE OCCLUSION OF LARGE ARTERIES

Ischemia of peripheral nerve in man can result from large artery occlusion. It produces either spontaneous activity in nerve fibers or loss of function. The degree of deficit varies with the duration of ischemia, location of the nerve fibers, age, and type of axon. The changes occur within 30 minutes, but recovery is relatively rapid after acute impairment. There may be a centrifugal effect, with proximal areas affected earlier, and a differential effect on myelinated fibers of different sizes; there is a relative sparing of unmyelinated fibers.

Arterial Embolism and Thrombosis

The classic features of acute arterial embolism and thrombosis are pain, pallor, coldness, weakness, numbness, and absence of pulses, all sudden in onset (Fairbairn et al., 1972). In a sizable group of cases of occlusion of large arteries, the clinical features were not classic (McKechnie and Allen, 1935; Haimovici, 1950). Of Haimovici's 330 cases, 40 per cent had no pain, and in only 33 per cent was numbness present. The disorder had a slow onset in 11 per cent and was silent in 6 per cent. The variability of the presenting symptoms and of the type and degree of deficit has been attributed to variability in the collateral circulation and vasospasm. Most of the emboli arise from cardiac disease such as rheumatic heart disease, myocardial infarction, atrial fibrillation, and arteriosclerotic heart disease. Intraarterial thrombosis usually occurs against a background of generalized atherosclerosis. The most commonly involved arteries are the femoral and iliac, although any of the major vessels may be involved, and the emboli may be multiple, as reported by Jones and Siekert (1968). These authors and Roberts (1948) described patients with subacute bacterial endocarditis and with neuropathy due to emboli. In two patients the neuropathy produced the presenting symptoms; in three, more than one nerve was involved.

Although common, the occurrence of neurologic signs and symptoms is seldom carefully analyzed. Haimovici reported that 22 per cent of his patients presented with sensory symptoms. Although this author did not provide frequency data, weakness, loss of reflexes, and demonstrable sensory loss also were common. A number of other reports also document neurologic deficits — motor in approximately 20 per cent and sensory in 50 per cent (Learmonth, 1948; Jacobs, 1958; Phelan and Young, 1958; Read et al., 1960). The motor and sensory deficit usually has a distal limb distribution, affecting all limb nerves equally. Welti and co-workers (1961), however, described three patients with selective peroneal palsy due to occlusion of the iliac or femoral vessels. Ferguson and Liversedge (1954) reported nine additional examples of ischemic mononeuropathy, all involving the lateral popliteal (common peroneal) nerve in association with a local vascular abnormality of the femoral or popliteal vessels. They drew attention to the susceptibility of this nerve to ischemic damage owing to its relatively poor blood supply in the region of the fibular head (Sunderland, 1945a, 1945b). Additional examples of mononeuropathies with vascular occlusion are found in a report by Blum (1957).

Detailed analysis of the sensory loss after vascular occlusion has only seldom been reported. Wortis, Stein, and Jolliffe (1942) described one patient with early loss of joint position and vibration sensations and later loss of touch and pricking pain sensations; sensation for delayed, unpleasant, diffuse, aching pain persisted. This pattern of sensation loss might result from sparing of the small ischemic resistant fibers. Assessment of the weakness due to ischemic nerve involvement is

complicated by the occurrence of ischemic muscle damage that results in local tenderness, swelling, and sometimes myoglobinuria (Haimovici, 1970). Although Lewis (1936) attributed most of the pain in acute occlusions to ischemic muscle damage, there may be a nerve involvement in its genesis. The neurologic deficit becomes permanent if arterial flow is not reestablished within a few hours. Of Haimovici's patients, 13.5 per cent had persistent neurologic deficits in the absence of gangrene. McKechnie and Allen (1935) linked the occurrence of severe, paroxysmal, sharp pain after embolism without gangrene to ischemic nerve damage and called it "ischemic neuritis," although there is no direct evidence associating this type of pain after embolism with nerve fiber damage. This term has subsequently been applied to the occurrence of similar pain in a number of other vascular disorders (Slessor and Learmonth, 1949).

Pathologic studies of nerves after acute occlusions of major vessels have been limited. Roberts (1948) studied the filling of vasa nervorum of amputated extremities by injection of contrast material and found nonfilling of many of the vessels, but in an extremely variable pattern. Histologic studies also have revealed a variability of involvement of nerve fibers. In studies by Pantchenko (1938; 1947) and Blackwood (1944), performed within approximately one week of the occlusion in patients with neurologic symptoms and signs, nerves showed prominent wallerian degeneration, but some viable axons could be found scattered among otherwise nonviable necrotic tissue. There also were areas of myelin breakdown without axonal destruction.

Trauma

The occurrence of ischemic damage of peripheral nerves with trauma of major blood vessels is well known. Two examples of this, Volkmann's ischemic contracture and the anterior tibial syndrome, are discussed separately in the following sections. In this section, the ischemic damage that occurs to nerves when major blood vessels are damaged without associated nerve injury is discussed. This type of damage was first defined by Tinel in 1918 in his studies of 639 patients with war injuries. Most of his examples of ischemic nerve damage were associated with trauma to the proximal portions of the major arteries of the limbs, although a few were due to radial or ulnar artery damage. There was an initial period of acute pain, swelling, and other distressing sensory symptoms that included numbness, paresthesias, and burning and that were increased with cold.

The sensory loss and associated weakness were located distally in the limbs. After a few weeks the edema and pain subsided, leaving an atrophic extremity with cutaneous anesthesia, smooth skin, and hard atrophic muscles. Persistent contractures of muscles were common, and recovery was generally slow and incomplete. The extent of these findings varied greatly from patient to patient, and a large percentage of patients who had had a major artery ligated developed no signs of ischemic neuropathy, apparently because of good collateral circulation.

A number of other cases of this type of neuropathy from the first and second world wars have been reported and are generally similar (Parkes, 1945; Wertheimer, 1946; Lyons and Woodhall, 1949; Woodhall and Davis, 1950; Sunderland, 1968). These reports include descriptions of patients with dissociation of sensory loss—loss of position and touch sensations with persistence of pain sensation. Such patients often exhibit a delayed response to painful stimulation. Histologic studies were limited, but axonal damage was commonly seen on standard light microscopy.

Traumatic ischemic neuropathies were reviewed in detail by Richards (1954), who reported 34 personal cases, and were summarized well by Sunderland (1968). At operation, many of these patients showed evidence of damage to collateral vessels or significant vasospasm in addition to the damage to the major artery. As earlier authors had noted, the sensory loss was generally distal, or a glove and stocking type, and the distal weakness was associated with severe wasting and late fibrosis and contracture. Many patients had persistent pain. In addition, of 44 cases of traumatic aneurysm with nerve damage, 4 were due to the ischemia resulting from the aneurysm. The ischemic paralysis in some of these cases was similar to Volkmann's ischemic contracture but occurred with arterial damage in both proximal and distal locations.

A single case report by Seddon and Holmes (1945), of a pilot who suffered severance of the median nerve and ligation of the anterior interosseous artery, provides evidence of the effection of destruction of both the regional and the longitudinal vascular supply to a nerve.

The median nerve in the forearm was severely atrophic and was replaced by dense connective tissue. There was no evidence of ischemic necrosis in surrounding muscle, and more distal portions of the nerve had only the appearance of wallerian degeneration.

Karnosh (1936) described another unique case in which trauma to the buttock was associated with bleeding from the inferior gluteal artery. This bleeding vessel was found two days after the injury, at operation, when there was no evidence of nerve damage. The vessel was ligated, and immediately thereafter the patient developed severe burning pain, hyperesthesia, absence of ankle jerk, and weakness of the leg. These findings were attributed to ischemic damage to the sciatic nerve, which receives much of its blood supply in the buttock from the inferior gluteal artery. Roberts (1948) also described a case of an apparent ischemic neuropathy after ligation of a major nutrient artery; in his case, the patient developed femoral palsy.

Two studies compared the effects of major vessel damage on the rate of nerve regeneration after nerve laceration and repair. Björkesten (1947) and Sunderland (1949) did not find differences in rate of recovery, suggesting that collateral circulation was adequate in these patients.

Volkmann's Ischemic Contracture

In 1881, Volkmann attributed the rapid, posttraumatic contracture of muscles of the arm and hand to ischemic damage to muscle. There have been many reports of this disorder since then, despite its relatively low rate of incidence (8 of 3782 patients with fractures in Griffiths's review and personal study, 1940). In Griffiths's view, the syndrome is due to ischemic damage to muscle as a result of arterial injury and spasm of the collateral circulation. The largest proportion of cases are associated with trauma, particularly supracondylar fractures of the humerus in children. It has a rapid onset (within a few hours of the injury) with the development of a burning pain in the hand and forearm. This is followed by cyanosis or pallor, loss of pulses, and swelling. Paralysis develops with or without sensory loss. As the swelling subsides, the muscles are left atrophic, fibrotic, and essentially useless. Among the most convincing pieces of evidence of the ischemic nature of the disorder are the cases of Volkmann's contracture that have occurred after arterial embolism (Jefferson, 1934; Griffiths, 1940).

In some cases there is associated evidence of direct nerve trauma, but in many there is not. Nonetheless, in the latter cases there often are symptoms and signs of impairment of peripheral nerve function, which consists of paresthesia or sensory loss usually in a distal distribution. It has been suggested from histologic studies that the nerves are damaged by ischemia and not by compression, stretching, or other mechanical processes (Tavernier et al., 1936; Griffiths, 1940).

Six patients with this disorder were studied by Holmes, Highet, and Seddon (1944) with arteriography and nerve biopsy. Spasm and occlusion of major vessels were found arteriographically, and loss of nerve fibers with endoneurial collagenation was seen in nerve biopsies.

Seddon (1956) has published additional studies of the pathology of this disorder, showing the extensive muscle necrosis in the region of ischemia, which appears to be an ellipsoid infarct. The muscle becomes densely fibrotic, and the nerves in the area of ischemia show severe loss of fibers, fibrosis, and atrophy. Seddon (1966, 1972), Owen and Tsimboukis (1967) and Mau (1969) have described the occurrence of a condition like Volkmann's contracture in the lower extremity with various types of injury and involving particularly the flexor hallucis longus muscle. Both the peroneal and tibial nerves are involved. Pain, particularly a severe, incapacitating pain, occurs much more frequently and is more persistent than in similar disorders in the upper extremity. The pain is similar to that of the "ischemic neuritis" noted in other sections of this chapter and probably has a similar pathophysiologic basis. The only electrophysiologic study reported in this disorder is by Kaeser (1965), who found slow median and ulnar nerve conduction velocities in two patients.

Anterior Tibial Syndrome

Closely related to Volkmann's ischemic contracture is the anterior tibial syndrome. Sirbu, Murphy, and White (1944) may have been the first to describe a case of this syndrome, which begins suddenly with local pain and tenderness over the anterior tibial muscle. The pretibial region is tense and erythematous, but the limb is cool. Paralysis of the muscles of the anterior compartment, particularly of the anterior tibial muscle, develops rapidly. The extensor digitorum brevis muscle also becomes weak; sensory loss sometimes occurs, and when it does, is usually limited to the distribution of the deep peroneal nerve but occasionally also extends into the distribution of the superficial peroneal nerve.

Hughes (1948) has shown that the histologic appearance of the muscles is like that of Volkmann's ischemic contracture, with severe necrosis and subsequent fibrosis of the muscles of the anterior compartment. Because of loss of arterial pulsations and abnormal vascular patterns, Hughes contended that the disorder was ischemic in origin. Others have disputed his contention, and these arguments are summarized by Carter, Richards, and Zachary (1949), who concluded that the disorder is brought on as a result of unaccustomed excessive walking or running, which triggers local trauma and swelling within the anterior compartment. Pressure increases within the tight compartment, the blood vessels become occluded, and secondary ischemic necrosis of the muscles and the deep peroneal nerve occurs. Evidence confirming this mechanism of production of the anterior tibial syndrome comes from experimental measurements of clearance and pressure in the anterior compartment (French and Price, 1962).

There have, however, been other reports not in agreement with these conclusions. Freedman and Knowles (1959) and Watson (1955) reported cases of this syndrome all due to embolism or thrombosis of the anterior tibial artery or its parent trunk. The anterior tibial artery was shown to be an end artery and unable to obtain adequate collateral circulation from other sources. These findings were confirmed by Mozes, Ramon, and Jake (1962), who demonstrated arterial occlusion in each of eight patients with this syndrome. Higgins (1961) described one case of this disorder with severe arteriosclerosis. The syndrome also has been reported for the lateral compartment with destruction of the peroneal group of muscles (Reszel et al., 1963; Lunceford, 1965).

From these reports it appears that the anterior tibial syndrome may have two mechanisms: (1) local swelling of muscle in response to local trauma with a secondary increase in pressure in the compartment and local vascular occlusion, and (2) acute occlusion, by embolus or thrombus, of the anterior tibial artery or one of its parent trunks, producing ischemic necrosis in its distribution. In either case there is ischemic destruction of the nerves in the anterior compartment—in particular, the deep peroneal nerve. If the occlusion is higher than the anterior tibial artery, there also may be evidence of damage to the superficial peroneal nerve.

Drug Injection

The occurrence of nerve damage as a result of injections of drugs directly into the nerve is well recognized, particularly with injections in the buttock; but the occurrence of a neuropathy due to nerve damage as a secondary result of injection into an artery is less well known. Among the earliest reports of such an event is that of Gammel (1928); in that case the neuropathy was the result of an injection of bismuth in the treatment of syphilis. The patient developed severe local pain with swelling, local skin mottling, and necrosis of the skin. This was associated with sensory loss, paresthesias and pain, and paralysis in the distribution of the sciatic nerve. Biopsy showed the presence of the bismuth crystals within the blood vessels. Gammel speculated that the injection was into the inferior gluteal artery and had caused secondary spasm and necrosis that produced the ischemic damage to the sciatic nerve.

Although the pathophysiologic mechanism in this case is not entirely certain, subsequent reports, as reviewed by Cohen (1948), include much more specific evidence of the ischemic origin of such neuropathies. In his review of the neuropathies that have been associated with the arterial injection of a wide variety of drugs, with thrombosis of the vessel into which they are injected in many cases, he presented 12 cases in which intraarterial injections of thiopental were made inadvertently at operation. All patients had immediate severe pain, vasoconstriction, mottling of the skin, edema of the arm, and, finally, necrosis of forearm and hand tissues, especially muscle. Two patients had anesthesia and atrophy due to ischemia of nerve, with little muscle damage; 6 of the 12 required amputation. Many had a clinical picture similar to that of Volkmann's contracture. Klatte, Brooks, and Rhamy (1969) demonstrated experimentally that the damage results from a severe endarteritis and diffuse thrombosis.

Mills (1949) first suggested an ischemic cause for sciatic palsy in neonates. He described eight cases of sciatic palsy with evidence of associated circulatory disturbance immediately after the umbilical injection of nikethamide for resuscitation. A number of additional reports of the same syndrome of sciatic palsy associated with edema and discoloration of the buttock region and followed by sloughing of tissue in this area in newborns, appeared in 1950 (Fahrni; Hudson et al.; McFarland). All these patients had had injections of analeptics into the umbilical vessels for resuscitation. At autopsy in one infant, small hemorrhages in the sciatic nerve were found at the level of the lesion. Additional cases and a review were published by Penn and Ross (1955) and Shaw (1960). It is argued that the sciatic nerve damage results from spasm of the umbilical (hypogastric), iliac, and inferior gluteal arteries produced by the intraarterial injection of the drug.

In recent years another type of ischemic nerve lesion from intraarterial injections has occurred. Reports by Morgan, Waugh, and Boback (1970), Ehringer and associates (1971), and Gaspar and Hare (1972) describe intraarterial injection of drugs by addicts. In each case the injection has been into the brachial artery at the elbow and has been followed immediately by severe pain in the arm and hand. Within a few hours, weakness or paralysis develops, and by 24 hours there is sensory loss distally, especially in the distribution of the median nerve. The muscle becomes necrotic and is infiltrated with inflammatory cells. As the swelling subsides, the muscle is left in contracture and fibrotic. If gangrene occurs, amputation may be required. The pathologic changes in nerve in this disorder have not been studied.

Tourniquet Paralysis

A bloodless field is considered a necessity for most surgical procedures on the limbs, and it is obtained by using a pneumatic tourniquet (Boyes, 1964). This practice is widely accepted and is thought to be safe for up to two hours of continuous use. Before the pneumatic tourniquet was developed, ligatures, tubing, or Esmarch bandage was used, but these were frequently associated with nerve damage (Klenerman, 1962). Early reports by Eckhoff (1931), by Allen (1938b), and by Speigel and Lewin (1945) described the clinical features of these tourniquet palsies and provided evidence that they were the result of local damage to nerves beneath the tourniquet, probably where the nerve was compressed against bone.

Sensory and motor symptoms are present immediately postoperatively. Signs are primarily in the distribution of the radial nerve in the upper extremity and of the sciatic nerve in the lower extremity. Motor function is more impaired than sensory, but little atrophy occurs. When sensation is impaired, touch, position, and vibration sensations are lost, but pain and temperature sensations remain intact. The duration of the deficit may be hours, weeks, or months.

Since the introduction of the pneumatic tourniquet, these complications are much less frequent and usually occur as a result of improper technique. Richards (1954) stated that no such complication occurs with proper use of the tourniquet. All of Moldaver's (1954) seven cases were due to improper technique. He described the presence of a local conduction block with normal electrical responses distally. In two recent reports by Bruner (1970) and Calderwood and Dickie (1972), the lesion also occurred through error; in both cases, improper reading of the manometer resulted in use of excessively high pressure. Electromyographic studies in one of these cases showed fibrillation potentials in a number of distal muscles, indicating that the lesion may be more than a simple local block of conduction and may be associated with wallerian degeneration. Kaeser (1965) also found denervation in one case with normal conduction velocities.

It is presumed that the nerve damage in tourniquet paralysis is primarily due to direct compression of the nerve. (For a discussion regarding the mechanism of nerve fiber damage from compression, see Chapter 34 by Aguayo.) However, studies by Paletta, Willman, and Ship (1960) and Martin and Paletta (1966) of tourniquet paralysis due to high pressures on dogs' legs, in which the damage was demonstrated to be in the sciatic nerve under the site of compression, are of interest in this regard. They found that heparin injected in the opposite extremity could significantly decrease the severity and duration of paralysis, and that cooling of the extremity during the compression could entirely prevent the occurrence of the paralysis. These studies suggest that vascular and local metabolic factors also play a significant role in producing nerve damage in tourniquet paralysis.

Other Neuropathies Attributed to Ischemia

Various other disorders have been reported in which peripheral nerve damage has been attributed to ischemia. These include neuropathies with coma, after perfusion, with decompression sickness, with renal dialysis ultrafiltration, and with exposure to cold. Mertens (1961) reported four cases of peripheral neuropathy that he attributed to hypoxia after barbiturate coma. Howse and Seddon (1966) described four similar cases of severe carbon monoxide and barbiturate poisoning with coma in which there was localized pain, swelling, and necrosis of soft tissue with associated motor and sensory paralysis of nerves in the region of the soft tissue damage. This was followed by hardening and contracture of the muscles in the region. The distribution was not that of a single nerve. At operation there was a dense fibrosis of muscle, and the nerves showed marked local narrowing with severe collagenation (two cases). The surgical findings were those of a sharply localized Volkmann's contracture. The authors speculated that the combination of shock, poor tissue perfusion, and the mild local pressure of the immobile body in one position produced localized ischemia and a secondary neuropathy. Kaeser (1965) reported one case of a neuropathy after coma; conduction velocity was normal.

Walsh (1968) described a patient who had mononeuritis multiplex of the axillary and radial nerves after open-heart surgery (postperfusion syndrome). Electromyographic and nerve conduction studies confirmed the clinical impression, and a radial nerve biopsy showed loss of myelinated fibers of all sizes, with wallerian degeneration and segmental demyelination. The etiology of the syndrome is not clear.

Akimov and co-workers (1969) described four patients with decompression sickness followed by transient isolated peripheral nerve impairment. No pathologic or electrical studies were performed. It was speculated that the abnormality was due to air emboli in the vasa nervorum.

Meyrier, Fardeau, and Richet (1972) reported three cases in which patients with chronic renal failure undergoing dialysis had an asymmetrical neuritis in association with rapid initial ultrafiltration. The clinical course and the electron microscopic findings on nerve biopsy suggested to the authors that the disorder was ischemic. They speculated that ultrafiltration produced a massive release of renin and catecholamines with vasoconstriction of arterioles and secondary ischemic damage to the nerves.

There are many reports of peripheral nerve damage due to cold, such as that seen in trench foot and frostbite. Experimental studies have not defined the mechanism of damage (Paintal, 1965). The neuropathy has similarities to ischemic damage clinically and pathologically, but an ischemic etiology is not generally accepted (Schaumburg et al., 1967).

CHRONIC OCCLUSION OF LARGE ARTERIES

Arteriosclerotic Occlusive Disease

The identification of neuropathic involvement in arteriosclerotic occlusive disease rests on finding neurologic or neurophysiologic signs of abnormality of nerves associated with symptoms of claudication, rest pain, decrease or absence of distal pulses, and trophic skin changes.

The term "ischemic neuritis" as used in textbooks refers to the syndrome of pain in the lower limbs associated with peripheral vascular disease (Richards, 1970; Fairbairn et al., 1972). The pain may be diffuse; then it is described as burning, as painful tingling, or as undue sensitivity, and may be especially bothersome at night. The pain also may be sharp and jabbing. These symptoms may, however, be seen in several neuropathies and are not distinctive for the neuropathy of peripheral vascular disease. In fact, there is no direct evidence to relate these symptoms in patients with arteriosclerotic occlusive disease to nerve fiber damage.

The frequency of occurrence of neurologic deficits in patients with peripheral vascular disease is difficult to ascertain because of incomplete data in reports on this subject. The association of neuropathy with arteriosclerotic occlusive vascular disease was made in case reports by Oppenheim (1893) and by Foerster-Breslau (1912) and was confirmed in large studies by Schlesinger (1933) and Hines (1938). Schlesinger found severe neurologic deficit in 4.7 per cent of 470 patients with intermittent claudication. Hines reported the presence of "ischemic neuritis" in 8 per cent of 280 patients with arteriosclerosis obliterans, but some of these patients had diabetes, and

of those with "neuritis" many showed no deficit on neurologic examination. Higher percentages of neurologic deficits have been reported in subsequent series of such patients. Mufson (1952) found sensory loss in 31 per cent of 145 patients and motor deficits in 5.5 per cent. Eleven per cent of these patients had anesthesia distally, often with causalgia-like symptoms or areas of hyperesthesia. All modalities of sensation were involved. The eight patients with severe motor deficit all had weakness in the distribution of the peroneal nerve.

Hutchinson and Liversedge (1956) also found a high frequency (59 per cent) of neurologic abnormalities, but they emphasized that the majority of these were minor. Sensory impairment was the most common finding, but reflex changes, muscle wasting, and muscle weakness also were found. The sensory disturbance usually was a distal tingling that, in some patients, increased with exertion. Three had severe hyperalgesia and hyperesthesia, and three had intermittent, severe, stabbing pain. The sensory loss was either in a stocking distribution or in patchy, localized areas. One patient with muscle weakness had what appeared to be acute peroneal palsy. The presence of neuropathy was directly related to the severity of the vascular disease.

Juergens, Barker, and Hines (1960) reported more "neuropathy" with femoral occlusion than with iliac or aortic occlusion. The incidence of neuropathy in his series was 16 per cent, but the criteria for the diagnosis of neuropathy were not specified. The highest rate of incidence of neurologic deficit was reported by Eames and Lange (1967), who found such abnormalities in 88 per cent of patients with severe vascular occlusive disease. The extent of deficit was proportional to the ischemia. Most of their patients had sensory deficits, although few complained of them. Fifty per cent had weakness, usually in the distribution of the peroneal nerve; 42 per cent had loss of reflexes. Some of the patients had neurologic deficits after only six months of symptomatic vascular disease.

Other reports of the neuropathic complications of peripheral vascular disease were based on the results of electrodiagnostic studies. Miglietta and Lowenthal (1962, 1966, 1967) found slowing of conduction velocity of motor fibers of peroneal nerve in patients who had severe peripheral vascular disease without neurologic signs (38 to 47 m per second in control subjects, 27 to 49 m per second in patients). They also noted an increase in residual latency, but did not comment on amplitudes of the compound action potentials. Thirty per cent of the patients were diabetic, but there was no difference in nerve conduction between these patients and those with vascular disease without diabetes. Chopra and Hurwitz (1968, 1969a, 1969b) also examined nerve conduction of motor fibers in median, ulnar, peroneal, and femoral nerves and of sensory fibers in median and peroneal nerves in patients with peripheral vascular disease. In contrast to the work of Miglietta, their study revealed little change except for some decrease in amplitude of sensory nerve action potentials from the median nerve. They stated that the severity of the disease in their patients was less than that in other series; 74 per cent of their patients had abnormal neurologic findings, mostly mild sensory loss.

Lipid analysis of sciatic, femoral, and tibial nerves of patients with occlusive vascular disease showed a decrease in phospholipid, cholesterol, and cerebroside, and an increase in neutral fats (Randall, 1938). The biochemical changes were more severe distally in the nerves and were thought to be due to wallerian degeneration.

The pathologic alterations in peripheral nerves associated with peripheral vascular disease have been reviewed by Krücke (1955; 1973). This author made the observation that, in comparison to the extensive physiologic and pathologic investigations of impaired circulation of the brain, such studies of peripheral nerve have been meager and monotonously incomplete. A few early studies of the pathologic changes in nerve, although incomplete, provide useful information. Joffroy and Achard (1889a, 1889b) evaluated a 63 year old man with pain in his extremities and sensory loss in his feet. Limb nerves of the lower extremities were unresponsive to galvanic and faradic stimulation. At autopsy they found marked degeneration of the large arteries in the lower limbs. Many of the vasa nervorum in the lower limbs had narrow or obliterated lumens. No pathologic change was observed in the sciatic nerve in the thigh. Marked degeneration of myelinated fibers was observed distally in the leg. The fibers lying in the center of a fascicle were "more or less degenerated," especially distally in the lower leg. Only the fibers adjacent to the edges of the fascicles were entirely normal. A similar central fascicular distribution of degenerating fibers has been noted in vascular occlusion of the third cranial nerve and in necrotizing angiitis (see

Chapter 57). This could result from preservation of circumferential fibers by the diffusion from surrounding tissues seen experimentally.

Early reports of pathologic studies of limb nerves from patients with peripheral vascular disease can be divided into those in which no changes were seen, reported by Fabre, Marinesco, Pitres and Vaillard, and Walkowitsch, and those in which changes were seen, reported by Goldflamm, Joffroy and Achard, Lapinsky, Murawier, Nikolsky and Lawrentjew, Pamas, Weiss, Winiwarter, and Zoge-Manteuffel (all cited by Krücke, 1955). Lapinsky (1899) attempted to make clinicopathologic correlations in eight patients, 26 to 55 years of age; seven had arterial disease confined to one leg and one had bilateral arterial disease. The initial symptom usually was an unpleasant sensation of coldness in the involved foot, followed by an itching and burning in the toes. At first the sensory symptoms occurred only with movement and disappeared with rest. Later they were persistent, and they were at their worst during the night but often disappeared when the position of the limb was changed. Sensory loss could be detected in the region of cutaneous burning. Pulsation was felt in the thigh but not in the leg or foot. Each patient had amputation because of gangrene of the toes. In five of the patients the arteries showed far-advanced atheroma with crystalline deposits or where obliterated. Nerve trunks were most altered near the foot. There was an increased amount of connective tissue in the epineurium, perineurium, and endoneurium, and the endoneurium appeared to spread the nerve fibers apart. Breakdown of myelinated fibers and myelinated fibers with thin myelin were observed.

Later, others — such as Priestley (1932); Kazmeier (1950), and Candela, Canazio, and Alonzo (1960)–also examined limbs amputated because of gangrene from patients with arteriosclerosis and found myelinated fibers undergoing wallerian degeneration. Fiber degeneration was proportional to the degree of arteriosclerosis and was more pronounced distally. Prolonged deficits were associated with fibrosis. Dible (1967) and Toporkov (1970), in reviews of the histologic changes in nerves of amputated legs, found marked nerve changes in 50 per cent and no abnormalities in 25 per cent. Amputated limbs from diabetics were included, but no difference between those with and those without diabetes were noted. The changes were most prominent distally but were quite variable from nerve to nerve.

Gairns and co-workers evaluated nerves from amputated limbs by determining the density and the frequency distribution of the diameters of myelinated fibers and comparing these with values from control nerves (Gairns et al., 1960; Garven et al., 1962). They found a significant loss of the large myelinated fibers. Chopra and Hurwitz (1967) studied sural nerve biopsies from six patients with severe peripheral vascular disease. Specific data on the neurologic examination were not presented, but the changes apparently were minimal. Their findings of variation in internodal length suggested that there had been demyelination and remyelination. There also was evidence of axonal degeneration in two of the biopsies. In a later report, Chopra and Hurwitz (1969b) described the fiber density and size in sural nerve biopsies from three patients with vascular disease, but they did not specify whether these were the same cases as those reported earlier, nor did they present the clinical findings. In contrast to the findings in their previous study, they found no definite differences in fiber density in nerves of patients as compared to controls.

A similar but more complete study was made by Eames and Lange (1967), who described the pathologic changes in sural nerve biopsies in eight patients with vascular disease and neurologic evidence of a neuropathy. They found evidence of segmental demyelination and remyelination, of axonal degeneration and regeneration, and of increase in endoneurial collagen. The unmyelinated fibers were normal except for some vacuoles and loss of neurofibrils.

Thromboangiitis Obliterans

Thromboangiitis obliterans or Buerger's disease is a migratory phlebitis of young men that produces the clinical picture of an obliterative vascular disease with many similarities to arteriosclerosis obliterans. Its cause is unknown, and it is characterized by relapsing episodes of pain, local skin changes, pallor, and, in severe cases, gangrene. It is due to intimal proliferation with cellular infiltrates and thrombi, particularly of larger vessels. The presence of neurologic symptoms and signs with damage to the peripheral nerves in this disorder was recognized early, even before Buerger's description of the disease. Dutil and Lamy (1893) and Schlesinger (1933) both described patients who probably had thromboangiitis obliterans.

The report by Dutil and Lamy was of a 40 year old man with intermittent claudication. A year after the onset of the claudication, a cold, burning pain developed in the first and second toes of the left foot. In the third year, the arterial pulses became diminished and a burning pain developed in the right foot. No bleeding occurred when the right leg was amputated. In the fifth year, pulses disappeared in the left foot, and sensation over the anterior half of the foot was lost. At amputation of this leg, the patient died. Autopsy revealed obliteration of leg arteries and periarteritis. The peripheral nerves were thickened and had degenerating fibers characteristic of wallerian degeneration. The authors wrote that the lack of nourishment from occluded arteries had produced wallerian degeneration. Buerger (1908) also described these changes in peripheral nerves and attributed the pain to the fibrosis found in the nerve trunks. Such fibrosis has been noted by others as well (Brown and Allen, 1928).

Goldsmith and Brown (1935) provided data on the clinical evidence of the involvement of peripheral nerves in a series of 100 consecutive cases of thromboangiitis obliterans. Twelve of the patients had the pain of "ischemic neuritis" — one in the distribution of the posterior tibial nerve, one in the distribution of the peroneal nerve, and the others not localized to a specific nerve. Three had decreased reflexes, and one had a loss of sensation. Most had hyperesthesia. Histologic studies of nerves of one of these patients showed both degeneration and loss of myelin.

These pathologic changes were confirmed in a study by Barker (1938), who also made an interesting clinicopathologic correlation. He studied the peripheral nerves of 20 patients with thromboangiitis obliterans; all but 1 patient had definite histologic abnormalities. Fibrosis of the nerves, especially distally, was the most prominent change and was present in 15 cases. Wallerian degeneration was present in 10 of the 17 amputated legs and usually was patchy. Changes in the vasa nervorum were found in only six cases and were not sufficient to explain the extent of wallerian degeneration. He therefore postulated that the changes were due to large-vessel disease. He also found that all the patients who complained of "neuritis type of pain" had wallerian degeneration in the proximal nerve trunks, and this was not present in those patients who had only local pain. The neuritis type of pain could not be correlated with any of the other histologic changes that he found.

There have been subsequent reports confirming these findings. Kazmeier (1950) found evidence of demyelination in a patient with a clinical picture of polyneuritis. Erbslöh and Kazmeier (1950) also found that the changes in the vasa nervorum were not sufficient to account for the extent of degeneration seen. There have been no well-defined electrophysiologic studies of the nerves in this disorder.

References

Abramson, D. I., Rickert, B. L., Alexis, J. T., Hlavova, A., Schwab, C., and Tandoc, J.: Effect of repeated periods of ischemia on motor nerve conduction velocity in forearm. J. Appl. Physiol., *30*:636, 1971.

Abramson, D. I., Hlavova, A., Rickert, B., Talso, J., Schwab, C., Feldman, J., and Chu, L. S. W.: Effect of ischemia on median and ulnar motor nerve conduction velocities at various temperatures. Arch. Phys. Med. Rehabil., *51*:463, 1970a.

Abramson, D. I., Hlavova, A., Rickert, B., Talso, J., Schwab, C., Feldman, J., and Chu, L. S. W.: Effect of ischemia on latencies of median nerve in the hand at various temperatures. Arch. Phys. Med. Rehabil., *51*:471, 1970b.

Adams, W. E.: Blood supply of nerves. I. Historical review. J. Anat., *76*:323, 1942.

Adams, W. E.: The blood supply of nerves. II. The effects of exclusion of its regional sources of supply on the sciatic nerve of the rabbit. J. Anat., *77*:243, 1943.

Akimov, G., Yelinsky, M., and Lvovskiy, A.: Disorders of the nervous system in decompression diseases. Zh. Nevropatol. Psikhiatr., *69*:979, 1969.

Allbrook, D. B., and Aitken, J. T.: Reinnervation of striated muscle after acute ischaemia. J. Anat., *85*:376, 1951.

Allen, F. M.: Effects of ligations on nerves of the extremities. Ann. Surg., *108*:1088, 1938a.

Allen, F. M.: The tourniquet and local asphyxia. Am. J. Surg., *41*:192, 1938b.

Asbury, A. K.: Ischemic disorders of peripheral nerve. *In* Vinken, P. J., and Bruyn, G. W. (eds.): Handbook of Clinical Neurology: Diseases of Nerves, Part II. Vol. 8. New York, Elsevier Publishing Co., 1970, pp. 154–164.

Bacsich, P., and Wyburn, G. M.: The vascular pattern of peripheral nerve during repair after experimental crush injury. J. Anat., *79*:9, 1945a.

Bacsich, P., and Wyburn, G. M.: The effect of interference with the blood supply on the regeneration of peripheral nerves. J. Anat., *79*:74, 1945b.

Barker, N. W.: Lesions of peripheral nerves in thrombo-angiitis obliterans. Arch. Intern. Med., *62*:271, 1938.

Bartholdy, K.: Die Arterien der Nerven. Morphol. Arbeit., *7*:393, 1897.

Bentley, F. H., and Schlapp, W.: Experiments on the blood supply of nerves. J. Physiol. (Lond.), *102*:62, 1943.

Björkesten, G.: Suture of war injuries to peripheral nerves: clinical studies of results. Acta Chir. Scand., *95*:Suppl. 119:1, 1947.

Blackwood, W.: A pathologist looks at ischaemia. Edinburgh Med. J., *51*:131, 1944.

Blackwood, W., and Holmes, W.: Histopathology of nerve injury. *In* Seddon, H. J. (ed.): Peripheral Nerve Injuries: Medical Research Council Special Report Series 282. London, Her Majesty's Stationery Office, 1954, pp. 88–134.

Blum, L.: The clinical entity of anterior crural ischemia: report of four cases. Arch. Surg., *74*:59, 1957.

Blunt, M. J.: Ischemic degeneration of nerve fibers. Arch. Neurol., *2*:528, 1960.

Blunt, M. J., and Stratton, K.: The immediate effects of ligature of vasa nervorum. J. Anat., *90*:204, 1956a.

Blunt, M. J., and Stratton, K.: The development of compensatory collateral circulation to nerve trunk. J. Anat., *90*:508, 1956b.

Boyes, J. H.: Bunnell's Surgery of the Hand. 4th Edition. Philadelphia, J. B. Lippincott Co., 1964, pp. 132–135.

Brobeck, J. R.: Best and Taylor's Physiological Basis of Medical Practice. 9th Edition. Baltimore, Williams & Wilkins Co., 1973, pp. 1–51.

Brown, G. E., and Allen, E. V.: Thrombo-angiitis Obliterans: Clinical, Physiologic and Pathologic Studies. Philadelphia, W. B. Saunders Co., 1928.

Bruner, J. M.: Time, pressure and temperature factors in the safe use of the tourniquet. Hand, *2*:39, 1970.

Buerger, L.: Thrombo-angiitis obliterans: a study of the vascular lesions leading to presenile spontaneous gangrene. Am. J. Med. Sci., *136*:567, 1908.

Bülbring, E., and Burn, J. H.: Vascular changes affecting the transmission of nervous impulses. J. Physiol. (Lond.), *97*:250, 1939.

Calderwood, J. W., and Dickie, W. R.: Tourniquet paresis complicating tendon grafting. Hand, *4*:53, 1972.

Calkins, E., Taylor, I. M., and Hastings, A. B.: Potassium exchange in the isolated rat diaphragm: effect of anoxia and cold. Am. J. Physiol., *177*:211, 1954.

Candela, F., Canazio, P., and Alonzo, M.: Studio sulle alterazioni dei nervi periferici in arteriopatie obstruttive. Rass. Int. Clin. Ter., *40*:1289, 1960.

Carter, A. B., Richards, R. L., and Zachary, R. B.: The anterior tibial syndrome. Lancet, *2*:928, 1949.

Caruso, G., Labianca, O., and Ferrannini, E.: Effect of ischaemia on sensory potentials of normal subjects of different ages. J. Neurol. Neurosurg. Psychiatry, *36*:455, 1973.

Cathala, H.-P., and Scherrer, J.: Modifications du potentiel de nerf, sous l'influence d'un brassard ischémiant, chez l'homme. Rev. Neurol. (Paris), *108*:201, 1963.

Causey, G., and Schoepfle, G. M.: Fatigue of mammalian nerve in relation to the cell body and vascular supply. J. Physiol. (Lond.), *115*:143, 1951.

Causey, G., and Stratmann, C. J.: The relative importance of the blood supply and the continuity of the axon in recovery after prolonged stimulation of mammalian nerve. J. Physiol. (Lond.), *120*:373, 1953.

Chopra, J. S., and Hurwitz, L. J.: Internodal length of sural nerve fibres in chronic occlusive vascular disease. J. Neurol. Neurosurg. Psychiatry, *30*:207, 1967.

Chopra, J. S., and Hurwitz, L. J.: Femoral nerve conduction in diabetes and chronic occlusive vascular disease. J. Neurol. Neurosurg. Psychiatry, *31*:28, 1968.

Chopra, J. S., and Hurwitz, L. J.: A comparative study of peripheral nerve conduction in diabetes and non-diabetic chronic occlusive peripheral vascular disease. Brain, *92*:83, 1969a.

Chopra, J. S., and Hurwitz, L. J.: Sural nerve myelinated

fibre density and size in diabetics. J. Neurol. Neurosurg. Psychiatry, 32:149, 1969b.

Clark, D., Hughes, J., and Gasser, H. S.: Afferent function in the group of nerve fibers of slowest conduction velocity. Am. J. Physiol., 114:69, 1935.

Cohen, S. M.: Accidental intra-arterial injection of drugs. Lancet, 2:409, 1948.

Creese, R., Scholes, N. W., and Whalen, W. J.: Resting potentials of diaphragm muscle after prolonged anoxia. J. Physiol. (Lond.), 140:301, 1958.

Dahlbäck, L.-O., Ekstedt, J., and Stålberg, E.: Ischemic effects of impulse transmission to muscle fibers in man. Electroencephalogr. Clin. Neurophysiol., 29:579, 1970.

Dible, J. H.: The Pathology of Limb Ischaemia. St. Louis, W. H. Green, 1967.

Durward, A.: The blood supply of nerves. Postgrad. Med. J., 24:11, 1948.

Dutil, A., and Lamy, H.: L'artérite oblitérante progressive: et des névrites d'origine vasculaire. Arch. Med. Exp. Anat. Pathol., 5:102, 1893.

Eames, R. A., and Lange, L. S.: Clinical and pathological study of ischaemic neuropathy. J. Neurol. Neurosurg. Psychiatry, 30:215, 1967.

Eckhoff, N. L.: Tourniquet paralysis: a plea for the extended use of the pneumatic tourniquet. Lancet, 2:343, 1931.

Ehringer, H., Fischer, M., Holzner, J. H., Imhof, H., Kubiena, K., Lechner, K., Pichler, H., Schnack, H., Seidl, K., and Staudacher, M.: Gangrän nach versehentlicher intraarterieller Injektion von Dicloxacillin. Dtsch. Med. Wochenschr., 96:1127, 1971.

Erbslöh, F., and Kazmeier, F.: Polyneuritis bei Thrombangiitis Obliterans. Arch. Psychiatr. Nervenkr., 183:703, 1950.

Fahrni, W. H.: Neonatal sciatic palsy. J. Bone Joint Surg. [Br.], 32:42, 1950.

Fairbairn, J. F., II, Juergens, J. L., and Spittell, J. A., Jr.: Allen-Barker-Hines Peripheral Vascular Diseases. 4th Edition. Philadelphia, W. B. Saunders Co., 1972.

Feng, T. P., and Liu, Y. M.: The connective tissue sheath of the nerve as effective diffusion barrier. J. Cell. Comp. Physiol., 34:1, 1949.

Ferguson, F. R., and Liversedge, L. A.: Ischaemic lateral popliteal nerve palsy. Br. Med. J., 2:333, 1954.

Foerster-Breslau, O.: Arteriosklerotische Neuritis und Radiculitis. Dtsch. Z. Nervenheilkd., 45:374, 1912.

Fox, J. L., and Kenmore, P. I.: The effect of ischemia on nerve conduction. Exp. Neurol., 17:403, 1967.

Frankenhaeuser, B.: Ischaemic paralysis of a uniform nerve. Acta Physiol. Scand., 18:75, 1949.

Frankenhaeuser, B., and Hodgkin, A. L.: The action of calcium on the electrical properties of squid axons. J. Physiol. (Lond.), 137:218, 1957.

Freedman, B. J., and Knowles, C. H. R.: Antbrior tibial syndrome due to arterial embolism and thrombosis: ischaemic necrosis of the anterior crural muscles. Br. Med. J., 2:270, 1959.

French, E. B., and Price, W. H.: Anterior tibial pain. Br. Med. J., 2:1290, 1962.

Fröhlich, F. W., and Tait, J.: Zur Kenntnis der Erstickung und Narkose des Warmblüternerven. Z. Allg. Physiol., 4:105, 1904.

Gairns, F. W., Garven, H. S. D., and Smith, G.: The digital nerves and the nerve endings in progressive obliterative vascular disease of the leg. Scott. Med. J., 5:382, 1960.

Gammel, J. A.: Local accidents following the intramuscular administration of salts of the heavy metals: report of two cases of embolia cutis medicamentosa. Arch. Dermatol. Syph., 18:210, 1928.

Garven, H. S. D., Gairns, F. W., and Smith, G.: The nerve fibre populations of the nerves of the leg in chronic occlusive arterial disease in man. Scott. Med. J., 7:250, 1962.

Gaspar, M. R., and Haire, R. R.: Gangrene due to intra-arterial injection of drugs by drug addicts. Surgery, 72:573, 1972.

Gelfan, S., and Tarlov, I. M.: Physiology of spinal cord, nerve root and peripheral nerve compression. Am. J. Physiol., 185:217, 1956.

Gerard, R. W.: Studies on nerve metabolism. II. Respiration in oxygen and nitrogen. Am. J. Physiol., 82:381, 1927.

Gerard, R. W.: The response of nerve to oxygen lack. Am. J. Physiol., 92:498, 1930.

Gerard, R. W.: Nerve metabolism. Physiol. Rev., 12:469, 1932.

Goldsmith, G. A., and Brown, G. E.: Pain in thromboangiitis obliterans: a clinical study of 100 consecutive cases. Am. J. Med. Sci., 189:819, 1935.

Griffiths, D. L.: Volkmann's ischaemic contracture. Br. J. Surg., 28:239, 1940.

Groat, R. A., and Koenig, H.: Centrifugal deterioration of asphyxiated peripheral nerve. J. Neurophysiol., 9:275, 1946.

Gutmann, E.: Factors affecting recovery of motor function after nerve lesions. J. Neurol. Psychiatry, 5:81, 1942.

Haimovici, H.: Peripheral arterial embolism: a study of 330 unselected cases of embolism of the extremities. Angiology, 1:20, 1950.

Haimovici, H.: Arterial embolism, myoglobinuria, and renal tubular necrosis. Arch. Surg., 100:639, 1970.

Heinbecker, P.: Effect of anoxemia, carbon dioxide and lactic acid on electrical phenomena of myelinated fibers of the peripheral nervous system. Am. J. Physiol., 89:58, 1929.

Hershey, W. N., and Wagman, I. H.: Effects of ischemia on range of conduction velocities and on facilitation in human motor nerves. Trans. Am. Neurol. Assoc., 91:246, 1966.

Hess, N.: Zur Frage der vaskulären ischämischen peripheren Neuropathie. Schweiz. Arch. Neurol. Neurochir. Psychiatr., 105:1, 1969.

Higgins, D. C.: Ischemic necrosis of anterior tibial muscles associated with arteriosclerosis obliterans. N. Y. State J. Med., 61:1583, 1961.

Hines, E. A., Jr.: Thrombo-arteriosclerosis obliterans: a clinical study of 280 cases. Proc. Staff Meet. Mayo Clin., 13:694, 1938.

Hodgkin, A. L., and Keynes, R. D.: Active transport of cations in giant axons from Sepia and Loligo. J. Physiol. (Lond.), 128:28, 1955.

Holmes, W., Highet, W. B., and Seddon, H. J.: Ischaemic nerve lesions occurring in Volkmann's contracture. Br. J. Surg., 32:259, 1944.

Howse, A. J. G., and Seddon, H.: Ischaemic contracture of muscle associated with carbon monoxide and barbiturate poisoning. Br. Med. J., 1:192, 1966.

Hubbard, J. I., and Løyning, Y.: The effects of hypoxia on neuromuscular transmission in a mammalian preparation. J. Physiol. (Lond.), 185:205, 1966.

Hudson, F. P., McCandless, A., and O'Malley, A. G.: Sciatic paralysis in newborn infants. Br. Med. J., 1:223, 1950.

Hughes, J. R.: Ischaemic necrosis of the anterior tibial muscles due to fatigue. J. Bone Joint Surg. [Br.], 30:581, 1948.

Hutchinson, E. C.: Ischaemic neuropathy and peripheral vascular disease. *In* Vinken, P. J., and Bruyn, G. W. (eds.): Handbook of Clinical Neurology: Diseases of Nerves, Part II. Vol. 8. New York, Elsevier Publishing Co., 1970, pp. 149–153.

Hutchinson, E. C., and Liversedge, L. A.: Neuropathy in peripheral vascular disease: its bearing on diabetic neuropathy. Q. J. Med., *25*:267, 1956.

Jacobs, A. L.: Arterial embolism in the limbs: clinical assessment and management. Postgrad. Med. J., *34*:464, 1958.

Jefferson, G.: Arterial embolectomy. Br. Med. J., *2*:1090, 1934.

Joffroy, A., and Achard, C.: Gaugréne cutanée du gros orteil: chez un ataxique. Arch. Med. Exp. Anat. Pathol., *1*:241, 1889a.

Joffroy, A., and Achard, C.: Névrite périphérique: d'origine vasculaire. Arch Med. Exp. Anat. Pathol., *1*:229, 1889b.

Jones, H. R., Jr., and Siekert, R. G.: Embolic mononeuropathy and bacterial endocarditis. Arch. Neurol., *19*: 535, 1968.

Juergens, J. L., Barker, N. W., and Hines, E. A., Jr.: Arteriosclerosis obliterans: review of 520 cases with special reference to pathogenic and prognostic factors. Circulation, *21*:188, 1960.

Kaeser, H. E.: Veränderungen der Leitgeschwindigkeit bei Neuropathien und Neuritiden. Fortschr. Neurol. Psychiatr., *33*:221, 1965.

Karnosh, L. J.: Sciatic causalgia due to nerve trunk ischemia. J. Nerv. Ment. Dis., *84*:283, 1936.

Kazmeier, F.: Der vasale Faktor bei Erkrankungen der peripheren Nerven. Nervenarzt, *21*:353, 1950.

Klatte, E. C., Brooks, A. L., and Rhamy, R. K.: Toxicity of intra-arterial barbiturates and tranquilizing drugs. Radiology, *92*:700, 1969.

Klenerman, L.: The tourniquet in surgery. J. Bone Joint Surg. [Br.], *44*:937, 1962.

Kline, D. G., Hackett, E. R., Davis, G. D., and Myers, M. B.: Effect of mobilization on the blood supply and regeneration of injured nerves. J. Surg. Res., *12*:254, 1972.

Koch, E.: Über den Einfluss vorübergehender Blutabsperrung auf den Längsquerschnittstrom des Warmblüternerven. Z. Gesamte Exp. Med., *50*:238, 1926.

Krnjević, K.: Some observations on perfused frog sciatic nerves. J. Physiol. (Lond.), *123*:338, 1954.

Krnjević, K., and Miledi, R.: Failure of neuromuscular propagation in rats. J. Physiol. (Lond), *140*:440, 1958.

Krnjević, K., and Miledi, R.: Presynaptic failure of neuromuscular propagation in rats. J. Physiol. (Lond.), *149*:1, 1959.

Krücke, W.: Erkrankungen der peripheren Nerven. *In* Henke, F. (ed.): Handbuch der speziellen pathologischen Anatomie und Histologie: Nervensystem. Vol. 13. Berlin, Springer-Verlag, 1955, pp. 1–203.

Krücke, W.: Pathologie der peripheren Nerven. *In* Handbuch der Neurochirurgie Bd. VII/3. Heidelberg, Springer-Verlag, 1973.

Kugelberg, E.: Accommodation in human nerves: and its significance for the symptoms in circulatory disturbances and tetany. Acta Physiol. Scand., Suppl. *24*:1, 1944.

Lapinsky, M.: Ueber Veränderungen der Nerven bei acuter Störung der Blutzufuhr. Dtsch. Z. Nervenheilkd., *15*:364, 1899.

Learmonth, J. R.: Arterial embolism. Edinburgh Med. J., *55*:449, 1948.

Lehmann, J. E.: The effect of asphyxia on mammalian A nerve fibers. Am. J. Physiol., *119*:111, 1937.

Lewis, T.: Pain as an early symptom in arterial embolism and its causation. Clin. Sci., *2*:237, 1936.

Lorente de Nó, R.: A study of nerve physiology. Stud. Rockefeller Inst. Med. Res., *131*:1; *132*:1, 1947.

Lunceford, E. M., Jr.: The peroneal compartment syndrome. South. Med. J., *58*:621, 1965.

Lyons, W. R., and Woodhall, B.: Atlas of Peripheral Nerve Injuries. Philadelphia, W. B. Saunders Co., 1949, pp. 205–219.

Magladery, J. W., McDougal, D. B., Jr., and Stoll, J.: Electrophysiological studies of nerve and reflex activity in normal man. II. Effects of ischemia. Johns Hopkins Hosp. Bull., *86*:291, 1950.

Martin, F. R., and Paletta, F. X.: Tourniquet paralysis: a primary vascular phenomenon. South. Med. J., *59*: 951, 1966.

Maruhashi, J., and Wright, E. B.: Effect of oxygen lack on the single isolated mammalian (rat) nerve fiber. J. Neurophysiol., *30*:434, 1967.

Mau, H.: Die ischämischen Kontrakturen der Unteren Extremitaten und das Tibialis-Anterior-Syndrome. Z. Orthop., Suppl. 105, 1969.

McFarland, B.: Comment on neonatal sciatic palsy. J. Bone Joint Surg. [Br.], *32*:47, 1950.

McKechnie, R. E., and Allen, E. V.: Sudden occlusion of the arteries of the extremities: a study of 100 cases of embolism and thrombosis. Proc. Staff Meet. Mayo Clin., *10*:678, 1935.

Mertens, H. G.: Die disseminierte Neuropathie nach Koma: zur Differenzierung der sogenannten toxischen Polyneuropathien. Nervenarzt, *32*:71, 1961.

Meyrier, A., Fardeau, M., and Richet, G.: Acute asymmetrical neuritis associated with rapid ultrafiltration dialysis. Br. Med. J., *2*:252, 1972.

Miglietta, O.: Nerve motor fiber characteristics in chronic ischemia. Arch. Neurol., *14*:448, 1966.

Miglietta, O.: Electrophysiologic studies in chronic occlusive peripheral vascular disease. Arch. Phys. Med. Rehabil., *48*:89, 1967.

Miglietta, O., and Lowenthal, M.: Nerve conduction velocity and refractory period in peripheral vascular disease. J. Appl. Physiol., *17*:837, 1962.

Mills, W. G.: A new neonatal syndrome. Br. Med. J., *2*:464, 1949.

Moldaver, J.: Tourniquet paralysis syndrome. Arch. Surg., *68*:136, 1954.

Morgan, N. R., Waugh, T. R., and Boback, M. D.: Volkmann's ischemic contracture after intra-arterial injection of secobarbital. J.A.M.A., *212*:476, 1970.

Mozes, M., Ramon, Y., and Jahr, J.: The anterior tibial syndrome. J. Bone Joint Surg. [Am.], *44*:730, 1962.

Mufson, I.: Diagnosis and treatment of neural complications of peripheral arterial obliterative disease. Angiology, *3*:392, 1952.

Ochs, S., and Hollingsworth, D.: Dependence of fast axoplasmic transport in nerve on oxidative metabolism. J. Neurochem., *18*:107, 1971.

Okada, E.: Experimentelle Untersuchungen über die vasculäre Trophik des peripheren Nerven. Arb. Neurol. Inst. Anat. Physiol. Zent. Nerv. Univ. Wien, *12*:59, 1905.

Ophenheim, H.: Ueber die senile Form der multiplen Nervitis. Berl. Klin. Wochenschr., *30*:589, 1893.

Owen, R., and Tsimboukis, B.: Ischaemia complicating closed tibial and fibular shaft fractures. J. Bone Joint Surg. [Br.], *49*:268, 1967.

Paintal, A. S.: Block of conduction in mammalian myelinated nerve fibres by low temperatures. J. Physiol. (Lond.), *180*:1, 1965.

Paletta, F. X., Willman, V., and Ship, A. G.: Prolonged tourniquet ischemia of extremities: an experimental study on dogs. J. Bone Joint Surg. [Am.], *42*:945, 1960.

Pantchenko, D.: Sur certaines particularités de la névrite au cours de la gangrène spontanée. Ann. Anat. Pathol. (Paris), *15*:1013, 1938.

Pantchenko, P.: Sur l'influence de l'ischémie sur les troncs nerveux périphériques. Ann. Anat. Pathol. (Paris), *17*:61, 1947.

Parkes, A. R.: Traumatic ischaemia of peripheral nerves with some observations on Volkmann's ischaemic contracture. Br. J. Surg., *32*:403, 1945.

Paul, D. H.: The effects of anoxia on the isolated rat phrenic-nerve-diaphragm preparation. J. Physiol. (Lond.), *155*:358, 1961.

Penn, A., and Ross, W. T.: Sciatic nerve palsy in newborn infants. South. Afr. Med. J., *29*:553, 1955.

Phelan, J. T., and Young, W. P.: Diagnosis of peripheral arterial emboli in the extremities. J.A.M.A., *168*:1299, 1958.

Porter, E. L., and Wharton, P. S.: Irritability of mammalian nerve following ischemia. J. Neurophysiol., *12*:109, 1949.

Priestley, J. B.: Histopathologic characteristics of peripheral nerves in amputated extremities of patients with arteriosclerosis. J. Nerv. Ment. Dis., *75*:137, 1932.

Quénu, M. M., and Lejars, M.: Étude anatomique sur les vaisseaux sanguins des nerfs. Arch. de Neurologie, *23*:1, 1892.

Randall, L. O.: Changes in lipid composition of nerves from arteriosclerotic and diabetic subjects. J. Biol. Chem., *125*:723, 1938.

Read, A. E. A., Ball, K. P., and Rob, C. G.: Embolic occlusion of the aorta in patients with mitral stenosis. Q. J. Med., *29*:459, 1960.

Reszel, P. A., Janes, J. M., and Spittell, J. A., Jr.: Ischemic necrosis of peroneal musculature, a lateral compartment syndrome: report of case. Proc. Staff Meet. Mayo Clin., *38*:130, 1963.

Richards, R. L.: Ischaemic lesions of peripheral nerves: a review. J. Neurol. Neurosurg. Psychiatry, *14*:76, 1951.

Richards, R. L.: Neurovascular lesions. *In* Seddon, H. J. (ed.): Peripheral Nerve Injuries: Medical Research Council Special Report Series 282. London, Her Majesty's Stationery Office, 1954, pp. 186–238.

Richards, R. L.: Peripheral Arterial Disease: A Physician's Approach. Edinburgh, E. & S. Livingstone Ltd., 1970.

Roberts, J. T.: The effect of occlusive arterial diseases of the extremities on the blood supply of nerves: experimental and clinical studies on the role of the vasa nervorum. Am. Heart J., *35*:369, 1948.

Ruskin, A. P., Tanyag-Jocson, A., and Rogoff, J. B.: Effect of ischemia on conduction of nerve fibers of varying diameters. Arch. Phys. Med. Rehabil., *48*:304, 1967.

Schaumburg, H., Dyck, R., Herman, R., and Rosengart, C.: Peripheral nerve damage by cold. Arch. Neurol., *16*:103, 1967.

Schlesinger, H.: Über eine wenig bekannte Form der vaskulären Neuritis. Wien. Med. Wochenschr., *83*:98, 1933.

Schoepfle, G. M., and Bloom, F. E.: Effects of cyanide and dinitrophenol on membrane properties of single nerve fibers. Am. J. Physiol., *197*:1131, 1959.

Seddon, H. J.: Volkmann's contracture: treatment by excision of the infarct. J. Bone Joint Surg. [Br.], *38*:152, 1956.

Seddon, H. J.: Volkmann's ischaemia in the lower limb. J. Bone Joint Surg. [Br.], *48*:627, 1966.

Seddon, H. J.: Surgical Disorders of the Peripheral Nerves. Baltimore, Williams & Wilkins Co., 1972.

Seddon, H. J., and Holmes, W.: Ischaemic damage in the peripheral stump of a divided nerve. Br. J. Surg., *32*:389, 1945.

Seneviratne, K. N. and Peiris, O. A.: The effect of ischaemia on the excitability of human sensory nerve. J. Neurol. Neurosurg. Psychiatry, *31*:338, 1968.

Shanes, A. M.: Potassium movement in relation to nerve activity. J. Gen. Physiol., *34*:795, 1951.

Shanes, A. M.: Electrochemical aspects of physiological and pharmacological action in excitable cells. Pharmacol. Rev., *10*:59, 1958.

Shaw, N. E.: Neonatal sciatic palsy from injection into the umbilical cord. J. Bone Joint Surg. [Br.], *42*:736, 1960.

Shumacker, H. B., Jr., and Stokes, G. E.: Studies of combined vascular and neurologic injuries. I. The effect of somatic and sympathetic denervation upon the results of arterial ligation in the rat. Ann. Surg., *132*:386, 1950.

Shumacker, H. B., Jr., Boone, R., and Kunkler, A.: Studies of combined vascular and neurologic injuries. III. The effect of arterial ligation and sympathetic denervation upon return of function after crushing of sciatic nerve of the cat. Arch. Surg., *67*:753, 1953.

Sirbu, A. B., Murphy, M. J., and White, A. S.: Soft tissue complications of fractures of the leg. Calif. West. Med., *60*:53, 1944.

Slessor, A. J., and Learmonth, J.: Pain in peripheral vascular disease. Practitioner, *164*:445, 1949.

Smith, J. W.: Factors influencing nerve repair. I. Blood supply of peripheral nerves. Arch. Surg., *93*:335, 1966a.

Smith, J. W.: Factors influencing nerve repair. II. Collateral circulation of peripheral nerves. Arch. Surg., *93*:433, 1966b.

Speigel, I. J., and Lewin, P.: Tourniquet paralysis: analysis of three cases of surgically proved peripheral nerve damage following use of rubber tourniquet. J.A.M.A., *129*:432, 1945.

Sunderland, S.: Blood supply of the nerves of the upper limb in man. Arch. Neurol. Psychiatr., *53*:91, 1945a.

Sunderland, S.: Blood supply of the sciatic nerve and its popliteal divisions in man. Arch. Neurol. Psychiatr., *54*:283, 1945b.

Sunderland, S.: Observations on the course of recovery and late end results in a series of cases of peripheral nerve suture. Aust. N.Z. J. Surg., *18*:264, 1949.

Sunderland, S.: Nerves and Nerve Injuries. Baltimore, Williams & Wilkins Co., 1968.

Tavernier, L., Dechaume, J., and Pouzet, F.: Infarctus musculaires et lésions nerveuses dans le syndrome de Volkmann. J. Méd. Lyon, *17*:815, 1936.

Thompson, I. M., and Kimball, H. S.: Effect of local ischemia upon human nerve fibers in vivo. Proc. Soc. Exp. Biol. Med., *34*:601, 1936.

Tinel, J.: Nerve Wounds: Symptomatology of Peripheral Nerve Lesions Caused by War Wounds. London, Bailliere, Tindall & Cox, 1918.

Tonkoff, W.: Die Arterien der Intervertebralganglien und der Cerebrospinalnerven des Menschen. Int. Monatsschr. Anat. Physiol., *15*:353, 1898.

Toporkov, I. A.: Vascular syndromes of the peripheral nervous system. Zh. Nevropatol. Psikhiatr., *70*:1070, 1970.

Volkmann, R.: Die ischaemischen Muskellähmungen und Kontrakturen. Centralbl. Chir., *8*:801, 1881.

Walsh, J. C.: Mononeuritis multiplex complicating the postperfusion syndrome. Australas. Ann. Med., *17*:327, 1968.

Watson, D. C.: Anterior tibial syndrome following arterial embolism. Br. Med. J., *1*:1412, 1955.

Webster, H., and Ames, A.: Reversible and irreversible changes in the fine structure of nervous tissue during oxygen or glucose deprivation. J. Cell. Biol., *26*:885, 1965.

Welti, J.-J., Melekian, B., and Reveillaud, M.: Paralysies périphériques ischémiques (paralysies périphériques provoquées par une embolie artérielle des membres). Presse Méd., *69*:333, 1961.

Wertheimer, P.: Effets des lésions vasculaires sur les lésions nerveuses périphériques. Lyon Chir., *41*:385, 1946.

Woodhall, B., and Davis, C., Jr.: Changes in the arteriae nervorum in peripheral nerve injuries in man. J. Neuropathol. Exp. Neurol., *9*:335, 1950.

Wortis, H., Stein, M. H., and Jolliffe, N.: Fiber dissociation in peripheral neuropathy. Arch. Intern. Med., *69*:222, 1942.

Wright, E. B.: A comparative study of the effects of oxygen lack on peripheral nerve. Am. J. Physiol., *147*:78, 1946.

Wright, E. B.: The effects of asphyxiation and narcosis on peripheral nerve polarization and conduction. Am. J. Physiol., *148*:174, 1947.

Chapter 36

NEUROPATHY DUE TO PHYSICAL AGENTS

P. K. Thomas *and* J. B. Cavanagh

The peripheral nerves constitute the most exposed portion of the nervous system and consequently are vulnerable to trauma or to damage by physical events such as chilling. Peripheral nerves may also be directly involved by electrical or thermal burns, acute x-radiation damage, or freezing. Of greater interest are the delayed consequences of x-irradiation and possible late sequelae of electrical injury.

MECHANICAL INJURY

Classification of Nerve Injury

It has been recognized since the time of Weir Mitchell (Mitchell et al., 1864) and Erb (1874, 1876) that mechanical injury can give rise to either temporary or persisting paralysis. Moreover, the degree of damage at the site of injury was known to have a profound influence on the quality of recovery.

Seddon (1943) proposed a classification of nerve injuries that categorized the different types of localized lesion of mechanical origin, although it must be realized that mixed lesions are frequent. The term "neurapraxia" was employed to designate a localized conduction block with preservation of conduction distal to the lesion. Signs of denervation do not develop. Full recovery occurs within days or weeks and takes place more or less simultaneously throughout the territory of the nerve. "Axonotmesis" described lesions that give rise to axonal interruption, but with preservation of the connective tissue frame-

work of the nerve. Wallerian degeneration occurs distal to the lesion, and signs of denervation develop. Recovery takes place by axonal regeneration in which the axons regain their former peripheral connections and is therefore satisfactory. Evidence of reinnervation is first detected in the territory of the nerve closest to the site of injury. The local pathologic changes in this type of lesion are considered in Chapter 9. Finally, "neurotmesis" denotes lesions in which the axons are interrupted and, additionally, the connective tissue components of the nerve are damaged or the nerve is completely transected. Recovery again has to take place by axonal regeneration but is always incomplete because of misrouting of fibers at the site of injury.

A more elaborate classification was devised by Sunderland (1951) in which five degrees of nerve injury were recognized. First- and second-degree injuries corresponded respectively to "neurapraxia" and "neurotmesis" in Seddon's classification. The third to fifth degrees consisted of subdivisions of "neurotmesis." In third-degree injuries, the fascicular architecture of the nerve is maintained, but there is disorganization within the fascicles involving rupture of the endoneurial connective tissue sheaths and hemorrhage. In fourth-degree injury, in addition to the changes of the previous categories, the perineurium is ruptured, but without loss of continuity of the nerve. In both third- and fourth-degree injury, regeneration is impeded by misrouting of regenerating axons because of rupture of endoneurial connective tissue sheaths and because of endoneurial scarring.

734

Fifth-degree injury consists of complete severence of the nerve trunk.

Types of Mechanical Injury

NERVE COMPRESSION

Damage to peripheral nerves by compression may occur for a variety of reasons, which include external compression by steady pressure or a blunt blow, entrapment within anatomical canals, compression by tumors or ganglia or inflammatory masses, and compression resulting from hemorrhage or edema within confined anatomical compartments. The clinical features, pathology, and pathophysiology of such lesions are considered in Chapter 34.

PENETRATING WOUNDS

Apart from nerve compression, the commonest type of nerve injury is related to open wounds, either incised wounds or less often lacerations. In a series of 385 nerve injuries from incised wounds recorded by Seddon (1972), 80 per cent were caused by glass, and in more than 90 per cent the nerve was partly or completely divided. In incised wounds that have caused nerve damage, the probability that surgical repair of the nerve will be necessary is therefore great. Exploration is thus desirable unless there is evidence of an only partial lesion, in which case spontaneous recovery is often good. The intact part of the nerve ensures that the cut ends of the severed portion do not retract too extensively so that regeneration can occur across the gap. If the patient is not seen until some time after the injury, and recovery, estimated by calculating the expected regeneration time from the site of injury to the denervated muscles, could occur within a few weeks, it would be justifiable to delay exploration for this period.

Lacerated wounds are less common, and the type of nerve damage is more variable. The probability of complete division is in the region of 75 per cent (Seddon, 1972) and may involve either a simple transection or loss of a segment of the nerve. Exploration is therefore again usually desirable, once the laceration has healed satisfactorily and any wound infection has been eradicated.

The question of the desirability of primary or delayed suture has given rise to much discussion and has not been finally resolved. The decision partly depends upon the availability of adequate surgical expertise. At three to four weeks after injury, because of epineurial thickening, suture may be technically easier, and Schwann cell activity is then near its maximum (Young, 1949). Prolonged delays are definitely undesirable because of the risk of irreversible changes developing in denervated muscles. More detailed surgical aspects of nerve repair are beyond the scope of this chapter.

NERVE INJURIES ASSOCIATED WITH FRACTURES

Nerves may be damaged directly by fractures (Seddon, 1947) or, as discussed in the succeeding section, a fracture or fracture-dislocation may result in a traction injury. In the large majority of nerve injuries associated with fractures, satisfactory spontaneous recovery occurs and exploration should usually be restricted to those cases in which recovery has failed to take place after the anticipated interval. The sciatic nerve provides an exception. Because of the length of time required for regeneration in this nerve, should it be injured in the region of the hip or upper thigh, early exploration is probably merited. The substantial amount of time lost should regeneration fail to occur means that the risk of irreversible denervation atrophy of the lower leg muscles would be significant.

STRETCH INJURY

The brachial plexus may be damaged by traction in a variety of ways: these are considered in Chapter 32. Joint dislocations may result in stretch injuries, examples of which are damage to the axillary nerve in dislocations of the shoulder, of the ulnar nerve in elbow dislocations, and of the sciatic nerve in dislocations at the hip or knee. With fractures of the limb bones and distraction of the limb, various nerve trunks may be affected, sometimes at a site remote from the injury. This can give rise to puzzling clinical consequences (Seddon, 1972). Nobel (1966) recorded examples of traction injury of the common peroneal nerve at its point of separation from the sciatic nerve that resulted from fractures of the tibia and fibula, or even from inversion sprains at the ankle.

Nerves may inadvertently be damaged by retraction during operations or by stretching during procedures for the correction of joint contractures. The cranial nerve palsies that may develop during halo-pelvic traction in the treatment of scoliosis are also presumably the result of stretching and usually recover in the course of a few weeks after release of the appliance (Nickel et al., 1968; O'Brien et al., 1971). Lesions of the cervical roots may also occur.

Except when nerves are directly involved in a missile wound, nerve damage occurs as the consequence of rapid displacement. High-velocity missiles or fragments from explosions produce rapid expansion around them as they traverse the tissues, the track then rapidly collapsing. Experimental studies employing very brief photographic (Black et al., 1941) or x-ray (Harvey et al., 1945) exposures, have demonstrated that the missile produces cavitation with explosive suddenness. The effects on the sciatic nerve of cats produced by bullets shot through the thigh were investigated by Puckett and co-workers (1946). The sciatic nerves were outlined by the injection of a radiopaque material. Microsecond x-ray exposures demonstrated that the nerve is rapidly displaced by the expansion of a large temporary cavity in the tissues by missiles that pass close to the nerve but do not strike it directly. Nerve stimulation showed interruption of conduction without severance of the nerve trunk.

Milder degrees of traction injury may produce no more than a reversible conduction block (Seddon, 1972). More severe injury tends to give rise to damage over a considerable length of the nerve (Highet and Holmes, 1943). In nerves that have remained in continuity, damage to vessels and intraneural hemorrhage presumably contribute to subsequent intraneural fibrosis (Highet and Holmes, 1943; Nobel, 1966). The considerable longitudinal extent of this damage poses substantial problems in nerve repair and grafting.

The sequence of events during traction injuries has been studied experimentally on a number of occasions with discordant findings. The studies of Liu, Benda, and Lewey (1948) and Sunderland and Bradley (1961) both yielded the conclusion that the nerve fibers become ruptured with intact perineurial sleeves, whereas Denny-Brown and Doherty (1945) concluded that the perineurium ruptured first. The more recent findings of Haftek (1970) have been considered in Chapter 9. He found that the first component of the nerve to break was the epineurium, followed by the perineurium, and finally the nerve fibers.

VIBRATION

Raynaud's phenomenon is a well-recognized occurrence in individuals who work with vibrating tools such as pneumatic hammers or road drills, but the mechanism of its production is uncertain (see Agate, 1949). Although it was specifically denied by Telford, McCann, and MacCormack (1945), Jepson (1951) considered that there were persistent sensory abnormalities in the fingers between attacks. This view was supported by Marshall, Poole, and Reynard (1954), who also detected weakness in the hands in such cases. They were inclined to the view that the neurologic signs and the Raynaud's phenomenon were secondary to damage to nerve fibers produced by the vibration.

Consequences of Nerve Injury

CONDUCTION BLOCK

Erb (1874) recognized that in lesions of the radial nerve that develop during heavy sleep, electrical stimulation of the nerve below the lesion may evoke a normal muscle response, whereas stimulation above the site of damage obtains none. A conduction block produced by mechanical injury may recover after minutes, days, or weeks. The more persistent instances are probably related to local demyelination (Denny-Brown and Brenner, 1944; Mayer and Denny-Brown, 1964; Ochoa et al., 1972).

Both with compressive lesions and with those resulting from gunshot wounds, the motor deficit is characteristically greater than the sensory loss (Mitchell et al., 1864). If such lesions produce a greater degree of damage to larger fibers, a sensory deficit would be less easy to detect in view of the substantial amount of cutaneous sensory information carried in smaller fibers.

The explanation of very transient conduction blocks caused by mechanical injury is unknown.

WALLERIAN DEGENERATION

Interruption of axons in a localized injury results in wallerian degeneration distal to the lesion. Conduction persists in the degenerating fibers for three to four days (Gutmann and Holubář, 1950) or even as long as eight days (Gilliatt and Hjorth, 1972). During this period there is little alteration in conduction velocity. Neuromuscular transmission fails slightly before conduction ceases in the nerve trunk, as reported by Lissak, Dempsey, and Rosenblueth (1939) and Birks, Katz, and Miledi (1960). Gilliatt and Hjorth (1972) showed that degenerative changes in the terminal branches of intramuscular nerve fibers preceded those in the nerve trunk. An evoked muscle response to electrical stimulation after nerve section in man can be obtained for three to five days (Landau, 1953; Gilliatt and Taylor, 1959).

The structural changes that occur in nerve during wallerian degeneration are detailed in Chapter 16.

CONSEQUENCES OF DENERVATION

Motor Function. Muscle paralysis consequent upon axonal interruption is not always easy to assess in cases of nerve injury, as the situation may be complicated by anomalous innervation, the adoption of "trick movements" by the patient, or the presence of superimposed hysterical or feigned weakness, particularly in cases in which compensation for injury is involved. In the management of cases of nerve injury it is often important to know whether the lesion is partial or complete and whether recovery is taking place at the appropriate time. Although nerve blocking by local anesthetic has been advocated by Highet (1942) in instances in which anomalous innervation may be involved, the use of electromyography combined with nerve stimulation usually suffices.

Loss of the motor innervation of muscle leads to denervation atrophy. The rate of muscle wasting is most rapid initially and is due to a reduction in the caliber of the muscle fibers. In man, loss of muscle fibers begins six to nine months following injury, and few fibers remain after three years (Bowden and Gutmann, 1944). Fibrotic contracture may occur in paralyzed muscles if they are immobilized in a shortened position or if there is associated damage to arteries (Volkmann's ischemic contracture). Shortening in unopposed antagonist muscles may develop in cases in which there is persisting paralysis.

Sensation. The margins of regions of cutaneous sensory loss are graded because of overlap from adjacent nerves. Sensory loss occurs in the "autonomous zone" of the nerve and is less for pain appreciation than for touch. Its area tends to shrink with time, even if regeneration does not occur, probably owing to the ingrowth of collateral branches from the surrounding innervated skin (Weddell et al., 1941). Paresthesias are not common after lesions causing axonal interruption, although they may appear during the recovery phase. They are felt throughout the distribution of the nerve, which will be greater than the area of sensory loss.

The "triple response" to mechanical stimulation of the skin or to the intradermal injection of histamine is due to an axon reflex in sensory fibers and is lost after peripheral nerve section. It is preserved with preganglionic lesions of the brachial plexus (Bonney, 1954).

Autonomic Function. Loss of sweating after peripheral nerve injuries that cause axonal interruption occurs in the autonomous zone of the distribution of the nerve. Vasomotor function and piloerection are also affected, but are less easily examined. Vascular changes tend to be most evident following lesions of the median, ulnar, and sciatic nerves. In a proportion of cases, the denervated skin becomes warm and reddened from loss of the sympathetic vasoconstrictor innervation. Later, after a matter of a few weeks, the affected skin tends to become cold, particularly if the ambient temperature is low. The normal vasodilator response to local mechanical stimulation or warmth is lost, and there may be hypersensitivity of the denervated vessels to cold, resulting in vasoconstriction (Doupe, 1943; Moorhouse et al., 1966). These factors tend to reduce the blood supply to denervated regions. A detailed review of the vascular changes following nerve injury has been made by Sunderland (1968).

Trophic Changes. The atrophy of denervated muscle fibers, to which reference has already been made, is due to the loss of a trophic influence of unknown nature that is normally provided by the motor axons. Most other alterations following nerve injury that are designated as "trophic" are the consequence of reduced muscle activity, of trauma secondary to sensory loss, or of reduced blood supply (see also Chapter 24).

In the early stages after nerve injury to a limb, if the affected limb is immobilized or not used, scaliness of the skin or hyperkeratosis of the sole of the foot or of the palm may develop. In persistent denervation, the skin may become thin and shiny, and the subcutaneous tissue atrophic. Nail growth may be retarded or accelerated (Sunderland and Ray, 1952), and hair growth also shows inconsistent changes.

Ulceration of the skin may be caused by badly fitting footwear and other inadvertent mechanical or thermal injury and is related to loss of pain sensation. Injury is probably more likely to occur if there is dependent edema or if the skin has become atrophic.

SENSORY DISTURBANCES FOLLOWING NERVE INJURY

Causalgia. The first clear description of this condition was given by Weir Mitchell, Morehouse, and Keen (1864) in their beautifully written monograph describing nerve injuries from the American Civil War. Its delineation from other painful syndromes that may follow nerve injury has given rise to some dispute. Barnes (1954), in a study of 48 cases derived from the Second World War listed its characteristic features. It is severe persistent pain, usually having a burning quality, which may spread beyond the territory of the injured nerve or nerves. Barnes considered that although it is "spontaneous," causalgic pain is invariably aggravated by both emotional and physical factors, the latter including touching of the affected skin and movement or jarring of the limb. Authoritative descriptions of causalgia have also been given by Ulmer and Mayfield (1946), Shumacker, Speigel, and Upjohn (1948b), White, Heroy, and Goodman (1948), Richards (1967), Seddon (1972), and others. It is most frequently related to injuries of the median nerve, the tibial division of the sciatic nerve, and the lowest trunk of the brachial plexus, and usually follows high-velocity missile wounds, less commonly traction injuries, and rarely other forms of nerve damage. The causative

lesions are usually but not always partial and are most often above the elbow or knee. Multiple involvement of nerves is frequent. The onset is most commonly within the first 24 hours after injury, but may be delayed for several weeks. It sometimes regresses spontaneously. The pain is most severe in the hand or foot. The affected extremity frequently exhibits redness and shininess of the skin, fixation of finger joints, and osteoporosis. These changes are probably mainly related to immobility and protection of the skin from contact. In some patients, the affected skin may sweat excessively, whereas in others sweating is diminished.

Causalgia may be relieved by sympathectomy (Freeman, 1947; Shumacker et al., 1948a; White et al., 1948; Barnes, 1954; and others); this has led some authorities to restrict the use of the term "causalgia" to cases that are relieved by this procedure. The results of sympathectomy in the various reported series have been reviewed by Richards (1967). Relief may be immediate or delayed for several days. Beneficial effects are obtained in 70 to 80 per cent of cases, and in general, although there has been some disagreement on this aspect, similar results are obtained for both upper and lower limb causalgia. A delay of several years after the original injury does not necessarily prevent a good response.

The explanation of causalgia is unknown. Nathan (1947) concluded that the pain arises in the region of the injury, but the mechanism that has received the widest measure of support is that of Doupe, Cullen, and Chance (1944). This sought to explain aggravation by emotional factors and the response to sympathectomy by postulating that efferent impulses in sympathetic fibers are able to activate sensory fibers in the lesion. The concept of "artificial synapses" produced by nerve injury has been widely accepted, but although cross excitation between fibers has been demonstrated in short-term experiments by Granit, Leksell, and Skoglund (1944), no convincing anatomical or physiologic corroboration of persisting contacts of this nature has been presented.

Other Painful Sequelae of Nerve Injury. Some authorities such as Seddon (1972) have drawn a clear distinction between causalgia and other painful sequelae of nerve injury, whereas others have failed to make such a rigid separation (e.g., Sunderland, 1968). The terminology is unsatisfactory. The clinical features of noncausalgic pain syndromes are less uniform. Seddon (1972) has grouped these conditions together as "irritative nerve lesions," although a reduced afferent input into the spinal cord might be a possible explanation if the views of Melzack and Wall (1966) and Wall and Sweet (1967) concerning the origin of pain are accepted. The group includes cutaneous hyperpathia (see Chapter 24) and also deep aching pain. These symptoms can occur together or independently and may arise following injuries, which may be either partial or complete, to any nerve. Sympathectomy is not beneficial. Spontaneous pain in some of these cases appears to be due to neuroma formation, either on the proximal stump of a completely severed nerve or laterally on a partially severed nerve. Resection of the neuroma or resection and nerve suture, both in digital and other cutaneous nerves and in mixed nerve trunks, can be curative (Seddon, 1972), but in quite a large proportion the symptoms ultimately subside spontaneously.

Phenomena Related to Limb Amputations. A "phantom limb" develops following almost all limb amputations, either of the arm or the leg. Henderson and Smyth (1948) found that only about 2 per cent of a series of 300 Second World War amputees denied ever having experienced this phenomenon. The phantom is described as a positive sensation of numbness or mild tingling. The peripheral parts of the limb, particularly the hand and foot, are more vividly appreciated than the more proximal regions. With time, the phantom gradually shortens, the hand and foot becoming "telescoped" toward the stump. The rate of regression is faster in younger individuals, and more rapid for the lower than the upper limb. Henderson and Smyth (1948) found that in their cases, lower limb phantoms had all disappeared within two years, whereas those for the upper limb were much more persistent, especially after proximal amputations. Apart from the study just cited, detailed considerations of the various intriguing aspects of phantom limbs and their possible explanations have been given by Riddoch (1941), Stone (1950), Cronholm (1951), and others.

Neuromas rapidly form at the ends of all divided nerves and continue to increase in size for up to three years. They are usually painless, although percussion produces a brief burst of tingling paresthesias in the distribution of the relevant nerve in the phantom. Exposed neuromas in the stump may be tender, and their excision abolishes such sensations but has no effect on the generalized tingling in the phantom (Henderson and Smyth, 1948). Neuromas constitute the commonest but by no means the only cause for stump pain.

Apart from this persistent mild tingling sensation in the phantom, more definite tingling or thermal paresthesias, or sudden lancinating or cramplike pains may also occur. These usually subside within a few months. Persistently painful phantoms can constitute an exceedingly difficult problem. Their incidence has varied greatly between different series, the reason for which is not entirely clear. They are commoner in older subjects and in cases in which the phantom is particularly distinct (Stone, 1950; Cronholm 1951). Phantoms do not regress if they are painful. The pain may be intermittent or continuous and is often described as having a burning quality. The cause of painful phantoms is obscure, although the emotive situation of a limb amputation undoubtedly results in the superimposition of psychogenic factors in a proportion of cases.

Factors Influencing Recovery After Nerve Injury

These have been extensively reviewed by Sunderland (1968) and are only briefly surveyed here. They can be subdivided into factors that affect the regenerative capacity of the neurons; those that are operative at the site of injury; those related to conditions in the portion of nerve distal to the site of injury; and those affecting peripheral structures.

REGENERATIVE CAPACITY

Transection of axons may lead to the death of the parent neuron as an immediate sequel to the injury. This is most likely to occur following proximal lesions and is greater in extent in young individuals. A continued slow loss of neurons takes place if effective regeneration fails to occur (for references, see Sunderland, 1968). A reduced number of axons in the central stump will obviously have a disadvantageous influence on functional recovery.

Experiments on laboratory animals have suggested that regenerative capacity is sustained virtually indefinitely (Duncan and Jarvis, 1943). This may not be true of man (Seddon, 1972). The capacity for recovery in children seems appreciably superior to that in adults, even allowing for factors such as shorter regeneration distances and more rapid axonal regeneration rates.

FACTORS AT THE SITE OF INJURY

Lesions in Continuity. In lesions in which the abnormality is strictly a local conduction block, recovery is uniformly satisfactory. As discussed earlier, it is presumed, on the basis of experimental models, that the conduction failure is due to localized demyelination (Denny-Brown and Brenner, 1944; Mayer and Denny-Brown, 1964; Ochoa et al., 1972). Recovery is associated with remyelination. When the axons have been interrupted but the endoneurial connective tissue sheaths of the nerve fibers have not been severed (axonotmesis), the regenerating axons are able to traverse the site of injury within the persisting basal laminal tubes of the Schwann cells to regain their former pathways in the nerve distal to the injury (Haftek and Thomas, 1968). Recovery is usually satisfactory, but involves a greater delay, related to the distance over which axonal regeneration has to take place.

Traction lesions, as has already been discussed, may give rise to damage distributed over a considerable length of the nerve and lead to extensive intraneural fibrosis. Consequently, recovery is often grossly defective.

Nerve Transection. When the nerve is either partially or completely interrupted, recovery is always more or less imperfect because of misrouting of regenerating axons. Should the cut not involve all the fascicles and the nerve remain partially in continuity, the outgrowths from the proximal and distal cut ends will have a fair chance of making contact, and reasonably good restoration of function may be possible. If the nerve is completely divided, the cut ends draw apart and recovery is not achieved unless the ends can be approximated. Particularly when the injury has led to the loss of a portion of the nerve, the variations in the fascicular pattern that occur along the length of the nerve trunk mean that mismatching between the cut ends will be inevitable (Sunderland, 1945; Sunderland and Ray, 1948). This will be greater if repair is delayed because of atrophy of the distal stump (Sunderland and Bradley, 1950).

When the nerve ends are separated by a gap, nerve suture may be achieved by mobilization of the stumps, but if this is too extensive, a poor result may ensue because of devascularization or because of subsequent traction on the nerve if it crosses a joint (Highet and Sanders, 1943). Repair of longer gaps requires grafting. Consideration of this aspect is beyond the scope of the present discussion, but the only method so far developed from which reasonably satisfactory results may be obtained is the use of autografts, usually derived from cutaneous nerves. Microsurgical techniques that involve the joining of individual fascicles, introduced in recent years by Millesi, Gangleberger, and Berger (1967), have yet to be adequately evaluated: in the repair of long gaps, the alterations that occur in the fascicular pattern along the length of the nerve may result in the regenerating fibers being directed toward inappropriate peripheral terminations. Only limited success has been achieved using homografts, including frozen irradiated grafts described by Campbell, Bassett, and Böhler (1963) and Marmor (1964), or by employing artificial materials such as Millipore (Campbell et al., 1956). The use of freeze-dried irradiated homografts protected by immunosuppressive drugs during the period of regeneration through the graft may have an application in particular circumstances (Guy et al., 1972).

THE NERVE DISTAL TO THE SITE OF INJURY

After a latent interval for the axons to reach the nerve distal to the lesion, which is related to the nature of the injury, the regenerating axons advance toward the periphery. The rate of axonal advance has been assessed both experimentally in animals, and in man, and has been reviewed by Bowden and Sholl (1954). It is evident that rates found in animal experiments cannot be transferred to man, in whom the distances over which regeneration may have to take place are considerably longer. Rates are faster after crush injuries producing an axonotmesis type of lesion than after transection and suture. Observations on laboratory animals suggest that, in general, the rate of regeneration is uniform. In man, it is clear that it declines with increasing distance and that there are considerable variations between individuals the reasons for which are not easy to understand. It is likely that regeneration rates decline the more peripheral is the lesion. The values obtained by Seddon, Medawar, and Smith (1943) for motor recovery, which were 1.4 mm per day after axonotmesis lesions and 1.5 mm per day after suture, can only be considered as rough approximations.

Maturation of the regenerating axons has been assessed by measurements of the diameter of myelinated fiber populations. It is only satisfactory if appropriate peripheral connections are achieved, (Weiss et al., 1945; Aitken et al., 1947). Cross anastomosis experiments by Simpson and Young (1945) indicate that if axons are made to regenerate into endoneurial tubes derived from fibers of smaller size, this imposes a restriction on the diameter that they are ultimately able to attain.

Conduction velocity in axons that have regenerated fully after crush lesions fails to return fully to normal, being reduced by approximately 25 per cent (Cragg and Thomas, 1964). Fiber diameter also never returns fully to normal.

PERIPHERAL FACTORS

The loss of muscle fibers that begins in denervated muscles after about six months means that delay in reinnervation after this period will lead to reduced functional recovery. Sunderland (1950) found that satisfactory motor function is obtainable for periods of up to a year of denervation. In partially denervated muscles, experimental studies showed that muscle power increases for some months after the injury (Van Harreveld, 1945). This has been demonstrated to be due mainly to collateral branching from the surviving motor axons that reinnervate denervated muscle fibers (Edds, 1950; Hoffman, 1950; Morris, 1953). The increase in motor unit size found in chronic denervating processes in man indicates that this is an important mechanism in functional recovery.

Failure to prevent the development of muscle contractures or joint fixation secondary to muscle paralysis may lead to impaired functional recovery when reinnervation occurs. The question of the use of electrical stimulation of denervated muscle to retard denervation atrophy is considered in Chapter 70.

COLD INJURY

Effects of Cooling on Nerve

COOLING AND NERVE CONDUCTION

Conduction velocity is reduced by cooling, transmission failing when it falls to 1 to 2 per cent of normal for myelinated axons and 4 to 5 per cent for unmyelinated axons (Franz and Iggo, 1968). These authors found a constant reduction with cooling for myelinated fibers in the cat saphenous nerve (3.16 per cent per degree centigrade), whereas for unmyelinated axons the rate of slowing decreased from 3.22 to 2.17 per cent per degree below 17° C.

It has generally been agreed that conduction is blocked at a lower temperature in unmyelinated axons than in myelinated fibers (Lundberg, 1948; Douglas and Malcolm, 1955). Franz and Iggo (1968) argued that the difference may depend upon their separate modes of conduction. Transmission presumably fails when the action current is reduced below a critical value required to excite either the next node or the adjacent part of the axon. Douglas and Malcolm (1955) found that, on cooling, small myelinated fibers ceased to conduct before larger fibers. Dodt (1953) had also reached a similar conclusion, whereas Torrance and Whitteridge (1948), Whitteridge (1948) and Widdicombe (1954) believed that larger fibers were more susceptible. Paintal (1965a, 1965b) later concluded that conduction became blocked in all myelinated fibers at approximately the same temperature and attributed the findings of Douglas and Malcolm to temporal dispersion causing apparent disappearance of the smaller peak of the gamma group before the larger alpha peak. A differential effect was demonstrated for trains of impulses: repetitive activity is interrupted at a higher temperature in smaller than in larger axons. These findings were confirmed by Franz and Iggo (1968). More recent studies by Byck and associates (1972) and Basbaum (1973) have reaffirmed that conduction fails earlier and recovers less readily in the smaller than in the larger myelinated fibers. Byck and his co-workers employed a collision technique to demonstrate blocking, which avoided the objections raised by Paintal.

Miller and Irving (1963) and Petajan (1968) have demonstrated in experiments on the caudal nerve of the rat tail that conduction velocity is reduced by exposing the animals to a cold environment for one to two weeks. With continued exposure, recovery occurs. Petajan suggested that a cold-induced neuropathy is produced and that the subsequent adaptation may be a response to initial pathologic changes in the tissues.

SENSATIONS INDUCED BY COLD

If a part of the body such as the hand is immersed in ice-cold water, it is a commonplace experience that the sensation of cold is rapidly replaced by pain. The nature of this pain has been studied by Wolf and Hardy (1941), Kellgren, McGowan, and Hughes (1948), and Marshall (1953). It appears if the hand is placed in water at 15° to 16° C and reaches a maximum after about one minute; it then changes in quality to an unpleasant deep-seated ache, which fluctuates in severity, but subsides again over the course of five to seven minutes. The lower the temperature, the more intense is the pain, although if the temperature is reduced gradually, pain does not occur. The fibers transmitting this pain are extremely resistant to ischemia: cold pain is still felt after 45 minutes of arterial occlusion by a pressure cuff at a stage when tactile and pinprick sensation are lost (Wolf and Hardy, 1941).

Tingling paresthesias are also experienced, felt as a diffuse vibratory sensation. They develop between one and two minutes after immersion at 15° C and disappear within five minutes of immersion. Marshall (1953) considered that they probably arise in the nerve trunk in fibers subserving touch sensibility. Experimental observations on mammalian nerves demonstrated the direct excitation of nerve fibers by cooling (Dodt, 1953). Matthews and Searle (1969) found that in the cat saphenous nerve only a small proportion of fibers respond to cold stimulation, but that at temperatures below 15° C excitation occurs in fibers with a conduction velocity range of 0.8 to 18 m per second.

Immersion in very cold water (less than 4° C) produces, after an interval of about three minutes, a further type of pain additional to that already described. It is felt as a severe burning sensation in the skin of the hand and was termed "skin pain" by Kellgren, McGowan, and Hughes (1948). This sensation was be-

lieved by Marshall (1953) to arise from pain receptors deep in the skin.

COLD BLOCK OF NERVE FIBERS IN MAN

Dissociated sensory loss produced by cooling a nerve trunk, originally described by Weber in 1847, was examined by Bickford (1939). Over the ulnar nerve, he applied a tubular cooling element through which a cooling solution was circulated by a mechanical pump. He found that appreciation of cold was lost first, that motor and vasomotor paralysis followed, and that later, loss of pain, touch, and warmth sensibility ensued. The possibility of direct pressure by the cooling element being responsible was eliminated by flushing warm water through the element, which led to prompt recovery of sensation. The sensory changes in nerve blocks induced by cooling were studied in more detail by Sinclair and Hinshaw (1951), who produced cooling of the ulnar nerve by immersing the elbow in brine at a temperature of 0° to −2° C, or of the peroneal nerve by a technique similar to that employed by Bickford. For the former, the order of sensory loss was cold, warm, pain, and touch; for the latter, touch, warm, pain, and cold. Glasgow and Sinclair (1962) later confirmed a failure of cold sensation before loss of appreciation of warmth. They concluded, however, that cold cannot produce its effects by a differential susceptibility of nerve fibers of different diameters and suggested that the results must depend upon factors related to the test situation other than the cold blocking.

Cold Injury Syndromes in Man

Observations on cold injury of nerve have largely stemmed from the exigencies of war. From experience with soldiers in Flanders during the 1914–1918 war, Smith, Ritchie, and Dawson (1915) clearly differentiated the the syndrome of "trench foot" from true frostbite that follows freezing of the tissues, and recognized that it results from prolonged chilling short of freezing. The different conditions in the Second World War led to the syndrome occurring mainly in shipwreck survivors in northern waters, who spent many hours clinging to rafts or sitting in waterlogged lifeboats. This came to be termed "immersion foot." The essential cause is prolonged exposure of the limbs to cold at temperatures insufficient to cause freezing of the tissues (Ungley et al., 1945). In the wartime cases following shipwreck, the temperatures were in the range between 15° and −1.9° C. Sea water freezes at −1.9° C, whereas the tissues freeze at −2.5° C. Frostbite therefore does not occur in limbs continuously immersed in sea water.

In frostbite, the tissues become frozen, with the formation of ice crystals. This subsequently leads to gangrene, involving necrosis of all tissue elements. Cutaneous sensory changes may be present in a narrow area surrounding the region of gangrene (Ungley and Blackwood, 1942).

Descriptions of the clinical features of the immersion foot (and immersion hand) syndrome were made in particular by Ungley and Blackwood (1942), Webster, Woolhouse, and Johnston (1942), White and Scoville (1945) and Ungley, Channell, and Richards (1945), and it is clear that they are closely similar to those in the cases of trench foot seen in the First World War and in the Spanish Civil War. The clinical features were divided by Ungley and co-workers (1945) into four stages.

1. Exposure. During exposure the limbs feel numb and powerless, swelling of the tissues develops, and various changes in skin color occur depending upon the external temperature.

2. Prehyperemic Stage. For some hours after rescue the limbs continue to feel numb and distal sensory loss affecting all modalities is demonstrable, sometimes extending as high as midcalf level. This is associated with distal muscular weakness or total paralysis. The limbs are cold and pale or blue in color and show a variable degree of swelling. The foot pulses are usually absent.

3. Hyperemic Stage. Two to five hours after rescue, the limbs become hot and red, with full bounding pulses. This is accompanied by severe burning or throbbing pain that reaches maximal intensity in 24 to 36 hours. The degree of swelling increases and cutaneous blisters and ecchymoses appear, particularly if rewarming is too rapid. Occasionally there are areas of tissue necrosis or gangrene that become apparent later. How far these may be due to pressure effects from constricting clothing or footwear, or to some degree of associated true frostbite, is uncertain. In experimental immersion foot in rabbits, gangrene is observed only if there is superimposed pressure or local infection (Lange et al., 1948).

As the hyperemic stage develops, there is a rapid return of sensation, although this may only be partial; a persisting sensory loss just affecting the feet may remain, associated with anhidrosis. The areas in which sensory recovery occurs become intensely hyperesthetic. Distal muscular weakness may persist, later possibly associated with muscle wasting and clawing of the toes.

The duration of this stage in cases of moderate severity varies from 6 to 10 weeks, but it may range from a few days to several months.

4. Posthyperemic Stage. Mild cases may recover fully after the hyperemic stage. In more severe cases, there is a gradual change to a stage in which the feet become at first intermittently and then persistently cold, sometimes with episodic feelings of heat that usually develop in bed or are provoked by exercise. Hyperhidrosis may also be troublesome, occurring especially at the margins of the analgesic and anhidrotic areas.

The distal sensory loss and weakness gradually recover, but permanent contractures of the toes may remain.

Pathology of Cold Injury of Nerve

Blackwood (1944) examined cases of the immersion foot syndrome. Except for one patient who died shortly before rescue, the material was obtained after intervals of several weeks to many months following exposure. Histologic study revealed that damage was present in all the tissues of the extremity, but was most evident in nerve and muscle. Nerve fiber damage was observed as far proximally as the knees in severe cases. In the later stages, evidence of regeneration was present. Muscle was available only at an interval of eight months after exposure: this showed changes of denervation with occasional small areas of fibrous replacement from earlier direct muscle damage. Figures 36–1 and 36–2 illustrate myelinated fiber damage in the sural nerve in a case of cold injury.

A number of attempts have been made to duplicate the immersion foot syndrome experimentally, including studies on rat tail by Blackwood and Russell (1943), and on the limbs of dogs by Large and Heinbecker (1944) and of rabbits by Lange, Weiner, and Boyd (1948) and Sayen and co-workers (1960) (see Montgomery, 1954). These reproduced the edema, subcutaneous hemorrhages, and mus-

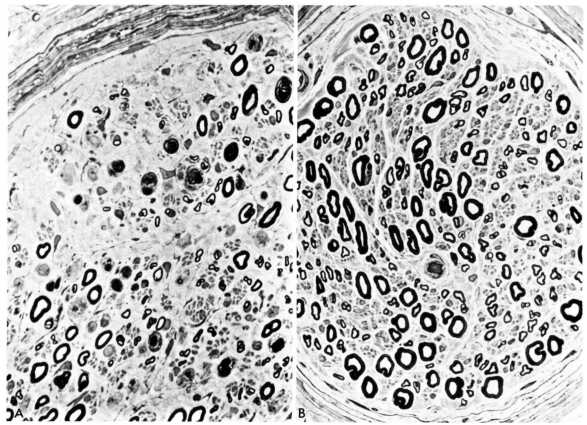

Figure 36–1 *A*. Human neuropathy due to accidental exposure to cold. A neuropathy developed after the patient, a 26 year old man, lay unconscious for several hours with his body partially immersed in icy water. A transverse section from a sural nerve biopsy obtained four weeks later displays a loss of myelinated fibers. Myelin debris is present. × 550. *B*. Control sural nerve. × 550. (Photomicrographs by courtesy of Dr. J. M. Peyronnard and Dr. A. J. Aguayo.)

cle paralysis; histologic examination confirmed the particular sensitivity of nerve and muscle. Sayen (1962) demonstrated that chilling of the hind limbs of rabbits in water at 2° C gave rise to early damage to motor nerve terminals in muscle, the innervation of muscle spindles and tendon organs being more resistant. The mechanism of the damage remains uncertain. Ungley and Blackwood (1942) originally considered it to be mediated through ischemia, whereas others favored the concept of direct injurious effect on the nerve fibers produced by the lowered temperature.

Experiments on the direct effect of cooling have yielded conflicting results that may not be directly relevant to the pathology of the immersion foot syndrome. Denny-Brown and co-workers (1945) examined cat sciatic nerve. The nerves were either frozen with carbon dioxide snow or chilled by means of a metal jacket through which a cooling solution was circulated. They found that the lesion selec-

tively affected the nerve fibers, with relative sparing of the connective tissue cells and blood vessels. In partial lesions, some axons were observed to be swollen; this could be associated with paranodal demyelination. In more severe lesions, axons and myelin degenerated simultaneously. They found that the largest fibers were most susceptible to damage and the smallest fibers least so, although this was not assessed quantitatively. Few macrophages were observed within the Schwann cell columns of degenerating fibers, which suggested to them that the myelin disappeared by lysis and diffusion. From these observations, Denny-Brown and his associates saw no reason to separate the effects of chilling and freezing except in degree. Pirozynski and Webster (1953) employed intravital methylene blue staining to study the nerve fiber damage caused by freezing rabbits' ears by immersion in fluid at −20° to 30° C. Under the circumstances of their investigation, they found that

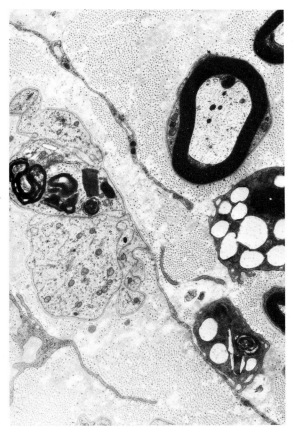

Figure 36–2 Electronmicrograph from sural nerve biopsy in Figure 36–1*A* shows a normal myelinated fiber (right upper corner) and a Schwann cell profile containing myelin remnants (left of center). × 9000. (By courtesy of Dr. J. M. Peyronnard and Dr. A. J. Aguayo.)

the larger axons were more resistant than smaller myelinated or unmyelinated axons. Schaumburg and co-workers (1967) cooled cat sciatic nerve by means of a cold probe. Cooling to 20° C produced no persisting effects. Damage to nerve fibers occurred below this level: the lower the temperature, the greater the severity of the changes. These involved both large and small myelinated fibers, no differential effect on fibers of different sizes being detected.

In a recent study, Basbaum (1973) cooled the rat sciatic nerve with a thermoelectric device. A reduction in the temperature of the nerve to 5° C resulted in a total block of conduction in myelinated fibers, and in all cases conduction recovered on rewarming. Nevertheless, a morphologic study showed that selective degeneration of larger myelinated fibers subsequently took place with a time course similar to that of wallerian degeneration. Schwann cells and macrophages both partici-

pated in the removal of the debris. Vasogenic edema of the endoneurium and enzymatic activation of the Schwann cell were observed within a few hours of cooling, and it was considered possible that they precipitated the fiber degeneration. A further mechanism considered was the disintegration of axonal microtubules that Rodriguez Echandía and Piezzi (1968) have shown to be produced by cold and that might disturb axoplasmic transport. It is of interest that the conduction block on cooling and the fiber degeneration bore an inverse relationship to one another with respect to fiber size; the smaller fibers displayed a greater susceptibility to conduction block, whereas it was the larger ones that degenerated.

RADIATION NEUROPATHY

Effects of X-Irradiation on Nervous Tissue

Little attention has been paid in the neurologic literature to the effects of x-rays and similar radiations upon peripheral nerves. The general impression has been gained, which is supported by the paucity of published instances of peripheral nerve damage due to x-irradiation, that peripheral nervous tissue is very insensitive to this type of trauma (Warren, 1944). In fact, this impression is only partly true, and any damage that may have, in fact, occurred, is only too often masked or confused by the presence on the one hand of the tumorous growth for which x-rays have been administered or on the other of the post-irradiation scarring of the tissue due to vascular damage (Sams, 1963). This impression has also been strengthened by the observations of Jansen and Warren (1942) that the sciatic nerves of rats locally radiated with 10,000 rads of 200 kv x-rays showed no structural or functional disturbances when examined over the subsequent two months by conventional techniques.

In one sense the insensitivity of mature stable peripheral nerves is true. The conductive function of nerve fibers is unaffected significantly by doses below 30,000 rads (Gaffey, 1962). With larger doses than these, which are far in excess of the therapeutic range, disturbances to the membrane functions of nerve can be detected (Bachofer and Gauteraux, 1959), but are probably not relevant to clinical problems. In another sense, however, the insensitivity of nerves to x-rays is only apparent. The principal cellular action of small doses, not more than 2000 rads, of x-rays is upon the DNA of the chromosomes of cells (Lea, 1946). If, therefore, the irradiated cells are nonmitotic in normal circumstances, even if their chromosomal material is damaged by the ionizing effects of x-rays, they will not express this damage in the same way as we see it expressed, for instance, by intestinal epithelium, by bone marrow, or by any other mitotically active population of cells. This latent damage is capable of being expressed, however, if for any reason the resting tissue is stimulated into mitotic activity. Such a situation occurs, and can be readily induced, in peripheral nerves.

There has been much discussion over the mechanism of production of postradiation necrosis of central nervous tissue that is germane to this theme. The arguments as to whether the primary fault lies with the glial cells (Bailey, 1962) or with the vascular bed (Scholtz and Hsu, 1938) probably have little substance in radiobiologic terms. All cells will be, or are statistically likely to be, affected to some degree in an area exposed to x-rays. Those with a minimal amount of damage to DNA will be capable in time of repairing this. The majority, however, will not do so successfully, but provided that the damaged part of the chromosome is not being used for the differentiated functions of the cell, there is no reason why ill effects need necessarily be shown by these cells. A few cells may be damaged at some vital point and will die; their numbers will be related to the dose given.

The cells of the vascular bed probably undergo slow mitotic replacement, and there is evidence that this turnover rate is influenced by fluctuations in the blood pressure and possibly by other causes (Crane and Dutta, 1963). The astrocytes also may normally be undergoing slow replacement, and certainly respond to local alterations in their environment by cell division (Cavanagh, 1970). Both these tissue components every now and then "switch" momentarily from their differentiated state to mitotic activity, and it is then that the latent damage caused by irradiation can be expressed. Minimally damaged cells may divide satisfactorily and continue their differentiated function. The greater the chromosomal derangement, however, the less likely they are to survive. Their weaknesses

are seen as chromosome "bridges" at anaphase, multiple micronuclei derived from reconstructed chromosome fragments, and polyploidy where DNA synthesis has occurred but cell division cannot for one reason or another be completed. Such aberrant products are unlikely to divide again should the necessity for this arise, and they will probably die. If a brain wound is made at any time after local x-irradiation of the brain with doses larger than 100 rads, all these aberrant mitotic forms will be met with in astrocytes, in microglial and vascular cells, and in meningeal cells (Cavanagh, 1968a), but not in neurons, in oligodendrocytes, or in ependymal cells, since none of these cell types responds to injury by cell division. No hint of abnormality can be seen earlier in unwounded but irradiated brains to suggest the widespread nature of the damage.

It is apparent, therefore, that delayed radiation necrosis in central nervous tissue is explicable in terms, first, of widespread potentially lethal, but latent, radiation damage to cells, and second, in terms of the time and extent of any demand for cell division subsequent to the irradiation. The occurrence of hypertension, experimentally induced, hastens the onset of delayed necrosis in rats (Assher and Anson, 1962), and it is known that cell turnover in the vascular tree is increased in hypertension (Crane and Dutta, 1963). It is known also that astrocytes respond actively to exudation of plasma into the brain extracellular space (Blakemore, 1971) and that this may be a mitotic stimulus for them. A vicious circle can thus be envisaged being set up in the brain in these circumstances that leads to the final state of delayed radiation necrosis.

Effects of Radiation Upon Peripheral Nerves

Given this sequence of events in central nervous tissue, the effects of radiation upon peripheral nerves can be looked at anew. The total absence of any effects of doses of less than 10,000 rads or so upon the structure and function, as might be found by using conventional histologic and electrophysiologic methods, is explicable since there is good evidence that nerve under normal circumstances is composed of nonmitotic tissue.

It is well established that neurons do not divide once settled into their mature locus, and axons, as we have seen from Jansen and Warren's (1942) findings, are not significantly altered by x-rays in the therapeutic dose range. The studies of Vizoso (1950) have shown that internodal lengths and fiber diameters in general persist unchanged in humans into the sixth or even the eighth decade of life. The final length of an internode is imposed by growth of the part subsequent to the onset of myelination (Shepherd, Sholl and Vizoso, 1949). Since in the adult state, repair of either selective demyelination or of axonal degeneration by the Schwann cell making new myelin can only result, in mammals, in internodes within the range of 200 to 300 μm because of the absence of the elongation caused by growth of the part, it is impossible to conceive of a constantly dividing Schwann cell. Indeed autoradiographic studies using ^{3}H-thymidine show no cells in the DNA synthesizing phase in normal adult nerve (Asbury, 1967). Equally, therefore, it is probable that Remak cells surrounding unmyelinated fibers, fibroblasts, vascular cells, and perineurial cells are also similarly nonmitotic under normal circumstances in the adult mammalian nerve.

So far as cell replacement goes, therefore, peripheral nerve is a static nonmitotic tissue. Any x-irradiation damage from doses in the therapeutic range and below must therefore remain latent until injury stimulates the cells to division. From an experimental standpoint, however, it is very easy to test whether damage has been produced; all that is necessary is to crush the nerve and study the mitotic activity of the schwannian and other cells and their population changes. It is also easy to determine whether repair of the radiation damage has occurred in individual cells with time by crushing the nerve at different times after x-irradiation. If repair has been effected, then any change induced by the x-rays in the population kinetics of the nerve would diminish with time.

Experiments have shown these deductions to be correct (Cavanagh, 1968b, 1968c). Crushing the sciatic nerves of rats shortly after doses of 200 to 2000 rads given at a dose rate of 100 rads per minute has shown that at all dose levels, the population increase at one week after crushing is detectably different from the normal response. At two weeks after crushing, the population depletion is restored to normal levels after 200 and 500 rads, but after 1000 rads it is still markedly less than control figures. After 2000 rads, the population

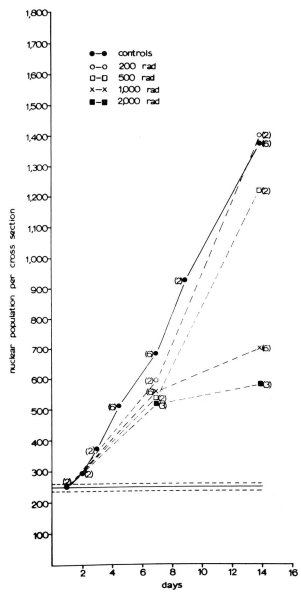

Figure 36–3 Nuclear populations of rat sciatic nerve below a crush lesion made three weeks after local irradiation of one leg with x-rays. Note that the figures at all dose levels are reduced below normal at the end of one week. By two weeks the population has recovered after 200 rads and almost recovered after 500 rads; following 1000 and 2000 rads there is only a marginal increase in cells beyond that found at one week. (From Cavanagh, J. B.: Effects of x-irradiation on the proliferation of cells in peripheral nerve during wallerian degeneration in the rat. Br. J. Radiol., *41*:275, 1968b. Reprinted by permission.)

hardly changes at two weeks from the level at one week (Fig. 36–3).

From a qualitative standpoint, abnormalities are present at one week after radiation in cells of all types with all doses, but are least numer-

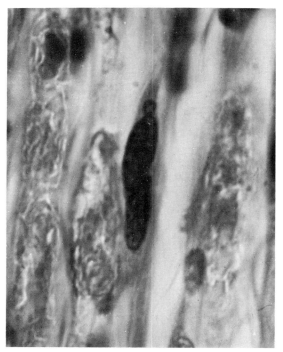

Figure 36–4 One week after crush following irradiation (200 rads). A Schwann cell with two nuclei and a micronucleus, the last having arisen probably from a fragmented chromosome. Hematoxylin and eosin stain. × 1600.

ous after 200 rads (Figs. 36–4, 36–5, and 36–6). They consist of multiple micronuclei in Schwann cells, chromosome "bridges" at anaphase, and chromosome fragmentation seen at metaphase. Greatly enlarged, probably polyploid nuclei are commonly seen, owing presumably to failure of division after DNA synthesis. While these alterations are more numerous and more obvious in the large

Schwann cells, they are also evident in endoneurial fibroblasts, in vascular cells, and occasionally in perineurial cells. They are not seen, however, in the mononuclear phagocytes that are of hematogenous origin, which would not have been affected by local irradiation of the limb.

From the point of view of effective recovery of the total cell population after crush of irradiated nerves, hematogenous macrophages play an important role, the magnitude of which is, however, difficult to evaluate from the figures gained from these experiments. Thus, after 2000 rads the population increase from the uncrushed state at the end of one week was × 1.95. This does not mean that almost all the indigenous cells have divided once, because within this population are an undefined number of macrophages that have newly entered the area. Nonetheless, it can be safely said that after 2000 rads the capacity of the cells within the nerve has been profoundly altered, and in general this is in accord with the radiobiologic findings in other tissues, for example, the liver, stimulated to division after x-irradiation (cf. Albert, 1958; Weinbren et al., 1960; Curtis, 1967). From the in vitro studies of Puck and Marcus (1956) and the in vivo studies of Hewitt and Wilson (1959), it would be expected that the number of cells capable of continued proliferation, i.e., that were viable, after 2000 rads would be in the region of 1 in 100,000 in well-oxygenated tissue. On this basis, therefore, the finding of so small an increase in the nuclear population in crushed nerves after 2000 rads should cause little surprise, and it is probable that most of the increase is due to incursive monocytic cells.

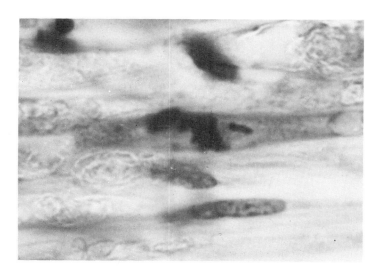

Figure 36–5 One week after crush following irradiation (200 rads). A Schwann cell is in metaphase; chromosome fragment is visible. Hematoxylin and eosin stain. × 1600.

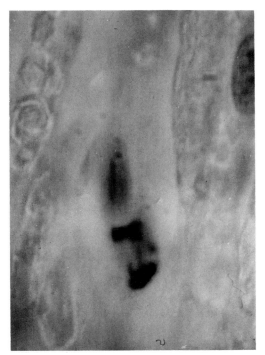

Figure 36–6 One week after crush following irradiation (500 rads). Endoneurial fibroblast is in anaphase. Note the "bridge" and chromosome fragments. Hematoxylin and eosin stain. × 1600.

The second question that this type of experiment aimed to answer was whether any evidence of repair could be found with time after irradiation (Cavanagh, 1968c). After a dose of 1000 rads, some evidence of recovery of the population toward normal two weeks after the crush was apparent. The effect of this dose was studied when the crush was made three weeks or nine months after irradiation. No statistically significant differences were found. Thus, at three weeks after irradiation the population was 49.8 per cent of the un-

TABLE 36–1 NUCLEAR POPULATIONS OF RAT SCIATIC NERVES FOLLOWING 1000 RADS OF X-RAYS AND AFTER CRUSHING*

Period Between Radiation and Crush	Number of Animals	Mean Nuclear Population (cells/unit vol.)	Per Cent of Control
3 weeks	6	700.6 ± 16.8	49.8
9 months	6	739.2 ± 50.1	52.6
Controls	6	1405.8 ± 41.4	

*Radiation preceded crushing by three weeks or nine months; controls had no irradiation. (From Cavanagh, J. B.: Prior x-irradiation and the cellular response to nerve crush: duration of effect. Exp. Neurol., 22:253, 1968. Reprinted by permission.)

irradiated nerves, while at nine months it was 52.6 per cent of the controls (Table 36–1). It is apparent, therefore, that the individual cells had not made any successful repair of the radiation damage during this long period.

Experimentally, it has been shown in mice that irradiation of a limb with only 2000 rads causes disturbances of the vascular architecture and leads commonly to necrosis of the distal parts of the limb (Sams, 1963). This does not happen apparently in the rat, and certainly no disturbances from this source can be found in the latter species.

Radiation Effects on Peripheral Nerves in Man

Very few papers indeed report careful studies of the effects of x-rays within the therapeutic range in man, and unless clinical and physiologic studies are correlated with later anatomical studies, the complicating factor of the invasive tumor is impossible to eliminate. One such example is the report of Greenfield and Stark (1948), who described three cases of muscular weakness of "motor neurone type" following one million volt x-ray treatment. The patients had been given 5000 to 6000 rads to the retroperitoneal lymph nodes as treatment for primary carcinoma of the testis. Muscular weakness in the legs developed three to five months later and became steadily worse until one year after irradiation. No postmortem studies were made, however, and these disturbances could have been due to recrudescence of the tumor, to vascular lesions in the irradiated field, or to direct action upon the lumbosacral plexus.

The paper of Stoll and Andrews (1966) is much more explicit. They studied 117 cases for 30 months after irradiation of the axilla for carcinoma of the breast with high-voltage small-field radiotherapy, using either 6300 rads or 5775 rads in divided doses. With the larger dose 73 per cent developed subsequent neurologic symptoms as compared with 15 per cent of those who had the smaller dose. These developed from 4 months to 30 months after treatment, most occurring after about one year. The presenting symptoms were hypoesthesia with or without some weakness of the hand or fingers. Mixed motor and sensory signs were elicitable, not related to any particular segmental innervation field. Two cases were studied postmortem. One patient, who had the larger dose, showed much fibrosis of the brachial plexus in the irradiation area. Above this region the nerves appeared normal, but in the fibrotic zone there was marked loss of myelin and of axons. Below this region there was also marked myelin and axon loss that implied widespread axonal degeneration. In the second patient, who received the smaller dose, some fibrosis was present, but this did not involve the brachial plexus, and the nerves did not show any significant degenerative changes.

Edema was thought to play some role in the genesis of the nerve changes, but clear relationship could not be established between these two events. The authors considered that an "entrapment" phenomenon might be operating here, but they should also have considered the possibility of a vascular factor, in view of the observations of Sams (1963) noted earlier. The nerve degeneration and the fibrosis is likely to be explicable on the basis of interactions between failure of vascular repair mechanisms on the one hand and failure of the neuronal repair mechanism on the other. Further studies along these lines would be very helpful in unraveling the causative mechanisms operating here.

Effects of Large Kilorad Doses of X-Rays on Nerve

The function and the structure of nerve fibers are undoubtedly interfered with by large doses of x-rays or gamma rays. Bachofer and co-workers (1964) in particular have been interested in these effects, but since this type of study deals with dose ranges of 100 to 1000 kilorads, it is more the concern of the biophysicist than of the clinician. Changes in resting potential are observable that are dependent upon dose rate, and alterations in the polarization state from hyperpolarization to depolarization occur that are also dose dependent. Basically this seems to be a problem concerned with the functions of cell membranes in relation to their ionic transfer properties and how these are disturbed by the sudden transfer of energy into the system. Its relevance to the clinical problems of peripheral nerves is dubious, for the studies of Bergström (1962) show that in the rat, high-energy protons in doses of 20 to 40 kilorads delivered through a narrow slit 2 to 4 mm wide

caused almost complete destruction of myelin and axons in this region, as though the nerve had been crushed. Later, mononuclear cells entered the lesion in a fashion similar to that seen in wallerian degeneration. It was not clear, however, whether the myelin bearing Schwann cells were killed by this dose or whether the myelin and axons were directly disorganized.

ELECTRICAL INJURIES

Peripheral nerves may be directly damaged at the time of electrical injury, either from lightning or from generated electrical supplies, by involvement in electrical burns (Dale, 1954; Panse, 1955; Di Vincenti et al., 1969). Delayed facial palsy, appearing after a few days, has been observed following electrical injuries to the head (Richards, 1973).

Amyotrophy developing after electrical injuries that have affected the spinal cord has been described with some frequency. These have been attributed to anterior horn cell damage, although this has not been substantiated by histologic study. Such cases, which are usually associated with other clinical evidence of spinal cord dysfunction, have been reviewed by Panse (1970). Interestingly, the onset of the amyotrophy may be delayed for several months, and subsequent improvement has been reported. There may be an associated segmental sensory loss. The mechanism of these delayed effects is unknown.

It has been suggested that a progressive disorder with the clinical features of motor neuron disease, with both lower and upper motor neuron involvement, may supervene upon an electrical injury. Such cases have also been collected by Panse (1970), but are not very numerous, raising the possibility of a chance association. On the other hand, an association with other types of progressive neurologic disorder apart from the occurrence of relapses of multiple sclerosis following electrical shocks has not been documented (see McAlpine et al., 1965). The possibility of electrical injury providing a trigger for the onset of motor neuron disease cannot therefore be entirely dismissed. Yet once such a relationship has been mooted, this fact in itself is likely to provide a bias in favor of this particular association being preferentially reported.

EFFECTS OF ULTRASOUND

Ultrasonic irradiation of peripheral nerve may give rise either to a reversible conduction block or to axonal destruction. Young and Henneman (1961) reported that the smaller fibers are more sensitive, so they could be selectively blocked without the larger fibers being affected. Lele (1963) could not confirm this. He found that after an initial period of enhancement when conduction velocity is increased, conduction is reversibly and then irreversibly depressed. Although the smaller fibers were observed to be affected earlier, it was not possible to block them separately, except for a brief period, without blocking the larger fibers. Lele considered that the effects are entirely due to heating. If the surface temperature of the irradiated nerve is not permitted to become elevated, even prolonged exposure to focused ultrasound has no physiologic or structural effects. If the temperature is allowed to rise, however, the effects are rapidly produced at much lower intensities of irradiation. Such effects were found to be entirely comparable to those produced by heating.

REFERENCES

Agate, J. N.: An outbreak of Raynaud's phenomenon of occupational origin. Br. J. Indust. Med., 6:144, 1949.

Aitken, J. T., Sharman, N., and Young, J. Z.: Maturation of regenerating nerve fibres with various peripheral connections. J. Anat., 81:1, 1947.

Albert, M. D.: X-irradiation induced mitotic abnormalities in mouse liver regenerating after carbon tetrachloride injury. I. Total body irradiation. J. Natl. Cancer Inst., 20:309, 1958.

Asbury, A. K.: Schwann cell proliferation in the developing mouse sciatic nerve. J. Cell Biol., 34:735, 1967.

Assher, A. W., and Anson, S. G.: Arterial hypertension and irradiation damage to the nervous system. Lancet, 2:1343, 1962.

Bachofer, C. S., and Gauteraux, M. E.: X-ray effects on single nerve fibers. J. Gen. Physiol., 42:723, 1959.

Bachofer, C. S., Gauteraux, M. E., and Kaack, S. M.: Relative sensitivity of isolated nerves to Co⁶⁰ gamma rays. In Haley, T. J., and Snider, R. S. (eds.): Response of the Nervous System to Ionizing Radiation. London, J. and A. Churchill Ltd., 1964.

Bailey, O. T.: Basic problems in the histopathology of radiation of the central nervous system. In Haley, T. J., and Snider, R. S. (eds.): The Response of the Nervous System to Ionizing Radiation. New York, Academic Press, 1962.

Barnes, R.: Causalgia: a review of 48 cases. In Seddon, H. J. (ed.): Peripheral Nerve Injuries, London, H.M.S.O., 1954.

Basbaum, C. B.: Induced hypothermia in peripheral nerve: electron microscopic and electrophysiological observations. J. Neurocytol. 2:171, 1973.

Bergström, R.: Changes in peripheral nerve tissue after irradiation with high energy protons. Acta Radiol. (Stockh.), 58:301, 1962.

Bickford, R. G.: The fibre dissociation produced by cooling human nerves. Clin. Sci., 4:159, 1939.

Birks, R., Katz, B., and Miledi, R.: Physiological and structural changes at the amphibian myoneural junction. J. Physiol. (Lond.), 150:145, 1960.

Black, A. N., Burns, B. D., and Zuckerman, S.: An experimental study of the wounding mechanism of high velocity missiles. Br. Med. J., 2:872, 1941.

Blackwood, W.: Studies in the pathology of human "immersion foot." Br. J. Surg., 31:329, 1944.

Blackwood, W., and Russell, H.: Experiments in the study of immersion foot. Edin. Med. J., 50:385, 1943.

Blakemore, W. F.: The ultrastructural appearance of astrocytes following thermal lesions of the rat cortex. J. Neurol. Sci., 12:312, 1971.

Bonney, G.: The value of the axon responses in determining the site of lesion in traction injuries of the brachial plexus. Brain, 77:588, 1954.

Bowden, R. E. M., and Gutmann, E.: Denervation and re-innervation of human voluntary muscle. Brain, 67:273, 1944.

Bowden, R. E. M., and Sholl, D. A.: Rates of regeneration. In Seddon, H. J. (ed.): Peripheral Nerve Injuries. London, Her Majesty's Stationery Office, 1954.

Byck, R., Goldfarb, J., Schaumberg, H. H., and Sharpless, S. K.: Reversible differential block of saphenous nerve by cold. J. Physiol. (Lond.), 222:17, 1972.

Campbell, J. B., Bassett, C. A. L., and Böhler, J.: Frozen irradiated homografts shielded with microfilter sheaths in peripheral nerve surgery. J. Trauma, 3:302, 1963.

Campbell, J. B., Bassett, C. A. L., Giraldo, J. M., Seymour, R. J., and Rossi, J. P.: Application of monomolecular filter tubes in bridging gaps in peripheral nerves and for prevention of neuroma formation. J. Neurosurg., 13:635, 1956.

Cavanagh, J. B.: Effects of previous x-irradiation on the cellular response of nervous tissue to injury. Nature (Lond.), 219:626, 1968a.

Cavanagh, J. B.: Effects of x-irradiation on the proliferation of cells in peripheral nerve during wallerian degeneration in the rat. Br. J. Radiol., 41:275, 1968b.

Cavanagh, J. B.: Prior x-irradiation and the cellular response to nerve crush: duration of effect. Exp. Neurol., 22:253, 1968c.

Cavanagh, J. B.: The proliferation of astrocytes around a brain needle wound in the rat brain. J. Anat., 106:471, 1970.

Cragg, B. G., and Thomas, P. K.: The conduction velocity of regenerated peripheral nerve fibres. J. Physiol. (Lond.), 171:164, 1964.

Crane, W. A. J., and Dutta, L. P.: The utilization of tritiated thymidine for deoxyribonucleic acid synthesis by lesions of experimental hypertension. J. Pathol. Bacteriol., 86:83, 1963.

Cronholm, B.: Phantom limbs in amputees; study of changes in integration of centripetal impulses with special reference to referred sensations. Acta Psychiatr. Scand. [Suppl.], 72:1, 1951.

Curtis, H. J.: Recovery of mammalian chromosomes from radiation injury. In Recovery and Repair Mechanisms in Radiobiology. Brookhaven Symp. Biol., 20:223, 1967.

Dale, R. H.: Electrical accidents. Br. J. Plast. Surg., 7:44, 1954.

Denny-Brown, D., and Brenner, G.: Paralysis of nerve induced by direct pressure and by tourniquet. Arch. Neurol. Psychiatry, 51:1, 1944.

Denny-Brown, D., and Doherty, M. M.: Effects of transient stretching of peripheral nerve. Arch. Neurol. Psychiatry, 54:116, 1945.

Denny-Brown, D., Adams, R. D., Brenner, C., and Doherty, M. M.: The pathology of injury to nerve induced by cold. J. Neuropathol. Exp. Neurol., 4:305, 1945.

Di Vincenti, F. C., Moncrief, J. A., and Pruitt, B. A.: Electrical injuries: a review of 65 cases. J. Trauma, 9:497, 1969.

Dodt, E.: Differential thermosensitivity of mammalian A-fibres. Acta Physiol. Scand., 29:19, 1953.

Douglas, W. W., and Malcolm, J. L.: Effect of localized cooling on conduction in cat nerves. J. Physiol. (Lond.), 130:63, 1955.

Doupe, J.: Studies in denervation: circulation in denervated digits. J. Neurol. Psychiatry, 6:97, 1943.

Doupe, J., Cullen, C. H., and Chance, G. Q.: Post-traumatic pain and causalgic syndrome. J. Neurol. Neurosurg. Psychiatry, 7:33, 1944.

Duncan, D., and Jarvis, W. H.: Observations on repeated regeneration of the facial nerve in cats. J. Comp. Neurol., 79:315, 1943.

Edds, M. V.: Collateral regeneration of residual axons in partially denervated muscles. J. Exp. Zool., 113:517, 1950.

Erb, W.: Handbuch der Krankheiten des Nervensystems II. In Ziemssen, H. von (ed.): Handbuch der speciellen Pathologie und Therapie. Vol. 12, Part 1. Leipzig, Vogel, 1874.

Erb, W. H.: Diseases of the Peripheral Cerebro-spinal Nerves. Trans. H. Power, New York, Wood, 1876.

Franz, D. N., and Iggo, A.: Conduction failure in myelinated and non-myelinated axons at low temperatures. J. Physiol. (Lond.), 199:319, 1968.

Freeman, N. E.: The treatment of causalgia arising from gunshot wounds of the peripheral nerves. Surgery, 22:68, 1947.

Gaffey, C. T.: Bioelectric effects of high energy irradiation on nerve. In Haley, T. J., and Snider, R. S. (eds.): Responses of the Nervous System to Ionizing Radiation. New York, Academic Press, 1962.

Gilliatt, R. W., and Hjorth, R. J.: Nerve conduction during wallerian degeneration in the baboon. J. Neurol. Neurosurg. Psychiatry, 35:335, 1972.

Gilliatt, R. W., and Taylor, J. C.: Electrical changes following section of the facial nerve. Proc. R. Soc. Med., 52:1080, 1959.

Glasgow, E. F., and Sinclair, D. C.: Dissociation of cold and warm sensibility in experimental blocks of the ulnar nerve. Brain, 85:67, 1962.

Granit, R., Leksell, L., and Skoglund, C. R.: Fibre interaction in injured or compressed region of peripheral nerve. Brain, 67:125, 1944.

Greenfield, M. M., and Stark, F. M.: Post irradiation neuropathy. Am. J. Roentgenol., 60:617, 1948.

Gutmann, E., and Holubář, J.: The degeneration of peripheral nerve fibres. J. Neurol. Neurosurg. Psychiatry, 13:89, 1950.

Guy, R. S., McLeod, J. G., Hargrave, J. Pollard, J. D., Loewenthall, J., and Booth, G.: The use of immunosuppressive agents in human nerve grafting. Lancet, 1:647, 1972.

Haftek, J.: Stretch injury of peripheral nerve. Acute

effects of stretching on rabbit peripheral nerve. J. Bone Joint Surg., 52B:354, 1970.

Haftek, J., and Thomas, P. K.: Electron-microscope observations on the effects of localized crush injuries on the connective tissues of peripheral nerve. J. Anat., 103:233, 1968.

Harreveld, A. van: Reinnervation of denervated muscle fibers by adjacent functioning motor units. Am. J. Physiol., 144:466, 1945.

Harvey, E. N., Butler, E. G., McMillen, J. H., and Puckett, W. O.: Mechanism of wounding. War Med. (Chicago), 8:91, 1945.

Henderson, W. R., and Smyth, G. E.: Phantom limbs. J. Neurol. Neurosurg. Psychiatry, 11:88, 1948.

Hewitt, H. B., and Wilson, C. W.: A survival curve for mammalian leukaemic cells irradiated in vivo (implications for the treatment of mouse leukaemia by whole body irradiation). Br. J. Cancer, 13:69, 1959.

Highet, W. B.: Procaine nerve block in investigation of peripheral nerve injuries. J. Neurol. Psychiatry, (Lond.), 5:101, 1942.

Highet, W. B., and Holmes, W.: Traction injuries to the lateral popliteal nerve and traction injuries to peripheral nerves after suture. Br. J. Surg., 30:212, 1943.

Highet, W. B., and Sanders, F. K.: The effect of stretching nerves after suture. Br. J. Surg., 30:355, 1943.

Hoffman, H.: Local re-innervation in partially denervated muscle: a histo-physiological study. Aust. J. Exp. Biol. Med. Sci., 28:383, 1950.

Jansen, A. H., and Warren, S.: Effect of roentgen rays on peripheral nerves of rat. Radiology, 38:333, 1942.

Jepson, R. P.: Raynaud's phenomenon: a review of the clinical problem. Ann. R. Coll. Surg. Engl., 9:35, 1951.

Kellgren, J. H., McGowan, A. J., and Hughes, E. S. R.: On deep hyperalgesia and cold pain. Clin. Sci., 7:13, 1948.

Lange, K., Weiner, D., and Boyd, L. J.: The functional pathology of experimental immersion foot. Am. Heart J., 35:238, 1948.

Landau, W. M.: The duration of neuromuscular function after nerve section in man. J. Neurosurg., 10:64, 1953.

Large, A., and Heinbecker, P.: Nerve degeneration following prolonged cooling of an extremity. Ann. Surg., 120:742, 1944.

Lea, D. E.: Actions of Radiations on Living Cells. London, Cambridge University Press, 1946.

Lele, P. P.: Effects of focussed ultrasonic radiation on peripheral nerve, with observations on local heating. Exp. Neurol., 8:47, 1963.

Lissak, K., Dempsey, E. W., and Rosenblueth, A.: The failure of transmission of motor nerve impulses in the course of wallerian degeneration. Am. J. Physiol., 128:45, 1939.

Liu, C. T., Benda, C. E., and Lewey, F. H.: Tensile strength of human nerves: experimental physical and histologic study. Arch. Neurol. Psychiatry, 59:322, 1948.

Lundberg, A.: Potassium and the differential thermosensitivity of membrane potential, spike and negative after potential in mammalian A and C fibres. Acta Physiol. Scand., Suppl. 50, 15:1, 1948.

Marmor, J.: Regeneration of peripheral nerves by irradiated homografts. J. Bone Joint Surg., 46A:383, 1964.

Marshall, J.: The paraesthesiae induced by cold. J. Neurol. Neurosurg. Psychiatry, 16:19, 1953.

Marshall, J., Poole, E. W., and Reynard, W. A.: Raynaud's

phenomenon due to vibrating tools. Lancet, *1*:1151, 1954.

Matthews, B., and Searle, B. N.: Excitation of peripheral nerve by direct cooling. J. Physiol. (Lond.), *203*:25P, 1969.

Mayer, R. F., and Denny-Brown, D.: Conduction velocity in peripheral nerve during experimental demyelination in the cat. Neurology (Minneap.), *14*:714, 1964.

McAlpine, D., Lumsden, C. E., and Acheson, E. D.: Multiple Sclerosis: a Reappraisal. Edinburgh and London, E. & S. Livingstone Ltd., 1965.

Melzack, R., and Wall, P. D.: Pain mechanisms: a new theory. Science, *150*:971, 1966.

Miller, L. K., and Irving, L.: Alteration of peripheral nerve function in the rat after prolonged outdoor cold exposure. Am. J. Physiol., *204*:359, 1963.

Millesi, H., Gangleberger, J., and Berger, A.: Erfarungen mit der Mikrochirurgie peripherer Nerven. Chir. Plast. Reconstr., *3*:47, 1967.

Mitchell, S. Weir, Morehouse, G. R., and Keen, W. W.: Gunshot wounds and other injuries of nerves. Philadelphia, J. B. Lippincott Co., 1864.

Montgomery, H.: Experimental immersion foot. Review of physiopathology. Physiol. Rev., *34*:127, 1954.

Moorhouse, J. A., Carter, S. A., and Doupe, J.: Vascular responses in diabetic peripheral neuropathy. Br. Med. J., *5492*:883, 1966.

Morris, D. D. B.: Recovery in partially paralysed muscles. J. Bone Joint Surg., *358*:650, 1953.

Nathan, P. W.: On the pathogenesis of causalgia in peripheral nerve injuries. Brain, *70*:145, 1947.

Nickel, V. L., Perry, J., Garrett, A., and Heppenstall, M.: The halo: a spinal skeletal traction fixation device. J. Bone Joint Surg., *50A*:1400, 1968.

Nobel, W.: Peroneal palsy due to hematoma at the common peroneal nerve sheath after distal torsional fractures and inversion ankle sprains. J. Bone Joint Surg., *48A*:1484, 1966.

O'Brien, J. P., Yan, A. C. M. C., Smith, T. K., and Hodgson, A. R.: Halopelvic traction: a preliminary report on a method of external skeletal fixation for correcting deformities and maintaining fixation of the spine. J. Bone Joint Surg., *53B*:217, 1971.

Ochoa, J., Fowler, T. J., and Gilliatt, R. W.: Anatomical changes in peripheral nerves compressed by a pneumatic tourniquet. J. Anat., *113*:433, 1972.

Paintal, A. S.: Block of conduction in mammalian myelinated nerve fibres by low temperatures. J. Physiol. (Lond.), *180*:1, 1965a.

Paintal, A. S.: Effects of temperature on conduction in single vagal and saphenous myelinated nerve fibres of the cat. J. Physiol. (Lond.), *180*:20, 1965b.

Panse, F.: Die Neurologie des elektrischen Unfalls und dès Blitzschlags, II. *In* Koeppen, S., and Panse, F. (eds.): Klinische Elektropathologie. Stuttgart, Thieme, 1955.

Panse, F.: Electrical lesions of the nervous system. *In* Vinken, P. J., and Bruyn, G. W. (eds.): Handbook of Clinical Neurology. Vol. 7. Amsterdam, North Holland Publishing Co., 1970, p. 344.

Petajan, J. H.: Changes in rat ventral caudal nerve conduction velocity during cold exposure. Am. J. Physiol., *214*:130, 1968.

Pirozynski, W. J., and Webster, D. R.: Experimental investigation of changes in axis cylinders of peripheral nerves following local cold injury. Am. J. Pathol., *29*:547, 1953.

Puck, T. T., and Marcus, P. I.: Action of x-rays on mammalian cells. J. Exp. Med., *103*:653, 1956.

Puckett, W. O., Grundfest, H., McElroy, W. D., and

McMillen, J. H.: Damage to peripheral nerves by high velocity missiles without a direct hit. J. Neurosurg., *3*:294, 1946.

Richards, A.: Traumatic facial palsy. Proc. R. Soc. Med., *66*:556, 1973.

Richards, R. L.: Causalgia, a centennial review. Arch. Neurol., *16*:339, 1967.

Riddoch, G.: Phantom limbs and body shapes. Brain, *64*:197, 1941.

Rodriguez Echandía, E. L., and Piezzi, R. S.: Microtubules in the nerve fibers of the toad *Bufo arenarum* Hensel. Effect of low temperature on the sciatic nerve. J. Cell Biol., *39*:491, 1968.

Sams, A.: Effect of x-irradiation on the circulatory system of the hind limb of the mouse. Int. J. Radiat. Biol., *7*:113, 1963.

Sayen, A.: Comparative histologic changes at myoneural junctions, terminal axons, spindles and tendon organs of muscle after local cold injury. J. Neuropathol. Exp. Neurol., *21*:348, 1962.

Sayen, A., Meloche, B. R., Tedeschi, G. C., and Montgomery, H.: Experimental immersion foot: observations in the chilled leg of the rabbit. Clin. Sci., *19*:243, 1960.

Schaumburg, H., Byck, R., Herman, R., and Rosengart, C.: Peripheral nerve damage by cold. Arch. Neurol., *16*:103, 1967.

Scholtz, W., and Hsu, Y. K.: Late damage from roentgen irradiation of the human brain. Arch. Neurol. Psychiatry, *40*:928, 1938.

Seddon, H. J.: Three types of nerve injury. Brain, *66*: 237, 1943.

Seddon, H. J.: Nerve lesions complicating certain closed bone injuries. J.A.M.A., *135*:691, 1947.

Seddon, H. J.: Surgical Disorders of the Peripheral Nerves. Edinburgh and London, Churchill Livingstone, 1972.

Seddon, H. J., Medawar, P. B., and Smith, H.: Rate of regeneration of peripheral nerve in man. J. Physiol. (Lond.), *102*:191, 1943.

Shepherd, R. H., Sholl, D. A., and Vizoso, A. D.: The size relationships subsisting between body length, limbs and jaws in man. J. Anat., *83*:296, 1949.

Shumacker, H. B., Speigel, I. J., and Upjohn, R. H.: Causalgia. I. The role of sympathetic interruption in treatment. Surg. Gynecol. Obstet., *86*:76, 1948a.

Shumacker, H. B., Speigel, I. J., and Upjohn, R. H.: Causalgia: signs and symptoms, with particular reference to vasomotor disturbances. Surg. Gynecol. Obstet., *86*:452, 1948b.

Simpson, S. A., and Young, J. Z.: Regeneration of fibre diameter after cross-unions of visceral and somatic nerves. J. Anat., *79*:48, 1945.

Sinclair, D. C., and Hinshaw, J. R.: Sensory changes in nerve blocks induced by cooling. Brain, *74*:318, 1951.

Smith, J. L., Ritchie, J., and Dawson, J.: Clinical and experimental observations on the pathology of trench frostbite. J. Pathol. Bacteriol. *20*:159, 1915.

Stoll, B. A., and Andrews, J. T.: Radiation induced peripheral neuropathy. Br. Med. J., *1*:834, 1966.

Stone, T. T.: Phantom limb pain and central pain; relief by ablation of portion of posterior central cerebral convolution. Arch. Neurol. Psychiatry, *63*:739, 1950.

Sunderland, S.: The intraneural topography of the radial, median and ulnar nerves. Brain, *68*:243, 1945.

Sunderland, S.: Capacity of reinnervated muscles to function efficiently after prolonged denervation. Arch. Neurol. Psychiatry, *64*:755, 1950.

Sunderland, S.: A classification of peripheral nerve injuries producing loss of function. Brain, *74*:491, 1951.

Sunderland, S.: Nerves and Nerve Injuries. Edinburgh and London, E. & S. Livingstone Ltd., 1968.

Sunderland, S., and Bradley, K. C.: Denervation atrophy of the distal stump of a severed nerve. J. Comp. Neurol., *93*:401, 1950.

Sunderland, S., and Bradley, K. C.: Stress-strain phenomena in human peripheral nerve trunks. Brain, *84*:102, 1961.

Sunderland, S., and Ray, L. J.: The intraneural topography of the sciatic nerve and its popliteal division in man. Brain, *71*:242, 1948.

Sunderland, S., and Ray, L. J.: The effect of denervation on nail growth. J. Neurol. Neurosurg. Psychiatry, *15*:50, 1952.

Telford, E. D., McCann, M. B., and MacCormack, D. H.: "Dead hand" in users of vibrating tools. Lancet, *2*:259, 1945.

Torrance, R. W., and Whitteridge, D.: Technical aids in the study of respiratory reflexes. J. Physiol. (Lond.), *107*:6P, 1948.

Ulmer, J. L., and Mayfield, F. H.: Causalgia: a study of 75 cases. Surg. Gynecol. Obstet., *83*:789, 1946.

Ungley, C. C., and Blackwood, W.: Peripheral vaso-neuropathy after chilling. "Immersion foot and immerson hand." Lancet, *2*:447, 1942.

Ungley, C. C., Channell, G. D., and Richards, R. L.: The immersion foot syndrome. Br. J. Surg., *33*:17, 1945.

Vizoso, A. D.: The relationship between internodal length and growth in human nerves. J. Anat., *84*:342, 1950.

Wall, P. D., and Sweet, W. H.: Temporary abolition of pain in man. Science, *155*:108, 1967.

Warren, S.: Histopathology of radiation lesions. Physiol. Rev., *24*:225, 1944.

Webster, D. R., Woolhouse, F. M., and Johnston, J. L.: Immersion foot. J. Bone Joint Surg., *24*:785, 1942.

Weddell, G., Guttmann, L., and Gutmann, E.: The local extension of nerve fibres into denervated areas of skin. J. Neurol. Psychiatry (Lond.), *4*:206, 1941.

Weinbren, K., Fitschen, W., and Cohen, M.: The unmasking by regeneration of latent irradiation effects in the rat liver. Br. J. Radiol., *33*:419, 1960.

Weiss, P., Edds, M. V., Jr., and Cavanaugh, M.: Effect of terminal connections on caliber of nerve fibers. Anat. Rec., *92*:215, 1945.

White, J. C., and Scoville, W. B.: Trench foot and immersion foot. N. Engl. J. Med., *232*:415, 1945.

White, J. C., Heroy, W. H., and Goodman, E. N.: Causalgia following gunshot injuries of nerves: role of emotional stimuli and surgical cure through interruption of diencephalic efferent discharge by sympathectomy. Ann. Surg., *128*:161, 1948.

Whitteridge, D.: Afferent nerve fibers from the heart and lungs in the cervical vagus. J. Physiol. (Lond.), *107*: 496, 1948.

Widdicombe, J. G.: Receptors in the trachea and bronchi of the cat. J. Physiol. (Lond.), *123*:71, 1954.

Wolf, S., and Hardy, J. D.: Studies on pain. Observations on pain due to local cooling and on factors involved in the "cold pressor" effect. J. Clin. Invest., *20*:521, 1941.

Young, J. Z.: Factors influencing the regeneration of nerves. Adv. Surg., *1*:65, 1949.

Young, R. R., and Henneman, E.: Reversible block of nerve conduction by ultrasound. Arch. Neurol., *4*:83, 1961.

INDEX

In this index page numbers in *italics* indicate
illustrations; those followed by (t) indicate tables.
The abbreviation vs. indicates differential diagnosis.